SECOND EDITION

Advanced Oncology Nursing Certification Review and Resource Manual

Edited by
Barbara Holmes Gobel, MS, RN, AOCN®
Shirley Triest-Robertson, PhD, AOCNS®, ACHPN, ACNSBC, RN-BC (Pain)
Wendy H. Vogel, MSN, FNP, AOCNP®

Oncology Nursing Society
Pittsburgh, Pennsylvania

ONS Publications Department

Publisher and Director of Publications: William A. Tony, BA, CQIA
Managing Editor: Lisa M. George, BA
Assistant Managing Editor: Amy Nicoletti, BA, JD
Acquisitions Editor: John Zaphyr, BA, MEd
Copy Editors: Vanessa Kattouf, BA, Andrew Petyak, BA
Graphic Designer: Dany Sjoen
Editorial Assistant: Judy Holmes

Library of Congress Cataloging-in-Publication Data

Advanced oncology nursing certification review and resource manual / edited by Barbara Holmes Gobel, Shirley Triest-Robertson, Wendy H. Vogel. -- 2nd edition.
　　p. ; cm.
　Includes bibliographical references and index.
　ISBN 978-1-935864-55-4
　I. Gobel, Barbara Holmes, editor. II. Triest-Robertson, Shirley, editor. III. Vogel, Wendy H., editor. IV. Oncology Nursing Society, issuing body.
　[DNLM: 1. Neoplasms--nursing. 2. Oncology Nursing--methods. 3. Advanced Practice Nursing--methods. WY 156]
　RC266
　616.99'40231076--dc23

2015026331

Publisher's Note

　　This book is published by the Oncology Nursing Society (ONS). ONS neither represents nor guarantees that the practices described herein will, if followed, ensure safe and effective patient care. The recommendations contained in this book reflect ONS's judgment regarding the state of general knowledge and practice in the field as of the date of publication. The recommendations may not be appropriate for use in all circumstances. Those who use this book should make their own determinations regarding specific safe and appropriate patient care practices, taking into account the personnel, equipment, and practices available at the hospital or other facility at which they are located. The editors and publisher cannot be held responsible for any liability incurred as a consequence from the use or application of any of the contents of this book. Figures and tables are used as examples only. They are not meant to be all-inclusive, nor do they represent endorsement of any particular institution by ONS. Mention of specific products and opinions related to those products do not indicate or imply endorsement by ONS. Websites mentioned are provided for information only; the hosts are responsible for their own content and availability. Unless otherwise indicated, dollar amounts reflect U.S. dollars.

　　ONS publications are originally published in English. Publishers wishing to translate ONS publications must contact ONS about licensing arrangements. ONS publications cannot be translated without obtaining written permission from ONS. (Individual tables and figures that are reprinted or adapted require additional permission from the original source.) Because translations from English may not always be accurate or precise, ONS disclaims any responsibility for inaccuracies in words or meaning that may occur as a result of the translation. Readers relying on precise information should check the original English version.

Printed in the United States of America

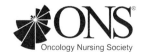

Innovation • Excellence • Advocacy

Contributors

Editors

Barbara Holmes Gobel, MS, RN, AOCN®
Director of Professional Practice and Development
Magnet Program Director
Northwestern Memorial Hospital
Chicago, Illinois
Adjunct Faculty
Rush University College of Nursing
Chicago, Illinois
Chapter 22. Test Questions

Shirley Triest-Robertson, PhD, AOCNS®, ACHPN, ACNSBC, RN-BC (Pain)
APNP Palliative Services
St. Vincent Hospital
Green Bay, Wisconsin
Chapter 22. Test Questions

Wendy H. Vogel, MSN, FNP, AOCNP®
Oncology Nurse Practitioner
Wellmont Cancer Institute
Kingsport, Tennessee
Chapter 20. Roles of the Oncology Advanced Practice Nurse; Chapter 22. Test Questions

Authors

Lisa Aiello-Laws, MSN, RN, AOCNS®
Assistant Clinical Professor
Drexel University College of Nursing and Health
  Professions
Philadelphia, Pennsylvania
Chapter 9. Clinical Research

Roberta H. Baron, MSN, RN, AOCN®
Clinical Nurse Specialist
Memorial Sloan Kettering Cancer Center
New York, New York
Chapter 17. Psychosocial Management

Diane G. Cope, PhD, ARNP-BC, AOCNP®
Oncology Nurse Practitioner
Florida Cancer Specialists and Research Institute
Fort Myers, Florida
Chapter 15. Metabolic Emergencies

Marianne J. Davies, DNP, MSN, APRN, ACNP, AOCNP®
Assistant Professor
Yale School of Nursing
Oncology Nurse Practitioner—Thoracic
Smilow Cancer Hospital at Yale–New Haven
New Haven, Connecticut
Chapter 12. Cardiac and Pulmonary Toxicities

Vanna M. Dest, MSN, APRN-BC, AOCN®
Manager, Oncology Advanced Practice Providers
Oncology Nurse Practitioner—Thoracic and Head/
  Neck Medical Oncology
Smilow Cancer Hospital at Yale–New Haven
New Haven, Connecticut
Chapter 14. Neurologic, Ocular, and Dermatologic Toxicities

Hollie Devine, MSN, ANP-BC
Adult Nurse Practitioner
Arthur G. James Cancer Hospital and Richard J.
  Solove Research Institute
The Ohio State University
Columbus, Ohio
Chapter 7. Blood and Marrow Stem Cell
Transplantation

Tracy K. Gosselin, PhD, RN, AOCN®
Associate Chief Nursing Officer and Assistant Vice
  President
Duke Cancer Institute
Durham, North Carolina
Chapter 6. Radiation Therapy

Heather Greene, MSN, RN, FNP, AOCNP®
Nurse Practitioner
West Cancer Center
Memphis, Tennessee
Chapter 1. Cancer Prevention, Screening, and Early
Detection

Debra E. Heidrich, MSN, RN, ACHPN
Palliative Care Nurse Consultant, Self-Employed
West Chester, Ohio
Chapter 19. Palliative and End-of-Life Care

Joyce Jackowski, MS, FNP-BC, AOCNP®
Nurse Practitioner
Florida Cancer Specialists
Venice, Florida
Chapter 18. Cancer Survivorship

Marcelle Kaplan, MS, RN, AOCN®, CBCN®
Oncology Nurse Consultant
Merrick, New York
Chapter 16. Structural Oncologic Emergencies

Colleen O. Lee, MS, ANP-BC, AOCN®, CLNC
Captain, U.S. Public Health Service
Senior Standards Advisor
Standards Management Staff
Center for Devices and Radiological Health
U.S. Food and Drug Administration
Silver Spring, Maryland
Chapter 8. Complementary and Integrative Therapies

Joanne Lester, PhD, CNP, ANP-BC, AOCN®
Clinical Research Nurse Practitioner
Division of Surgical Oncology
The Ohio State University
Columbus, Ohio
Chapter 5. Surgery

Suzanne M. Mahon, DNSc, RN, AOCN®, APNG
Professor, Internal Medicine
Professor, School of Nursing
Saint Louis University
St. Louis, Missouri
Chapter 2. Genetic Risk

Kimberly Noonan, RN, ANP-BC, AOCN®
Nurse Practitioner
Dana-Farber Cancer Institute
Boston, Massachusetts
Chapter 10. Pain, Fatigue, and Cognitive Impairment

Colleen M. O'Leary, MSN, RN, AOCNS®
Associate Director, Nursing Education
Associate Director, Evidence-Based Practice
Arthur G. James Cancer Hospital and Richard J.
  Solove Research Institute
The Ohio State University Comprehensive Cancer
  Institute and Wexner Medical Center
Columbus, Ohio
Chapter 13. Gastrointestinal, Genitourinary, and
Hepatic Toxicities

Kathy Sharp, MSN, FNP-BC, AOCNP®, CCD
Oncology Nurse Practitioner
Wellmont Cancer Institute
Bristol, Virginia
Chapter 21. Professional Practice of Advanced
Practice Nurses

Brenda K. Shelton, DNP, RN, APRN-CNS, CCRN,
AOCN®
Clinical Nurse Specialist
The Sidney Kimmel Comprehensive Cancer Center
  at Johns Hopkins Hospital
Faculty, The Johns Hopkins University School of
  Nursing
Baltimore, Maryland
Chapter 11. Myelosuppression and Second
Malignancies

Gail M. Wilkes, APRN-BC, MS, AOCN®
Oncology Nursing Consultant
Kilauea, Hawaii
Chapter 4. Chemotherapy, Targeted Biotherapy, and
Molecular Therapy

Laura J. Zitella, MS, RN, ACNP-BC, AOCN®
Lead Advanced Practice Provider/Hematology and
  Oncology Nurse Practitioner
Stanford Health Care
Stanford, California
Chapter 3. Cancer Diagnosis and Staging

Disclosure

Editors and authors of books and guidelines provided by the Oncology Nursing Society are expected to disclose to the readers any significant financial interest or other relationships with the manufacturer(s) of any commercial products.

A vested interest may be considered to exist if a contributor is affiliated with or has a financial interest in commercial organizations that may have a direct or indirect interest in the subject matter. A "financial interest" may include, but is not limited to, being a shareholder in the organization; being an employee of the commercial organization; serving on an organization's speakers bureau; or receiving research funding from the organization. An "affiliation" may be holding a position on an advisory board or some other role of benefit to the commercial organization. Vested interest statements appear in the front matter for each publication.

Contributors are expected to disclose any unlabeled or investigational use of products discussed in their content. This information is acknowledged solely for the information of the readers.

The contributors provided the following disclosure and vested interest information:

Wendy H. Vogel, MSN, FNP, AOCNP®: Celgene, Genentech, Novartis, Onyx, honoraria

Marianne J. Davies, DNP, MSN, APRN, ACNP, AOCNP®: Bristol-Myers Squibb, Merck, advisory role; Bristol-Myers Squibb, Eisai, Genentech, Novartis, honoraria

Vanna M. Dest, MSN, APRN-BC, AOCN®: Jazz Pharmaceuticals, ProStrakan, honoraria

Tracy K. Gosselin, PhD, RN, AOCN®: Oncology Nursing Society, leadership position and honoraria

Joanne Lester, PhD, CNP, ANP-BC, AOCN®: National Comprehensive Cancer Network, research funding

Laura J. Zitella, MS, RN, ACNP-BC, AOCN®: On Q Health, Teva, consultant and/or advisory role

Contents

Preface

The inspiration for the development of the first edition of the *Advanced Oncology Nursing Certification Review and Resource Manual* was in response to requests from Oncology Nursing Society (ONS) advanced oncology certification review course participants seeking additional study resources. Since its publication, it has been a valuable resource for thousands of oncology practitioners. The goals of this manual are threefold. The first is to provide a comprehensive review for oncology advanced practice nurses (APNs) who are preparing to sit for an Oncology Nursing Certification Corporation (ONCC) advanced oncology certified clinical nurse specialist (AOCNS®) or advanced oncology certified nurse practitioner (AOCNP®) examination. The second goal is to provide a comprehensive clinical resource for oncology APNs. The third is to provide a comprehensive overview of oncology advanced practice for faculty and students in graduate oncology nursing education.

The editors of this book have served as faculty for advanced oncology review courses. This educational experience, feedback from course participants, and the ONCC test bulletins have contributed to the development of the content of each chapter. Authors were selected based on expertise in their respective areas, their experience in clinical practice, and their advanced oncology certification status. This book provides a foundation for a comprehensive review of advanced oncology nursing content.

Each chapter includes content on topics pertinent to APNs, key points to emphasize important concepts for readers to review, and a case study with questions relevant to the most important topics within the chapter, which gives readers an opportunity to affirm their understanding of the content. In addition, practice test questions are provided in Chapter 22. These multiple-choice questions are similar in structure to questions used in the oncology advanced practice nursing certification examinations. These varied methods of instruction are intended to address current adult learning principles.

Chapter content is correlated to the weighting assigned to specific topics in the ONCC certification tests. The number of review questions per topic in Chapter 22 also is reflective of this weighting. These topic percentages may change periodically; therefore, test candidates are advised to refer to the most current test bulletin when preparing for a certification examination.

Authors consulted the most current oncology clinical evidence in the preparation of this book. Although it is beyond the scope of any review or resource book to completely cover the entire field of advanced oncology nursing, the editors believe the mastery of the content presented herein will give the readers a broader understanding of advanced oncology nursing. The use of this book does not guarantee successful completion of an advanced oncology nursing examination; however, readers will be better prepared to identify areas where more in-depth study is required.

This book also serves as a valuable resource to oncology APNs, graduate nursing students, medical residents, physician assistants, and oncology nurses in clinical practice.

To achieve this goal, advanced oncology APN topics have been expanded beyond the scope of a review course to include the most current literature and clinical evidence available at the time of this writing. Certification examination questions generally are developed over a long period of time and may not always reflect the most current evidence. Each chapter contains useful, important, and timely references recommended by the expert and practicing APN authors, making this review book a valued resource for oncology clinicians.

It is our hope that this revised edition of the *Advanced Oncology Nursing Certification Review and Resource Manual* will be a timely addition to the oncology nursing literature. We would like to acknowledge and thank our expert authors. We also are indebted and grateful to the dedicated staff of the ONS Publications Department.

Barbara Holmes Gobel
Shirley Triest-Robertson
Wendy H. Vogel

CHAPTER 1

Cancer Prevention, Screening, and Early Detection

Heather Greene, MSN, RN, FNP, AOCNP®

Introduction

In 2015, an estimated 1,658,370 new cases of cancer are expected to be diagnosed in the United States, and 589,430 cancer deaths are expected (American Cancer Society [ACS], 2015). One-quarter to one-third of these cancer deaths will be related to tobacco use, poor nutrition, physical inactivity, and obesity (World Cancer Research Fund & American Institute for Cancer Research, 2009). All cancer deaths related to tobacco and alcohol abuse are entirely preventable. Additionally, any of the more than two million new cases of skin cancer diagnosed annually could be prevented by avoiding overexposure to ultraviolet light. Cancers related to viral or bacterial infections, such as the hepatitis B virus, human papillomavirus (HPV), HIV, and *Helicobacter*, also can be prevented through lifestyle changes and use of vaccines or antibiotics (ACS, 2015).

In addition to avoidance of risk factors, routine use of screening modalities can aid in prevention and early detection of cancer. Screening tests for cancers of the colon, rectum, and cervix can help prevent cancer by enabling removal of precancerous growths. In addition to reducing incidence, greater use of screening tests could decrease deaths related to breast, colorectal, and cervical cancers (ACS, 2015). Despite this, even mammography use has not increased since 2010. Half of all new cases of cancer are considered preventable or could be detected at an earlier stage (ACS, 2015).

Role of the Advanced Practice Nurse

Oncology advanced practice nurses (APNs) are in a unique position to educate their patients and the public regarding recommended cancer risk reduction and screening guidelines. The scope of practice for nurse practitioners includes an emphasis on health promotion and disease prevention (American Association of Nurse Practitioners, 2013). Therefore, cancer prevention and early detection are clearly responsibilities of the oncology APN.

In the Oncology Nursing Society's *Scope and Standards of Oncology Nursing Practice: Generalist and Advanced Practice* (Brant & Wickham, 2013), oncology APNs are encouraged to receive educational preparation in the principles of cancer prevention and early detection. Oncology specialty certification examinations (such as the advanced oncology certified nurse practitioner [AOCNP®] and advanced oncology certified clinical nurse specialist [AOCNS®] examinations) cover this topic. In accordance with their state's scope of practice, nurse practice act, and requirements for educational preparation, oncology APNs must be able to assess, evaluate, and interpret cancer risk assessments and recommend appropriate strategies related to cancer prevention and screening. All oncology nurses must be able to provide culturally sensitive cancer prevention and early detection services and participate in the development of resources that focus on wellness and primary prevention throughout the life span. Research on cancer prevention and early detection requires integration into current practice.

Cancer Risk Assessment

Cancer risk assessment is a vital part of the oncology APN's role in cancer prevention and early detection. To provide accurate counseling on cancer risk reduction strategies (e.g., tobacco cessation, lifestyle modifications, dietary changes, chemoprevention agents), cancer screening recommendations, and genetic testing (if appropriate), oncology APNs must first perform a comprehensive risk assessment. A cancer risk assessment is an individualized evaluation of a patient's risk for cancer based on a variety of both intrinsic and extrinsic factors and begins with a detailed history. This includes thorough past medical, social, obstetric/gynecologic, and surgical histories and documentation of recent age-appropriate screening tests, or lack thereof. Family history is a critical part of cancer risk assessment and includes at least a three-generation pedigree, particularly if a hereditary cancer syndrome is suspected (see Chapter 2). Medication history (such as hormone use), dietary history, level of physical activity, environmental exposures, history of tobacco and alcohol use, and other lifestyle choices also are important factors to assess when determining cancer risk. A thorough physical examination concludes the cancer risk assessment and includes a breast, pelvic or testicular, and rectal examination.

Multiple cancer risk assessment tools and models are available to help APNs convey this risk to patients, such as the Gail model, Tyrer-Cuzick model, and BRCAPRO for breast cancer risk (Quante, Whittemore, Shriver, Strauch, & Terry, 2012; Warner, 2011) and the MMRpro model for hereditary colon cancer risk (Greco, 2007). Each of these tools has its strengths and weaknesses. The Gail model is the most commonly used general breast cancer risk assessment tool and is used to estimate a woman's five-year risk and overall lifetime risk for breast cancer. Scores are calculated based on a variety of risk factors, including age, age at menarche, age at first live birth, race, number of first-degree relatives with breast cancer, and number of previous breast biopsies. The score is based on a comparison to that of a woman of average risk and of the same race and age, with elevated risk considered greater than 1.7%. However, this model fails to take into account the age at breast cancer diagnosis in affected family members, history of bilateral breast cancer, second-degree relatives affected with breast cancer, and history of ovarian cancer or lobular carcinoma in situ (Quante et al., 2012; Warner, 2011).

The National Cancer Institute (NCI) has several cancer risk assessment tools available online, most prominently those for breast (www.cancer.gov/bcrisktool) and colon cancer (www.cancer.gov/colorectalcancerrisk) risk assessment. All of these models are best used in conjunction with an individualized, comprehensive cancer risk assessment by the APN to best estimate and counsel patients on their overall cancer risk and on interventions to decrease that risk.

Primary Prevention and Risk Reduction

Cancer prevention is achieved through primary, secondary, and tertiary methods. Primary cancer prevention consists of interventions aimed at keeping the carcinogenic process from beginning. Examples include smoking cessation interventions and chemoprophylaxis in women at high risk for breast cancer. Secondary cancer prevention is the discovery of cancerous or precancerous conditions while still in their earliest stage, when the disease is most likely to be treated successfully (Spratt, 1981). Examples include mammography to detect and remove premalignant changes in the breast and colonoscopy to remove polyps in the colon. Tertiary cancer prevention is applied to those individuals who have already been diagnosed with a malignancy with the intent of keeping the original disease in remission as long as possible.

Tobacco Use

Smoking has long been established as a detriment to overall health. As early as 1928, studies have referred to smoking and its association with cancer (Lombard & Doering, 1928). Research culminated with the 1964 U.S. Department of Health, Education, and Welfare's Surgeon General's report, which concluded that smoking was the major cause of lung cancer and was associated with oral and laryngeal cancers in men. Since then, thousands of additional studies and subsequent reports of the Surgeon General have confirmed tobacco's detrimental health effects. More than 4,000 chemicals have been identified in tobacco products and tobacco smoke, 55 of which are identified as carcinogens by the International Agency for Research on Cancer. These carcinogens may induce genetic mutations and ultimately lead to cancer development. In 2015, nearly 171,000 deaths will be attributable to tobacco (ACS, 2015). Tobacco use is considered a contributing or causative agent in a multitude of malignancies, including lung, nasal cavity, larynx, pharynx, esophagus, stomach, colon, rectum, liver, pancreas, kidney, bladder, uterine cervix, ovary (mucinous), and myeloid leukemia (ACS, 2015; Centers for Disease Control and Prevention [CDC], 2004). Smoking is thought to cause up to 90% of lung cancers and is the leading cause of preventable cancer-related and non–cancer-related deaths in the United States (ACS, 2015). Lung cancer is estimated to be diagnosed in close to 221,200 Americans in 2015, of which approximately 158,040 will die, encompassing nearly 30% of all cancer deaths (ACS, 2015).

Tobacco abuse and addiction is perhaps one of the greatest public health concerns of our time, particularly as cancer is concerned. According to CDC's National Health Interview Survey, cigarette smoking prevalence in U.S. adults declined between 2005 and 2011 from 20.9% to 19%. In addition, heavy smoking declined significantly during this time, reflecting long-term historical trends toward lower cigarette consumption in smokers (CDC, 2012a). Most adult smokers today began smoking in their youth. According to the 2011 National Youth Tobacco Survey, about 23.2% of high school students reported current use of any tobacco product (CDC, 2012b). Data from the Youth Risk Behavior Survey showed that in 2011, 18.1% of high school students reported current cigarette smoking (smoking on at least one day in the past 30 days), and 6.4% reported frequent smoking (smoking on 20 or more days in the past

30 days) (CDC, 2012b). Results from that survey also showed a 40% decline in cigarette smoking prevalence in high school students between 1997 and 2003 (from 36.4% to 22%) (CDC, 2012b). However, between 2003 and 2011, the percentage decline was about half as much, showing an 18% drop, from 22% to 18.1% (Eaton et al., 2012).

Primary prevention measures for tobacco-related cancers and tobacco deterrent programs must be aimed at children and adolescents. Recent research shows that adolescents are three times more sensitive to tobacco advertising than adults and are more likely to be influenced to smoke by advertisements for cigarettes than by peer pressure (Campaign for Tobacco-Free Kids, 2014). Tobacco prevention efforts include increased tobacco prices and taxes, public smoking restrictions, and anti-tobacco advertisements. For example, since the state of California implemented a comprehensive tobacco control program, a documented drop has occurred in adolescent smoking initiation. This program, which included excise tax increases, also resulted in greater reductions in cigarette smoking among smokers age 35 or older and cessation rates among adult smokers age 35 or younger, compared to states without such measures (Messer & Pierce, 2010). Furthermore, compared to other parts of the country, lung cancer incidence is declining faster in the Western states, including California (CDC, 2011).

Smoking Cessation

Despite the known consequences of tobacco use on health and society and the proven benefits of smoking cessation (see Table 1-1), most clinicians fail to identify and counsel patients on this topic (Fiore et al., 2008). Reasons for this include inability to quickly identify current tobacco users and a knowledge deficit about what treatments are effective, how they are delivered, and the associated side effects of treatment. Time constraints and lack of institutional support for tobacco cessation counseling also may contribute to the fact that only 21% of clinic visits with current smokers included smoking cessation counseling (Fiore et al., 2008).

Clinicians can identify current tobacco users by asking all patients at every visit about their smoking status and whether they are interested in quitting. It also may be beneficial to document tobacco use as an additional vital sign in the medical record. It is estimated that up to 70% of current smokers want to quit, but more than a third of those are never asked about their smoking status or desire to quit (Fiore et al., 2008). Even if patients have attempted cessation in the past and failed, several attempts are common before long-term abstinence is achieved (Fiore et al., 2008).

The U.S. Department of Health and Human Services' *Treating Tobacco Use and Dependence* clinical practice guideline (Fiore et al., 2008) thoroughly outlines instructions for clinicians to use in identifying and treating nicotine dependence. The first step in treating tobacco dependence is identifying tobacco users. The "5 A's" outlined in this guideline can be useful in guiding patients through this process: *Ask* about tobacco use at every visit. Once identified, *advise* tobacco users to quit. Next, *assess* whether the patient is ready to make a quit attempt. Smokers can be categorized into one of two groups—those who are interested in making a quit attempt and those who are not. APNs can then *assist* patients in tobacco cessation either at the current visit or, for those unwilling to quit, with a brief intervention to assist cessation at future visits. Lastly, *arrange* follow-up after the quit attempt or to discuss tobacco cessation again at another visit. These steps are outlined in Table 1-2 (Fiore et al., 2008).

Often, inadequate knowledge of tobacco cessation therapy inhibits clinicians' ability to assist patients in their quit attempt (Barr, Houston-Miller, Hasan, & Makinson, 2013). Successful smoking cessation interventions contain two components: behavioral counseling and pharmacotherapy. The combined use of these approaches has been shown to improve smoking cessation rates (Fiore et al., 2008; Harrill-Smith, Moffitt, & Goldstein, 2013). Most studies esti-

Table 1-1. Health Benefits of Smoking Cessation

Elapsed Time After Smoking Cessation	Health Benefits
2 weeks–3 months	Circulation, skin tone, oral hygiene, and pulmonary function improve.
1–9 months	Ciliary function in the lungs is restored.
12 months	Risk for coronary heart disease is reduced by 50% compared to persistent smokers.
5–15 years	Risk of stroke is decreased to that of nonsmokers.
10 years	Risk of death from lung cancer is reduced by 50% compared to persistent smokers.
15 years	Risk of coronary heart disease is reduced to that of nonsmokers.

Note. Based on information from Fiore et al., 2008.

Table 1-2. The 5 A's of Smoking Cessation Counseling

"A"	Intervention
Ask	Ask about the tobacco status of every patient at every visit.
Advise	Advise tobacco users to quit in a strong, clear, and personalized manner.
Assess	Assess patients' readiness to quit.
Assist	Assist patients who are willing to quit with individualized counseling and pharmacotherapy. Assist patients who are unwilling to quit with a brief intervention to assist future cessation.
Arrange	Arrange follow-up within one week of the stated quit date for patients who are willing to quit. Arrange to discuss tobacco use again at the next visit for patients who are unwilling to quit.

Note. Based on information from Fiore et al., 2008.

mate successful smoking cessation rates to be 40%–60% using this combination. This drops to 25%–30% after one year, but it is still higher than the less than 10% of smokers who attain long-term abstinence on their own (Fiore et al., 2008).

Behavioral counseling begins by identifying triggers and stressors unique to each individual smoker. These can be moods, feelings, places, or activities. Some of the most common stressors and triggers include feeling stressed or depressed, talking on the phone or watching television, drinking alcohol or coffee, driving, finishing a meal, managing work and family issues, taking a work break, being with other smokers or seeing someone else smoke, cooling off after a fight, feeling lonely, and having sex (Fiore et al., 2008). Making patients aware of their triggers is a valuable method of assisting them to stay in control. Once the patient-specific triggers and stressors have been identified, teaching patients to cope involves avoiding these triggering situations and replacing old habits with new ones (Fiore et al., 2008).

Nurses should advise all tobacco users to quit smoking at every encounter (Fiore et al., 2008; Quinn et al., 2009). Even if individuals are uninterested in making a quit attempt at that particular time, discussing the process, benefits, and perceived barriers to smoking cessation can propel them closer to seriously contemplating quitting. For tobacco users who are not willing to attempt cessation, APNs can offer motivational support using the "5 R's" listed in Table 1-3 (Fiore et al., 2008). These steps allow patients to identify the relevance of smoking cessation and assist in identifying the risks, rewards, and barriers of smoking cessation as it pertains to them personally.

In addition to behavioral counseling, pharmacotherapy may benefit all smokers ready to make a quit attempt (with the exception of certain populations, such as adolescents, those with specific medical contraindications, and pregnant women) (Chaney & Sheriff, 2012; Fiore et al., 2008; Harrill-Smith et al., 2013). Currently, seven U.S. Food and Drug Administration (FDA)-approved first-line therapies are available: five types of nicotine replacement therapy (NRT) (transdermal, oral lozenges, gum, nasal spray, and oral inhaler) and two non-nicotine medications, bupropion sustained-release (SR) and varenicline (Chaney & Sheriff, 2012; Fiore et al., 2008). Studies show that NRT with or without the use of other FDA-approved medications increases smoking cessation success (Chaney & Sheriff, 2012; Fiore et al., 2008; Harrill-Smith et al., 2013). Studies have shown a twofold increase in cessation rates with NRT alone over placebo (Fiore et al., 2008). Most forms of NRT are easy to use and available over the counter, with prices equivalent to or less than cigarettes, depending on the patient's habit. Pharmacotherapy dosing, common side effects, contraindications, and costs are listed in Table 1-4. As noted in this table, the most common side effect of NRT is local irritation of the involved surface (mouth, nose, skin), and caution is advised in patients immediately post–myocardial infarction or with other serious cardiovascular events.

A newer form of NRT not listed in this table is the electronic cigarette, or e-cigarette. The use of e-cigarettes in smoking cessation is not entirely clear at this point, and more research is needed to evaluate its place in this arena. However, early studies are suggesting cessation rates similar to nicotine patches and few adverse effects (Bullen et al., 2013).

Whether through routine office visits or in clinics designed specifically for smoking cessation therapy, the role of the APN in smoking cessation interventions is critical (Barr et al., 2013). In addition to using the Department of Health and Human Services clinical practice guideline, APNs can take other steps to improve smoking cessation awareness and therapy.

Table 1-3. The 5 R's of Smoking Cessation Counseling

"R"	Intervention
Relevance	Encourage personal relevance of smoking cessation (i.e., health status, impact on family members, economic impact).
Risks	Ask patients to identify risks of continued tobacco use that are pertinent to them, including those that are acute (shortness of breath), chronic (cancer, chronic obstructive pulmonary disease), and environmental (cancers and lung diseases in their spouse and children).
Rewards	Ask patients to identify potential rewards of smoking cessation, both immediate and long term (e.g., improved overall health for individual and family, money saved).
Roadblocks	Ask patients to identify potential or actual barriers to smoking cessation (e.g., withdrawal symptoms, weight gain).
Repetition	Repeat the 5 R's at every encounter with patients. Also, repeated attempts at smoking cessation are common among smokers.

Note. Based on information from Fiore et al., 2008.

Table 1-4. First-Line Therapy for Treating Tobacco Abuse

Drug	Dose	Common Side Effects	Precautions/ Contraindications	Cost
Bupropion SR	Start 1–2 weeks before quit date at a dose of 150 mg daily for 3 days, then BID for up to 7–12 weeks (can consider up to 6 months after quitting)	Insomnia, dry mouth	Contraindicated in patients with history of seizure or eating disorder Pregnancy class C	Prescription; ~$3.33/day
Nicotine gum	2 mg (< 25 cig/day); 4 mg (≥ 25 cig/day) Use at least one piece every 1–2 hours for first 6 weeks; use up to 12 weeks; do not exceed 24 pieces/ day.	Dyspepsia, mouth sore- ness, hiccups, jaw ache	Caution is advised among patients immediately post– myocardial infarction (MI) (2 weeks) or with serious arrhythmias or unstable chest pain. Dentures may prohibit proper use; patients should avoid eating or drinking 15 min- utes prior to and dur- ing use. Pregnancy class D	Over the counter; 2 mg: ~$48/box of 100–170 pieces; 4 mg: ~$63/box of 100–110 pieces
Nicotine inhaler	6–16 cartridges/ day for 6 months, tapering over last 3 months	Mouth or throat irritation, cough, rhinitis	Caution is advised among patients immediately post-MI (2 weeks) or with seri- ous arrhythmias or unstable chest pain. Patients should avoid eating or drinking 15 minutes prior to and during use. Pregnancy class D	Prescription; ~$196/box of 168 cartridges
Nicotine lozenges	2 mg (patients smoking first ciga- rette > 30 minutes after waking); 4 mg (patients smoking < 30 minutes after waking) Use at least 9 loz- enges/day for first 6 weeks and continue up to 12 weeks; do not exceed 20 loz- enges/day.	Mouth irritation, hiccups, nau- sea, dyspepsia	Patients should not chew or swallow loz- enges. Caution is advised among patients immediately post-MI (2 weeks), with seri- ous arrhythmias or unstable chest pain Patients should avoid eating or drinking 15 minutes prior to and during use.	Over the counter; 2 mg: ~$34/box of 72 lozenges; 4 mg: ~$39/box of 72 loz- enges

(Continued on next page)

Table 1-4. First-Line Therapy for Treating Tobacco Abuse *(Continued)*

Drug	Dose	Common Side Effects	Precautions/ Contraindications	Cost
Nicotine nasal spray	Initially 1–2 doses/ hour and minimum of 8 doses/day; no more than 40 doses/ day for 3–6 months	Nasal irritation	Caution is advised among patients immediately post-MI (2 weeks) or with serious arrhythmias or unstable chest pain. Pregnancy class D	Prescription; ~$49/ bottle
Nicotine patch	Step-down dosing: 21 mg/24 hours for 4 weeks, then 14 mg/24 hours for 2 weeks, then 7 mg/24 hours for 2 weeks Single-patch dosing: 22 mg/24 hours (heavy smokers); 11 mg/24 hours (light smokers)	Local skin irritation	Caution is advised among patients immediately post-MI (2 weeks) or with serious arrhythmias or unstable chest pain. Pregnancy class D	Prescription or over the counter; 1 box of any dose ranges from $37–$48
Varenicline	0.5 mg once a day for 3 days, then BID for 4 days, then 1 mg BID for total of 12 weeks	Insomnia, nausea	Caution is advised in patients with creatinine clearance < 30 ml/min. Monitor for changes in mood or behavior in all patients, and consider psychiatric history before use. Pregnancy class D	Prescription; ~$130 for a 30-day supply

Note. Based on information from Chaney & Sheriff, 2012; Fiore et al., 2008.

For instance, studies have shown that longer, more intensive and individualized interventions result in higher abstinence rates, up to 40% in some cases (Chaney & Sheriff, 2012; Fiore et al., 2008). APNs can have patients set a quit date and sign a smoking cessation contract to facilitate ongoing commitment to their quit attempt. The Fagerström Test for Nicotine Dependence (Heatherton, Kozlowski, Frecker, & Fagerström, 1991) is a tool used to identify levels of nicotine dependence and thus gear the intensity of interventions accordingly. Oncology APNs are in a unique position to guide patients along the continuum of nicotine dependence—from identifying tobacco users to providing behavioral counseling and pharmacotherapy and aiding in relapse prevention or treatment.

Sun Exposure

Overexposure to ultraviolet radiation (UVR) is the greatest risk factor for all types of skin cancer, including melanoma and basal and squamous cell cancers. Most skin cancers are highly treatable, but the most deadly form of skin cancer, melanoma, is rising (ACS, 2015). More than 73,000 will be diagnosed in 2015, and close to 10,000 will die (ACS, 2015).

UVR is a known carcinogen, and two types can affect the skin—UVA and UVB. UVA rays penetrate deeper layers of the skin and are responsible for premature aging effects on the skin, whereas UVB rays mainly affect the epidermis and are the primary cause of sunburn (Brannon, n.d.; U.S. Environmental Protection Agency [EPA], 2006). UVB rays vary depending on the season and time of day. Engaging in regular activities to decrease exposure and protect the skin from UVR can significantly reduce the risk of skin cancer (ACS, 2013b). Primary prevention of skin cancer includes avoiding UVR as much as possible. ACS (2013b) recommends avoiding exposure to direct sunlight from 10 am to 4 pm, when UV rays are known to be most intense. Avoiding artificial sources of UVR, such as tanning beds, also is crucial in reducing the risk of skin cancer (ACS, 2013b). The International Agency for Research on Cancer Working Group on Artificial Ultraviolet Light and Skin Cancer (2007) listed these types of UVR-emitting devices as carcinogenic to humans, noting that melanoma risk was increased by 75% in those who used tanning beds as young adults (Cust et al., 2011).

In addition to minimizing sun exposure, other protective behaviors include protecting the skin with proper clothing and sunscreen. ACS (2013b) recommends the following four sun protective measures.
• Slip on a shirt.
• Slop on sunscreen.
• Slap on a hat.
• Wrap on sunglasses.

Wearing hats with wide brims, shirts and pants that adequately cover the extremities, and sunglasses to protect the eyes and covering exposed skin with sunscreen with a sun protection factor (SPF) of 15 or higher are all pertinent sun protective behaviors (ACS, 2013b, 2015). Broad-spectrum sunscreens contain ingredients that block or absorb both UVA and UVB rays with chemicals such as avobenzone, titanium dioxide, and zinc oxide (ACS, 2013b; Brannon, n.d.; U.S. EPA, 2006). FDA requires that all sunscreens contain an SPF, which correlates to the level of protection from UVB rays. For example, a sunscreen with an SPF of 15 protects against 93% of the sun's UVB rays, and every 15 minutes of wearing sunscreen with an SPF of 15 is equivalent to one minute of UVB exposure without sunscreen (ACS, 2013b; U.S. EPA, 2006).

In general, approximately 1 oz of sunscreen should be used to cover all exposed areas of skin, enough to form a thin film when first applied (ACS, 2013b; Brannon, n.d.). Sunscreen should be applied 30 minutes before exposure to the sun and reapplied every two hours and again after swimming, sweating, or toweling off (ACS, 2013b; Brannon, n.d.; U.S. EPA, 2006). Sunscreens labeled *water resistant* maintain their SPF for 40 minutes of water immersion, and those that are *very water resistant* maintain their SPF for 80 minutes (ACS, 2013b; U.S. EPA, 2006), but both need routine reapplication. Sunscreen should be applied before makeup. When used in combination with insect repellant, sunscreen with a higher SPF should be applied because repellants can reduce sunscreen's effectiveness by up to one-third (ACS, 2013b; Brannon, n.d.).

Diet and Exercise

The combination of obesity, physical inactivity, and poor nutrition is the second major risk factor for cancer behind tobacco use (ACS, 2015). Obesity is linked with a higher risk of cancer of the esophagus, pancreas, colon and rectum, breast (postmenopausal), endometrium, kidney, thyroid, gallbladder, liver, cervix, and ovaries (ACS, 2015; NCI, 2012). According to NCI (2012) Surveillance, Epidemiology, and End Results data, the percentage of cases attributed to obesity was as high as 40% in some cancers, such as esophageal and endometrial. Obesity is linked to 14%–20% of all cancer deaths in the United States (Kushi et al., 2012).

Obesity increases the risk for cancer in several possible ways. For example, excess amounts of estrogen are stored in fat cells, increasing the risk for female malignancies such as breast and endometrial cancers. Additionally, obesity increases levels of insulin and insulin-like growth factor-1, which may promote the development of certain tumors by inhibiting programmed cell death. Fat cells may also have direct and indirect effects on other tumor growth regulators, including mammalian target of rapamycin and adenosine monophosphate–activated protein kinase (NCI, 2012).

While obesity levels in the United States are staggering, with two-thirds of Americans overweight or obese (body mass index greater than 25) (ACS, 2015; NCI, 2012), less than one-quarter exercise or eat enough fruits or vegetables to be in accordance with ACS's guidelines on nutrition and physical activity for cancer prevention (Kushi et al., 2012). Most of the calories consumed by Americans come from foods high in fat, sugar, and refined carbohydrates. In 2011, only 20% of adults reported engaging in moderate or vigorous levels of physical activity, and only 15% ate three or more servings of vegetables. Increased intake of fruits and vegetables (nonstarchy) is associated with a lower risk of lung, esophageal, gastric, and colorectal cancers (ACS, 2015).

Physical activity can reduce the risk of several types of cancer, including breast, colon, endometrial, and prostate, and also can promote healthy body weight by matching energy output with caloric input (ACS, 2015). Examples of moderate everyday exercise include walking, dancing, and yoga. More vigorous activities include jogging or running, martial arts, and swimming. Moderate-intensity sports include baseball, volleyball, and golf, whereas soccer, basketball, and racquetball are considered vigorous activities. Even workplace activities can be sources of exercise, such as farming and custodial work. Forms of heavy manual labor, such as forestry, construction work, and firefighting, are considered vigorous activities (ACS, 2015).

Recommendations for diet and exercise to promote physical activity and combat obesity are outlined in Table 1-5. In general, to maintain lean body weight, people should engage in regular physical activity and limited consumption of high-calorie foods and drinks. For cancer prevention, recommendations include limiting intake of processed and/or red meats and alcohol, consuming at least 2.5 cups of vegetables and fruits per day, and choosing whole grains over refined grains (ACS, 2015).

Chemoprevention

Chemoprevention is defined as the use of natural, synthetic, or biologic agents to reverse, suppress, or prevent carcinogenic progression (NCI, 2014a). A variety of agents are being studied, and some have been approved for the prevention of prostate, colon, and breast cancer. However, certain risks are associated with chemopreventive drugs, such as unwanted side effects and the potential to cause more harm or even higher rates of malignancy, which occurred with the Alpha-Tocopherol, Beta-Carotene Cancer Prevention (ATBC) Trial and the Beta-Carotene and Retinol Efficacy Trial (CARET) (NCI, 2003). In these two studies, no benefit was seen from supplements in men at high risk for lung cancer. In fact, in participants taking beta-carotene in the ATBC Trial, 18% more lung cancers were diagnosed, and 8% more deaths occurred. In CARET, 28% more lung cancers were diagnosed, and 17% more deaths occurred in participants taking beta-carotene and vitamin A than in those taking placebos (Clark et al., 1996; Heinonen et al., 1998).

Oncology APNs play an important role in chemoprevention, either through risk assessments that lead to identification of potential candidates for chemopreventive agents, referral

---

Table 1-5. Guidelines on Nutrition and Physical Activity for Cancer Prevention

Topic	Recommendations
Diet	Consume a healthy diet with an emphasis on plant sources. • Consume foods and beverages in smaller portion sizes to help maintain healthy weight. • Consume whole grain rather than refined grain foods. • Consume at least 2.5 cups of fruits and vegetables/day. • Limit intake of processed and red meats. • Limit alcohol consumption to less than 1 drink/day for women and less than 2 drinks/day for men.
Exercise	Adopt a physically active lifestyle. • Adults: Engage in at least 150 minutes of moderate-intensity activity or 75 minutes of vigorous activity per week. • Children and adolescents: Engage in at least 60 minutes of moderate-intensity or vigorous activity every day with vigorous activity at least 3 days/week. • Limit sedentary activities such as watching television or other screen-related activities (e.g., computers, video games).
Weight	Achieve and maintain a healthy weight throughout life. • Maintain a lean body weight. • Avoid excess weight gain at all ages. • Even small amounts of weight loss can be beneficial in those who are overweight or obese.

Note. Based on information from American Cancer Society, 2015.

---

to appropriate clinical trials, or referral to qualified colleagues for further evaluation and management. Certain oncology APNs have subspecialized in the area of risk assessment, genetic counseling, and chemoprevention and are excellent sources of referral or collaboration (Swiderski, 2011; Vogel, 2003).

Tamoxifen and Raloxifene

In 1998, FDA approved tamoxifen, a selective estrogen receptor modulator (SERM), for the prevention of invasive breast cancer after results from the Breast Cancer Prevention Trial showed a 49% reduction in invasive breast cancer in more than 13,000 high-risk pre- and postmenopausal women (Fisher et al., 2005). Tamoxifen was approved for the prevention of invasive breast cancer for women with a history of noninvasive breast cancer (ductal carcinoma in situ and lobular carcinoma in situ) (Fisher et al., 2005). It is most effective in preventing estrogen receptor–positive breast cancers. Women who benefited most were those with a known genetic predisposition for *BRCA1/2* mutation, history of lobular carcinoma in situ, or atypical ductal hyperplasia (Fisher et al., 2005). Additional benefits yielded from the study included a 29% decrease in the risk of osteoporotic bone fractures in women aged 50 and older and a 53% decrease in women younger than 50 (Fisher et al., 2005). Risks associated with tamoxifen use include a higher incidence of thromboembolic events and endometrial cancer (Fisher et al., 2005). Because of these and other risks, the use of tamoxifen is individualized.

Results from the National Surgical Adjuvant Breast and Bowel Project Study of Tamoxifen and Raloxifene revealed that raloxifene, a second-generation SERM, has similar effects as tamoxifen in reducing invasive breast cancer in high-risk, postmenopausal women (Vogel et al., 2006). Additionally, fewer cases of uterine cancer, thromboembolic events, and cataracts were seen with raloxifene. Raloxifene was associated with an insignificantly higher number of patients with noninvasive breast cancer compared to tamoxifen (Vogel et al., 2006). Raloxifene is approved for breast cancer risk reduction in postmenopausal women at high risk for invasive breast cancer. While these drugs only prevent estrogen-driven breast cancer, studies are underway that are aimed at prevention of HER2-positive and triple-negative breast cancer—breast cancer that does not express estrogen, progesterone, or HER2 receptors (den Hollander, Savage, & Brown, 2013).

Celecoxib

Aspirin and nonsteroidal anti-inflammatory drugs (NSAIDs) have shown activity in the treatment and prevention of colon cancer; however, their gastrointestinal side effects have limited their applicability (Cuzick et al., 2009). Newer NSAIDs, such as celecoxib, selectively inhibit cyclooxygenase-2 (COX-2), a catalytic enzyme in prostaglandin synthesis that is induced in inflammatory conditions, including those involved with tumor proliferation. COX-2 is not normally found in the epithelium of the colon but is overexpressed in a majority of adenocarcinomas and less so in adenomatous polyps of the colon (Bertagnolli et al., 2006). Celecoxib, at 400 mg BID, has received approval from FDA for the prevention of adenomatous polyps in patients with familial adenomatous polyposis, a hereditary colon cancer syndrome associated with hundreds of thousands of colon polyps and a 100% risk of colorectal cancer if untreated. Celecoxib is not approved for chemoprevention in the general public (Bertagnolli et al., 2006).

Human Papillomavirus Vaccines

Three FDA-approved vaccines are available for the prevention of cervical cancer, precancerous or dysplastic cervical and vaginal lesions, and genital warts associated with HPV. Gardasil® (human papillomavirus quadrivalent [types 6, 11, 16, and 18] vaccine, recombinant) received approval in 2006 and protects against HPV types 6, 11, 16, and 18 (U.S. FDA, 2006). This was the first vaccine approved for cervical cancer prevention, and in clinical trials it showed nearly 100% effectiveness in preventing precancerous cervical, vaginal, and vulvar lesions and genital warts caused by HPV in women who had not yet been infected (U.S. FDA, 2006). In 2014, a newer version of the vaccine, Gardasil® 9, was approved for five additional subtypes of HPV (for a total of nine). Its indications and uses are similar to the original vaccine. However, Gardasil is approved for use in females ages 9–26 and also has an indication for prevention of anal cancer and genital warts in males in the same age group, whereas Gardasil 9 has a similar indication for females but is only approved for use in males ages 9–18 (U.S. FDA 2006, 2015). Another vaccine, Cervarix® (HPV bivalent [types 16 and 18] vaccine, recombinant), received approval in early 2009 and protects against HPV types 16 and 18 only (U.S. FDA, 2009) and is approved for use in females ages 9–25 only. All of these vaccines should be given before a patient is sexually active to be most effective (ACS, 2015; U.S. FDA, 2015). These vaccines are not approved to treat cervical or anal cancer and are not intended to replace cervical cancer screening.

Secondary Prevention and Screening

According to NCI (2014b), screening for cancer in the general population refers to detecting cancer when no apparent symptoms are present, with an overall goal of decreasing cancer-related morbidity and mortality. Estimates of early deaths that have the potential to be avoided through the use of screening tests vary from 3% to 35%. For almost all types of cancer, improved outcomes are seen when treatment is initiated at the earliest stage possible, hence the importance of early detection. For cancer screening to be effective, screening tests must meet two criteria. First, the screening test must be able to detect cancer at an earlier stage than if it were detected as a result of symptom development. Second, evidence must support that treatment given at an earlier stage results in improved outcomes (NCI, 2014b). The sensitivity and specificity of all screening tests must be considered. *Sensitivity* refers to the proportion of people with cancer that are found to have a positive test—a higher sensitivity means fewer false-negative results. Conversely, *specificity* refers to the proportion of people without cancer that have negative results (NCI, n.d.); in other words, the higher the specificity, the fewer false-positive results. Potential harms from screening tests also must be weighed against potential benefits. Some screening tests are invasive, such as colonoscopy for colon cancer, and carry risks associated with any invasive procedure, including some serious if not life-threatening complications (such as bowel perforation with colonoscopy). Other potential harms include the emotional anxiety associated with false-positive results and the dangers of missing an early malignancy with false-negative test results (NCI, 2014b). The financial cost of different screening tests varies widely.

Multiple organizations have published screening guidelines for a variety of malignancies, both for average-risk and high-risk populations. Oncology APNs must have an understanding of each organization's guidelines and appreciate the differences among them. In general, consensus exists among screening recommendations for the most common malignancies, including breast, cervical, colorectal, lung, and prostate cancer. Variances in screening intervals and ages for screening initiation and cessation vary from minute to major differences. The recommended routine screening guidelines from ACS, the National Comprehensive Cancer Network® (NCCN®), and the U.S. Preventive Services Task Force (USPSTF) are outlined in Table 1-6.

Breast Cancer

Breast cancer is the most common female malignancy and the second most common cause of cancer death in women. In 2015, an estimated 234,190 new cases of breast cancer are expected to be diagnosed. The lifetime risk of developing breast cancer in an average-risk woman is one in eight. This risk increases with age, and the disease occurs most commonly in women; however, approximately 2,350 cases of breast cancer are expected to be diagnosed in men in 2015. The five-year survival rate for localized breast cancer is 98%, hence the importance of early diagnosis and treatment (ACS, 2015).

Risk factors for breast cancer are generally well known and linked to genetic, reproductive, and lifestyle factors. Modifiable risk factors include weight gain after age 18, postmenopausal obesity, menopausal hormone replacement therapy, physical inactivity, and alcohol consumption. Nonmodifiable risk factors and medical conditions that increase risk for breast cancer include high breast tissue density, high bone mineral density, breast biopsy positive for hyperplasia, high-dose radiation therapy to the chest (such as mantle radiation for Hodgkin lymphoma), early menarche, late menopause, nulliparity, primiparity after age 30, family history of breast cancer (particularly one or more first-degree relative), and *BRCA1* or *BRCA2* deleterious mutations (ACS, 2015).

In 2015, more than 40,000 women will die from breast cancer. Breast cancer screening has been shown to decrease mortality from breast cancer (ACS, 2015). As listed in Table 1-6, the general consensus for breast cancer screening in average-risk women includes counseling regarding breast awareness, clinical breast examination (CBE) beginning at various ages and continued at various intervals, and annual mammography beginning at age 40 (ACS, 2013a; NCCN, 2014a). Most organizations no longer specifically recommend a breast self-

Table 1-6. Selected Cancer Screening Recommendations for Average-Risk Population

Organization	Breast Cancer	Cervical Cancer	Colorectal Cancer	Lung Cancer	Prostate Cancer
National Comprehensive Cancer Network	Women aged 25–39: • CBE every 1–3 years and breast awareness Women aged ≥ 40: • Annual MMG • Annual CBE and breast awareness	Women aged 21–29: • Pap test every 3 years • No HPV testing Women aged 30–65: • Pap test and HPV testing every 5 years (preferred) **OR** Pap test alone every 3 years Women > age 65: • No screening if there is no history of CIN2+ in the past 20 years **OR** 3 consecutive negative Pap tests (or 2 consecutive Pap and HPV cotests) in the last 10 years and the most recent test within the last 5 years No screening at any age for women with a history of total hysterectomy and no history of CIN2+	Men and women aged ≥ 50 (with no history of inflammatory bowel disease and no personal or family history of adenoma or colon cancer): • Colonoscopy every 10 years (preferred) **OR** • FOBT or FIT annually **AND** flexible sigmoidoscopy every 5 years **OR** • Flexible sigmoidoscopy every 5 years	Men and women aged 55–74, current or former smokers **AND** ≥ 30 pack-year smoking history **AND** smoking cessation < 15 years, **AND** Men and women aged ≥ 50, current or former smokers **AND** ≥ 20-pack-year smoking history **AND** one additional risk factor other than secondhand smoke exposure (radon, occupational exposure, personal or family history of cancer, COPD, or pulmonary fibrosis) • Baseline LDCT and for at least 2 years and until no longer eligible for treatment No routine lung cancer screening for low- or moderate-risk patients	Men aged ≥ 40: • Risk-benefit discussion about baseline PSA testing and DRE

(Continued on next page)

Table 1-6. Selected Cancer Screening Recommendations for Average-Risk Population *(Continued)*

Organization	Breast Cancer	Cervical Cancer	Colorectal Cancer	Lung Cancer	Prostate Cancer
American Cancer Society	Women aged 20–39: • BSE (optional) • CBE at least every 3 years Women aged ≥ 40: • BSE (optional) • CBE annually • MMG annually	Women aged 21–29: • Pap test (conventional or liquid-based) every 3 years Women aged 30–65: • Pap and HPV DNA test every 5 years **OR** Pap alone every 3 years Women aged > 65: • No screening if ≥ 3 negative Pap tests or ≥ 2 negative HPV and Pap co-tests within the last 10 years (and the most recent occurring within the last 5 years) No screening for women with a history of total hysterectomy	Men and women starting at age 50: • FOBT or FIT annually **OR** • Flexible sigmoidoscopy every 5 years **OR** • DCBE every 5 years **OR** • Colonoscopy every 10 years • CT colonography every 5 years	Men and women aged 55–74, current or former smokers (quit < 15 years ago), in good health, and ≥ 30 pack-year smoking history: • Discussion with healthcare provider about screening with low-dose helical chest CT scan	Men aged ≥ 50 with at least 10-year life expectancy: • Consideration of DRE and PSA after informed clinical decision making process with healthcare provider

(Continued on next page)

Table 1-6. Selected Cancer Screening Recommendations for Average-Risk Population (Continued)

Organization	Breast Cancer	Cervical Cancer	Colorectal Cancer	Lung Cancer	Prostate Cancer
U.S. Preventive Services Task Force	Women aged 40–49: • Individualized discussion and consideration of biennial MMG Women aged 50–74: • MMG every 2 years Women aged ≥ 75: • No recommendation for MMG Women with dense breasts: • Insufficient evidence to recommend adjunctive screening with other methods BSE not recommended for any age group, and no recommendation for CBE	Women aged 21–65: • Pap test every 3 years or every 5 years with HPV co-testing Women aged > 65: • May opt to discontinue screening if 3 consecutive negative Pap tests or 2 negative consecutive Pap tests with HPV co-testing within the previous 10 years (and the most recent test within previous 5 years) No screening for women with a history of hysterectomy (with removal of cervix) and no history of CIN2 or 3	Men and women aged 50–75: • Routine screening with use of FOBT, flexible sigmoidoscopy, and colonoscopy (no specific intervals given) Men and women aged 76–85: • Clinical considerations may warrant individualized screening; otherwise, routine screening not recommended Men and women aged > 85: • Routine screening not recommended No recommendation on fecal DNA testing or CT colonography	Men and women of any age: • No recommendation for routine screening with chest x-ray, LDCT, or sputum cytology	Men of any age: • Recommends against PSA-based screening

BSE—breast self-examination; CBE—clinical breast exam; CIN—cervical intraepithelial neoplasia; COPD—chronic obstructive pulmonary disease; CT—computed tomography; DCBE—double-contrast barium enema; DRE—digital rectal examination; FIT—fecal immunochemical test; FOBT—fecal occult blood test; HPV—human papillomavirus; LDCT—low-dose computed tomography; MMG—mammogram; PSA—prostate-specific antigen

Note. Based on information from American Cancer Society, 2013a, 2015; National Comprehensive Cancer Network, 2014a, 2014b, 2014c, 2015a, 2015b; Saslow et al., 2012; U.S. Preventive Services Task Force, 2008, 2009, 2012a, 2012b, 2013, 2016.

examination but rather breast awareness with an emphasis on reporting any changes in the breasts immediately to a healthcare provider. Breastcancer.org (2014) offers an easy, patient-friendly guide to breast self-examination. Premenopausal women may find breast examination to be most effective at the end of menses (NCCN, 2015a). When performing a CBE, clinicians should inspect and palpate women's breasts in upright and supine positions, documenting any changes in breast color, symmetry, and thickness or the presence of masses (Grethlein, 2013).

However, ongoing controversy exists regarding the sensitivity and cost-effectiveness of mammography in women between ages 40 and 50. In 2009, USPSTF recommended against screening mammography in women younger than age 50. According to USPSTF, the over-all reduced mortality from breast cancer with biennial screening mammography was greatest in women ages 50–59. In younger women, those ages 40–49, the relative risk reduction was lower, and USPSTF felt that little additional benefit was attained. Thus, its recommendation was to start mammography at age 50 and then continue only every two years. The task force's data projected that biennial screening achieved 70%–99% of the benefit of annual screening and with fewer harms. Most other organizations have not changed their recommendations for breast cancer screening because they felt that the data from USPSTF overemphasized the harms of mammography (Smith, Cokkinides, Brooks, Saslow, & Brawley, 2010).

As with all screening tests, mammography has risks and benefits. Risks include false-positive results, potentially leading to more testing and invasive procedures such as biopsy. False negatives are also a concern, as not all breast cancers are detected with mammography. Mammographic sensitivity reaches up to 96% but is lower in women aged 40–49 and those with denser breasts (Smith et al., 2011). According to the Digital Mammographic Imaging Screening Trial, digital mammography proved to be more accurate than film mammography in women with dense breasts who were younger than 50 years of age and who were pre- or peri-menopausal (ACS, 2015).

Magnetic resonance imaging (MRI) may be superior to mammography in high-risk women (ACS, 2013a; Warner, 2011). Several studies using MRI screening in high-risk populations are ongoing, but MRI screening has not yet been found to reduce mortality in any group of women. ACS and NCCN recommend annual breast screening with MRI as an adjunct to mammography in women at high risk for breast cancer. This includes women with a 20%–25% or greater lifetime risk of developing breast cancer, *BRCA1* or *BRCA2* mutation carriers, women with a first-degree family member with *BRCA1* or *BRCA2* mutation, and women with Li-Fraumeni (p53 mutation) or Cowden syndromes (*PTEN* mutation), significant family history of breast or ovarian cancer, or history of mantle radiation therapy associated with treatment for Hodgkin lymphoma (NCCN, 2014a; Saslow et al., 2007).

Cervical Cancer

Cervical cancer is the third most common female gynecologic cancer. Since the introduction of the Pap test more than 50 years ago, cervical cancer incidence and mortality rates have declined steadily (ACS, 2015). In 2015, approximately 12,900 new cases of cervical cancer are expected to be diagnosed, and 4,100 deaths from the disease are estimated to occur. When detected early, localized cervical cancer is one of the most successfully treated cancers, boasting a five-year survival rate of 91% (ACS, 2015).

The most significant risk factor for cervical cancer is HPV infection. HPV, a sexually transmitted infection, is the most common cause of and greatest risk factor for premalignant and malignant cervical lesions (ACS, 2015). More than 200 types of HPV have been identified, 20 of which have been associated with cancer. Benign cervical lesions (genital warts and cervical intraepithelial neoplasia) are most commonly associated with HPV types 6, 11, 42, 43, and 44.

HPV strains 16 and 18 are most commonly associated with cervical cancer and are targeted by the HPV vaccines Gardasil, Gardasil 9, and Cervarix (Dunne et al., 2007; U.S. FDA, 2009, 2015). An estimated 26.8% of women aged 14–59 are infected with HPV, according to data from the National Health and Nutrition Examination Survey. HPV infection was highest in women aged 20–24, and 15.2% of women overall were infected with high-risk strains 16 and 18 (Dunne et al., 2007). Additionally, other risk factors for cervical cancer include those related to sexual history and gynecologic history, smoking, and immunosuppression (ACS, 2015).

Routine screening recommendations for cervical cancer are outlined in Table 1-6. Recommendations generally include initiation of Pap test alone by age 21. By age 30, co-testing with Pap and HPV testing every five years is preferred over Pap testing alone every three years. Annual screening with any test in any age group is not recommended (ACS, 2013a; Saslow et al., 2012).

Colorectal Cancer

Colorectal cancer is both the third most common cancer and the third leading cause of cancer death in the United States. In 2015, an estimated 132,700 new cases of colorectal cancer are expected to be diagnosed, with 49,700 deaths expected to occur (ACS, 2015). Colorectal cancer incidence and mortality rates have been declining over the past 20 years, mainly as a result of increased use of early detection and screening tests (Haggar & Boushey, 2009).

When colorectal cancer is detected early, the five-year survival rate is 90%. However, less than half of colorectal cancers are diagnosed this early. As with most malignancies, a more advanced stage at diagnosis is associated with decreased survival. The five-year survival rate for locally advanced colorectal cancer (involvement of regional lymph nodes) is 70%, and those with distant metastases have even poorer outcomes, with only a 12% five-year survival (ACS, 2015).

Several known risk factors exist for colorectal cancer, although up to 70% of cases have no identifiable risk factors (Haggar & Boushey, 2009). The most common risk factor for the development of colorectal cancer is age, with more than 90% of cases found in those older than age 50 (ACS, 2015). Other risk factors include lifestyle factors, such as physical inactivity, obesity, alcohol intake, type 2 diabetes, smoking, and diets high in red meat and low in fiber, fruits, and vegetables (ACS, 2015). Other conditions of the colon, such as inflammatory bowel disease, colon adenomas, and a genetic predisposition or hereditary polyposis syndrome, increase the risk of colorectal cancer (see Table 1-7) (ACS, 2015; Haggar & Boushey, 2009). Conversely, protective factors include diets high in calcium, higher serum vitamin D levels, and regular use of aspirin or other NSAIDs (ACS, 2015).

The purpose of screening for colorectal cancer is to identify adenomatous or precancerous polyps and remove them before they progress to malignancy, thereby resulting in decreased mortality and better outcomes. Polypectomy and subsequent surveillance with colonoscopy can reduce colorectal cancer incidence by 90% (Haggar & Boushey, 2009). Guidelines for screening average-risk populations (age 50 or older, no history of adenoma or inflammatory bowel disease, and negative family history) are outlined in Table 1-6. In general, recommendations include screening beginning at age 50 and include either annual fecal occult blood test (FOBT) or fecal immunochemical testing (FIT), sigmoidoscopy every five years, annual FOBT or FIT in combination with sigmoidoscopy every five years, or a full colonoscopy every 10 years (ACS, 2013a; NCCN, 2014b).

Lung Cancer

Lung cancer is the most fatal malignancy and the second most commonly occurring cancer in both men and women. In 2015, an approximate 221,200 new cases and 158,040 deaths are

Table 1-7. Diseases of the Colon and Colorectal Cancer Risk

Risk Factor	Risk of Colorectal Cancer (CRC)
Ulcerative colitis	• Causes 1% of all cases of CRC • Increases with age at onset, extent of disease, and duration of active disease • Cumulative risk is 3% at 15 years, 5% at 20 years, and 9% at 25 years.
Crohn disease	• Twofold increased risk of CRC
Polyps	• 70% of polyps are adenomatous or neoplastic: 75%–85% tubular adenomas (lowest risk), 10%–25% tubulovillous adenomas (intermediate risk), ≤ 5% villous adenomas (highest risk) • > 1 cm in size: 2–4-fold increased risk of CRC • Multiple polyps: 5–7-fold increased risk • Time to malignant progression: 3.5 years for severely dysplastic polyps and 11.5 years for mild atypia
Family history of CRC	• One first-degree relative: Relative risk increased to 1.72 • Two first-degree relatives: Relative risk increased to 2.75

Hereditary nonpolyposis colorectal cancer	Lynch syndromes
	• Lynch I (colonic syndrome)
	  – Autosomal dominant trait associated with proximal mucinous or poorly differentiated synchronous or metachronous colonic tumors
	  – Usual development of CRC by age 50; 75% overall lifetime risk
	• Lynch II
	  – Associated with extracolonic tumors in the ovaries, endometrium, stomach, small intestine, and genitourinary and hepatobiliary tracts

Familial adenomatous polyposis	• Autosomal dominant inherited syndrome (germ-line mutation in adenomatous polyposis coli gene on chromosome 5q21) consisting of hundreds of colonic polyps developed by late adolescence • 100% lifetime risk of developing CRC

Note. Based on information from American Cancer Society, 2015; Haggar & Boushey, 2009.

to be expected. Cigarette smoking is the main risk factor in lung cancer development, with risk increasing based on duration and quantity smoked (expressed in pack-years). Additional risk factors include radon exposure and other occupational or environmental exposures, including secondhand smoke (ACS, 2015).

Only 15% of lung cancers are diagnosed at an early stage, where the five-year survival rate is 54% (ACS, 2015). Until recently, no routine screening for lung cancer had shown effectiveness in reducing lung cancer deaths. In 2011, results from the National Lung Screening Trial were published, citing a 20% reduction in lung cancer deaths with annual low-dose computed tomography (LDCT) in smokers with at least a 30 pack-year smoking history (one pack per day for 30 years) (National Lung Screening Trial Research Team, 2011). Since then, ACS and NCCN have updated their lung cancer screening guidelines (see Table 1-6). ACS (2013a) and NCCN (2015b) recommend screening for lung cancer with annual LDCT in patients ages 55–74 who are current or former smokers (greater than or equal to 30 pack years) and are otherwise in good health. NCCN guidelines also include screening recommendations for those who smoke less but have additional risk factors. It is noted that smoking cessation counseling should not be eliminated in lieu of lung cancer screening.

Prostate Cancer

Prostate cancer is the most commonly diagnosed cancer in men and the second leading cause of cancer-related death in men in the United States. In 2015, close to 220,800 new cases of prostate cancer will be diagnosed, and 27,540 deaths are expected to occur. The most common risk factor for prostate cancer is age, with 97% of prostate cancer diagnosed in men older than age 50. African American men have a higher incidence and mortality from prostate cancer compared to Caucasian men (ACS, 2015).

The majority (93%) of prostate cancers are diagnosed in an early stage, and the five-year survival rate for localized disease approaches 100%. However, the data surrounding regular screening for prostate cancer with prostate-specific antigen (PSA) have become a controversial issue over the past several years (ACS, 2015). The issue is that although PSA screening clearly detects prostate cancer in its earliest stage, it is largely debatable as to whether screening asymptomatic men with PSA testing reduces mortality. Studies have documented that more than half of the prostate cancers diagnosed early with PSA screening are low risk and would likely never have caused clinically significant problems. Thus, routine screening may lead to overdiagnosis and overtreatment in a large part of the screened population. This was noted in the large U.S. randomized Prostate, Lung, Colorectal and Ovarian Cancer Screening Trial: the early detection of low-risk disease may ultimately result in increased morbidity and diminished quality of life if these men are treated with aggressive therapy (Croswell, Kramer, & Crawford, 2011).

Another issue is the reliability of the PSA test itself. Data suggest that although one out of every three prostate biopsies is positive because of an elevated PSA, two out of three are not (high false-positive results). Additionally, it is suggested that one in seven men with a normal PSA have prostate cancer (high false-negative results) (Smith et al., 2011). PSA results may be low with very aggressive prostate cancer, and benign conditions such as prostatitis can result in markedly elevated levels (Hoffman, 2011). Research is ongoing to find newer biologic markers for screening, different screening modalities, and initiation and interval of screening, with the aim to detect those high-risk prostate cancers and reduce unnecessary testing and treatment of men with low risk of mortality from the disease (ACS, 2015; Hoffman, 2011).

Most experts agree that individualized risk assessments and evaluation for screening should be determined by the patient and provider (ACS, 2015). Screening guidelines for average-risk men are outlined in Table 1-6 and generally consist of initiating PSA screening between ages 40 and 50 with discussion regarding risk-benefit ratio. In keeping with controversial results surrounding PSA testing, USPSTF (2012b) specifically recommends against screening with PSA for any man at any time.

Skin Cancer

In 2015, an estimated 73,870 cases of malignant melanoma are expected to be diagnosed. This is in addition to the millions of nonmelanoma skin cancers diagnosed each year, such as basal and squamous cell skin cancers. These are difficult to accurately account for because they are not reported to tumor registries. Nonmelanoma skin cancers are mostly highly curable, but melanoma, which accounts for less than 2% of skin cancers, has the highest mortality rate. In 2015, an expected 9,940 people will die from melanoma (ACS, 2015).

Most cases of skin cancer are caused by unprotected or excessive exposure of the skin to UVR (ACS, 2015). UVR exposure can come from natural sources or artificial sources, such as tanning beds, and both result in skin damage ranging from wrinkling and premature aging to skin cancer (ACS, 2015). Risk factors for melanoma and nonmelanoma skin cancers differ. The greatest risk factors for melanoma include a personal or family history of melanoma and the presence of multiple atypical nevi (greater than 50). Risk factors for all skin cancers, including nonmelanoma skin cancers, include lighter skin tone (lifetime risk of melanoma is 25 times higher among Caucasians compared to African Americans), high sun sensitivity (e.g., having difficulty tanning or easily sunburning, red or blond hair, previous sunburns), immunosuppression, and previous history of skin cancer (ACS, 2015).

Melanoma is highly curable if treated early, with a 98% five-year survival rate. Melanoma is more likely to metastasize than other skin cancers, and the five-year survival rate drops to 16% for late-stage disease (ACS, 2015). The most effective way to detect skin cancer early, including melanoma, is to recognize new or changing skin lesions. The ABCD rule—asymmetry, border, color, and diameter—is an easy, patient-friendly tool to help remember the warning signs for suspicious skin lesions or melanoma (see Figure 1-1).

- **A** is for **Asymmetry**: One half of the mole does not match the other half.
- **B** is for **Border** irregularity: The edges of the mole are irregular, blurred, jagged, or notched.
- **C** is for **Color**: The color of the mole is not uniform, with varying degrees of tan, brown, or black.
- **D** is for **Diameter**: The diameter of the mole is greater than 6 mm, or the size of a pencil eraser.

Figure 1-1. ABCD Rule for Melanoma

Note. Based on information from American Cancer Society, 2015.

Other Cancers

Although established screening tests and guidelines exist for several cancers, the majority of malignancies do not have screening recommendations, as insufficient evidence exists to suggest that screening would affect mortality rates. No standard screening tests are recommended for cancers of the kidney, pancreas, thyroid, or urinary bladder. For cancers of the liver and ovary, no screening tests are recommended for average-risk individuals, but those at high risk for these cancers are often screened despite no proven reduction in mortality. As such, no standard screening testing is recommended for women at average risk for endometrial cancer, but those with known or suspected Lynch syndrome should have annual screening with endometrial biopsy or transvaginal ultrasound beginning at age 35 (ACS, 2015). More research is needed in identifying beneficial screening modalities and recommendations for these and other malignancies. The National Institutes of Health lists almost 1,000 clinical trials across the United States that are actively recruiting for cancer screening trial participants.

Implications for Oncology Advanced Practice Nurses

The role of oncology APNs encompasses cancer risk reduction, screening, and early detection. Oncology APNs are able to assess, evaluate, and interpret cancer risk assessments and recommend appropriate interventions. Familiarity with known risk factors for various cancers alerts APNs to patients who would benefit from evidence-based interventions to reduce cancer risk. Guidelines are available to guide APN interventions. Strategies are modified based on individual characteristics, population risk variances, and cultural diversities. It is imperative that oncology APNs master these topics to provide comprehensive, thorough oncology care that begins with risk assessment to reach the goal of cancer prevention.

Conclusion

Cancer prevention and early detection are integral parts of the cancer care continuum. Ideally, primary cancer prevention in the form of risk reduction is the best way to decrease morbidity and mortality related to cancer. Certain populations are considered to be at high risk for some malignancies, and the screening and management of these populations differs from that of the general population. Risk models are available to assist APNs in assessment for certain cancers. Evidence-based pharmacologic, nonpharmacologic, and behavioral interventions are available. Education of both individuals and populations is crucial. Education encompasses information about exercise, dietary habits, sun protection, smoking cessation, and recommended screening practices. Early detection achieved by adhering to routine screening guidelines facilitates diagnosis at the earliest stage, when the cancer is most likely to be treated successfully and is associated with the best patient outcomes. Oncology APNs have the opportunity and obligation to offer risk-reduction care and appropriate screening to both individual patients and populations.

Case Study

A.K. is a 55-year-old African American woman seen in the oncology clinic by the oncology APN for follow-up care for anemia. A.K. states that she receives health care at a walk-in clinic only when she is ill and that she had previously been out of work for some time and had not had insurance to cover routine medical care until recently. Review of her family history confirms colon cancer in her 70-year-old mother, diagnosed at age 65. Her 73-year-old father has heart disease and hypertension and was diagnosed with prostate cancer at age 72. She has two brothers, who also have hypertension. She is married and has no children or any pregnancies. She smokes less than one half pack of cigarettes per day for 15 years and is interested in quitting but admits she needs help. She denies alcohol use. A.K. works 40–50 hours a week, does not engage in regular exercise, and eats fast food frequently.

Her review of systems is negative except for fatigue and intermittent arthralgia with a previous history of osteoarthritis, for which she takes occasional acetaminophen. She is postmenopausal; her last menstrual cycle was more than two years ago. Other past medical and surgical history is negative. The physical examination (including CBE, pelvic examination, and Pap/HPV test) is also negative, vital signs are stable, and no gross abnormalities are apparent on examination except for moderate obesity and pale oral mucosal membranes.

1. What risk factors for malignancy can be identified based on this history?
   - Her risks for cancer include tobacco use, sedentary lifestyle, obesity, and poor nutrition. She is nulliparous and has one first-degree relative with a history of colon cancer. Her father's recent diagnosis of prostate cancer at age 72 is noted but does not necessarily affect A.K.'s risk factors at this point.
2. What screening tests does A.K. need, and what cancer risk–reduction strategies can the oncology APN discuss with A.K.?
   - As A.K. has not received routine medical care in several years, she has neglected the recommended cancer screening tests. Recommendations include smoking cessation, and because she is willing to make a quit attempt, NRT may be offered in the form of transdermal nicotine. Counseling regarding smoking cessation will increase effective-

ness of the intervention. Physical activity of moderate intensity for at least 150 minutes per week is a behavioral goal. Dietary counseling is necessary, focusing on eating fewer high-fat foods and consuming at least 2.5 cups of fruits and vegetables per day. Counseling on the techniques, benefits, and limitations of breast self-examination will increase the patient's confidence in performing this examination.

- A screening mammogram is appropriate, along with a referral to a gastroenterologist for a screening colonoscopy. Informational needs include screening recommendations for mammogram and CBE annually, pelvic examination with Pap and HPV co-testing every five years, and colonoscopy every five years, given her positive family history (assuming initial colonoscopy results are benign). She is not a candidate for LDCT because of her low risk for lung cancer at this point. Smoking cessation should still be advised.

3. Before she leaves, A.K. inquires about a television commercial for a vaccine for cervical cancer and wants to know if that is an option for her. How does the oncology APN respond?

- The oncology APN tells A.K. that three vaccines are available, Gardasil, Gardasil 9, and Cervarix, and are for the prevention of cervical cancer associated with HPV infection in females 9–26 years of age. Therefore, A.K. is not a candidate for this vaccination, and the APN recommends she continue with Pap and HPV co-testing for early detection of cervical cancer as discussed previously.

Key Points

- Primary prevention of cancer is achieved through promotion of wellness and reduction of known risks for cancer.
- Cancer risk assessment involves an individualized, comprehensive patient history and examination to provide accurate cancer risk–reduction counseling and screening recommendations.
- Major components of cancer risk reduction for the general population include
  - Avoid or cease cigarette smoking.
  - Minimize UVR exposure, and use sunscreen with an SPF of at least 15 on sun-exposed skin.
  - Maintain an active lifestyle with regular physical activity.
  - Maintain a healthy weight (avoid obesity).
  - Eat a diet high in fiber, fruits, and vegetables and low in red or processed meats, fats, and sugars.
- Chemoprevention is an option for certain high-risk patients.
- Secondary prevention includes screening and early detection of cancer.
- Screening tests require specificity (few false positives) and sensitivity (few false negatives) for the disease being screened for.
- Screening guidelines exist for the general population and for populations at high risk for various cancers, including those with a genetic predisposition for certain cancers.

Recommended Resources for Oncology Advanced Practice Nurses

- Breast Cancer Risk Assessment Tool (www.cancer.gov/bcrisktool): This tool was developed to estimate a woman's risk for breast cancer. The model has been updated to include risk for racial differences. Mobile access is available.

- Colorectal Cancer Risk Assessment Tool (www.cancer.gov/colorectalcancerrisk): This tool was developed for risk estimation in men and women of multiple racial backgrounds and with a variety of other gastrointestinal precursors. Mobile access is available.
- Melanoma Risk Assessment Tool (www.cancer.gov/melanomarisktool): An interactive tool developed to estimate absolute risk of developing invasive melanoma. Mobile access is available.
- NCCN guidelines for detection, prevention, and risk reduction (www.nccn.org): Guidelines are available on breast, hereditary breast and ovarian, cervical, colorectal, lung, and prostate cancer screening or early detection.
- NCI's *Dictionary of Cancer Terms* (www.cancer.gov/dictionary): This resource contains more than 7,000 terms related to cancer and medicine and is available in Spanish.

References

American Association of Nurse Practitioners. (2013). *Scope of practice for nurse practitioners.* Retrieved from http://www.aanp.org/images/documents/publications/scopeofpractice.pdf

American Cancer Society. (2013a). American Cancer Society guidelines for the early detection of cancer. Retrieved from http://www.cancer.org/healthy/findcancerearly/cancerscreeningguidelines/american-cancer-society-guidelines-for-the-early-detection-of-cancer

American Cancer Society. (2013b). Skin cancer prevention and early detection. Retrieved from http://www.cancer.org/acs/groups/cid/documents/webcontent/003184-pdf.pdf

American Cancer Society. (2015). *Cancer facts and figures 2015.* Retrieved from http://www.cancer.org/research/cancerfactsstatistics/cancerfactsfigures2015/index

Barr, G., Houston-Miller, N., Hasan, I., & Makinson, G. (2013). Nurse practitioners, wake up and smell the smoke. *Journal of the American Association of Nurse Practitioners, 25,* 362–367. doi:10.1002/2327-6924.12049

Bertagnolli, M.M., Eagle, C.J., Zauber, A.G., Redston, M., Solomon, S.D., Kim, K., … Hawk, E.T. (2006). Celecoxib for the prevention of sporadic colorectal adenomas. *New England Journal of Medicine, 355,* 873–884. doi:10.1056/NEJMoa061355

Brannon, H. (n.d.). Proper use of sunscreen. Retrieved from http://dermatology.about.com/cs/skincareproducts/l/blsunscreen.htm

Brant, J.M., & Wickham, R. (2013). *Statement on the scope and standards of oncology nursing practice: Generalist and advanced practice.* Pittsburgh, PA: Oncology Nursing Society.

Breastcancer.org. (2014). The five steps of a breast self-exam. Retrieved from http://www.breastcancer.org/symptoms/testing/types/self_exam/bse_steps

Bullen, C., Howe, C., Laugesen, M., McRobbie, H., Parag, V., Williman, J., & Walker, N. (2013). Electronic cigarettes for smoking cessation: A randomised controlled trial. *Lancet, 382,* 1629–1637. doi:10.1016/S0140-6736(13)61842-5

Campaign for Tobacco-Free Kids. (2014, December 30). Toll of tobacco in the United States of America. Retrieved from http://www.tobaccofreekids.org/research/factsheets/pdf/0072.pdf

Centers for Disease Control and Prevention. (2004). *The health consequences of smoking: A report of the surgeon general.* Atlanta, GA: Author.

Centers for Disease Control and Prevention. (2011). State-specific trends in lung cancer incidence and smoking—United States, 1999–2008. *Morbidity and Mortality Weekly Report, 60,* 1243–1247. Retrieved from http://www.cdc.gov/mmwr/preview/mmwrhtml/mm6036a3.htm

Centers for Disease Control and Prevention. (2012a). Current cigarette smoking among adults—United States, 2011. *Morbidity and Mortality Weekly Report, 61,* 889–894. Retrieved from http://www.cdc.gov/mmwr/preview/mmwrhtml/mm6144a2.htm

Centers for Disease Control and Prevention. (2012b). Current tobacco use among middle and high school students—United States, 2011. *Morbidity and Mortality Weekly Report, 61,* 581–585. Retrieved from http://www.cdc.gov/mmwr/preview/mmwrhtml/mm6131a1.htm

Chaney, S.E., & Sheriff, S. (2012). Evidence-based treatments for smoking cessation. *Nurse Practitioner, 37*(4), 24–31. doi:10.1097/01.NPR.0000412892.27557.e8

Clark, L.C., Combs, G.F., Jr., Turnbull, B.W., Slate, E.H., Chalker, D.K., Chow, J., … Taylor, J.R. (1996). Effects of selenium supplementation for cancer prevention in patients with carcinoma of the skin: A randomized controlled trial. *JAMA, 276,* 1957–1963. doi:10.1001/jama.1996.03540240035027

Croswell, J.M., Kramer, B.S., & Crawford, E.D. (2011). Screening for prostate cancer with PSA testing: Current status and future directions. *Oncology, 25*, 452–460, 463. Retrieved from http://www.cancernetwork.com/oncology -journal/screening-prostate-cancer-psa-testing-current-status-and-future-directions

Cust, A.E., Armstrong, B.K., Goumas, C., Jenkins, M.A., Schmid, H., Hopper, J.L., … Mann, G.J. (2011). Sunbed use during adolescence and early adulthood is associated with increased risk of early-onset melanoma. *International Journal of Cancer, 128*, 2425–2435. doi:10.1002/ijc.25576

Cuzick, J., Otto, F., Baron, J.A., Brown, P.H., Burn, J., Greenwald, P., … Thun, M. (2009). Aspirin and non-steroidal anti-inflammatory drugs for cancer prevention: An international consensus statement. *Lancet Oncology, 10*, 501–507. doi:10.1016/S1470-2045(09)70035-X

den Hollander, P., Savage, M.I., & Brown, P.H. (2013). Targeted therapy for breast cancer prevention. *Frontiers in Oncology, 3*, 250. doi:10.3389/fonc.2013.00250

Dunne, E.F., Unger, E.R., Sternberg, M., McQuillan, G., Swan, D.C., Patel, S.S., & Markowitz, L.E. (2007). Prevalence of HPV infection among females in the United States. *JAMA, 297*, 813–819. doi:10.1001/jama.297.8.813

Eaton, D.K., Kann, L., Kinchen, S., Shanklin, S., Flint, K.H., Hawkins, J., … Wechsler, H. (2012). Youth risk behavior surveillance—United States, 2011. *Morbidity and Mortality Weekly Report Surveillance Summaries, 61*(4), 1–162. Retrieved from http://www.cdc.gov/mmwr/preview/mmwrhtml/ss6104a1.htm

Fiore, M.C., Jaén, C.R., Baker, T.B., Bailey, W.C., Benowitz, N.L., Curry, S.J., … Wewers, M.E. (2008). *Treating tobacco use and dependence: 2008 update. Clinical practice guideline.* Rockville, MD: U.S. Department of Health and Human Services.

Fisher, B., Costantino, J.P., Wickerham, D.L., Cecchini, R.S., Cronin, W.M., Robidoux, A., … Wolmark, N. (2005). Tamoxifen for the prevention of breast cancer: Current status of the National Surgical Adjuvant Breast and Bowel Project P-1 study. *Journal of the National Cancer Institute, 97*, 1652–1662. doi:10.1093/jnci/dji372

Greco, K. (2007). Caring for patients at risk for hereditary colorectal cancer. *Oncology, 21*(Suppl. 2), 29–38.

Grethlein, S.J. (2013, February 11). Breast examination. Retrieved from http://emedicine.medscape.com/ article/1909276-overview

Haggar, F.A., & Boushey, R.P. (2009). Colorectal cancer epidemiology: Incidence, mortality, survival, and risk factors. *Clinics in Colon and Rectal Surgery, 22*, 191–197. doi:10.1055/s-0029-1242458

Harrill-Smith, C., Ripley-Moffitt, C., & Goldstein, A.O. (2013). Tobacco cessation in 2013: What every clinician should know. *North Carolina Medical Journal, 74*, 401–405. Retrieved from http://www.ncmedicaljournal.com/ archives/?74508

Heatherton, T.F., Kozlowski, L.T., Frecker, R.C., & Fagerström, K. (1991). The Fagerström test for nicotine dependence: A revision of the Fagerström tolerance questionnaire. *British Journal of Addiction, 86*, 1119–1127. doi:10.1111/j.1360-0443.1991.tb01879.x

Heinonen, O.P., Albanes, D., Virtamo, J., Taylor, P.R., Huttunen, J.K., Hartman, A.M., … Edwards, B.K. (1998). Prostate cancer and supplementation with alpha-tocopherol and beta-carotene: Incidence and mortality in a controlled trial. *Journal of the National Cancer Institute, 90*, 440–446. doi:10.1093/jnci/90.6.440

Hoffman, R.M. (2011). Screening for prostate cancer. *New England Journal of Medicine, 365*, 2013–2019. doi:10.1056/ NEJMcp1103642

International Agency for Research on Cancer Working Group on Artificial Ultraviolet Light and Skin Cancer. (2007). The association of use of sunbeds with cutaneous malignant melanoma and other skin cancers: A systematic review. *International Journal of Cancer, 120*, 1116–1122. doi:10.1002/ijc.22453

Kushi, L.H., Doyle, C., McCullough, M., Rock, C.L., Demark-Wahnefried, W., Bandera, E.V., … Gansler, T. (2012). American Cancer Society guidelines on nutrition and physical activity for cancer prevention: Reducing the risk of cancer with healthy food choices and physical activity. *CA: A Cancer Journal for Clinicians, 62*, 30–67. doi:10.3322/ caac.20140

Lombard, H.L., & Doering, C.R. (1928). Cancer studies in Massachusetts: Habits, characteristics and environment of individuals with and without cancer. *New England Journal of Medicine, 198*, 481–487. doi:10.1056/ NEJM192804261981002

Messer, K., & Pierce, J.P. (2010). Changes in age trajectories of smoking experimentation during the California Tobacco Control Program. *American Journal of Public Health, 100*, 1298–1306. doi:10.2105/AJPH.2009.160416

National Cancer Institute. (n.d.). Specificity. In *Dictionary of cancer terms.* Retrieved from http://www.cancer.gov/ dictionary

National Cancer Institute. (2003). Alpha-Tocopherol, Beta Carotene Cancer Prevention (ATBC) Trial. Retrieved from http://www.cancer.gov/newscenter/qa/2003/atbcfollowupqa

National Cancer Institute. (2012). Obesity and cancer risk. Retrieved from http://www.cancer.gov/about-cancer/ causes-prevention/risk/obesity/obesity-fact-sheet

National Cancer Institute. (2014a). Cancer prevention overview (PDQ®). Retrieved from http://www.cancer.gov/ cancertopics/pdq/prevention/overview/HealthProfessional

National Cancer Institute. (2014b). Cancer screening overview (PDQ®). Retrieved from http://www.cancer.gov/cancertopics/pdq/screening/overview/healthprofessional

National Comprehensive Cancer Network. (2014a). *NCCN Clinical Practice Guidelines in Oncology (NCCN Guidelines®): Breast cancer screening and diagnosis* [v.1.2014]. Retrieved from http://www.nccn.org/professionals/physician_gls/pdf/breast-screening.pdf

National Comprehensive Cancer Network. (2014b). *NCCN Clinical Practice Guidelines in Oncology (NCCN Guidelines®): Colorectal cancer screening* [v.1.2014]. Retrieved from http://www.nccn.org/professionals/physician_gls/pdf/colorectal_screening.pdf

National Comprehensive Cancer Network. (2014c). *NCCN Clinical Practice Guidelines in Oncology (NCCN Guidelines®): Prostate cancer early detection* [v.1.2014]. Retrieved from http://www.nccn.org/professionals/physician_gls/pdf/prostate_detection.pdf

National Comprehensive Cancer Network. (2015a). *NCCN Clinical Practice Guidelines in Oncology (NCCN Guidelines®): Genetic/familial high-risk assessment: Breast and ovarian* [v.1.2015]. Retrieved from http://www.nccn.org/professionals/physician_gls/pdf/genetics_screening.pdf

National Comprehensive Cancer Network. (2015b). *NCCN Clinical Practice Guidelines in Oncology (NCCN Guidelines®): Lung cancer screening* [v.2.2015]. Retrieved from http://www.nccn.org/professionals/physician_gls/pdf/lung_screening.pdf

National Lung Screening Trial Research Team. (2011). Reduced lung-cancer mortality with low-dose computed tomographic screening. *New England Journal of Medicine, 365,* 395–409. doi:10.1056/NEJMoa1102873

Quante, A.S., Whittemore, A.S., Shriver, T., Strauch, K., & Terry, M.B. (2012). Breast cancer risk assessment across the risk continuum: Genetic and nongenetic risk factors contributing to differential model performance. *Breast Cancer Research, 14,* R144. doi:10.1186/bcr3352

Quinn, V.P., Hollis, J.F., Smith, K.S., Rigotti, N.A., Solberg, L.I., Hu, W., & Stevens, V.J. (2009). Effectiveness of the 5-As tobacco cessation treatments in nine HMOs. *Journal of General Internal Medicine, 24,* 149–154. doi:10.1007/s11606-008-0865-9

Saslow, D., Boetes, C., Burke, W., Harms, S., Leach, M.O., Lehman, C.D., … Russell, C.A. (2007). American Cancer Society guidelines for breast screening with MRI as an adjunct to mammography. *CA: A Cancer Journal for Clinicians, 57,* 75–89. doi:10.3322/canjclin.57.2.75

Saslow, D., Solomon, D., Lawson, H.W., Killackey, M., Kulasingam, S.L., Cain, J., … Myers, E.R. (2012). American Cancer Society, American Society for Colposcopy and Cervical Pathology, and American Society for Clinical Pathology screening guidelines for the prevention and early detection of cervical cancer. *American Journal of Clinical Pathology, 137,* 516–542. doi:10.1309/AJCPTGD94EVRSJCG

Smith, R.A., Cokkinides, V., Brooks, D., Saslow, D., & Brawley, O.W. (2010). Cancer screening in the United States, 2010: A review of current American Cancer Society guidelines and issues in cancer screening. *CA: A Cancer Journal for Clinicians, 60,* 99–119. doi:10.3322/caac.20063

Smith, R.A., Cokkinides, V., Brooks, D., Saslow, D., Shah, M., & Brawley, O.W. (2011). Cancer screening in the United States, 2011. *CA: A Cancer Journal for Clinicians, 61,* 8–30. doi:10.3322/caac.20096

Spratt, J.S. (1981). The primary and secondary prevention of cancer. *Journal of Surgical Oncology, 18,* 219–230. doi:10.1002/jso.2930180302

Swiderski, M. (2011). Predictive genetic testing: Can specialized advanced practitioners quell consumer confusion? *Journal of the Advanced Practitioner in Oncology, 2,* 71–85.

U.S. Department of Health, Education, and Welfare. (1964). *Smoking and health: Report of the advisory committee to the surgeon general of the public health service.* Washington, DC: Author.

U.S. Environmental Protection Agency. (2006, September). *Sunscreen: The burning facts.* Washington, DC: Author.

U.S. Food and Drug Administration. (2006, June 8). Approval letter—Human papillomavirus quadrivalent (types 6, 11, 16, 18) vaccine, recombinant. Retrieved from http://www.fda.gov/biologicsbloodvaccines/vaccines/approvedproducts/ucm111283.htm

U.S. Food and Drug Administration. (2009, October 16). FDA approves new vaccine for prevention of cervical cancer [Press release]. Retrieved from http://www.fda.gov/NewsEvents/Newsroom/PressAnnouncements/ucm187048.htm

U.S. Food and Drug Administration. (2015, January 9). Gardasil 9. Retrieved from http://www.fda.gov/BiologicsBloodVaccines/Vaccines/ApprovedProducts/ucm426445.htm

U.S. Preventive Services Task Force. (2008). Colorectal cancer: Screening. Retrieved from http://www.uspreventiveservicestaskforce.org/uspstf/uspscolo.htm

U.S. Preventive Services Task Force. (2009). Breast cancer: Screening. Retrieved from http://www.uspreventiveservicestaskforce.org/uspstf/uspsbrca.htm

U.S. Preventive Services Task Force. (2012a). Cervical cancer: Screening. Retrieved from http://www.uspreventiveservicestaskforce.org/uspstf/uspscerv.htm

U.S. Preventive Services Task Force. (2012b). Prostate cancer: Screening. Retrieved from http://www.uspreventive servicestaskforce.org/Page/Topic/recommendation-summary/prostate-cancer-screening

U.S. Preventive Services Task Force. (2013). Lung cancer: Screening. Retrieved from http://www.uspreventive servicestaskforce.org/uspstf/uspslung.htm

U.S. Preventive Services Task Force. (2016). Breast cancer: Screening. Retrieved from http://www.uspreventive servicestaskforce.org/Page/Document/UpdateSummaryFinal/breast-cancer-screening1

Vogel, V.G., Costantino, J.P., Wickerham, D.L., Cronin, W.M., Cecchini, R.S., Atkins, J.N., … Wolmark, N. (2006). Effects of tamoxifen vs raloxifene on the risk of developing invasive breast cancer and other disease outcomes. *JAMA, 295,* 2727–2741. doi:10.1001/jama.295.23.joc60074

Vogel, W. (2003). The advanced practice nursing role in a high-risk breast cancer clinic. *Oncology Nursing Forum, 30,* 115–122. doi:10.1188/03.ONF.115-122

Warner, E. (2011). Breast-cancer screening. *New England Journal of Medicine, 365,* 1025–1032. doi:10.1056/ NEJMcp1101540

World Cancer Research Fund & American Institute for Cancer Research. (2009). *Policy and action for cancer prevention: Food, nutrition, and physical activity: A global perspective.* Retrieved from http://www.dietandcancerreport .org/policy_report/index.php

CHAPTER 2

Genetic Risk

Suzanne M. Mahon, DNSc, RN, AOCN®, APNG

Introduction

The evolution of the Human Genome Project has greatly changed the scope of advanced oncology nursing practice. An estimated 5%–10% of all cancers have a hereditary basis (American Cancer Society [ACS], 2015; Pyeritz, 2011). The field of genetics is continually and rapidly growing with many changing implications for oncology advanced practice nurses (APNs), including an emphasis on identification of at-risk populations, basic cancer risk assessment, referrals for hereditary cancer evaluation to credentialed genetics providers, assistance with implementing cancer prevention and detection measures, and management of the psychosocial ramifications of testing (Mahon, 2012a). The expansion of genetic knowledge will also undoubtedly change the focus and priorities in nursing research and education.

The magnitude of change in genetics practice has been extensive over the past fifteen years. The perspectives of credentialed genetics professionals who are most familiar with cancer genetic counseling and testing issues have changed radically since genetic testing for *BRCA1/2* became commercially available in 1996 (Matloff, Bonadies, Moyer, & Brierley, 2014). Today it is possible, and in many instances routine, to use cancer predisposition genetic testing to identify individuals who are at increased risk for developing cancer because of an inherited mutated cancer predisposition gene. Emerging legal and ethical ramifications of risk assessment and genetic testing include identifying high-risk individuals and families and informing them about the option for testing; disclosing the risks, benefits, and limitations of testing and follow-up; maintaining confidentiality; and warning other relatives who are at risk (Robson, Storm, Weitzel, Wollins, & Offit, 2010).

Because of genetic advances, a new population of patients with cancer is emerging. *Previvors* are individuals who are survivors of having an inherited genetic predisposition for developing cancer (Hoskins, Roy, & Greene, 2012). Although they do not have a cancer diagnosis, previvors are often confronted with difficult decisions about risk management, which might include aggressive screening and prophylactic surgery. Affected individuals, their partners, and offspring face psychosocial challenges. APNs must be aware of the complex and special needs of this growing population.

Genetic testing is now readily and commercially available for hereditary breast and ovarian cancer (HBOC), hereditary nonpolyposis colorectal cancer (HNPCC or Lynch syndrome), familial adenosis polypcos (FAP) syndromes, hereditary melanoma, and hereditary pancreatic cancer. Also, predisposition genes for many unique or rare syndromes exist for which testing is available as part of some of the newer next-generation sequencing panels or through research studies (Biesecker, Burke, Kohane, Plon, & Zimmern, 2012). Examples of rarer syndromes sometimes encountered in clinical practice include Cowden syndrome, hereditary retinoblastoma, multiple endocrine neoplasia (MEN), von Hippel-Lindau (VHL) syndrome, Wilms tumor, and Li-Fraumeni syndrome. With the increasing availability of predisposition testing for malignancy and the emergence of next-generation sequencing panels, oncology APNs need a fundamental understanding of the science of genetics and the ramifications of genetic predisposition testing (Mahon, 2013c).

Basic Competencies

Although genetic testing is employed more frequently in oncology practice, genetic testing is best used to help individuals at high risk for developing cancer make good decisions about cancer screening and prevention strategies. It is not a tool to be used in routine population screening because of the expense of testing and the complex counseling needs associated with it. Because of the increasing availability of testing, individuals with expertise in cancer genetics are needed to educate at-risk individuals about the strengths, limitations, and risks associated with genetic testing. The Oncology Nursing Society (ONS) position "Oncology Nursing: The Application of Cancer Genetics and Genomics Throughout the Oncology Care Continuum" emphasizes the need for oncology APNs to provide care and education to at-risk families, which might include performing comprehensive cancer genetic risk assessments, providing education, ordering and interpreting genetic tests, providing pre- and post-test counseling, and delivering personally tailored recommendations for cancer prevention and early detection and necessary supportive services (ONS, 2014). The position notes that although genetic testing has many benefits, the very process of testing can lead to ethical, legal, and social issues, and nurses need to safeguard patients and families from these potential risks. A recent Cochrane review suggested that cancer genetic risk assessment is beneficial for families with hereditary risk for developing breast cancer, but clearly more studies are required to assess the best means of delivering cancer risk assessment services (Hilgart, Coles, & Iredale, 2012). To provide effective cancer genetics care, oncology APNs need ongoing education in this rapidly changing field.

In the United States, the *Essentials of Genetic and Genomic Nursing: Competencies, Curricula Guidelines, and Outcome Indicators* (Jenkins, 2009) define the minimum genetic and genomic competencies for all nurses in the United States. These widely accepted competencies, which were first published in 2006, have been endorsed by more than 50 different nursing organizations and have promoted recent efforts to increase genomics material in undergraduate nursing programs.

In 2012, the *Essential Genetic and Genomic Competencies for Nurses With Graduate Degrees* (Greco, Tinley, & Seibert, 2012) were published. These focus on the following areas: (a) risk assessment and interpretation, (b) genetic education, counseling, testing, and results interpretation, (c) clinical management, (d) ethical, legal, and social implications, (e) professional roles, (f) leadership, and (g) research. According to these competencies, nurses with graduate degrees functioning in APN roles should be able to perform a more detailed evaluation; gather an expanded history; complete risk assessments; collect, confirm, and update reported family health histories; analyze a pedigree to identify potential inherited predisposition to disease; use family history and pedigree information to plan and conduct a targeted physical assessment; interpret the findings from the physical assessment, family history, and screening tests;

and refer at-risk family members for assessment of an inherited predisposition to disease to a genetic professional.

Nurses have a professional responsibility to be familiar with these guidelines. They are all free and readily accessible. These competencies and position statements challenge nurses to obtain the necessary skills and training to provide genomic health care in practice, as well as to know when to refer clients to providers with expertise in the provision of genetic and genomic health services.

Genetic Professionals

Different types of credentialed genetics professionals exist. In many cases, APNs will work with these professionals in a multidisciplinary setting. This often depends on the practice setting.

Geneticists are physicians with board certification in genetics from the American Board of Medical Genetics. They complete a fellowship in genetics and pass a board examination. An active list of board-certified geneticists that is searchable by name or location is available from the American Board of Medical Genetics (www.abmg.org/pages/searchmem.shtml).

Licensed genetic counselors are healthcare professionals with specialized graduate degrees in the areas of medical genetics and counseling. More than 30 accredited programs in genetic counseling exist in the United States. The American Board of Genetic Counseling certifies genetic counselors. The National Society of Genetic Counselors (NSGC) maintains an active website in which healthcare professionals and the public can identify credentialed genetics professionals by zip code (www.nsgc.org/FindaGeneticCounselor).

Credentialed genetic nurses have specialized education and training in genetics and are credentialed by the American Nurses Credentialing Center after evaluation of a portfolio (www.nursecredentialing.org/Certification/NurseSpecialties/AdvancedGenetics). Nurses who are prepared with a master's in nursing may complete specialized education and training to qualify for the advanced genetics credential (AGN-BC) following submission of an acceptable portfolio (Monsen, 2005). The portfolio includes documentation of 1,500 hours of genetic practicum experience in the last three years that reflects genetic expertise in the areas of professional development, ethical practice, teamwork and collaboration, and quality and safety; at least 30 hours of genetic content in the past three years through academic courses or continuing education; and peer and supervisor evaluations, as well as additional supporting data in the areas of presentations, publications, research, preceptorships, and professional service.

Definitions

An understanding of basic cancer cell biology is essential when providing cancer genetic care. The evolution of the Human Genome Project led to the development and more widespread use of genetic terms. For many, these terms were not addressed in basic nursing education (Greco, Tinley, & Seibert, 2011). An understanding of types of risk, risk assessment strategies, and basic biologic and genetic terms, as well as terms specific to genetic testing, is essential. Table 2-1 contains a list of terms with definitions commonly encountered in genetic nursing practice. Oncology APNs not only need to understand these terms to read literature and research reports, but they also must be able to explain this complex and often technical scientific information to patients and families, tailoring teaching to meet varying educational and individual needs of patients and families. The biology of cancer and cancer genetics can be overwhelming to patients and families, especially if they have limited educa-

Table 2-1. Definitions of Terms Commonly Used in Cancer Genetics

Term	Definition
Types of Risk	
Absolute risk	Refers to the occurrence of the cancer in the general population (either incidence or mortality)
Attributable risk	Refers to the number of cancer cases that could be prevented with the manipulation of a known risk factor
Incidence	Refers to the number of cancer cases that develop in a defined population in a specified period of time (such as one year)
Population	Refers to the number of people in a defined group who are capable of developing cancer
Prevalence	Refers to the actual number of cancers in a defined population at a given time Typically expressed as the number of cases per 100,000 people
Relative risk	Refers to a statistical estimate, which is a comparison of the likelihood of a person with a specific risk factor developing a cancer with the likelihood of a person who does not have the specific risk factor
Risk factor	A trait, characteristic, or lifestyle factor that is associated with a statistically significant increased likelihood of developing a particular cancer
Types of Cancer Prevention	
Primary	Implementing direct measures to avoid carcinogen exposure or begin a healthy practice May include chemoprevention agents or prophylactic surgery
Secondary	Identifying individuals who are at risk for development of a particular cancer and implementing appropriate screening modalities Goal of detecting cancer at the earliest possible stage, when treatment is easiest and most likely to be effective
Tertiary	Monitoring for recurrence and second primary tumors in people who have previously been diagnosed with and treated for cancer
Basic Genetic Terminology	
Allele	One of the various forms of a gene at a particular location on a chromosome
Autosomal dominant	Mendelian inheritance in which an affected individual possesses one copy of a mutant allele and one normal copy A statistical 50% chance exists that the allele and associated disorder or disease will be passed to offspring.
Autosome	Any chromosome other than a sex chromosome Humans have 22 pairs of autosomal chromosomes (46 chromosomes in all).
Biallelic	Both alleles of a gene Biallelic mutations are mutations that occur on both alleles (or versions) of the same gene.
Chromosome	A thread-like package in the nucleus of the cell that contains genes Humans have 23 pairs of chromosomes; 22 pairs are autosomes, and one pair is sex chromosomes.

(Continued on next page)

Table 2-1. Definitions of Terms Commonly Used in Cancer Genetics *(Continued)*

Term	Definition
Gene	Functional and physical unit of heredity Passed from parent to offspring Contains information necessary for making a specific protein
Genome	The entire DNA contained in an organism
Genotype	Genetic identity May or may not be manifested in outward characteristics
Germ-line	Inherited material that comes from the egg or sperm
Heterozygous	Possessing two different forms of a particular gene One is inherited from each parent.
Homozygous	Possessing two identical forms of a particular gene One is inherited from each parent.
Mutation	A permanent structural change in DNA
Oncogene	Gene that leads to transformation of normal cells into cancer cells
Penetrance	The portion of a population with a particular genotype or mutation that expresses the corresponding phenotype of disorder
Phenotype	Characteristics or traits in an organism that are observable
Proband	Family member who serves as the "spokesperson" Risks are calculated based on an individual's relationship to the proband.
Promoter	The part of the gene that contains the information to turn the gene on or off Transcription is initiated in the promoter part of the gene.
Recessive	A trait or disorder that only appears in people who have received two copies of a mutant or altered gene (one from each parent)
Somatic cells	Any cell in the body except the reproductive cells
Tumor suppressor gene	A protective gene that usually limits the growth of tumors If mutated, it may not be able to keep a cancer from growing, for example, *BRCA* genes.
Terms That Apply to Genetic Testing	
Accuracy	The degree to which a measurement represents the true value of the characteristic being measured
Deletion	A type of chromosomal abnormality in which a piece of DNA is removed or omitted from a gene Results in the disruption of the normal structure and function of that gene
DNA sequencing	Determining the exact order of the base pairs in a segment of DNA (adenine, guanine, cytosine, and thymine)
False negative	A test result indicating that the tested person does not have a particular characteristic, but the person actually does have the characteristic Example: A negative mammogram in a woman with early-stage breast cancer

(Continued on next page)

Table 2-1. Definitions of Terms Commonly Used in Cancer Genetics *(Continued)*

Term	Definition
False positive	A test result indicating that the tested person has a particular characteristic, but the person actually does not have the characteristic Example: A very suspicious mammogram in a woman who does not have breast cancer
Fluorescence in situ hybridization (FISH)	Lab process that involves painting chromosomes or sections of chromosomes with fluorescent molecules Useful technique for identification of chromosomal abnormalities and gene mapping
Insertion	Type of chromosomal abnormality in which an extra piece of DNA is inserted into a gene Results in the disruption of the normal structure and function of that gene
Karyotype	The chromosomal complement of an individual, including all chromosomes and abnormalities Also used to refer to a photograph of an individual's chromosomes
Microsatellite	A repetitive short sequence of DNA that is used as a genetic marker to track inheritance in families
Next-generation sequencing	Sequencing in which many strands of DNA are sequenced at once, generating far more data per instrument run than the Sanger method
Polymerase chain reaction	Fast, relatively inexpensive means for making an unlimited number of copies of any piece of DNA
Sanger sequencing	Original sequencing technology that helped scientists determine the human genetic code. Now automated, it is still used to sequence short pieces of DNA. It relies on a technique known as capillary electrophoresis, which separates fragments of DNA by size and then sequences them by detecting the final fluorescent base on each fragment.
Sensitivity	The ability of a screening test to detect individuals with the characteristic being screened for Calculated by dividing the total number of true positives by the total number of the population
Single nucleotide polymorphisms (SNPs)	Each SNP ("snip") represents a difference in a single nucleotide and occurs normally throughout a person's DNA, usually about once every 300 nucleotides. Typically these variations are found in the DNA between genes functioning as biologic markers, helping scientists locate genes associated with disease. About 10 million SNPs are present in the human genome.
Specificity	The ability of a screening test to detect individuals without the characteristic being screened for Calculated by dividing the total number of true negatives by the sum of the true-negative and false-positive results
True negative	A test result indicating that the tested person does not have the trait tested for, and the person does not have it Example: A woman has a negative mammogram and does not develop cancer in the next 12–24 months.

(Continued on next page)

Table 2-1. Definitions of Terms Commonly Used in Cancer Genetics *(Continued)*

Term	Definition
True positive	A test result indicating that the tested person has the characteristic tested for, and the person does have it Example: A woman has a suspicious mammogram, and a biopsy demonstrates that the area is a malignancy.
Validity	A measure of how well a test measures what it is supposed to measure

Note. Based on information from Biesecker et al., 2012; Brown, 2009; Gunder & Martin, 2011; Ross & Cronin, 2011; Wiggs, 2009.

tion or background in science (Gaff & Bylund, 2010). Furthermore, many oncology APNs, especially those with expertise in genetics, provide education about hereditary predisposition for developing cancer to other nurses, healthcare providers, and physicians. This education is important to help ensure that those with a hereditary predisposition for developing cancer are referred for further evaluation to a credentialed genetic provider.

The Genetic Basis of Cancer

Humans carry an estimated 20,000 to 25,000 genes, which are composed of DNA (Brown, 2009). DNA is composed of four chemicals: adenine (A), thymine (T), cytosine (C), and guanine (G). The specific order of these chemicals ultimately determines physical characteristics, growth and development, and predisposition for a wide variety of attributes and diseases. Within the human genome, these four chemicals are repeated billions of times in a specific sequence within 23 pairs of chromosomes. Twenty-two of these pairs are autosomes, and one pair is a sex chromosome (Wiggs, 2009).

All cancer results from a process of genetic mutations, or a change in the arrangement of the four basic chemicals of A, T, C, and G. Mutations that predispose a human to developing a disease such as cancer can occur any time during the lifetime, particularly during growth and development of a tissue or organ (*somatic mutations*) or at conception in the ova or sperm (*germ-line mutations*). Hereditary mutations are carried in the DNA of the reproductive cells (germ-line mutations). When reproductive germ cells containing mutations combine to produce offspring, the mutation will be present in all of the offspring's body cells (Gunder & Martin, 2011; Wiggs, 2009). An accurate family history combined with predisposition genetic testing differentiates between somatic and germ-line mutations (see Table 2-2). Identifying individuals with germ-line mutations is important because of their increased risk for second primary cancers and the potential risk for other close relatives.

Sporadic cancers occur from multiple somatic mutations in a cell (Gunder & Martin, 2011). Acquired somatic mutations develop in DNA during a person's lifetime. If the mutation arises in a body cell, copies of the mutation will exist only in descendants of that particular cell. Some mutations are changes in genetic material but do not cause disease or problems; these are referred to as *polymorphisms*. Other mutations, referred to as *deleterious*, can result in disease or other significant changes because of sequence changes that result in alterations of the protein (Brown, 2009).

As noted, genes come in pairs, with one copy inherited from each parent. Many genes come in a number of variant forms, known as *alleles*. A dominant allele prevails over a recessive allele.

Table 2-2. Differences Between Somatic and Germ-Line Mutations

Characteristic	Somatic Mutations	Germ-Line Mutations
Proportion of all cancers	85%	10%–15%
Type of cancer	Sporadic cancer	Hereditary cancer predisposition syndromes
Timing of mutation	After conception	In the egg or sperm
Transmission of mutation	Cannot be passed to subsequent generations	Can be passed to subsequent generations
Number of cells affected	One cell and the cells that come from that cell's division	All cells in an offspring
Examples	HER2/neu amplification in breast cancer, Philadelphia chromosome in chronic leukemia	Mutations in *BRCA1/2*, *MSH2*, *MLH1*, *p16*, *FAP* genes
Role of genetic testing	Genetic testing may drive treatment decisions. It will not help other relatives to determine their risk for developing the cancer.	Genetic testing may alter treatment strategies and often alters prevention and screening strategies. Testing may be able to determine other relatives who are at risk.

Note. Based on information from Brown, 2009; Euhus & Robinson, 2013; Gunder & Martin, 2011; Weitzel et al., 2011.

A recessive gene becomes apparent if its counterpart allele on the other chromosome becomes inactivated or lost. Not all mutated alleles invariably lead to disease. For example, even with a dominant allele such as the *BRCA1* breast cancer susceptibility gene, the risk of developing breast cancer by age 80 may be as high as 90%, not 100% (Petrucelli, Daly, & Feldman, 2013). An indication of the probability that a given gene mutation will produce disease is referred to as *penetrance*.

A number of mutations occur in malignant cells (Fisher, Pusztai, & Swanton, 2013). Many malignancies develop as a result of the conversion of proto-oncogenes to oncogenes. Proto-oncogenes regulate normal cell growth, whereas oncogenes are associated with abnormal cell growth, leading to increased cellular proliferation and uncontrolled growth (Wiggs, 2009). Other tumors arise because of the inactivation of both alleles of tumor suppressor cells, which play an important role in slowing or stopping abnormal cell growth. Tumor suppressor cells include caretaker genes, which maintain integrity of the genetic material, and gatekeeper genes, which regulate proliferation and cell life (Gunder & Martin, 2011). Mismatch repair (MMR) genes repair mistakes that occur during DNA replication (Brown, 2009). When MMR genes are damaged, genetic stability is altered, and tumor cells replicate. Some mutations interfere with apoptosis (normal programmed cell death). Certain genetic patterns or syndromes occur as a result of some of the mutations described here, and a brief discussion of the more common ones follows.

Common Genetic Cancer Predisposition Syndromes

Oncology APNs will encounter some hereditary cancer predisposition syndromes fairly regularly in their practice. Commercial testing is readily available for these syndromes, which include

HBOC, HNPCC, FAP, hereditary pancreatic cancer, and hereditary melanoma. It is important to identify families who are at risk for these predisposition syndromes, to know how to refer them for cancer genetic education services, and to provide support for these families as they make complex and often difficult decisions about genetic testing and treatment measures. Some of the less common syndromes that APNs may encounter in their practice are shown in Table 2-3.

Hereditary Breast Cancer Syndromes

An estimated 70% of breast cancer is sporadic, and another 15%–20% is familial, meaning that one or two family members have breast cancer but no obvious pattern of autosomal dominant transmission is present (Shannon & Chittenden, 2012). Among women, an estimated 5%–10% of breast cancers and 10%–15% of ovarian cancers are caused by inherited mutations in the *BRCA1* and *BRCA2* genes (Petrucelli et al., 2013). Mutations in these genes occur in about 1 in every 300–500 individuals (Christinat & Pagani, 2013). Other hereditary syndromes associated with breast cancer include Li-Fraumeni, Cowden, Peutz-Jeghers, and diffuse hereditary gastric syndromes (Christinat & Pagani, 2013; Shannon & Chittenden, 2012).

Many studies have estimated the risk of those with *BRCA1/2* mutations developing cancer. The risk for younger women is estimated to be 33%–50% by age 50 (Euhus & Robinson, 2013; Lindor, McMaster, Lindor, & Greene, 2008; Petrucelli et al., 2013). The cumulative risk for developing breast cancer by age 70 is estimated to be about 87%, and the risk is as high as 44% for ovarian cancer. The risk of developing a second primary cancer (breast or ovarian) also increases (Petrucelli et al., 2013). The degree of risk depends on the first primary malignancy, as well as the current age and other comorbidities of the proband (see Table 2-1) (Lindor et al., 2008). *BRCA1*-related tumors show an excess of medullary histopathology, are of higher histologic grade, and are more likely than sporadic tumors to be estrogen receptor, progesterone receptor, and HER2/neu negative (triple negative), but there is not a definitive pathologic type (Petrucelli et al., 2013). Mutations in the *BRCA1/2* genes also are associated with melanoma and prostate, gastric, pancreatic, and male breast cancers (Petrucelli et al., 2013). The relative risk for pancreatic cancer is approximately 3.1 in *BRCA1* mutation carriers and 6.6 in *BRCA2* mutation carriers (Iqbal et al., 2012; Lindor et al., 2008). Key indicators of HBOC syndrome are shown in Figure 2-1.

Men who have a mutation in *BRCA1/2* have been shown to have an increased risk for developing prostate cancer that might be more aggressive, have nodal involvement, and be associated with a poorer survival rate than men who do not have a mutation (Euhus & Robinson, 2013). The risk of prostate cancer in *BRCA1* carriers has been estimated to be approximately double that observed in the general population for men younger than 65 years old and five to seven times as high in *BRCA2* carriers based on results from the international IMPACT (Identification of Men with a genetic predisposition to ProstAte Cancer: Targeted screening in men at a higher genetic risk and controls) study (Mitra et al., 2011). Lifetime breast cancer risk is estimated at 1.8% for men with *BRCA1* mutations and 8.3% for those with *BRCA2* mutations (Euhus & Robinson, 2013).

Membership in some populations infers increased risk for having a *BRCA1/2* mutation. Founder mutations have been noted in those of Ashkenazi Jewish, Dutch, and Icelandic descent. An estimated 1 in 40 Ashkenazi women carries one of three mutations (185delAG and 5382insC on *BRCA1* and 6174delT on *BRCA2*) (National Comprehensive Cancer Network® [NCCN®], 2014c; Shannon et al., 2011).

These autosomal dominant genes, which are highly penetrant, predispose individuals to significant risk for developing breast and/or ovarian cancer. The loss of the wild-type allele on chromosomes 17q (*BRCA1*) and 13q (*BRCA2*) suggests that these genes function as tumor

Table 2-3. Less Common Hereditary Cancer Syndromes

Characteristic	Neurofibromatosis (NF)	Multiple Endocrine Neoplasia (MEN)	Von Hippel-Lindau (VHL) Syndrome	Cowden Syndrome	Li-Fraumeni Syndrome	Peutz-Jeghers Syndrome
Genetic location	*NF1* at 17q11.2 *NF2* at 22q12.2	*MEN1* is at 11q13 *MEN2* is at RET 10q11.2	*VHL* at 3p25–p26	*PTEN* at 10q23.3	*TP53* at 17p13.1, commonly called p53	*STK11/LKB1* at 19p13.3
Incidence	*NF1*: 1 in 3,000; one-third to one-half of cases represent a new germ-line mutation *NF2*: 1 in 35,000; one-half of cases represent a new germ-line mutation	*MEN1*: 1 in 5,000–50,000 *MEN2*: 1 in 30,000	1 in 30,000–40,000	1 in 200,000–250,000	Very rare—approximately 400 unrelated families	1 in 8,300–280,000
Penetrance/cancer risk	*NF1*: 100% by the end of childhood *NF2*: Nearly 100% develop bilateral vestibular schwannomas by age 30.	*MEN1*: For all clinical features, rises above 50% by age 20 and above 95% by age 40 *MEN2*: Nearly 100%	Nearly 100% penetrant with at least some symptoms by age 65	Lifetime risk of female breast cancer is 30%–67%. Male breast cancer can also occur. Lifetime risk of thyroid cancer is 5%–10% (usually follicular). Lifetime risk of endometrial cancer is 5%–10%.	Cancer risks are estimated to be 50% by age 40 and up to 90% by age 60. An estimated 15% will develop a second cancer. Age-specific cancer risks are not known.	93% for all cancers combined • 54% breast • 39% colon • 36% pancreas • 29% stomach • 21% ovary • 15% lung • 13% small intestine • 9% uterus

(Continued on next page)

Table 2-3. Less Common Hereditary Cancer Syndromes (Continued)

Characteristic	Neurofibromatosis (NF)	Multiple Endocrine Neoplasia (MEN)	Von Hippel-Lindau (VHL) Syndrome	Cowden Syndrome	Li-Fraumeni Syndrome	Peutz-Jeghers Syndrome
Key indicators	*NF1*: Multiple café au lait spots, axillary and inguinal freckling, multiple cutaneous neurofibromas, iris Lisch nodules Learning disabilities are present in at least 50% of individuals with NF1. *NF2*: Bilateral vestibular schwannomas	*MEN1*: High frequency of disorders of the pituitary (30%–55%), parathyroid (95%), pancreatic (50%–75%), and adrenal (16%) glands *MEN2*: Medullary thyroid cancer, pheochromocytoma, parathyroid disease	An individual with no known family history of VHL syndrome presenting with two or more characteristic lesions: • Hemangioblastomas • Kidney or pancreatic cysts • Renal cell carcinoma • Adrenal or extra-adrenal pheochromocytomas	Major criteria: • Breast cancer • Thyroid cancer • Mucocutaneous lesions • Trichilemmomas • Papillomatous mucosal lesions • Macrocephaly (circumference ≥ 97th percentile) • Endometrial carcinoma Minor criteria: • Other thyroid lesions • Mental retardation (IQ ≤ 75) • Hamartomatous intestinal polyps • Fibrocystic disease of the breast • Uterine fibroids • Lipomas • Fibromas • Genitourinary tumors (especially renal cell carcinoma) • Genitourinary malformations	Diagnostic criteria: • One person with sarcoma diagnosed before age 45 • A first-degree relative diagnosed with cancer (of any kind) before age 45 • A third affected family member (first- or second-degree relative) with either sarcoma at any age or cancer (type not specified) before age 45	Clinical suspicion with the presence of numerous pigmented spots on the lips and the buccal mucosa and multiple gastrointestinal hamartomatous polyps (especially in the jejunum). The most common clinical signs associated with intestinal polyps are obstruction, abdominal pain, rectal bleeding, and rectal extrusion of the polyp.

(Continued on next page)

Table 2-3. Less Common Hereditary Cancer Syndromes (Continued)

Characteristic	Neurofibromatosis (NF)	Multiple Endocrine Neoplasia (MEN)	Von Hippel-Lindau (VHL) Syndrome	Cowden Syndrome	Li-Fraumeni Syndrome	Peutz-Jeghers Syndrome
Risk reduction measures	NF1: Referral to specialists for treatment of complications involving the eye, central or peripheral nervous system, cardiovascular system, spine, or long bones; surgical removal of disfiguring or uncomfortable discrete cutaneous or subcutaneous neurofibromas. Surveillance: Annual physical exam by a physician familiar with the disorder; annual ophthalmologic exam; regular developmental assessment of children; regular blood pressure monitoring; MRI for follow-up of clinically suspected intracranial tumors and other internal tumors	MEN1: Surveillance including biochemical testing of serum concentrations of calcium (from age 8), gastrin (from age 20), pancreatic polypeptide (from age 10), and prolactin (from age 5) Imaging: • Abdominal CT or MRI (from age 20) • Head MRI (from age 5) Because early detection affects medical management, molecular genetic testing is offered to at-risk members of a family in which a germline MEN1 mutation has been identified as early as age 3–5. MEN2: Prophylactic thyroidectomy is recommended by age 5–10.	Starting by age 5: • Annual physical exam, including blood pressure (pheochromocytoma) and neurologic evaluation for signs of cerebellar or spinal cord lesions • Imaging of CNS and spinal cord by MRI starting at approximately age 11. Biennial imaging is recommended. • Annual CBC (polycythemia caused by EPO secretion from renal cysts and cerebellar hemangioblastoma) and annual urinalysis • Annual urine and/or plasma fractionated metanephrines starting between ages 2 and 5 when relatives have pheochromocytomas or chromocytoma or	Breast self-awareness beginning at age 18 Biannual breast exam beginning at age 20–25 Annual mammography and breast MRI starting at age 25–30 Consider prophylactic mastectomy. Annual gynecologic exam Annual thyroid exam beginning at age 18 Annual dermatologic exam Annual urinalysis Consider annual cytology and renal ultrasound examination if family history is positive for renal cell carcinoma. Baseline colonoscopy at age 50 (unless symptoms arise earlier). If only hamartomas are found, follow routine guidelines	Complete physical exam every 12 months Dermatologic exam every 12 months Urinalysis and CBC every 12 months Clinical breast exam every 6 months Consider annual breast MRI starting at age 25.	Upper and lower endoscopy (preferably wireless capsule endoscopy) plus radiographic exam of the small bowel beginning at age 8 or when symptoms occur Annual gynecologic and breast exams including mammogram beginning at age 20–25 Consider prophylactic hysterectomy and bilateral salpingo-oophorectomy after age 35 or after childbearing has been completed.

(Continued on next page)

Table 2-3. Less Common Hereditary Cancer Syndromes *(Continued)*

Characteristic	Neurofibromatosis (NF)	Multiple Endocrine Neoplasia (MEN)	Von Hippel-Lindau (VHL) Syndrome	Cowden Syndrome	Li-Fraumeni Syndrome	Peutz-Jeghers Syndrome
Risk reduction measures *(cont.)*	*NF2:* Vestibular schwannomas are treated primarily by surgery; stereotactic radiosurgery may be an alternative.	Screening for pheochromocytoma includes annual biochemical screening followed by MRI if the biochemical results are abnormal.	at age 16 in those without history • Annual ultrasound imaging of the kidneys and pancreas, beginning no later than age 16	for colon cancer screening (i.e., colonoscopy every 5–10 years).		

CBC—complete blood count; CNS—central nervous system; CT—computed tomography; EPO—erythropoietin; MRI—magnetic resonance imaging

Note. Based on information from Daniels, 2012; Frantzen et al., 2012; Gunder & Martin, 2011; Jasperson, 2012; Lindor et al., 2008; Mahon & Waldman, 2010a, 2010b, 2012; Pilarski & Nagy, 2012; Shannon & Chittenden, 2012; Shinagare et al., 2011.

- Personal and/or family history of breast cancer diagnosed before age 50
- Personal and/or family history of ovarian cancer diagnosed at any age
- Women of Ashkenazi Jewish ancestry diagnosed with breast and/or ovarian cancer at any age, regardless of family history
- Personal and/or family history of male breast cancer
- Personal history of triple-negative breast cancer diagnosed before age 60
- Affected first-degree relative with a known *BRCA1* or *BRCA2* mutation
- Bilateral breast cancer, especially if diagnosed at an early age
- Breast and ovarian cancer in the same woman
- Known *BRCA1/2* mutation in a first- or second-degree relative

The presence of one or more of these factors in an individual or family history is suggestive of hereditary breast and ovarian cancer syndrome and warrants further evaluation.

Figure 2-1. Key Indicators of Hereditary Breast and Ovarian Cancer Syndrome

---

Note. Based on information from National Comprehensive Cancer Network, 2014c; Petrucelli et al., 2013; Shannon et al., 2011.

---

suppressor genes (Christinat & Pagani, 2013). *BRCA1* and *BRCA2* are considered caretaker genes and help maintain genomic stability by recognizing and repairing DNA damage as well as having a role in cell cycle checkpoint control (Murray & Davies, 2013).

In late 2012, NCCN updated its hereditary breast and ovarian cancer guidelines to support the inclusion of comprehensive large rearrangement testing for all patients undergoing genetic testing for the *BRCA1* and *BRCA2* genes, as the rearrangement panel accounts for 6%–10% of all mutations in these two genes (NCCN, 2014c). Many women have undergone *BRCA1/2* testing but have not had comprehensive rearrangement testing; some of these individuals may have a large rearrangement mutation that has not been identified (Hartman et al., 2012; Shannon et al., 2011). APNs need to identify individuals who have had comprehensive testing (especially if genetic testing was done before 2013) and facilitate large rearrangement testing when appropriate (Mahon, 2013b).

Hereditary Nonpolyposis Colorectal Cancer Syndrome

The autosomal dominant syndrome HNPCC syndrome (also known as Lynch syndrome) accounts for 3%–5% of all colorectal cancers (Lindor et al., 2008). It also is associated with endometrial, ovarian, gastric, bile duct, small bowel, renal pelvis, and ureter cancers (Barrow, Hill, & Evans, 2013; Kohlmann & Gruber, 2012). The majority of mutations responsible for HNPCC syndrome occur in four MMR genes: *MSH2, MLH1, PMS2,* and *MSH6* (Martín-López & Fishel, 2013; Weissman et al., 2012). The *EPCAM* gene is a recently discovered contributor to Lynch syndrome, accounting for an estimated 1%–3% of all detectable HNPCC mutations because of large deletions in the end of this gene, which is located directly upstream of *MSH2* and can lead to a loss of *MSH2* expression, resulting in HNPCC syndrome (Gala & Chung, 2011; Ligtenberg, Kuiper, van Kessel, & Hoogerbrugge, 2013). Patients with a mutation associated with HNPCC syndrome have an 80% lifetime risk of developing colorectal cancer as compared with a 6% risk in the general population. Women with mutations in these genes have a 60% lifetime risk for developing endometrial cancer and a 12% lifetime risk for developing ovarian cancer (Lindor et al., 2008). Lifetime risk of stomach cancer is 1%–13% as compared to 1% in the general population (NCCN, 2014b). Risk of ovarian cancer is 4%–24% as compared to 1% in the general population (NCCN, 2014b).

Individuals with HNPCC-related cancers are more likely to have poorly differentiated tumors with an excess of mucoid and signet-cell features (Barrow et al., 2013; Kohlmann & Gruber, 2012). Although HNPCC syndrome is not associated with large numbers of polyps, people with the syndrome who form adenomatous polyps are more likely to do so at an earlier age, are more likely to develop right-sided colon cancer, and tend to exhibit a very rapid progression to malignancy in 1–3 years instead of the 5–10-year pattern seen in the general population (Weissman et al., 2012).

Risk assessment for HNPCC syndrome is approached in several ways. The Bethesda criteria assess the number of relatives affected by colorectal cancer or other HNPCC-related cancers with particular emphasis on the age at onset (Vasen et al., 2013). The Bethesda guidelines (see Figure 2-2) assist in identification of tumors that should undergo microsatellite instability (MSI) and immunohistochemical (IHC) testing for one of the four MMR genes (NCCN, 2014b). Germ-line analysis of MMR genes is very complex and time consuming. It cannot be offered to every patient diagnosed with colorectal or HNPCC-associated cancer but should be restricted to patients with MSI tumors because this molecular phenotype is a landmark of HNPCC cancers.

IHC staining and MSI testing may be done to predict an MMR defect and thereby avoid unnecessary, expensive, and time-consuming DNA analyses. IHC staining can be done on tumor tissue from individuals who fulfill the Bethesda criteria to determine the presence or absence of MLH1, MSH2, MSH6, and PMS2 proteins (Schneider, Schneider, Kloor, Fürst, & Möslein, 2012). If IHC is abnormal, this indicates that one of the proteins is not expressed, and an inherited mutation may be present (NCCN, 2014b). Alternatively, an MSI assay could be performed. In HNPCC, mutations in the DNA repair genes result in the phenomenon of MSI. Microsatellites are repeated sequences of DNA that are a defined length for each individual. Because of the accumulation of errors, these sequences can become abnormally longer or shorter, which is referred to as *microsatellite instability* (Kastrinos & Syngal, 2012). An MSI-high phenotype is reported in 85%–92% of HNPCC colon cancers and approximately 15% of sporadic cancers (NCCN, 2014b). If either of these tests is abnormal, then further testing with DNA analysis would be appropriate. Key indicators of HNPCC syndrome are shown in Figure 2-3.

Familial Adenomatous Polyposis Syndromes

FAP, an autosomal dominant trait, is characterized by numerous (usually more than 100) adenomatous colonic polyps and accounts for about 1% of colorectal cancer cases (Jasperson & Burt,

---

Revised Bethesda Criteria
- Colorectal carcinoma diagnosed before age 50
- Presence of synchronous or metachronous HNPCC-related carcinomas, regardless of age[a]
- Colorectal carcinoma with specific pathologic features diagnosed before age 60[b]
- Colorectal carcinoma diagnosed in one or more first-degree relatives with an HNPCC-related tumor, with one diagnosed before age 50
- Colorectal carcinoma in two or more first- or second-degree relatives with an HNPCC-related tumor, regardless of age

Only one of these criteria must be met to proceed with MSI or IHC testing. If positive by MSI or IHC, then mismatch repair testing may begin.

Figure 2-2. Criteria to Proceed With Microsatellite Instability (MSI) or Immunohistochemical (IHC) Testing for Hereditary Nonpolyposis Colorectal Cancer (HNPCC) Syndrome

---

[a] Colorectal, endometrial, stomach, ovarian, pancreas, ureter and renal pelvis, biliary tract, brain, sebaceous gland, and small bowel carcinomas

[b] Tumor-infiltrating lymphocytes, Crohn-like lymphocyte reaction, mucinous/signet-ring differentiation, or medullary growth pattern

Note. Based on information from National Comprehensive Cancer Network, 2014b; Vasen et al., 2013; Weissman et al., 2012.

- Personal history of colorectal and/or endometrial cancer diagnosed before age 50
- First-degree relative with colorectal cancer diagnosed before age 50
- Two or more relatives with colorectal cancer or an HNPCC-associated cancer, which includes endometrial, ovarian, gastric, hepatobiliary, small bowel, renal pelvis, sebaceous adenomas, or ureter cancers; at least one relative must be a first-degree relative of another.
- Colorectal cancer occurring in two or more generations on the same side of the family
- A personal history of colorectal cancer and a first-degree relative with adenomas diagnosed before age 40
- An affected relative with a known HNPCC mutation

The presence of one or more of these factors in an individual or family history is suggestive of HNPCC syndrome and warrants further evaluation.

Figure 2-3. Key Indicators of Hereditary Nonpolyposis Colorectal Cancer (HNPCC) Syndrome

Note. Based on information from Barrow et al., 2013; Jasperson, 2012; Shia et al., 2013; Weissman et al., 2012.

2011). The *FAP* gene is nearly 100% penetrant; so, if a person is not treated, he or she will develop colorectal cancer because of the sheer number of polyps. The mean age at onset of cancer is 39, although as many as 75% will have developed adenomas by age 20 (Lindor et al., 2008). A less severe form of FAP called *attenuated familial adenomatous polyposis* (AFAP) is characterized by fewer than 100 polyps (usually about 20) at presentation and later onset of colorectal cancer. More than 800 mutations in the *APC* gene are associated with FAP (Senter, 2012). Deleterious mutations in this tumor suppressor gene result in the premature truncation of the APC protein (Jasperson & Burt, 2011). An autosomal recessive gene on chromosome 1 also exists, called *MYH*, which is associated with polyposis. Approximately 25% of individuals with FAP have a de novo mutation (Jasperson & Burt, 2011). Figure 2-4 provides an overview of key indicators of FAP and AFAP.

MUTYH-associated polyposis (MAP) is an autosomal recessive colon cancer syndrome. MAP is thought to account for 0.5%–1% of all colorectal cancers. Biallelic (both alleles affected) mutations of the *MUTYH* (also known as *MYH*) gene have been found in 22%–29% of North Europeans with more than 10 adenomatous polyps, as well as 28% of *APC* germ-line negative patients with 10–100 polyps (NCCN, 2014b). Although more research is needed, the estimated risk of developing colon cancer in MAP is 19% by age 50 and 43% by age 60 with an overall lifetime risk of colon cancer estimated to be 80% (Gala & Chung, 2011). The cumulative lifetime risk of duodenal cancer is 4%, as well as a 38% lifetime risk of any extraintestinal cancer including ovarian, bladder, and skin cancers (Patel & Ahnen, 2012). The risk of colon cancer in heterozygote carriers appears to be slightly elevated and similar to that of individuals with a first-degree relative with colon cancer (Jasperson & Burt, 2011).

Hereditary Melanoma

Hereditary melanoma is an autosomal dominant disease that accounts for about 10% of all melanomas. Germ-line mutations in the tumor suppressor *p16* (*CDKN2A*) gene account for 25%–40% of hereditary melanomas (Lindor et al., 2008). Mutations in the *p16* gene also have been associated with pancreatic cancer. Those with germ-line mutations in *p16* are at substantial risk for developing melanoma; the lifetime risk approaches 60% (Lindor et al., 2008). The lifetime risk of developing pancreatic cancer for these individuals approaches 17%. Other genes implicated in hereditary melanoma include the *CDK4* gene (Gabree & Seidel, 2012). Figure 2-5 shows the key indicators of hereditary melanoma.

Genetic testing for hereditary melanoma is controversial because individuals with a family history of melanoma can be managed with regular full body screening for cutaneous changes

- Patient has a clinical diagnosis of FAP (100 or more polyps).
- Patient has suspected FAP or AFAP (15–99 polyps).
- Patient is a first-degree relative of an individual with FAP or AFAP.
- Patient has an affected relative with a known *FAP* or *MYH* mutation.
- Patient has any number of adenomas in a family with FAP.

The presence of one or more of these factors in an individual or family history is suggestive of hereditary FAP/AFAP and warrants further evaluation.

Figure 2-4. Key Indicators of Familial Adenomatous Polyposis (FAP) and Attenuated Familial Adenomatous Polyposis (AFAP)

Note. Based on information from Jasperson, 2012; Jasperson & Burt, 2011; Patel & Ahnen, 2012.

- Three or more primary melanomas in an individual
- A patient with melanoma with three or more melanomas in the family
- Melanoma and pancreatic cancer in an individual and/or family
- First-degree relative of a *p16* mutation carrier

The presence of one or more of these factors in an individual or family history is suggestive of hereditary melanoma and warrants further evaluation.

Figure 2-5. Key Indicators of Hereditary Melanoma

Note. Based on information from Gabree & Seidel, 2012; Weitzel et al., 2011.

and insurance coverage for this testing is often limited. However, identification of such a mutation can be very helpful in providing recommendations for aggressive surveillance for pancreatic cancer, which should be reserved for those with documented elevated risk of developing melanoma. Families with suspected hereditary melanoma syndromes benefit from intensive education about their risks, how to avoid ultraviolet exposure, and the risks and benefits of genetic testing. Once they have been fully informed of these issues, they can make a decision regarding genetic testing.

Hereditary Pancreatic Cancer

Pancreatic cancer can be seen in different hereditary cancer syndromes. When predominantly pancreatic cancer is seen, the most common mutations are in the *PALB2* and *BRCA2* genes. The *PALB2* gene, named because it is a "Partner and Localizer of *BRCA2*," produces a protein that interacts with *BRCA2* and is also involved in DNA repair as a tumor suppressor gene (Axilbund & Wiley, 2012). It is located on chromosome 16p12.2. Mutations in *PALB2* are inherited in an autosomal dominant manner (Lindor et al., 2008). When APNs are assessing hereditary cancer risk, they should collect patients' personal and family history to investigate the risk for hereditary pancreatic cancer (see Figure 2-6). If predominantly pancreatic cancer is seen, genetic testing for *PALB2* and *BRCA2* may be appropriate (Jones et al., 2009). Mutations in *PALB2* have been identified in families with multiple cases of pancreatic cancer, but the exact risk for pancreatic cancer conferred by *PALB2* mutations has not yet been established (Axilbund & Wiley, 2012). The cumulative breast cancer risk among female *PALB2* mutation carriers is estimated to be 18%–35% by age 70 (Axilbund & Wiley, 2012).

Other genes are associated with pancreatic cancer risk, including *BRCA1*, *BRCA2*, *CDKN2A*, and those associated with Lynch syndrome (*MLH1*, *MSH2*, *MSH6*, *PMS2*, and *EPCAM*) (Axil-

• Patient with pancreatic cancer with at least one close relative with pancreatic cancer
• Individual with two or more close relatives with pancreatic cancer
• Individual of Ashkenazi Jewish descent with a personal history of pancreatic cancer or a first-degree relative with pancreatic cancer
• A previously identified *PALB2* mutation in the family

Figure 2-6. Key Indicators of Hereditary Pancreatic Cancer

Note. Based on information from Axilbund & Wiley, 2012; Jones et al., 2009; Larghi et al., 2009.

bund & Wiley, 2012). APNs should consider and discuss these potential syndromes and genetic mutations when evaluating families with a history of pancreatic cancer. An emerging trend is to consider next-generation panel testing for these families because often these syndromes have similar presentations (Mahon, 2013c).

Indications for Genetic Assessment

Identifying and managing people who are at risk for hereditary cancer syndromes is now an integral part of cancer prevention and treatment. With proper assessment, testing, and implementation of aggressive screening and prevention measures, healthcare providers can significantly affect the future health of patients and their families who have a hereditary risk for cancer. APNs are increasingly assuming responsibility for the management of these families with an emphasis on wellness and cancer prevention.

Identification of individuals who are at risk for hereditary cancer syndromes is the first critical step in providing effective, comprehensive genetic care. In addition to the indicators described in Figures 2-1, 2-3, 2-4, 2-5, and 2-6, the general factors shown in Figure 2-7 might suggest a person is at risk for a hereditary cancer syndrome. Some family histories do not suggest a specific syndrome, such as HBOC or HNPCC, but may include a larger number of malignancies than would be expected by chance or that could be explained by environmental exposures. An unusual constellation of cancer types also may be present. When this occurs, it is best to refer to a healthcare provider with expertise in genetics to consider rare syndromes and possible testing strategies or research studies available to help the family better define their risk (Brierley et al., 2012; Mahon, 2013d).

Genetic testing for germ-line hereditary predisposition syndromes usually uses traditional Sanger DNA sequencing (see Table 2-1). More recently, efforts have been undertaken to increase efficiency and analyze massive numbers of different DNA sequences in a single reaction, which is called a parallel reaction. This is referred to as *next-generation sequencing* (Desmedt, Voet, Sotiriou, & Campbell, 2012; Rizzo & Buck, 2012) (see Table 2-1). Next-generation sequencing has led to reduced cost and turnaround time with the simultaneous testing of multiple genes. Next-generation sequencing panels analyze less common high- and intermediate-penetrance cancer susceptibility genes. The American College of Medical Genetics and Genomics has issued a policy statement on the use of next-generation sequencing, emphasizing the importance of correctly identifying families who are likely to benefit from testing, comprehensive pretest counseling, post-test considerations, and the role of genetics professionals (American College of Medical Genetics and Genomics, 2012). When combined with comprehensive genetic counseling, next-generation sequencing can be helpful for families who have confusing histories or who have tested negative for the more common syndromes (Ku et al., 2013; Mahon, 2013c).

- A cluster of the same cancer in close relatives
- Cancer occurring at a younger age than expected in the general population
- More than one primary cancer in one person
- Evidence of autosomal dominant inheritance (two or more generations affected, with both males and females affected)
- Bilateral cancer in any paired organ
- Cancers in an organ that are multifocal
- Any pattern of cancer associated with a known cancer syndrome
- Cancers that are occurring more frequently in a family than are expected by chance in the absence of known environmental and lifestyle risk factors

These factors are considered after gathering a family history, and if one or more criteria are present, it may be prudent to refer to a healthcare provider with expertise in cancer genetics.

Figure 2-7. General Indicators of a Hereditary Predisposition for Developing Cancer

Note. Based on information from Lynch et al., 2009; Mai et al., 2011; Robson et al., 2010; Weitzel et al., 2011.

Standards for Genetic Testing

Family history and mathematical models are used to calculate a person's risk of developing cancer and carrying a mutation, but ultimately, genetic testing is the only means available to determine who has inherited a germ-line mutation. A number of professional and government agencies have issued position statements regarding genetic testing. Some are more general, but many identify conditions for offering specific cancer predisposition testing, most often *BRCA1/2* testing. These recommendations are updated frequently, and APNs should consult the individual agencies for updates. Many of these recommendations and guidelines are available at the National Guideline Clearinghouse website (www.guideline.gov). A summary of these position statements is shown in Table 2-4. Most of the agencies emphasize that testing should be done in high-risk people where there is a reasonable likelihood of finding a mutation, where qualified personnel are available to provide informed consent in the context of pre- and post-test counseling, and when the knowledge of mutation status will influence care.

Provision of Cancer Genetics Education and Counseling

Providing education, counseling, and support is a central responsibility for APNs who are caring for people with a hereditary predisposition for developing cancer. Education must be tailored to the individual needs and learning capabilities of each family member. This usually is a labor-intensive process, and families should anticipate at least one to three sessions lasting 60–90 minutes prior to testing to ensure that they truly have informed consent and adequate information to make a good decision that is congruent with their individual needs (Mahon, 2013a). Additional counseling sessions following testing also will be needed; how many often depends on the outcome of testing and the person's psychological response to the results.

Assessment of Hereditary Risk

During the assessment for hereditary risk, families are asked to provide detailed information about family history and cancer diagnoses. It often is helpful to inform patients of the need for a detailed family history prior to the appointment. Typically, the proband for the family is instructed to gather information about all cancer diagnoses, ages at diagnosis, and current ages or ages at death for all first- and second-degree relatives. Gathering this information frequently requires the proband to communicate with multiple family members. When

Table 2-4. Standards for Genetic Testing

Agency/ Organization	Position

American Society of Clinical Oncology	• Genetic testing is offered when
	  – Personal or family history features suggest a genetic cancer susceptibility condition.
	  – The test can be adequately interpreted.
	  – Results will aid in diagnosis or influence the medical or surgical management of the patient and/or at-risk family members.
	• Testing is only done in the setting of pre- and post-test counseling, which includes discussions of possible risks and benefits of cancer early detection and prevention modalities.
	• Efforts should be made to ensure that all individuals at significantly increased risk have access to appropriate genetic counseling, testing, screening, surveillance, and all related medical and surgical interventions, which should be covered without penalty by public and private third-party payers.
	• Providers make direct efforts to protect the confidentiality of genetic information.
	• Educational opportunities for physicians and other healthcare providers are available regarding
	  – Methods of cancer risk assessment
	  – Clinical characteristics of hereditary cancer susceptibility syndromes
	  – Pre- and post-test genetic counseling
	  – Risk management.

National Society of Genetic Counselors	• Genetic testing for hereditary cancer susceptibility is offered only when
	  – A client has a significant personal and/or family history of cancer.
	  – The test can be adequately interpreted.
	  – The results will affect medical management.
	  – The clinician can provide or make available adequate genetic education and counseling.
	  – The client can provide informed consent.
	• Informed consent is a necessary component of genetic testing in both clinical and research settings.
	• The process of informed consent includes
	  – A thorough discussion of the possible outcomes of testing
	  – A review of the possible benefits, risks, and limitations
	  – A discussion of alternatives to molecular testing.

Oncology Nursing Society	• Risk assessment counseling and cancer predisposition genetic testing are essential components of comprehensive cancer care.
	• Healthcare providers offering these services must have educational preparation in both human genetic principles and oncology.
	• Cancer predisposition genetic testing requires informed consent and must include
	  – Pre- and post-test counseling
	  – Follow-up by qualified individuals.
	• Legislation exists that provides protection from
	  – Genetic discrimination in both employment and insurance arenas
	  – Reimbursement for and access to genetic counseling, cancer predisposition genetic testing services, and appropriate medical management.
	• Ongoing educational resources for healthcare providers, individuals at increased risk, and the lay public are developed, evaluated, and disseminated.

(Continued on next page)

Table 2-4. Standards for Genetic Testing *(Continued)*

Agency/ Organization	Position
U.S. Preventive Services Task Force	• Fair evidence exists that women with certain specific family history patterns ("increased risk family history") have an increased risk for developing breast or ovarian cancer associated with *BRCA1/2* and may benefit from genetic testing. • These women would benefit from genetic counseling that allows informed decision making about testing and prophylactic treatment. • Counseling is performed by suitably trained healthcare providers.

Note. Based on information from Oncology Nursing Society, 2014; Riley et al., 2012; Robson et al., 2010; U.S. Preventive Services Task Force, 2005.

the proband obtains this information before the appointment, it saves time and allows APNs to perform some preliminary risk calculations and identify areas where more information is needed. This usually is organized into a pedigree format, as shown in Figure 2-8. This information is confirmed by pathology reports and/or death certificates whenever possible because families often have incomplete or incorrect information about cancer diagnoses. Without accurate information regarding the cancer diagnoses, APNs cannot accurately assess risk and select the correct genetic test to order. This visual presentation also is very helpful for explaining risk to families. A variety of computerized programs are available to facilitate the drawing of pedigrees. Programs also are available that help to calculate statistical risk for developing cancer and for carrying a mutation for hereditary predisposition (see Figure 2-9).

Families deserve basic information on how risk assessments are completed, what the models imply, and a summary of their risk. Frequently, this includes a statistical discussion of risk. Patients need to understand the risk for developing the disease in the general population

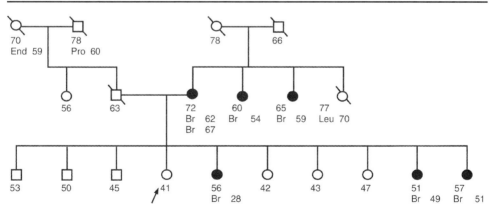

This pedigree represents a typical presentation of family history. Squares represent males, and circles represent females. A slash represents a deceased person. Filled-in circles and squares represent diagnoses confirmed with pathology reports. The family member's current age or age at death is shown as well as the age at any cancer diagnosis. The arrow represents the proband or spokesperson for the family. There are three generations, showing both maternal and paternal sides. If information is known about ethnicity, it can also be included. Ideally, all cancer diagnoses are verified by pathology reports and/or death certificates.

Figure 2-8. Example of a Pedigree

Gail Model
Purpose: Estimates breast cancer risk in women without a diagnosis of cancer
Target: Women with a minimal to moderate family history of breast cancer
Advantages: Readily available; considers commonly collected risk factors; provides risk estimates for next five years and lifetime
Disadvantage: Does not consider family history of ovarian cancer, age at diagnosis, affected second-degree relatives, or paternal family history

Pedigree Assessment Tool
Purpose: Identifies women at increased risk for hereditary breast or ovarian cancer
Target: Women being seen in primary care settings with multiple family members diagnosed with breast cancer
Advantage: Simple point scoring system based on family history with points weighted according to features associated with *BRCA1/2* mutations
Disadvantage: May over-refer some women for genetic counseling

Claus Model
Purpose: Estimates risk of developing breast cancer over time in 10-year increments
Target: Women with multiple family members diagnosed with breast cancer
Advantage: Considers maternal and paternal history of breast cancer as well as age at diagnosis
Disadvantage: Does not consider history of ovarian cancer or ethnicity

Shattuck-Eidens Model
Purpose: Estimates risk of carrying a *BRCA1* mutation
Target: Women with substantial family history of breast cancer or early-onset breast cancer
Advantage: Considers early-onset breast cancer, bilateral breast cancer, and ovarian cancer history
Disadvantage: Does not consider ethnicity or *BRCA2* mutations

Couch Model
Purpose: Estimates risk of carrying a *BRCA1* mutation
Target: Women with a substantial family history of breast cancer
Advantage: Considers the average age at diagnosis in the family and ethnicity
Disadvantage: Is relatively insensitive in small families or those with few cancers

Berry Model
Purpose: Estimates risk of carrying a *BRCA1* or *BRCA2* mutation
Target: Women with a family history of breast and/or ovarian cancer
Advantage: Considers first- and second-degree relatives, age at diagnosis, and breast and ovarian cancer history
Disadvantage: Has limited utility in some ethnic groups

Frank Model
Purpose: Estimates risk of carrying a *BRCA1* or *BRCA2* mutation
Target: Women diagnosed with breast cancer before age 50
Advantage: Considers first- and second-degree relatives, age at diagnosis, and breast and ovarian cancer history
Disadvantage: May not be as sensitive in families with older age at onset

Manchester Model
Purpose: Estimates risk of carrying a *BRCA1* or *BRCA2* mutation
Target: Non-Jewish women with a family history of breast and/or ovarian cancer
Advantage: Useful in identifying women who have *BRCA2* mutations
Disadvantage: May be less useful in identifying women who have *BRCA1* mutations

Figure 2-9. Risk Models Commonly Used When Counseling About Hereditary Cancer Syndromes

(Continued on next page)

Tyrer-Cuzick Model

Purpose: Establishes risk of developing breast cancer over a lifetime and risk of carrying a *BRCA1* or *BRCA2* mutation

Target: Women with a family history of breast and/or ovarian cancer

Advantages: Considers both maternal and paternal family history as well as history of ovarian and breast cancer; calculates both risk of a mutation and risk of developing breast cancer

Disadvantage: Requires some time to enter all of the data into the software program

Wijnen Model

Purpose: Estimates the risk of carrying an *MSH2* or *MLH1* mutation

Target: People with a family history of colon and/or endometrial cancer

Advantages: Considers history of colon and endometrial cancer; may be more useful when used in conjunction with Amsterdam criteria and microsatellite instability testing

Disadvantage: Does not consider ovarian cancer or other gastrointestinal cancers

PREMM Model

Purpose: Estimates the risk of carrying an *MSH2* or *MLH1* mutation

Target: People with a family history of colorectal and gynecologic cancers

Advantages: Considers both colorectal and gynecologic cancers as well as personal risk factors; easy to complete with a Web-based model

Disadvantage: May not be able to incorporate complex combinations of diagnoses

MMRpro Model

Purpose: Predicts people who may benefit from genetic testing for *MSH2* or *MLH1* mutations

Target: People with a personal and/or family history of colorectal or endometrial cancer

Advantage: May be useful in small families, families with older ages at diagnosis, and families that do not meet Bethesda criteria

Disadvantage: Does not consider other cancers associated with hereditary nonpolyposis colorectal cancer

Figure 2-9. Risk Models Commonly Used When Counseling About Hereditary Cancer Syndromes *(Continued)*

Note. Based on information from Amir et al., 2003; Balmaña et al., 2006; Evans et al., 2004; Kastrinos et al., 2013; Parmigiani et al., 2007; Ståhlbom et al., 2012; Tyrer et al., 2004; van Zitteren et al., 2011; Weitzel et al., 2011.

(absolute risk), as well as the relative risk for developing the cancer when compared to people who do not have risk factors. Using relative risk is complicated in people with a family history of cancer. If the individual did not inherit the predisposition gene, the person's relative risk score will overestimate his or her risk. If the individual did inherit the gene, it will probably underestimate the risk (Domchek & Antoniou, 2007; Freedman et al., 2005). Patients need to be informed of these potential and significant limitations.

Performing a risk calculation as to whether the individual has a genetic mutation is necessary. If no testing has been done in a family, this calculation usually is based on the number of family members diagnosed with a specific constellation of cancers, the family's ethnicity, and family members' ages at diagnosis (see Figure 2-9). Usually several different models are used, and the patient receives the risk estimate in a range. Each of these methods has distinct strengths and limitations. It is especially important to note that if the family is small with few affected individuals, these models usually will underestimate the risk of having a mutation (Domchek & Antoniou, 2007; Wiseman, Dancyger, & Michie, 2010). In the case of HBOC, additional criteria that may influence a decision to offer testing in a small family might include a diagnosis of both breast and ovarian cancer in one member, male breast cancer, bilateral breast cancer (especially if diagnosed before age 45), ovarian cancer diagnosed before age 40, or breast cancer diagnosed before age 35 (NCCN, 2014c). Once a mutation is detected in a family, APNs can determine the statistical risk based on Mendelian patterns of inheritance: in the case of autosomal dominance, first-degree relatives have a statistical 50% chance of having inherited the predisposition gene.

Basic Genetic Information

For families to make an informed decision about testing, they need to receive basic genetic information. At the minimum, this includes information about autosomal dominant transmission, penetrance, statistical risks, and the difference between germ-line and somatic mutations. Pictures and diagrams are useful when conveying this information, and APNs or genetic counselors might use a brochure or handout with this information so that patients can review the information at a later date. Sharing a copy of the pedigree with the family will facilitate their understanding of the principles of autosomal dominant transmission. Other materials that might be shared with families include copies of risk calculations, especially if these calculations help the family to understand how their risk compares with the risk in the general population and estimates of risk over time. These calculations may also be important to provide insurance justification for aggressive or altered screening such as breast magnetic resonance imaging (MRI) in women with a greater than 20% calculated lifetime risk of breast cancer (NCCN, 2014a).

Prevention Strategies

Prior to genetic testing, patients need a clear understanding of the recommendations and guidelines for management of risk if they test positive and if they do not. This anticipatory guidance helps them to prepare for all potential ramifications so they can make a choice about testing that is congruent with their values and needs.

Patients usually are interested in prevention, but it can lead to very difficult choices. For many cancers with a hereditary predisposition, prevention is best achieved by prophylactic surgery such as mastectomy, hysterectomy, colectomy, or oophorectomy. Each of these procedures carries not only the risks associated with surgery and anesthesia but also psychosocial concerns, significant body image changes, and alterations in body function. It is important to explore patients' feelings, concerns, and openness regarding these preventive measures prior to testing.

Prevention measures also may include chemoprevention if a strategy exists. Patients need to be aware of the risks, side effects, and potential benefits of such agents. This usually requires a discussion of current research. It is important to explore whether individuals are willing to commit to taking such an agent long term when the effectiveness may not be immediately evident and potential side effects exist.

Finally, prevention measures may include lifestyle measures such as a healthy diet, weight management, exercise, smoking cessation, and application of sunscreen and other measures that protect against ultraviolet light exposure (ACS, 2013). Patients need more than a simple recommendation. For prevention strategies to be effective, most patients will need specific information, planning, and approaches to such behavior. Chapter 1 provides more information on prevention and screening.

Early Detection Strategies

Families and individuals with hereditary predisposition need specific information regarding how to detect cancer in the earliest stages, when treatment is most likely to be effective.

This includes signs and symptoms to report promptly, as well as screening measures. For each recommended screening measure, there needs to be a discussion of the sensitivity and specificity of the screening tests and the expected benefits and risks. Guidelines given to the general population may require modification in high-risk families. It is important that families clearly understand that screening will not prevent cancer but rather that it can result in sufficiently early detection for the disease to be treated with limited morbidity and mortality.

Genetic Testing Process

The process of genetic testing is relatively straightforward once the proper test is selected and the patient has been informed of the potential risks, benefits, and limitations of testing. The patient usually must sign a consent to ensure that he or she understands the ramifications of testing and that he or she is not being coerced. A number of agencies, including American Society of Clinical Oncology (ASCO), International Society of Nurses in Genetics (ISONG), NSGC, NCCN, and ONS, have developed recommendations about the need for informed consent (see Figure 2-10) and consultation with a qualified health professional with expertise in genetics (ISONG, 2009; NCCN, 2014c; ONS, 2010, 2014; Robson et al., 2010). Other components of the genetic testing process are shown in Figure 2-11.

Because testing is usually expensive and insurance reimbursement can vary, preauthorization often is desirable so that patients understand their potential financial responsibilities. Preauthorization frequently requires a letter of medical necessity. Typical components of a letter of medical necessity include the test being ordered, why it is appropriate, and how the results will influence the care and management of the patient's risk.

Once preauthorization has been obtained, a blood specimen or a buccal (saliva) sample is obtained from the patient and sent to the testing laboratory. Some laboratories will hold the specimen until preauthorization is final. Each laboratory has specific rules for collecting and transporting the specimen. In most cases, results are available in two to four weeks; next-generation sequencing may take six to eight weeks. Results are best disclosed in person, and this policy is addressed in pretest counseling. In some cases, phone disclosure may be acceptable and be associated with an equally acceptable outcome, but this needs to be discussed and determined during the pretest phase (Baumanis, Evans, Callanan, & Susswein, 2009; Bradbury et al., 2011). Depending on the outcome, additional sessions may be needed to discuss management strategies.

Because genetic testing for a hereditary cancer syndrome has implications for other family members, a clear plan needs to be made prior to testing regarding how other family members will be informed of their risk. Genetic test results are confidential medical information. The proband will need to inform other at-risk relatives. The focus in genetic risk assessment is on the family, not the individual. Genetic information has not only profound effects on an individual, but also far-reaching implications for other family members who may or may not be prepared to learn they have risk and need coordination of care. Discussions should include information on why genetic information is unique and how it will be stored in the medical record. Also to be addressed is that the proband or individuals being tested, with the assistance of the genetic professional, will be responsible for informing other family members of potential risk.

Perhaps one of the biggest risks and liabilities that occurs when genetic testing is ordered outside of the formal genetic testing process by a credentialed genetic provider is that care may not be appropriately coordinated and offered to the entire family at risk. When genetic testing moves away from a credentialed genetic professional, the ordering provider often interprets the test for an individual, and it is unclear who should care for the rest of the family (Bri-

Pretest Visit
Discuss purpose and agenda of visit.
Assess patient concerns, motivations, and expectations regarding genetic testing.
Clarify misconceptions about the process or concepts.
Construct pedigree.
Document lifestyle and medical history risk factors.
Perform targeted physical examination for features associated with hereditary cancer syndromes.
Discuss factors that limit interpretation and assessment.
Present basic risk information for developing cancer(s).
Present risk calculations of having a mutation.
Discuss principles of cancer genetics.
Discuss and identify the best individual(s) to test in the family.
Discuss alternatives to testing.
Prioritize order of tests if more than one test or strategy is considered.
Discuss specimen collection.
Discuss potential test outcomes of testing.
Discuss possible management strategies for each outcome.
Discuss testing costs and insurance issues.
Discuss possible discrimination issues.
Offer opportunities to ask questions for clarification.

Testing Ordered

Testing Declined

Post-Test Counseling
Disclose and interpret test results.
Identify other at-risk family members.
Coordinate testing for other family members.
Provide psychological support as needed.

Management
Increased surveillance and screening
Prophylactic surgery
Clinical trials
Chemoprevention

Figure 2-10. Algorithm for Providing Genetic Testing Services

Note. Based on information from Christinat & Pagani, 2013; Riley et al., 2012; Weitzel et al., 2011; Wiseman et al., 2010.

erley et al., 2012). Even if the primary care provider orders the correct test, it is not usually the practice of primary care providers to identify and coordinate genetic testing for all members at risk, including those who live outside of the geographic region they serve. Credentialed genetic professionals are trained in using the pedigree to identify those at risk and coordinating care for the entire family. Many instances exist when a mutation has been identified in a family and other family members were not informed and therefore missed the opportunity to

- Basic information on the mode of transmission and penetrance
- Genetic test being performed; sensitivity, specificity, and technical aspects of the test
- Likelihood of having a positive test based on risk assessment
- Discussion of how testing may clarify risks in a family
- Implications of a positive test, including prophylactic surgical procedures, chemoprevention, and screening measures
- Benefits of testing an affected person first
- Implications of a negative test if a mutation has not been identified in the family
- Implications of a negative test for a known mutation, including population risks for developing cancer
- Discussion of Mendelian patterns of transmission and risks for children, siblings, and other first-degree relatives
- Discussion of fees for counseling and testing and coverage for prophylactic procedures and screening
- Exploration of feelings about testing
- Discussion of potential negative and positive psychological outcomes associated with testing
- Discussion of potential risks of employer and insurance discrimination, as well as risks of loss of privacy, including how confidentiality will be maintained during the testing process
- Discussion of alternatives to testing
- Discussion of policies for storage or reuse of genetic material by the testing laboratory
- Importance of sharing genetic testing results with at-risk relatives and healthcare providers

Figure 2-11. Recommended Components of Informed Consent

Note. Based on information from International Society of Nurses in Genetics & American Nurses Association, 2007; Oncology Nursing Society, 2014; Riley et al., 2012; Robson et al., 2010.

prevent or detect a malignancy, potentially resulting in the liability of an early death (Mahon, 2011). Sharing information within families is often complicated (Menko et al., 2013). Consequently, genetic professionals will inform the patient, work with the patient to identify other family members at risk, and send a follow-up letter that informs the patient about the risk and how family members can access genetic care. This education begins in the pretest counseling and is continued through the follow-up phase.

A related issue that families sometimes encounter deals with testing of minor children. Because test results may change prevention and screening behaviors, it is important to consider the implications of testing for minor children. In the case of HBOC, HNPCC, and hereditary melanoma, knowledge of mutation status will not alter screening or prophylactic surgical decisions because in most cases these maneuvers do not begin until early adulthood. Children would probably not be candidates for mammography, ultrasonography, or chemoprevention (Sie, Prins, Spruijt, Kets, & Hoogerbrugge, 2013). Families at risk should be counseled about the benefits of healthy lifestyle behaviors for the prevention of cancer (ACS, 2013). It would not be necessary to know an individual's mutation status to make recommendations regarding a low-fat, high-fiber diet or reduction in ultraviolet light exposure. These recommendations would be appropriate for any member of the population. When minors reach an age with maturity to consent and have received adequate counseling, they can make their own decision about testing. One exception sometimes encountered in cancer genetics is individuals from families with a known mutation associated with FAP. Because these individuals begin forming polyps early in their teenage years, colonoscopy often is initiated before the individuals reach the legal age to provide consent. In this case, with careful counseling of both the minor child and the parents, a decision sometimes is made to test a minor child. In this case, the parents would consent because knowing the results of mutation status may provide support for regular colonoscopy at a young age or may eliminate the need for this invasive screening procedure. Similarly, because screening and perhaps prophylactic surgery may be indicated in children or adolescents, genetic testing, with counseling by a credentialed genetic professional, may be appropriate for those with genetic predisposition syndromes such as MEN or VHL syndrome (Mahon & Waldman, 2010a, 2010b, 2012).

Potential Risks, Benefits, and Limitations of Testing

The biggest risks of testing involve loss of privacy and psychosocial distress. In most cases, pretest counseling aids in the identification of potential problems so that these may be addressed before testing. Efforts need to be made to protect confidentiality. Concerns about confidentiality and potential discrimination often are paramount for patients and, in some cases, make it difficult for patients to even begin to learn about the ramifications of testing. Clearly, these fears keep some individuals and families from seeking genetic services or participating in genetic research (Twomey, 2011). The Genetic Information Nondiscrimination Act of 2008 (GINA) is a federal law designed to protect patients' genetic information. Group health insurance plans cannot use genetic information to deny or limit eligibility for coverage or to increase premiums, and genetic information cannot be considered a preexisting condition. However, this protection has gaps and does not apply to people who have individual or self-insured plans. This lack of confidence demonstrated by both healthcare providers and the public may stem from the fact that no real test cases of actual enforcement have occurred. Employment discrimination is also prohibited under GINA. Patients need to be counseled about how to manage questions about risk in the workplace.

Prior to testing, patients also are counseled about risks and potential problems with obtaining life or disability insurance. Failure to disclose a genetic condition may result in cancellation of a policy. Some people may opt to purchase or increase coverage prior to testing to avoid possible problems. More controversy exists with life insurance because individuals fear that if they have a mutation and desire increased coverage, it will be unaffordable, which often limits or discourages them from obtaining genetic testing that might provide health benefits. Conversely, life insurance providers argue that they need access to genetic testing information to prevent excessive financial loss.

As part of the informed consent process, patients and families need to understand how their genetic risk and test results will be handled. Some genetics programs will use a specific consent to release genetic information (Twomey, 2011). Information about genetic testing is important to many primary care providers and other subspecialists so that they can order proper cancer prevention and early detection measures. As part of the informed consent process, APNs need to discuss with patients and families how and whether they intend to release genetic test results to healthcare providers and the implications of these decisions. Many commercial laboratories that perform genetic testing provide a copy of results intended to be given to the patients. Some patients opt to share this directly with their primary healthcare provider rather than having the genetic healthcare provider release the results.

One of the biggest threats to confidentiality is unintentional disclosures from the medical record, such as one healthcare provider dictating a note that the reason for a prophylactic procedure or screening modality was a positive genetic test. That healthcare provider inadvertently and unintentionally released confidential information without authorization from the patient to whoever reads the note (Twomey, 2011). This also occurs when an entire medical record is copied, including the genetic testing records, even if they were not ordered by the healthcare provider.

Patients and families need assurance that their records will be maintained in a confidential way. Some practices keep genetic records separate from the regular medical record. Practices vary in how records are stored and copied. If the information is not in the regular medical record, it may be difficult for the healthcare provider to provide proper care and recommendations. Conversely, putting genetic information in the regular medical record increases the risk that it could be disclosed to third parties without proper authorization (Plutynski, 2012). Genetic records also contain information about other family members, such as pathology reports, medical notes, or death certificates, and these are never to be released to third parties. Any third party desiring this information needs to go to the source to obtain this information.

Outcomes of Testing

Three outcomes of testing are possible: negative results, positive results, or results of a variant of indeterminate significance (see Figure 2-12). Following disclosure, most patients want

---

Positive Result
- A mutation is detected; individual is at increased risk for developing cancer(s).
- Other relatives can undergo single-site testing to clarify their risk.
- Results do not inform about what cancer will develop or when, only that the risk is higher.
- Results assist in making informed decisions about cancer prevention and early detection strategies.
- Risks include psychological distress, fears of being isolated, and concerns regarding transmission to offspring.

True-Negative Result
- No mutation was detected in a person with a known mutation in the family.
- Individual will not need screening greater than that recommended for the general population.
- Patient will not need to consider prophylactic surgery or chemoprevention.
- Patient has a more accurate cancer risk assessment.
- The individual experiences psychological relief regarding risk for developing cancer.
- The individual experiences psychological relief that offspring will not inherit mutation.
- Risks include a false sense of security for the patient that he or she will not develop cancer.
- The individual may feel guilty that he or she "escaped" the mutation (i.e., "survivor guilt").

Negative Result—No Mutation Identified in Family
- No mutation is detected in an individual from a family with no known mutation.
- This result usually occurs when the first individual in a family is tested. It may occur because the person did not inherit a mutation, the cancer is due to a different mutation than the one tested, or the cancer seen in the family is due to nonhereditary reasons.
- Results are difficult to interpret and must be considered in conjunction with personal risk factors and family history.
- Testing is not available to other unaffected members in the family.
- Disappointment that results are inconclusive can occur.
- Uncertainty exists about the usefulness of cancer risk reduction strategies.
- Patient can consider participating in research studies or high-risk registries.

Variant of Indeterminate Significance
- Test identifies a mutation; it is not clear if it is a polymorphism or deleterious.
- Results do not provide meaningful information.
- This result may be anxiety provoking.
- Meaningful testing will not be available to other family members.
- Uncertainty exists about the usefulness of cancer risk reduction strategies.
- Recommendations for cancer prevention and detection need to be formulated based on personal risk factors and family history with careful information about potential benefits and risks.
- Patient can consider participating in a research study or hereditary cancer registry.

Figure 2-12. Implications of Genetic Testing Results

Note. Based on information from Lachance et al., 2010; Riley et al., 2012; Robson et al., 2010; U.S. Preventive Services Task Force, 2005; Weitzel et al., 2011.

to know the implications of the results. Recommendations for follow-up, prevention, and early detection are based on the results of testing and, in many cases, the personal and family history. For individuals who test positive for a mutation, aggressive screening and prevention measures are indicated. For those who test negative for a known mutation in a family, recommendations for screening and prevention that would be appropriate for the general population are given. For those who test negative and there is not a known mutation in the family, recommendations for prevention are provided following a balanced discussion of the potential risks and benefits of such recommendations. These families also may benefit from enrollment in a hereditary cancer research registry with the hope of identifying a mutation in the family through research. For those who have a variant of indeterminate significance, results can bring confusion and disappointment because risk has not been clarified (Culver et al., 2013). Often the laboratory will want to test other family members; if this is an option, testing can be offered to families. Some of these families may be able to enroll in a research registry but may not receive useful information in a timely fashion. These families also will need recommendations for prevention and early detection based on a discussion of the potential risks and benefits of these recommendations.

Psychosocial Concerns

A primary objective of genetic counseling and education is to help each individual and family in weighing the options, risks, and benefits of testing in their unique life situation. Identifying potential psychosocial concerns is a substantial component of the counseling process. Testing is not in itself good or bad, or right or wrong. However, for some people, testing is appropriate and will have positive outcomes, whereas for others, the risk is significant that the information will result in considerable psychosocial distress (Vadaparampil, Miree, Wilson, & Jacobsen, 2006–2007).

Patients may experience anxiety and fear while waiting for their test results (Rew, Kaur, McMillan, Mackert, & Bonevac, 2010). Increased support may be needed during this time period. Patients also have reported finding it helpful to have written brochures, a letter summarizing recommendations, and guidance about how to share risk information and testing outcomes with other relatives and healthcare professionals (Kardashian, Fehniger, Creasman, Cheung, & Beattie, 2012).

Perceptions of genetic risk are influenced by prior experiences with cancer. People who have experienced loss related to cancer often find it particularly difficult to learn about the risks and benefits of genetic testing (Lapointe et al., 2012). APNs need to explore not only the motivations for testing or not testing but also how the individual has coped with past cancer experiences. Individuals who have lost a relative and then test positive often have difficulty coping, as they fear the same outcome and that their children will lose a parent early. For those who test negative after having lost a parent, it often is difficult to accept a negative result because they assume they will have the same outcome. For these patients, it can take time to reframe their personal identity.

Some patients who receive positive results feel empowered and relieved because they can make appropriate decisions about prevention strategies with confidence and feel as though they can exercise some control. Other patients who felt they were prepared for positive results can be overwhelmed by the outcome and require much counseling and support. Many people who test positive are not concerned as much for their own health conditions and fears but rather experience feelings of guilt if a child inherits the gene (Bjorvatn, Eide, Hanestad, Hamang, & Havik, 2009; Wevers et al., 2011).

Those who have a true-negative result often feel a huge sense of relief. This is especially true for parents who carry a mutation and learn that a child does not. A true-negative result, however, can sometimes be accompanied by a phenomenon referred to as *survivor guilt*. This occurs when the person who tests negative feels guilty and questions why he or she was fortunate enough to test negative when another sibling or relative tests positive (Hoskins et al., 2012; Tercyak, O'Neill, Roter, & McBride, 2012).

Individuals with a variant of indeterminate significance or an inconclusive negative result may experience a wide range of feelings. Many are frustrated because they feel they must make decisions about prevention and early detection without clear information. Others with an inconclusive result feel relief because they believe the malignancy may not be related to a hereditary cause.

Overall, research suggests that patients may be slightly distressed immediately following risk communication and genetic testing (den Heijer et al., 2012). Many patients will experience generalized anxiety during the counseling, testing, and short-term follow-up periods even with counseling (Wevers et al., 2011). These patients may need more intense psychosocial support during the testing process and in the short term during the follow-up period. Long-term follow-up and support usually are associated with improved knowledge of cancer risks and improved knowledge about testing, which, in most cases, ultimately leads to improved satisfaction with testing decisions and adjustment to the diagnosis of a genetic predisposition to malignancy (Metcalfe et al., 2012; Tilburt et al., 2011). These researchers also noted that providing anticipatory guidance prior to the visit is associated with lower feelings of anxiety and an increased sense of control. For patients undergoing prophylactic surgical procedures, the need for psychosocial support may persist longer. Additional support may be required if other family members are diagnosed with malignancy. For this reason, many genetic counselors and educators will encourage people to contact them again if questions or concerns arise (Mahon, 2013d). Families with children may contact the counselor for additional care as teenagers become old enough to consider their own risks and options for testing. Because of these long-term needs, families may be followed intermittently for years with some periods of more intense service.

Many genetic professionals generally disclose testing results in person because it provides a structured plan for providing education on recommended screening modalities and any other education and support as needed (Pal et al., 2014). Results disclosure probably takes more time when it is done in person; phone disclosure may take as little as 15 minutes (Rice, Ruschman, Martin, Manders, & Miller, 2010). Providing patients with a choice on how to receive results can be associated with positive outcomes (Baumanis et al., 2009). A concern with phone disclosure is that patients may have more difficulty understanding the meaning of the results regardless of whether they are negative or positive, although some genetics professionals believe that disclosing negative results over the phone is satisfactory (Bradbury et al., 2011).

Direct-to-Consumer Genetic Testing

Direct-to-consumer (DTC) genetic testing offers individuals the ability to acquire certain genetic information about themselves without the opportunity to discuss it with a credentialed genetic healthcare professional. In most cases, the individual selects and purchases the desired testing from an Internet-based company, obtains a collection kit, submits a sample (usually saliva), and obtains the results via a secure website. Several professional organizations have issued position statements that warn about the risks of DTC genetic testing. These include NSGC (2011), American Society of Human Genetics (2007), American College of Obstetricians and Gynecologists (2008), American College of Medical Genetics and Genomics (2004), European Society of Human Genetics (2010), and ASCO (Robson et al., 2010). Potential harms that may result if genetic professionals are not involved include misused tests, misinterpreted results, and misguided follow-up, as well as individuals being unprepared for the test results, being uninformed of the recommended screening or follow-up based on the results, or experiencing psychosocial distress when genetic testing occurs without informed pre- and post-test genetic counseling (Mahon, 2012b). APNs may be confronted with questions about DTC genetic testing and must be prepared to discuss its strengths and limitations.

Prevention and Screening Strategies for Those With Hereditary Risk

Hereditary Breast and Ovarian Cancer

Because the risks for both breast and ovarian cancer are significant, recommendations for prevention and screening made by the U.S. Preventive Services Task Force (Nelson, Huffman, Fu, & Harris, 2005), ASCO (Robson et al., 2010), and NCCN (2014c) are summarized in Table 2-5.

Screening recommendations for those at risk for HBOC are initiated at a much earlier age than in the general population because of the early age of cancer onset seen in this population (Lowry et al., 2012). Women from these families need education about the signs and symptoms of breast cancer (presence of a lump, thickening, change in breast skin or color, change in nipple direction, or nipple discharge) and ovarian cancer (vague abdominal pain or gastrointestinal symptoms, weight loss, or bloating). Training in breast self-examination (BSE) (often now referred to as breast self-awareness) may offer women some sense of control and ideally begins at age 18. Mammography typically is initiated at age 25. Women need to be clearly

---

Table 2-5. Recommendations for Prevention and Early Detection in Women With a Known *BRCA1/2* Mutation

Organ	Surveillance	Prevention
Breast	Instruct patient to perform monthly breast self-exam beginning at age 18. Perform clinical breast exam every 6 months beginning at age 20. Perform annual mammography and magnetic resonance imaging beginning at age 25.[a]	Consider prophylactic mastectomy (risk reduction of up to 95%). Consider chemoprevention. Consider prophylactic oophorectomy (risk reduction of up to 50%).
Ovary	Perform pelvic exam every 6 months beginning at age 25. Screen with transvaginal ultrasound[b] with color Doppler beginning at age 25 every 6–12 months.[a] Perform serum CA 125 testing every 6–12 months starting at age 25.	Consider prophylactic oophorectomy between ages 35–40 (risk reduction of up to 85%–96%).

[a] Age to begin screening can vary based on the youngest age at which breast or ovarian cancer was diagnosed in the family.

[b] Testing in premenopausal women should occur during days 1–10 of the menstrual cycle.

Note. Based on information from National Comprehensive Cancer Network, 2014c; Petrucelli et al., 2013; Shannon & Chittenden, 2012; U.S. Preventive Services Task Force, 2005.

instructed on the limitations of mammography in younger age groups because of the density of breast tissue. NCCN (2014c) and ACS (2015) recommend breast MRI in women with a known mutation associated with HBOC or who are found to have a lifetime risk of developing breast cancer of at least 20%.

Surveillance for ovarian cancer has been shown to be of limited benefit and is not associated with decrease in morbidity or mortality associated with ovarian cancer (Finch et al., 2013). Current screening recommendations include annual or semiannual concurrent transvaginal ultrasonography and CA 125 level beginning at age 25–35 or 5–10 years earlier than the youngest age at which ovarian cancer was first diagnosed in the family (NCCN, 2014c). The patient needs to clearly understand that these screening procedures are limited in their ability to detect ovarian cancer at a curable stage, and a prophylactic bilateral salpingo-oophorectomy (BSO) should be seriously considered (Gadducci, Biglia, Cosio, Sismondi, & Genazzani, 2010).

Chemoprevention is a potential strategy for women at risk for HBOC. Recent epidemiologic evidence suggests it may be an appropriate option for all women at risk for HBOC (Brauch & Jordan, 2009; Davies et al., 2013). Typically, the oral agent tamoxifen is initiated 5–10 years before the youngest age at onset of breast cancer in the family and is continued for five years (NCCN, 2014a, 2014c). Women who take tamoxifen, especially premenopausal women, need careful counseling about pregnancy prevention, and all women need to be aware of potential side effects, including risk of embolism (Bevers et al., 2010). In postmenopausal women, raloxifene also may be considered (NCCN, 2014c).

The use of oral contraceptive pills (OCPs) appears to reduce the risk of ovarian cancer by up to 50%, but data are very inconsistent regarding the use of OCPs and breast cancer risk in mutation-positive women (NCCN, 2014c). Given the controversy over breast cancer risk and the fact that oophorectomy often is recommended between ages 35–40, many clinicians are reluctant to use OCPs in this population. Woman who desire to use OCPs need a balanced discussion of the pros and cons of OCPs ("Oral Contraceptives and Ovarian Cancer Risk," 2008). An oophorectomy is associated with an earlier menopause, and some women experience significant hot flashes and other menopausal side effects such as vaginal dryness (Kaplan et al., 2011; Sturdee & Panay, 2010). These issues need to be addressed during counseling sessions. Several smaller studies suggest that women who undergo a prophylactic oophorectomy have less ovarian cancer worry without associated deterioration in physical and mental health-related quality of life (Finch, Evans, & Narod, 2012; Finch et al., 2013; Howard, Balneaves, Bottorff, & Rodney, 2011).

Mammography, even when combined with ultrasound, still may be ineffective in detecting breast cancer early in women with HBOC, especially those younger than age 35 or those with extremely dense breasts. Recent studies suggest that breast MRI results in higher sensitivity, especially when combined with mammography in high-risk women (Berg et al., 2012; Morrow, Waters, & Morris, 2011). MRI sensitivity can be as high as 70% in women with HBOC (Saslow et al., 2007). However, screening MRIs are limited if there is not a dedicated breast coil, the ability to perform a biopsy under MRI guidance, and an experienced radiologist to read the test (NCCN, 2014a, 2014c). When MRI, mammography, and breast ultrasound are used together with clinical breast examination (CBE), sensitivity rises to 95% (Berg et al., 2012). NCCN guidelines recommend that a screening breast MRI and mammography be performed annually on women with a mutated BRCA gene (NCCN, 2014c). Breast MRI can be offered to patients along with a balanced discussion of potential risks, including an increased number of false-positive readings necessitating biopsy, and benefits, including earlier detection of malignancy (NCCN, 2014c). It also may be recommended for individuals considered to be at risk for HBOC even in the absence of a confirmed mutation because of its increased sensitivity (NCCN, 2014c; Saslow et al., 2007).

Prophylactic mastectomy can result in a 90%–95% reduction in breast cancer (Petrucelli et al., 2013). This is an option for many women, especially those who have already been diagnosed with cancer, have undergone multiple breast biopsies, have abnormalities on CBE or mammography, or have breasts that are difficult to examine clinically or on mammography. Prophylactic mastectomy may lead to significant overall survival in mutation carriers diagnosed with cancer and is associated with an approximate 90%–97% reduction in the risk of developing breast cancer (Bevers et al., 2010; Euhus, 2012; Evans et al., 2013; Zagouri et al., 2013). However, it is an irreversible procedure that can be emotionally difficult for many women (Gopie et al., 2013). In most cases, a prophylactic mastectomy includes total mastectomy without axillary node dissection. Skin-sparing and nipple-sparing procedures sometimes are offered with informed consent, emphasizing that when more breast tissue is left, the effectiveness of the procedure decreases (Tokin, Weiss, Wang-Rodriguez, & Blair, 2012). Women who undergo a prophylactic mastectomy can opt for immediate reconstruction with a flap or implant or can choose to use prostheses. Detailed information about breast prostheses is available (see Mahon & Casey, 2003). This is a difficult decision for a woman and requires much support and education. Some women find the online resources from Facing Our Risk of Cancer Empowered (www.facingourrisk.org) especially helpful. The message boards and chat room on this site, in addition to the organization's telephone helpline, allow patients to communicate with women who have made this choice and who can serve as a source of peer support.

Prophylactic BSO may be a prudent choice because of the limited effectiveness of ovarian cancer screening (Finch et al., 2013). It also has been proved to be a cost-effective measure in this population (Gadducci et al., 2010). A BSO is associated with as much as a 90% reduction in ovarian cancer risk and a 50% reduction in breast cancer risk (Finch et al., 2012). The ideal time frame seems to be between ages 35 and 40 if childbearing is complete. Approximately 2%–18% of mutation-positive women in this age group will have occult ovarian cancers at the time of prophylactic surgery depending on the age at which the surgery is performed and the rigor of the pathologic review (Finch et al., 2012). Careful peritoneal washing and specific pathologic sectioning and review have been recommended; for this reason, this surgery may best be carried out by a gynecologic oncologist with expertise in these areas (Finch et al., 2012; NCCN, 2014c). This primary prevention strategy is considered after a careful discussion of the potential benefits of reduced breast and ovarian cancer risk with the consequences of early menopause associated with increased vasomotor symptoms and potential bone loss (Matloff, Barnett, & Bober, 2009). Preliminary data suggest it might be safe to offer short-term hormone replacement therapy following BSO to decrease vasomotor symptoms without negating the protective effect of the surgery (Howard, Balneaves, & Bottorff, 2009). Women at substantial risk for cervical and uterine problems and malignancies may want to consider a total abdominal hysterectomy (Gadducci et al., 2010).

Men who test positive for a *BRCA* mutation are recommended to undergo CBE every six months and perform BSE monthly, and mammography can be considered (NCCN, 2014c). Mammography sometimes is offered to men with gynecomastia. Prostate screening, including a digital rectal examination and prostate-specific antigen testing, is initiated at age 40 (NCCN, 2014c; Weitzel, Blazer, MacDonald, Culver, & Offit, 2011).

Hereditary Nonpolyposis Colorectal Cancer

Individuals who test positive for a Lynch syndrome mutation need a careful plan for screening and prevention of colorectal and gynecologic cancers. Current recommendations are summarized in Table 2-6.

HNPCC is associated with an accelerated carcinogenesis in which polyps can develop into carcinomas in 2–3 years instead of the typical 8–10 years seen in the general population (Kohl-

Table 2-6. Recommendations for Prevention and Early Detection in People With a Known *MLH1* or *MSH2* Mutation

Organ	Screening	Prevention
Colon	Perform colonoscopy with prompt removal of polyps annually starting between ages 20–25.[a] Consider gastroscopy and upper endoscopy.	Consider chemoprevention. Consider colectomy in patients who cannot or will not undergo regular colonoscopy.
Uterus/ovaries	Perform biannual pelvic exam beginning at age 25.[a] Screen with transvaginal ultrasound with color Doppler beginning at age 30–35[a] every 6–12 months.[b] Perform serum CA 125 testing every 6–12 months.	Consider chemoprevention with oral contraceptives. Consider prophylactic hysterectomy including bilateral salpingo-oophorectomy between ages 35–40 or when childbearing is complete.
Urogenital	Consider annual urinalysis with cytology and renal imaging.	–

[a] Age to begin screening may vary according to youngest age at which cancer was diagnosed in the family.

[b] Testing in premenopausal women should occur sometime during days 1–10 of the menstrual cycle.

Note. Based on information from Bernstein & Myrhøj, 2013; Kohlmann & Gruber, 2012; National Comprehensive Cancer Network, 2014b; Shia et al., 2013; Vasen et al., 2013.

mann & Gruber, 2012). Because of this potentially rapid development of malignancy, annual colonoscopy is recommended after age 20–25 (Kohlmann & Gruber, 2012; NCCN, 2014b). Research clearly shows that regular colonoscopy decreases the overall mortality rate by about 65% (Lastra et al., 2012; Patel & Ahnen, 2012; de Vos tot Nederveen Cappel et al., 2013).

Because HNPCC also is associated with increased risks to the endometrium and ovaries, women with this mutation require careful surveillance. This usually includes annual or semi-annual transvaginal ultrasound of the endometrium and ovaries with concurrent endometrial aspiration for pathologic evaluation and CA 125 testing (Weitzel et al., 2011). Women need to be informed about the low sensitivity and specificity of ultrasound and CA 125 testing for ovarian cancer (Senter, 2012). Ultrasound also has limited utility in evaluating endometrial thickness in premenopausal women because of cyclic changes (Lu & Daniels, 2013). Because of this, NCCN recommends that transvaginal ultrasound be performed within the first 10 days of the woman's menstrual cycle (NCCN, 2014b). Although individuals with HNPCC may be at risk for other cancers, no other standard screening recommendations exist at this time (Kohlmann & Gruber, 2012). Some families with an increased number of urinary tract malignancies might consider adding ultrasound and urine cytology, but more clinical trials are needed to determine the optimal interval, age to start, and modalities (Bernstein & Myrhøj, 2013; NCCN, 2014b). Similarly, many clinicians also will recommend upper endoscopy and gastroscopy (Kohlmann & Gruber, 2012).

Chemoprevention is another strategy sometimes considered in these families. The exact efficacy of daily aspirin in decreasing incidence of gastrointestinal cancers is not known (Barton, 2012). These measures are based largely on information gained from people with FAP. Because taking OCPs has been associated with decreased risk of developing ovarian and endometrial cancers, some women choose to consider this strategy (Lindor et al., 2008). People who are considering chemoprevention strategies for colon or gynecologic cancers need a carefully balanced discussion of the potential benefits and risks associated with the proposed agent. These individuals also may want to consider enrolling in a research study. Similarly, minimal data are available regarding the impact of a healthy diet and exercise in reducing risk of cancer development in people with an HNPCC-related mutation (Lindor et al., 2008). Such behaviors, however, may contribute to overall health and well-being and are recommended.

Prophylactic colectomy in HNPCC is controversial. It is not associated with a large increase in life expectancy over annual colonoscopy (Rodriguez-Bigas & Möeslein, 2013). It generally is reserved for individuals in whom colonoscopy is not technically possible or in individuals who refuse to undergo regular screening (Kohlmann & Gruber, 2012).

As the risks for endometrial and ovarian cancer are substantial and screening may be ineffective, many women will consider a total abdominal hysterectomy with BSO at age 35 or older if childbearing is complete (Lu & Daniels, 2013). These women need to be aware of the risks of premature menopause and that this surgery typically requires four to eight weeks of recuperation.

Familial Adenomatous Polyposis Syndromes

Medical and surgical management of FAP syndromes is complex because the risk of developing colorectal cancer is virtually 100% and the onset can occur before age 20. In general, it is recommended that people with FAP begin screening with colonoscopy and often upper endoscopy at puberty and undergo colectomy when symptomatic or when the number of adenomas is considered worrisome or not manageable with polypectomy (Jasperson, 2012; U.S. Preventive Services Task Force, 2008). Some patients will consider a total proctocolectomy with an ileal pouch anal anastomosis because the risks of developing rectal cancer after this surgery are small and a permanent stoma is not necessary. This procedure is very complex, requires a temporary stoma, and carries a small risk for bladder and sexual dysfunction (Rodriguez-Bigas & Möeslein, 2013). Other patients will choose a total abdominal colectomy with an ileorectal anastomosis, but this requires regular endoscopy of the rectum following surgery because of the higher risk of rectal cancer. If many rectal polyps are present prior to surgery, this is not the recommended choice. This surgery carries little to no risk for bowel or bladder dysfunction. A total proctocolectomy with ileostomy is another choice of surgery. However, this choice leaves the patient with a permanent stoma, unlike the first two options. It removes all risk of colorectal cancer, but bladder or sexual dysfunction is a possible result (Rodriguez-Bigas & Möeslein, 2013). Patients and families need much education and support when making decisions about colectomy.

Nonsteroidal anti-inflammatory drugs (NSAIDs), including the cyclooxygenase-2 (COX-2) inhibitor celecoxib, which has a U.S. Food and Drug Administration indication, and aspirin are sometimes used to prevent or delay polyp formation (Dupont, Arguedas, & Wilcox, 2007; Kohlmann & Gruber, 2012). Because COX-2 inhibitors are associated with an increased risk of cardiovascular problems, careful assessment of comorbid conditions is needed. NSAIDs may be particularly useful in patients with an ileorectal anastomosis and an increased risk for rectal cancer (Kohlmann & Gruber, 2012).

Hereditary Melanoma

Early detection and prevention measures are critical in families at risk for hereditary melanoma. Currently, no clear consensus exists on the utility of genetic testing in this population because it does not dramatically influence surveillance and prevention measures (Gabree & Seidel, 2012). Early detection of melanoma is particularly important, as the five-year survival rate is 98% when the disease is detected in stage I (ACS, 2015). Prevention and early detection measures for skin cancer are listed in Figure 2-13, which are similar to those recommended for the general population. Individuals from families at risk for hereditary melanoma need to be followed by a dermatologist with expertise in melanoma and biopsy technique. Follow-up must occur on a regular basis (typically every three to six months). It also may be prudent to recommend to those who test positive to consider entering a pancreatic cancer screening trial because of the 17% lifetime risk of developing this disease (Axilbund & Wiley, 2012; Gabree & Seidel, 2012).

Hereditary Pancreatic Cancer

Pancreatic screening is not typically offered to the general population, but screening has been used in high-risk patients from families with two or more cases of pancreatic cancer and in patients with inherited cancer syndromes such as *BRCA2* with family history of pancreatic cancer, *PALB2*, and *CDKN2A* mutations (Jones et al., 2009). Pancreatic cancer surveillance modalities include serum biomarkers (such as CA 19-9 and carcinoembryonic antigen), external imaging (including MRI and computed tomography scan), and internal imaging (such as endoscopic ultrasound, endoscopic retrograde cholangiopancreatography, and magnetic resonance cholangiopancreatography, with or without fine needle aspiration) (Shin & Canto, 2012).

At this time, no standardized guidelines exist for managing patients at high risk for developing pancreatic cancer, including the age at which screening should be initiated, the modalities used, and how often screening should be conducted (Templeton & Brentnall, 2013). Further studies are needed to determine the risk threshold at which various screening protocols are cost-effective and beneficial to patients (Jones et al., 2009). Some experts recommend that individuals at high risk for developing pancreatic cancer initiate screening at age 35–45 or 10–15 years before the earliest diagnosis of pancreatic cancer in the family. This may be adjusted based on the presence of other risk factors, such as smoking, alcohol intake, diabetes, and pancreatitis (Larghi, Verna, Lecca, & Costamagna, 2009). Patients should also be counseled regarding how these lifestyle factors may increase their risk of pancreatic cancer.

Data suggest that in high-risk individuals (those with at least 16% lifetime risk for developing pancreatic cancer), endoscopic ultrasound and MRI/magnetic resonance cholangiopancreatography can detect asymptomatic precursor benign and early invasive malignant pancre-

---

Early Detection
- Perform regular monthly full-body skin self-examination using full-length and handheld mirrors.
- Obtain a clinical skin examination every six months beginning at age 10. The frequency of this examination may need to be increased during pregnancy and puberty.
- Take full-body photographs every six months to monitor moles for changes.
- Obtain a prompt biopsy and removal of any suspicious lesions.

Prevention
- Limit ultraviolet light exposure, especially between the hours of 10 am and 3 pm.
- Wear protective clothing when outside. This includes long-sleeved shirts with a dense weave, sunglasses that provide ultraviolet A and B protection, and wide-brimmed hats.
- Use a broad-spectrum sunscreen with ultraviolet A and B protection with a sun protection factor of at least 30 daily and consistently.

Figure 2-13. Recommendations for Prevention and Early Detection in People With a Hereditary Predisposition for Developing Melanoma

Note. Based on information from American Cancer Society, 2015; Gabree & Seidel, 2012.

atic neoplasms that are more likely to be resectable compared to symptomatic tumors (Shin & Canto, 2012; Templeton & Brentnall, 2013).

Implications for Oncology Advanced Practice Nurses

Several considerations exist for APNs with expertise in genetics. Specialty credentialing is available through the American Nurses Credentialing Center. The credentialing process involves submission of a professional portfolio that demonstrates advanced nursing education in genetics, as well as evidence of clinical expertise and knowledge. Many nurses choose to obtain this credential to enhance their credibility and professional practice. To maintain the credential, APNs must pursue continuing education in genetics and develop professional skills in research, publication, and professional and lay presentations. Detailed information about the credentialing process is available at the American Nurses Credentialing Center website at www.nursecredentialing.org/Certification/NurseSpecialties/AdvancedGenetics and in Monsen (2005). In addition to ISONG, other opportunities exist for networking with oncology nurses who are interested in cancer genetics, such as the Cancer Genetics Special Interest Group (SIG) of ONS and the Cancer Genetics SIG of NSGC.

ISONG and the American Nurses Association have defined roles for basic and advanced practice nurses. They also have published standards for genetics and genomics nursing (ISONG & American Nurses Association, 2007). This document includes information about roles in risk and physical assessment, diagnostic testing, outcomes identification, and planning, implementation, and evaluation of genetics care. These standards address issues related to quality practice indicators, professional and continuing education, collegiality, collaboration, ethics, research, resource utilization, and leadership. APNs who practice in cancer genetics will find these standards to be a valuable resource when developing and improving cancer genetics programs. Additional helpful resources for patients and healthcare providers are listed at the end of this chapter.

All oncology APNs, regardless of practice setting, have a responsibility to refer to genetic healthcare providers and understand the influence of genetics in health care. The practice of oncology is greatly influenced by genetics in not only the evaluation and referral of families with a hereditary predisposition, but also in pharmacogenetics and evaluation of tumor characteristics. A growing need and role for oncology APNs exists in the area of cancer genetics research. Some of these potential areas include conducting research, disseminating research findings to colleagues, and keeping current with genetics research. Because the field is ever growing, some APNs find it helpful to subscribe to an email distribution list of genetic clinicians available through ISONG or NSGC. These email lists link colleagues who practice in geographically diverse areas, thereby allowing collaboration on studies and sharing of ideas.

One area in which oncology APNs often participate is referral of families to clinical trials at universities and laboratories that are studying families who test negative in standard or commercially available testing. Many families desire to participate in such research not only to contribute to science but also in hopes of gaining information about their personal and family risks, especially risk to children and siblings. APNs identify such studies for families, assist with the coordination of care, and provide follow-up as needed.

In many cases, oncology APNs will assist in the management of people with hereditary risk after they have undergone genetic testing or consultation with a genetic healthcare professional. Often APNs are responsible for ensuring that recommendations for screening are carried out. They also may assist with the care, education, and support of people who are considering prevention measures, especially prophylactic surgery.

When an appropriate comprehensive prevention/risk-reduction plan is incorporated into the care of a person with a hereditary high risk for cancer, morbidity and mortality associated with cancer can potentially be decreased. Unfortunately, current criteria and risk models do not always correctly categorize those who might be at risk for having a deleterious germ-line mutation (Kwon et al., 2010). In addition, family history information changes and evolves over time. A patient may initially present with a history that does not meet the criteria for genetic testing, but if the personal or family history changes (maternal or paternal), the patient may become eligible for genetic testing or be considered for testing of mutations on other less common genes. Updates in genetic testing technology also necessitate the need to reevaluate whether a patient or family might benefit from additional genetic testing.

Families with suspected or known hereditary susceptibility to developing malignancy have many psychosocial needs. These are ongoing and often change over time. Regular assessment to determine how families are managing their risk and the associated uncertainty, body image changes, and pregnancy concerns is important to address concerns promptly and appropriately and to help these families to have the best possible outcome (Bleiker, Esplen, Meiser, Petersen, & Patenaude, 2013). Oncology nurses have a major role in identifying reputable resources, including written materials, support groups, and Internet sites.

Lifestyle factors may indeed affect cancer risk in people with hereditary risk. The full impact is not fully understood. More prospective studies with confirmed gene mutation carriers should be performed to better clarify the role of all lifestyle factors in at-risk families, with the goal of establishing lifestyle and dietary recommendations to decrease or delay the development of malignancy (van Duijnhoven et al., 2013). ACS has recommendations for nutrition and physical activity that may be appropriate to share with these families, who are often motivated to engage in such behaviors (Kushi et al., 2012).

Conclusion

APNs' roles in cancer genetics include direct care of patients and families, including risk assessment and interpretation, education regarding testing and treatment options, and provision of psychosocial support. Often, APNs coordinate complex care with other disciplines and subspecialties, as well as serve as consultants. APNs have roles as staff educators, researchers, and administrators of programs that specialize in the care of individuals with a hereditary predisposition for developing cancer. With continuing advances in cancer genetics, this is an ever-growing and challenging area for APNs that requires not only an in-depth understanding of the science of genetics but also patient education skills and psychosocial skills to help patients manage their risk of hereditary cancer.

Case Study

M.B. presented for education and information about hereditary risk for cancer at the request of her primary care physician. She is a 32-year-old Caucasian woman with concerns about her personal risk of cancer. She reports she is certain that she has the "breast cancer gene." She presents with several pathology reports and death certificates from affected family members as requested by the APN prior to the appointment. M.B. is recently married and desires to have children. She is concerned not only about her personal risks but also about potential risks to her offspring. Additionally, M.B. reports that she had a child at age 24, which she gave up for adoption.

M.B. has three sisters. Two are affected with premenopausal breast cancer; one of these sisters has bilateral breast cancer. The APN constructed a pedigree (see Figure 2-14). Maternal ethnicity is Irish/English. M.B.'s mother is alive and reported to be healthy. Her only maternal uncle died in a motor vehicle accident. Her maternal grandparents did not have a malignancy. Paternal ethnicity is German/Ashkenazi Jewish. M.B.'s paternal family history is significant for ovarian cancer (paternal aunt), breast cancer (paternal grandmother), prostate cancer (father), and pancreatic cancer (paternal grandfather) (see Figure 2-14).

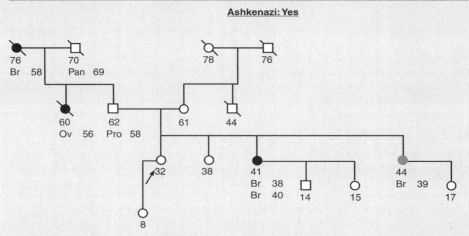

This pedigree shows M.B. as the proband (designated by the arrow).

Figure 2-14. Case Study Pedigree

M.B.'s past medical history reports menarche at age 12. She is gravida 1, para 1 (first complete pregnancy at age 24). She reports no hormonal therapy use but reports a past history of more than five years of OCP use from age 24 to about age 30. Her last Pap test/pelvic examination was within the past three months and negative. She has never had a mammogram. Her last breast examination was negative and was done at the time of the gynecologic examination. She denies having problems with depression or coping with difficult information. M.B. has had two breast biopsies for palpable masses, one at age 26 and one at age 30. The first biopsy was a fibroadenoma; the second one showed ductal hyperplasia with moderate atypia. Both biopsies were confirmed with pathology reports.

M.B. works as an elementary school teacher. She denies use of tobacco or recreational drugs and states she occasionally drinks socially but has less than one or two drinks per month. She walks approximately five miles per day and consumes three to five servings of fruits and vegetables daily. Her height is 5 foot 6 inches and weight is 136 pounds. She has disclosed to her husband that she had given up a child for adoption.

M.B. reports being concerned about her personal health as well as risks to potential offspring. She would like to consider prevention strategies and would like recommendations for screening. Her gynecologist recommended that she consider genetic testing, and M.B. believes she will test positive because of her sisters' histories. She has not discussed her desire for testing with her husband despite that a positive test could potentially have a significant impact on their relationship and marriage. She has discussed it with her affected sisters, who report they have not had testing or counseling for testing.

1. What in M.B.'s history is suggestive of HBOC syndrome?
    • M.B.'s paternal family history is significant for ovarian cancer in a paternal aunt, breast cancer in her paternal grandmother, prostate cancer in her father, and pancreatic cancer in her paternal grandfather. She has two first-degree relatives (sisters)

with premenopausal breast cancer, one of which was bilateral. Her father's family is also of Ashkenazi Jewish descent.

2. Which of the risk calculation models would be most appropriate for M.B. (see Table 2-7)?

  • The Gail model would underestimate her risk and would not take into account second-degree relatives, ovarian cancer in her family, or age of her relatives at diagnosis. The Claus model considers women with multiple family members diagnosed with breast cancer, as well as maternal and paternal history of breast cancer. It also considers age at diagnosis, which is important considering her sisters were premenopausal at diagnosis. Neither the Claus nor the Gail model considers the history of ovarian cancer. The Tyrer-Cuzick model considers both maternal and paternal family histories as well as the breast and ovarian cancer histories, which might make it the most appropriate model to use with this particular family. Other models (see Figure 2-9) will provide more information, and each model has disadvantages and advantages. BRCAPRO is a tool that constructs a pedigree and calculates risk using several statistical models that predict breast and colon cancer risk, as well as risk of carrying other hereditary predisposition mutations (see Table 2-7).

  • M.B.'s risk of having a mutation in *BRCA1/2* also was calculated. A range of risk figures was provided (see Table 2-8), but almost all are greater than a 10% risk (and most were much higher), suggesting it is appropriate to offer testing. The patient received copies of the pedigree and all risk calculations.

Table 2-7. Gail, Claus, and Tyrer-Cuzick Model Calculations for Case Study (% Risk)

M.B.'s Age	Claus Model	Gail Model	Tyrer-Cuzick Model	Population	No Risk Factors
37	5.6	2.27	Not calculated	0.3	0.2
42	11.2	5.84	13.8	0.6	0.3
52	35.2	15.68	Not calculated	2.3	1.3
62	52	27.42	Not calculated	5.1	7.6
Lifetime	77.8	41.89	54.5	13.2	12.8

Table 2-8. *BRCA* Mutation Probability Models for Case Study (Based on Ashkenazi Background, 15 Family Members)

Mutation	Proband Probability
BRCA1	
• Couch	28.6%
• Shattuck-Eidens	39.6%
• BRCAPRO	49.9%
• Tyrer-Cuzick	30.07%
BRCA2	
• BRCAPRO	1.7%
• Tyrer-Cuzick	17.58%
BRCA1 or *BRCA2*	
• Manchester	5.27%
• Frank	28.7%
• BRCAPRO	50.8%

3. Who would be the most appropriate person to test first in this case study?
   - Ideally, the person to test would be the youngest person in the family with cancer that is suspected to be part of a cancer syndrome. In this case, it would be M.B.'s youngest sister with breast cancer. If she tested negative, then most likely this family would not have this hereditary syndrome but could still be at risk for other less common hereditary cancer syndromes. If she tests positive, and M.B. then tests negative, that would be considered a true negative, and M.B.'s risk would then be considered to be that of the general population.
   - M.B.'s sister with bilateral breast cancer decided to test following genetic counseling and discussion of the benefits and limitations of testing. She tested positive for a mutation in *BRCA1*. Her other affected sister also tested positive. Both underwent oophorectomy. Her sister with unilateral breast cancer completed a prophylactic mastectomy on the unaffected side. They both began formulating a plan on how to educate their daughters about risks. M.B. underwent testing and also tested positive.
4. Because M.B. tested positive, what screening recommendations could the APN give?
   - In women with an inherited mutation of *BRCA1* or *BRCA2*, screening recommendations include
     - Monthly BSE
     - CBE every six months
     - Annual mammography and MRI (each alternating every six months)
     - Pelvic examination every six months
     - Transvaginal ultrasound every 6–12 months
     - Serum CA 125 testing every 6–12 months.
5. What preventive strategies are available?
   - Prophylactic mastectomy
   - Chemoprevention with tamoxifen
   - Prophylactic oophorectomy between ages 35 and 40 or after childbearing
   - Would chemoprevention with raloxifene be appropriate?
   - No, raloxifene is only appropriate in postmenopausal women. Tamoxifen could be prescribed for five years following discussion of the benefits of chemoprevention and the risk of toxicities.

M.B. completed a prophylactic double mastectomy and reconstruction with implants. She hopes to soon become pregnant. She is exploring how to inform the adoption agency about the potential risk to her daughter. She reports that she is gradually adjusting to the changes in her life and is satisfied with her decisions. After childbearing, between ages 35 and 40, M.B. plans to undergo a prophylactic BSO. She states that her only regrets are that she is not certain how her adopted child will handle the information and that her unaffected sister decided not to test. The oncology APN's recommendations were summarized in a letter that M.B. could share with her primary care providers as needed.

Key Points

- Approximately 10% of all cancers are attributable to hereditary predisposition. Genetic testing is increasingly available to identify individuals with this heightened risk. Genetic testing is readily available for HBOC, HNPCC, FAP and AFAP, hereditary pancreatic, and hereditary melanoma syndromes. Many unusual syndromes have testing available on a more limited or research basis.
- Most agencies recommend that testing be offered when a positive test result is a reasonable likelihood, the knowledge of test results will influence care, and a qualified healthcare provider is available to provide informed consent and psychosocial support in the context of pre- and post-test counseling.

- Risk assessment includes assessment of risk for developing cancer and risk of carrying a mutation for hereditary risk. Typically, a pedigree is constructed, risk is calculated, and then the risk is interpreted to the patient and family.
- Possible outcomes of testing include a positive result, a true-negative result, a negative inconclusive result, and a variant of indeterminate significance.
- Individuals may have a variety of psychosocial responses to test results. Family members are encouraged to share the results of testing with other family members.
- Prevention and early detection measures are based on the outcome of testing, family history, and personal history. Those who test positive often will receive recommendations for prophylactic surgery.
- APNs have professional responsibilities related to cancer genetics, including protecting privacy, conducting further research, and serving as leaders in the field of cancer genetics.

Recommended Resources for Oncology Advanced Practice Nurses

- Tools
  - American Medical Association Family History Tools (www.ama-assn.org/ama/pub/physician-resources/medical-science/genetics-molecular-medicine.page): Family history form, sample pedigree, and free online courses
  - BRCAPRO software (www4.utsouthwestern.edu/breasthealth/cagene): Free computer software for computer construction of pedigrees and calculation of statistical models that predict breast and colon cancer risk, as well as risk of carrying other hereditary predisposition mutations
  - Breast Cancer Risk Assessment Tool (www.cancer.gov/bcrisktool/default.aspx): Computerized tool for mobile devices and desktop computers
  - Tyrer-Cuzick Risk Assessment Tool (www.ems-trials.org/riskevaluator): Provides the software download for the Tyrer-Cuzick Risk Assessment Tool
- Organizations and websites
  - American Board of Medical Genetics (www.abmg.org/pages/searchmem.shtml): Searchable database of credentialed providers
  - GeneReviews® (www.ncbi.nlm.nih.gov/books/NBK1116): Extensive information on genetic syndromes through a searchable database
  - GeneTests™ (www.genetests.org): Directory of inherited diseases; clinical overview of management of affected or at-risk individuals and family
  - Genetics Professionals Directory (www.cancer.gov/cancertopics/genetics/directory): National Cancer Institute database of cancer genetic providers nationwide
  - ISONG (www.isong.org): Professional networking site for nurses interested in genetics; educational resources
  - National Institutes of Health Genetics Home Reference (http://ghr.nlm.nih.gov): Genetic education modules, glossary of genetic terms and conditions, and an overview of gene therapy and genetic testing
  - NCCN (www.nccn.org): Downloadable guidelines including genetics/familial high-risk assessment, breast cancer risk reduction, and screening for breast, colon, melanoma, and other cancers
  - NSGC (www.nsgc.org): Educational resources for patients and professionals and a search page for finding credentialed genetic professionals

– ONS (www.ons.org): Position statements, educational resources, SIGs, and free and fee-based online courses related to genetic testing
• Books
    – Calzone, K.A., Masny, A., & Jenkins, J. (Eds.). (2010). *Genetics and genomics in oncology nursing practice.* Pittsburgh, PA: Oncology Nursing Society.
    – Greco, K.E., Tinley, S., & Seibert, D. (2011). *Essential genetic and genomic competencies for nurses with graduate degrees.* Retrieved from http://nursingworld.org/MainMenu Categories/EthicsStandards/Genetics-1/Essential-Genetic-and-Genomic-Competencies -for-Nurses-With-Graduate-Degrees.pdf
    – Jenkins, J.F. (2009). *Essentials of genetic and genomic nursing: Competencies, curricula guidelines, and outcome indicators* (2nd ed.). Retrieved from www.genome.gov/Pages/ Careers/HealthProfessionalEducation/geneticscompetency.pdf
    – Monsen, R.B. (2005). *Genetics nursing portfolios: A new model for credentialing.* Silver Spring, MD: American Nurses Association.
    – National Coalition for Health Professional Education in Genetics. (2007). *Core competencies in genetics for health professionals* (3rd ed.). Retrieved from www.nchpeg.org/index. php?option=com_content&view=article&id=237&Itemid=84

References

American Cancer Society. (2013). *Cancer prevention and early detection facts and figures 2013.* Atlanta, GA: Author.

American Cancer Society. (2015). *Cancer facts and figures 2015.* Atlanta, GA: Author.

American College of Medical Genetics and Genomics. (2004). ACMG statement on direct-to-consumer genetic testing. *Genetics in Medicine, 6*(1), 60. doi:10.1097/01.GIM.0000106164.59722.CE

American College of Medical Genetics and Genomics. (2012). Policy statement: Points to consider in the clinical application of genomic sequencing. Retrieved from http://www.acmg.net/StaticContent/PPG/Clinical_Application _of_Genomic_Sequencing.pdf

American College of Obstetricians and Gynecologists. (2008). ACOG Committee Opinion No. 409: Direct-to-consumer marketing of genetic testing. *Obstetrics and Gynecology, 111,* 1493–1494. doi:10.1097/AOG.0b013e3181 7d250e

American Society of Human Genetics. (2007). ASHG statement on direct-to-consumer genetic testing in the United States. *American Journal of Human Genetics, 81,* 635–637. doi:10.1086/521634

Amir, E., Evans, D.G., Shenton, A., Lalloo, F., Moran, A., Boggis, C., ... Howell, A. (2003). Evaluation of breast cancer risk assessment packages in the family history evaluation and screening programme. *Journal of Medical Genetics, 40,* 807–814. doi:10.1136/jmg.40.11.807

Axilbund, J.E., & Wiley, E.A. (2012). Genetic testing by cancer site: Pancreas. *Cancer Journal, 18,* 350–354. doi:10.1097/ PPO.0b013e3182624694

Balmaña, J., Stockwell, D.H., Steyerberg, E.W., Stoffel, E.M., Deffenbaugh, A.M., Reid, J.E., ... Syngal, S. (2006). Prediction of *MLH1* and *MSH2* mutations in Lynch syndrome. *JAMA, 296,* 1469–1478. doi:10.1001/jama.296.12.1469

Barrow, E., Hill, J., & Evans, D.G. (2013). Cancer risk in Lynch syndrome. *Familial Cancer, 12,* 229–240. doi:10.1007/ s10689-013-9615-1

Barton, M.K. (2012). Daily aspirin reduces colorectal cancer incidence in patients with Lynch syndrome. *CA: A Cancer Journal for Clinicians, 62,* 143–144. doi:10.3322/caac.21136

Baumanis, L., Evans, J.P., Callanan, N., & Susswein, L.R. (2009). Telephoned *BRCA1/2* genetic test results: Prevalence, practice, and patient satisfaction. *Journal of Genetic Counseling, 18,* 447–463. doi:10.1007/s10897-009-9238-8

Berg, W.A., Zhang, Z., Lehrer, D., Jong, R.A., Pisano, E.D., Barr, R.G., ... Gabrielli, G. (2012). Detection of breast cancer with addition of annual screening ultrasound or a single screening MRI to mammography in women with elevated breast cancer risk. *JAMA, 307,* 1394–1404. doi:10.1001/jama.2012.388

Bernstein, I.T., & Myrhøj, T. (2013). Surveillance for urinary tract cancer in Lynch syndrome. *Familial Cancer, 12,* 279–284. doi:10.1007/s10689-013-9634-y

Bevers, T.B., Armstrong, D.K., Arun, B., Carlson, R.W., Cowan, K.H., Daly, M.B., ... Ward, J.H. (2010). Breast cancer risk reduction. *Journal of the National Comprehensive Cancer Network, 8,* 1112–1146. Retrieved from http://www .jnccn.org/content/8/10/1112.long

Biesecker, L.G., Burke, W., Kohane, I., Plon, S.E., & Zimmern, R. (2012). Next-generation sequencing in the clinic: Are we ready? *Nature Reviews Genetics, 13,* 818–824. doi:10.1038/nrg3357

Bjorvatn, C., Eide, G.E., Hanestad, B.R., Hamang, A., & Havik, O.E. (2009). Intrusion and avoidance in subjects undergoing genetic investigation and counseling for hereditary cancer. *Supportive Care in Cancer, 17,* 1371–1381. doi:10.1007/s00520-009-0594-6

Bleiker, E.M.A., Esplen, M.J., Meiser, B., Petersen, H.V., & Patenaude, A.F. (2013). 100 years Lynch syndrome: What have we learned about psychosocial issues? *Familial Cancer, 12,* 325–339. doi:10.1007/s10689-013-9653-8

Bradbury, A.R., Patrick-Miller, L., Fetzer, D., Egleston, B., Cummings, S.A., Forman, A., … Daly, M.B. (2011). Genetic counselor opinions of, and experiences with telephone communication of *BRCA1/2* test results. *Clinical Genetics, 79,* 125–131. doi:10.1111/j.1399-0004.2010.01540.x

Brauch, H., & Jordan, V.C. (2009). Targeting of tamoxifen to enhance antitumour action for the treatment and prevention of breast cancer: The "personalised" approach? *European Journal of Cancer, 45,* 2274–2283. doi:10.1016/j.ejca.2009.05.032

Brierley, K.L., Blouch, E., Cogswell, W., Homer, J.P., Pencarinha, D., Stanislaw, C.L., & Matloff, E.T. (2012). Adverse events in cancer genetic testing: Medical, ethical, legal, and financial implications. *Cancer Journal, 18,* 303–309. doi:10.1097/PPO.1090b1013e3182609490

Brown, S.M. (2009). *Essentials of medical genomics* (2nd ed.). Hoboken, NJ: John Wiley & Sons.

Christinat, A., & Pagani, O. (2013). Practical aspects of genetic counseling in breast cancer: Lights and shadows. *Breast, 22,* 375–382. doi:10.1016/j.breast.2013.04.006

Culver, J.O., Brinkerhoff, C.D., Clague, J., Yang, K., Singh, K.E., Sand, S.R., & Weitzel, J.N. (2013). Variants of uncertain significance in *BRCA* testing: Evaluation of surgical decisions, risk perception, and cancer distress. *Clinical Genetics, 84,* 464–472. doi:10.1111/cge.12097

Daniels, M.S. (2012). Genetic testing by cancer site: Uterus. *Cancer Journal, 18,* 338–342 doi:10.1097/PPO.0b013e3182610cc2

Davies, C., Pan, H., Godwin, J., Gray, R., Arriagada, R., Raina, V., … Peto, R. (2013). Long-term effects of continuing adjuvant tamoxifen to 10 years versus stopping at 5 years after diagnosis of oestrogen receptor-positive breast cancer: ATLAS, a randomised trial. *Lancet, 381,* 805–816. doi:10.1016/S0140-6736(12)61963-1

den Heijer, M., Vos, J., Seynaeve, C., Vanheusden, K., Duivenvoorden, H.J., Tilanus-Linthorst, M., … Tibben, A. (2012). The impact of social and personal resources on psychological distress in women at risk for hereditary breast cancer. *Psycho-Oncology, 21,* 153–160. doi:10.1002/pon.1879

Desmedt, C., Voet, T., Sotiriou, C., & Campbell, P.J. (2012). Next-generation sequencing in breast cancer: First take home messages. *Current Opinion in Oncology, 24,* 597–604. doi:10.1097/CCO.0b013e328359554e

de Vos tot Nederveen Cappel, W.H., Järvinen, H.J., Lynch, P.M., Engel, C., Mecklin, J.-P., & Vasen, H.F.A. (2013). Colorectal surveillance in Lynch syndrome families. *Familial Cancer, 12,* 261–265. doi:10.1007/s10689-013-9631-1

Domchek, S.M., & Antoniou, A. (2007). Cancer risk models: Translating family history into clinical management. *Annals of Internal Medicine, 147,* 515–517. doi:10.7326/0003-4819-147-7-200710020-00009

Dupont, A.W., Arguedas, M.R., & Wilcox, C.M. (2007). Aspirin chemoprevention in patients with increased risk for colorectal cancer: A cost-effectiveness analysis. *Alimentary Pharmacology and Therapeutics, 26,* 431–441. doi:10.1111/j.1365-2036.2007.03380.x

Euhus, D. (2012). Managing the breast in patients who test positive for hereditary breast cancer. *Annals of Surgical Oncology, 19,* 1738–1744. doi:10.1245/s10434-012-2258-x

Euhus, D.M., & Robinson, L. (2013). Genetic predisposition syndromes and their management. *Surgical Clinics of North America, 93,* 341–362. doi:10.1016/j.suc.2013.01.005

European Society of Human Genetics. (2010). Statement of the ESHG on direct-to-consumer genetic testing for health-related purposes. *European Journal of Human Genetics, 18,* 1271–1273. doi:10.1038/ejhg.2010.129

Evans, D.G.R., Eccles, D.M., Rahman, N., Young, K., Bulman, M., Amir, E., … Lalloo, F. (2004). A new scoring system for the chances of identifying a *BRCA1/2* mutation outperforms existing models including BRCAPRO. *Journal of Medical Genetics, 41,* 474–480. doi:10.1136/jmg.2003.017996

Evans, D.G.R., Ingham, S.L., Baildam, A., Ross, G.L., Lalloo, F., Buchan, I., & Howell, A. (2013). Contralateral mastectomy improves survival in women with *BRCA1/2*-associated breast cancer. *Breast Cancer Research and Treatment, 140,* 135–142. doi:10.1007/s10549-013-2583-1

Finch, A., Evans, G., & Narod, S.A. (2012). *BRCA* carriers, prophylactic salpingo-oophorectomy and menopause: Clinical management considerations and recommendations. *Women's Health, 8,* 543–555. doi:10.2217/whe.12.41

Finch, A., Metcalfe, K.A., Chiang, J., Elit, L., McLaughlin, J., Springate, C., … Narod, S.A. (2013). The impact of prophylactic salpingo-oophorectomy on quality of life and psychological distress in women with a *BRCA* mutation. *Psycho-Oncology, 22,* 212–219. doi:10.1002/pon.2041

Fisher, R., Pusztai, L., & Swanton, C. (2013). Cancer heterogeneity: Implications for targeted therapeutics. *British Journal of Cancer, 108,* 479–485. doi:10.1038/bjc.2012.581

Frantzen, C., Links, T.P., & Giles, R.H. (2012). Von Hippel-Lindau disease. *GeneReviews*. Retrieved from http://www.ncbi.nlm.nih.gov/books/NBK1463

Freedman, A.N., Seminara, D., Gail, M.H., Hartge, P., Colditz, G.A., Ballard-Barbash, R., & Pfeiffer, R.M. (2005). Cancer risk prediction models: A workshop on development, evaluation, and application. *Journal of the National Cancer Institute, 97,* 715–723. doi:10.1093/jnci/dji128

Gabree, M., & Seidel, M. (2012). Genetic testing by cancer site: Skin. *Cancer Journal, 18,* 372–380 doi:10.1097/PPO.0b013e3182624664

Gadducci, A., Biglia, N., Cosio, S., Sismondi, P., & Genazzani, A.R. (2010). Gynaecologic challenging issues in the management of *BRCA* mutation carriers: Oral contraceptives, prophylactic salpingo-oophorectomy and hormone replacement therapy. *Gynecological Endocrinology, 26,* 568–577. doi:10.3109/09513590.2010.487609

Gaff, C.L., & Bylund, C.L. (2010). *Family communication about genetics: Theory and practice.* New York, NY: Oxford University Press.

Gala, M., & Chung, D.C. (2011). Hereditary colon cancer syndromes. *Seminars in Oncology, 38,* 490–499. doi:10.1053/j.seminoncol.2011.05.003

Genetic Information Nondiscrimination Act of 2008, Pub. L. No. 110-233, 122 Stat. 881.

Gopie, J.P., Mureau, M.A.M., Seynaeve, C., ter Kuile, M.M., Menke-Pluymers, M.B.E., Timman, R., & Tibben, A. (2013). Body image issues after bilateral prophylactic mastectomy with breast reconstruction in healthy women at risk for hereditary breast cancer. *Familial Cancer, 12,* 479–487. doi:10.1007/s10689-012-9588-5

Greco, K.E., Tinley, S., & Seibert, D. (2011). Development of the essential genetic and genomic competencies for nurses with graduate degrees. *Annual Review of Nursing Research, 29,* 173–190. doi:10.1891/0739-6686.29.173

Greco, K.E., Tinley, S., & Seibert, D. (2012). *Essential genetic and genomic competencies for nurses with graduate degrees.* Retrieved from http://www.genome.gov/Pages/Health/HealthCareProvidersInfo/Grad_Gen_Comp.pdf

Gunder, L.M., & Martin, S.A. (2011). *Essentials of medical genetics for health professionals.* Burlington, MA: Jones & Bartlett Learning.

Hartman, A.R., Kaldate, R.R., Sailer, L.M., Painter, L., Grier, C.E., Endsley, R.R., … Sandbach, J.F. (2012). Prevalence of *BRCA* mutations in an unselected population of triple-negative breast cancer. *Cancer, 118,* 2787–2795. doi:10.1002/cncr.26576

Hilgart, J.S., Coles, B., & Iredale, R. (2012). Cancer genetic risk assessment for individuals at risk of familial breast cancer. *Cochrane Database of Systematic Reviews, 2012*(2). doi:10.1002/14651858.CD003721.pub3

Hoskins, L.M., Roy, K.M., & Greene, M.H. (2012). Toward a new understanding of risk perception among young female *BRCA1/2* "previvors". *Families, Systems, and Health, 30,* 32–46. doi:10.1037/a0027276

Howard, A.F., Balneaves, L., & Bottorff, J. (2009). Women's decision making about risk-reducing strategies in the context of hereditary breast and ovarian cancer: A systematic review. *Journal of Genetic Counseling, 18,* 578–597. doi:10.1007/s10897-009-9245-9

Howard, A.F., Balneaves, L.G., Bottorff, J.L., & Rodney, P. (2011). Preserving the self: The process of decision making about hereditary breast cancer and ovarian cancer risk reduction. *Qualitative Health Research, 21,* 502–519. doi:10.1177/1049732310387798

International Society of Nurses in Genetics. (2009). Direct-to-consumer marketing of genetic tests [Position statement]. Retrieved from http://www.isong.org/pdfs2013/PS_Marketing_Genetic_Tests.pdf

International Society of Nurses in Genetics & American Nurses Association. (2007). *Genetics/genomics nursing: Scope and standards of practice.* Retrieved from http://www.nursingworld.org/MainMenuCategories/EthicsStandards/Genetics-1/Genetics-and-Genomics-Nursing-Scope-and-Standards.pdf

Iqbal, J., Ragone, A., Lubinski, J., Lynch, H.T., Moller, P., Ghadirian, P., … Narod, S.A. (2012). The incidence of pancreatic cancer in *BRCA1* and *BRCA2* mutation carriers. *British Journal of Cancer, 107,* 2005–2009. doi:10.1038/bjc.2012.483

Jasperson, K.W. (2012). Genetic testing by cancer site: Colon (polyposis syndromes). *Cancer Journal, 18,* 328–333. doi:10.1097/PPO.0b013e3182609300

Jasperson, K.W., & Burt, R.W. (2011). *APC*-associated polyposis conditions. *GeneReviews*. Retrieved from http://www.ncbi.nlm.nih.gov/books/NBK1345

Jenkins, J.F. (2009). *Essentials of genetic and genomic nursing: Competencies, curricula guidelines, and outcome indicators* (2nd ed.). Retrieved from http://www.aacn.nche.edu/education-resources/Genetics__Genomics_Nursing_Competencies_09-22-06.pdf

Jones, S., Hruban, R.H., Kamiyama, M., Borges, M., Zhang, X., Parsons, D.W., … Klein, A.P. (2009). Exomic sequencing identifies *PALB2* as a pancreatic cancer susceptibility gene. *Science, 324*(5924), 217. doi:10.1126/science.1171202

Kaplan, M., Mahon, S., Cope, D., Keating, E., Hill, S., & Jacobson, M. (2011). Putting evidence into practice: Evidence-based interventions for hot flashes resulting from cancer therapies. *Clinical Journal of Oncology Nursing, 15,* 149–157. doi:10.1188/11.CJON.149-157

Kardashian, A., Fehniger, J., Creasman, J., Cheung, E., & Beattie, M.S. (2012). A pilot study of the Sharing Risk Information Tool (ShaRIT) for families with hereditary breast and ovarian cancer syndrome. *Hereditary Cancer in Clinical Practice, 10*(1), 4. doi:10.1186/1897-4287-10-4

Kastrinos, F., Balmaña, J., & Syngal, S. (2013). Prediction models in Lynch syndrome. *Familial Cancer, 12,* 217–228. doi:10.1007/s10689-013-9632-0

Kastrinos, F., & Syngal, S. (2012). Screening patients with colorectal cancer for Lynch Syndrome: What are we waiting for? *Journal of Clinical Oncology, 30,* 1024–1027. doi:10.1200/jco.2011.40.7171

Kohlmann, W., & Gruber, S.B. (2012). Lynch syndrome. *GeneReviews.* Retrieved from http://www.ncbi.nlm.nih.gov/books/NBK1211

Ku, C.S., Cooper, D.N., Ziogas, D.E., Halkia, E., Tzaphlidou, M., & Roukos, D.H. (2013). Research and clinical applications of cancer genome sequencing. *Current Opinion in Obstetrics and Gynecology, 25,* 3–10. doi:10.1097/GCO.0b013e32835af17c

Kushi, L.H., Doyle, C., McCullough, M., Rock, C.L., Demark-Wahnefried, W., Bandera, E.V., … Gansler, T. (2012). American Cancer Society guidelines on nutrition and physical activity for cancer prevention. *CA: A Cancer Journal for Clinicians, 62,* 30–67. doi:10.3322/caac.20140

Kwon, J.S., Gutierrez-Barrera, A.M., Young, D., Sun, C.C., Daniels, M.S., Lu, K.H., & Arun, B. (2010). Expanding the criteria for *BRCA* mutation testing in breast cancer survivors. *Journal of Clinical Oncology, 28,* 4214–4220. doi:10.1200/jco.2010.28.0719

Lachance, C.R., Erby, L.A.H., Ford, B.M., Allen, V.C., Jr., & Kaphingst, K.A. (2010). Informational content, literacy demands, and usability of websites offering health-related genetic tests directly to consumers. *Genetics in Medicine, 12,* 304–312. doi:10.1097/GIM.0b013e3181dbd8b2

Lapointe, J., Abdous, B., Camden, S., Bouchard, K., Goldgar, D., Simard, J., & Dorval, M. (2012). Influence of the family cluster effect on psychosocial variables in families undergoing *BRCA1/2* genetic testing for cancer susceptibility. *Psycho-Oncology, 21,* 515–523. doi:10.1002/pon.19 6

Larghi, A., Verna, E.C., Lecca, P.G., & Costamagna, G. (2009). Screening for pancreatic cancer in high-risk individuals: A call for endoscopic ultrasound. *Clinical Cancer Research, 15,* 1907–1914. doi:10.1158/1078-0432.ccr-08-1966

Lastra, E., García-González, M., Llorente, B., Bernuy, C., Barrio, M.J., Pérez-Cabornero, L., … García-Girón, C. (2012). Lynch syndrome diagnostics: Decision-making process for germ-line testing. *Clinical and Translational Oncology, 14,* 254–262. doi:10.1007/s12094-012-0793-3

Ligtenberg, M.J.L., Kuiper, R.P., van Kessel, A.G., & Hoogerbrugge, N. (2013). *EPCAM* deletion carriers constitute a unique subgroup of Lynch syndrome patients. *Familial Cancer, 12,* 169–174. doi:10.1007/s10689-012-9591-x

Lindor, N.M., McMaster, M.L., Lindor, C.J., & Greene, M.H. (2008). Concise handbook of familial cancer susceptibility syndromes—second edition. *Journal of the National Cancer Institute Monographs, 2008*(38), 1–93. doi:10.1093/jncimonographs/lgn001

Lowry, K.P., Lee, J.M., Kong, C.Y., McMahon, P.M., Gilmore, M.E., Chubiz, J.E.C., … Gazelle, G.S. (2012). Annual screening strategies in *BRCA1* and *BRCA2* gene mutation carriers. *Cancer, 118,* 2021–2030. doi:10.1002/cncr.26424

Lu, K., & Daniels, M. (2013). Endometrial and ovarian cancer in women with Lynch syndrome: Update in screening and prevention. *Familial Cancer, 12,* 273–277. doi:10.1007/s10689-013-9664-5

Lynch, H.T., Lynch, J.F., & Attard, T.A. (2009). Diagnosis and management of hereditary colorectal cancer syndromes: Lynch syndrome as a model. *Canadian Medical Association Journal, 181,* 273–280. doi:10.1503/cmaj.071574

Mahon, S.M. (2011). Managing families with a hereditary cancer syndrome. *Oncology Nursing Forum, 38,* 641–644. doi:10.1188/11.ONF.641-644

Mahon, S.M. (2012a). Complexities of genetic care: Implications for advanced practice nurses. *Journal for Nurse Practitioners, 8*(8), e23–e27. doi:10.1016/j.nurpra.2012.04.020

Mahon, S.M. (2012b). Impact of direct-to-consumer genetic testing. *Journal of Oncology Practice, 8,* 260. doi:10.1200/jop.2012.000653

Mahon, S.M. (2013a). Allocation of work activities in a comprehensive cancer genetics program. *Clinical Journal of Oncology Nursing, 17,* 397–404. doi:10.1188/13.cjon.397-404

Mahon, S.M. (2013b). Large genomic rearrangements in *BRCA1* and *BRCA2*: Implications for patient care. *Oncology Nursing Forum, 40,* 220–222. doi:10.1188/13.onf.220-222

Mahon, S.M. (2013c). Next-generation DNA sequencing: Implications for oncology care. *Oncology Nursing Forum, 40,* 437–439. doi:10.1188/13.ONF.437-439

Mahon, S.M. (2013d). Ordering the correct genetic test: Implications for oncology and primary care healthcare professionals. *Clinical Journal of Oncology Nursing, 17,* 128–131. doi:10.1188/13.CJON.128-131

Mahon, S.M., & Casey, M. (2003). Patient education for women being fitted for breast prostheses. *Clinical Journal of Oncology Nursing, 7,* 194–199. doi:10.1188/03.CJON.194-199

Mahon, S.M., & Waldman, L. (2010a). Multiple endocrine neoplasia 1: Providing care for the family. *Clinical Journal of Oncology Nursing, 14,* 657–660. doi:10.1188/10.CJON.657-660

Mahon, S.M., & Waldman, L. (2010b). Multiple endocrine neoplasia 2: Providing care for the family. *Clinical Journal of Oncology Nursing, 14,* 803–806. doi:10.1188/10.CJON.803-806

Mahon, S.M., & Waldman, L. (2012). Von Hippel-Lindau syndrome: Implications for nursing care. *Oncology Nursing Forum, 39,* 533–536. doi:10.1188/12.ONF.533-536

Mai, P.L., Garceau, A.O., Graubard, B.I., Dunn, M., McNeel, T.S., Gonsalves, L., … Wideroff, L. (2011). Confirmation of family cancer history reported in a population-based survey. *Journal of the National Cancer Institute, 103,* 788–797. doi:10.1093/jnci/djr114

Martín-López, J., & Fishel, R. (2013). The mechanism of mismatch repair and the functional analysis of mismatch repair defects in Lynch syndrome. *Familial Cancer, 12,* 159–168. doi:10.1007/s10689-013-9635-x

Matloff, E.T., Barnett, R.E., & Bober, S.L. (2009). Unraveling the next chapter: Sexual development, body image, and sexual functioning in female *BRCA* carriers. *Cancer Journal, 15,* 15–18. doi:10.1097/PPO.1090b1013e31819585f31819581

Matloff, E.T., Bonadies, D.C., Moyer, A., & Brierley, K.L. (2014). Changes in specialists' perspectives on cancer genetic testing, prophylactic surgery and insurance discrimination: Then and now. *Journal of Genetic Counseling, 23,* 164–171. doi:10.1007/s10897-013-9625-z

Menko, F.H., Aalfs, C.M., Henneman, L., Stol, Y., Wijdenes, M., Otten, E., … Tibben, A. (2013). Informing family members of individuals with Lynch syndrome: A guideline for clinical geneticists. *Familial Cancer, 12,* 319–324. doi:10.1007/s10689-013-9636-9

Metcalfe, K.A., Mian, N., Enmore, M., Poll, A., Llacuachaqui, M., Nanda, S., … Narod, S.A. (2012). Long-term follow-up of Jewish women with a *BRCA1* and *BRCA2* mutation who underwent population genetic screening. *Breast Cancer Research and Treatment, 133,* 735–740. doi:10.1007/s10549-011-1941-0

Mitra, A.V., Bancroft, E.K., Barbachano, Y., Page, E.C., Foster, C.S., Jameson, C., … Eeles, R.A. (2011). Targeted prostate cancer screening in men with mutations in *BRCA1* and *BRCA2* detects aggressive prostate cancer: Preliminary analysis of the results of the IMPACT study. *BJU International, 107,* 28–39. doi:10.1111/j.1464-410X.2010.09648.x

Monsen, R.B. (Ed.). (2005). Introduction: Using portfolios in genetics nursing: A model for the profession. In R.B. Monsen (Ed.), *Genetics nursing portfolios: A new model for credentialing* (pp. 1–7). Silver Spring, MD: American Nurses Association.

Morrow, M., Waters, J., & Morris, E. (2011). MRI for breast cancer screening, diagnosis, and treatment. *Lancet, 378,* 1804–1811. doi:10.1016/s0140-6736(11)61350-0

Murray, A.J., & Davies, D.M. (2013). The genetics of breast cancer. *Surgery, 31*(1), 1–3. doi:10.1016/j.mpsur.2012.10.019

National Comprehensive Cancer Network. (2014a). *NCCN Clinical Practice Guidelines in Oncology (NCCN Guidelines®): Breast cancer risk reduction* [v.1.2014]. Retrieved from http://www.nccn.org/professionals/physician_gls/pdf/breast_risk.pdf

National Comprehensive Cancer Network. (2014b). *NCCN Clinical Practice Guidelines in Oncology (NCCN Guidelines®): Colorectal cancer screening* [v.1.2014]. Retrieved from http://www.nccn.org/professionals/physician_gls/pdf/colorectal_screening.pdf

National Comprehensive Cancer Network. (2014c). *NCCN Clinical Practice Guidelines in Oncology (NCCN Guidelines®): Genetic/familial high-risk assessment: Breast and ovarian* [v.2.2014]. Retrieved from http://www.nccn.org/professionals/physician_gls/pdf/genetics_screening.pdf

National Society of Genetic Counselors. (2011, June 1). *Direct to consumer genetic testing* Retrieved from http://nsgc.org/p/bl/et/blogid=47&blogaid=22

Nelson, H.D., Huffman, L.H., Fu, R., & Harris, E.L. (2005). Genetic risk assessment and *BRCA* mutation testing for breast and ovarian cancer susceptibility: Recommendation statement. *Annals of Internal Medicine, 143,* 355–361. doi:10.7326/0003-4819-143-5-200509060-00011

Oncology Nursing Society. (2014). Oncology nursing: The application of cancer genetics and genomics throughout the oncology care continuum [Position statement]. Retrieved from https://www.ons.org/advocacy-policy/positions/education/genetics

Oral contraceptives and ovarian cancer risk. (2008). *CA: A Cancer Journal for Clinicians, 58,* 127–128. doi:10.3322/ca.2008.0004

Pal, T., Lee, J.-H., Besharat, A., Thompson, Z., Monteiro, A.N.A., Phelan, C., … Narod, S.A. (2014). Modes of delivery of genetic testing services and the uptake of cancer risk management strategies in *BRCA1* and *BRCA2* carriers. *Clinical Genetics, 85,* 49–53. doi:10.1111/cge.12130

Parmigiani, G., Chen, S., Iversen, E.S., Jr., Friebel, T.M., Finkelstein, D.M., Anton-Culver, H., … Euhus, D.M. (2007). Validity of models for predicting *BRCA1* and *BRCA2* mutations. *Annals of Internal Medicine, 147,* 441–450. doi:10.7326/0003-4819-147-7-200710020-00002

Patel, S.G., & Ahnen, D.J. (2012). Familial colon cancer syndromes: An update of a rapidly evolving field. *Current Gastroenterology Reports, 14,* 428–438. doi:10.1007/s11894-012-0280-6

Petrucelli, N., Daly, M.B., & Feldman, G.L. (2013). *BRCA1* and *BRCA2* hereditary breast and ovarian cancer. *GeneReviews.* Retrieved from http://www.ncbi.nlm.nih.gov/books/NBK1247

Pilarski, R., & Nagy, R. (2012). Genetic testing by cancer site: Endocrine system. *Cancer Journal, 18,* 364–371. doi:10.1097/PPO.0b013e3182609458

Plutynski, A. (2012). Ethical issues in cancer screening and prevention. *Journal of Medicine and Philosophy, 37,* 310–323. doi:10.1093/jmp/jhs017

Pyeritz, R.E. (2011). The coming explosion in genetic testing—Is there a duty to recontact? *New England Journal of Medicine, 365,* 1367–1369. doi:10.1056/NEJMp1107564

Rew, L., Kaur, M., McMillan, A., Mackert, M., & Bonevac, D. (2010). Systematic review of psychosocial benefits and harms of genetic testing. *Issues in Mental Health Nursing, 31,* 631–645. doi:10.3109/01612840.2010.510618

Rice, C.D., Ruschman, J.G., Martin, L.J., Manders, J.B., & Miller, E. (2010). Retrospective comparison of patient outcomes after in-person and telephone results disclosure counseling for *BRCA1/2* genetic testing. *Familial Cancer, 9,* 203–212. doi:10.1007/s10689-009-9303-3

Riley, B., Culver, J., Skrzynia, C., Senter, L., Peters, J., Costalas, J., … Trepanier, A. (2012). Essential elements of genetic cancer risk assessment, counseling, and testing: Updated recommendations of the National Society of Genetic Counselors. *Journal of Genetic Counseling, 21,* 151–161. doi:10.1007/s10897-011-9462-x

Rizzo, J.M., & Buck, M.J. (2012). Key principles and clinical applications of "*next-generation*" DNA sequencing. *Cancer Prevention Research, 5,* 887–900. doi:10.1158/1940-6207.capr-11-0432

Robson, M.E., Storm, C.D., Weitzel, J., Wollins, D.S., & Offit, K. (2010). American Society of Clinical Oncology policy statement update: Genetic and genomic testing for cancer susceptibility. *Journal of Clinical Oncology, 28,* 893–901. doi:10.1200/jco.2009.27.0660

Rodriguez-Bigas, M.A., & Möeslein, G. (2013). Surgical treatment of hereditary nonpolyposis colorectal cancer (HNPCC, Lynch syndrome). *Familial Cancer, 12,* 295–300. doi:10.1007/s10689-013-9626-y

Ross, J.S., & Cronin, M. (2011). Whole cancer genome sequencing by next-generation methods. *American Journal of Clinical Pathology, 136,* 527–539. doi:10.1309/ajcpr1svt1vhugxw

Saslow, D., Boetes, C., Burke, W., Harms, S., Leach, M.O., Lehman, C.D., … Russell, C.A. (2007). American Cancer Society guidelines for breast screening with MRI as an adjunct to mammography. *CA: A Cancer Journal for Clinicians, 57,* 75–89. doi:10.3322/canjclin.57.2.75

Schneider, R., Schneider, C., Kloor, M., Fürst, A., & Möslein, G. (2012). Lynch syndrome: Clinical, pathological, and genetic insights. *Langenbeck's Archives of Surgery, 397,* 513–525. doi:10.1007/s00423-012-0918-8

Senter, L. (2012). Genetic testing by cancer site: Colon (nonpolyposis syndromes). *Cancer Journal, 18,* 334–337. doi:10.1097/PPO.0b013e31826094b2

Shannon, K.M., & Chittenden, A. (2012). Genetic testing by cancer site: Breast. *Cancer Journal, 18,* 310–319. doi:10.1097/PPO.0b013e318260946f

Shannon, K.M., Rodgers, L.H., Chan-Smutko, G., Patel, D., Gabree, M., & Ryan, P.D. (2011). Which individuals undergoing BRACAnalysis need BART testing? *Cancer Genetics, 204,* 416–422. doi:10.1016/j.cancergen.2011.07.005

Shia, J., Holck, S., DePetris, G., Greenson, J., & Klimstra, D. (2013). Lynch syndrome-associated neoplasms: A discussion on histopathology and immunohistochemistry. *Familial Cancer, 12,* 241–260. doi:10.1007/s10689-013-9612-4

Shin, E.J., & Canto, M.I. (2012). Pancreatic cancer screening. *Gastroenterology Clinics of North America, 41,* 143–157. doi:10.1016/j.gtc.2011.12.001

Shinagare, A.B., Giardino, A.A., Jagannathan, J.P., Van den Abbeele, A.D., & Ramaiya, N.H. (2011). Hereditary cancer syndromes: A radiologist's perspective. *American Journal of Roentgenology, 197,* W1001–W1007. doi:10.2214/ajr.11.6465

Sie, A.S., Prins, J.B., Spruijt, L., Kets, C.M., & Hoogerbrugge, N. (2013). Can we test for hereditary cancer at 18 years when we start surveillance at 25? Patient reported outcomes. *Familial Cancer, 12,* 675–682. doi:10.1007/s10689-013-9644-9

Ståhlbom, A., Johansson, H., Liljegren, A., Wachenfeldt, A., & Arver, B. (2012). Evaluation of the BOADICEA risk assessment model in women with a family history of breast cancer. *Familial Cancer, 11,* 33–40. doi:10.1007/s10689-011-9495-1

Sturdee, D.W., & Panay, N. (2010). Recommendations for the management of postmenopausal vaginal atrophy. *Climacteric, 13,* 509–522. doi:10.3109/13697137.2010.522875

Templeton, A.W., & Brentnall, T.A. (2013). Screening and surgical outcomes of familial pancreatic cancer. *Surgical Clinics of North America, 93,* 629–645. doi:10.1016/j.suc.2013.02.002

Tercyak, K.P., O'Neill, S.C., Roter, D.L., & McBride, C.M. (2012). Bridging the communication divide: A role for health psychology in the genomic era. *Professional Psychology: Research and Practice, 43,* 568–575. doi:10.1037/a0028971

Tilburt, J.C., James, K.M., Sinicrope, P.S., Eton, D.T., Costello, B.A., Carey, J., … Murad, M.H. (2011). Factors influencing cancer risk perception in high risk populations: A systematic review. *Hereditary Cancer in Clinical Practice, 9,* 2. doi:10.1186/1897-4287-9-2

Tokin, C., Weiss, A., Wang-Rodriguez, J., & Blair, S.L. (2012). Oncologic safety of skin-sparing and nipple-sparing mastectomy: A discussion and review of the literature. *International Journal of Surgical Oncology, 2012,* Article ID 921821. doi:10.1155/2012/921821

Twomey, J. (2011). Ethical, legal, psychosocial, and cultural implications of genomics for oncology nurses. *Seminars in Oncology Nursing, 27,* 54–63. doi:10.1016/j.soncn.2010.11.007

Tyrer, J., Duffy, S.W., & Cuzick, J. (2004). A breast cancer prediction model incorporating familial and personal risk factors. *Statistics in Medicine, 23,* 1111–1130. doi:10.1002/sim.1668

U.S. Preventive Services Task Force. (2005). Genetic risk assessment and *BRCA* mutation testing for breast and ovarian cancer susceptibility: Recommendation statement. *Annals of Internal Medicine, 143,* 355–361. doi:10.7326/0003-4819-143-5-200509060-00011

U.S. Preventive Services Task Force. (2008). Screening for colorectal cancer: U.S. Preventive Services Task Force recommendation statement. *Annals of Internal Medicine, 149,* 627–637. doi:10.7326/0003-4819-149-9-200811040-00243

Vadaparampil, S.T., Miree, C.A., Wilson, C., & Jacobsen, P.B. (2006–2007). Psychosocial and behavioral impact of genetic counseling and testing. *Breast Disease, 27,* 97–108.

van Duijnhoven, F.B., Botma, A., Winkels, R., Nagengast, F., Vasen, H.A., & Kampman, E. (2013). Do lifestyle factors influence colorectal cancer risk in Lynch syndrome? *Familial Cancer, 12,* 285–293. doi:10.1007/s10689-013-9645-8

van Zitteren, M., van der Net, J.B., Kundu, S., Freedman, A.N., van Duijn, C.M., & Janssens, A.C.J.W. (2011). Genome-based prediction of breast cancer risk in the general population: A modeling study based on meta-analyses of genetic associations. *Cancer Epidemiology, Biomarkers and Prevention, 20,* 9–22. doi:10.1158/1055-9965.epi-10-0329

Vasen, H.F.A., Blanco, I., Aktan-Collan, K., Gopie, J.P., Alonso, A., Aretz, S., … Möslein, G. (2013). Revised guidelines for the clinical management of Lynch syndrome (HNPCC): Recommendations by a group of European experts. *Gut, 62,* 812–823. doi:10.1136/gutjnl-2012-304356

Weissman, S.M., Burt, R., Church, J., Erdman, S., Hampel, H., Holter, S., … Senter, L. (2012). Identification of individuals at risk for Lynch syndrome using targeted evaluations and genetic testing: National Society of Genetic Counselors and the Collaborative Group of the Americas on Inherited Colorectal Cancer joint practice guideline. *Journal of Genetic Counseling, 21,* 484–493. doi:10.1007/s10897-011-9465-7

Weitzel, J.N., Blazer, K.R., MacDonald, D.J., Culver, J.O., & Offit, K. (2011). Genetics, genomics, and cancer risk assessment. *CA: A Cancer Journal for Clinicians, 61,* 327–359. doi:10.3322/caac.20128

Wevers, M.R., Ausems, M.G.E.M., Verhoef, S., Bleiker, E.M.A., Hahn, D.E.E., Hogervorst, F.B.L., … Aaronson, N.K. (2011). Behavioral and psychosocial effects of rapid genetic counseling and testing in newly diagnosed breast cancer patients: Design of a multicenter randomized clinical trial. *BMC Cancer, 11,* 6. doi:10.1186/1471-2407-11-6

Wiggs, J. (2009). Fundamentals of genetics. In M. Yanoff (Ed.), *Ophthalmology* (pp. 1–9). St. Louis, MO: Elsevier.

Wiseman, M., Dancyger, C., & Michie, S. (2010). Communicating genetic risk information within families: A review. *Familial Cancer, 9,* 691–703. doi:10.1007/s10689-010-9380-3

Zagouri, F., Chrysikos, D.T., Sergentanis, T.N., Giannakopoulou, G., Zografos, C.G., Papadimitriou, C.A., & Zografos, G.C. (2013). Prophylactic mastectomy: An appraisal. *American Surgeon, 79,* 205–212.

CHAPTER 3

Cancer Diagnosis and Staging

Laura J. Zitella, MS, RN, ACNP-BC, AOCN®

Introduction

Malignancy can arise in any organ or tissue in the body with the exception of the fingernails, hair, and teeth. The diagnosis of cancer involves histopathologic or cytologic examination of tissues or cells to identify malignancy, the anatomic site of origin of the malignancy, and the type of cells involved (National Cancer Institute [NCI], 2012). In most cases, a biopsy or surgical resection of the tissue is required to render a diagnosis of cancer. *Histopathology* refers to examination of diseased tissue under a microscope by a pathologist, whereas *cytopathology* refers to examination of cells under a microscope by a pathologist.

In addition to microscopic examination, cells and tissues can be evaluated by the antigens expressed on or in the cell and specific chromosomal or genetic abnormalities. Molecular and tumor markers are playing a more significant role in cancer diagnosis, prognosis, and treatment. Tumor markers generally are substances secreted by the tumor. Molecular markers include gene expression levels, proteins, and genetic mutations.

The extent of the cancer at diagnosis is a key variable that defines prognosis and treatment. Cancer staging consists of comprehensive evaluation of the burden of disease, sites of involvement, and assessment of nonanatomic prognostic factors, such as tumor markers. A specific staging system exists for nearly every type of cancer. Staging occurs at the time of initial diagnosis, and restaging occurs at specific intervals in the disease process to determine response to therapy.

This chapter will present an overview of the cancer diagnosis and staging process as well as the specific staging systems used for several of the most common malignancies.

Signs and Symptoms of Cancer

A *symptom* is a subjective indication of disease that may be experienced by an individual but is not necessarily noticeable by others, for example, prolonged constipation. A *sign* is an objective indication of disease experienced by an individual that is noted by the healthcare professional, for example, abnormal breath sounds. Cancer causes a multitude of signs and symptoms, depending on the type and location of the cancer, the extent of the disease, and the presence and location of metastases.

Prompt recognition of early signs and symptoms of cancer allows diagnosis when cancer is most curable—in the early stages. The cardinal signs and symptoms of cancer are remembered using the mnemonic CAUTION: **C**hange in bowel or bladder habits; **A** sore that does not heal; **U**nusual bleeding or discharge, **T**hickening or lump in the breast, testicles, or elsewhere; **I**ndigestion or difficulty swallowing; **O**bvious change in the size, color, shape, or thickness of a wart, mole, or mouth sore; and **N**agging cough or hoarseness (American Cancer Society [ACS], 2014b). Other nonspecific signs and symptoms include unexplained weight loss, fevers, fatigue, pain, and skin changes, such as hyperpigmentation, jaundice, erythema, pruritus, or excessive hair growth (ACS, 2014b). Most symptoms related to cancer are attributed to the effect of a tumor's increasing mass, skin manifestations, or organ dysfunction.

History and Physical Examination

Patient History

The clinical evaluation of patients with cancer begins with a history and physical examination. The history includes the chief complaint, related in the patient's own words. The history of the present illness incorporates a chronologic account of the complaint, including symptoms and their manifestations (Bickley, 2013). The family, social, and past medical history is ascertained. When advanced practice nurses (APNs) are evaluating patients with a potential malignancy, the history includes determining predisposing factors for cancer, including familial cancers (e.g., breast, ovarian, prostate, or colorectal cancers), exposure to environmental mutagens (such as tobacco use and alcohol intake), and previous illnesses. Exploration of symptoms of cancer such as hemoptysis, blood in emesis or stool, abnormal vaginal bleeding, palpable masses or lumps, or any persistent or unexplained pain will be part of the comprehensive physical examination.

Clues obtained in the history can guide APNs toward a diagnosis of malignancy. For example, a history of immunosuppression could lead to the development of cancer (as seen with organ transplant, autoimmune disease, or HIV). Recipients of organ transplants have a twofold increased risk of cancer, and HIV-infected individuals have a 10-fold increased risk of cancer (Serraino et al., 2007). The increased risk in HIV-infected individuals may be a result of chronic immunosuppression as well as chronic viral infection. Chronic infections have also been linked to the development of human cancer, and it is estimated that 16% of all cancers globally are attributable to infection (de Martel et al., 2012). Infectious agents that are classified by the International Agency for Research on Cancer as carcinogenic to humans are listed in Table 3-1.

Work history is evaluated for occupational exposure to certain chemicals that have been implicated in the development of specific cancers, such as the association of benzene exposure with the development of acute myeloid leukemia and the association of formaldehyde exposure with the development of nasopharyngeal cancer and leukemia (Baan et al., 2009). Medication history is reviewed carefully to determine risk factors for specific cancers. For example, data from randomized controlled trials have shown that the risk of invasive breast cancer is slightly increased with estrogen-progestin use and slightly decreased with use of estrogen alone; therefore, a history of estrogen-progestin use may contribute to the development of breast cancer in some patients (Manson et al., 2013).

Table 3-1. Infectious Agents Carcinogenic to Humans

Infectious Agent	Cancers
Helicobacter pylori (H. pylori)	Gastric carcinoma Gastric lymphoma
Hepatitis B and C viruses	Hepatocellular carcinoma Non-Hodgkin lymphoma
Human papillomavirus	Cervical cancer Anogenital cancers (penile, vulva, vagina, anus) Oropharyngeal cancers
Epstein-Barr virus	Nasopharyngeal cancer Hodgkin lymphoma Burkitt lymphoma Non-Hodgkin lymphoma
Human T-cell lymphotropic virus type 1	Adult T-cell leukemia and lymphoma
Human herpesvirus type 8 (also known as Kaposi sarcoma herpesvirus)	Kaposi sarcoma
HIV	Cervical cancer Kaposi sarcoma Non-Hodgkin lymphoma Ocular cancers
Opisthorchis viverrini and *Clonorchis sinensis* (liver flukes)	Cholangiocarcinoma
Schistosoma haematobium	Bladder cancer

Note. Based on information from de Martel et al., 2012; International Agency for Research on Cancer, 2011.

Physical Examination

Clues taken from the history will lead to a more focused physical examination. If patients present with specific physical complaints, APNs should pay careful attention to those areas of involvement. Vital signs may provide information that leads to diagnosis. For example, a fever of unknown origin often is related to infection or inflammatory disease; however, malignancy also is in the differential diagnosis if fever remains undiagnosed after one week of investigation. Fever is a common symptom of hematologic malignancies (Goodrich, McNally, Ridgeway, & Zitella, 2013).

The skin is carefully inspected, and masses or ulcerations are noted. Enlarged or suspicious moles are examined carefully for signs of skin cancer, including melanoma. All lymphatic areas (including epitrochlear, axillary, infraclavicular, supraclavicular, cervical, and inguinal) are examined. Enlarged lymph nodes may indicate the presence of lymphoma or metastatic disease.

Examination of the chest includes percussion and auscultation, with specific attention to lung sounds. Coarse breath sounds, wheezing, and rhonchi are assessed. Absence of breath sounds or dullness to percussion could indicate fluid or even a mass (Bickley, 2013). Breast examination includes inspection of the breast skin and assessment for erythema or thickening, which could indicate an inflammatory carcinoma (Bickley, 2013). Changes in the breast contour and appearance of the nipple are noted. Palpation of the entire breast tissue is performed to evaluate for changes, including masses. Although breast cancer is rare in men, this examination is still important.

Abdominal examination includes assessment for hepatomegaly or splenomegaly. Tenderness of the abdominal area is evaluated, and any sign of ascites is noted. Masses in the abdominal area may be harder to discern because of their location (Bickley, 2013).

Male patients undergo a testicular examination, including assessment for any abnormalities in the scrotum or testicles. Examination of the healthy prostate normally reveals a rubbery, smooth, and nontender gland. Abnormalities of the prostate may manifest as hard nodules that feel irregular (Bickley, 2013). The female examination includes inspection of the vulva for any suspicious masses or lesions and a vaginal and adnexal examination, including cervical cytology. Digital rectal examination (DRE) is recommended for both males and females.

The musculoskeletal system is assessed, including range of motion and vertebral percussion tenderness. Pulses are evaluated for strength and symmetry. Any edema, clubbing, or cyanosis is recorded.

A full neurologic examination should be performed to assess for focal deficits, cranial nerve function, strength of reflexes, mental status and cognition, coordination, and gait (Bickley, 2013).

Evaluation of Patient Performance Status

Once the history and physical examination are completed, patients may be evaluated by their performance status. Performance status has both prognostic and therapeutic implications. Although performance status grading of patients is standard practice while on clinical trials, it is often overlooked during routine documentation. By grading patients' baseline performance status, clinicians are able to monitor subsequent changes resulting from disease and therapy. This allows clinicians to make treatment modifications as appropriate.

The Karnofsky Performance Scale and the Eastern Cooperative Oncology Group (ECOG) performance scale (also called Zubrod) are the two most commonly used scales in clinical practice and trials. The Karnofsky scale was developed in the 1940s by David Karnofsky and colleagues (Karnofsky, Abelmann, Craver, & Burchenal, 1948). The 11 levels evaluate functional status from death to perfect health, with a percentage score (0–100) assigned to each level. The ECOG performance scale has six levels (0–5); level 0 indicates fully ambulatory and functional and level 5 indicates death (Oken et al., 1982) (see Table 3-2). Modified versions of these scales are available for specific patient populations.

After evaluation of performance status, APNs may order diagnostic tests to continue the assessment for the presence and extent of cancer. These may include laboratory tests, imaging, and other procedures to facilitate obtaining tissue, tumor markers, molecular markers, and immunohistochemistry (IHC).

Diagnostic Evaluation

Laboratory Tests

Specific tests are conducted to further assess patients with a suspected malignancy. Initial laboratory tests for patients suspected of cancer usually include complete blood count (CBC), chemistry panel with renal and liver function, and coagulation studies. Assessment of blood counts will give valuable information in the workup of patients suspected of having a hematologic malignancy along with important baseline information prior to treatment for neoplastic disease. Liver function tests (LFTs) and coagulation panels can provide important data

Table 3-2. Comparison of Eastern Cooperative Oncology Group (ECOG) and Karnofsky Performance Scales

ECOG Grade	ECOG	Karnofsky Criteria	%
0	Fully active, able to carry on all predisease performance without restriction	Normal; no complaints; no evidence of disease	100
1	Restricted in physically strenuous activity but ambulatory and able to carry out work of a light or sedentary nature (e.g., light housework, office work)	Able to carry on normal activity; minor signs or symptoms of disease	90
		Normal activity with effort; some signs or symptoms of disease	80
2	Ambulatory and capable of all self-care but unable to carry out any work activities; up and about more than 50% of waking hours	Cares for self; unable to carry on normal activity or to do active work	70
		Requires occasional assistance but is able to care for most personal needs	60
3	Capable of only limited self-care; confined to bed or chair more than 50% of waking hours	Requires considerable assistance and frequent medical care	50
		Disabled; requires special care and assistance	40
4	Completely disabled; cannot carry on any self-care; totally confined to bed or chair	Severely disabled; hospital admission indicated although death not imminent	30
		Very sick; hospital admission necessary; active supportive treatment necessary	20
		Moribund; rapid progression of fatal processes	10
5	Dead	Dead	0

Note. Based on information from Karnofsky et al., 1948; Oken et al., 1982.

regarding the functional status of the liver, and electrolyte assessment allows a critical look at the renal system. Specific additional laboratory tests may be required based on patient presentation.

Imaging Tests

Imaging tests such as plain radiographs or x-rays, computed tomography (CT) scans, magnetic resonance imaging (MRI), or positron-emission tomography (PET) scans are ordered to assist clinicians in determining the location and extent of disease, staging the disease, or detecting recurrence. The American College of Radiology (ACR) developed Appropriateness Criteria for Diagnostic Imaging to assist clinicians with the identification of appropriate imaging modalities for specific clinical conditions (ACR, n.d.). ACR adopted the AQA definition of appropriateness:

> The concept of appropriateness, as applied to health care, balances risk and benefit of a treatment, test, or procedure in the context of available resources for an individual patient with specific characteristics. Appropriateness cri-

teria should provide guidance to supplement the clinician's judgment as to whether a patient is a reasonable candidate for the given treatment, test or procedure. (AQA, 2009, para. 2)

The factors to consider when selecting the appropriate imaging modality include tumor characteristics, sensitivity and specificity of the imaging modality, radiation dose, and cost-effectiveness (Mohammed et al., 2013). *Sensitivity* refers to the ability of the test to accurately identify a particular disease and is expressed as a percentage. This is calculated by dividing the number of patients who test positive for the disease by the total number of tested patients who actually have the disease. Sensitivity can vary in some diseases based on the stage or volume of disease. *Specificity* refers to the ability of the test to accurately identify the absence of a particular disease and also is expressed as a percentage. It is calculated by dividing the number of patients who test negative for the disease by the number of tested patients who do not have the disease. In general, highly sensitive tests are used to rule out a particular suspected disease, and highly specific tests are used to confirm or eliminate a suspected disease. The ideal diagnostic test would result in a positive result for affected individuals and a negative result for unaffected individuals. A *false positive* means that a positive result occurred in an individual who does not have the disease, and a *false negative* means that a negative result occurred in an individual who does have the disease. Diagnostic tests that have the greatest clinical utility are tests that have the greatest percentage of true-positive and true-negative results and the lowest percentage of false-positive and false-negative results.

APNs should consult with a radiologist if they have questions regarding the appropriateness of a certain imaging study. Although plain radiographs are one of the oldest and most common imaging tests, many additional imaging modalities are useful in the diagnosis and staging of cancer. Some of the more common tests will be discussed in the following section.

Plain radiographs: Conventional x-rays were discovered by William Roentgen in 1895 by exposing x-ray film to ionizing radiation that penetrated the body (Chen & Whitlow, 2011). During development of the x-ray film, the image of a body part with various densities ranges in color from black to white based on the amount of absorption of the x-ray radiation. For example, gas or air appears black, fat appears gray-black, soft tissue appears gray, and bone appears white (Chen & Whitlow, 2011).

Plain radiographs are most useful for evaluation of the bones but also are recommended for the initial evaluation of a soft tissue mass (Zoga et al., 2012). If a patient presents with bone pain, plain radiographs can visualize metastatic disease to the bone and are useful in ruling out impending or current fractures (see Figure 3-1). While a bone scan is generally a more sensitive assessment of osseous metastases, malignancies with purely lytic bone metastases, such as in multiple myeloma, are best evaluated by a skeletal survey of plain bone films (Roberts et al., 2012).

Chest radiographs are a relatively inexpensive, low-risk procedure to evaluate for cardiopulmonary disease (Mohammed et al., 2011). Most primary lung cancers are detected by routine chest radiograph (Ravenel et al., 2013). Chest radiographs should also be obtained as part of the initial staging evaluation of patients with malignancies that have a propensity to metastasize to the lungs, such as bone and soft tissue sarcomas, renal cell carcinoma, testicular carcinoma, melanoma, and head and neck carcinomas (Mohammed et al., 2013). Chest CT is more sensitive than chest radiograph to identify metastatic disease in the lungs and is indicated when the chest x-ray is negative or equivocal in a patient with a malignancy that has a high propensity for lung metastases (Mohammed et al., 2013).

Ultrasonography: Ultrasound is a noninvasive diagnostic test that uses sound waves with high frequencies that humans are unable to hear (Chen & Whitlow, 2011). A transducer probe that emits and receives sound waves is placed against the patient's skin with a thin layer of

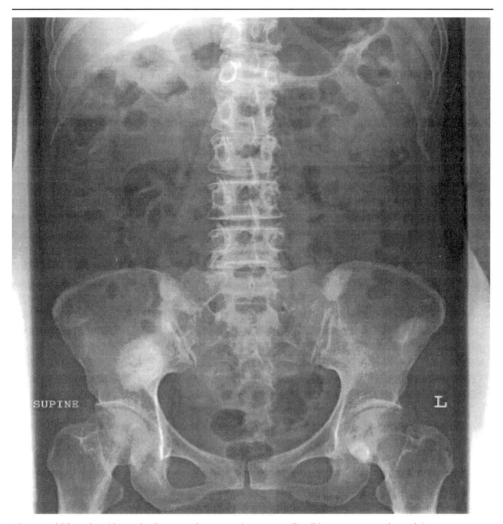

45-year-old female with newly diagnosed metastatic non-small cell lung cancer to the pelvis

Figure 3-1. Plain X-Ray Example of Metastatic Disease

Note. Figure courtesy of Pamela Hallquist Viale. Used with permission.

gel. As the sound waves encounter tissues and organs of varying density, they are reflected and "echo" back to the transducer, where they are converted into electric signals. The intensity of the echo influences the amplitude of the returning wave, which is depicted on a grayscale (or color) image. Tissues and organs are described by their echogenicity. Strong echoes, such as the liver or bone, appear a lighter gray-white. Soft tissue has moderate echogenicity and appears medium gray. Fluid is considered to have no echoes and appears black (Caserta, Chaudhry, & Bechtold, 2011). Ultrasound can be used to calculate the depth of the tissue (Chen & Whitlow, 2011).

Ultrasonography is commonly used to image abdominal organs (liver, gallbladder, pancreas, kidneys), reproductive organs, breasts, and heart and to evaluate fluid collections (pericardial, pleural, ascites) or deep vein thrombosis. In addition, ultrasound often is used to guide procedures such as thoracentesis, paracentesis, lesion biopsy, abscess drainage, and radiofrequency ablation (Chen & Whitlow, 2011). The utility of ultrasound is limited by its inability to penetrate through bone or air (bowel or lung) and its lower soft tissue resolution compared to CT. For example, there is variable visualization of midline abdominal organs when obscured by bowel gas (Chen & Whitlow, 2011).

Endoscopic ultrasonography (EUS) has become the standard of care for the staging of esophageal, gastric, pancreatic, and rectal cancers and often is used adjunctively to image lymphoma and lung, renal, and adrenal cancers (Kaul & Kothari, 2014). EUS provides the additional advantage of allowing a safe, minimally invasive method of histologic diagnosis with fine needle aspiration or core biopsy (Kaul & Kothari, 2014). EUS uses a flexible videoendoscope combined with a high-resolution ultrasound probe to image the histologic layers of the gastrointestinal (GI) tract. EUS is an outpatient procedure performed under moderate sedation and has a low rate of complications (Kaul & Kothari, 2014).

In rectal cancer, EUS is the preferred test for tumor staging (T stage) because it has a sensitivity of 88%–95% and specificity of 99% (Puli et al., 2009). In comparison, the accuracy of T staging is 65%–75% with abdominal CT and 75%–85% with MRI (Puli et al., 2009). EUS is also a highly sensitive method of determining T stage and node stage (N stage) in esophageal cancer, and recent data suggest that it is more accurate than CT (Kaul & Kothari, 2014). The reported accuracy of EUS in pancreatic cancer is 63%–94% for T staging and 44%–82% for N staging (Kaul & Kothari, 2014). Accurate preoperative staging assists in driving treatment decisions. EUS, similar to CT and PET, is limited in staging accuracy after neoadjuvant therapy because it is difficult to differentiate between tumor and post-treatment edema, inflammation, and fibrosis (Kaul & Kothari, 2014).

One of the best uses of ultrasonography is in guiding interventional procedures. EUS-guided fine needle aspiration is highly sensitive for malignancy and is very safe with a low risk of tumor seeding and a reported complication rate of 0%–6% (Puli et al., 2014). The procedure has a sensitivity of 80%–90% and a specificity of 100% in diagnosing pancreatic cancer (Kaul & Kothari, 2014). In lung cancer, EUS-guided fine needle aspiration has a median sensitivity of 89% and a specificity of 100% for the detection of malignant mediastinal (N2 or N3) lymph nodes (Silvestri et al., 2013). Transrectal ultrasound (TRUS) is the most frequently used initial imaging test performed in patients with suspected prostate cancer (Ghai & Toi, 2012). If an abnormality is found in the prostate-specific antigen (PSA) level or by DRE, the patient will undergo TRUS-guided biopsy. TRUS provides excellent imaging of the prostate, yet only 50%–70% of prostate cancers are visible on TRUS and 50% of hypoechoic lesions seen on TRUS are not malignant. Therefore, systematic biopsies are necessary to accurately detect malignancy. Typically, 12 core biopsy samples are obtained from the medial and lateral aspects of the peripheral zone of the prostate, and additional biopsies can be obtained if other suspicious areas are noted (Ghai & Toi, 2012).

Barium studies: Barium studies (e.g., esophagography, upper GI series, small bowel series, barium enema) are conducted to examine the esophagus, stomach, and small or large bowel (Freeman, 2008). Barium is radiopaque and therefore enhances the contrast between tissues. Barium studies are simple to perform, inexpensive, and highly sensitive; however, they are being superseded by endoscopy because of its advantages of direct visualization of the mucosa and opportunity to obtain a biopsy of suspicious tissue (Freeman, 2008).

Barium swallow or esophagography is useful in evaluating oropharyngeal and pharyngeal function, motility, and mucosal abnormalities (Freeman, 2008). The upper GI series includes the esophagus, stomach, and duodenum. Barium enema can screen the colon for suspected neoplasms, diverticular disease, or inflammatory bowel disease. Single-contrast barium studies use barium alone, whereas double-contrast studies use a combination of barium suspension and air to distend the GI tract so that no segment is obscured by a barium pool or coated poorly (Chen & Whitlow, 2011). In the upper GI double-contrast study, air is introduced into the GI lumen by administration of oral effervescent agents. For double-contrast evaluation of the lower GI tract with barium enema, barium is instilled into the colon per rectal tube, and air is introduced through the rectal tube to distend the colon (Bartram & Taylor, 2008). The diagnostic accuracy of double-contrast barium enemas to detect carcinoma is reported to be 75%–100%; however, it is limited to detection of luminal mucosal abnormalities and also requires skilled radiologic technique (Bartram & Taylor, 2008). CT colonography and colonoscopy are more accurate, particularly for smaller lesions or plaque-like lesions, and have largely replaced barium enemas for screening and diagnostic evaluation of colon cancer (Bartram & Taylor, 2008).

Computed tomography: CT is one of the most common diagnostic imaging techniques in oncology because it is the diagnostic imaging tool of choice for the chest, abdomen, and pelvis. CT shows cross-sectional views of the body as though looking up at it from the patient's feet. The CT scanner rotates around the patient to generate multidirectional x-rays that create cross-sectional two-dimensional images or computer-assisted construction of three-dimensional images (Chen & Whitlow, 2011). This examination may be obtained with or without contrast given orally, rectally, or intravenously. The specificity and sensitivity of CT vary with the type of tissue or organ being evaluated; for example, the sensitivity for contrast-enhanced CT to distinguish benign from malignant pulmonary nodules is 98% with a specificity of 58% (Kanne et al., 2012). These data suggest that nonenhancement is a strong predictor that the nodule is benign. In the staging of ovarian cancers, the accuracy is 94%, and the major limitation is in detection of small bowel surface, mesenteric, or peritoneal tumor implants (Mitchell et al., 2012).

CT is commonly used for staging malignant melanoma, bone and soft tissue sarcoma, and lung, ovarian, head and neck, GI, testicular, bladder, and renal cell cancers (Mohammed et al., 2013). It is particularly helpful for assessment of metastatic disease to the liver, and potential extrahepatic sites of disease in the abdomen and lung bases can be imaged during the same examination (Blake et al., 2011). CT is not ideal for differentiating tissue types in the evaluation of musculoskeletal malignancies because MRI is more sensitive to characterize soft tissue masses and bone involvement (Zoga et al., 2012). Both CT and MRI are imperfect in distinguishing between malignant and benign lesions, as well as between inflammation and neoplastic bone infiltration (Zoga et al., 2012).

Multislice CT and multidetector CT (MDCT) have significantly improved the speed of examination, increased diagnostic accuracy, allowed for decreased contrast load, reduced respiratory and cardiac motion artifact, and enhanced three-dimensional reconstruction capabilities (Chen & Whitlow, 2011). The spiral or helical CT scan is produced by an x-ray tube that continuously rotates around the patient, and the data from the x-ray beams is collected by multiple rows of detectors. MDCT has led to the development of CT angiography, which has replaced some of the more invasive imaging studies such as arteriography and other vascular studies (Chen & Whitlow, 2011). Likewise, MDCT can be used to perform arterial phase imaging for hypervascular liver lesions seen in metastases form renal cell, carcinoid, islet cell, thyroid, melanoma, and neuroendocrine tumors (Blake et al., 2011).

Another example of MDCT is CT colonography, which provides two-dimensional and three-dimensional images of the colon (Chen & Whitlow, 2011). CT colonography can image the mucosal surface of the colon as well as the bowel wall and other abdominal and pelvic structures. For this reason, it often is used instead of barium enemas, which are limited to images of the mucosal surface of the colon, or colonoscopy, which is a more invasive procedure (Chen & Whitlow, 2011). More than 95% of patients prefer CT colonography over colonoscopy, and it has a sensitivity of 93% and a specificity of 97% for detecting polyps larger than 1 cm (Dewhurst et al., 2011). In addition, its cross-sectional depiction allows characterization of tumors using the tumor-node-metastasis (TNM) staging system with reasonable T- and N-stage accuracies of 83% and 80%, respectively (Akin et al., 2012).

Most CT tables have a weight limit, thus limiting access for some patients. Also, CT scanners are not portable. Patients are required to lie still, sometimes for extended periods. For chest studies, patients must be able to hold their breath. Other limitations include the potential for anaphylactic reactions to the contrast medium, contrast-induced nephropathy, and radiation exposure (Chen & Whitlow, 2011).

Magnetic resonance imaging: MRI uses radiofrequency waves in the presence of a strong magnetic field, which detects different frequency emissions in the cells of the body to generate high-resolution, multiplanar images (Chen & Whitlow, 2011). The contrast most commonly used for MRI is gadolinium, which provides the additional advantage of absence of ionizing radiation (Chen & Whitlow, 2011). MRI can give valuable information regarding the specific characterization of tissues, function, and perfusion to provide three-dimensional images. MRI is commonly the diagnostic imaging technique of choice for brain, spinal cord, and musculoskeletal conditions. It also has a prominent role in imaging cardiac, hepatic, biliary, pancreatic, adrenal, renal, breast, and female pelvic conditions (Chen & Whitlow, 2011).

MRI is more sensitive than CT in determining soft tissue involvement, although MRI is generally performed following a plain x-ray because of its cost and limited availability in some settings (Zoga et al., 2012). For individual cancers, MRI is useful in tumors of the thorax, central nervous system, spinal cord, head and neck, kidneys, cervix, ovaries, endometrium, breast, and abdomen, as well as cancer of unknown primary (Chen & Whitlow, 2011). Magnetic resonance cholangiopancreatography is a specific MRI technique used to image pancreatobiliary malignancies in patients who are unable to tolerate endoscopic retrograde cholangiopancreatography (Chen & Whitlow, 2011).

Other MRI techniques: MRI spectroscopy, diffusion-weighted MRI, and dynamic contrast-enhanced MRI are three imaging modalities that combine functional imaging techniques with MRI to improve specificity (Akin et al., 2012). MRI spectroscopy produces three-dimensional graphs showing the relative concentrations of tissue metabolites within specified volumes of tissue (Akin et al., 2012). For example, large amounts of citrate are produced by healthy prostate tissue, and choline is elevated in prostate cancer; consequently, calculation of the ratio of choline plus creatine to citrate can be used to identify prostate cancer (Akin et al., 2012). Magnetic resonance spectroscopy can detect cellular metabolites before any change in tumor volume can be detected (Akin et al., 2012). Diffusion-weighted MRI measures the random movement of water molecules in tissue that allows for calculation of apparent diffusion coefficients (ADCs) for individual pixels that can be displayed as an image. Low ADCs are associated with malignancy because cancer cells are tightly and randomly packed together; thus, the diffusion of water molecules is more restricted than in normal tissues (Akin et al., 2012). Dynamic contrast-enhanced MRI evaluates tissue microvascular and perfusion properties based on the repeated acquisition of images during the passage of an intravenously administered contrast agent (Akin et al., 2012). Malignant tissue is distinguished from benign tissue by assessing the variation of the distribution of the contrast agent between vascular and extravascular spaces over time. For example, prostate cancer usually shows early, rapid, and intense enhancement with quick washout of contrast compared to noncancerous prostate tissue. Dynamic contrast-enhanced MRI has shown potential in assessing prostate cancer in preliminary studies, but further research is necessary to establish its clinical value and address technical challenges (Akin et al., 2012).

The disadvantages of MRI include cost, availability, length of time required, uncooperative patients, and small tube size, which limits its utility for obese or claustrophobic patients. MRI may be contraindicated in patients with certain pacemakers or other implanted metal devices.

Radionuclide imaging technique: Radionuclide imaging frequently is used in oncology. The technique involves administration of a radioactive material (or radiopharmaceutical), which is then detected by gamma camera. Images of body tissues that have taken up the radio-isotope are produced (Chen & Whitlow, 2011). Bone scans (or scintigraphy) and PET scans are the most common imaging modalities in this category. Images are useful in terms of functionality but less useful in the description of anatomy. Because of this, these scans often are completed in conjunction with an anatomic scan.

Positron-emission tomography scans: PET scans provide a noninvasive, quantitative assessment of biochemical and functional processes (Akin et al., 2012). A positron-labeled (radioactive) tracer, usually glucose (^{18}F-fluorodeoxyglucose [FDG]), is injected into the patient prior to scanning. Metabolically active areas will take up the glucose and will show up as "hot" spots on images produced by gamma camera tomography, giving specific information regarding malignant tissues (Chen & Whitlow, 2011). Figure 3-2 depicts a PET scan in a patient with non-Hodgkin lymphoma (NHL), and the sites of metabolic activity appear black. FDG uptake is reported as the standardized uptake value (SUV), which measures uptake of the tracer while controlling for variations in body weight (Podoloff et al., 2009). Therefore, a higher SUV correlates with increased levels of glucose metabolism and a greater intensity of PET images. Because the hallmark of cancer is elevated glucose metabolism, PET scanning is useful for the staging of many cancers, improves the accuracy of assessment for metastatic disease, and is used to assess treatment response (Akin et al., 2012).

In particular, PET scans are used for the staging of lung cancer, lymphoma, melanoma, colorectal cancer, and breast cancer (Chen & Whitlow, 2011). PET imaging often can differentiate between benign and malignant processes; tissue necrosis from recurrent tumor; and low-grade from high-grade tumors. For this reason, PET is used to evaluate a solitary pulmonary nodule or mass that is indeterminate by CT and has a sensitivity of 83%–97% and a specificity of 69%–100% (Kanne et al., 2012). However, certain tissues, such as kidney and brain, take up glucose, which limits the evaluation by PET scanning. False-positive results may occur for benign processes, such as muscle uptake after exercise and selective cardiac conditions, because of physiologic uptake of FDG. Nonmalignant conditions, such as infection or inflammation, can also result in false-positive results due to FDG uptake (Podoloff et al., 2009). For example, PET is generally not clinically useful to distinguish low-grade prostate cancers from benign conditions, such as benign prostatic hyperplasia and chronic inflammation, because the

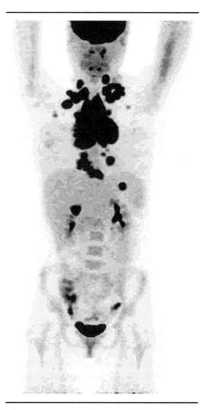

Figure 3-2. Positron-Emission Tomography Scan of a Patient With Non-Hodgkin Lymphoma

Note. Figure courtesy of Laura J. Zitella. Used with permission.

degree of FDG uptake is similar (Akin et al., 2012). False-negative results may occur in slow-growing or low-grade malignancies because of limited glucose uptake.

Combined PET-CT has enhanced the clinical value of PET, as increased glucose metabolism, or FDG uptake, associated with a suspicious mass is highly suggestive of malignancy (Podoloff et al., 2009). PET-CT is now one of the most accurate, routinely used imaging tools for detecting, staging, and assessing treatment response in several cancers. The accuracy of PET-CT in tumor staging for patients with a variety of cancers was 84%, compared to side-by-side PET and CT (76%), CT alone (63%), or PET alone (64%) (Podoloff et al., 2009). In fact, PET-CT scan is the most sensitive and specific radiologic test in lymphoma and improves staging accuracy and assessment of treatment response (Cheson, 2011). Likewise, PET-CT is recommended for routine staging in non-small cell lung cancer because it significantly increases the accuracy of tumor staging by improving the detection of chest wall involvement, mediastinal invasion, and distant metastases (Ravenel et al., 2013).

One of the biggest limitations of PET scanning is cost and insurance coverage. Other limitations of PET include diminished resolution when compared to CT and that combined PET-CT typically employs a noncontrast CT rather than a diagnostic CT (Podoloff et al., 2009). Because PET cannot distinguish FDG uptake due to benign causes versus malignancy, false-positive results occur (Podoloff et al., 2009). Alternatively, false-negative results can occur when the malignancy is not sufficiently metabolically active (Podoloff et al., 2009). The high concentration of FDG found in the normal brain limits the sensitivity of PET for detection of brain metastases; therefore, MRI remains the preferred modality for brain imaging (Akin et al., 2012).

Patients are required to fast for at least eight hours prior to the procedure, and the fasting blood glucose must be within a normal range. Diabetic patients are not to take oral hypoglycemic agents or insulin after midnight.

Scans for Specific Situations

Breast imaging: Mammograms, which are essentially plain x-rays of the breasts, are performed to detect and characterize abnormalities of the breast suggestive of breast cancer or other breast diseases (ACR, 2014a, 2014b). Abnormalities of the breast that are concerning for malignancy include masses, calcifications, and architectural distortion or asymmetry. Malignant lesions are usually irregular and heterogeneous, hypervascular masses, whereas benign lesions are more frequently smooth (Akin et al., 2012). In addition, cancer often has necrotic sites that undergo calcification, so identification of these microcalcifications allows mammography to detect small and noninvasive cancers (Akin et al., 2012).

Mammography detects 86%–91% of all breast malignancies, and early detection of breast cancer and advances in treatment are estimated to have resulted in a 30% decrease in breast cancer mortality (Akin et al., 2012; Harvey et al., 2012). Almost half of all breast cancers can be seen on mammogram before they are palpable. When a biopsy is recommended based on mammography, breast cancer will be diagnosed in 25%–45% of cases (Akin et al., 2012). However, a negative mammogram should not exclude biopsy if a palpable mass is present (Harvey et al., 2012).

Two types of mammograms exist: a screening mammogram and a diagnostic mammogram. A screening mammogram is an x-ray examination of the breast of an asymptomatic woman, whereas a diagnostic mammogram is performed in a patient with signs or symptoms of breast disease or who has had prior imaging findings requiring follow-up (ACR, 2014b). During a screening mammogram, two x-ray images are obtained from each breast: a craniocaudal image (taken from the top of the breast) and a mediolateral oblique image (taken from the side of the breast) (National Comprehensive Cancer Network® [NCCN®], 2014a). If a diagnostic mammogram is ordered, it should be performed under the supervision of the interpreting radiologist, who will review the images while the patient is still present so that additional images can be obtained if necessary (Harvey et al., 2012). Specialized views, such as spot compression or magnified views, may be necessary for closer evaluation of nodules, architecture, or microcalcifications (Harvey et al., 2012). Comparison of new findings to previous mammographic results is important to enhance detection of malignancy. All mammography in the United States must be performed according to the regulations published by the U.S. Food and Drug Administration (FDA) in the Mammography Quality Standards Act (U.S. FDA, 2006). Mammography findings are reported in a standardized manner as defined by the ACR Breast Imaging Reporting and Data System (BI-RADS®) (Sickles et al., 2013). The BI-RADS system uses the following categories to describe imaging findings: 0 = incomplete study, 1 = negative (no abnormalities noted), 2 = benign, 3 = probably benign, 4 = suspicious, 5 = highly suggestive of malignancy, or 6 = known biopsy-proven malignancy. Repeat imaging or biopsy may be recommended based on the BI-RADS category.

Ultrasonography is used as an adjunct test for high-risk women with dense breast tissue or when a lesion found on mammography cannot be determined to be cystic or solid. The negative predictive value is more than 97% when both mammography and ultrasound are negative or show a benign-appearing lesion (Harvey et al., 2012). The addition of ultrasound to mammography detects 93%–100% of breast cancers (Harvey et al., 2012). In young women (younger than age 40), ultrasound is the initial imaging modality of choice to evaluate a palpable breast mass because the sensitivity is higher than mammogram (95.7% compared to 60.9%) with similar specificity (89.2% and 94.4%, respectively) (Harvey et al., 2012). Ultrasound is also useful for directing accurate fine needle aspiration or core biopsy, especially if the mass is difficult to palpate, mobile, small, or deep, or if multiple masses are present (Harvey et al., 2012).

MRI of the breast serves as an adjunct to mammography for patients at high risk for breast cancer (ACR, 2014a; NCCN, 2014a). MRI of the breast is more sensitive for the detection and characterization of breast disease than mammography and can be used to guide biopsy (ACR, 2014a). Evidence supports annual breast MRI for individuals with a lifetime risk of breast cancer of 20% or greater, such as those with a *BRCA1* or *BRCA2* mutation or a strong family history (ACR, 2014a; NCCN, 2014a). In addition, experts recommend annual breast MRI in individuals who were treated with chest irradiation between ages 10 and 30; individuals with Li-Fraumeni syndrome, Cowden syndrome, or Bannayan-Riley-Ruvalcaba syndrome; or individuals with a first-degree relative with any of these syndromes (NCCN, 2014a). MRI also is useful in multifocal or multicentric disease (ACR, 2014a).

Detection of bone metastasis: Radionuclide bone scanning is the primary imaging test to detect osseous metastasis for most tumor types because it is highly sensitive for osseous abnormalities and allows for a total body survey (Roberts et al., 2012). Bone scanning involves the injection of a radiopharmaceutical agent (usually technetium-99m methylene diphosphonate) that is taken up by osteoblasts followed by a scan within several hours, which usually reflects osteoblastic activity in the bone (see Figure 3-3). Currently, bone scans are generally used for staging lung cancer, high-risk prostate cancer, and stage II–IV breast cancer (Roberts et al., 2012). They are particularly useful in patients with multifocal or extensive disease, but a single suspicious lesion may be due to benign causes; thus, additional diagnostic evaluation with CT or MRI is recommended (Roberts et al., 2012). CT can show axial bone metastasis, and both CT and MRI show more detail than bone scan (Roberts et al., 2012).

Bone scans are highly sensitive but are not very specific, so the use of PET and MRI is increasing, as studies have shown equivalent or improved sensitivity and specificity (Roberts et al., 2012). The utility of a bone scan also varies based on the type of malignancy. For exam-

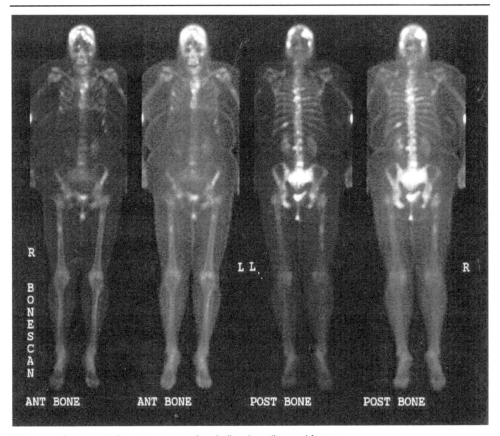

Widespread metastatic breast cancer to the skull, spine, ribs, and femur

Figure 3-3. Bone Scan of a Patient With Breast Cancer With Metastatic Disease

Note. Figure courtesy of Pamela Hallquist Viale. Used with permission.

ple, malignancies with purely lytic bone metastases, such as multiple myeloma, generally do not take up the radionuclide and result in a negative bone scan, whereas MRI is very sensitive.

Diagnostic Procedures

Endoscopy

Multiple studies or procedures may be conducted to facilitate biopsies, including procedures that provide direct visualization and access to suspicious tissue. Upper GI endoscopy, also called upper esophagogastroduodenoscopy (EGD), is the diagnostic procedure of choice for upper GI cancers. EGD uses a thin, easily maneuvered endoscope to visualize and biopsy suspicious lesions of the larynx, upper airways, esophagus, stomach, and upper duodenum (Kaul & Kothari, 2014). Most patients require only mild sedation.

Sigmoidoscopy

Flexible sigmoidoscopy can be used to visualize the distal colon. A flexible scope is inserted through the anus and advanced approximately 50 cm into the lower large intestine after cleansing with a small enema (Holme, Bretthauer, Fretheim, Odgaard-Jensen, & Hoff, 2013). The interior wall of the intestine can be inspected for benign lesions and malignant tumors, and sigmoidoscopy allows for removal of lesions or biopsy during the procedure (Holme et al., 2013). The modality is both sensitive and specific and can be performed by either physicians or APNs trained in the procedure. It is a relatively safe procedure with a rate of complications less than 1% (Holme et al., 2013).

In a meta-analysis, flexible sigmoidoscopy reduced the risk of death from colorectal cancer by 28% (95% confidence interval [CI] [21%, 35%]) (Holme et al., 2013). However, because of the length of the scope, malignancies located in the proximal colon may be missed, so it is not as sensitive as colonoscopy. If an abnormality, such as a polyp, is found on sigmoidoscopy, a follow-up colonoscopy should be performed.

Colonoscopy

Colonoscopy visualizes the entire colon with a flexible scope and can facilitate biopsy of any suspicious areas, removal of polyps, and collection of stool specimens. For this reason, it is the preferred screening procedure for the colon (NCCN, 2015d). An estimated 40% of colorectal cancers could be prevented with colonoscopy screening, particularly cancers of the proximal colon, which are more likely to be missed with flexible sigmoidoscopy (Nishihara et al., 2013). Quality indicators for colonoscopy include imaging from the rectum to the cecum, rectal retroflexion, thorough patient preparation to remove residual stool, sufficient distension of the colon to facilitate inspection, withdrawal time, and complete excision of polyps (NCCN, 2015d). (See Chapter 1 for further information regarding screening for colon cancer.)

However, this test is invasive and requires total cleansing of the colon as well as sedation during the examination. Possible complications include bowel perforation and hemorrhage. Contraindications to colonoscopy include acute diverticulitis, significant adhesions in the pelvis or abdomen, acute exacerbations of inflammatory bowel disease, suspected bowel perforation, recent pulmonary embolus or myocardial infarction, and blood coagulation abnormalities.

Laparoscopy

Laparoscopy allows clinicians to visualize the abdominal cavity and is useful for the staging and diagnosis of intra-abdominal malignancies. In traditional laparoscopy, a thin telescope is inserted through a small incision or puncture in the anterior abdominal wall while the patient is under local anesthesia and mild sedation. Using this method, clinicians may diagnose intra-abdominal metastases. This may prevent certain patients from undergoing a major surgery only to find metastatic or unresectable disease.

Enhanced sensitivity of imaging has decreased the need for laparoscopy for staging and evaluation. However, laparoscopy has become quite common as a minimally invasive surgical method. For example, laparoscopic-assisted colon resection is preferred over open colectomy because it results in earlier return of bowel function, decreased postoperative pain, decreased length of stay, decreased morbidity, and improved cosmesis (Kumar & Lee, 2013). Likewise, laparoscopic surgical staging of early ovarian cancer has been shown to be safe and feasible with decreased morbidity and length of stay compared with laparotomy (Park et al., 2013). Complications of laparoscopy include intestinal injury from the trocar, bleeding, and port-site tumor seeding (Kumar & Lee, 2013; Park et al., 2013).

Bronchoscopy

Bronchoscopy is a diagnostic procedure that involves insertion of a flexible bronchoscope to directly visualize bronchial tissue and obtain cells or tissue for cytologic or pathologic examination (Du Rand et al., 2013). It is a well-tolerated procedure that is performed on an out-patient basis with conscious sedation and topical anesthesia. Bronchoscopy is used to diagnose lung cancer, interstitial lung disease, and pulmonary infection. The diagnostic yield from bronchoscopy is 85% or greater if the tumor is visible within the bronchial tree; therefore, it is preferred for central tumors (Du Rand et al., 2013). Complications of bronchoscopy are rare (1%) but may include cardiac arrhythmias, bleeding, bronchospasm, cough, dyspnea, sore throat, respiratory failure, pneumothorax, and pulmonary edema (Du Rand et al., 2013).

Mediastinoscopy

Mediastinoscopy is most commonly used to assess mediastinal lymph node involvement for the staging of lung cancer. The examination is conducted by a thoracic surgeon in the operating room while the patient is under general anesthesia. The surgeon makes an incision in the suprasternal area and inserts the mediastinoscope alongside the trachea, which provides visualization of the superior mediastinum to enable biopsy of the mediastinal lymph nodes (Silvestri et al., 2013). Most patients are discharged the same day, and the rates of morbidity and mortality as a result of this procedure are low (2% and 0.08%, respectively) (Silvestri et al., 2013). A videomediastinoscope allows better visualization, more extensive lymph node sampling, and the performance of a lymph node dissection (Silvestri et al., 2013). Complications of mediastinoscopy may include hemorrhage, pneumothorax, recurrent or phrenic nerve injury, tracheal or esophageal injury, wound infection, or difficulties with anesthesia (Silvestri et al., 2013).

Thoracoscopy

Thoracoscopy, also known as video-assisted thoracic surgery, involves a small incision for the insertion of an open-tube scope for removal of fluid and biopsy of the pleural surface. It is a minimally invasive procedure and is done while the patient is under general anesthesia. It involves the creation of a pneumothorax and allows for visualization of the total visceral and parietal pleural surfaces, as well as biopsy of suspicious areas. The average rate of complications is 2% and includes hemorrhage, respiratory failure, prolonged air leak, intercostal neuritis, and port-site metastases (Silvestri et al., 2013).

Biopsy and Histopathology

Almost without exception, a tissue biopsy must be obtained for the clinician to make a diagnosis of malignancy. Histopathology is an assessment that categorizes the tumor according to its corresponding normal tissue type or the cell type that it most closely resembles (Compton et al., 2012). For example, hepatocellular carcinoma is derived from liver tissue, breast carcinoma from breast tissue, and osteosarcoma from bone.

Biopsy techniques may vary among differing tumor types and include fine needle aspiration, core needle biopsy, incisional biopsy, and excisional biopsy. Often, a diagnostic test such as colonoscopy or imaging such as CT is necessary to locate the tumor for biopsy. Methods of biopsies are discussed in Chapter 5. The clinician obtaining the biopsy tissue must ensure that the specimen is adequate in quantity, representative of the suspicious tissue, and well preserved.

A pathologist evaluates the tissue by various means to determine whether malignancy exists. For most specimens, microscopy with histochemical stains is adequate to make a diagnosis. Tissue removed during a biopsy or surgery must be cut into thin sections, placed on slides, and stained with dyes in order for it to be examined under a microscope (NCI, 2010). The tissue must be frozen or embedded in paraffin to make it firm enough to be cut into thin sections.

Permanent (paraffin-embedded) sections are prepared by placing the tissue in fixative (usually formalin) to preserve the tissue, processing it with additional solutions, and then placing it in paraffin wax. After the wax has hardened, the tissue is cut into very thin slices, which are placed on slides and stained. A permanent section provides the best quality for examination by the pathologist and produces more accurate results than a frozen section, but the process usually takes several days (NCI, 2010). All tissue samples are prepared as permanent sections, but sometimes frozen sections are also prepared.

Frozen sections are prepared by freezing the sample and slicing the frozen tissue into thin slices. They can be done in about 15–20 minutes, so they are used during surgery when an immediate answer is needed to ascertain if a malignancy is present to determine the course of an operation (NCI, 2010).

The pathologist examines the prepared slides under a microscope and renders a histologic assessment based on the size, shape, and appearance of the cells (NCI, 2010). Figure 3-4 depicts a slide from a patient with Hodgkin lymphoma, which is diagnosed by the presence of the characteristic Reed-Sternberg cell. In addition to microscopy, other diagnostic tests to assess biochemical, molecular, genetic, immunologic, or functional characteristics of the tumor or normal tissues have become important or essential to precisely classify malignancies (Compton et al., 2012). These include IHC, cytogenetics, fluorescence in situ hybridization (FISH), flow cytometry, polymerase chain reaction, and serum tumor markers. Table 3-3 describes these techniques and their use in diagnosis.

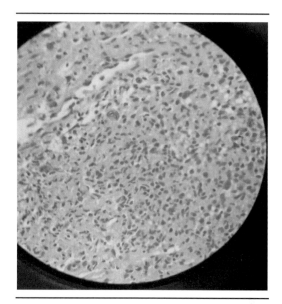

Figure 3-4. Microscopy of a Reed-Sternberg Cell in a Patient With Hodgkin Lymphoma

Note. Figure courtesy of Laura J. Zitella. Used with permission.

Cancer Biomarkers

Biomarkers are molecules found in blood, body fluids, or tissues that are a sign of a normal process, an abnormal process, a condition, or a disease (Research Advocacy Network, 2010). A cancer biomarker is a biomarker that can identify and measure aspects of malignant growth, contributing to the detection, diagnosis, classification, prognosis, or monitoring of a specific cancer or response to therapy. Cancer biomarkers (or tumor markers) include proteins, genetic markers (abnormal chromosomes or oncogenes), hormones, hormone receptors, oncofetal antigens, enzymes, or other substances produced by tumor cells or in response to tumor growth (Febbo et al., 2011). The ideal tumor marker would be specific for the suspected malignancy as well as sensitive to changes in tumor growth and response (Febbo et al., 2011). Cancer biomarkers used to play a limited role in patients with cancer because early serum tumor markers had limited sensitivity and specificity for malignancy. However, with advances in the understanding of the molecular basis of cancer, cancer biomarkers are playing a more prominent role in the detection, diagnosis, prognosis, and

Table 3-3. Diagnostic Tests Used in Oncology

Test	Description
Microscopy	Microscopy uses magnification to visualize cells to determine morphology and staining characteristics. It is the oldest and most commonly used diagnostic technique in pathology but is limited by its inability to distinguish cells that look the same yet are molecularly different.
Immunohistochemistry (IHC)	IHC is a technique used to identify specific antigens in different kinds of tissue. The tissue is treated with an antibody that binds to the specific antigen. The antibody is tagged with a radioisotope, a fluorescent dye, or an enzyme that produces a color reaction so that the antibody-antigen complex is visible under a microscope. IHC is used to help diagnose cancer, identify biomarkers, and detect the presence of microorganisms.
Flow cytometry	Flow cytometry is a technique that measures cellular properties while the individual cells move in a fluid stream through an electronic detector that is capable of rapidly analyzing multiple physical and chemical properties. Cells can be sorted so that additional analysis can be performed on a subset of cells using monoclonal antibodies that bind to intracellular proteins or proteins expressed on the cell surface. For example, if a monoclonal population of cells is identified, a panel of antibodies can be used to identify the proteins expressed by those cells to determine their phenotype and assist with diagnosis. When flow cytometry is used to determine the phenotype of a population of cells, it is referred to as *immunophenotyping*.
Cytogenetics	Cytogenetics is the microscopic analysis of chromosomes during metaphase when they align in the midline of the cell. Typically, 20 cells in metaphase are analyzed by staining them to produce specific bands, which can be viewed under a microscope. Cytogenetics is also known as conventional cytogenetics, chromosome analysis, or karyotyping. Cytogenetics identifies the complete karyotype, including the number of chromosomes in the cell as well as chromosomal abnormalities, such as translocations, inversions, and deletions. The disadvantages of this test are that it requires live, dividing cells and it cannot detect genetic mutations unless there is a large structural chromosomal abnormality.
Fluorescence in situ hybridization (FISH)	FISH combines standard microscopic cytogenetic analysis with molecular methods to detect specific DNA sequences or RNA targets using fluorescent probes. The advantage of FISH over conventional cytogenetics is that it does not require actively dividing cells and is more sensitive for specific chromosomal or genetic mutations. The disadvantage is that each FISH test is specific for one target (e.g., *HER2*), whereas conventional cytogenetics evaluates all of the chromosomes in the cell.
Polymerase chain reaction (PCR)	PCR can be performed with DNA or RNA. Very small amounts of DNA or RNA are needed because DNA sequences are amplified and copied to produce enough DNA to be tested (DNA-PCR). For RNA, the enzyme reverse transcriptase is used to synthesize DNA from the RNA. The resulting DNA copy (cDNA) is then amplified as in conventional DNA-PCR. This technique is known as the reverse-transcriptase polymerase chain reaction, or RT-PCR. Because small amounts of DNA and RNA are needed, this is a highly sensitive test to detect specific genes and mutations.
Gene expression profiling	Uses DNA or RNA microarrays to analyze the genome for expression of multiple genes at the same time.

Note. Based on information from Craig & Foon, 2008; Igbokwe & Lopez-Terrada, 2011; Olsen, 2013.

treatment of malignancy (Febbo et al., 2011). Biomarkers are measured in the serum or tissue of origin.

Types of Cancer Biomarkers

Many types of biomarkers exist, and an individual biomarker may be associated with more than one indication. Diagnostic markers are biomarkers that aid in the diagnosis or classification of a malignancy. For example, FISH can identify the presence of the Philadelphia chromosome, which is pathognomonic for chronic myeloid leukemia (Febbo et al., 2011).

Prognostic markers are cancer biomarkers that predict a clinical outcome, such as overall survival or progression-free survival, regardless of the treatment administered (Febbo et al., 2011). Examples of prognostic markers in breast cancer include *HER2* gene overexpression, which portends a poorer prognosis, and estrogen receptor (ER) positivity, which predicts a longer disease-free survival (Hammond et al., 2010).

Predictive markers predict the likely benefit of a specific class or type of therapy for an individual patient and are used to guide treatment decisions (Febbo et al., 2011). *HER2* gene overexpression is not only a prognostic factor but also a predictive biomarker because *HER2*-positive malignancies respond to trastuzumab, and *HER2*-negative malignancies do not (Febbo et al., 2011). Similarly, ER and progesterone receptor (PR) status predicts the response of breast cancer to hormone therapy, thereby guiding the clinician in choice of therapy (Hammond et al., 2010).

Companion diagnostic markers may be diagnostic, prognostic, or predictive. A companion diagnostic biomarker is a biomarker that has been proved to be associated with a beneficial response to a particular therapy (Febbo et al., 2011). An example of a companion diagnostic biomarker is the *BRAF* V600E mutation, found in 30%–60% of melanomas, which confers sensitivity to BRAF inhibitors, such as vemurafenib or dabrafenib (Febbo et al., 2011).

Clinical Utility

Numerous cancer biomarkers are FDA-approved, yet most lack clinical utility. *Clinical utility* means that the biomarker provides significant clinical information that is not available from histopathologic or other data to improve clinical decision making and patient outcomes (Febbo et al., 2011). Table 3-4 lists common cancer biomarkers with clinical utility. For example, the use of alpha-fetoprotein and beta human chorionic gonadotropin is routine in the staging, diagnosis, and prognosis of testicular cancer. Alpha-fetoprotein can also help distinguish seminomatous from nonseminomatous testicular cancer, as seminomatous testicular cancers do no excrete alpha-fetoprotein. In contrast, carcinoembryonic antigen (CEA) is positive in many patients with colorectal cancer but cannot be used as a screening test because elevated CEA levels are possible in the absence of colon cancer and also may occur in other types of malignancy such as breast cancer (NCCN, 2015a, 2015c). Another example is PSA, a cancer biomarker for prostate cancer that is not diagnostic, prognostic, or predictive. Diagnosis of prostate cancer relies on pathology, the Gleason score remains the single most prognostic feature of localized cancer, and PSA does not predict response to treatment (Febbo et al., 2011).

Although most serum tumor markers lack the sensitivity and specificity to be useful in screening for primary disease, they can be useful to monitor treatment efficacy and may indicate progression or regression of disease. Examples of serum tumor markers that may be used for surveillance of disease progression or recurrence include CA 27.29 in breast cancer, CEA for colorectal cancer, CA 125 in ovarian cancer, and PSA for prostate cancer (NCCN, 2014b, 2015a, 2015c, 2015d, 2015g).

Table 3-4. Common Cancer Biomarkers With Accepted Clinical Utility or Emerging Evidence for Clinical Utility

Biomarker	Molecular Type	Test	Cancer Type	Clinical Use
ER, PR	Tumor protein	IHC	Breast	Diagnostic Prognostic (positive) Predictive for hormonal therapy (tamoxifen, aromatase inhibitors)
HER2	Tumor protein or gene amplification or overexpression	FISH, IHC	Breast Gastric	Breast cancer: • Diagnostic • Prognostic (negative) • Predictive for anti-HER2 therapy (trastuzumab, lapatinib, pertuzumab)
Oncotype DX®	Tumor RNA	21-gene RT-PCR expression assay	Breast	Prognostic Predictive
Mamma-Print®*	Tumor RNA	70-gene microarray expression assay	Breast	Prognostic
CTCs*	Serum CTCs	Cell surface staining and magnetic separation	Breast Colorectal Prostate	Breast cancer: Surveillance of patients with metastatic disease Colorectal and prostate cancer: Prognostic
KRAS mutation	Tumor DNA	PCR, multiplex assays, or direct sequencing	Colorectal Non-small cell lung*	Predictive for anti-EGFR therapy (cetuximab, panitumumab) Prognostic (negative)
MSI and/or MMR protein loss	Tumor DNA for MSI testing with PCR; tumor IHC for MMR proteins	PCR, IHC	Colorectal	Screening Prognostic (positive) Predictive for lack of benefit with adjuvant single-agent fluoropyrimidine therapy
CEA	Serum protein	Immunoassay	Colorectal Breast	Surveillance
ColoPrint®*	Tumor mRNA	18-gene microarray assay	Colorectal	Prognostic in stage II
Oncotype DX Colon®*	Tumor mRNA	12-gene RT-PCR gene expression assay	Colorectal	Prognostic in stage II
EGFR mutation	Tumor DNA	PCR, multiplex assays, or direct sequencing	Non-small cell lung	Predictive for anti-EGFR therapy (gefitinib, erlotinib)

(Continued on next page)

Table 3-4. Common Cancer Biomarkers With Accepted Clinical Utility or Emerging Evidence for Clinical Utility *(Continued)*

Biomarker	Molecular Type	Test	Cancer Type	Clinical Use
BRAF mutation	Tumor DNA	PCR, multiplex assays, or direct sequencing	Melanoma	Melanoma: Predictive for anti-*BRAF* therapy (vemurafenib, dabrafenib) Colorectal cancer: • Prognostic • Predictive for anti-*BRAF* therapy (vemurafenib, dabrafenib)
EML4-ALK gene fusion	Tumor DNA	FISH	Non-small cell lung	Predictive for anti-*ALK* therapy (crizotinib)
ERCC1	Tumor protein	IHC, FISH	Non-small cell lung	Predictive for poor response to platinum chemotherapy
PSA	Serum protein	Immunoassay	Prostate	Diagnostic
FLT3-ITD mutation	Tumor DNA	PCR, multiplex assays, or direct sequencing	AML	Predictive Prognostic (negative)
CEBPA mutation	Tumor DNA	PCR, multiplex assays, or direct sequencing	AML	Predictive Prognostic (positive if normal cytogenetics and in absence of *FLT3*-ITD)
NPM1 mutation	Tumor DNA	PCR, multiplex assays, or direct sequencing	AML	Predictive Prognostic (positive if normal cytogenetics and in absence of *FLT3*-ITD)
KIT mutation	Tumor DNA	PCR, multiplex assays, or direct sequencing	AML GIST	AML: Prognostic (negative if present with t(8;21), inv(16), or t(16;16) mutations) AML and GIST: Predictive for anti-*KIT* therapy (imatinib)
BCR-ABL mutation	Tumor DNA	PCR, multiplex assays, or direct sequencing	CML ALL	CML and ALL: Predictive for anti-*BCR-ABL* therapy (imatinib, dasatinib, nilotinib) ALL: Prognostic (negative)
Alpha-fetoprotein	Serum protein	Immunoassay	Nonseminomatous testicular	Diagnostic Prognostic Surveillance
Human chorionic gonadotropin-beta	Serum protein	Immunoassay	Nonseminomatous or seminomatous testicular	Prognostic Surveillance
CA 19-9	Serum carbohydrate	Immunoassay	Pancreatic	Surveillance

(Continued on next page)

Table 3-4. Common Cancer Biomarkers With Accepted Clinical Utility or Emerging Evidence for Clinical Utility *(Continued)*

Biomarker	Molecular Type	Test	Cancer Type	Clinical Use
CA 125	Serum protein	Immunoassay	Ovarian	Surveillance
Thyroglob-ulin	Serum protein	Immunoassay	Thyroid	Surveillance

* Biomarkers with emerging evidence; not established

ALL—acute lymphoblastic leukemia/lymphoma; AML—acute myeloid leukemia; CA—cancer antigen; CEA—carcinoembryonic antigen; CML—chronic myeloid leukemia; CTC—circulating tumor cell; EGFR—epidermal growth factor receptor; ER—estrogen receptor; FISH—fluorescence in situ hybridization; GIST—gastrointestinal stromal tumor; IHC—immunohistochemistry; MMR—mismatch repair; mRNA—messenger RNA; MSI—microsatellite instability; PCR—polymerase chain reaction; PR—progesterone receptor; PSA—prostate-specific antigen; RT-PCR—reverse-transcriptase polymerase chain reaction

Note. Based on information from Duffy & Crown, 2013; Febbo et al., 2011; National Cancer Institute, 2011; National Comprehensive Cancer Network, 2015a.

Overview of Staging and Grading

Staging is a process that determines the location and extent of the primary cancer. Stage is a significant factor in determination of prognosis and selection of treatment (Compton et al., 2012). The goal of staging is to provide a common language for all clinicians to use in the care and treatment of cancer; therefore, accuracy is essential (Compton et al., 2012). Historically, staging was primarily anatomic, but other factors are increasingly being incorporated into staging systems.

The TNM staging system is used for most solid cancers. It was developed and is maintained by the American Joint Committee on Cancer (AJCC) and the International Union Against Cancer (Compton et al., 2012). This system undergoes continual evaluation and revision. In the TNM staging system, the stage is determined by T, the size or extent of tumor; N, the extent of lymph node involvement; and M, metastases (Compton et al., 2012). Each malignancy has staging criteria unique to the features of the disease. For example, the size of the tumor is prognostic in breast cancer, whereas the depth of invasion is important in colon cancer. Therefore, the T in breast cancer is based on the size of the tumor, and the T in colon cancer is based on the depth of invasion. T, N, and M are defined specifically for each tumor type and then grouped into stages based on prognosis (Compton et al., 2012). Because hematologic malignancies have different features than solid tumors, they are staged with disease-specific systems rather than TNM staging.

Stage may be defined at several points after diagnosis. *Clinical staging* refers to assessment of the extent of the cancer before initiation of treatment (surgery, systemic or radiation therapy, active surveillance, or palliative care) or within four months after the date of diagnosis, whichever is shorter, as long as the cancer has not clearly progressed during that time frame (Compton et al., 2012). Clinical staging incorporates information obtained from symptoms; physical examination; endoscopic examinations; imaging studies of the tumor, regional lymph nodes, and metastases; biopsies of the primary tumor; and surgical exploration without resection. *Pathologic staging* refers to assessment of the extent of the cancer based on surgical specimens (Compton et al., 2012). Stage also may be determined after neoadjuvant therapy before surgery; at the time of recurrence; and for cancers identified at autopsy (Compton et al., 2012). It is important to identify the type of staging: clinical, pathologic, postneoadjuvant, or recurrent. The nomenclature for clinical staging is cT, cN, and cM, and pathologic staging is denoted as pT, pN, and pM. Postneoadjuvant therapy can be clinical staging, denoted as "yc," or pathologic, denoted as "yp." However, the postneoadjuvant therapy stage is not used for cancer registry purposes because it would not accurately depict the stage at diagnosis if the patient had a response to therapy. Staging at the time of recurrence is documented as rTNM, and staging at the time of autopsy is documented as aTNM (Compton et al., 2012).

Stage groups are based on the TNM assessments, and the stage group correlates with prognosis. There are four stage groups from I to IV, where stage I is early-stage disease and each subsequent stage indicates increasing severity of the disease (Compton et al., 2012). Stage I generally denotes cancers that are smaller or less deeply invasive without spread to the lymph nodes. Stage II and III are cancers with increasing tumor burden or nodal extent. Stage IV indicates presence of distant metastases at diagnosis. The primary TNM groupings are purely clinical or pathologic; however, clinical and pathologic information can be combined to determine stage (Compton et al., 2012). For example, a patient with colon cancer may undergo colon resection with lymph node sampling for a pathologic T and N, and CT scan to assess for metastases for a clinical M.

The grade of a tumor is distinct from the stage. Grading indicates the degree of differentiation of a tumor (Compton et al., 2012). In plain terms, low-grade tumors are well differentiated, which means that the tumor cells closely resemble the tissue of origin. Low-grade tumors generally are associated with a favorable prognosis (Compton et al., 2012). High-grade tumors are minimally differentiated or undifferentiated, which means the tumor cells have become significantly different from the tissue of origin. For example, a well-differentiated breast cancer can easily be recognized as breast tissue; whereas an undifferentiated tumor may have become so abnormal that it is impossible to discern the tissue of origin. Poorly differentiated or undifferentiated tumors carry a poorer prognosis (Compton et al., 2012).

Diagnostic Evaluation of Common Malignancies

Breast Cancer

The initial evaluation of a patient with breast cancer should include a thorough history and physical examination, bilateral diagnostic mammography, basic laboratory tests, determination of ER, PR, and HER2 tumor status, selective testing for distant metastases, referral for genetic counseling in high-risk individuals, and fertility counseling in appropriate individuals.

History

History and current complaints: Breast symptoms are common, and recognition and evaluation of these symptoms can result in timely breast cancer detection. The most common breast symptoms are a palpable breast mass, breast pain, and nipple discharge (Salzman, Fleegle, & Tully, 2012). Although most causes of breast symptoms are usually benign, patients should be evaluated with a detailed clinical history and physical examination to determine the degree of suspicion for breast cancer. The characteristics of breast masses should be noted, including the location, method of discovery, and duration; change in size over time or in relation to the menstrual cycle; and presence of pain, redness, fever, skin thickening, or nipple discharge (Salzman et al., 2012). Nipple discharge is classified as pathologic if it is spontaneous, unilateral, bloody, serous, clear, or associated with a mass (Salzman et al., 2012). Although pain is one of the most frequent breast symptoms presenting to clinicians, it is not usually the presenting symptom of cancer and may represent benign findings. A breast mass is the most frequent presenting symptom associated with breast cancer (Salzman et al., 2012).

Risk factors: The history includes assessment of risk factors that increase the likelihood of breast cancer. These include increasing age, overweight or obesity in a postmenopausal woman, Caucasian or Ashkenazi Jewish descent, alcohol consumption (more than one drink per day), current or prior use of hormonal therapy or oral contraceptives, menarche prior to age 12, menopause after age 55, nulliparity or first live birth after age 35, and higher breast density on mammogram (NCCN, 2015b; Salzman et al., 2012).

Family history: Family history includes information about all relatives (both paternal and maternal) over three generations, documenting all cancer occurrences, with a special focus on breast cancer. The degree of excess risk of breast cancer increases with the number of affected family members, the proximity of the relationship to the affected family members (i.e., first-degree confers greater risk than second-degree), and the earlier the age of the affected family members at diagnosis (NCCN, 2015b). Factors associated with an increased risk of breast cancer include a family member with *BRCA1*, *BRCA2*, *TP53*, or *PTEN* mutation(s); two or more breast primaries in a single individual; two or more individuals with primary breast cancer on the same side of the family (maternal or paternal); one or more family members with male breast cancer or ovarian, fallopian tube, or primary peritoneal cancer; a first- or second-degree relative with breast cancer diagnosed at age 45 or younger; and a personal or family history of three or more of the following: pancreatic cancer, prostate cancer (Gleason score of 7 or higher), sarcoma, adrenocortical carcinoma, brain tumors, endometrial cancer, thyroid cancer, kidney cancer, dermatologic manifestations, and/or macrocephaly, hamartomatous polyps of the GI tract, or diffuse gastric cancer (NCCN, 2015b).

Past medical history: A complete past medical history is obtained. Patients with a known *BRCA1* or *BRCA2* mutation are at significantly higher risk for developing breast cancer than the general population. Other elements of the past medical history that increase the risk of breast cancer include previous breast biopsies (regardless of results), atypical hyperplasia or lobular carcinoma in situ, and breast or ovarian cancer (NCCN, 2015b; Salzman et al., 2012).

Physical Examination

The clinical breast examination (CBE) is ideally conducted the week after menses, when breast tissue is least dense (Salzman et al., 2012). CBE is performed with the patient in both the supine and sitting position. With the patient in the sitting position, the clinician inspects the breasts with the patient raising arms overhead, relaxed at the patient's side, and with hands on hips. The breast should be inspected for size, skin contour, and asymmetry; nipple discharge; obvious masses; and skin changes such as dimpling, peau d'orange, skin color changes, ulcers, inflammation, rashes, or retraction of the nipple. After careful inspection, the clinician palpates the breasts, chest wall, axillary lymph nodes, and supraclavicular lymph nodes with the patient in the sitting position. In the supine position, the patient raises arms overhead to flatten the breast, and the clinical again inspects the breasts followed by a thorough and systematic palpation of all of the breast tissue, including the nipple areolar complex as well as the axillae, supraclavicular area, and chest wall (Salzman et al., 2012). Several techniques exist for palpating the breast; one method is to use the pads of the middle three fingers, moving in dime-sized circular motions while applying light, medium, and deep pressure at each point along a vertical strip pattern (Salzman et al., 2012). The most important aspect of the breast examination is that it is systematic and includes all of the pertinent areas. If a mass is noted, the location is described as the position on a clock face and distance from the nipple (Salzman et al., 2012).

Identification and characterization of a mass by CBE can be difficult because breasts have varying amounts of glandular tissue, fibrosis, and fat (Harvey et al., 2012). Although clinical findings are inadequate to distinguish between benign and malignant masses, benign masses generally are smooth, soft to firm, mobile, and have discrete margins without any associated skin changes. Conversely, malignant masses are generally hard, immobile, and fixed to surrounding tissue with poorly defined margins (Harvey et al., 2012; Salzman et al., 2012). Any breast mass that is a three-dimensional lesion distinct from the surrounding tissues with asymmetry relative to the other breast is considered to be a "dominant mass" that raises the suspicion for malignancy and warrants further investigation with imaging (Harvey et al., 2012; Salzman et al., 2012).

Differential Diagnosis

The differential diagnosis includes changes from fibrocystic disease (often symmetric and located in the upper outer quadrants in areas of increased glandular tissue), fibroadenoma, hyperplastic changes with or without atypia, and mammary duct ectasia (Salzman et al., 2012). Any palpable mass, however, is considered malignant until proved otherwise and must be carefully evaluated (Salzman et al., 2012). Anatomically, tumors originate in the terminal duct lobular unit; thus, half of all breast cancers occur in the upper outer quadrant of the breast, where concentration of glandular tissue is greatest (Compton et al., 2012).

Diagnostic Tests

Radiologic examinations: A bilateral diagnostic mammogram is recommended for breast cancer workup and staging (NCCN, 2015a). If needed, an ultrasound can help distinguish a cystic mass from a solid mass (NCCN, 2015a). Breast MRI should be performed for patients whose breasts cannot adequately be imaged with mammogram or ultrasound, but it is not recommended for routine staging because of the high rate of false-positive results (NCCN, 2015a). Breast MRI is particularly useful to image dense breast tissue or suspected mammographic occult primary breast tumors because it provides a three-dimensional view of tissue with a higher sensitivity than mammogram (Lehman, DeMartini, Anderson, & Edge, 2009).

For stage I–IIB disease, no additional imaging is recommended in an asymptomatic patient (Moy et al., 2014; NCCN, 2015a). Additional imaging tests should be directed by signs and symptoms, keeping in mind that the most common sites of distant metastases in breast cancer are the bone, lung, liver, and brain (Moy et al., 2014). For example, a bone scan should be obtained in patients with localized bone pain or elevated alkaline phosphatase (NCCN, 2015a). A diagnostic CT or MRI of the abdomen is indicated if the patient has abdominal symptoms, an elevated alkaline phosphatase, abnormal LFTs, or abnormal physical examination of the abdomen. A diagnostic chest CT is recommended if pulmonary symptoms are present (NCCN, 2015a). The NCCN panel specifically recommends against PET-CT in early-stage breast cancer because of its limited sensitivity to detect lesions smaller than 1 cm or nodal metastases, the low probability that these patients have distant metastases, and the high rate of false-positive results (NCCN, 2015a).

For patients with clinical stage IIIA disease, chest imaging with plain x-ray or CT typically is obtained. Additional imaging may be considered to definitively rule out metastatic disease, including bone scan and diagnostic CT or MRI of the abdomen (NCCN, 2015a). PET-CT is generally reserved for situations where the standard imaging results are equivocal. If PET-CT shows bone metastases, an additional bone scan is not necessary because there is a high concordance between the two studies (NCCN, 2015a).

Patients with stage IV invasive breast cancer require comprehensive assessment of the extent of disease with diagnostic CT of the chest, abdomen, and pelvis; bone scan; and radiographs of any weight-bearing bone that is painful or appears abnormal on bone scan (NCCN, 2015a). Additional imaging is directed by symptoms.

Laboratory studies: Routine laboratory studies include CBC and LFTs. Other laboratory studies are ordered as clinically indicated.

Biopsy: A biopsy is performed to obtain cells for examination and to determine the type of breast cancer. Fine needle aspiration, core needle biopsy, and incisional or excisional biopsy are equally reasonable methods to retrieve cells from a palpable mass for pathologic examination. Stereotactic MRI or ultrasound-guided core needle biopsy are alternatives to excisional biopsy for nonpalpable lesions (Compton et al., 2012; NCCN, 2015a). Fine needle aspiration has shown to be very useful in the diagnosis of breast cancer, with a sensitivity of 92.7% (95% CI [0.921, 0.933]) and specificity of 94.8% (95% CI [0.943, 0.952]) (Yu, Wei, & Liu, 2012).

Pathology: The pathologic classification of invasive breast cancer includes the following histologic types: not otherwise specified (NOS); ductal; inflammatory; medullary, NOS; medullary with lymphoid stroma; mucinous; papillary (predominantly micropapillary pattern); tubular; lobular; Paget disease and infiltrating; undifferentiated; squamous cell; adenoid cystic; secretory; and cribriform carcinomas (Edge et al., 2010). In situ carcinomas include NOS, intraductal, and Paget disease and intraductal (Edge et al., 2010). Invasive breast carcinomas are graded using the Nottingham combined histologic grade (Elston-Ellis modification of Scarff-Bloom-Richardson grading system) (Edge et al., 2010). The grade is determined by assessing three morphologic features: tubule formation, nuclear polymorphism, and mitotic count. A value of 1 (favorable) to 3 (unfavorable) is assigned to each feature, and the scores are added together to determine the histologic grade. The histologic grade can be GX (grade cannot be assessed), G1 (low combined histologic grade with a score of 3–5 [favorable]), G2 (intermediate combined histologic grade with a score of 6–7 [moderately favorable]), or G3 (high combined histologic grade with a score of 8–9 [unfavorable]) (Compton et al., 2012).

Biologic information plays an important role in accurate breast cancer staging, and ER, PR, and HER2 statuses are the most significant biomarkers for prognosis and treatment decisions (NCCN, 2015a; Wolff et al., 2013). The American Society of Clinical Oncology (ASCO) and NCCN recommend that all newly diagnosed and recurrent invasive breast cancers are assessed by IHC for tumor ER and PR status (NCCN, 2015a; Wolff et al., 2013). In addition, ASCO, NCCN, and the College of American Pathologists recommend testing for HER2 status in all patients diagnosed with invasive primary, recurrent, or metastatic breast cancer (Wolff et al., 2013). If the IHC score is 2+ rather than 3+ (which represents uniform, intense membrane staining of more than 10% of invasive tumor cells), then FISH should be performed on the same specimen, if possible (Wolff et al., 2013). The threshold for an IHC score of 3+ changed from uniform, intense staining of greater than 30% of tumor cells to greater than 10% of tumor cells in 2013 (Wolff et al., 2013).

Staging

Breast cancer is staged by AJCC using the TNM staging system (see Tables 3-5 and 3-6). After a tissue diagnosis is made, other imaging studies based on individual patient's clinical presentation are ordered to complete staging (NCCN, 2015a). Both clinical staging (physical examination of skin, mammary gland, lymph nodes, and imaging) and pathologic staging (examination of surgical specimens from tumor resection, lymph nodes, and metastatic sites) are generally used to determine breast cancer stage (Edge et al., 2010).

Patients with clinically negative axillary lymph nodes are candidates for sentinel lymph node biopsy (NCCN, 2015a). Clinically suspicious axillary lymph nodes should be biopsied by fine needle aspiration or core biopsy; sentinel lymph node biopsy can be consid-

Table 3-5. Tumor-Node-Metastasis (TNM) Definitions for Breast Cancer

Primary Tumor (T)

Definitions for classifying the primary tumor (T) are the same for clinical and pathologic classification. Tumors should be measured to the nearest 0.1 cm increment. For example, if a tumor is 2.01 cm in size, it is reported as 2.0 cm. The subscript "c" should be used for clinical measurements using clinical and radiographic findings and the subscript "p" should be used for pathologic measurements. Pathologic measurements should take precedence over clinical measurements of T size.

Postneoadjuvant pathologic measurement of T is denoted by ypT and will be measured as the largest single focus of invasive tumor, with the modifier "m" indicating multiple foci. The measurement of the largest tumor focus should not include areas of fibrosis within the tumor bed. The inclusion of additional information in the pathology report such as the distance over which tumor foci extend, the number of tumor foci present, or the number of slides/blocks in which tumor appears may assist the clinician in estimating the extent of disease. A comparison of the cellularity in the initial biopsy to that in the post-treatment specimen may also aid in the assessment of response.

TX	Primary tumor cannot be assessed
T0	No evidence of primary tumor
Tis	Carcinoma in situ
Tis (DCIS)	Ductal carcinoma in situ
Tis (LCIS)	Lobular carcinoma in situ
Tis (Paget's)	Paget's disease of the nipple NOT associated with invasive carcinoma and/or carcinoma in situ (DCIS and/or LCIS) in the underlying breast parenchyma. Carcinomas in the breast parenchyma associated with Paget's disease are categorized based on the size and characteristics of the parenchymal disease, although the presence of Paget's disease should still be noted.
T1	Tumor 2 cm or less in greatest dimension
T1mi	Tumor 0.1 cm or less in greatest dimension
T1a	Tumor more than 0.1 cm but not more than 0.5 cm in greatest dimension
T1b	Tumor more than 0.5 cm but not more than 1 cm in greatest dimension
T1c	Tumor more than 1 cm but not more than 2 cm in greatest dimension
T2	Tumor more than 2 cm but not more than 5 cm in greatest dimension
T3	Tumor more than 5 cm in greatest dimension
T4	Tumor of any size with direct extension to chest wall and/or to the skin (ulceration or skin nodules) *Note*. Invasion of the dermis alone does not qualify as T4.
T4a	Extension to chest wall, not including only pectoralis muscle adherence/invasion
T4b	Ulceration of the skin of the breast and/or satellite skin nodules confined to the same breast and/or edema (including peau d'orange) of the skin, which do not meet criteria for inflammatory carcinoma
T4c	Both T4a and T4b
T4d	Inflammatory carcinoma

(Continued on next page)

Table 3-5. Tumor-Node-Metastasis (TNM) Definitions for Breast Cancer *(Continued)*

Regional Lymph Nodes (N)

Clinical

NX	Regional lymph nodes cannot be assessed (e.g., previously removed)
N0	No regional lymph node metastases
N1	Metastases to movable ipsilateral level I, II axillary lymph node(s)
N2	Metastases in ipsilateral level I, II axillary lymph nodes that are clinically fixed or matted; or in clinically detected* ipsilateral internal mammary nodes in the absence of clinically evident axillary lymph node metastases
N2a	Metastases in ipsilateral level I, II axillary lymph nodes fixed to one another (matted) or to other structures
N2b	Metastases only in clinically detected* ipsilateral internal mammary nodes and in the absence of clinically evident axillary lymph node metastases
N3	Metastases in ipsilateral infraclavicular (level III axillary) lymph node(s) with or without level I, II axillary lymph node involvement, or in clinically detected* ipsilateral internal mammary lymph node(s) with clinically evident level I, II axillary lymph node metastases; or metastases in ipsilateral supraclavicular lymph node(s) with or without axillary or internal mammary lymph node involvement
N3a	Metastases in ipsilateral infraclavicular lymph node(s)
N3b	Metastases in ipsilateral internal mammary lymph node(s) and axillary lymph node(s)
N3c	Metastases in ipsilateral supraclavicular lymph node(s)

* *Clinically detected* is defined as detected by imaging studies (excluding lymphoscintigraphy) or by clinical examination and having characteristics highly suspicious for malignancy or a presumed pathologic macrometastasis based on fine needle aspiration biopsy with cytologic examination. Confirmation of clinically detected metastatic disease by fine needle aspiration without excision biopsy is designated with an (f) suffix, for example, cN3a(f). Excisional biopsy of a lymph node or biopsy of a sentinel node, in the absence of assignment of a pT, is classified as a clinical N, for example, cN1. Information regarding the confirmation of the nodal status will be designated in site-specific factors as clinical, fine needle aspiration, core biopsy, or sentinel lymph node biopsy. Pathologic classification (pN) is used for excision or sentinel lymph node biopsy only in conjunction with a pathologic T assignment.

Pathologic (pN)*

pNX	Regional lymph nodes cannot be assessed (e.g., previously removed, or not removed for pathologic study)
pN0	No regional lymph node metastasis histologically
pN0(i–)	No regional lymph node metastases identified histologically, negative IHC
pN0(i+)	Malignant cells in regional lymph node(s) no greater than 0.2 mm (detected by H&E or IHC including ITC)

Note: Isolated tumor cells (ITC) are defined as single tumor cells or small clusters of cells not greater than 0.2 mm, or a cluster of fewer than 200 cells in a single histologic cross-section. ITCs may be detected by routine histology or by immunohistochemical (IHC) methods. Nodes containing only ITCs are excluded from the total positive node count for purposes of N classification but should be included in the number of nodes evaluated.

(Continued on next page)

Table 3-5. Tumor-Node-Metastasis (TNM) Definitions for Breast Cancer *(Continued)*

pN0(mol–)	No regional lymph node metastases histologically, negative molecular findings (RT-PCR)**
pN0(mol+)	No regional lymph node metastases detected histologically or by IHC, positive molecular findings (RT-PCR)**
pN1	Micrometastases; or metastases in 1 to 3 axillary lymph nodes; and/or internal mammary nodes with metastases detected by sentinel lymph node biopsy but not clinically detected***
pN1mi	Micrometastases (greater than 0.2 mm and/or more than 200 cells, none greater than 2.0 mm)
pN1a	Metastases in 1 to 3 axillary lymph nodes, at least one metastasis greater than 2.0 mm
pN1b	Metastases in internal mammary nodes with micrometastases or macrometastases detected by sentinel lymph node biopsy but not clinically detected***
pN1c	Metastases in 1 to 3 axillary lymph nodes and in internal mammary lymph nodes with micrometastases or macrometastases detected by sentinel lymph node biopsy but not clinically detected***
pN2	Metastases in 4 to 9 axillary lymph nodes; or in clinically detected**** internal mammary lymph nodes in the absence of axillary lymph node metastases
pN2a	Metastases in 4 to 9 axillary lymph nodes (at least one tumor deposit greater than 2.0 mm)
pN2b	Metastases in clinically detected**** internal mammary lymph nodes in the absence of axillary lymph node metastasis
pN3	Metastases in 10 or more axillary lymph nodes; or in infraclavicular (level III axillary) lymph nodes; or in clinically detected**** ipsilateral internal mammary lymph nodes in the presence of 1 or more positive level I, II axillary lymph nodes; or in more than 3 axillary lymph nodes and in internal mammary lymph nodes with micrometastases or macrometastases detected by sentinel lymph node biopsy but not clinically detected***; or in ipsilateral supraclavicular lymph nodes
pN3a	Metastases in 10 or more axillary lymph nodes (at least one tumor deposit greater than 2.0 mm); or metastases to the infraclavicular (level III axillary) lymph nodes
pN3b	Metastases in clinically detected**** ipsilateral internal mammary lymph nodes in the presence of 1 or more positive axillary lymph nodes; or in more than 3 axillary lymph nodes and in internal mammary lymph nodes with micrometastases or macrometastases detected by sentinel lymph node biopsy but not clinically detected****
pN3c	Metastases in ipsilateral supraclavicular lymph nodes

* Classification is based on axillary lymph node dissection with or without sentinel lymph node biopsy. Classification based solely on sentinel lymph node biopsy without subsequent axillary lymph node dissection is designated (sn) for "sentinel node," e.g., pN0(sn).

** RT-PCR: reverse transcriptase/polymerase chain reaction.

*** *Not clinically detected* is defined as not detected by imaging studies (excluding lymphoscintigraphy) or not detected by clinical examination.

**** *Clinically detected* is defined as detected by imaging studies (excluding lymphoscintigraphy) or by clinical examination and having characteristics highly suspicious for malignancy or a presumed pathologic micrometastasis based on fine needle aspiration biopsy with cytologic examination.

(Continued on next page)

Table 3-5. Tumor-Node-Metastasis (TNM) Definitions for Breast Cancer *(Continued)*

Post-treatment ypN

• Post-treatment yp "N" should be evaluated as for clinical (pretreatment) "N" methods above. The modifier "sn" is used only if a sentinel node evaluation was performed after treatment. If no subscript is attached, it is assumed that the axillary nodal evaluation was by axillary node dissection (AND).
• The X classification will be used (ypNX) if no yp post-treatment SN or AND was performed.
• N categories are the same as those used for pN.

Distant Metastasis (M)

MX	Distant metastasis cannot be assessed
M0	No clinical or radiographic evidence of distant metastases
cM0(i+)	No clinical or radiographic evidence of distant metastases, but deposits of molecularly or microscopically detected tumor cells in circulating blood, bone marrow, or other non-regional nodal tissue that are no larger than 0.2 mm in a patient without symptoms or signs of metastases
M1	Distant detectable metastases as determined by classic clinical and radiographic means and/or histologically proven larger than 0.2 mm

Post-treatment yp M classification: The M category for patients treated with neoadjuvant therapy is the category assigned in the clinical stage, prior to initiation of neoadjuvant therapy. Identification of distant metastases after the start of therapy in cases where pretherapy evaluation showed no metastases is considered progression of disease. If a patient was designated to have detectable distant metastases (M1) before chemotherapy, the patient will be designated as M1 throughout.

DCIS—ductal carcinoma in situ; LCIS—lobular carcinoma in situ

Note. From *AJCC Cancer Staging Manual* (7th ed.), by S.B. Edge, D.R. Byrd, C.C. Compton, A.G. Fritz, F.L. Greene, and A. Trotti III (Eds.), 2010, New York, NY: Springer, www.springeronline.com. Used with permission of the American Joint Committee on Cancer (AJCC), Chicago, Illinois.

---

ered if the lymph node biopsy results are negative. Sentinel lymph node biopsy is preferred over axillary lymph node dissection in patients with clinical stage I–II breast cancer because it has a lower risk of arm and shoulder morbidity (e.g., pain, lymphedema, sensory loss) (NCCN, 2015a). Axillary lymph node dissection is reserved for patients with stage III breast cancer or patients with more than two positive axillary lymph nodes on sentinel lymph node excision. At least 10 lymph nodes should be excised to accurately stage the axilla with axillary lymph node dissection, and all suspicious lymph nodes should be removed (NCCN, 2015a).

Breast cancer may metastasize via the blood or the lymphatic system. The four major sites of metastases are the bone, lung, brain, and liver (Compton et al., 2012). However, tumor cells can metastasize to many other sites, including micrometastases to the bone marrow or circulating tumor cells. Although M1 disease is defined as clinical or radiographic evidence of disease, microscopic evidence of metastases may be prognostic for recurrence and is denoted as M0(i+) (Compton et al., 2012).

Prognosis

Once patients diagnosed with breast cancer are staged, the stage, biologic characteristics of the disease, and characteristics of the patients determine prognosis and guide the choice of treatment. Prognostic factors for breast cancer include age, comorbidity, tumor size, hormone receptor status, HER2 status, grade and histology of tumor, and lymph node involve-

Table 3-6. Stage Grouping for Breast Cancer

Stage	T	N	M
Stage 0	Tis	N0	M0
Stage IA	T1*	N0	M0
Stage IB	T0	N1mi	M0
	T1*	N1mi	M0
Stage IIA	T0	N1**	M0
	T1*	N1**	M0
	T2	N0	M0
Stage IIB	T2	N1	M0
	T3	N0	M0
Stage IIIA	T0	N2	M0
	T1*	N2	M0
	T2	N2	M0
	T3	N1	M0
	T3	N2	M0
Stage IIIB	T4	N0	M0
	T4	N1	M0
	T4	N2	M0
Stage IIIC	Any T	N3	M0
Stage IV	Any T	Any N	M1

* T1 includes T1mi

** T0 and T1 tumors with nodal micrometastases only are excluded from Stage IIA and are classified Stage IB.

Notes:
- M0 includes M0(i+).
- The designation pM0 is not valid; any M0 should be clinical.
- If a patient presents with M1 prior to neoadjuvant systemic therapy, the stage is considered Stage IV and remains Stage IV regardless of response to neoadjuvant therapy. Stage designation may be changed if postsurgical imaging studies reveal the presence of distant metastases, provided that the studies are carried out within 4 months of diagnosis in the absence of disease progression and provided that the patient has not received neoadjuvant therapy.
- Postneoadjuvant therapy is designated with "yc" or "yp" prefix. Of note, no stage group is assigned if there is a complete pathologic response (CR) to neoadjuvant therapy, for example, ypT0ypN0cM0.

Note. From *AJCC Cancer Staging Manual* (7th ed.), by S.B. Edge, D.R. Byrd, C.C. Compton, A.G. Fritz, F.L. Greene, and A. Trotti III (Eds.), 2010, New York, NY: Springer, www.springeronline.com. Used with permission of the American Joint Committee on Cancer (AJCC), Chicago, Illinois.

ment (NCCN, 2015a). Tools are available to help clinicians to individualize therapy by assessing the risk for recurrence more accurately.

A computer-based model, Adjuvant! Online (www.adjuvantonline.com), is a commonly used algorithm to estimate 10-year disease-free and overall survival in patients with invasive breast cancer who have undergone primary resection of the tumor. Users of the program assess clinical components such as the patient's age, comorbidities, tumor size, tumor grade, and number of affected lymph nodes. Based on these factors, the tool calculates the estimated mortality risk and treatment efficacy of selected adjuvant hormonal and/or systemic chemotherapy. This information is useful for providing patients with an estimate of the net benefit of pursuing additional therapy. Adjuvant! was validated in a study of 4,083 women with breast cancer and was found to predict outcomes reliably except in a few specific subgroups of patients (Olivotto et al., 2005). The major limitation of the program is that it does not include HER2 status as a prognostic factor.

Oncotype DX® and MammaPrint® are gene assays that may assist clinicians in determining prognosis in specific patients with breast cancer and in predicting which patients will benefit from further therapy or have increased risk of metastasis. Oncotype DX is a 21-gene reverse transcriptase–polymerase chain reaction assay and recurrence score algorithm that can quantify the risk of recurrence and predict the responsiveness to tamoxifen and chemotherapy (Harris et al., 2007; Paik et al., 2004). Newly diagnosed patients with stage I, node-negative, ER-positive, HER2-negative breast cancer have a very favorable risk profile, and the use of adjuvant chemotherapy may not provide additional survival benefit in many of these patients. For this subpopulation, the Oncotype DX assay is more accurate than Adjuvant! in predicting the risk of recurrence and identifying patients who may benefit from adjuvant chemotherapy in addition to tamoxifen (Harris et al., 2007). The assay is performed on formalin-fixed, paraffin-embedded tumor tissue. Analysis of the gene panel provides a Recurrence Score™ that is reported as a value between 0 and 100. A recurrence score below 18 places the patient in a low-risk range, whereas scores ranging 18–30 constitute the intermediate-risk range. A recurrence score of 31 or higher places the patient in a high-risk range (NCCN, 2015a). A calculation of the average rate of distant recurrence at 10 years also is reported.

MammaPrint is a 70-gene assay that is FDA-approved to determine the risk of recurrence for patients with stage I or II invasive breast cancer (ER positive or negative) with lymph node–negative disease; it is not indicated to predict benefit from systemic adjuvant therapy (Harris et al., 2007; NCCN, 2015a). MammaPrint requires a punch biopsy sample of fresh tumor (at least 3 mm in diameter) (Agendia, n.d.). MammaPrint was validated in a trial of 326 patients with node-negative breast cancer and was found to add independent prognostic information to clinical and pathologic risk information in patients with early-stage breast cancer (Buyse et al., 2006). However, both ASCO and NCCN consider MammaPrint to be investigational, and current, prospective trials are underway (Harris et al., 2007; NCCN, 2015a).

Survival

Using 2002–2008 data, ACS statistics for breast cancer in the United States reported five-year survival rates of 99% for localized disease, 85% for women with regional disease, and 25% for those with distant metastases (Siegel, Miller, & Jemal, 2015).

Colorectal Cancer

The initial evaluation of a patient with colorectal cancer includes a comprehensive history and physical examination; laboratory tests; colonoscopy; CT of the chest, abdomen, and pelvis; and referral for genetic counseling in high-risk individuals.

History

History and current complaints: Colorectal cancer typically is diagnosed after the onset of symptoms; only 30% of cancers are diagnosed in asymptomatic patients through screening methods (Moiel & Thompson, 2011). The symptoms that raise concern for colorectal cancer are not particularly sensitive or specific (John, George, Primrose, & Fozard, 2011; Olde Bekkink et al., 2010). The most common symptom of colorectal cancer is rectal bleeding, yet rectal bleeding usually has a benign etiology, with the probability of colorectal cancer rang-ing from 2.4% to 11% (John et al., 2011; Olde Bekkink et al., 2010). Bright red streaking of the stool and dark red blood are associated with a greater likelihood of colorectal cancer than bright red blood dripping into the toilet at the end of defecation or on the toilet paper, which is associated with hemorrhoids (John et al., 2011). Other signs and symptoms include a change in bowel habits, abdominal pain, unexpected weight loss (at least 5% of body weight in 6–12 months), abdominal mass, and anemia. Changes in bowel habit are broadly defined as consti-pation or diarrhea but can be described more specifically as a change in the frequency of defe-cation, consistency of stool, or shape of stool, and/or difficulty in evacuation (John et al., 2011).

The presenting symptoms of colorectal cancer may suggest the location of the tumor. Changes in bowel habit and rectal bleeding are more common with left-sided cancers, whereas iron-deficiency anemia is more common in right-sided cancers (John et al., 2011; Kent, Woolf, McCue, & Greenfield, 2010). Weight loss, pain, and obstruction were not associated with can-cer site. Left-sided or rectal tumors are more likely to be symptomatic than right-sided tumors (Kent et al., 2010).

Patients may present with partial or complete bowel obstruction or even perforation. These are poor prognostic factors and, in patients with stage II disease, can be used to determine the need for chemotherapy treatment (NCCN, 2015c). Up to 34% of patients have metastatic dis-ease at presentation (NCCN, 2015c). The most common sites of metastatic disease are the liver and lungs (Compton et al., 2012).

Risk factors: The most striking risk factor when assessing for colorectal cancer is age; 90% of new cases of colorectal cancer are found in those older than age 50 (ACS, 2014a). Nonmod-ifiable risk factors for colorectal cancer include a personal or family history of colorectal can-cer, a personal or family history of adenomatous polyps, and/or a personal history of inflam-matory bowel disease (ACS, 2014a). Modifiable risk factors for this disease include a diet high in red or processed meats, lack of exercise, obesity, smoking, and moderate to heavy alcohol consumption (ACS, 2014a).

Family history: Approximately 20% of colorectal cancer is associated with familial clus-tering, meaning that patients have at least one close relative with a history of colon cancer (ACS, 2014a; NCCN, 2015c). A comprehensive family history for colorectal cancer should span four generations, including parents, siblings, and children; aunts, uncles, grandparents, and half-siblings; and nieces, nephews, cousins, and great-grandparents (NCCN, 2015d). For each affected individual in the family, the following information should be collected: current age, age at diagnosis of cancer, type of cancer, availability of tumor sample, cause of death (if applicable), ethnicity and country of origin, suspected colon cancer syndromes, the occur-rence of multiple primary tumors, and all other inherited conditions and birth defects (NCCN, 2015d). Individuals with a first-degree relative (parent, sibling, or children) with a history of colorectal cancer have two to three times the risk of developing the disease compared to indi-viduals with no family history; the risk increases to three to six times that of the general pop-ulation if the relative was diagnosed at a young age or if there is more than one affected rela-tive (ACS, 2014a).

The two major hereditary colorectal cancer syndromes are familial adenomatous polyp-osis and hereditary nonpolyposis colorectal cancer (Lynch syndrome) (ACS, 2014a; NCCN, 2015d) (see Chapter 2 for more comprehensive information). Lynch syndrome is the most common, accounting for 2%–4% of colorectal cases, and is the result of inherited mutations in DNA mismatch repair (MMR) genes. Individuals with Lynch syndrome are predisposed to numerous types of cancer, yet risk of colorectal cancer is highest, with lifetime risks of 66% in men and 43% in women. The median age at diagnosis of colorectal cancer in people with Lynch syndrome is 42 years in men and 47 years in women, compared to 67 years for men and

71 years for women in the general population (ACS, 2014a). Individuals with familial adenomatous polyposis have a lifetime risk of colorectal cancer that approaches 100% by age 40 without intervention (ACS, 2014a).

Past medical history: A comprehensive medical and surgical history should be obtained that includes all previous cancers and the age at diagnosis. In addition, previously diagnosed adenomatous polyps or history of inflammatory bowel disease should be noted, as these individuals have an increased risk of colorectal cancer (ACS, 2014a; NCCN, 2015d). Evidence is emerging that suggests a possible association between diabetes and colorectal cancer (ACS, 2014a). Lastly, all inherited syndromes should be documented because many are associated with an increased risk of colon cancer (NCCN, 2015d).

Physical Examination

The workup for patients suspected of colorectal cancer includes a complete physical with rectal examination. However, in patients with early-stage disease, examination may yield no physical findings. As the disease progresses, physical findings may reveal abdominal tenderness or discomfort, a palpable liver mass, adenopathy, hepatomegaly, icterus, jaundice, abdominal mass, bleeding on rectal examination, or the general appearance of cachexia. As with presenting symptoms, the clinical findings may vary depending on the location of the cancer. Abdominal distension and constipation may be palpated in patients with sigmoid or left-sided colon cancers. Right-sided colon cancers may not have palpable masses upon examination. Bowel sounds may suggest hypermotility or a bowel obstruction. The liver is palpated carefully to assess for hepatomegaly. Lymphatics are carefully assessed. Rectal examination might detect an anorectal mass. Female patients also should undergo pelvic examination.

Differential Diagnosis

The differential diagnosis includes inflammatory or other bowel disease, adenomatous polyps, metastatic disease from another primary cancer, or other tumors of the GI tract.

Diagnostic Tests

Radiologic examinations: Imaging studies depend on the patient's clinical presentation. If a rectal cancer is present, TRUS is the standard imaging test because it can visualize the rectal wall layers and measure tumor depth and perirectal spread (Dewhurst et al., 2011). To complete staging assessment for metastases, the clinician also should perform CTs of the chest, abdomen, and pelvis (Dewhurst et al., 2011). When colonic polyps are found, NCCN guidelines recommend marking the suspected cancerous polyp site (either at the time of the colonoscopy or within two weeks of polypectomy if deemed necessary by the surgeon) (NCCN, 2015c). If the polyps are completely resected and have favorable features, no further surgery is required. Alternatively, if invasive colon cancer is found, the patient should have a colonoscopy, followed by a CT scan of the chest, abdomen, and pelvis with IV and oral contrast (Dewhurst et al., 2011; NCCN, 2015c). The use of PET is not routinely recommended unless synchronous metastatic disease exists that is potentially surgically curable.

Laboratory studies: Laboratory evaluation includes CBC, chemistry profile with LFTs, and CEA (NCCN, 2015c). CEA is not useful in detecting early colorectal cancer, thus limiting its usefulness as a screening tumor marker. However, serial measurements of CEA are able to detect recurrent or progressive colorectal cancer (NCCN, 2015c). CEA is the marker of choice for monitoring the response of metastatic disease to treatment (Locker et al., 2006).

Biopsy: Patients undergo colonoscopy for visualization and biopsy of suspected lesions or masses.

Pathology: The pathology of colorectal cancer is primarily adenocarcinoma (96%) (ACS, 2014a). Most adenocarcinomas are thought to arise from adenomatous polyps over a period of 10–20 years (ACS, 2014a). Other histopathologic classifications of colorectal tumors include adenocarcinoma in situ, medullary carcinoma, mucinous carcinoma (colloid type), signet cell carcinoma, squamous cell (epidermoid) carcinoma, adenosquamous, small cell carcinoma, undifferentiated carcinoma, or carcinoma NOS (Edge et al., 2010). The histologic grade is assigned from GX to G4 (Edge et al., 2010). GX means that the grade cannot be assessed. Grade 1 is a well-differentiated tumor; grade 2 is a moderately differentiated tumor; grade 3 is a poorly differentiated tumor; and grade 4 is an undifferentiated tumor (Compton et al., 2012).

Biomarkers: Some molecular markers of colorectal cancer predict the likelihood of sensitivity to certain treatments, thus helping clinicians to target treatments more effectively. Epidermal growth factor receptor (EGFR) is overexpressed in 49%–82% of colorectal tumors, but EGFR testing has no proven predictive value for anti-EGFR therapy (NCCN, 2015c). Therefore, NCCN does not recommend routine EGFR testing (NCCN, 2015c). Instead, *KRAS* mutations, present in approximately 40% of colorectal cancers, are predictive of response to anti-EGFR therapy. The RAS/RAF/MAK pathway is downstream from *EGFR*, and *KRAS* mutations predict a lack of benefit from anti-EGFR therapy (e.g., cetuximab, panitumumab) (NCCN, 2015c). All patients diagnosed with metastatic colorectal cancer should have *KRAS* genotyping performed, and anti-EGFR therapy should not be administered if a *KRAS* mutation is present (Allegra et al., 2009; NCCN, 2015c). *BRAF* mutations also appear to confer resistance to anti-EGFR therapy and appear to occur only in patients who do not have the *KRAS* mutation, so they identify another subset of patients unlikely to benefit from cetuximab or panitumumab. In addition, *BRAF* mutation is a strong prognostic marker that is associated with decreased overall survival (NCCN, 2015c).

Other markers studied in colorectal cancer include *TP53* (tumor suppressor gene), CA 19-9, thymidine synthase, dihydropyrimidine dehydrogenase, thymidine phosphorylase, 18q loss of heterozygosity, or deleted-in-colorectal-cancer protein (Locker et al., 2006). Currently, ASCO does not recommend these for screening, diagnosis, staging, surveillance, prognostic determination, or treatment monitoring and prognostication, as published data are insufficient (Locker et al., 2006).

Staging

Colon cancer is staged using the TNM staging system, which essentially replaced the historically used Dukes staging system or Astler-Coller modifications (see Tables 3-7 and 3-8). The staging system for colon cancer is based on the depth of mucosal invasion, regional lymph involvement, and distant metastasis. Surgery usually is performed for all patients who can be successfully resected with colectomy and lymphadenectomy; a minimum of 12 lymph nodes should be examined for accurate staging (NCCN, 2015c). The number of lymph nodes examined correlates with survival for unclear reasons; one possible explanation is that extent and quality of the surgical resection allows for retrieval of more lymph nodes (NCCN, 2015c).

Prognosis

The most important prognostic factor for colorectal cancer is the stage of disease at diagnosis (NCCN, 2015c). Additional prognostic factors include lymphovascular invasion, inadequate sampling of lymph nodes, high-grade tumors, and presentation with obstruction or perforation (NCCN, 2015c).

For stage II–III disease, microsatellite instability (MSI) and multigene assays may provide prognostic and predictive information. Mutations of MMR genes can result in MMR protein deficiency or MSI, which is associated with a low frequency of distant metastasis and a

---

Table 3-7. Tumor-Node-Metastasis (TNM) Definitions for Colorectal Cancer

---

The same classification is used for both clinical and pathologic staging.

Primary Tumor (T)

TX   Primary tumor cannot be assessed

T0   No evidence of primary tumor

Tis   Carcinoma in situ: intraepithelial or invasion of lamina propria*

T1   Tumor invades submucosa

T2   Tumor invades muscularis propria

T3   Tumor invades through the muscularis propria into pericolorectal tissues

T4a   Tumor penetrates to the surface of the visceral peritoneum**

T4b   Tumor directly invades or is adherent to other organs or structures**,***

* Tis includes cancer cells confined within the glandular basement membrane (intraepithelial) or mucosal lamina propria (intramucosal) with no extension through the muscularis mucosae into the submucosa.

** Direct invasion in T4 includes invasion of other organs or other segments of the colorectum as a result of direct extension through the serosa, as confirmed on microscopic examination (for example, invasion of the sigmoid colon by a carcinoma of the cecum) or, for cancers in a retroperitoneal or sub-peritoneal location, direct invasion of other organs or structures by virtue of extension beyond the muscularis propria (i.e., respectively, a tumor on the posterior wall of the descending colon invading the left kidney or lateral abdominal wall; or a mid or distal rectal cancer with invasion of prostate, seminal vesicles, cervix, or vagina).

*** Tumor that is adherent to other organs or structures, grossly, is classified cT4b. However, if no tumor is present in the adhesion, microscopically, the classification should be pT1–4a depending on the anatomical depth of wall invasion. The V and L classifications should be used to identify the presence or absence of vascular or lymphatic invasion whereas the PN site-specific factor should be used for perineural invasion.

Regional Lymph Nodes (N)

NX   Regional lymph nodes cannot be assessed

N0   No regional lymph node metastasis

N1   Metastasis in 1–3 regional lymph nodes

N1a   Metastasis in one regional lymph node

N1b   Metastasis in 2–3 regional lymph nodes

N1c   Tumor deposit(s) in the subserosa, mesentery, or nonperitonealized pericolic or perirectal tissues without regional nodal metastasis

N2   Metastasis in 4 or more regional lymph nodes

N2a   Metastasis in 4–6 regional lymph nodes

N2b   Metastasis in 7 or more regional lymph nodes

Note. A satellite peritumoral nodule in the pericolorectal adipose tissue of a primary carcinoma without histologic evidence of residual lymph node in the nodule may represent discontinuous spread, venous invasion with extravascular spread (V1/2), or a totally replaced lymph node (N1/2). Replaced nodes should be counted separately as positive nodes in the N category, whereas discontinuous spread or venous invasion should be classified and counted in the Site-Specific Factor category Tumor Deposits (TD).

(Continued on next page)

Table 3-7. Tumor-Node-Metastasis (TNM) Definitions for Colorectal Cancer
(Continued)

Distant Metastasis (M)

MX	Distant metastasis cannot be assessed
M0	No distant metastasis
M1	Distant metastasis
M1a	Metastasis confined to one organ or site (e.g., liver, lung, ovary, nonregional node)
M1b	Metastases in more than one organ/site or the peritoneum

Note. From *AJCC Cancer Staging Manual* (7th ed.), by S.B. Edge, D.R. Byrd, C.C. Compton, A.G. Fritz, F.L. Greene, and A. Trotti III (Eds.), 2010, New York, NY: Springer, www.springeronline.com. Used with permission of the American Joint Committee on Cancer (AJCC), Chicago, Illinois.

Table 3-8. Stage Grouping for Colorectal Cancer

Stage	T	N	M	Dukes*	MAC*
0	Tis	N0	M0	–	–
I	T1	N0	M0	A	A
	T2	N0	M0	A	B1
IIA	T3	N0	M0	B	B2
IIB	T4a	N0	M0	B	B2
IIC	T4b	N0	M0	B	B3
IIIA	T1–T2	N1/N1c	M0	C	C1
	T1	N2a	M0	C	C1
IIIB	T3–T4a	N1/N1c	M0	C	C2
	T2–T3	N2a	M0	C	C1/C2
	T1–T2	N2b	M0	C	C1
IIIC	T4a	N2a	M0	C	C2
	T3–T4a	N2b	M0	C	C2
	T4b	N1–N2	M0	C	C3
IVA	Any T	Any N	M1a	–	–
IVB	Any T	Any N	M1b	–	–

Note. cTNM is the clinical classification; pTNM is the pathologic classification. The "y" prefix is used for those cancers that are classified after neoadjuvant pretreatment (e.g., ypTNM). Patients who have a complete pathologic response are ypT0N0cM0 that may be similar to Stage Group 0 or I. The "r" prefix is to be used for those cancers that have recurred after a disease-free interval (rTNM).

* Dukes B is a composite of better (T3 N0 M0) and worse (T4 N0 M0) prognostic groups, as is Dukes C (Any TN1 M0 and Any T N2 M0). MAC is the modified Astler-Coller classification.

Note. From *AJCC Cancer Staging Manual* (7th ed.), by S.B. Edge, D.R. Byrd, C.C. Compton, A.G. Fritz, F.L. Greene, and A. Trotti III (Eds.), 2010, New York, NY: Springer, www.springeronline.com. Used with permission of the American Joint Committee on Cancer (AJCC), Chicago, Illinois.

favorable outcome (NCCN, 2015c). NCCN recommends that all patients with stage II disease undergo MSI/MMR testing because patients with MSI-H (high) and MMR defects are unlikely to benefit from adjuvant therapy and may be cured by surgical resection alone (NCCN, 2015c). In addition, MMR mutations are associated with Lynch syndrome; thus, all patients diagnosed before age 70 should be tested (NCCN, 2015c).

The Oncotype DX colon cancer assay is a 12-gene assay to determine the risk of recurrence in stage II–III colon cancer (NCCN, 2015c). ColoPrint® is an 18-gene assay to determine the risk of recurrence that is currently undergoing further validation in a prospective trial of patients with stage II colon cancer (NCCN, 2015c). Neither of these tests has sufficient data to validate its clinical utility at this time.

Survival

The five-year survival rate in the United States for colorectal cancer is 90% for patients with localized disease, 70% for patients with regional disease, and 12% for patients with distant metastases (Siegel et al., 2015).

Lung Cancer

The initial evaluation of patients with lung cancer should include a thorough history and physical examination, assessment of performance status, pulmonary function tests, CT imaging, PET scan, basic laboratory tests, and selective testing for distant metastases and paraneoplastic syndromes. All patients should be counseled on tobacco cessation. Patients with metastatic disease should be referred to palliative care at diagnosis even if they will be treated with anticancer therapy (NCCN, 2015f).

History

History and current complaints: Nearly all patients diagnosed with lung cancer present with symptoms (Ellis & Vandermeer, 2011). The most common symptoms at presentation are cough, shortness of breath, chest pain, and hemoptysis (Ellis & Vandermeer, 2011). Other symptoms may include fatigue, lung infection, weight loss, malaise, pain, loss of appetite, or hoarse voice (Ellis & Vandermeer, 2011). There is often a delay in the diagnosis of lung cancer because most patients present with respiratory symptoms that are similar to those of other chronic respiratory conditions, such as chronic obstructive pulmonary disease (COPD) (Ellis & Vandermeer, 2011).

Symptoms may be associated with regional spread, the location of the tumor, or metastatic disease. For example, patients may present with cough or dyspnea due to pleural effusions, localized pain from chest wall invasion, hoarseness from left recurrent laryngeal nerve palsy, or dysphagia from subcarinal lymphadenopathy or direct invasion of tumor (Saeed & Anderson, 2011). Pancoast tumors are defined as apical lung cancer tumors that invade structures of the apical chest wall, such as the thoracic inlet structures, the brachial plexus, and the cervical sympathetic nerves (Kozower, Larner, Detterbeck, & Jones, 2013). These tumors are associated with Pancoast syndrome, which is characterized by Horner syndrome (a constellation of signs including ptosis, slow pupillary dilation, and impaired flushing and perspiration on the ipsilateral side of the face) from invasion of the sympathetic chain and stellate ganglion; pain and atrophy of the muscles of the hand from invasion of the brachial plexus; and shoulder, arm, or neck pain from invasion of the chest wall and ribs (Saeed & Anderson, 2011).

The most common sites of metastatic disease are the brain, bone, adrenal glands, contralateral lung, liver, pericardium, kidneys, and subcutaneous tissues (Compton et al., 2012). Approximately 25% of patients with stage IV non-small cell lung cancer (NSCLC) have a brain metastasis (Kozower et al., 2013). Symptoms of metastatic disease are related to the site of metastasis. Superior vena cava obstruction is more common in small cell lung cancer (SCLC) and may present as facial and upper extremity swelling (particularly in the right upper extremity), dilated neck veins, headache, dizziness, and cough (NCCN, 2015h). Pleuritic pain may indicate metastasis to the pleura with or without effusion.

Paraneoplastic syndromes can be seen with NSCLC but are more common in SCLC (NCCN, 2015h; Ost, Yeung, Tanoue, & Gould, 2013). Paraneoplastic syndromes cause effects unrelated to metastasis because of autoimmune mechanisms or hormonal mechanisms (from the production of substances such as adrenocorticotropic hormone, antidiuretic hormone, growth hormone, and parathyroid hormone) (Ost et al., 2013; Saeed & Anderson, 2011). Some of the paraneoplastic syndromes commonly seen in lung cancer include hypercalcemia, syndrome of inappropriate antidiuretic hormone secretion, Cushing syndrome, digital clubbing, and hypertrophic osteoarthropathy and other neurologic syndromes, such as Lambert-Eaton myasthenic syndrome or peripheral neuropathy (Ost et al., 2013).

Risk factors: Smoking accounts for approximately 85%–90% of all cases of lung cancer (NCCN, 2015f). Exposure to secondhand smoke is also believed to increase the risk of lung cancer. Other risk factors include age, previous cancer history, family history, chemical exposures (e.g., radon, asbestos, arsenic, chromium, nickel, cadmium, beryllium, silica, diesel fumes), other lung disease (e.g., COPD, pulmonary fibrosis), exposure to infectious agents (e.g., tuberculosis, fungal infections), and immunosuppression (NCCN, 2015f).

Family history: Family history is not a predominant risk factor for lung cancer. However, a genetic predisposition may be partially responsible for the development of the disease in some individuals, as not all smokers develop lung cancer (NCCN, 2015f).

Physical Examination

A complete physical examination should be performed with particular attention to the lungs, lymph nodes, central nervous system, liver, and musculoskeletal system. The cervical, supraclavicular, and scalene lymph nodes are examined carefully, and axillary regions are assessed for masses or signs of adenopathy (Ost et al., 2013). A thorough chest evaluation includes auscultation, percussion, and observation for signs of obstruction or effusions (Ost et al., 2013). Superior vena cava syndrome is characterized by edema of the face, neck, and upper arm and venous distension in the neck, upper chest, and arms. The abdomen is assessed for pain on palpation and organ enlargement (Ost et al., 2013). Bone tenderness, focal neurologic signs, and soft tissue masses are noted (Ost et al., 2013).

Differential Diagnosis

Presenting symptoms of lung cancer are similar to those that may be attributed to other respiratory conditions, such as COPD or pneumonia (Ellis & Vandermeer, 2011). The differential diagnosis of SCLC includes other neuroendocrine tumors (NCCN, 2015h).

Diagnostic Tests

Radiologic examinations: A chest CT with contrast is recommended for patients with known or suspected lung cancer (Ravenel et al., 2013; Silvestri et al., 2013). The typical radiologic appearance of lung carcinoma is a solitary pulmonary nodule or mass with a well-marginated, lobulated, irregular, or poorly defined border (Akin et al., 2012). The lesions of adenocarcinomas tend to be located in the peripheral lung zones and may invade the pleura or be associated with air bronchograms (Akin et al., 2012). Because squamous cell carcinomas are strongly associated with smoking, the majority of lesions are found in the central to mid-lung zones, where the larger airways, such as the main, lobar, and segmental bronchi, are located (Akin et al., 2012). SCLC is characterized by large, lobulated lesions located centrally, often invading the mediastinum and hila (Akin et al., 2012; NCCN, 2015h).

In patients with a known lung malignancy, a PET scan is recommended for staging to evaluate for nodal and extrathoracic metastases (Ravenel et al., 2013; Silvestri et al., 2013). PET scanning is more sensitive than CT in detecting mediastinal lymph node involvement; up to 30% of patients with a negative CT have mediastinal lymph node involvement (Ravenel et al., 2013). Accurate assessment of the mediastinal lymph nodes is particularly important because mediastinal involvement determines whether the disease can be surgically resected (Silvestri et al., 2013). If PET cannot be obtained, bone scan and abdominal CT are reasonable alternatives (Silvestri et al., 2013). MRI of the brain is recommended for all patients except for those with stage IA NSCLC (NCCN, 2015f).

Laboratory studies: A CBC and chemistries, including renal function, liver function, calcium, and serum alkaline phosphatase, are recommended (NCCN, 2015f).

Biopsy: Histologic confirmation of malignancy is necessary to rule out other causes of respiratory symptoms. Depending on the location of the tumor, clinicians may use bronchoscopy with transbronchial needle aspiration (TBNA), radial endobronchial ultrasound (EBUS), transthoracic needle aspiration (TTNA), mediastinoscopy, or thoracoscopy to obtain tissue for diagnosis (NCCN, 2015f). NCCN recommends basing the choice of biopsy on a multidisciplinary review that takes into account the clinical suspicion of lung cancer, the location of the tumor, and patient characteristics (NCCN, 2015f). For example, bronchoscopy with TBNA is recommended for central tumors, whereas navigational bronchoscopy, radial EBUS, or TTNA is recommended for patients with peripheral nodules (NCCN, 2015f). Patients who have no evidence of mediastinal disease by imaging should undergo pathologic evaluation of the mediastinum for accurate staging (NCCN, 2015f; Silvestri et al., 2013).

Pathology: The two major classes of lung cancer are NSCLC and SCLC. More than 85% of lung cancer cases are NSCLC, which includes the broad histologic categories of nonsquamous (including adenocarcinoma, large-cell carcinoma, and others) and squamous cell carcinoma. These histologies are subtyped by the pattern of growth observed (e.g., acinar, papillary, micropapillary, or lepidic) (NCCN, 2015f). Adenocarcinoma is the most common type of lung cancer overall and is the most frequently occurring type in nonsmokers (NCCN, 2015f). It is particularly important to distinguish squamous cell carcinoma from adenocarcinoma and other NSCLCs in patients with advanced lung cancer because this distinction significantly influences treatment decisions. Research has demonstrated that pemetrexed may be preferable to other agents for treatment of patients with nonsquamous NSCLC, whereas patients with squamous cell carcinoma are unlikely to benefit from treatment with pemetrexed and are at risk for life-threatening hemorrhage from treatment with bevacizumab (Travis et al., 2011).

IHC staining is a valuable tool to differentiate various types of NSCLC. The two main IHC tests used are TTF-1 and p63. TTF-1 is a diagnostic immunohistochemical marker present in 70%–85% of pulmonary adenocarcinomas, whereas p63 is the best diagnostic marker for squamous cell carcinoma (Travis et al., 2011). TTF-1 also can be useful to distinguish primary pulmonary adenocarcinoma from pulmonary metastases from another primary adenocarcinoma (NCCN, 2015f). Metastatic adenocarcinoma from another adenocarcinoma, such as breast or colon, is nearly always negative for TTF-1 with the exception of metastatic thyroid malignancies, which can be diagnosed by a positive thyroglobulin (NCCN, 2015f).

The classification for adenocarcinoma was updated in 2011 by the International Association for the Study of Lung Cancer, American Thoracic Society, and European Respiratory Society to address advances in oncology, molecular biology, pathology, radiology, and surgery (Travis et al., 2011). This new adenocarcinoma classification is based on the 2004 World Health Organization (WHO) classification but eliminated the terms *bronchioloalveolar carcinoma (BAC)* and *mixed subtype adenocarcinoma.* The subtypes that replaced BAC and mixed subtype adeno-carcinoma are adenocarcinoma in situ; minimally invasive adenocarcinoma; lepidic predom-inant adenocarcinoma (nonmucinous); adenocarcinoma, predominantly invasive with some nonmucinous lepidic component (includes some resected tumors, formerly classified as mixed subtype) and some clinically advanced adenocarcinomas (formerly classified as nonmucinous BAC); and invasive mucinous adenocarcinoma (formerly mucinous BAC) (Travis et al., 2011). Most mucinous tumors (approximately 76%) have a *KRAS* mutation, whereas approximately 45% of nonmucinous adenocarcinomas have an *EGFR* mutation, which has implications for prognosis and treatment options (Travis et al., 2011).

The histologic grading for lung cancer ranges from GX to G4 (undifferentiated) (Edge et al., 2010). Grade 1 (G1) is well differentiated; G2 is moderately differentiated; and G3 is poorly differentiated (Edge et al., 2010).

Biomarkers: The biomarkers of significance in lung cancer include EGFR, ERCC1 (the 5' endonuclease of the nucleotide excision repair complex), *KRAS* oncogene, and *ALK* onco-gene (NCCN, 2015f). ERCC1 and *KRAS* are prognostic biomarkers for NSCLC: high levels of ERCC1 expression are associated with improved overall survival, and *KRAS* mutations are associated with poorer overall survival (NCCN, 2015f). *EGFR* and the *ALK* oncogene are pre-dictive biomarkers that predict response to EGFR tyrosine kinase inhibitors and *ALK* tyrosine kinase inhibitors, respectively (NCCN, 2015f; Travis et al., 2011). Testing for *EGFR* and *ALK* should guide treatment decisions with regard to the use of *EGFR* and *ALK* tyrosine kinase inhibitors (Lindeman et al., 2013). *EGFR* mutations may also be prognostic as they have been associated with a more indolent clinical course, and *EGFR* and *KRAS* mutations are virtu-ally mutually exclusive (Travis et al., 2011). The frequency of either *KRAS* or *EGFR* mutation is 10%–30% with a greater incidence of *EGFR* mutation in Asians, never-smokers, and those with nonmucinous tumors and a greater incidence of *KRAS* mutations in non-Asians, smok-ers, and those with invasive mucinous adenocarcinomas (Travis et al., 2011). *ALK* gene rear-rangements occur in 2%–7% of patients with NSCLC and confer resistance to EGFR tyrosine kinase inhibitors (NCCN, 2015f). *ALK* mutations are more likely to be present in patients who are male, are younger, have adenocarcinoma histology, and are nonsmokers (NCCN, 2015f).

Staging

The staging for lung cancer is performed using the TNM system (see Tables 3-9 and 3-10). The staging system is based on the size of the lung mass, extension to surrounding structures, regional lymph node involvement, and distant metastasis. The Veterans Administration Lung Study Group two-stage system was traditionally used for SCLC. This system classified SCLC as limited- or extensive-stage disease. Limited-stage disease was defined as tumors confined to one hemithorax that could be encompassed by one radiation port (Compton et al., 2012). All other patients were classified as extensive-stage disease, and the majority of patients with SCLC present with extensive-stage disease. However, an analysis of a large database of patients with SCLC showed that the TNM staging system is applicable to SCLC; therefore, AJCC rec-ommends use of the TNM staging system for both NSCLC and SCLC (Compton et al., 2012).

Prognosis

Favorable prognostic factors include early stage at diagnosis, good performance status (ECOG 0–2), absence of weight loss of more than 5% of body weight, and female gender (NCCN, 2015f).

Survival

The five-year survival rate for lung and bronchus cancer (all types) is 54% for localized dis-ease, 27% for regional disease, and 4% for metastatic disease (Siegel et al., 2015).

Table 3-9. Definition of Tumor-Node-Metastasis (TNM) Staging for Lung Cancer

Primary Tumor (T)

TX	Primary tumor cannot be assessed, or tumor proven by the presence of malignant cells in sputum or bronchial washings but not visualized by imaging or bronchoscopy
T0	No evidence of primary tumor
Tis	Carcinoma in situ
T1	Tumor 3 cm or less in greatest dimension, surrounded by lung or visceral pleura, without bronchoscopic evidence of invasion more proximal than the lobar bronchus (i.e., not in the main bronchus)*
T1a	Tumor 2 cm or less in greatest dimension
T1b	Tumor more than 2cm but 3 cm or less in greatest dimension
T2	Tumor more than 3 cm but 7 cm or less Or tumor with any of the following features (T2 tumors with these features are classified as T2a if 5 cm or less): • Involves main bronchus, 2 cm or more distal to the carina • Invades the visceral pleura (PL1 or PL2) • Associated with atelectasis or obstructive pneumonitis that extends to the hilar region but does not involve the entire lung
T2a	Tumor more than 3 cm but 5 cm or less in greatest dimension
T2b	Tumor more than 5 cm but 7 cm or less in greatest dimension
T3	Tumor more than 7 cm or tumor of any size that directly invades any of the following: parietal pleural (PL3) chest wall (including superior sulcus tumors), diaphragm, phrenic nerve, mediastinal pleura, parietal pericardium; or tumor in the main bronchus (less than 2 cm distal to the carina*, but without involvement of the carina); or associated atelectasis or obstructive pneumonitis of the entire lung or separate tumor nodules in the same lobe
T4	Tumor of any size that invades any of the following: mediastinum, heart, great vessels, trachea, recurrent laryngeal nerve, esophagus, vertebral body, carina; or separate tumor nodules in a different ipsilateral lobe

* The uncommon superficial spreading tumor of any size with its invasive component limited to the bronchial wall, which may extend proximal to the main bronchus, is also classified T1a.

Regional Lymph Nodes (N)

NX	Regional lymph nodes cannot be assessed
N0	No regional lymph node metastases
N1	Metastasis in ipsilateral peribronchial and/or ipsilateral hilar lymph nodes, and intrapulmonary nodes, including involvement by direct extension of the primary tumor
N2	Metastasis in ipsilateral mediastinal and/or subcarinal lymph node(s)
N3	Metastasis in contralateral mediastinal, contralateral hilar, ipsilateral or contralateral scalene, or supraclavicular lymph node(s)

(Continued on next page)

Table 3-9. Definition of Tumor-Node-Metastasis (TNM) Staging for Lung Cancer
(Continued)

Distant Metastasis (M)

MX   Distant metastasis cannot be assessed

M0   No distant metastasis

M1   Distant metastasis (in extrathoracic organs)

M1a   Separate tumor nodule(s) in a contralateral lobe tumor with pleural nodules or malignant pleural (or pericardial) effusion*

M1b   Distant metastasis

---

* Most pleural (and pericardial) effusions with lung cancer are due to tumor. In a few patients, however, multiple cyto-pathologic examinations of pleural (pericardial) fluid are negative for tumor, and the fluid is nonbloody and is not an exudate. Where these elements and clinical judgment dictate that the effusion is not related to the tumor, the effusion should be excluded as a staging element and the patient should be classified as M0.

Note. From *AJCC Cancer Staging Manual* (7th ed.), by S.B. Edge, D.R. Byrd, C.C. Compton, A.G. Fritz, F.L. Greene, and A. Trotti III (Eds.), 2010, New York, NY: Springer, www.springeronline.com. Used with permission of the American Joint Committee on Cancer (AJCC), Chicago, Illinois.

Non-Hodgkin Lymphoma

The initial evaluation of patients with NHL should include a thorough history and physical examination, assessment of performance status, PET-CT imaging, basic laboratory tests, and, in most cases, a bone marrow biopsy (NCCN, 2015e).

History and current complaints: A comprehensive health history should include assessment of "B" symptoms, including fever, night sweats (often soaking), and unexplained weight loss. Other symptoms include fatigue, abdominal fullness, or early satiety (may indicate splenomegaly). Providers should inquire about the presence of enlarged lymph nodes of the neck, axilla, and inguinal areas, including how long they have been present and whether they grow and shrink (Goodrich et al., 2013). Often, in low-grade lymphomas, patients report that they have had enlarged lymph nodes that wax and wane in size.

Risk factors: Known risk factors associated with NHL include exposure to chemicals or radiation, history of immunosuppressive therapy, history of autoimmune disorders, and history of infection with specific viruses or bacteria (e.g., Epstein-Barr virus, HIV, *Helicobacter pylori*) (Goodrich et al., 2013).

Physical Examination

When performing a physical assessment on a person with suspected lymphoma, it is critical to assess all lymph nodes, the spleen, and the liver. Lymphoma can spread to extranodal sites, including the GI tract, lungs, bones, skin, liver, central nervous system, and testes (Goodrich et al., 2013).

Diagnosis

Laboratory testing: Laboratory testing should include CBC with differential, comprehensive metabolic panel, and lactate dehydrogenase (LDH) (Goodrich et al., 2013; NCCN, 2015e). Other laboratory parameters may be appropriate depending on disease and patient characteristics.

Table 3-10. Stage Grouping for Lung Cancer

Stage	T	N	M
Occult carcinoma	TX	N0	M0
Stage 0	Tis	N0	M0
Stage IA	T1a	N0	M0
	T1b	N0	M0
Stage IB	T2a	N0	M0
Stage IIA	T2b	N0	M0
	T1a	N1	M0
	T1b	N1	M0
	T2a	N1	M0
Stage IIB	T2b	N1	M0
	T3	N0	M0
Stage IIIA	T1a	N2	M0
	T1b	N2	M0
	T2a	N2	M0
	T2b	N2	M0
	T3	N1	M0
	T3	N2	M0
	T4	N0	M0
	T4	N1	M0
Stage IIIB	T1a	N3	M0
	T1b	N3	M0
	T2a	N3	M0
	T2b	N3	M0
	T3	N3	M0
	T4	N2	M0
	T4	N3	M0
Stage IV	Any T	Any N	M1a
	Any T	Any N	M1b

Note. From *AJCC Cancer Staging Manual* (7th ed.), by S.B. Edge, D.R. Byrd, C.C. Compton, A.G. Fritz, F.L. Greene, and A. Trotti III (Eds.), 2010, New York, NY: Springer, www.springeronline.com. Used with permission of the American Joint Committee on Cancer (AJCC), Chicago, Illinois.

Radiographic examinations: Imaging to determine the extent of disease includes chest radiographs; CT scan of the chest, abdomen, pelvis, and/or neck; and PET or combined PET-CT scan (NCCN, 2015e). Of these imaging modalities, PET-CT is the most important radiologic examination for pretreatment staging, restaging, and assessment of response to therapy (Cheson, 2011). Additional studies, such as bone scan, lumbar puncture, cardiac function studies, MRI, or endoscopy/colonoscopy, may be appropriate for certain NHL subtypes or based on clinical presentation (NCCN, 2015e).

Biopsy
The diagnosis of lymphoma is made by excisional lymph node biopsy of an affected lymph node with immunophenotyping and examination by a skilled hematopathologist (Goodrich

et al., 2013). Fine needle aspiration is considered insufficient to render a definitive diagnosis (NCCN, 2015e). However, an incisional or core needle biopsy may be obtained from a lymph node or other involved organ, and flow cytometry, IHC, and molecular testing may assist with precise diagnosis (Goodrich et al., 2013).

Bone marrow biopsy is critical for comprehensive staging and optimal patient management for most NHL subtypes because bone marrow involvement denotes stage IV disease, which may have significant prognostic and therapeutic implications (Goodrich et al., 2013; NCCN, 2015e). The bone marrow biopsy specimen should be 1.6–2 cm or greater for adequate evaluation. Bone marrow aspiration is typically not necessary unless certain molecular tests or cytogenetics are indicated (NCCN, 2015e).

Pathology

The pathologic classification of NHL is complex, as more than 50 specific subtypes exist. The current classification system is the 2008 WHO classification of haematopoietic and lymphoid tissue tumors (Swerdlow et al., 2008). Broadly, lymphoid neoplasms are divided into mature B-cell neoplasms and mature T-cell and natural killer (NK)-cell neoplasms. The various subtypes of NHLs fall into one of these categories based on their derivation from B-cell, T-cell, or NK-cell origin (Swerdlow et al., 2008). B-cell lymphoma is the most common NHL, and diffuse large B-cell lymphoma is the most common subtype (Goodrich et al., 2013).

The distinction among the various subtypes of NHL can be difficult to diagnose; therefore, IHC, flow cytometry, and molecular and cytogenetic testing have become increasingly important for accurate classification (NCCN, 2015e). In addition, Ki-67 mitotic index is a measure of proliferation that has prognostic value in certain NHL subtypes, such as mantle cell lymphoma (Goodrich et al., 2013).

Grade

Grading varies by the subtype of NHL. Clinically, NHL can be classified as low grade, intermediate grade, and high grade (Goodrich et al., 2013). Low-grade lymphomas tend to be chronic, indolent lymphomas that are treatable but not curable, as they respond to treatment but invariably recur and continue to require retreatment (Goodrich et al., 2013). Intermediate-grade and high-grade lymphomas are more aggressive and tend to be fatal if left untreated, but are potentially curable with treatment (Goodrich et al., 2013).

Staging

The staging system for non-Hodgkin and Hodgkin lymphomas is the Cotswolds-Modified Ann Arbor staging system (Lister et al., 1989) as outlined in Table 3-11. Lymphomas are staged from stage I to IV, based on lymph node involvement and extranodal sites of disease. Stage I is defined as involvement of a single lymph node region; stage II is defined as involvement of more than one lymph node region on the same side of the diaphragm; and stage III disease is defined as lymph node involvement on both sides of the diaphragm (Lister et al., 1989). Stage IV indicates disseminated disease to the bone marrow, central nervous system, or more than one extranodal site.

The stage is assigned a subscript(s) to represent special features of the disease. The subscripts A and B indicate the presence or absence of B symptoms. B symptoms are defined as unexplained weight loss of more than 10% of body weight during the six months before initial staging investigation; unexplained, persistent, or recurrent fever with temperatures above 38°C (100.4°F) during the previous month; and/or recurrent drenching night sweats during the previous month (Lister et al., 1989). The absence of B symptoms is represented with the subscript A, such that a patient with stage IV disease and no B symptoms would be staged as IVA. The

Table 3-11. Cotswolds-Modified Ann Arbor Staging System for Non-Hodgkin and Hodgkin Lymphomas

Stage	Description
I	Involvement of a single lymph node region (e.g., cervical, axillary, inguinal, mediastinal) or lymphoid structure (e.g., spleen, thymus, Waldeyer ring)
II	Involvement of 2 or more lymph node regions or lymph node structures on the same side of the diaphragm. Hilar nodes should be considered "lateralized," and when involved on both sides, constitute stage II disease.
III	Involvement of lymph node regions or lymphoid structures on both sides of the diaphragm
IV	Disseminated disease (e.g., bone marrow or central nervous system involvement) or more than 1 extranodal site
Subscripts	
A	The subscript *A* denotes absence of B symptoms.
B	The subscript *B* indicates the presence of B symptoms, which include one or more of the following. • Unexplained weight loss of more than 10% of the body weight during the 6 months before initial staging investigation • Unexplained, persistent, or recurrent fever with temperatures above 38°C (100.4°F) during the previous month • Recurrent drenching night sweats during the previous month.
X	The subscript *X* refers to bulky disease. No subscripts will be used in the absence of bulk. Bulky disease is defined as • A node or nodal mass ≥ 10 cm, or • A mediastinal mass with a maximum width ≥ one-third of the internal transverse diameter of the thorax at the level of T5–6 on a posteroanterior chest radiograph taken 6 ft from the patient.
E	The subscript *E* refers to limited extranodal extension. Limited extranodal extension is defined as involvement of extralymphatic tissue on one side of the diaphragm by limited direct extension from an adjacent nodal site. This is traditionally regarded as extranodal involvement that could be encompassed within a radiation field. A single extralymphatic site as the only site of disease is classified as IE. More than one extranodal site is designated stage IV.
Other considerations	The term *mediastinal* includes the following nodal subgroups. • Prevascular, aortopulmonary • Paratracheal, pretracheal, subcarinal • Posterior mediastinal Hilar (bronchopulmonary) nodes are considered to be outside the mediastinum.

Note. Based on information from Lister et al., 1989.

presence of B symptoms is represented with the subscript *B*, and similarly, a patient with stage IV disease and one or more B symptoms would be staged as IVB. Staging can be further refined by designating bulky disease with the subscript *X*, which is defined as a mediastinal mass ratio greater than 0.33 or a lymph node mass larger than 10 cm (Lister et al., 1989). The mediastinal mass ratio is the ratio of the maximum width of the mass and the maximum intrathoracic diameter measured at T5–6 on a posteroanterior chest radiograph taken 6 ft from the patient. For example, a patient with stage II NHL with a mediastinal mass that has a mediastinal mass ratio greater than 0.33 and B symptoms would be staged as stage IIXB. Extranodal extension is represented with an "E." One extranodal site as the sole measurable disease is staged IE, whereas more than one extranodal site is considered stage IV disease (Lister et al., 1989).

Prognosis

Specific prognostic indices exist for several subtypes of NHL, including diffuse large B-cell lymphoma, follicular lymphoma, primary central nervous system lymphoma, and mantle cell lymphoma (Goodrich et al., 2013). In general, unfavorable prognostic factors include older age, advanced stage, elevated LDH, extranodal involvement, and poor performance status (Goodrich et al., 2013).

Survival

Survival varies widely by cell type and stage of disease. Early-stage disease with favorable subtypes are associated with a five-year overall survival of 80%–90% (Goodrich et al., 2013). For all NHL diagnoses combined, the five-year relative survival rates are 82% for localized disease, 73% for regional disease, and 62% for distant involvement (Siegel et al., 2015).

Ovarian Cancer

The initial evaluation of patients with ovarian cancer should include a thorough history and physical examination with abdominal/pelvic examination, chest imaging, CT and/or ultrasound of the abdomen/pelvis, basic laboratory tests, CA 125, and selective testing for distant metastases. High-risk patients should be referred for genetic counseling (NCCN, 2015g).

History

History and current complaints: More than 70% of patients with ovarian cancer will present with disease that has spread beyond the ovaries at diagnosis because the early symptoms, such as abdominal discomfort and bloating, are vague and difficult to attribute to cancer (Rubin, Sabbatini, & Viswanathan, 2013). Ovarian cancer has been called the "silent killer" because symptoms often occur only when the disease is advanced. Clusters of symptoms are more likely to yield a diagnosis than the presence of a single symptom. The specificity for a diagnosis of ovarian cancer was 90% for women older than age 50 if any of the following symptoms were present more than 12 times in a given month but with overall duration of less than one year: pelvic/abdominal pain, urinary urgency or frequency, increased abdominal size or bloating, and difficulty eating or feeling full quickly (NCCN, 2015g; Rubin et al., 2013). Patients with advanced disease may experience swelling or bloating of the abdomen due to ascites, bladder or rectal symptoms from a large pelvic mass, respiratory symptoms from a pleural effusion (more common on the right side), and, rarely, vaginal bleeding (Rubin et al., 2013).

Risk factors: Older age (age 35 and older) at first pregnancy or birth and nulliparity are associated with an increased risk of ovarian cancer (NCCN, 2015g). Evidence is emerging suggesting that hormone therapy, pelvic inflammatory disease, and ovarian stimulation for in vitro fertilization are also associated with an increased risk of ovarian cancer (NCCN, 2015g).

Family history: Although most epithelial ovarian cancer occurs sporadically, hereditary ovarian cancer occurs in approximately 5% of malignancies (NCCN, 2015g). Individuals with *BRCA1* and *BRCA2* mutations, Lynch syndrome, and a family history of two or more first-degree relatives with ovarian cancer are at increased risk for developing the disease (NCCN,

2015g). These cancers occur at earlier ages than the nonhereditary tumors. Patients with a family history of two first-degree relatives with ovarian cancer have a higher risk, as do those with hereditary nonpolyposis colorectal cancer. A three-generation maternal and paternal family history should be obtained. More information on hereditary cancer is discussed in Chapter 2.

Physical Examination

Although the pelvic examination is the most widely used examination for a patient suspected of ovarian cancer, it is not very sensitive to early forms of the disease (Rubin et al., 2013). The examination assesses for ascites and a pelvic mass located in the cul-de-sac, which may feel hard and fixed with multiple nodularities (Rubin et al., 2013). Lymph nodes are examined carefully. Breast examination is performed to assess for a possible synchronous breast cancer or metastatic disease. The rest of the physical examination is directed at symptomatology and suspicion of metastatic disease.

Differential Diagnosis

The differential diagnosis includes abdominal or pelvic infections, GI disorders or malignancy, metastases from another primary cancer, pregnancy, ovarian cysts, ectopic pregnancy, gestational trophoblastic disease, and uterine conditions such as fibroids or benign tumors of the reproductive tract (Rubin et al., 2013).

Diagnostic Tests

Radiologic examinations: Transvaginal ultrasound or abdominal/pelvic ultrasound may be used in some settings to evaluate a pelvic mass in the initial workup for suspected ovarian cancer. CT of the chest, abdomen, and pelvis with contrast or MRI of the abdomen and pelvis is recommended for preoperative staging of ovarian cancer (Mitchell et al., 2012). These scans are useful in evaluating involvement of the pelvic ureter, uterine serosa, lymph nodes, peritoneum, mesentery, omentum, liver, spleen, and lung (Mitchell et al., 2012). However, CT is limited in detection of involvement of the bowel surface, as well as mesenteric or peritoneal implants smaller than 5 mm in size (Mitchell et al., 2012).

Laboratory studies: Laboratory studies include CBC, chemistries with LFTs, and CA 125 (NCCN, 2015g). CA 125 is elevated in approximately 50% of patients with early ovarian cancers and approximately 80% of patients with advanced ovarian cancer (Rubin et al., 2013).

CA 125 is neither sensitive nor specific enough to use in screening or for a definitive diagnosis; however, it may be used for surveillance for disease recurrence. The median time to clinical relapse following documentation of an increased CA 125 level is two to six months (NCCN, 2015g).

Biopsy: Referral to a gynecologic oncologist is recommended for surgical staging with exploratory laparotomy (NCCN, 2015g; Rubin et al., 2013). Paracentesis or needle biopsy of a pelvic mass may lead to seeding of tumor cells along needle tracks and is not recommended (Rubin et al., 2013).

Pathology: Ovarian tumors are classified according to the structures of origin within the ovary itself, and approximately 90% of ovarian cancer has an epithelial histology (NCCN, 2015g). The main histologic types of epithelial tumors include serous (approximately 70%), mucinous, endometrioid, and clear cell (NCCN, 2015g). The histologic grades for ovarian cancer range from GX to G4 (Edge et al., 2010).

Staging

Comprehensive surgical staging is recommended for ovarian cancer. The TNM and the FIGO systems are used for staging (see Tables 3-12 and 3-13). Staging is based on involvement of one

Table 3-12. Definition of Tumor-Node-Metastasis (TNM) Staging for Ovarian Cancer

Primary Tumor (T)

TNM Categories	FIGO Stages	
TX		Primary tumor cannot be assessed
T0		No evidence of primary tumor
T1	I	Tumor limited to ovaries (one or both)
T1a	IA	Tumor limited to one ovary; capsule intact, no tumor on ovarian surface. No malignant cells in ascites or peritoneal washings
T1b	IB	Tumor limited to both ovaries; capsules intact, no tumor on ovarian surface. No malignant cells in ascites or peritoneal washings
T1c	IC	Tumor limited to one or both ovaries with any of the following: capsule ruptured, tumor on ovarian surface, malignant cells in ascites or peritoneal washings
T2	II	Tumor involves one or both ovaries with pelvic extension
T2a	IIA	Extension and/or implants on uterus and/or tube(s). No malignant cells in ascites or peritoneal washings
T2b	IIB	Extension to and/or implants on other pelvic tissues. No malignant cells in ascites or peritoneal washings
T2c	IIC	Pelvic extension and/or implants (T2a or T2b) with malignant cells in ascites or peritoneal washings
T3	III	Tumor involves one or both ovaries with microscopically confirmed peritoneal metastasis outside the pelvis
T3a	IIIA	Microscopic peritoneal metastasis beyond pelvis (no macroscopic tumor)
T3b	IIIB	Macroscopic peritoneal metastasis beyond pelvis 2 cm or less in greatest dimension
T3c	IIIC	Peritoneal metastasis beyond pelvis more than 2 cm in greatest dimension and/or regional lymph node metastasis

Note. Liver capsule metastasis T3/Stage III; liver parenchymal metastasis M1/Stage IV. Pleural effusion must have positive cytology for M1/Stage IV.

Regional Lymph Nodes (N)

NX		Regional lymph nodes cannot be assessed
N0		No regional lymph node metastasis
N1	IIIC	Regional lymph node metastasis

Distant Metastasis (M)

MX		Distant metastasis cannot be assessed
M0		No distant metastasis
M1	IV	Distant metastasis (excludes peritoneal metastasis)

Note. From *AJCC Cancer Staging Manual* (7th ed.), by S.B. Edge, D.R. Byrd, C.C. Compton, A.G. Fritz, F.L. Greene, and A. Trotti III (Eds.), 2010, New York, NY: Springer, www.springeronline.com. Used with permission of the American Joint Committee on Cancer (AJCC), Chicago, Illinois.

Table 3-13. Stage Grouping for Ovarian Cancer

Stage	T	N	M
Stage I	T1	N0	M0
Stage IA	T1a	N0	M0
Stage IB	T1b	N0	M0
Stage IC	T1c	N0	M0
Stage II	T2	N0	M0
Stage IIA	T2a	N0	M0
Stage IIB	T2b	N0	M0
Stage IIC	T2c	N0	M0
Stage III	T3	N0	M0
Stage IIIA	T3a	N0	M0
Stage IIIB	T3b	N0	M0
Stage IIIC	T3c	N0	M0
	Any T	N1	M0
Stage IV	Any T	Any N	M1

Note. From *AJCC Cancer Staging Manual* (7th ed.), by S.B. Edge, D.R. Byrd, C.C. Compton, A.G. Fritz, F.L. Greene, and A. Trotti III (Eds.), 2010, New York, NY: Springer, www.springeronline.com. Used with permission of the American Joint Committee on Cancer (AJCC), Chicago, Illinois.

or both ovaries; extension to the uterus, other pelvic tissues, or peritoneum; regional lymph node metastases; and distant metastases. The initial surgery for staging and cytoreduction includes a staging laparotomy, total abdominal hysterectomy, and bilateral salpingo-oophorectomy (NCCN, 2015g). Aspiration of ascites or peritoneal lavage should be obtained for cytology. All obvious disease (e.g., involving the omentum or lymph nodes) should be resected. Approximately 30% of ovarian cancer will be upstaged based on clinically occult surgical findings (NCCN, 2015g).

Survival and Prognosis

The most significant prognostic factor is the stage of disease (Rubin et al., 2013). The five-year survival rate in the United States for ovarian cancer is 92% for localized disease, 72% for regional disease, and 27% for metastatic disease (Siegel et al., 2015).

Prostate Cancer

The initial evaluation of patients with prostate cancer should include a thorough history and physical examination, assessment of performance status, DRE, and PSA. For patients with a life expectancy of five years or longer or patients with symptoms, a bone scan and pelvic CT or MRI may be indicated (NCCN, 2014b).

History

History and current complaints: Most men are asymptomatic from the disease; approximately 90% of all cases of prostate cancer are diagnosed through PSA screening (Hoffman,

2011). In patients who have symptoms, the most common are difficulty in voiding or change in the force of the urinary stream as a result of prostate enlargement.

Risk factors: The three risk factors for prostate cancer are older age, family history, and African American race (Hoffman, 2011). Age is one of the most significant risk factors, and the median age at diagnosis is 67 years (Hoffman, 2011). However, the great majority of men diagnosed with prostate cancer die of other causes, and 30% of men older than age 50 and 70% of men older than age 70 have evidence of undiagnosed prostate cancer on autopsy (Hoffman, 2011). African American men have the highest incidence of prostate cancer and are more likely to be diagnosed with advanced-stage disease than any other racial or ethnic group (Hoffman, 2011). The risk of prostate cancer is lower for individuals with a history of negative prostate biopsy (Wolf et al., 2010).

Family history: A comprehensive family history should be obtained because individuals with a first-degree relative with prostate cancer have a twofold higher risk of the disease (Heidenreich et al., 2011; Hoffman, 2011). If more than one first-degree relative has prostate cancer, the risk increases to 5–11-fold (Heidenreich et al., 2011). Hereditary prostate cancer accounts for 9% of cases and is defined as three or more relatives affected or two or more relatives who developed early-onset prostate cancer (before age 55) (Heidenreich et al., 2011).

Physical Examination

PSA and DRE are essential in the workup for patients suspected of having prostate cancer. DRE detects approximately 18% of prostate cancer, irrespective of PSA (Heidenreich et al., 2011). Although an irregular and firm prostate usually is considered an abnormal rectal finding, symptoms could be the result of an overdistended bladder, lymphedema of the lower extremities, deep vein thrombosis, or even cancer cachexia. Finding areas of induration may indicate direct extension of the disease. DRE is unlikely to find anterior or midline prostate tumors. Percussion and palpation of the pelvis are performed to assess for bladder distention. Inguinal nodes are assessed carefully as well.

Differential Diagnosis

The differential diagnosis of prostate cancer includes benign prostatic hyperplasia, prostatitis or cystitis, perineal trauma, or recent instrumentation for testing or surgery in the urinary tract (Heidenreich et al., 2011; Hoffman, 2011).

Diagnostic Tests

Radiologic examinations: Following an abnormal DRE or PSA finding, the first study ordered usually is TRUS, which is used to guide biopsy sites (Heidenreich et al., 2011). Additional studies are ordered based on clinical criteria. A bone scan is performed in symptomatic patients with T1 disease and PSA greater than 20 ng/ml; T2 disease and PSA greater than 10 ng/ml; Gleason score of 8 or higher; or any T3 or T4 disease (NCCN, 2014b). Pelvic CT or MRI is performed in symptomatic patients with T1–T2 disease and greater than 10% nomogram-indicated probability of lymph node involvement or any T3–T4 disease (NCCN, 2014b).

Laboratory values: Laboratory values include a measurement of PSA. It is a very specific test; however, elevated PSA levels are found in nonmalignant conditions such as benign prostatic hyperplasia or prostatitis (Heidenreich et al., 2012; Hoffman, 2011).

Biopsy: A biopsy must be performed to make a definitive diagnosis. TRUS-guided systematic core biopsy is the recommended method (Heidenreich et al., 2011; NCCN, 2014b). Many prostate cancers are not palpable or able to be seen by ultrasound; thus, the standard practice is to systematically obtain a minimum of 10 core biopsies from the medial and lateral aspects of the peripheral zone of the prostate (Heidenreich et al., 2011; NCCN, 2014b). Additional biopsies can be obtained if other suspicious areas are noted.

Pathology: Nearly all prostate cancers are adenocarcinomas. They tend to be multifocal, and 80%–85% arise from the peripheral zone, 10%–15% from the transitional zone, and 5%–10% from the central zone (Compton et al., 2012). The Gleason scoring system was developed to grade this specific tumor type. The pathologist assigns a Gleason score of 1–5 on the two most common growth patterns identified based on the morphology of the specimen. The final score is the sum of these two numbers (as in the example of 2 + 4 = 6) (Gleason & Mellinger, 1974; NCCN, 2014b). Most newly diagnosed patients have a Gleason score of 6 or higher (NCCN, 2014b).

Staging

Staging of prostate cancer uses the TNM system (see Tables 3-14 and 3-15). Staging information for prostate cancer includes the PSA level and Gleason score (Edge et al., 2010). Pathologic lymph node status (N staging) is only considered important for patients who will be treated with potentially curative therapy and have 2% or greater probability of nomogram-predicted lymph node involvement (NCCN, 2014b). Patients with stage T1–T2, PSA less than 10 ng/ml, a Gleason score of 6 or lower, and less than 50% positive biopsy cores have less than 10% probability of lymph node metastases (Heidenreich et al., 2011).

Table 3-14. Definition of Tumor-Node-Metastasis (TNM) Staging for Prostate Cancer

Primary Tumor (T)

Clinical

TX	Primary tumor cannot be assessed
T0	No evidence of primary tumor
T1	Clinically inapparent tumor neither palpable nor visible by imaging
T1a	Tumor incidental histologic finding in 5% or less of tissue resected
T1b	Tumor incidental histologic finding in more than 5% of tissue resected
T1c	Tumor identified by needle biopsy (e.g., because of elevated PSA)
T2	Tumor confined within prostate*
T2a	Tumor involves one-half of one lobe or less
T2b	Tumor involves more than one-half of one lobe but not both lobes
T2c	Tumor involves both lobes
T3	Tumor extends through the prostate capsule**
T3a	Extracapsular extension (unilateral or bilateral)
T3b	Tumor invades seminal vesicle(s)
T4	Tumor is fixed or invades adjacent structures other than seminal vesicles: bladder neck, external sphincter, rectum, levator muscles, and/or pelvic wall

* Tumor found in one or both lobes by needle biopsy, but not palpable or reliably visible by imaging, is classified as T1c.

** Invasion into the prostatic apex or into (but not beyond) the prostatic capsule is classified not as T3 but as T2.

(Continued on next page)

Table 3-14. Definition of Tumor-Node-Metastasis (TNM) Staging for Prostate Cancer
(Continued)

Pathologic (pT)*

pT2   Organ confined

pT2a   Unilateral, involving one-half of one lobe or less

pT2b   Unilateral, involving more than one-half of one lobe but not both lobes

pT2c   Bilateral disease

pT3   Extraprostatic extension

pT3a   Extraprostatic extension or microscopic invasion of bladder neck**

pT3b   Seminal vesicle invasion

pT4   Invasion of rectum, levator muscles, and/or pelvic wall

* There is no pathologic T1 classification.
** Positive surgical margin should be indicated by an R1 descriptor (residual microscopic disease).

Regional Lymph Nodes (N)

Clinical

NX   Regional lymph nodes were not assessed

N0   No regional lymph node metastasis

N1   Metastasis in regional lymph nodes(s)

Pathologic

pNX   Regional nodes not sampled

pN0   No positive regional nodes

pN1   Metastases in regional node(s)

Distant Metastasis (M)*

MX   Distant metastasis cannot be assessed

M0   No distant metastasis

M1   Distant metastasis

M1a   Non-regional lymph node(s)

M1b   Bone(s)

M1c   Other site(s) with or without bone disease

* When more than one site of metastasis is present, the most advanced category is used. pM1c is most advanced.

PSA—prostate-specific antigen

Note. From *AJCC Cancer Staging Manual* (7th ed.), by S.B. Edge, D.R. Byrd, C.C. Compton, A.G. Fritz, F.L. Greene, and A. Trotti III (Eds.), 2010, New York, NY: Springer, www.springeronline.com. Used with permission of the American Joint Committee on Cancer (AJCC), Chicago, Illinois.

Table 3-15. Stage Grouping for Prostate Cancer

Stage	T	N	M	PSA	Gleason
Stage I	T1a–c	N0	M0	PSA < 10	Gleason ≤ 6
	T2a	N0	M0	PSA ≥ 10 < 20	Gleason ≤ 6
	T2a	N0	M0	PSA < 20	Gleason 7
	T1–2a	N0	M0	PSA X	Gleason X
Stage IIA	T1a–c	N0	M0	PSA < 20	Gleason 7
	T1a–c	N0	M0	PSA ≥ 10 < 20	Gleason ≤ 6
	T2a	N0	M0	PSA < 20	Gleason ≤ 7
	T2b	N0	M0	PSA < 20	Gleason ≤ 7
	T2b	N0	M0	PSA X	Gleason X
Stage IIB	T2c	N0	M0	Any PSA	Any Gleason
	T1–2	N0	M0	PSA ≥ 20	Any Gleason
	T1–2	N0	M0	Any PSA	Gleason ≥ 8
Stage III	T3a–b	N0	M0	Any PSA	Any Gleason
Stage IV	T4	N0	M0	Any PSA	Any Gleason
	Any T	N1	M0	Any PSA	Any Gleason
	Any T	Any N	M1	Any PSA	Any Gleason

PSA—prostate-specific antigen

* When either PSA or Gleason is not available, grouping should be determined by T stage and/or either PSA or Gleason as available.

Note. From *AJCC Cancer Staging Manual* (7th ed.), by S.B. Edge, D.R. Byrd, C.C. Compton, A.G. Fritz, F.L. Greene, and A. Trotti III (Eds.), 2010, New York, NY: Springer, www.springeronline.com. Used with permission of the American Joint Committee on Cancer (AJCC), Chicago, Illinois.

Survival and Prognosis

Prognostic factors in prostate cancer include stage, PSA levels, and Gleason score (Compton et al., 2012; NCCN, 2014b). The natural history of the disease is poorly understood and has variable survival times. Patients with lower-grade tumors may have disease that is slow growing, whereas others with high-grade lesions may progress to metastatic disease quite quickly (NCCN, 2014b). Nomograms often are used in making an assessment about prognosis to assist with treatment decision making. The Partin tables are commonly used to predict the pathologic stage of a prostate cancer based on the clinical stage, biopsy Gleason grade, and preoperative PSA level (NCCN, 2014b). Another model, the Epstein criteria, uses clinical criteria to predict which prostate cancers are likely to be clinically insignificant. According to the Epstein criteria, a prostate cancer is likely to be clinically insignificant if the following factors are present: clinical stage T1c, biopsy Gleason score of 6 or lower, prostate cancer present in fewer than three biopsy cores, prostate cancer involvement of 50% or less in any core, and PSA density less than 0.15 ng/ml/g (NCCN, 2014b).

The five-year survival rate in the United States for prostate cancer is 100% for patients with localized disease and 28% for patients with distant metastasis (Siegel et al., 2015).

Implications for Oncology Advanced Practice Nurses

Many oncology APNs are directly involved in cancer diagnosis and staging. Accurate diagnosis and staging are essential prior to beginning treatment for cancer. APNs may be involved in the initial examination of patients with a suspected cancer and/or the ordering of imaging studies, laboratory reports, or biopsies. APNs may review the collected pathologic data and stage patients once a malignancy is found; restaging may be performed in certain cancers. The APN role varies among different practice settings, but in every setting, an understanding of the diagnosis and staging of cancer is critical to comprehensive, evidence-based care of patients with cancer.

Conclusion

The diagnosis of cancer is made using a variety of tools, including examination techniques, diagnostic and laboratory tests, and histopathologic data. This information gives clinicians data regarding the type, location, and extent of neoplastic disease. The use of biomarkers provides more specific information regarding tumor substances excreted or shed by some tumor types. The role of biomarkers is expected to expand as more is learned about the molecular processes of various cancers. Correct staging is essential to describe the extent of disease so that appropriate treatment options can be considered. APNs are well qualified to participate in the diagnosis and staging of cancer, using these tools and tumor markers or biomarkers for the initial evaluation of patients suspected of having a cancer. As the science continues to evolve, APNs must keep abreast of the latest information regarding cancer diagnosis and staging in order to provide the most up-to-date and comprehensive care possible.

Case Study

C.M. is a 67-year-old widowed male with complaints of progressively severe obstipation persisting over two weeks. He tried many over-the-counter remedies to treat his bowel complaints, but he was unsuccessful and finally came to the emergency department for management. He states that his bowels have always been fairly normal with occasional constipation relieved by prunes or over-the-counter laxatives. He reports new onset of frequent rectal bleeding over the past year and describes this as bright red streaking in the stool. He has mild abdominal pain, some nausea, and weight loss of 10 pounds over the past three years. He admits to increasing fatigue and arthritic complaints over the past year.

Past medical history is significant for acute myocardial infarction at age 58 and subsequent placement of two coronary artery stents. He denies other comorbidities. He walks regularly and gardens in his backyard. He admits to mild alcohol use and denies smoking. C.M.'s family history is negative for colon cancer in his immediate family, but he has a grandfather who was thought to have died of stomach cancer in his 70s. His mother died at age 72 of diabetic complications thought to be cardiac related, and his father died of an acute myocardial infarction at age 54. He has two healthy children. C.M. denies having any major surgeries. A screening colonoscopy seven years ago showed several small noncancerous polyps, which were successfully removed.

On physical examination, C.M. looks generally well and has an ECOG performance status of 0. Chest and abdominal examination are unremarkable except for mild tenderness at the area of the umbilicus with deep palpation. Liver edge is palpable with deep inspiration; the edge is smooth and without nodules. No masses are appreciated during the rectal examination. Stool is trace guaiac positive, and prostate examination reveals slightly enlarged prostate gland with rubbery consistency.

C.M. is scheduled for a colonoscopy, and a large mass is found in his transverse colon, as well as two other large (2.2 cm and 1.4 cm) adenomatous polyps in the descending colon. A biopsy reveals moderately differentiated adenocarcinoma of the colon.

1. What further diagnostic testing may be indicated in the staging of this patient?
    *   CT of the chest, abdomen, and pelvis is recommended to assess for distant metastases.
    *   C.M. has a chest, abdominal, and pelvic CT that shows two metastatic liver lesions. Preoperative CEA is elevated at 77.8 ng/ml. C.M. undergoes partial colectomy for relief of partial obstruction. Pathology showed moderately differentiated adenocarcinoma of the colon that invaded through the muscularis propria into the pericolorectal tissues and 4 out of 14 positive lymph nodes.
2. What is the final stage for this patient?
    *   Final staging was determined to be stage IVA disease (T3 N2a M1a). M stage was determined to be M1a because the metastatic disease was confined to one organ. Neoadjuvant chemotherapy is considered to enable surgical resection of the liver metastases. FOLFOX (5-fluorouracil, oxaliplatin, and leucovorin) with bevacizumab is administered over three months, and serial measurements show a steady decrease in CEA.

Following chemotherapy, C.M. is reevaluated. One liver lesion had completely resolved, and the other was decreased to 2.1 cm. He undergoes successful surgical resection of his liver metastases. The pathology report from this surgery reveals a 2.6 cm poorly differentiated tumor from the right lobe of the liver. No further lymph node involvement is discerned during resection. His postoperative CEA decreases to 7.5 approximately one month after his surgery.

Following liver resection, C.M. completes a total of six months of adjuvant therapy with FOLFIRI (5-fluorouracil, leucovorin, and irinotecan) with bevacizumab. Three years after his original diagnosis, he is without evidence of disease, his CEA is 2, and his scans are negative for recurrence.

3. Because the CEA was elevated at diagnosis and decreased following surgery, might this have been a screening tool for him along with colonoscopy?
    *   No, CEA may be used as a convenient marker for evaluation of disease recurrence and treatment efficacy, but it is neither sensitive nor specific enough to use in general population screening. However, because it was elevated preoperatively and postoperatively, it should be monitored every three to six months for the first two years and then every six months for three to five years.
4. If C.M. develops recurrent disease, what biomarker would be helpful to guide treatment decisions?
    *   *KRAS* mutations are predictive for lack of response to anti-EGFR therapy. All recurrent tumors should be tested for *KRAS* mutations to determine if anti-EGFR therapy may be of benefit.

Key Points

*   Cancer is considered a microscopic diagnosis.
*   One of the most important diagnostic tools is the patient history.
*   Tumor markers are substances secreted by the tumor and are used in the workup of many different cancers and play a significant role in staging and diagnosis.
*   Molecular markers include expression levels, structures of proteins, and alterations in gene sequences and assist in determining treatments and predicting response to therapy.
*   Selection of diagnostic tests is based on the type of abnormality suspected and consideration of the value of information obtained and how it will affect decision making.

- Cancer biomarkers include proteins, genetic markers, hormones, hormone receptors, onco-fetal antigens, enzymes, and other substances produced by tumor cells or in response to tumor growth.
- Accurate staging is essential to guide treatment decisions and determine prognosis.

Recommended Resources for Oncology Advanced Practice Nurses

- ACR (www.acr.org): Guidelines on the appropriateness of various imaging tests for the workup of certain conditions
- Adjuvant! Online (www.adjuvantonline.com): Algorithm to estimate 10-year disease-free and overall survival in patients with invasive breast cancer who have undergone primary resection of the tumor
- ASCO (www.asco.org): Clinical practice guidelines on assays and predictive markers
- National Guideline Clearinghouse (www.guideline.gov): Public resource for evidence-based clinical practice guidelines, including guidelines for diagnostic testing
- NCCN (www.nccn.org): Clinical practice guidelines on cancer screening and treatment for specific cancers, as well as guidelines on supportive care
- NCI (www.cancer.gov): Information for patients, and also education for healthcare providers (www.cancer.gov/cancertopics/cancerlibrary/health-professional-training-tools/page2)
- Research Advocacy Group (www.researchadvocacy.org): Nonprofit organization dedicated to advancing cancer research through advocacy and education

The author would like to acknowledge Pamela Hallquist Viale, RN, MS, ANP, CS, AOCNP®, for her contribution to this chapter that remains unchanged from the first edition of this book.

References

Agendia. (n.d.). Breast specimen sampling instructions. Retrieved from http://www.agendia.com/media/Specimen-sampling-FRESH.pdf

Akin, O., Brennan, S.B., Dershaw, D.D., Ginsberg, M.S., Gollub, M.J., Schöder, H., … Hricak, H. (2012). Advances in oncologic imaging: Update on 5 common cancers. *CA: A Cancer Journal for Clinicians, 62,* 364–393. doi:10.3322/caac.21156

Allegra, C.J., Jessup, J.M., Somerfield, M.R., Hamilton, S.R., Hammond, E.H., Hayes, D.F., … Schilsky, R.L. (2009). American Society of Clinical Oncology provisional clinical opinion: Testing for *KRAS* gene mutations in patients with metastatic colorectal carcinoma to predict response to anti-epidermal growth factor receptor monoclonal antibody therapy. *Journal of Clinical Oncology, 27,* 2091–2096. doi:10.1200/JCO.2009.21.9170

American Cancer Society. (2014a). *Colorectal cancer facts and figures 2014–2016.* Retrieved from http://www.cancer.org/acs/groups/content/documents/document/acspc-042280.pdf

American Cancer Society. (2014b). Signs and symptoms of cancer. Retrieved from http://www.cancer.org/cancer/cancerbasics/signs-and-symptoms-of-cancer

American College of Radiology. (n.d.). ACR Appropriateness Criteria®. Retrieved from http://www.acr.org/ac

American College of Radiology. (2014a). *ACR practice parameter for the performance of contrast-enhanced magnetic resonance imaging (MRI) of the breast.* Retrieved from http://www.acr.org/~/media/ACR/Documents/PGTS/guidelines/MRI_Breast.pdf

American College of Radiology. (2014b). *ACR practice parameter for the performance of screening and diagnostic mammography.* Retrieved from http://www.acr.org/~/media/ACR/Documents/PGTS/guidelines/Screening_Mammography.pdf

AQA. (2009). AQA principles for appropriateness criteria. Retrieved from http://www.aqaalliance.org/files/AppropriatenessCriteriaPrinciples.pdf

Baan, R., Grosse, Y., Straif, K., Secretan, B., El Ghissassi, F., Bouvard, V., … Cogliano, V. (2009). A review of human carcinogens—Part F: Chemical agents and related occupations. *Lancet Oncology, 10,* 1143–1144. doi:10.1016/S1470-2045(09)70358-4

Bartram, C.I., & Taylor, S. (2008). The large bowel. In A. Adam, A.K. Dixon, R.G. Grainger, & D.J. Allison (Eds.), *Grainger and Allison's diagnostic radiology: A textbook of medical imaging* (5th ed., pp. 679–705). New York, NY: Elsevier Churchill Livingstone.

Bickley, L.S. (2013). *Bates' guide to physical examination and history taking* (11th ed.). Philadelphia, PA: Wolters Kluwer Health/Lippincott Williams & Wilkins.

Blake, M.A., McDermott, S., Rosen, M.P., Baker, M.E., Fidler, J.L., Greene, F.L., … Yee, J. (2011). American College of Radiology ACR Appropriateness Criteria®: Suspected liver metastases. Retrieved from http://www.acr.org/~/media/ACR/Documents/AppCriteria/Diagnostic/SuspectedLiverMetastases.pdf

Buyse, M., Loi, S., van't Veer, L., Viale, G., Delorenzi, M., Glas, A.M., … Piccart, M.J. (2006). Validation and clinical utility of a 70-gene prognostic signature for women with node-negative breast cancer. *Journal of the National Cancer Institute, 98,* 1183–1192. doi:10.1093/jnci/djj329

Caserta, M.P., Chaudhry, F., & Bechtold, R.E. (2011). Liver, biliary tract, and pancreas. In M.Y.M. Chen, T.L. Pope, & D.J. Ott (Eds.), *Basic radiology* (2nd ed.). Retrieved from http://www.accessmedicine.com

Chen, M.Y.M., & Whitlow, C.T. (2011). Scope of diagnostic imaging. In M.Y.M. Chen, T.L. Pope, & D.J. Ott (Eds.), *Basic radiology* (2nd ed.). Retrieved from http://www.accessmedicine.com

Cheson, B.D. (2011). Role of functional imaging in the management of lymphoma. *Journal of Clinical Oncology, 29,* 1844–1854. doi:10.1200/JCO.2010.32.5225

Compton, C.C., Byrd, D.R., Garcia-Aguilar, J., Kurtzman, S.H., Olawaiye, A., & Washington, M.K. (Eds.). (2012). *AJCC cancer staging atlas: A companion to the seventh editions of the AJCC cancer staging manual and handbook* (2nd ed.). doi:10.1007/978-1-4614-2080-4

Craig, F.E., & Foon, K.A. (2008). Flow cytometric immunophenotyping for hematologic neoplasms. *Blood, 111,* 3941–3967. doi:10.1182/blood-2007-11-120535

de Martel, C., Ferlay, J., Franceschi, S., Vignat, J., Bray, F., Forman, D., & Plummer, M. (2012). Global burden of cancers attributable to infections in 2008: A review and synthetic analysis. *Lancet Oncology, 13,* 607–615. doi:10.1016/S1470-2045(12)70137-7

Dewhurst, C., Rosen, M.P., Blake, M.A., Baker, M.E., Cash, B.D., Fidler, J.L., … Yee, J. (2011). American College of Radiology ACR Appropriateness Criteria®: Pretreatment staging of colorectal cancer. Retrieved from http://www.acr.org/~/media/ACR/Documents/AppCriteria/Diagnostic/PretreatmentStagingColorectalCancer.pdf

Duffy, M.J., & Crown, J. (2013). Companion biomarkers: Paving the pathway to personalized treatment for cancer. *Clinical Chemistry, 59,* 1447–1456. doi:10.1373/clinchem.2012.200047

Du Rand, I.A., Blaikley, J., Booton, R., Chaudhuri, N., Gupta, V., Khalid, S., … Munavvar, M. (2013). British Thoracic Society guideline for diagnostic flexible bronchoscopy in adults: Accredited by NICE. *Thorax, 68*(Suppl. 1), i1–i44. doi:10.1136/thoraxjnl-2013-203618

Edge, S.B., Byrd, D.R., Compton, C.C., Fritz, A.G., Greene, F.L., & Trotti, A., III. (Eds.). (2010). *AJCC cancer staging manual* (7th ed.). New York, NY: Springer.

Ellis, P.M., & Vandermeer, R. (2011). Delays in the diagnosis of lung cancer. *Journal of Thoracic Disease, 3,* 183–188. doi:10.3978/j.issn.2072-1439.2011.01.01

Febbo, P.G., Ladanyi, M., Aldape, K.D., De Marzo, A.M., Hammond, M.E., Hayes, D.F., … Birkeland, M.L. (2011). NCCN task force report: Evaluating the clinical utility of tumor markers in oncology. *Journal of the National Comprehensive Cancer Network, 9*(Suppl. 5), S1–S32. Retrieved from http://www.jnccn.org/content/9/Suppl_5/S-1.long

Freeman, A.H. (2008). The oesophagus. In A. Adam, A.K. Dixon, R.G. Grainger, & D.J. Allison (Eds.), *Grainger and Allison's diagnostic radiology: A textbook of medical imaging* (5th ed., pp. 609–626). New York, NY: Elsevier Churchill Livingstone.

Ghai, S., & Toi, A. (2012). Role of transrectal ultrasonography in prostate cancer. *Radiologic Clinics of North America, 50,* 1061–1073. doi:10.1016/j.rcl.2012.08.007

Gleason, D.F., & Mellinger, G.T. (1974). Prediction of prognosis for prostatic adenocarcinoma by combined histological grading and clinical staging. *Journal of Urology, 111,* 58–64.

Goodrich, A., McNally, G.A., Ridgeway, J., & Zitella, L.J. (2013). Mature B-cell neoplasms. In M. Olsen & L.J. Zitella (Eds.), *Hematologic malignancies in adults* (pp. 201–361). Pittsburgh, PA: Oncology Nursing Society

Hammond, M.E.H., Hayes, D.F., Dowsett, M., Allred, D.C., Hagerty, K.L., Badve, S., … Wolff, A.C. (2010). American Society of Clinical Oncology/College of American Pathologists guideline recommendations for immunohistochemical testing of estrogen and progesterone receptors in breast cancer. *Journal of Clinical Oncology, 28,* 2784–2795. doi:10.1200/JCO.2009.25.6529

Harris, L., Fritsche, H., Mennel, R., Norton, L., Ravdin, P., Taube, S., … Bast, R.C., Jr. (2007). American Society of Clinical Oncology 2007 update of recommendations for the use of tumor markers in breast cancer. *Journal of Clinical Oncology, 25,* 5287–5312. doi:10.1200/JCO.2007.14.2364

Harvey, J.A., Mahoney, M.C., Newell, M.S., Bailey, L., Barke, L.D., D'Orsi, C., … Haffty, B.G. (2012). American College of Radiology ACR Appropriateness Criteria®: Palpable breast masses. Retrieved from http://www.acr.org/~/media/ACR/Documents/AppCriteria/Diagnostic/PalpableBreastMasses.pdf

Heidenreich, A., Bellmunt, J., Bolla, M., Joniau, S., Mason, M., Matveev, V., … Zattoni, F. (2011). EAU guidelines on prostate cancer. Part 1: Screening, diagnosis, and treatment of clinically localised disease. *European Urology, 59,* 61–71. doi:10.1016/j.eururo.2010.10.039

Hoffman, R.M. (2011). Screening for prostate cancer. *New England Journal of Medicine, 365,* 2013–2019. doi:10.1056/NEJMcp1103642

Holme, Ø., Bretthauer, M., Fretheim, A., Odgaard-Jensen, J., & Hoff, G. (2013). Flexible sigmoidoscopy versus faecal occult blood testing for colorectal cancer screening in asymptomatic individuals. *Cochrane Database of Systematic Reviews, 2013*(9). doi:10.1002/14651858.CD009259.pub2

Igbokwe, A., & Lopez-Terrada, D.H. (2011). Molecular testing of solid tumors. *Archives of Pathology and Laboratory Medicine, 135,* 67–82. doi:10.1043/2010-0413-RAR.1

International Agency for Research on Cancer. (2011). *IARC monographs on the evaluation of carcinogenic risks to humans, volume 100: A review of carcinogen—Part B: Biological agents.* Retrieved from http://monographs.iarc.fr/ENG/Monographs/vol100B/mono100B-1.pdf

John, S.K.P., George, S., Primrose, J.N., & Fozard, J.B.J. (2011). Symptoms and signs in patients with colorectal cancer. *Colorectal Disease, 13,* 17–25. doi:10.1111/j.1463-1318.2010.02221.x

Kanne, J.P., Jensen, L.E., Mohammed, T.-L.H., Kirsch, J., Amorosa, J.K., Brown, K., … Shah, R.D. (2012). American College of Radiology ACR Appropriateness Criteria®: Radiographically detected solitary pulmonary nodule. Retrieved from http://www.acr.org/~/media/ACR/Documents/AppCriteria/Diagnostic/SolitaryPulmonaryNodule.pdf

Karnofsky, D.A., Abelmann, W.H., Craver, L.F., & Burchenal, J.H. (1948). The use of the nitrogen mustards in the palliative treatment of carcinoma. With particular reference to bronchogenic carcinoma. *Cancer, 1,* 634–656. doi:10.1002/1097-0142(194811)1:4<634::aid-cncr2820010410>3.0.co;2-l

Kaul, V., & Kothari, S. (2014). Endoscopic ultrasound in oncology. *Ultrasound Clinics, 9,* 43–52. doi:10.1016/j.cult.2013.08.004

Kent, A.J., Woolf, D., McCue, J., & Greenfield, S.M. (2010). The use of symptoms to predict colorectal cancer site: Can we reduce the pressure on our endoscopy services? *Colorectal Disease, 12,* 114–118. doi:10.1111/j.1463-1318.2009.01770.x

Kozower, B.D., Larner, J.M., Detterbeck, F.C., & Jones, D.R. (2013). Special treatment issues in non-small cell lung cancer: Diagnosis and management of lung cancer, 3rd ed: American College of Chest Physicians evidence-based clinical practice guidelines. *Chest, 143*(Suppl. 5), e369S–e399S. doi:10.1378/chest.12-2362

Kumar, A.S., & Lee, S.W. (2013). Laparoscopy in colorectal surgery. *Surgical Clinics of North America, 93,* 217–230. doi:10.1016/j.suc.2012.09.006

Lehman, C.D., DeMartini, W., Anderson, B.O., & Edge, S.B. (2009). Indications for breast MRI in the patient with newly diagnosed breast cancer. *Journal of National Comprehensive Cancer Network, 7,* 193–201. Retrieved from http://www.jnccn.org/content/7/2/193.long

Lindeman, N.I., Cagle, P.T., Beasley, M.B., Chitale, D.A., Dacic, S., Giaccone, G., … Ladanyi, M. (2013). Molecular testing guideline for selection of lung cancer patients for EGFR and ALK tyrosine kinase inhibitors: Guideline from the College of American Pathologists, International Association for the Study of Lung Cancer, and Association for Molecular Pathology. *Journal of Thoracic Oncology, 8,* 823–859. doi:10.1097/JTO.0b013e318290868f

Lister, T.A., Crowther, D., Sutcliffe, S.B., Glatstein, E., Canellos, G.P., Young, R.C., … Tubiana, M. (1989). Report of a committee convened to discuss the evaluation and staging of patients with Hodgkin's disease: Cotswolds meeting. *Journal of Clinical Oncology, 7,* 1630–1636. Retrieved from http://jco.ascopubs.org/content/7/11/1630.abstract

Locker, G.Y., Hamilton, S., Harris, J., Jessup, J.M., Kemeny, N., Macdonald, J.S., … Bast, R.C., Jr. (2006). ASCO 2006 update of recommendations for the use of tumor markers in gastrointestinal cancer. *Journal of Clinical Oncology, 24,* 5313–5327. doi:10.1200/JCO.2006.08.2644

Manson, J.E., Chlebowski, R.T., Stefanick, M.L., Aragaki, A.K., Rossouw, J.E., Prentice, R.L., … Wallace, R.B. (2013). Menopausal hormone therapy and health outcomes during the intervention and extended post stopping phases of the Women's Health Initiative randomized trials. *JAMA, 310,* 1353–1368. doi:10.1001/jama.2013.278040

Mitchell, D.G., Javitt, M.C., Glanc, P., Bennett, G.L., Brown, D.L., Dubinsky, T., … Zelop, C.M. (2012). American College of Radiology ACR Appropriateness Criteria®: Staging and follow-up of ovarian cancer. Retrieved from http://www.acr.org/~/media/ACR/Documents/AppCriteria/Diagnostic/StagingAndFollowUpOvarianCancer.pdf

Mohammed, T.-L.H., Kirsch, J., Amorosa, J.K., Brown, K., Chung, J.H., Dyer, D.S., … Shah, R.D. (2011). American College of Radiology ACR Appropriateness Criteria®: Routine admission and preoperative chest radiography. Retrieved from http://www.acr.org/~/media/ACR/Documents/AppCriteria/Diagnostic/RoutineAdmissionAnd PreoperativeChestRadiography.pdf

Mohammed, T.-L.H., Kirsch, J., Brown, K., Chung, J.H., Dyer, D.S., Ginsburg, M.E., … Suh, R.D. (2013). American College of Radiology ACR Appropriateness Criteria®: Screening for pulmonary metastases. Retrieved from http://www.acr.org/~/media/ACR/Documents/AppCriteria/Diagnostic/ScreeningForPulmonaryMetastases.pdf

Moiel, D., & Thompson, J. (2011). Early detection of colon cancer—The Kaiser Permanente Northwest 30-year history: How do we measure success? Is it the test, the number of tests, the stage, or the percentage of screen-detected patients? *Permanente Journal, 15*(4), 30–38. Retrieved from http://www.ncbi.nlm.nih.gov/pmc/articles/PMC3267557

Moy, L., Newell, M.S., Bailey, L., Barke, L.D., Carkaci, S., D'Orsi, C., … Mahoney, M.C. (2014). American College of Radiology (ACR) Appropriateness Criteria® Clinical Condition: Stage I breast cancer: Initial workup and surveillance for local recurrence and distant metastases in asymptomatic women: rule out metastases. Retrieved from https://acsearch.acr.org/docs/69496/Narrative

National Cancer Institute. (2010). National Cancer Institute fact sheet: Pathology reports. Retrieved from http://www.cancer.gov/cancertopics/factsheet/detection/pathology-reports

National Cancer Institute. (2011). National Cancer Institute fact sheet: Tumor markers. Retrieved from http://www.cancer.gov/cancertopics/factsheet/detection/tumor-markers

National Cancer Institute. (2012). SEER training modules: Cancer diagnosis. Retrieved from http://training.seer.cancer.gov/disease/diagnosis

National Comprehensive Cancer Network. (2014a). *NCCN Clinical Practice Guidelines in Oncology (NCCN Guidelines®): Breast cancer screening and diagnosis* [v.1.2014]. Retrieved from http://www.nccn.org/professionals/physician_gls/pdf/breast-screening.pdf

National Comprehensive Cancer Network. (2014b). *NCCN Clinical Practice Guidelines in Oncology (NCCN Guidelines®): Prostate cancer* [v.1.2015]. Retrieved from http://www.nccn.org/professionals/physician_gls/pdf/prostate.pdf

National Comprehensive Cancer Network. (2015a). *NCCN Clinical Practice Guidelines in Oncology (NCCN Guidelines®): Breast cancer* [v.2.2015]. Retrieved from http://www.nccn.org/professionals/physician_gls/pdf/breast.pdf

National Comprehensive Cancer Network. (2015b). *NCCN Clinical Practice Guidelines in Oncology (NCCN Guidelines®): Breast cancer risk reduction* [v.1.2015]. http://www.nccn.org/professionals/physician_gls/pdf/breast_risk.pdf

National Comprehensive Cancer Network. (2015c). *NCCN Clinical Practice Guidelines in Oncology (NCCN Guidelines®): Colon cancer* [v.2.2015]. Retrieved from http://www.nccn.org/professionals/physician_gls/pdf/colon.pdf

National Comprehensive Cancer Network. (2015d). *NCCN Clinical Practice Guidelines in Oncology (NCCN Guidelines®): Colorectal cancer screening* [v.1.2015]. Retrieved from http://www.nccn.org/professionals/physician_gls/pdf/colorectal_screening.pdf

National Comprehensive Cancer Network. (2015e). *NCCN Clinical Practice Guidelines in Oncology (NCCN Guidelines®): Non-Hodgkin's lymphomas* [v.2.2015]. http://www.nccn.org/professionals/physician_gls/pdf/nhl.pdf

National Comprehensive Cancer Network. (2015f). *NCCN Clinical Practice Guidelines in Oncology (NCCN Guidelines®): Non-small cell lung cancer* [v.7.2015]. Retrieved from http://www.nccn.org/professionals/physician_gls/pdf/nscl.pdf

National Comprehensive Cancer Network. (2015g). *NCCN Clinical Practice Guidelines in Oncology (NCCN Guidelines®): Ovarian cancer* [v.1.2015]. Retrieved from http://www.nccn.org/professionals/physician_gls/pdf/ovarian.pdf

National Comprehensive Cancer Network. (2015h). *NCCN Clinical Practice Guidelines in Oncology (NCCN Guidelines®): Small cell lung cancer* [v.1.2016]. Retrieved from http://www.nccn.org/professionals/physician_gls/pdf/sclc.pdf

Nishihara, R., Wu, K., Lochhead, P., Morikawa, T., Liao, X., Qian, Z.R., … Chan, A.T. (2013). Long-term colorectal-cancer incidence and mortality after lower endoscopy. *New England Journal of Medicine, 369,* 1095–1105. doi:10.1056/NEJMoa1301969

Oken, M.M., Creech, R.H., Tormey, D.C., Horton, J., Davis, T.E., McFadden, E.T., & Carbone, P.P. (1982). Toxicity and response criteria of the Eastern Cooperative Oncology Group. *American Journal of Clinical Oncology, 5,* 649–656. Retrieved from http://journals.lww.com/amjclinicaloncology/Fulltext/1982/12000/Toxicity_and_response_criteria_of_the_Eastern.14.aspx

Olde Bekkink, M., McCowan, C., Falk, G.A., Teljeur, C., Van de Laar, F.A., & Fahey, T. (2010). Diagnostic accuracy systematic review of rectal bleeding in combination with other symptoms, signs and tests in relation to colorectal cancer. *British Journal of Cancer, 102,* 48–58. doi:10.1038/sj.bjc.6605426

Olivotto, I.A., Bajdik, C.D., Ravdin, P.M., Speers, C.H., Coldman, A.J., Norris, B.D., … Gelmon, K.A. (2005). Population-based validation of the prognostic model ADJUVANT! for early breast cancer. *Journal of Clinical Oncology, 23,* 2716–2725. doi:10.1200/JCO.2005.06.178

Olsen, M. (2013). Overview of hematologic malignancies. In M. Olsen & L.J. Zitella (Eds.), *Hematologic malignancies in adults* (pp. 1–17). Pittsburgh, PA: Oncology Nursing Society.

Ost, D.E., Yeung, S.-C.J., Tanoue, L.T., & Gould, M.K. (2013). Clinical and organizational factors in the initial evaluation of patients with lung cancer: Diagnosis and management of lung cancer, 3rd ed: American College of Chest Physicians evidence-based clinical practice guidelines. *Chest, 143*(Suppl. 5), e121S–e141S. doi:10.1378/chest.12 -2352

Paik, S., Shak, S., Tang, G., Kim, C., Baker, J., Cronin, M., … Wolmark, N. (2004). A multigene assay to predict recurrence of tamoxifen-treated, node-negative breast cancer. *New England Journal of Medicine, 351,* 2817–2826. doi:10.1056/NEJMoa041588

Park, H.J., Kim, D.W., Yim, G.W., Nam, E.J., Kim, S., & Kim, Y.T. (2013). Staging laparoscopy for the management of early-stage ovarian cancer: A metaanalysis. *American Journal of Obstetrics and Gynecology, 209,* 58.e1–58.e8. doi:10.1016/j.ajog.2013.04.013

Podoloff, D.A., Ball, D.W., Ben-Josef, E., Benson, A.B., III, Cohen, S.J., Coleman, R.E., … Wong, R.J. (2009). NCCN task force: Clinical utility of PET in a variety of tumor types. *Journal of the National Comprehensive Cancer Network, 7*(Suppl. 2), S1–S23. Retrieved from http://www.jnccn.org/content/7/Suppl_2/S-1.full.pdf+html

Puli, S., Bechtold, M., Reddy, J.K., Choudhary, A., Antillon, M., & Brugge, W. (2009). How good is endoscopic ultrasound in differentiating various T stages of rectal cancer? Meta-analysis and systematic review. *Annals of Surgical Oncology, 16,* 254–265. doi:10.1245/s10434-008-0231-5

Ravenel, J.G., Mohammed, T.-L.H., Rosenzweig, K.E., Ginsburg, M.E., Kanne, J.P., Kestin, L.L., … Saleh, A.G. (2013). American College of Radiology ACR Appropriateness Criteria®: Non-invasive clinical staging of bronchogenic carcinoma. Retrieved from http://www.acr.org/Quality-Safety/~/~/media/91B2DBA77F3048CBAE117E82AAC5D9FF .pdf

Research Advocacy Network. (2010). *Biomarkers in cancer: An introductory guide for advocates.* Retrieved from http:// researchadvocacy.org/general-resources/tutorialbiomarkers-cancer

Roberts, C.C., Weissman, B.N., Appel, M., Bancroft, L.W., Bennett, D.L., Bruno, M.A., … Lutz, S.T. (2012). American College of Radiology ACR Appropriateness Criteria®: Metastatic bone disease. Retrieved from http://www.acr .org/~/media/ACR/Documents/AppCriteria/Diagnostic/MetastaticBoneDisease.pdf

Rubin, S.C., Sabbatini, P., & Viswanathan, A.N. (2013). Ovarian cancer. In D.G. Haller, L.D. Wagman, K.A. Camphausen, & W.J. Hoskins (Eds.), *Cancer management: A multidisciplinary approach.* Retrieved from http://www .cancernetwork.com/cancer-management

Saeed, I., & Anderson, J. (2011). Cancer of the lung: Staging, radiology, surgery. *Surgery, 29,* 221–226. doi:10.1016/ j.mpsur.2011.02.003

Salzman, B., Fleegle, S., & Tully, A.S. (2012). Common breast problems. *American Family Physician, 86,* 343–349. Retrieved from http://www.aafp.org/afp/2012/0815/p343.html

Serraino, D., Piselli, P., Busnach, G., Burra, P., Citterio, F., Arbustini, E., … Franceschi, S. (2007). Risk of cancer following immunosuppression in organ transplant recipients and in HIV-positive individuals in southern Europe. *European Journal of Cancer, 43,* 2117–2123. doi:10.1016/j.ejca.2007.07.015

Sickles, E.A., D'Orsi, C.J., Bassett, L.W., et al. (2013). BI-RADS: Mammography. In C.J. D'Orsi, E.A. Sickles, E.B. Mendelson, & E.A. Morris (Eds.), *Breast Imaging Reporting and Data System: ACR BI-RADS®—Breast imaging atlas* (5th ed.) [Electronic version]. Reston, VA: American College of Radiology.

Siegel, R.L., Miller, K.D., & Jemal, A. (2015). Cancer statistics, 2015. *CA: A Cancer Journal for Clinicians, 65,* 5–29. doi:10.3322/caac.21254

Silvestri, G.A., Gonzalez, A.V., Jantz, M.A., Margolis, M.L., Gould, M.K., Tanoue, L.T., … Detterbeck, F.C. (2013). Methods for staging non-small cell lung cancer: Diagnosis and management of lung cancer, 3rd ed: American College of Chest Physicians evidence-based clinical practice guidelines. *Chest, 143*(Suppl. 5), e211S–e250S. doi:10.1378/chest.12-2355

Swerdlow, S.H., Campo, E., Harris, N.L., Jaffe, E.S., Pileri, S.A., Stein, H., … Vardiman, J.W. (Eds.). (2008). *WHO classification of tumours of haematopoietic and lymphoid tissues* (4th ed.). Lyon, France: IARC Press.

Travis, W.D., Brambilla, E., Noguchi, M., Nicholson, A.G., Geisinger, K.R., Yatabe, Y., … Yankelewitz, D. (2011). International Association for the Study of Lung Cancer/American Thoracic Society/European Respiratory Society international multidisciplinary classification of lung adenocarcinoma. *Journal of Thoracic Oncology, 6,* 244–285. doi:10.1097/JTO.0b013e318206a221

U.S. Food and Drug Administration. (2006). Guidance for industry and FDA staff: The Mammography Quality Standards Act final regulations and additions to policy guidance help system #9. Retrieved from http://www.fda.gov/Radiation -EmittingProducts/MammographyQualityStandardsActandProgram/DocumentArchives/ucm114207.htm

Wolf, A.M.D., Wender, R.C., Etzioni, R.B., Thompson, I.M., D'Amico, A.V., Volk, R.J., … Smith, R.A. (2010). American Cancer Society guideline for the early detection of prostate cancer: Update 2010. *CA: A Cancer Journal for Clinicians, 60,* 70–98. doi:10.3322/caac.20066

Wolff, A.C., Hammond, M.E.H., Hicks, D.G., Dowsett, M., McShane, L.M., Allison, K.H., … Hayes, D.F. (2013). Recommendations for human epidermal growth factor receptor 2 testing in breast cancer: American Society of Clinical Oncology/College of American Pathologists clinical practice guideline update. *Journal of Clinical Oncology, 31,* 3997–4013. doi:10.1200/JCO.2013.50.9984

Yu, Y.-H., Wei, W., & Liu, J.-L. (2012). Diagnostic value of fine-needle aspiration biopsy for breast mass: A systematic review and meta-analysis. *BMC Cancer, 12,* 41. doi:10.1186/1471-2407-12-41

Zoga, A.C., Weissman, B.N., Kransdorf, M.J., Adler, R., Appel, M., Bancroft, L.W., … Ward, R.J. (2012). American College of Radiology ACR Appropriateness Criteria®: Soft-tissue masses. Retrieved from http://www.acr.org/~/media/ACR/Documents/AppCriteria/Diagnostic/SoftTissueMasses.pdf

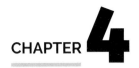

CHAPTER **4**

Chemotherapy, Targeted Biotherapy, and Molecular Therapy

Gail M. Wilkes, APRN-BC, MS, AOCN®

Introduction

This past decade has brought many advances in the treatment of cancer using chemotherapy and targeted therapy, both biologic and molecular. This chapter will review the principles of chemotherapy, biologic therapy, and molecular-targeted therapy, along with implications for oncology advanced practice nurses (APNs).

Cancer is a disease of cellular mutations. In 2006, Andrew von Eschenbach, then director of the National Cancer Institute (NCI), declared that by 2015, suffering and death from cancer would be eliminated, in part, by advances in molecular-targeted therapy (National Institutes of Health, 2006; Von Eschenbach, 2006). While this goal will not be achieved, much has been learned about cancer biology, targets of therapy, targeted therapy, and personalized or precision cancer patient care. Classic hallmarks of cancer give direction to finding the molecular targets to stop cancer growth and cell proliferation. These hallmarks result from genomic instability and include (a) sustained signaling for cell proliferation, (b) evasion of growth suppressors, (c) avoidance of cell death (apoptosis), (d) activation of tissue invasion and metastases, (e) limitless replication, (f) sustained angiogenesis, (g) reprogramming of energy metabolism, (h) evasion of the immune system, (i) commandeering of normal cells to create a microenvironment that supports tumor growth, and (j) inflammation (Hanahan & Weinberg, 2011).

Chemotherapy has been used for more than 60 years to disrupt genetic functions within the cell and cause cell death (cytotoxic) or alter regulation of growth and division to prevent cell division (cytostatic, such as tamoxifen). As understanding of the many molecular flaws in cancer biology increases, it is clear that multitargeted therapies are required to more precisely target multiple cancer pathways. For example, epidermal growth factor receptor (EGFR) is known to be overexpressed in many solid tumors, and a number of agents blocking this pathway have been approved by the U.S. Food and Drug Administration (FDA), such as cetuximab, panitumumab, and erlotinib. Inhibition of this pathway theoretically results in decreased cell proliferation, decreased stimulation of angiogenesis, increased sensitivity to apoptosis, and reduced stimulation of invasion and metastases. Other agents target angiogenesis directly, either by neutralization of the ligand (growth factor or hormone that activates the receptor on the cell membrane) vascular endothelial growth factor (VEGF), such as with bevacizumab, or inhibition of the endothelial cell receptor (on cells lining the nearest blood vessel) for VEGF receptors, such as with sunitinib or sorafenib. Several targeted biologic agents have been used for many years, such as the monoclonal antibody (mAb) rituximab, a CD20-specific mAb that causes death of CD20-positive lymphocytes. Toxicities related to targeted molecular or biologic therapy are drug and class specific (Wilkes, 2011b).

In contrast, chemotherapy generally is nonspecific, targeting frequently dividing cancer cell populations. Although normal, frequently dividing cell populations are more capable of repairing the cellular damage and surviving; severe, often life-threatening side effects can occur, including febrile neutropenia, thrombocytopenia, and organ damage. Among the few targeted agents under the chemotherapy umbrella are the antiestrogen agents, such as tamoxifen, which are targeted against estrogen receptors in breast cancer cells.

Chemotherapy

General Principles

Chemotherapy is the use of cellular toxins that block cell replication and commonly lead to apoptosis, or programmed cell death, in frequently dividing cancer cell populations. Chemotherapy agents are classified by their action during the cell cycle that leads to cell replication as either cell cycle specific or cell cycle nonspecific. The cell cycle consists of five phases: G_0, G_1, G_2, S, and M (see Figure 4-1). The G stands for *gap*, as scientists were able to see the S and M phases clearly but were not sure what occurred during the time gaps before and after.

G_0 is the resting phase, where cells will remain until recruited back into the cell cycle. A few cell types remain in G_0 indefinitely, such as neurons. Normal cells have a finite life span, and once the life span expires, the cells are replaced by new cells. To accomplish this, a certain percentage of cells are recruited into the cell cycle; this is referred to as the *growth fraction*. Once recruited into the cell cycle, the cell enters G_1. The cell cycle is one of the most highly controlled cellular processes because of key restriction points, or checkpoints, that theoretically prevent subversion. Unfortunately, in malignancies, mutations are present in the genes that make proteins to control the cell cycle checkpoints and enzymes moving the cell through the cell cycle (cyclin-dependent kinases [CDKs]). At the G_1 checkpoint, a decision is required for the cell to commit to cell division. The checkpoint determines whether the cell is large enough, whether adequate nutrition exists in the environment, and whether the cell's DNA is intact in order to avoid replication of damaged DNA (Weinberg, 2013). If the conditions are met, the cell commits to cell division, and in late G_1, the nucleus enlarges and the materials needed for DNA duplication are made.

During the S, or synthesis, phase, the cell actively replicates the DNA, forming a complementary set of chromatids (a chromatid is one daughter strand of DNA). During this time, both DNA strands are examined to ensure that they are exact and without errors; if errors are found, they are repaired. If they cannot be repaired, the cell undergoes apoptosis to prevent duplication of mutated DNA. If the DNA strands are intact and pass inspection, they proceed to the G_2 phase. *TP53* is the "guardian of the genome" and is responsible for checkpoint inspections and ensuring that irreparably damaged DNA is destroyed by apoptosis (Weinberg,

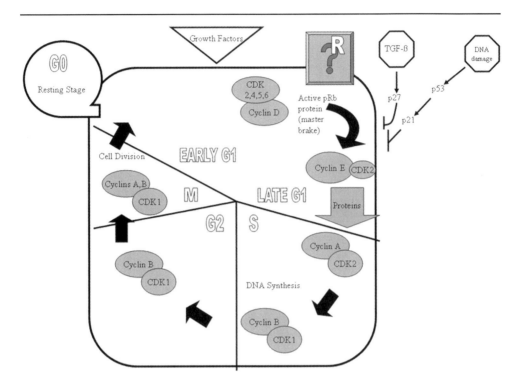

The cell cycle consists of four stages (G1, S, G2, M) that are controlled by proteins called cyclins. The cyclins (D, E, A, B) are activated when complexed with enzymes called cyclin-dependent kinases (CDKs). Upon activation, the cyclin-CDK complex allows the cell to progress through each specific cell cycle stage. Present throughout the cell cycle, the cyclin-CDK complexes serve as checkpoints or monitors of the cell cycle. Inhibitory proteins prevent progression through the cell cycle if DNA damage is present or there is a lack of nutrients or oxygen to support cellular proliferation. Examples of inhibitory proteins include p21 p27, p53. The inhibitory proteins in turn are regulated by the presence of inhibitory growth factors and TGF-β. Once past R (the restriction point) the cell cycle is turned "on" and progression through the cell cycle is inevitable. Cyclin-CDK complexes and pRB (the "master brake") tightly regulate the R point. The stability of the inhibitory proteins and cyclin-CDK complexes are altered in cancer, thereby altering control of the cell cycle and uncontrolled cellular proliferation prevails.

Figure 4-1. Chemotherapy Drug Action During Cell Cycle

Note. From "Biology of Cancer" (p. 14), by C.J. Merkle in C.H. Yarbro, D. Wujcik, and B.H. Gobel (Eds.), *Cancer Nursing: Principles and Practice* (7th ed.), 2011, Burlington, MA: Jones & Bartlett Learning. Copyright 2011 by Jones & Bartlett Learning. Reprinted with permission.

2013). Unfortunately, *TP53* is the most frequently mutated gene in solid tumors (Vogelstein, Sur, & Prives, 2010). In G_2, the cell prepares for mitosis and synthesizes the materials for the mitotic spindle. At the end of the G_2/beginning of the M, or mitosis, phase, the cell is inspected again for damaged or unduplicated DNA and unduplicated centrosomes (small areas of cytoplasm next to the nucleus that contain and organize the microtubules), which are key in mitosis (Weinberg, 2013). If all conditions are met, the cell moves into the M phase.

During the M phase, the chromosomes line up at the centromere (area joining the two chromatids) and are attached by mitotic spindle fibers. An M phase checkpoint delays the segregation of chromosomes if they are not attached to the spindle fibers, and the cell undergoes metaphase arrest unless it is repaired (Merkle, 2011). Otherwise, the daughter cells may have the wrong number of chromosomes. Once repaired, the cell undergoes the completion of mitosis, and two identical daughter cells are formed. Depending on the need for additional cells, the daughter cells may enter G_0 or be recruited back into the cycle. In cancer, a mutation often occurs in the M checkpoint, resulting in completion of mitosis, but the daughter cells may have too few or too many chromosomes (aneuploidy) (Ricke & van Deursen, 2011).

Cancer chemotherapy is intended to either prevent cell division (cytostatic) or cause cell death (cytocidal). Most chemotherapy agents are cytocidal and bring about cell death by interfering with cellular processes, such as DNA replication, RNA function, and mitosis.

Two fundamental principles of chemotherapy are the "cell kill model" and Gompertzian tumor growth kinetics. Skipper (1971) postulated that a certain percentage of cancer cells will be killed ("cell kill model") with each cycle of chemotherapy (first-order kinetics), assuming that all the cells are actively dividing, consistently sensitive to treatment, and growing at a constant rate. However, all tumor cells are not actively dividing, and cells can become insensitive to chemotherapy; so, the cell kill model has limitations. A second principle is the Norton-Simon hypothesis (Gompertzian tumor growth kinetics), which states that tumors grow fastest when small, and tumors given less time to recover can be more effectively destroyed (Norton & Simon, 1977). This principle has led to the use of dose-dense chemotherapy that includes shorter cycle intervals so that the actively dividing cells can be killed before they have a chance to divide. In breast cancer, when treatment with standard chemotherapy with doxorubicin and cyclophosphamide (AC regimen) given every three weeks was compared with every-two-week AC "dose dense" therapy, overall survival was higher with the dose-dense treatment (Citron et al., 2003). Although the risk for myelosuppression is greater, the use of hematopoietic growth factors to stimulate production and differentiation of neutrophils can prevent febrile neutropenia.

Factors that affect response to treatment include tumor burden, rate of tumor growth, combination versus single-agent therapy, dose or dose intensity, hormone receptor status in hormone-sensitive tumors, and drug resistance (Polovich, Olsen, & LeFebvre, 2014). Combination chemotherapy provides a strategy to maximize cell kill. Drug regimens combine drugs that have synergy but minimal overlapping toxicities, such as the CHOP regimen, which consists of cyclophosphamide, doxorubicin, vincristine, and prednisone. The myelosuppression with cyclophosphamide occurs in 7–10 days, whereas that of doxorubicin occurs in 10–14 days. Vincristine and prednisone are nonmyelosuppressive, but vincristine is neurotoxic, and prednisone causes hyperglycemia and other side effects. The regimens were developed to be given in the ambulatory setting and commonly are dosed on schedules with a cycle every 21 days so that normal cells can recover before the next cycle (Wilkes, 2011a).

Unfortunately, normal, frequently dividing cell populations are affected by chemotherapy as well, including the bone marrow, gastrointestinal mucosa, gonads, and hair follicles. In addition, chemotherapy agents have drug-specific toxicities, including organ toxicities, such as cardiomyopathy, which is associated with the anthracycline antibiotics. Table 4-1 outlines chemotherapy agents, their activity during the cell cycle, and toxicities. Many of the severe toxicities, including specific organ toxicities and cognitive dysfunction, are discussed in greater detail in other chapters. Because of the narrow therapeutic window and anticipated toxicities that would not be tolerated with other drugs, it is imperative to employ practices that reduce the chance for prescription error. Errors involving drug overdose, wrong dose, or inappropriate route (e.g., vincristine given intrathecally) have resulted in patient deaths (Noble & Donaldson, 2010).

One strategy to reduce damage to normal cells and improve delivery to malignant cells involves nanotechnology. Liposomal doxorubicin uses stealth technology to evade the immune system and takes advantage of the leaky capillaries supplying tumors so that the drug leaks into the tumor; in addition, the drug has a long half-life of 54 hours (Janssen Products, LP, 2013).

A second example is the use of albumin to wrap paclitaxel, which is preferentially taken up by tumor cells (paclitaxel protein-bound particles for injectable suspension).

Drugs that interfere with a specific phase of the cell cycle are called *cell cycle–specific* agents and include the antimetabolites, antimitotic agents, and topoisomerase inhibitors. Drugs that are active throughout all phases of the cell cycle are called *cell cycle–nonspecific* agents and include alkylating agents and antitumor antibiotics. *Miscellaneous* agents include those with indeterminate or unusual activity that are unlike others in its class, such as procarbazine. Because of the extensive scope of this topic, this section will highlight one or two commonly used agents in each class. The reader is referred to chemotherapy texts or drug package inserts for a full discussion of each drug. In addition, the drug or manufacturer websites provide patient and provider resources. All chemotherapy agents pose reproductive hazards, so patients should avoid becoming pregnant and breast-feeding, and nurses should wear personal protective equipment (PPE) when preparing and administering the drugs and handling

Table 4-1. Chemotherapy Agents by Class

Class	FDA-Approved Drugs	Common Toxicities and Comments
Cell Cycle Nonspecific		
Alkylating agents	Altretamine (Hexalen®) BCNU (carmustine, BiCNU®) Busulfan (Myleran®) Carboplatin (Paraplatin®) Chlorambucil (Leukeran®) Cisplatin (Platinol®) Cyclophosphamide (Cytoxan®) Dacarbazine (DTIC-DOME®) Ifosfamide (Ifex®) Lomustine (CeeNU®) Mechlorethamine (nitrogen mustard, Mustargen®) Melphalan (Alkeran®) Oxaliplatin (Eloxatin®) Streptozocin (Zanosar®) Temozolomide (Temodar®) Thiotepa (Thioplex®)	Alopecia Fatigue Gonadal suppression (azoospermia, amenorrhea) Hemorrhagic cystitis (ifosfamide, cyclophosphamide) Myelosuppression Nausea and vomiting Neuropathy (cisplatin analogs) Secondary malignancies Comments: Nitrosoureas: Carmustine and lomustine are lipid soluble and cross BBB; temozolomide crosses BBB and is a radiosensitizer. Cisplatin and analogs are radiosensitizers.
Antitumor antibiotics	Actinomycin D (dactinomycin, Cosmegen®) Bleomycin (Blenoxane®) Mitomycin (Mutamycin®) Mitoxantrone (Novantrone®) Anthracycline antibiotics • Doxorubicin (Adriamycin®) • Daunorubicin (Cerubidine®) • Epirubicin (Ellence®) • Idarubicin (Idamycin®) • Liposomal daunorubicin (DaunoXome®) • Liposomal doxorubicin (Doxil®) • Valrubicin (Valstar®)	Actinomycin D, mitomycin, and anthracycline antibiotics (except for liposomal formulations) are vesicants.* Alopecia Bone marrow suppression (except for bleomycin) Cardiotoxicity (anthracycline antibiotics, dose dependent) Fatigue Gonadal suppression Mucositis Nausea and vomiting Pulmonary fibrosis (bleomycin) Radiation recall

(Continued on next page)

Table 4-1. Chemotherapy Agents by Class *(Continued)*

Class	FDA-Approved Drugs	Common Toxicities and Comments
Cell Cycle Specific		
Antimetabolites	Capecitabine (Xeloda®) Cladribine (Leustatin®) Clofarabine (Clolar®) Cytarabine (cytosine arabinoside, Cytosar-U®) Floxuridine (FUDR®) Fludarabine (Fludara®) Fluorouracil (5-FU, Adrucil®) Gemcitabine (Gemzar®) Hydroxyurea (Hydrea®) Liposomal cytarabine (DepoCyt®) Mercaptopurine (6-MP, Purinethol®) Methotrexate (MTX, Mexate®) Pemetrexed (Alimta®) Pentostatin (Nipent®) Thioguanine (6-TG, Tabloid®) Trimetrexate (Neutrexin®)	Anorexia Bone marrow suppression Fatigue Nausea and vomiting Stomatitis, diarrhea 5-FU, capecitabine, and gemcitabine are radiosensitizers.
Miscellaneous agents	Asparaginase (Elspar®) Pegaspargase (Oncaspar®)	Hepatotoxicity Hyperglycemia Hypersensitivity reactions including anaphylaxis (which can be greatly reduced by intramuscular administration) Nausea and vomiting Pancreatitis
	Arsenic trioxide (Trisenox®)	Acute promyelocytic leukemia differentiation syndrome (fever, dyspnea, weight gain, pulmonary infiltrates, pleural/pericardial effusions, leukocytosis) Fatigue Fever, anemia, disseminated intravascular coagulation, bleeding Nausea, vomiting, diarrhea Paresthesia, dizziness, tremor, insomnia QTc interval prolongation, with risk of torsades de pointes if serum magnesium and potassium are low Comment: Causes degradation of fusion protein PML/RARα, characteristic of acute promyelocytic leukemia
Mitotic inhibitors, vinca alkaloids	Vinblastine (Velban®) Vincristine (Oncovin®) Vinorelbine (Navelbine®)	All agents are vesicants.* Alopecia Nausea and vomiting, myelosuppression (vinblastine, vinorelbine) Neurotoxicity (vincristine > vinblastine > vinorelbine)

(Continued on next page)

Table 4-1. Chemotherapy Agents by Class *(Continued)*

Class	FDA-Approved Drugs	Common Toxicities and Comments
Mitotic inhibitors, taxanes	Docetaxel (Taxotere®) Paclitaxel (Taxol®) Paclitaxel protein-bound particles (Abraxane®) Eribulin mesylate (Halaven®)	Alopecia Arthralgias and myalgias Hypersensitivity reactions (paclitaxel, docetaxel) Myelosuppression Nausea and vomiting Sensory-motor peripheral neuropathy
Topoisomerase I inhibitors	Irinotecan (Camptosar®) Topotecan (Hycamtin®)	Alopecia Cross the BBB Diarrhea Myelosuppression Nausea and vomiting
Topoisomerase II inhibitors	Daunorubicin (Cerubidine®) Doxorubicin (Adriamycin®) Etoposide (VP-16, VePesid®)	Hypersensitivity Hypotension Myelosuppression Nausea and vomiting (See antitumor antibiotics for doxorubicin and daunorubicin.)
Hormones		
Antiandrogens (nonsteroidal)	Bicalutamide (Casodex®) Flutamide (Eulexin®) Nilutamide (Nilandron®)	Decreased libido, impotence Edema, fatigue Hot flashes, gynecomastia, breast tenderness Nausea, diarrhea, or constipation Rare hepatitis Usually given with an LHRH agonist or prior to an LHRH agonist to prevent tumor flare
Androgen receptor inhibitor	Enzalutamide (Xtandi®)	Asthenia/fatigue, diarrhea, back pain, arthralgia, hot flashes, peripheral edema, musculoskeletal pain, muscle weakness Dizziness, rare seizures Drug interactions Teach patient safety measures to avoid falls.
LHRH analogs; LHRH agonists	Goserelin acetate (Zoladex®) Histrelin (Vantas® implant) Leuprolide acetate (Lupron®, Lupron Depot®; Viadur®; Eligard®) Triptorelin (Trelstar®)	Decreased libido, erectile impotence Depression, decreased mental acuity, loss of muscle mass, weight gain Edema, osteoporosis, fatigue Hot flashes, gynecomastia Initial increase in testosterone before decreasing to very low levels Rare anorexia, nausea, vomiting Tumor flare, bone pain (prevent by giving antiandrogen before starting LHRH analog)

(Continued on next page)

Table 4-1. Chemotherapy Agents by Class *(Continued)*

Class	FDA-Approved Drugs	Common Toxicities and Comments
LHRH antagonist	Degarelix (Firmagon®)	Increased liver function tests Injection-site reactions (pain, redness, swelling) Possible side effects: Decreased libido, impotence, hot flashes, breast tenderness, osteoporosis, anemia, decreased mental acuity, loss of muscle mass, weight gain, fatigue, increased cholesterol, depression Reduce testosterone levels quickly, do not cause tumor flare compared to LHRH agonists
CYP17 enzyme inhibitor (blocks other sources of androgen [e.g., prostate cancer cells, adrenals])	Abiraterone (Zytiga®)	Bone or muscle pain, hypertension, edema, hot flashes, diarrhea, upset stomach, dyspnea, joint swelling or discomfort, hot flashes, vomiting, urinary tract infection, confusion Possible drug interactions Adrenocortical insufficiency; administer with prednisone.
Antiestrogens (non-steroidal)	Tamoxifen (Nolvadex®) Toremifene (Fareston®)	Depression Edema Hot flashes, vaginal discharge, endometrial hyperplasia, increased risk of endometrial cancer (tamoxifen) Hypercalcemia with tumor flare Nausea, vomiting Rare but increased risk of thromboembolic events, vaginal bleeding Toremifene: Prolonged QTc interval; contraindicated in patients with QTc prolongation, uncorrected hypomagnesemia/hypokalemia
Antiestrogen (receptor antagonist)	Fulvestrant (Faslodex®)	Depression Edema Flu-like syndrome Hot flashes, insomnia, nausea, vomiting Rare but increased risk of thromboembolic events
Antiestrogens (non-steroidal aromatase inhibitor, reversible) Postmenopausal women only	Anastrozole (Arimidex®) Letrozole (Femara®)	Hot flashes Increased risk for osteoporosis Joint stiffness or pain Nausea, fatigue, dizziness Peripheral edema

(Continued on next page)

Table 4-1. Chemotherapy Agents by Class *(Continued)*

Class	FDA-Approved Drugs	Common Toxicities and Comments
Antiestrogen (steroidal aromatase inhibitor, irreversible) Postmenopausal women only	Exemestane (Aromasin®)	Diaphoresis Fatigue Hot flashes Nausea

* Vesicants cause tissue necrosis if the drug escapes into tissue during IV administration.

BBB—blood-brain barrier; FDA—U.S. Food and Drug Administration; LHRH—luteinizing hormone-releasing hormone

Note. Based on information from manufacturers' prescribing information. Please consult the manufacturer's product information as well as the FDA's Center for Drug Evaluation and Research website (www.accessdata.fda.gov/scripts/cder/drugsatfda/index.cfm), which offers an email service that alerts subscribers when a new drug or new indication is approved by FDA, for updated information.

patient excreta. Patients receiving home chemotherapy and their families should be instructed in safe handling of hazardous drugs, as well as handling of patient excreta. In addition, they must understand how to use the chemotherapy spill kit provided.

Cell Cycle–Specific Agents

Antimetabolite Agents

These agents prevent the synthesis of the complementary DNA strand during the S phase to make an exact copy of DNA for the daughter cell. The agent acts as a false cellular nutrient, such as a purine, pyrimidine, or enzyme, when inserted into the DNA strand or when the enzyme tries to function, and cell replication is prevented and the cell undergoes apoptosis. In addition, a false metabolite may be inserted in the RNA strand, making it unable to function. Common side effects of antimetabolites include bone marrow depression, with nadir (lowest blood counts) in 7–10 days after administration and recovery within 21 days, and mucositis (e.g., stomatitis, esophagitis, diarrhea).

Gemcitabine (Gemzar®) is a prodrug that must be metabolized within the cell into metabolites: the active metabolite is gemcitabine triphosphate. It inhibits DNA synthesis by blocking an enzyme necessary for making deoxynucleoside triphosphate that is needed for DNA synthesis. Gemcitabine triphosphate is instead taken up into DNA, forcing the cell into apoptosis. It also halts cells as they move from the G_1 phase into the S phase. It is given intravenously and is metabolized by the liver with almost all drug excreted in the urine within one week of administration. Women and older adults have lower drug clearance, with increased half-life and plasma concentrations, which becomes significant if the infusion is longer than 70 minutes (Eli Lilly and Co., 2014). Toxicity is schedule dependent, and the drug should be given IV by a 60-minute infusion, no more frequently than once weekly. This drug should be used cautiously in patients with renal or hepatic insufficiency. Gemcitabine is a radiosensitizer and can exacerbate radiation therapy toxicity (Eli Lilly and Co., 2014). Potential side effects include bone marrow suppression (dose-limiting toxicity), nausea, vomiting, flu-like symptoms with fever on the day of administration, rash, hepatic transaminitis, increased alkaline phosphatase, dyspnea, and peripheral edema. Less commonly, diarrhea, stomatitis, alopecia, and esophagitis (especially in patients with lung cancer receiving radiation therapy to the chest) may occur. Rarely, pulmonary fibrosis, interstitial pneumonia, capillary leak syndrome, or pulmonary edema can occur, as can hemolytic uremic syndrome (Eli Lilly and Co., 2014).

Antimitotic Agents

Antimitotic agents are active during the mitosis phase (M phase) and include the plant-derived vinca alkaloids, the taxanes, and eribulin mesylate. The vinca alkaloid group includes vincristine (Oncovin®), vinblastine (Velban®), and vinorelbine (Navelbine®); all are vesicant agents, causing tissue necrosis if allowed to extravasate outside the vein during administration. Hence, scrupulous technique must be used to administer the drug. If extravasation is suspected, the drug should be stopped, an IV should be started in another noncontiguous vein to avoid extravasation from the venipuncture hole in the blood vessel proximal to it, and the suspected site should be treated as an extravasation. Nurses should be familiar with extravasation management, such as aspiration of any remaining drug from the tubing, administration of antidote (recommended hyaluronidase, manufactured by specialty pharmacies), and application of heat at least four times a day. Patients should be taught to elevate the extremity, be reassessed the next day, and given specific management instructions (Polovich et al., 2014). Special care must be taken to ensure that drugs such as vincristine are not administered intrathecally by accident, as this is usually fatal (Noble & Donaldson, 2010). The taxanes include paclitaxel and docetaxel. All these agents are given IV and cause differing degrees of peripheral neuropathy because the drugs interfere with microtubular function and the axons are made up of microtubules.

The taxanes affect mitosis in a different way. Whereas the vinca alkaloids prevent the formation of the mitotic spindle, paclitaxel promotes early microtubule assembly and prevents disassembling, while docetaxel stabilizes the microtubules so that they cannot move. Both result in arrest of mitosis and cell death.

Paclitaxel (Taxol®) is derived using a semisynthetic process from the Pacific Yew tree (*Taxus brevifolia*). It is extensively protein bound, metabolized in the liver, and excreted in the bile. The solvent used to make the drug soluble in blood, polyoxyethylated castor oil (Cremophor® EL), increases the risk of hypersensitivity reactions and requires premedication. Because Cremophor EL can leach the plasticizer di(2-ethylhexyl) phthalate (DEHP) from polyvinyl chloride IV sets, the drug must be administered with non-DEHP tubing and IV bags. This drug should be given by IV infusion following premedication with dexamethasone (usually 20 mg PO 12 and 6 hours prior to the infusion), and right before the drug infusion, diphenhydramine and a histamine-2 antagonist. Paclitaxel also may be given intraperitoneally. This drug is a radiosensitizer. It causes cardiotoxicity when given concomitantly with either doxorubicin or trastuzumab. Other potential toxicities include bone marrow suppression with nadir in 7–10 days, sensory-motor peripheral neuropathy, hypersensitivity reactions, alopecia, mild nausea and vomiting, diarrhea, stomatitis, hepatotoxicity, hypotension, arrhythmia, fatigue, arthralgia, and myalgia. When administered in combination with cisplatin, paclitaxel should be administered first, as cisplatin may decrease renal clearance of the drug and increase neutropenia (Rowinsky et al., 1991).

Paclitaxel protein-bound particle for injectable suspension albumin-bound (Abraxane®) was engineered to take advantage of tumor cells' thirst for albumin. Using nanotechnology, paclitaxel is surrounded by albumin, and the tumor cells preferentially uptake the albumin-bound drug. This obviates the need to use Cremophor EL, so the risk of hypersensitivity is significantly reduced, as is the risk for persistent neurotoxicity. In addition, higher doses of paclitaxel bound to albumin can be given, as paclitaxel with Cremophor EL is incorporated into micelles (trapped in Cremophor lipid globules) once a certain dose is reached (Sparreboom et al., 1999), so there is a ceiling effect (Mould, Fleming, Darcy, & Spriggs, 2006). Potential side effects are similar to paclitaxel; however, the incidence of peripheral neuropathy is higher related to a higher dose of paclitaxel (71% vs. 56%) but is more quickly reversible (Celgene Corp., 2014). Peripheral neuropathy is sensory only. Because the drug contains albumin derived from human blood, there is a theoretical risk of viral transmission. Similar to paclitaxel, the drug should be used cautiously in patients with hepatic dysfunction. If severe hypersensitivity occurs, the drug should be discontinued. Men, as well as women of reproductive age, receiving the drug should also be counseled to use effective contraception because the drug demonstrates reduced fertility in laboratory animals, as well as embryo loss and fetal abnormalities (Celgene Corp., 2014).

Eribulin mesylate (Halaven®) inhibits mitosis by another mechanism (Eisai Inc., 2013). The drug binds to the ends of the microtubules, preventing their growth and causing them to clump. This disrupts the mitotic spindle, stops the cell cycle at the G_2/M phase, and forces the cell into apoptosis. The drug is administered by slow IV push over two to five minutes, and the dose should be reduced in patients with hepatic or renal impairment. Potential side effects are neutropenia, anemia, asthenia/fatigue, peripheral neuropathy, nausea, and constipation. Peripheral neuropathy is primarily grade 1 or 2. The drug can prolong the QTc interval. Patients with congestive heart failure (CHF) or those with bradyarrhythmias, taking drugs known to prolong the QTc interval, or with electrolyte abnormalities should have their QTc interval monitored closely and electrolyte serum levels corrected to normal (e.g., magnesium and potassium).

Topoisomerase Inhibitors

Irinotecan (Camptosar®), topotecan (Hycamptin®), doxorubicin (Adriamycin®), daunorubicin (Cerubidine®), mitoxantrone (Novantrone®), and etoposide (Vepesid®) are included among the topoisomerase inhibitors. Topoisomerase I and II are critical to allow unwinding and then rewinding of the DNA helix during cell replication so that the DNA can be copied and a complementary strand assembled during the synthesis phase of the cell cycle. Topoisomerase I (makes one strand cut and then subsequent relegation of the DNA break) is inhibited by irinotecan and topotecan, whereas topoisomerase II (causes double-stranded breaks) is inhibited by etoposide, doxorubicin, daunorubicin, and mitoxantrone. The action of these agents prevents DNA and RNA synthesis in dividing cells. Topoisomerase I is found in higher than normal concentrations in certain malignancies, such as adenocarcinoma of the colon. These drugs are given IV, and topotecan and irinotecan can cross the blood-brain barrier (Haddadin & Perry, 2012; Pharmacia & Upjohn Co., 2014). Doxorubicin and daunorubicin are vesicants, causing tissue necrosis if the drug is extravasated (Polovich et al., 2014).

Irinotecan is a semisynthetic agent derived from camptothecin, a plant alkaloid. The drug and its active metabolite SN-38 bind to topoisomerase I. Irinotecan is metabolized in the liver to the metabolite SN-38, which then is conjugated by an enzyme UGT1A1 to form a glucuronide metabolite. A UGT1A1*28 polymorphism (variation in a gene copy) exists in 10% of Americans, resulting in impaired metabolism of SN-38 (Walko & McLeod, 2009). Patients can be tested for this polymorphism, and if positive, they should receive a dose reduction. Otherwise, a higher serum level of SN-38 results in increased toxicity, especially grade 4 febrile neutropenia. In addition, in older adults, the terminal half-life of the drug is longer (6 hours vs. 5.5 hours in people younger than age 65) (Pharmacia & Upjohn Co., 2014). Therefore, patients should be monitored closely for toxicity. Significant drug interactions exist with CYP3A4 inducers (i.e., phenytoin or St. John's wort), as they induce the cytochrome P450 microenzyme system responsible for metabolizing irinotecan; either of these drugs can significantly lower levels of SN-38. These drugs should not be coadministered, and the anticonvulsant should be changed to another, noninteracting agent two weeks before irinotecan is administered. CYP3A4 inhibitors, such as ketoconazole, should not be given concurrently and should be stopped one week before irinotecan dosing (Pharmacia & Upjohn Co., 2014).

The dose-limiting drug toxicity of irinotecan is persistent, delayed diarrhea, which can be fatal. Two types of diarrhea exist. One type of diarrhea is early onset, with a cholinergic etiology and manifested as abdominal cramping, diarrhea, diaphoresis, lacrimation, flushing, miosis, and rhinitis during the drug administration. This can be rapidly reversed with IV atropine. The second type of diarrhea, which is delayed from a motility origin, occurs at least 24 hours after the drug is given. This delayed diarrhea may be refractory and can lead to dehydration and electrolyte imbalance or sepsis, often simultaneously with the occurrence of the nadir. Patients should be taught to take an aggressive regimen of loperamide: 4 mg at the first sign of diarrhea and then 2 mg every two hours until 12 hours have passed without any diarrhea (should not exceed 48 hours of loperamide at these doses), with close patient monitoring. Patients should receive IV hydration if they are unable to maintain oral hydration, should be given antidiarrheals for grade 3 or 4 diarrhea (i.e., octreotide), and should be started on antibiotics if the diarrhea persists after 24 hours or if ileus, fever, or neutropenia develops. The drug is emetic, so aggressive antiemetics are given prior to drug administration. Other potential significant side effects are neutropenia, anemia, abdominal pain, anorexia, asthenia, weight loss, and alopecia. In combination therapy, mucositis/stomatitis may occur. Rarely, pulmonary infiltrates or renal impairment or failure may occur, especially in patients dehydrated from severe vomiting or diarrhea. The drug should not be used in combination with a regimen of 5-fluorouracil (5-FU) and leucovorin administered for four to five consecutive days outside of a clinical trial because of the risk of severe toxicity. Caution should be used in patients with either hepatic or renal impairment, and the drug should not be administered to patients with a serum bilirubin level greater than 2 mg/dl, or on renal dialysis. Irinotecan dose must be reduced depending on the severity of side effects experienced (Pharmacia & Upjohn Co., 2014).

Cell Cycle–Specific Antitumor Antibiotics

Doxorubicin causes myelosuppression, with nadir in 10–14 days and recovery by day 21. The myofibrils take up the drug, so a key side effect is cardiotoxicity, principally decreased left ventricular ejection fraction (LVEF), with the development of CHF if the drug is continued. A multigated acquisition (MUGA) scan or echocardiogram should be performed to obtain a baseline LVEF, and the same test repeated periodically during therapy. The drug should be stopped if LVEF decreases to below normal or the maximum recommended dose is reached. Common side effects are nausea, vomiting, anorexia, and, less commonly, stomatitis. The drug is red in color, so following administration, the patient's urine is pink for one to two days. In addition, doxorubicin causes hyperpigmentation (darkening) of the veins and soft palate, especially in dark-skinned patients. The drug is excreted in the urine and bile; thus, the dose must be modified in patients with renal or hepatic dysfunction.

Cell Cycle–Nonspecific Agents

Antitumor Antibiotics

These are cytotoxic antibiotics that end in the suffix -mycin. All except for bleomycin are vesicant agents. Bleomycin, along with doxorubicin and daunomycin (daunorubicin), are the only agents that are cell cycle specific, with the remaining drugs being cell cycle nonspecific. These drugs often are radiosensitizers.

Alkylating Agents

This class includes many agents, such as nitrogen mustard (Mustargen®), its derivatives cyclophosphamide (Cytoxan®) and ifosfamide (Ifex®), and others listed in Table 4-1. Also included in this class are the platinum analogs cisplatin, carboplatin, and oxaliplatin and the nitrosourea carmustine, which crosses the blood-brain barrier.

Oxaliplatin (Eloxatin®) is a third-generation platinum analog that is unique in that it has efficacy in colon and rectal cancers. It is synergistic with 5-FU/LV, and the drug is indicated for the treatment of patients with colorectal cancers in combination with 5-FU/leucovorin by FDA. The dose-limiting toxicity is cumulative, persistent peripheral neuropathy that increases in risk at cumulative doses of 750–800 mg/m^2. This is reversible in many cases but may take a long time. In addition, oxaliplatin causes a very common, reversible, acute neuropathy that lasts less than 14 days and often is precipitated by exposure to cold (Wilkes, 2011a). An uncommon manifestation is pharyngolaryngeal dysesthesia, which can be very frightening. The patient senses that no air is being moved into the lungs and becomes anxious (Wilkes, 2011a). Oncology APNs first rule out a hypersensitivity reaction by assessing vital signs, including oxygen saturation. In addition, patients may experience acute peripheral neuropathy that reverses within two weeks. Acute neuropathy appears to be related to voltage-gated channelopathy (dysfunction of an ion channel—in this case, calcium) and decreased extracellular calcium. Although the benefit of IV calcium and magnesium infusions to reduce the incidence of oxaliplatin-induced peripheral neuropathy has been debated for many years, a contemporary phase III randomized, placebo-controlled, double-blind study has shown no benefit (Loprinzi et al., 2014). Other common toxicities are neutropenia (very low incidence of febrile neutropenia), nausea and vomiting that are easily preventable with serotonin-antagonist/dexamethasone combinations, diarrhea, and transient, elevated liver transaminases. Anaphylaxis may occur during the infusion but also may occur as a delayed hypersensitivity reaction after 10–12 cycles of therapy, similar to carboplatin. Rarely, pulmonary toxicity (characterized by nonproductive cough, dyspnea, and crackles with or without pulmonary infiltrates) and reversible posterior leukoencephalopathy syndrome, characterized by headache, altered mental functioning, seizures, and visual abnormalities, with or without hypertension, may occur (Sanofi-Aventis U.S. LLC, 2014).

Hormones

These agents alter the hormonal milieu in tumors that are stimulated by hormones, such as certain breast and prostate cancers. **Tamoxifen** (Nolvadex®) is an oral, nonsteroidal, selective estrogen receptor modulator and is an estrogen antagonist in breast tissue, whereas it is an agonist in other tissues (e.g., endometrium, bone). The drug is a prodrug and is metabolized primarily by the CYP2D6 microenzyme system in the liver, into metabolites having a high affinity for the estrogen receptor and which compete with estrogen for binding. Without estrogen binding to the estrogen receptor, there is no activation of breast cancer growth-stimulating genes. This causes cancer cells to be arrested in the G_0 or G_1 phase, so the drug is cytostatic rather than cytocidal. It is indicated for the treatment of estrogen receptor–positive breast cancer and for the prevention of breast cancer in high-risk women. Patients who have a specific single nucleotide polymorphism (SNP) of the metabolizing enzyme CYP2D6 may metabolize tamoxifen very slowly and thus have a decreased response (Singh, Francis, & Michael, 2011). A SNP is a single change in a nucleotide in DNA so that the sequence is slightly different from people in the general population (like a point mutation), but which occurs in a certain percentage of the population. However, in patients with breast cancer with a CYP2D6 SNP, no data currently exist to show a significant decrease in response to tamoxifen (Lum, Perel, Hingorani, & Holmes, 2013). Thus, genotyping of CYP2D6 is not routinely recommended. Drugs such as the antidepressants paroxetine and fluoxetine that inhibit the CYP2D6 enzyme pathway may also potentially inhibit tamoxifen's metabolism and should be used cautiously, if at all, in patients receiving tamoxifen. Tamoxifen's toxicity profile includes hot flashes, menstrual irregularities in premenopausal women, endometrial changes including endometrial cancer, risk of thromboembolic events, and, rarely, leukopenia and thrombocytopenia. Endometrial biopsy should be performed annually, and patients should be taught the signs and symptoms to report related to a venous thromboembolism (e.g., pain in the calf, changes in breathing, chest pain). When the drug is started in patients with metastatic breast cancer, patients may experience a flare reaction with transient bone and tumor pain.

Prostate cancer hormonal therapies are based on tumor response to androgens. Prostate cancer cells can be (a) androgen dependent, when androgen is blocked, the cell dies; (b) androgen sensitive, when androgen is blocked, the cell stops dividing; or (c) androgen independent, when tumor cells do not respond to loss of hormones (Kazar & Harmon, 2011).

Enzalutamide (Xtandi®) is an oral inhibitor of the androgen receptor, causing decreased proliferation and death of prostate cancer cells. It is indicated for the treatment of patients with metastatic castration-resistant prostate cancer who have previously received docetaxel (Astellas Pharma, Inc., 2014). The drug's metabolism can be affected by a number of drugs. For example, concurrent administration with a strong CYP2C8 inhibitor, such as gemfibrozil, increases the serum plasma level of enzalutamide, so coadministration is not advised. If they must be given concurrently, the dose of enzalutamide should be reduced (Astellas Pharma Inc., 2014). Most common side effects are fatigue, diarrhea, arthralgia, and hot flashes. Enzalutamide may rarely cause seizures; thus, patients should be advised to avoid performing any activity where sudden loss of consciousness could be harmful to self or others. Classes of these agents are summarized in Table 4-1.

Biologic- and Molecular-Targeted Agents

Targeted agents can be either biologic or molecular and contribute to personalized or precision cancer treatment. The many different types of cancer can best be defined by their genetic mutations and other cellular abnormalities. Although it was once thought that breast cancer was simply defined by the presence or absence of estrogen or progesterone and HER2 receptors, today it is known that at least 10 different subtypes of breast cancer exist (Baird & Caldas, 2013; Curtis et al., 2012). Biologic therapies offer a targeted approach to treating cancer and, together with an improved understanding of the molecular changes that accompany malignant transformation and growth, have made the 21st century the century of targeted therapy.

Biologic-Targeted Therapy

Biologic-targeted therapy may be given alone or in combination with chemotherapy and/or radiation therapy. This type of therapy takes advantage of normal immune mechanisms to stop the growth of or destroy cancer cells. Targeted biotherapy is directed toward an identifiable target on the malignant cell with the hope of reducing collateral damage to normal cells. These agents can be reviewed in terms of their classes as well, although some agents fall into more than one class because of their activity. Biologic-targeted agents and their side effects are shown in Table 4-2 (mAbs), Table 4-3 (immune checkpoint inhibitor toxicities), and Table 4-4 (immunomodulatory agents, vaccines, and miscellaneous agents). As knowledge of the immune system and malignant cells' evasion of immunosurveillance evolves, a new class of agents showing promise are immune checkpoint inhibitors. These include ipilimumab (Yervoy®), nivolumab (Opdivo®) and pembrolizumab (Keytruda®), although all three are also mAbs. Almost all of these agents are fetotoxic or embryotoxic; therefore, pregnancy and breast-feeding should be avoided, and women of childbearing age and men should be counseled to use effective contraception. In some cases, mandatory monitoring is required to prevent pregnancy.

Monoclonal Antibodies

Monoclonal antibodies (mAbs) are antibodies that have been cloned from a single antibody. Originally, mAbs were made from a hybrid of a myeloma cell (antibody factory) that had lost its ability to make antibody and a healthy B cell that had been exposed to the antigen against which the antibody was to be developed (Scott, Wolchok, & Old, 2012). Today, mAbs are made using DNA recombinant (genetically engineered) technology. As with any antibody, the mAb has an Fc (constant) portion, which is responsible for the immune function against the antigen. It can bind to complement and initiate the complement cascade, and it can bind

Table 4-2. Biologic-Targeted Therapies

Drug Class	Target	Drugs and Indications[a]	Side Effects[b]
Unconjugated mAbs	CD19 Drug is a bispecific CD19-directed T-cell engager	Blinatumomab (Blincyto®) Indicated for treatment of Philadelphia chromosome–negative relapsed or refractory B-cell precursor acute lymphoblastic leukemia	Most common are pyrexia, headache, peripheral edema, febrile neutropenia, nausea, hypokalemia, tremor, rash, and constipation. Cytokine release syndrome may occur and be life threatening or fatal; monitor patients closely and manage. Neurologic toxicities occurred in 50% of patients and included encephalopathy, seizures, speech disorder, change in consciousness, confusion, disorientation, and disorder of coordination/balance. Teach patients to avoid driving or performing hazardous activities while drug is being administered. Infections (including sepsis, pneumonia, opportunistic infections, and catheter site): Monitor patients closely for signs and symptoms and treat promptly. Tumor lysis syndrome may occur; prevent by prophylaxis. Neutropenia and febrile neutropenia: Monitor complete blood count/differential during drug infusion and interrupt drug for prolonged neutropenia. Elevated liver enzymes: monitor AST, ALT, GGT, and total bilirubin at baseline and during drug therapy. Leukoencephalopathy may occur as shown on MRI, especially in patients who had prior cranial irradiation and antileukemic therapy. Preparation and administration errors have occurred; follow instructions for preparation and administration in package insert.

(Continued on next page)

Table 4-2. Biologic-Targeted Therapies *(Continued)*

Drug Class	Target	Drugs and Indications[a]	Side Effects[b]

Unconjugated mAbs *(cont.)*	CD20	Rituximab (Rituxan®) Indicated for treatment of patients with
		• CD20-positive
		  – Relapsed or refractory, low-grade or follicular, B-cell NHL
		  – Previously untreated follicular B-cell NHL with chemotherapy, and if response, maintenance
		  – Nonprogressing low-grade NHL after CVP chemotherapy
		  – Previously untreated diffuse large B-cell NHL with CHOP chemotherapy
		• CD20-positive CLL
		• Rheumatoid arthritis
		• Wegener granulomatosis, microscopic polyangiitis
			Rare, fatal infusion reaction within 24 hours of drug infusion (characterized by hypoxia, pulmonary infiltrates, ARDS, MI, VF, or cardiogenic shock); 80% occur after first infusion.
			Fever, chills
			Infections
			Cytopenias
			Bowel obstruction and/or perforation (abdominal pain, vomiting, associated symptoms)
			In new patients with high tumor burden, tumor lysis syndrome may occur following rapid lysis of lymphocytes
			Severe mucocutaneous (e.g., Stevens-Johnson syndrome) reactions; reactivation of hepatitis B and fulminating hepatitis
			Posterior multifocal leukoencephalopathy syndrome (headache, lethargy, confusion, seizure, visual changes)

	CD20	Ofatumumab (Arzerra®) Indicated for treatment of patients with CLL • Previously untreated and in whom fludarabine is inappropriate, in combination with chlorambucil • Refractory to fludarabine and alemtuzumab	Neutropenia, anemia Infusion reactions Neutropenia, anemia, thrombocytopenia Nausea, diarrhea Infection, pyrexia, cough, dyspnea Fatigue, rash Tumor lysis syndrome in new patients with high tumor burden
	CD20	Obinutuzumab (Gazyva®) Indicated in combination with chlorambucil for treatment of patients with previously untreated CLL	Infusion reactions Neutropenia, thrombocytopenia, anemia Nausea Diarrhea Tumor lysis syndrome in patients with high tumor burden or high circulating lymphocyte count Bleeding, hemorrhage with thrombocytopenia

(Continued on next page)

Table 4-2. Biologic-Targeted Therapies *(Continued)*

Drug Class	Target	Drugs and Indications[a]	Side Effects[b]
Unconjugated mAbs *(cont.)*	CD52	Alemtuzumab (Campath®-1H) Indicated for treatment of patients with B-cell CLL Given with Pneumocystis jiroveci pneumonia and herpes virus infection prophylaxis	Infusion reactions (rash, fever, rigors, hypotension); premedication required Myelosuppression Prolonged and severe lymphopenia with increased risk of opportunistic infection Nausea, vomiting, diarrhea Insomnia
EGFR inhibitors mAbs	EGFR1	Cetuximab (Erbitux®) Indicated for treatment of patients with • Locally or regionally advanced, recurrent or metastatic squamous cell head and neck cancer in combination with RT, platinum-based therapy with 5-FU, or monotherapy after progression following platinum-based therapy • *KRAS* mutation–negative (wild type) EGFR-expressing metastatic CRC in combination with FOLFIRI chemotherapy for first-line treatment, in combination with irinotecan in patients refractory to irinotecan-based chemotherapy, or as a single agent in refractory disease	Sterile, inflammatory rash that may be severe; increased hair growth of eyelashes and eyebrows; alopecia; hypomagnesemia 3% severe hypersensitivity reaction (90% occur during first infusion) Nausea, vomiting, diarrhea, stomatitis; rare ILD Use of cetuximab with radiation and cisplatin increased the incidence of grade 3–4 mucositis toxicity without improvement in progression-free survival (endpoint of study).
		Panitumumab (Vectibix®) Indicated for treatment of patients with wild-type *KRAS* (exon 2) metastatic colorectal cancer • In combination with FOLFOX for first-line treatment • As a single agent after disease progression after prior therapy with fluoropyrimidine, oxaliplatin, and irinotecan-containing chemotherapy	Rash (which may be severe); monitor patients with dermatologic or soft tissue toxicities closely for infection, as necrotizing fasciitis, sepsis, and death have occurred. Infusion reactions (4%), severe in 1% Paronychia, pruritus, diarrhea, nausea, vomiting, stomatitis, hypomagnesemia, hypocalcemia; rare ILD Keratitis and ulcerative keratitis

(Continued on next page)

Table 4-2. Biologic-Targeted Therapies *(Continued)*

Drug Class	Target	Drugs and Indications[a]	Side Effects[b]
EGFR inhibitors mAbs *(cont.)*	EGFR2 (HER2/neu receptor)	Trastuzumab (Herceptin®) Indicated for treatment of HER2-positive patients with • Breast cancer • Metastatic gastric or gastroesophageal junction adenocarcinoma	Most common: Headache, diarrhea, nausea, chills Decreased LVEF and cardiomyopathy (increased risk when receiving anthracycline chemotherapy) Infusion reactions, with sequelae including rare pulmonary toxicity (e.g., pneumonitis, ARDS), especially in patients with lung disease or pulmonary metastases Increased risk of neutropenia and anemia when receiving chemotherapy; increased risk of thrombotic events Rare nephritic syndrome Embryo-fetal toxicity
	EGFR2 (HER2) (HER2 dimerization inhibitor)	Pertuzumab (Perjeta®) Indicated for treatment of patients with HER2-positive • Metastatic breast cancer who have not received prior anti-HER2 therapy or chemotherapy for metastatic disease, in combination with trastuzumab and docetaxel • Locally advanced, inflammatory, or early-stage breast cancer (> 2 cm, or node positive), in combination with trastuzumab and docetaxel as neoadjuvant therapy	Left ventricular dysfunction Infusion reactions Hypersensitivity reactions/anaphylaxis In combination with chemotherapy and trastuzumab, most common were diarrhea, alopecia, neutropenia, fatigue, nausea, vomiting, rash, and peripheral neuropathy.
Immune checkpoint inhibitors	Cytotoxic T-lymphocyte–associated antigen 4 (CTLA-4)	Ipilimumab (Yervoy®) Indicated for treatment of patients with unresectable or metastatic melanoma	Immune-related side effects that are potentially severe Enterocolitis, hepatitis Neuropathy Endocrinopathies Most common: Fatigue, diarrhea, pruritus, rash Less common: Infusion reactions, Stevens-Johnson syndrome
	PD-1 blocking antibody	Nivolumab (Opdivo®) Indicated for treatment of patients with unresectable or metastatic melanoma and disease progression following ipilimumab and, if *BRAF V600*–mutation positive, a BRAF inhibitor	Most common adverse effect was rash. Immune-related adverse reactions: Pneumonitis, colitis, hepatitis, nephritis and renal dysfunction, hypothyroidism and hyperthyroidism Embryo-fetal toxicity

(Continued on next page)

Table 4-2. Biologic-Targeted Therapies *(Continued)*

Drug Class	Target	Drugs and Indications[a]	Side Effects[b]
Immune checkpoint inhibitors *(cont.)*	PD-1 blocking antibody	Pembrolizumab (Keytruda®) Indicated for treatment of patients with unresectable or metastatic melanoma and disease progression following ipilimumab and, if *BRAF V600*–mutation positive, a BRAF inhibitor	Most common included fatigue, cough, nausea, pruritus, rash, decreased appetite, constipation, diarrhea, and arthralgia. Immune-related adverse reactions: Pneumonitis, colitis, hepatitis, hypophysitis, nephritis, hyperthyroidism and hypothyroidism Embryo-fetal toxicity
Antiangiogenesis agents	VEGF (ligand)	Bevacizumab (Avastin®) Indicated for treatment of patients with • Metastatic CRC (mCRC) with 5-FU–based chemotherapy • mCRC with fluoropyrimidine-irinotecan or fluoropyrimidine-oxaliplatin–based chemotherapy for second-line treatment in patients who have progressed on first-line bevacizumab-containing regimen • Nonsquamous cell NSCLC with carboplatin and paclitaxel for first-line treatment of unresectable, locally advanced, recurrent, or metastatic • Glioblastoma, as a single agent, in adult patients with progressive disease after prior therapy • Metastatic renal cell carcinoma with interferon alfa • Cervical cancer, in combination with paclitaxel and cisplatin, or paclitaxel and topotecan in persistent, recurrent, or metastatic disease • Platinum-resistant, recurrent epithelial ovarian, fallopian tube, or primary peritoneal cancer, in combination with paclitaxel, pegylated liposomal doxorubicin, or topotecan	Hypertension Bleeding (epistaxis, rectal bleeding), rare hemorrhage Delayed wound healing (do not give within 28 days of major surgery, resume after wound has healed) GI perforation or fistula, non-GI fistula Proteinuria; dipstick urine for protein prior to treatment, if 2+ or higher, assess 24-hour urine for protein; if ≥ 2 g/24 hr, temporarily suspend until 24-hour protein < 2 g/24 hr. Venous and arterial thromboembolic complications Common adverse effects include headache, rhinitis, proteinuria, taste alterations, dry skin, lacrimation disorder, back pain, and exfoliative dermatitis. Uncommon infusion reactions Rare CHF in patients who have received anthracyclines, rare nasal septum perforation, rare posterior reversible encephalopathy syndrome (headache, lethargy, confusion, seizure, visual changes), ovarian failure Fetal harm

(Continued on next page)

Table 4-2. Biologic-Targeted Therapies *(Continued)*

Drug Class	Target	Drugs and Indications[a]	Side Effects[b]
Antiangiogenesis agents *(cont.)*	VEGFR2 antagonist	Ramucirumab (Cyramza®) Indicated for treatment of patients with • Advanced gastric or gastroesophageal junction adenocarcinoma, with disease progression on or after prior fluoropyrimidine- or platinum-containing chemotherapy, as a single agent • Metastatic NSCLC with disease progression on or after platinum-based chemotherapy; if EGFR or ALK mutations, patient should have progressed on FDA-approved, in combination with docetaxel	Most common adverse effects when drug is given as a single agent are hypertension and diarrhea; when combined with chemotherapy, effects included fatigue, neutropenia, epistaxis, and stomatitis/mucosal inflammation. Arterial thrombotic events Infusion-related reactions GI perforation Impaired wound healing Clinical deterioration in patients with cirrhosis Reversible posterior leukoencephalopathy syndrome
Antibody-drug conjugate, mAb conjugated to a cytotoxic agent	HER2	Ado-trastuzumab emtansine for injection (Kadcyla®) Indicated for treatment of patients with HER2-positive metastatic breast cancer after prior treatment with trastuzumab and a taxane separately or in combination Patients should have received prior therapy for metastatic disease, or developed disease recurrence during or within 6 months of completing adjuvant therapy.	Infusion or hypersensitivity reactions Nausea, constipation, increased transaminases Musculoskeletal pain, headache, fatigue Left ventricular dysfunction Thrombocytopenia, hemorrhage, epistaxis Pulmonary toxicity Peripheral neuropathy
mAb conjugated to cytotoxic agent	CD30	Brentuximab vedotin (Adcetris®) Indicated for treatment of patients with • Hodgkin disease, after failure ASCT or after failure of at least 2 prior multiagent chemotherapy regimens in non-ASCT candidates • Systemic anaplastic large cell lymphoma, after failure of at least one prior multiagent regimen	Anaphylaxis and infusion reactions Neutropenia, thrombocytopenia, anemia Serious infections and opportunistic infections Peripheral sensory neuropathy Nausea, vomiting, diarrhea, hepatotoxicity Fatigue Pyrexia, rash, URI, cough Tumor lysis syndrome Pulmonary toxicity Stevens-Johnson syndrome (rare) Embryo-fetal toxicity

(Continued on next page)

Table 4-2. Biologic-Targeted Therapies *(Continued)*

Drug Class	Target	Drugs and Indications[a]	Side Effects[b]
mAb conjugated with radioisotope	CD20	^{90}Y ibritumomab tiuxetan (Zevalin®) Indicated for treatment of patients with • Relapsed or refractory, low-grade or follicular B-cell NHL • Previously untreated follicular NHL who achieved a partial or complete response to first-line chemotherapy	Rare, fatal infusion reactions reported within 24 hours of rituximab infusion (hypoxia, pulmonary infiltrates, ARDS, MI, VF, cardiogenic shock); 80% occurred during first infusion of rituximab. Prolonged and severe cytopenias; severe cutaneous and mucosal reactions (e.g., Stevens-Johnson syndrome); fetotoxicity (avoid pregnancy) Rare secondary malignancies (AML, MDS) Contraindicated: Patients with > 25% bone marrow occupied by lymphoma, impaired bone marrow reserve Hypersensitivity reaction to murine antibody; altered biodistribution

[a] This table includes indications, but they change frequently. Please consult the manufacturer's product information as well as the FDA's Center for Drug Evaluation and Research website (www.accessdata.fda.gov/scripts/cder/drugsatfda/index.cfm), which offers an email service to alert subscribers when a new drug or new indication is approved by FDA, for updated information. Every effort has been made to ensure drug data are consistent with the most recent package insert, but typographical errors may occur, and drug information may be updated by the manufacturer. Please see drug package insert for complete prescribing information.

[b] Almost all the drugs are potentially fetotoxic, so women and men should be counseled to use effective contraception to avoid pregnancy.

ALK—anaplastic lymphoma kinase; ALL—acute lymphoblastic leukemia; ALT—alanine aminotransferase; AML—acute myeloid leukemia; ARDS—acute respiratory distress syndrome; ASCT—autologous stem cell transplant; AST—aspartate aminotransferase; CD—cluster of differentiation antigen on lymphocytes; CHF—congestive heart failure; CHOP—cyclophosphamide, doxorubicin, vincristine, and prednisone; CLL—chronic lymphocytic leukemia; CML—chronic myeloid leukemia; CRC—colorectal cancer; CVP—cyclophosphamide, vincristine, and prednisone; EGFR—epidermal growth factor receptor; EGFR1—epidermal growth factor receptor 1; EGFR2—epidermal growth factor receptor 2, also known as HER2/neu; FDA—U.S. Food and Drug Administration; FOLFIRI—chemotherapy regimen with folinic acid, infusional 5-fluorouracil, and irinotecan; FOLFOX—chemotherapy regimen with folinic acid, infusional 5-fluorouracil, and oxaliplatin; GGT—gamma-glutamyl transferase; GI—gastrointestinal; ILD—interstitial lung disease; LFTs—liver function tests; LVEF—left ventricular ejection fraction; mAb—monoclonal antibody; mCRC—metastatic colorectal cancer; MDS—myelodysplastic syndrome; MI—myocardial infarction; MRI—magnetic resonance imaging; NHL—non-Hodgkin lymphoma; NSCLC—non-small cell lung cancer; PD-1—programmed death receptor-1; PDGFR—platelet-derived growth factor receptor; RT—radiation therapy; TKI—tyrosine kinase inhibitor; URI—upper respiratory tract infection; VEGF—vascular endothelial growth factor; VEGFR—vascular endothelial growth factor receptor; VF—ventricular fibrillation

Note. Based on information from manufacturers' prescribing information.

to receptors on effector immunomodulatory cells such as macrophages, resulting in phagocytosis as well as stimulation of cytokine release that orchestrates the immune response, leading to destruction of the cell expressing the antigen (Hansel, Kropshofer, Singer, Mitchell, & George, 2010). The two most effective processes for killing cancer cells are antibody-dependent cell-mediated cytotoxicity (ADCC) and complement-dependent cellular cytotoxicity (CDC). The Fab (variable) fragment is the antigen-binding portion, and it will bind to only one antigen. The IgG core of the mAb theoretically makes a difference; mAbs derived from IgG1 are believed to have the strongest ADCC response, and they also have complement activation compared to IgG2 mAbs, which bind with weaker activation of host immune function (Adams

Table 4-3. Toxicities of Immune Checkpoint Inhibitors

Immune-Related Adverse Event	Signs and Symptoms	Assessment and Management
Gastrointestinal: Diarrhea, entero-colitis	Diarrhea, abdominal pain, blood or mucus in the stool, bowel perforation, peritoneal signs, ileus	Teach patient to report any diarrhea and take antidiarrheal medicine. Grade 1: Symptomatic treatment Grade 2: Hold drug; oral steroids Grade 3–4: Hold drug; IV steroids, see algorithm
Skin	Erythematous and/or maculopapular rash, dry skin, pruritus, blisters, ulceration Stevens-Johnson syndrome or toxic epidermal necrolysis	Most are mild and do not require drug interruption. Hold for severe rashes; consider rehospitalization for workup, dermatology consult, and systemic steroids.
Hepatitis	Elevated LFTs	Monitor LFTs baseline and prior to each dose. Hold drug for moderate elevations of LFTs, and discontinue for severe elevations.
Endocrinopathy: Hypophysitis, thyroid dysfunction (e.g., autoimmune thyroiditis)	Vague symptoms such as fatigue, headaches, myalgias, anorexia, nausea/vomiting, eye pain, diplopia, other visual changes Less commonly, hyponatremia due to syndrome of inappropriate antidiuretic hormone secretion or diabetes insipidus	Obtain brain MRI. Assess TFTs, cortisol, ACTH, luteinizing hormone, FSH, and testosterone in men. Hypophysitis with adrenal insufficiency/crisis is a medical emergency; start corticosteroids and thyroid replacement therapy as needed. Try to set up endocrine resource prior to starting drug in case hypophysitis develops. Assess baseline TSH, free T4, and monitor every 3 weeks during ipilimumab, then every 2–3 months after treatment.

ACTH—adrenocorticotropic hormone; FSH—follicle-stimulating hormone; LFT—liver function test; TFT—thyroid function test; TSH—thyroid-stimulating hormone

Note. Based on information from Fecher et al., 2013.

& Weiner, 2005). IgG1 mAbs include ado-trastuzumab emtansine (Kadcyla®), bevacizumab (Avastin®), brentuximab vedotin (Adcetris®), cetuximab (Erbitux®), ofatumumab (Arzerra®), pertuzumab (Perjeta®), rituximab (Rituxan®), trastuzumab (Herceptin®), and yttrium-90 ibritumomab tiuxetan (Zevalin®), whereas panitumumab (Vectibix®) is an IgG2 mAb.

Monoclonal antibodies are made to be totally human (human, suffix -umab), mostly human and only a small part mouse (humanized, suffix -zumab), some mouse and some human (chimeric, suffix -ximab), or entirely mouse protein (murine, suffix -momab) (see Figure 4-2). Although murine antibodies are better at finding their target because their Fab portion of the antibody is more efficient than the human Fab, significant difficulties exist as well. These include hypersensitivity reactions and development of neutralizing antibodies against the mouse antibody (human anti-mouse antibodies). Chemotherapy and mAbs differ in a number of ways, including the fact that mAbs may have long half-lives. For example, rituximab can

Table 4-4. Immunomodulatory Drugs, Vaccines, and Miscellaneous Drugs

Class	Target	Drugs and Indications[a]	Side Effects and Comments[b]
Immunomodulatory agents	Tumor microenvironment; antiangiogenesis activity	Thalidomide (Thalomid®) Indicated for treatment of patients with • Newly diagnosed myeloma with dexamethasone • Cutaneous manifestations of moderate to severe erythema nodosum leprosum (acute treatment)	Drug is available through Thalomid REMS® program with prescriber, patient, and pharmacist requirements. Drug is a teratogen and pregnancy is an absolute contraindication; pregnancy testing beginning 4 weeks prior to and during drug therapy is mandatory (repeated every 4 weeks in women with regular menses, and every 2 weeks in those with irregular menses). Women must be taught to use 2 highly effective forms of contraception. Drug is excreted in semen: Men must agree to wear latex or synthetic condom during and up to 28 days after drug is stopped and not to donate sperm. Common side effects are fatigue, hypocalcemia, edema, drowsiness, constipation, neuropathy (sensory and motor), dyspnea, muscle weakness, neutropenia, rash, confusion, anorexia, nausea, anxiety, asthenia, tremor, fever, somnolence, and headache. Drowsiness, orthostatic hypotension, and somnolence: Teach patients not to take other drugs that may cause drowsiness. Increased risk of thromboembolism may occur when combined with dexamethasone. Increased HIV viral load: Assess viral load after months 1 and 3, then every 3 months in HIV-positive patients. Bradycardia and syncope may occur. Stevens-Johnson syndrome and toxic epidermal necrolysis may occur; stop drug. Seizures may occur in patients with history of seizures. TLS (if high tumor burden) may occur; take appropriate precautions. Patients must not donate blood during and for 1 month after treatment. Ischemic heart disease has been observed when combined with dexamethasone. Neutropenia may necessitate dose interruption and/or reduction. Hypersensitivity may occur.

(Continued on next page)

Table 4-4. Immunomodulatory Drugs, Vaccines, and Miscellaneous Drugs *(Continued)*

Class	Target	Drugs and Indications[a]	Side Effects and Comments[b]
Immunomodulatory agents *(cont.)*		Lenalidomide (Revlimid®) Indicated for treatment of patients with • Multiple myeloma with dexamethasone • Transfusion-dependent anemia as a result of low- or intermediate-1-risk MDS associated with a deletion 5q • Mantle cell lymphoma whose disease has relapsed or progressed after 2 prior therapies, one of which included bortezomib	Drug is available through Revlimid REMS® program with prescriber, patient, and pharmacist requirements. Drug is a teratogen, and pregnancy is an absolute contraindication. Pregnancy testing beginning 4 weeks prior to and during drug therapy is mandatory (repeated every 4 weeks in women with regular menses, and every 2 weeks in those with irregular menses). Women must be taught to use 2 highly effective forms of contraception. Drug is excreted in semen: Men must agree to wear latex or synthetic condom during and up to 28 days after drug is stopped and not to donate sperm. Significant neutropenia and thrombocytopenia may occur. Most common adverse effects include diarrhea, fatigue, constipation, neutropenia, nausea, dizziness, dyspnea, and thrombocytopenia. Risk for venous and arterial thromboembolism is increased when combined with dexamethasone; antithrombotic prophylaxis should be considered. Risk is also elevated in patients taking concomitant erythropoiesis-stimulating agents or estrogen-containing therapy. Drug can cause hypersensitivity reactions (rare). TLS (high tumor burden) may occur. Tumor flare reaction may occur in patients with chronic lymphocytic leukemia and lymphoma (not approved for chronic lymphocytic leukemia). Hepatotoxicity with hepatic failure may rarely occur. Second primary malignancy has been reported in patients with multiple myeloma. Impairs stem cell mobilization (decreased number of CD34+ cells collected), so early referral to a transplant center should be considered. Patients must not donate blood during and for 1 month after treatment.

(Continued on next page)

Table 4-4. Immunomodulatory Drugs, Vaccines, and Miscellaneous Drugs *(Continued)*

Class	Target	Drugs and Indications[a]	Side Effects and Comments[b]
Immunomodulatory agents *(cont.)*		Pomalidomide (Pomalyst®) Indicated for treatment of patients with multiple myeloma previously treated with at least 2 prior therapies including lenalidomide and bortezomib and who progressed within 60 days of last therapy	Drug is available only through Pomalyst REMS® program with prescriber, patient, and pharmacist requirements. Drug is a teratogen and pregnancy is an absolute contraindication. Pregnancy testing beginning 4 weeks prior to and during drug therapy is mandatory (repeated every 4 weeks in women with regular menses, and every 2 weeks in those with irregular menses). Women must be taught to use 2 highly effective forms of contraception. Drug is excreted in semen. Men must agree to wear latex or synthetic condom during and up to 28 days after drug is stopped and not to donate sperm. Most common side effects are fatigue, asthenia, neutropenia, anemia, constipation, nausea, diarrhea, dyspnea, URI, back pain, and pyrexia. Deep vein thrombosis and pulmonary embolism may occur in patients with multiple myeloma receiving concomitant dexamethasone. In clinical trials, prophylaxis was used (81% aspirin, 16% warfarin, 3% clopidogrel). Grade 3–4 neutropenia was the most frequent grade 3–4 adverse event (43%), followed by anemia and thrombocytopenia. Monitor complete blood count and differential weekly for first 2 months, then monthly. Dizziness and confusional state may occur; patients should be taught to avoid situations when this might cause a problem and to avoid other medications that cause dizziness or confusion. Neuropathy occurred in 18% of patients (no grade 3 or 4). Risk of second primary malignancies (e.g., AML) is increased. TLS may occur in patients with high tumor burden; institute precautionary measures to prevent TLS. Patients must not donate blood during and for 1 month after treatment.

(Continued on next page)

Table 4-4. Immunomodulatory Drugs, Vaccines, and Miscellaneous Drugs *(Continued)*

Class	Target	Drugs and Indications[a]	Side Effects and Comments[b]
Vaccine	Prostate tumor antigen	Sipuleucel-T (Provenge®) Autologous cellular immunotherapy indicated for treatment of asymptomatic or minimally symptomatic metastatic castrate-resistant (hormone-refractory) prostate cancer	Most common include chills, fatigue, fever, back pain, nausea, joint ache, and headache. Acute infusion reactions, which may be severe, may occur. Syncope and hypotension may also occur. Three doses are given, about 2 weeks apart. Autologous cellular immunotherapy uses patient immune cells, which are obtained by leukapheresis. Dendritic, T and B lymphocytes are then cultured with tumor antigen preparation, forming primed antigen-presenting cells (CD54+), which are then reinfused into the patient. These will activate and lead immune cells to tumor cells with that antigen and kill them. Ensure correct patient and correct vaccine prior to administering vaccine. Use cautiously in patients at risk for thromboembolic events. Concomitant use of chemotherapy and immunosuppressive medications with vaccine has not been studied.
Miscellaneous	Primitive promyelocytes in APL; promoting maturation followed by repopulation of the bone marrow and peripheral blood with normal myeloid cell line in patients who achieve a complete remission	Tretinoin (all-trans-retinoic acid, ATRA, Vesanoid®) Indicated for induction of remission in patients with APL (IV formulation, liposomal tretinoin [Atragen®] is investigational.)	Retinoic acid-APL syndrome (rapid leukocytosis, fever, dyspnea, weight gain, pulmonary infiltrates, effusions) may occur and may be fatal. Treat with high-dose steroids. Vitamin A toxicity (headaches, fever, skin/mucous membrane dryness, bone pain, nausea, vomiting, rash, mucositis, pruritus, diaphoresis, visual disturbances, skin changes, alopecia) may occur. Other side effects include arrhythmia, flushing, earache, hypercholesterolemia and/or hypertriglyceridemia, and rare pseudotumor cerebri. Drug is teratogenic and embryotoxic (avoid pregnancy).

(Continued on next page)

Table 4-4. Immunomodulatory Drugs, Vaccines, and Miscellaneous Drugs (Continued)

Class	Target	Drugs and Indications[a]	Side Effects and Comments[b]
Miscellaneous (cont.)	Retinoid X receptor: Selectively binds and activates retinoid X receptor (RXRα, RXRβ, RXRγ), thus inhibiting transcription factors that regulate gene expression controlling differentiation and proliferation	Bexarotene (Targretin®) Indicated for treatment of cutaneous manifestations of cutaneous T-cell lymphoma	Clinical hypothyroidism; cataracts; diarrhea, fatigue/lethargy, headache, rash, nausea, anemia, muscle spasm; elevated fasting triglycerides and cholesterol; liver function test abnormalities; leukopenia; and pancreatitis may occur. Drug is teratogenic and embryotoxic (avoid pregnancy).
Hypomethylating agents (epigenetic)	DNA; drug inhibits methyltransferase, causing hypomethylation of DNA, cellular differentiation, or apoptosis. Hypomethylation may restore normal function to genes controlling cellular differentiation and proliferation.	Decitabine (Dacogen®) Indicated for treatment of patients MDS, and intermediate-1, -2, and high-risk International Prognostic Scoring System groups	Neutropenia (including febrile neutropenia), thrombocytopenia, anemia, nausea, diarrhea, constipation, hyperglycemia, cough, and pyrexia may occur. Drug is teratogenic. Women of childbearing potential and men with female partners of childbearing potential should use effective contraception and avoid pregnancy.
	DNA; drug inhibits methyltransferase, causing hypomethylation of DNA, and direct cytotoxicity to rapidly proliferating cells. Hypomethylation may restore normal function to genes controlling cellular differentiation and proliferation.	Azacitidine (Vidaza®) Indicated for treatment of patients with MDS subtypes: RA, RARS, RAEB, RAEB-T, and CMML	Neutropenia, thrombocytopenia, and anemia occur in > 50% of patients; monitor CBC/differential frequently. Nausea, vomiting, diarrhea, pyrexia, constipation, weakness, rigors, and anorexia may occur. Dose adjustment is made for decreased serum bicarbonate, and dose is interrupted and decreased for unexplained increases in BUN or serum creatinine. Injection-site reactions (erythema) and ecchymosis may develop when drug is given subcutaneously. Teach women and men to avoid pregnancy, as drug may cause fetal harm.

(Continued on next page)

Table 4-4. Immunomodulatory Drugs, Vaccines, and Miscellaneous Drugs *(Continued)*

Class	Target	Drugs and Indications[a]	Side Effects and Comments[b]
HDAC inhibitors (epigenetic)	HDAC, an enzyme that prevents uncoiling of DNA strands, thus suppressing transcription of tumor suppressor genes (turns them off); HDAC inhibitors block the enzyme, thus allowing the DNA strands to uncoil, expressing the genes, and the tumor suppressor genes are turned back on	Belinostat (Beleodaq®) Indicated for treatment of patients with relapsed or refractory PTCL	Most common adverse reactions include nausea, vomiting, fatigue, pyrexia, and anemia. Thrombocytopenia, neutropenia, lymphopenia, anemia occur: Monitor CBC/differential, and modify dose according to package insert. Infection, including sepsis, may occur. TLS may occur in patients with advanced-stage disease and/or high tumor burden; administer prophylaxis to prevent. Teach women of reproductive potential to use effective contraception to avoid pregnancy, as drug is embryo-fetal toxic.
	HDAC	Panobinostat (Farydak®) Indicated for treatment of patients with multiple myeloma who have received at least 2 prior therapies (including bortezomib and an immunomodulatory agent), in combination with bortezomib and dexamethasone	Severe diarrhea occurred in 25% in clinical studies and can be fatal; teach patients to stop drug, begin antidiarrheal medications, and call provider right away. When diarrhea resolves, drug dose should be reduced. Severe and potentially fatal cardiac ischemic events, severe arrhythmias, and ECG changes have occurred. Arrhythmias may be exacerbated by abnormal electrolyte levels. ECG should be performed at baseline for all, and during therapy for those at risk. ECG abnormalities are ST-segment depression, T-wave abnormalities, and QTc prolongation. Drug should be not be started in patients with QTc > 450 ms and should be interrupted if QTc is ≥ 480 ms after a normal baseline. Severe and frequent thrombocytopenia, neutropenia, lymphopenia, leukopenia, and anemia may occur. Monitor CBC/differential closely. Most common adverse effects were diarrhea, fatigue, nausea, peripheral edema, decreased appetite, pyrexia, and vomiting. Hepatotoxicity may occur; monitor LFTs and adjust dose as necessary. Nonhematologic lab abnormalities include hypophosphatemia, hypokalemia, hyponatremia, and increased serum creatinine.

(Continued on next page)

Table 4-4. Immunomodulatory Drugs, Vaccines, and Miscellaneous Drugs *(Continued)*

Class	Target	Drugs and Indications[a]	Side Effects and Comments[b]
HDAC inhibitors (epigenetic) *(cont.)*	HDAC *(cont.)*	Panobinostat (Farydak®) *(cont.)*	Teach patient to report bleeding, as GI and pulmonary hemorrhage have been reported. Drug interactions can occur with strong CYP3A4 inhibitors and inducers. Avoid concomitant use of antiarrhythmic drugs that can prolong the QTc interval. Teach women of reproductive potential to use effective contraception to avoid pregnancy, as drug is embryo-fetal toxic.
	HDAC	Romidepsin (Istodax®) Indicated for treatment of patients who have received at least 1 prior therapy, with • Cutaneous T-cell lymphoma • PTCL	Most common are neutropenia, lymphopenia, thrombocytopenia, anemia, infections, nausea, vomiting, anorexia, and ECG T-wave changes. Myelosuppression: Monitor CBC/differential at baseline and during treatment. Refer to package insert for dose interruption and modification doses. Infections are serious and may be fatal; reactivation of Epstein-Barr virus and hepatitis B can occur; monitor patients with prior hepatitis B closely and consider prophylaxis. QTc prolongation is possible; ensure patients' serum potassium and magnesium are within normal limits. Monitor cardiovascular system in patients at risk (e.g., significant cardiovascular disease, congenital long QT syndrome, taking medicines that prolong the QTc interval). TLS may occur in patients with a high tumor burden. Avoid coadministration with strong CYP3A4 inhibitors or inducers. Monitor prothrombin time and international normalized ratio closely in patients taking warfarin.

(Continued on next page)

Table 4-4. Immunomodulatory Drugs, Vaccines, and Miscellaneous Drugs *(Continued)*

Class	Target	Drugs and Indications[a]	Side Effects and Comments[b]
HDAC inhibitors (epigenetic) *(cont.)*	HDAC	Vorinostat (Zolinza®) Indicated for treatment of cutaneous manifestations of cutaneous T-cell lymphoma in patients who have progressed or have persistent or recurrent disease, on or after 2 prior systemic therapies	Most common side effects are diarrhea, fatigue, nausea, thrombocytopenia, anorexia, and dysgeusia. Deep vein thrombosis and pulmonary embolism may occur. Thrombocytopenia and anemia may occur; monitor complete blood count every 2 weeks for first 8 weeks, then monthly. Nausea, vomiting, and diarrhea may occur. Prevent/manage with antiemetics, antidiarrheals, and fluid and electrolyte replacement. Prevent dehydration. Electrolyte imbalance may develop: Assess electrolytes, including magnesium and calcium, at baseline, then every 2 weeks, during first 2 months of therapy, then at least monthly. Correct imbalances. Hyperglycemia: Monitor blood glucose at baseline and every 2 weeks during first 2 months of therapy, then monthly. If combined with other HDAC inhibitors (e.g., valproic acid), severe thrombocytopenia and GI bleeding may occur; monitor platelet counts more frequently and teach patients to report any signs/symptoms of bleeding. Prothrombin time and international normalized ratio may be prolonged in patients receiving concomitant warfarin. Teach women of reproductive potential to use effective contraception to avoid pregnancy, as drug can cause fetal harm.

(Continued on next page)

Table 4-4. Immunomodulatory Drugs, Vaccines, and Miscellaneous Drugs (Continued)

Class	Target	Drugs and Indications[a]	Side Effects and Comments[b]
Fusion protein	CD25 component of inter-leukin (IL)-2 recep-tor found on cutaneous T-cell lymphoma cells Drug is recombinant DNA-derived fusion pro-tein containing diphthe-ria toxin fragments plus IL-2 receptor. The pro-tein attaches to the IL-2 receptor of cells carry-ing CD25 proteins and internalizes the diphthe-ria fragments; this stops protein synthesis and kills the cell.	Denileukin diftitox (Ontak®) Indicated for treatment of patients with cutaneous T-cell lymphoma, persistent or recur-rent, that expresses the CD25 component of the IL-2 receptor	Acute hypersensitivity reactions (hypotension, back pain, dyspnea, vasodila-tion, rash, chest pain/tightness, chills/fever, tachycardia with rare anaphy-laxis) may occur. Premedicate patients with antihistamine and acetamino-phen before dose. Capillary leak syndrome (hypotension, serum albumin < 3 g/dl, edema) may develop. Onset may be delayed for up to 2 weeks after an infusion. Assess patients for weight gain, new or worsening edema, and hypotension, and correct serum albumin to ≥ 3 g/dl. Peripheral edema, pyrexia, fatigue, rigors, headache, cough, pruritus, nau-sea, vomiting, diarrhea, anorexia, and loss of visual acuity with loss of color vision may occur. Patients must avoid pregnancy, as fetotoxicity tests have not been done.
PARP inhibitor	PARP, a DNA repair enzyme BRCA1/2 is a tumor sup-pressor that repairs DNA; if BRCA1/2 is mutated and PARP is inhibited, the cancer cell dies.	Olaparib (Lynparza®) Indicated as monotherapy in patients with advanced ovar-ian cancer with germ-line BRCA mutation as determined by an FDA-approved test and who have been treated with 3 or more prior lines of chemotherapy	Most common are anemia, nausea, fatigue, vomiting, diarrhea, dysgeusia, dyspepsia, headache, decreased appetite; nasopharyngitis, pharyngitis, URI, cough; arthralgia, musculoskeletal pain, myalgia, back pain; dermatitis/rash; and abdominal pain/discomfort. Most common laboratory abnormalities are increased creatinine and MCV and decreased hemoglobin, lymphocytes, ANC, and platelets. MDS/AML may occur; monitor patients for hematologic toxicity baseline, and monthly thereafter. Pneumonitis may occur; interrupt drug if suspected, and discontinue if diag-nosis confirmed. Drug is embryo-fetal toxic. Drug interactions may occur with CYP3A4 inhibitors and inducers.

(Continued on next page)

Table 4-4. Immunomodulatory Drugs, Vaccines, and Miscellaneous Drugs (Continued)

Class	Target	Drugs and Indications[a]	Side Effects and Comments[b]
Alkaloid translation inhibitor	Inhibits expression of *BCR-ABL* oncogene, so suppresses Bcr-Abl protein kinase formation; mechanism is not well understood but it is a different mechanism of action from the TKIs.	Omacetaxine (Synribo®) Indicated for treatment of adult patients with chronic- or accelerated-phase chronic myeloid leukemia with resistance or intolerance to 2 or more tyrosine kinase inhibitors. Induction and maintenance dosing are modified for toxicity.	Most common are thrombocytopenia, anemia, neutropenia, diarrhea, nausea, fatigue, asthenia, injection-site reaction, pyrexia, infection, and lymphopenia. Severe and fatal thrombocytopenia and risk of bleeding, neutropenia, and anemia may occur; monitor closely. Fatal cerebral hemorrhage and nonfatal GI hemorrhage have occurred. Hyperglycemia and glucose intolerance, including hyperosmolar nonketotic hyperglycemia, are possible. Teach women of reproductive potential to use effective contraception to avoid pregnancy, as drug is embryo-fetal toxic.
Hedgehog pathway inhibitor	Smoothened, a transmembrane protein in the Hedgehog pathway, responsible for signal transduction	Vismodegib (Erivedge®) Indicated for treatment of adults with metastatic basal cell carcinoma or with locally advanced basal cell carcinoma that has recurred after surgery or who are not candidates for either surgery or radiation	Most common are muscle spasms, alopecia, dysgeusia, ageusia, weight loss, fatigue, nausea, vomiting, diarrhea, constipation, decreased appetite, and arthralgias. Drug causes death to embryo and severe birth defects; men and women must avoid pregnancy. Patients must not donate blood during and for 7 months after the drug has been stopped.

[a] This table includes indications, but they change frequently. Please consult the manufacturer's product information as well as the FDA's Center for Drug Evaluation and Research website (www.accessdata.fda.gov/scripts/cder/drugsatfda/index.cfm), which offers an email service to alert subscribers when a new drug or new indication is approved by FDA, for updated information. Every effort has been made to ensure drug data are consistent with the most recent package insert, but typographical errors may occur, and drug information may be updated by the manufacturer. Please see drug package insert for complete prescribing information.

[b] Most of the drugs are potentially fetotoxic, so women and men should be counseled use effective contraception to avoid pregnancy. In addition, most TKIs are metabolized by the CYP3A4 hepatic microenzyme system and require a review of the patient's medication profile for possible interactions.

AML—acute myeloid leukemia; ANC—absolute neutrophil count; APL—acute promyelocytic leukemia; BUN—blood urea nitrogen; CBC—complete blood count; CMML—chronic myelomonocytic leukemia; ECG—electrocardiogram; FDA—U.S. Food and Drug Administration; GI—gastrointestinal; HDAC—histone deacetylase; LFTs—liver function tests; MCV—mean corpuscular volume; MDS—myelodysplastic syndrome; PARP—poly (ADP-ribose) polymerase; PTCL—peripheral T-cell lymphoma; QTc—QT interval, corrected, measure of time from start of Q wave and end of T wave on electrocardiogram (depolarization and repolarization of the cardiac ventricles, normal is ≤ 450 msec); RA—refractory anemia; RAEB—refractory anemia with excess blasts; RAEB-T—refractory anemia with excess blasts in transformation; RARS—refractory anemia with ringed sideroblasts; TKI—tyrosine kinase inhibitor; TLS—tumor lysis syndrome; URI—upper respiratory tract infection

Note. Based on information from manufacturers' prescribing information.

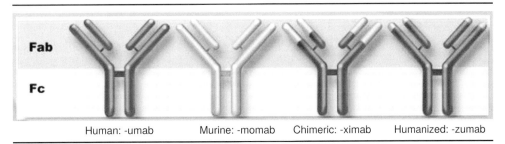

Human: -umab   Murine: -momab   Chimeric: -ximab   Humanized: -zumab

Figure 4-2. Types of Monoclonal Antibodies

Note. From *Biomolecular Targeted Therapies in Cancer Treatment* [Slide Kit], by Oncology Education Services, Inc., 2003, Pittsburgh, PA: Author. Copyright 2003 by Oncology Education Services, Inc. Reprinted with permission.

remain in the blood six months after the dose was administered, after which time B-cell lymphocytes begin to recover (Biogen Idec, Inc., & Genentech, Inc., 2014).

Monoclonal antibodies can be unconjugated (naked) or conjugated (attached to a toxin or radionuclide). The unconjugated mAb kills tumor cells by first attaching to the antigen, such as the CD20 B lymphocyte. (*CD* represents "cluster of differentiation.") It then has five biologic activities that can injure or kill the cell (Hansel et al., 2010).

- Direct interference with cell signaling of target cell (cytostatic, e.g., block receptor)
- ADCC, in which cytokines recruit phagocytes, T cells, and natural killer cells, which destroy the target cell
- CDC, in which the complement system is activated to destroy the target cell
- Direct induction of apoptosis in antibody-bound cell
- Release of inhibitory checkpoints so that target cell is attacked by immune system (antibodies against cytotoxic T-lymphocytic antigen-4, antibodies against T-regulatory cells)

Unconjugated Monoclonal Antibodies, Including Immune Checkpoint Inhibitors

This category of unconjugated, or naked, mAbs includes alemtuzumab (Campath®), bevacizumab, blinatumomab (Blincyto®), cetuximab, ipilimumab, nivolumab, obinutuzumab (Gazyva®), ofatumumab, panitumumab, pertuzumab, ramucirumab (Cyramza®), rituximab, and trastuzumab. Rituximab is perhaps the most well known, as it was the first mAb approved for treatment of cancer, is a cornerstone for the treatment of patients with CD20-positive lymphoma, and has found application in a number of non-oncology settings, such as rheumatoid arthritis (see Table 4-2 for indications).

Rituximab is an IgG1 mAb that targets the CD20 antigen, found on both malignant and normal B lymphocytes (pre-B and mature, but not on hematopoietic stem cells). This antigen is expressed on more than 90% of B-cell non-Hodgkin lymphoma (NHL) cells, and B lymphocytes are implicated in rheumatoid arthritis. The Fab portion of the mAb binds to the CD20 antigen, and the Fc fragment calls in immune effector cells, which bring about cell lysis. This is believed to be due to induction of ADCC as well as CDC with activation of complement that coats the antigen-bearing cell, causing cell lysis and induction of apoptosis (Biogen Idec, Inc., & Genentech, Inc., 2014). Rituximab is indicated for the treatment of CD20 antigen–positive NHL, including low-grade or follicular lymphoma, diffuse large cell lymphoma (in combination with CHOP), CD20-positive chronic lymphocytic leukemia (CLL), rheumatoid arthritis, Wegener granulomatosis, and microscopic polyangiitis. (See Table 4-2 for full indications.) The drug's half-life varies with the dose and frequency of schedule, and when it was used to treat NHL, the estimated median terminal elimination half-life was 22 days (range 6.1–52 days) (Biogen Idec, Inc., & Genentech, Inc., 2014). The NHL dose is 375 mg/m^2 as a weekly IV infusion for four to eight doses, whereas for rheumatoid arthritis, the dose is 1,000 mg IV infusion every two weeks for two doses only, together with glucocorticoid premedication (Biogen Idec, Inc., & Genentech, Inc., 2014). Rituximab also is given in combination with yttrium-90 ibritumomab tiuxetan or other chemotherapy regimens such as CHOP.

Potential side effects include infusion reactions (chills, rigors, severe hypersensitivity reaction of hypotension, bronchospasm, and anaphylaxis requiring emergency intervention) and rare severe mucocutaneous reactions. An increased risk of tumor lysis syndrome (TLS) exists in newly diagnosed patients with lymphoma with a high tumor burden because of the dramatic lysis of lymphocytes during their first rituximab treatment. Rarely, the drug has been associated with bowel obstruction and perforation, renal failure, cardiac arrhythmias, and hepatitis B reactivation with fulminant hepatitis. Rituximab has been associated with severe and sometimes fatal infusion reactions within 24 hours of infusion; 80% occurred in association with the first infusion (Biogen Idec, Inc., & Genentech, Inc., 2014). Patients should be monitored closely, rituximab discontinued for severe reactions (grade 3–4), and immediate medical intervention instituted. Infusion reactions may include urticaria, hypotension, angioedema, hypoxia, bronchospasm, pulmonary infiltrates, acute respiratory distress syndrome (ARDS), myocardial infarction, ventricular fibrillation, cardiogenic shock, anaphylactoid events, or death (Biogen Idec, Inc., & Genentech, Inc., 2014). In addition, progressive multifocal leukoencephalopathy related to reactivation of viral infection caused by John Cunningham virus (referred to as the JC virus), a type of human polyomavirus, rarely occurs. Progressive multifocal leukoencephalopathy principally occurs in patients who have received combination chemotherapy or stem cell transplant, in patients with autoimmune disease, or in those receiving concurrent immunosuppressive therapy. Most cases occurred within 12 months of the patient's last dose of rituximab. If the patient presents with new-onset neurologic signs and symptoms, the drug should be discontinued, along with concomitant chemotherapy or immunosuppressive therapy, and a neurology consult obtained, along with magnetic resonance imaging of the brain and lumbar puncture (Biogen Idec, Inc., & Genentech, Inc., 2014; Clifford et al., 2011).

A number of mAbs block EGFR, also known as the human epidermal receptor (HER). The EGFR family consists of four receptors: EGFR1 (HER1), EGFR2 (HER2), EGFR3 (HER3), and EGFR4 (HER4) (see Figure 4-3). EGFR1 and EGFR2 may be mutated or overexpressed in a number of solid tumors. Figure 4-4 depicts the activity of the EGFRs when overexpressed, leading to cell survival (avoidance of apoptosis), growth and proliferation, release of VEGF to begin angiogenesis, and metastases. Blocking the receptor results in interruption of signal transduction, so the message for the cell to proliferate, make VEGF, become invasive, and ignore death signals (apoptosis) never reaches the cell nucleus. EGFR inhibitors represent a powerful group of agents in molecular-targeted therapy and include the mAbs cetuximab, panitumumab, pertuzumab, and trastuzumab.

Trastuzumab is an IgG1 mAb that targets the HER2 receptor, also known as EGFR2. The HER2 receptor has extracellular, transmembrane, and intracellular domains; trastuzumab targets the extracellular domain. In 20%–25% of patients with breast cancer, the *HER2* gene can be amplified (too many copies of the *HER2* gene) or the receptor can be overexpressed (too many HER2 receptors on the cell surface) (Luoh et al., 2013). Although *HER2* overexpression confers a more aggressive disease with a less favorable prognosis, success with trastuzumab has improved survival, especially in the adjuvant setting. *HER2* is also overexpressed in other cancers such as gastric and gastroesophageal junction cancers.

The HER2 receptor is involved in complex cell signaling, resulting in cell cycle progression, cell proliferation, survival, and motility transduction (Gravalos & Jimeno, 2008). The HER2 receptor does not have a ligand; however, it is most commonly the partner with any of

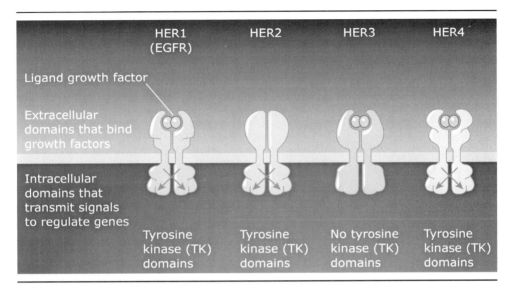

Figure 4-3. Epidermal Growth Factor Receptor Family of Receptors

Note. From *Clinical Breakthroughs in EGFR Inhibition: Applying the Science to Your Clinical Practice* (Slide 14), by T. Knoop, M. Morse, and L. Tyson, May 2006. Presentation given at the Oncology Nursing Society 31st Annual Congress, Boston, MA. Copyright 2006 by Oncology Nursing Society. Reprinted with permission.

the other EGFRs to dimerize. Once trastuzumab binds to the HER2 receptor on the cell surface, it is believed to interrupt dimerization (two surface receptors must come together or dimerize to initiate the signal for proliferation), thus bringing about G_1 phase cell cycle arrest, decreased cell proliferation, antiangiogenic factor release, suppression of VEGF secretion, and enhancement of ADCC immune function (Sliwkowski et al., 1999). Patients must have significant overexpression of HER2 to benefit from trastuzumab, so the National Comprehensive Cancer Network® (NCCN®) guidelines recommend confirming HER2 positivity by in situ hybridization (ISH) testing or 3+ by immunohistochemistry (IHC) (NCCN, 2015). The dual ISH is available, offering chromogenic ISH genetic information with visualization and interpretation of IHC (LabCorp, 2013). Accurate HER2 testing is critical to effectively plan therapy for women who are HER2 positive.

Once a patient has been determined to be HER2 positive, discussion about treatment with an HER2 receptor antagonist takes place. Trastuzumab is the most thoroughly studied agent to date. When given in the adjuvant setting, trastuzumab can be given for 52 weeks, either (a) weekly, with a 4 mg/kg IV loading dose given over 90 minutes, and if well tolerated, subsequent weekly doses of 2 mg/kg IV given over 30 minutes, or (b) as an initial loading dose of 8 mg/kg IV over 90 minutes, then 6 mg/kg IV over 30–90 minutes, every three weeks (Genentech, Inc., 2014b). In the metastatic HER2-overexpressing setting, patients with metastatic breast cancer receive the regimen identified in (a), while patients with metastatic gastric cancer receive the regimen in (b). If the patient develops mild to moderate infusion reactions, the infusion rate should be reduced and the drug administered over a longer time. Signs of infusion reaction characteristically include fever and chills, which respond to acetaminophen, diphenhydramine, and meperidine. Less commonly, nausea, vomiting, pain (related to tumor), headache, dizziness, dyspnea, hypotension, rash, and asthenia also may occur. Rarely, more serious infusion reactions may include bronchospasm, hypoxia, dyspnea, and severe hypotension, which may develop during or immediately following drug infusion. For these responses, the drug

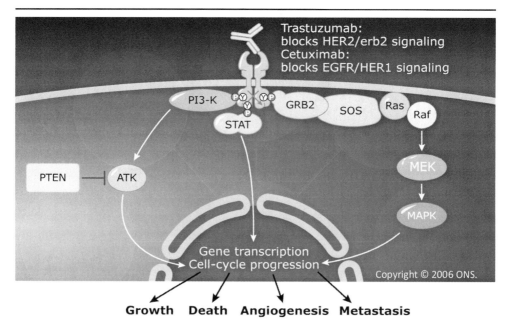

A growth factor (ligand) binds to the EGFR, causing dimerization or pairing of receptors, and this initiates the signaling cascade telling the nucleus what to do. Many pathways to reach the nucleus exist: shown in this slide are the mitogen-activated protein kinase (MAPK) pathway and the PI3-K/ATK pathway (phosphoinositide 3 kinase/protein kinase B). The monoclonal antibody cetuximab blocks the EGFR1 from initiating a message, while trastuzumab blocks the HER-2 receptor from initiating the signal. This prevents the signaling cascade and subsequent proliferation and angiogenesis and encourages the cell to die.

Figure 4-4. Trastuzumab and Cetuximab Mechanism of Action as Anti-Epidermal Growth Factor Receptor (EGFR) Antibodies

ATK—protein kinase B; GRB2—growth factor receptor-binding protein 2; MAPK—mitogen-activated protein kinase; MEK—Map erk kinase; P—phosphorylation of EGFR tyrosine kinase; PI3-K—phosphoinositide 3 kinase; PTEN—phosphatase and tensin homolog; Raf—protein kinase that is a Ras effector (carries out its work); Ras—protein product from *ras* family of oncogenes; SOS—son of sevenless protein; STAT—signal transducer and activator of transcription; Y—yes, phosphorylation occurs and the signal activates the indicated pathways

Note. From *Clinical Breakthroughs in EGFR Inhibition: Applying the Science to Your Clinical Practice* (Slide 29), by T. Knoop, M. Morse, and L. Tyson, May 2006. Presentation given at the Oncology Nursing Society 31st Annual Congress, Boston, MA. Copyright 2006 by Oncology Nursing Society. Reprinted with permission.

should be interrupted until symptoms completely resolve. If severe or life-threatening infusion reactions occur, such as anaphylaxis, angioedema, pneumonitis, or ARDS, the drug should be discontinued (Genentech, Inc., 2014b). However, there are reports of successful desensitization protocols for hypersensitivity reactions (Hong, Bankova, Cahill, Kyin, & Castells, 2012).

In a number of adjuvant studies, the relative risk of recurrence decreased by 52% when trastuzumab was added to chemotherapy, and the absolute difference in disease-free survival was 12% at three years and 18% at four years in favor of the trastuzumab plus chemotherapy group (Baselga, Perez, Pienkowski, & Bell, 2006; Romond et al., 2005). However, because up to a 4.1% incidence of cardiotoxicity was found in the group receiving trastuzumab, Slamon et al. (2011) studied the efficacy and safety of the nonanthracycline regimen of docetaxel, carboplatin, and trastuzumab (TCH regimen) for 52 weeks. The authors found that at a median follow-up of 65 months, the estimated five-year disease-free survival rate was 75% for patients receiving doxorubicin, cyclophosphamide, and docetaxel (AC-T regimen), 84% for patients receiving AC-T plus trastuzumab, and 81% for patients receiving TCH. Estimated overall survival was 87%, 92%, and 91%, respectively. In a risk-benefit analysis, the TCH regimen was preferred over AC-T plus trastuzumab because it had a significantly lower risk of cardiotoxicity compared to the anthracycline groups (containing doxorubicin). Trastuzumab also improves survival in patients with metastatic HER2-positive breast cancer in first-line therapy, compared to chemotherapy alone (Slamon et al., 2011), as well as after disease progression (von Minckwitz et al., 2008). More recently, Swain et al. (2013) found that the addition of pertuzumab to trastuzumab, plus docetaxel in the first-line metastatic setting, significantly improved median overall survival, compared to trastuzumab and docetaxel alone.

HER2 signaling is important for cardiac repair. Trastuzumab is associated with cardiomyopathy, with increased risk when given with an anthracycline drug, such as doxorubicin, or within three weeks of doxorubicin administration (Bowles et al., 2012). Anthracyclines kill myocytes, whereas trastuzumab has a different and reversible mechanism of action related to HER2 signaling interruption (Ewer & Ewer, 2010). The risk decreases when there is a greater interval between the anthracycline dosing and the administration of trastuzumab. In the National Surgical Adjuvant Breast and Bowel Project (NSABP) B-31 and Breast Cancer International Research Group (BCIRG) 006 trials, trastuzumab was administered 30 days after the anthracycline, with 3.8% and 1.8% of patients developing heart failure (NSABP B-31 and BCIRG 006, respectively) (Slamon et al., 2009; Tan-Chiu et al., 2005). When trastuzumab was administered 60 days after the anthracycline, 3.3% of patients developed heart failure (North Central Cancer Treatment Group N9831) (Perez et al., 2008). However, when trastuzumab was administered 90 days after the anthracycline, the incidence of heart failure was 0.6% (HER2-positive Adjuvant [HERA] trial evaluating 1 year vs. 2 years of trastuzumab) (Suter et al., 2007).

In a recent population-based, retrospective cohort study of 12,500 women with breast cancer, Bowles et al. (2012) found the cumulative risk of cardiomyopathy at one year versus five years was (a) 1.2% at one year and 4.3% at five years in women receiving anthracycline alone, (b) 3.6% at one year and 12.1% at five years in women receiving trastuzumab alone, (c) 6.2% at one year and 20.1% at five years in women receiving anthracycline plus trastuzumab, and (d) 0.9% at one year and 3.1% at five years in women receiving no chemotherapy or biotherapy. This has led to the replacement of doxorubicin with docetaxel as an option in adjuvant breast cancer therapy.

Baseline LVEF should be determined just before treatment begins and repeated every three months during and upon completion of trastuzumab (in the adjuvant setting), using the same test (echocardiogram or MUGA scan). Normal baseline LVEF is 50% or greater (Genentech, Inc., 2014b). The drug should be held for at least four weeks for (a) 16% or greater absolute decrease in LVEF from pretreatment values, or (b) an LVEF value below institutional limits of normal and 10% or greater absolute decrease in LVEF from pretreatment values. The drug should be resumed if within four to eight weeks, the LVEF returns to within normal limits and the absolute decrease from baseline is 15% or less. Trastuzumab should be permanently discontinued for persistent (longer than eight weeks) decline in LVEF or for suspension of trastuzumab dosing on more than three occasions for cardiomyopathy (Genentech, Inc., 2014b).

Pulmonary toxicity has been reported with trastuzumab and has led to death. Patients with existing lung disease or extensive lung metastases that cause dyspnea at rest appear to be at risk. Toxicity includes dyspnea, pneumonitis, hypoxia, ARDS, and pulmonary fibrosis, which may occur during or after the infusion as part of an infusion reaction (Genentech, Inc., 2014b). Pronounced neutropenia, especially febrile neutropenia, may occur when trastuzumab is combined with myelosuppressive chemotherapy. Other side effects include nausea, vomiting, diarrhea, infections, increased cough, headache, fatigue, rash, and myalgia. Rarely, thrombosis and embolism may occur. During drug administration, only normal saline should be used so as to avoid incompatibilities with 5% dextrose solutions (Genentech, Inc., 2014b).

Cetuximab is a mAb that targets the extracellular domain of EGFR1, as shown in Figure 4-4. Cetuximab is FDA-approved for treatment of patients with advanced colorectal cancer or head and neck cancer as described in Table 4-2. Colorectal tumors must be *KRAS* gene wild-type (not mutated) to respond to the drug; thus, *KRAS* determination must be done prior to starting the drug. It also appears that a wild-type *BRAF* gene is required for a response to either EGFR inhibitor mAb (cetuximab or panitumumab) (Di Nicolantonio et al., 2008). The initial loading dose is 400 mg/m^2 IV over two hours, followed by weekly maintenance treatments of 250 mg/m^2 over 60 minutes. When given with radiation therapy for patients with head and neck cancer, the drug should be started one week prior to starting radiation therapy. Cetuximab infusion should be completed one hour prior to platinum-based therapy with 5-FU and with FOLFIRI (folinic acid, 5-FU, irinotecan) chemotherapy. Premedications should be given before each treatment and include H$_1$ antagonists such as diphenhydramine. Cetuximab is a chimeric mAb that may cause infusion reactions, including severe reactions in 3% of patients, such as symptomatic bronchospasm, hypotension, and anaphylaxis (ImClone LLC & Bristol-Myers Squibb Co., 2013). Ninety percent of these reactions occur during the first infusion (ImClone LLC & Bristol-Myers Squibb Co., 2013). Chung et al. (2008) showed that certain patients living in distinct geographical areas developed antibodies to the cetuximab molecule (epitope), with up to 21% of patients receiving the drug in Tennessee experiencing anaphylaxis and 6.1% of patients treated in Northern California experiencing anaphylaxis, compared to 0.6% of patients treated in Boston, Massachusetts.

EGFRs are located in the skin, hair follicles, and gastric mucosa; therefore, toxicities are manifested in these areas and include a sterile, inflammatory skin rash (follicular or maculopapular); alopecia; increased hair growth on face, eyebrows, and eyelashes; paronychia (periungual irritation) and skin fissures; and xerosis (dry skin) and pruritus. EGFR signaling in the loop of Henle in the kidneys is necessary for resorption of magnesium and calcium, so that when inhibited by mAb EGFR inhibitors, hypomagnesemia and hypocalcemia may occur (Fakih & Vincent, 2010). EGFR signaling is also important in the healing of pulmonary injury, so when it is blocked, interstitial lung disease (pneumonitis) may rarely occur (Finigan, Downey, & Kern, 2012).

Managing skin toxicity is a major challenge, as few evidence-based interventions exist and the available grading scales are inadequate to fully characterize the rash or its subjective effect on patients. Although it is often called an *acneform* rash, it is not acne and must not be treated as such, as this will exacerbate the rash. The rash typically is on the face, back, and chest. EGFR inhibition results in abnormal proliferation, migration, and differentiation of keratinocytes, leading to disruption of skin integrity and recruitment of inflammatory cells (Melosky et al., 2009). Because the rash is associated with a tumor response, it is important to support patients so that they can tolerate full-dose therapy if possible (Fakih & Vincent, 2010). The rash is predictable and usually involves four phases: (a) sunburn-like erythema in weeks 0–1, with sensory changes, (b) development of papulopustules in weeks 1–3, especially in sun-exposed areas, (c) crusting of lesions in weeks 3–5, and (d) persistent dry skin and erythema in weeks 5–8. This is followed by healing, formation of telangiectasias (dilated capillaries), and hyperpigmentation (Lacouture et al., 2011; Lynch et al., 2007). The skin becomes thin and loses its ability to retain moisture. Within several months of starting therapy, changes in the hair and nails occur: Diffuse, reversible alopecia may occur, along with increased growth (hypertrichosis) with distortion of facial hair and eyelashes (trichomegaly). The long eyelashes may irritate and cause conjunctivitis (Borkar, Lacouture, & Basti, 2013). Paronychia may result in crusting on the nail folds and nails, especially on the thumbs, which can become tender and interfere with function. Finally, skin fissures may occur on the fingers.

Recommendations have been provided in multiple guidelines, including those from Lynch et al. (2007), the Multinational Association of Supportive Care in Cancer (MASCC) (Lacouture et al., 2011), and Alberta Health Services (2012). The goal for skin management related to mAbs is to support patients and to prevent infection until the rash resolves. Please refer to these articles for more in-depth discussions. Although little prospective data are available to guide management, consensus guidelines and recommendations are summarized below. In addition, the Skin Toxicity Evaluation Protocol With Panitumumab (STEPP) trial, reported by Lacouture et al. (2010), shows that a regimen of daily moisturizer, sunscreen, topical 1% hydrocortisone, and oral doxycycline reduced the incidence of grade 2 or higher rash and other skin changes, compared to a control group. Tumor response was no different between groups.

Nursing priorities are to teach patients strategies to maintain skin integrity (to prevent infection), as the rash will ultimately regress. Teach patients to use cool water for bathing, water-based moisturizing creams for skin, and sunscreen (with sun protection factor [SPF] of at least 30, containing zinc or titanium), and to wear protective clothing when in the sun, apply moisturizer to hands and feet, keep nails clean and short, and stay well hydrated. Management of rash is based on severity. If the rash is mild to moderate, recommendations include topical 2% clindamycin plus 1% hydrocortisone lotion BID until rash resolves (Alberta Health Services, 2012; Lynch et al., 2007). For moderate to severe rash, recommendations include topical 2% clindamycin plus 1% hydrocortisone lotion BID plus oral minocycline 100 mg BID for four weeks, then until rash resolves (Alberta Health Services, 2012; Lynch et al., 2007); MASCC recommends topical (e.g., clindamycin 1%) and systemic therapy (e.g., doxycycline 100 mg BID). Severe rash, one that is extensive, painful, or intolerable and which interferes with daily life, requires a treatment delay of one to two weeks, and drug discontinuation if no improvement (ImClone LLC & Bristol-Myers Squibb Co., 2013). Other considerations are using topical clindamycin 2% plus hydrocortisone lotion BID, plus oral minocycline 100 mg BID or doxycycline 100 mg daily or BID. Lynch et al. (2007) recommends the use of hydrocortisone 2.5% cream or clindamycin 1% gel, plus doxycycline 100 mg BID, plus methylprednisolone dose pack and dose reduce the EGFR inhibitor; Alberta Health Services (2012) adds a methylprednisolone dose pack to treatment.

It is important to culture any lesion that looks suspicious (e.g., vesicular rash, oozing, yellow crusting), and treat patients based on culture and sensitivity. For paronychia or skin fissures, steroid tape may be prescribed. Patients should be referred to a dermatologist when the rash is progressive or treatment is ineffective.

Patients may develop very long eyelashes (trichomegaly). Refer patients to an ophthalmologist for conjunctivitis related to long, irritating eyelashes or other ocular issues (Balagula et al., 2011).

If patients develop acute or worsening pulmonary symptoms, hold the drug and rule out interstitial lung disease. Finally, serum magnesium and calcium levels should be assessed before each treatment and repleted as needed. Recently, it has been found that cetuximab in combination with radiation and cisplatin results in increased grades 3–4 mucositis, radiation recall syndrome, rash, cardiac events, and electrolyte disturbances without an improvement in progression-free survival (endpoint of study) (ImClone LLC & Bristol-Myers Squibb Co., 2013).

Bevacizumab is a humanized mAb directed against the ligand VEGF (see Figure 4-4). A tumor cannot grow larger than 1–2 mm, the diffusion distance of oxygen, without developing a new blood supply (Folkman, 1971). The tumor cells must then release VEGF, and as mentioned earlier, EGFR overexpression stimulates the release of VEGF as it drives cell proliferation. If VEGF is inactivated and cannot bind to its receptors on the endothelial cell, then angiogenesis is halted. Bevacizumab binds to VEGF so that the growth factor cannot bind to the VEGF receptors on the endothelial cells.

The drug is indicated for the primary treatment of metastatic colorectal cancer (not adjuvant), nonsquamous non-small cell lung cancer, glioblastoma, metastatic renal cell cancer, persistent cervical cancer, and platinum-resistant ovarian cancer, fallopian tube cancer, or primary peritoneal cancer. The dose is 5–10 mg/kg every two weeks or 7.5 mg/kg every three weeks, together with 5-FU-irinotecan– or 5-FU-oxaliplatin–based regimens, as an IV infusion for metastatic colorectal cancer. For nonsquamous NSCLC, the dose is 15 mg/kg every three weeks with carboplatin/paclitaxel. For glioblastoma and metastatic renal cell cancer (with interferon alfa), the dose is 10 mg/kg every two weeks. The dosing of patients with persistent or metastatic cervical cancer is 15 mg/kg IV every three weeks with paclitaxel/cisplatin or paclitaxel/topotecan, whereas dosing for patients with platinum-resistant epithelial ovarian cancer is 10 mg/kg IV every two weeks with paclitaxel, pegylated liposomal doxorubicin, or weekly topotecan, or 15 mg/kg IV every three weeks with topotecan given every three weeks (Genentech, Inc., 2014a).

The most serious but uncommon side effects of bevacizumab are hemorrhage, gastrointestinal perforation, arterial thrombotic events, non-gastrointestinal fistula formation, delayed wound healing complications, and rare necrotizing fasciitis, usually secondary to wound healing perforation or fistula. Fatal hemorrhage occurred during a study of patients with squamous cell lung cancer, thus making the drug contraindicated in this patient population. The half-life of bevacizumab is 20 days, so this drug should not be given sooner than 28 days after major surgery or until healing has occurred (Genentech, Inc., 2014a). In addition, the incidence of severe neutropenia, febrile neutropenia, and infection is increased in patients receiving both bevacizumab and chemotherapy. More common side effects are mild and easily managed, including epistaxis, asthenia, hypertension, constipation or diarrhea, and headache. Less commonly experienced side effects include infusion reaction, proteinuria and nephritic syndrome, reversible posterior leukoencephalopathy syndrome, CHF in patients who have previously received anthracycline chemotherapy, ovarian failure, and perforation of the nasal septum. Urine protein should be monitored prior to each treatment, and if it is 2+ or greater, a 24-hour urine for proteinuria should be done. If there is 2 grams or higher of proteinuria in 24 hours, bevacizumab should be held until the urine protein is less than 2 grams in 24 hours. The drug should be discontinued if patients develop nephritic syndrome.

Hypertension with VEGF inhibition is a class effect of antiangiogenesis agents. Fortunately, the resulting hypertension develops over time and generally is well controlled with available antihypertensives such as diuretics, angiotensin-converting enzyme (ACE) inhibitors, or calcium channel blockers as recommended by the Joint National Committee 7 guidelines (Chobanian et al., 2003; Woods, Lech, & Fadol, 2013). Some clinicians assert that ACE inhibitors may be preferable because these drugs also help to manage proteinuria (Escalante & Zalpour, 2011). Patients in clinical trials were excluded if they had brain metastases. Clinical trials are ongoing to study the safety of bevacizumab in this population.

Recently, **immune checkpoint inhibitors** (see Table 4-4) have brought cancer immunotherapy back to center stage. The immune system, especially T lymphocytes, is able to recognize and kill cells displaying tumor antigens. However, somehow cancer cells and their antigens are able to evade immune surveillance. It now looks like one of the ways tumor cells do this is by "co-opting" normal immune protective measures used to keep the immune system from hurting "self" (Pardoll, 2012). Two immune checkpoints that tumor cells "co-opt" have been identified. These involve cell surface molecules that help the immune system regulate the immune response, but also protect the self from being attacked by mediating co-inhibitory signals (Naidoo, Page, & Wolchok, 2014).

First, CTLA-4 (cytotoxic T-lymphocyte–associated antigen 4) is a protein expressed on activated and regulatory T lymphocytes. It is a negative regulator of the immune system and is upregulated in cancer (Fecher, Agarwala, Hodi, & Weber, 2013). Its purpose is to turn off the immune system once activated T cells have killed the antigen so that normal body cells are not injured. However, by co-opting this normal process, cancer cells are able to turn off activation of T cells so that they are not attacked (immune tolerance). CTLA-4 is an immune checkpoint target.

Ipilimumab is FDA-approved for the treatment of unresectable or metastatic melanoma. Ipilimumab was approved with a risk evaluation and mitigation strategy (REMS) because the drug can result in severe and potentially fatal immune-related reactions due to T-lymphocyte activation and proliferation. As a part of the REMS package, a nursing assessment and management guide and checklist are available, as well as a patient wallet card. Although some of the drug's side effects are similar to other mAbs, because ipilimumab targets the immune system (CTLA-4), its most concerning side effects are immune mediated. Because the drug blocks the protective dampening of the immune system, the activated and proliferating T lymphocytes attack both tumor antigen and some normal tissue, resulting in the immune-related adverse effects. Ipilimumab is given intravenously over 90 minutes, every three weeks, for a total of four doses, which must be given within 16 weeks. The drug is very expensive ($120,000 for full regimen), so APNs must ensure that patients have access to financial resources as needed (Fellner, 2012). Most patients (70%–88%) experience side effects, and these are dose related. Early side effects that begin during or up to 24–72 or more hours after the infusion are fatigue, nausea, vomiting, diarrhea, fever, headache, dizziness, rash, and pruritus (Fecher et al., 2013). Symptomatic treatment with antihistamines, antipyretics, IV or oral fluid hydration, and anti-pruritics usually is effective.

Although any organ can be affected, the most common immune-mediated adverse reactions are enterocolitis, hepatitis, dermatitis, neuropathy, and endocrinopathy (Bristol-Myers Squibb Co., 2013). Most reactions begin during treatment, but some may occur weeks to months after the drug has been stopped. Early identification of toxicity is critical so that early intervention can follow and minimize the effect. Enterocolitis is rare, with signs and symptoms of diarrhea, abdominal pain, and blood or mucus in the stool. If bowel perforation occurs, peritoneal signs and ileus may be seen. Liver function tests (LFTs) should be monitored prior to each dose to detect hepatitis. Endocrinopathies are vague in onset; thus, a neurologic evaluation should be performed before each dose to detect signs and symptoms of hypophysitis, along with appropriate laboratory evaluations as shown in Table 4-3. Most low-grade immune-related adverse effects are managed with supportive care, whereas moderate or severe toxicity is managed by drug interruption and high-dose steroids followed by a taper (Bristol-Myers Squibb Co., 2013; Fecher et al., 2013). Algorithms are available for toxicity management (Fecher et al., 2013). The drug is discontinued if steroids cannot be tapered to 7.5 mg prednisone or equivalent per day or if the full treatment course is not completed within 16 weeks from the first dose. Baseline laboratory assessment includes a baseline metabolic panel, complete blood count with differential, thyroid-stimulating hormone and free T4, LFTs, and amylase and lipase levels (Fecher et al., 2013).

A second immune checkpoint protein that is co-opted by tumor cells is the programmed cell death protein 1 (PD-1), as well as its ligand (PD-L1). Normally, T lymphocytes become activated and express the PD-1 receptor. To turn off the immune system once the cells bearing the invading antigen are destroyed, PD-L1 binds to the PD-1 receptor and shuts off the T lymphocytes so that normal "self" tissue is not damaged. Tumors upregulate this ligand to block the immune system response (Pardoll, 2012). Thus, tumor cells develop an invisible shield protecting them from the immune system by expressing the ligand PD-L1 on their cells. Nivolumab and pembrolizumab, both anti-PD-1 receptor mAbs, have been FDA-approved for treatment of patients with unresectable or metastatic melanoma or disease progression after ipilimumab, and if *BRAF V600*–mutation positive, a *BRAF* inhibitor (Bristol-Myers Squibb Co., 2014a; Merck & Co., Inc., 2015).

Conjugated Monoclonal Antibodies (Antibody Drug Conjugates)

Antibody drug conjugates have an attached toxin or radioisotope. The Fab portion recognizes the target antigen and brings the attached toxin or radioisotope to the target cell to destroy it. An example of a conjugated mAb is the radioisotope conjugated mAb yttrium-90 ibritumomab tiuxetan that is directed against the CD20 antigen on malignant B lymphocytes. Chemotherapy is often the toxin conjugated or attached by a linker molecule to a mAb, such as with ado-trastuzumab emtansine for injection and brentuximab vedotin.

Ado-trastuzumab emtansine for injection is an HER2-targeted mAb with an attached microtubular poison emtansine, indicated as a single agent for the treatment of patients with HER2-positive metastatic breast cancer previously treated with trastuzumab and a taxane, separately or in combination. Complete blood count and differential (due to thrombocytopenia) and LFTs should be assessed prior to each treatment. LVEF should be assessed at baseline and then every three months during treatment.

The drug is administered by IV infusion every three weeks (21-day cycle) until disease progression or unacceptable toxicity occurs. The drug is incompatible with dextrose (5%) solutions. Although ado-trastuzumab emtansine is not a known vesicant, extravasation should be avoided. Extravasation that has been observed was mild (erythema, skin irritation, tenderness, pain, or swelling at the infusion site). Ado-trastuzumab emtansine is administered IV over 90 minutes initially, then if well tolerated, over 30 minutes during subsequent infusions. Patients should be observed for at least 90 minutes after the initial infusion and 30 minutes after subsequent treatments. Assess patients for signs and symptoms of an infusion reaction (e.g., flushing, fever, chills, dyspnea, hypotension, wheezing, bronchospasm, tachycardia). Although uncommon (incidence is 1.4%), if it occurs during the infusion, the infusion should be slowed or stopped, and appropriate medications administered to reverse the symptoms. The drug should be discontinued for severe reactions. The drug should be interrupted or the dose modified for adverse events (e.g., hepatotoxicity, left ventricular cardiac dysfunction, thrombocytopenia, pulmonary toxicity, peripheral neuropathy). Most common side effects are fatigue, nausea, musculoskeletal pain, thrombocytopenia, headache, increased liver transaminases, and constipation. Although uncommon (incidence is 1.8%–3.3% in combination with lapatinib), the drug may reduce LVEF (Genentech, Inc., 2014c). LVEF should be assessed at baseline and then every three months during treatment. If LVEF falls to less than 40% or is 40%–45% with a 10% or greater absolute decrease below the pretreatment value, hold ado-trastuzumab emtansine and repeat the LVEF assessment within three weeks. If the LVEF has not improved or is further reduced, the drug should be permanently discontinued (Genentech Inc., 2014c). Rarely, the drug may cause interstitial lung disease or pneumonitis (incidence is 1.2%) that may be severe. Nurses should assess for dyspnea, cough, fatigue, and pulmonary infiltrates, and if interstitial lung disease or pneumonitis is diagnosed, the drug should be permanently discontinued. Thrombocytopenia occurs in about a third of patients, with grade 3 occurring in 14.5% of patients (45.1% in Asian patients) (Genentech, Inc., 2014c). The platelet nadir occurs on day 8, with recovery by day 21. The drug should not be given if the platelet count is less than 50,000/mm³. Fatal cases of hemorrhage were reported in clinical trials in patients without known risk factors, as well as those receiving anticoagulants or antiplatelet therapy, or who had thrombocytopenia (Genentech, Inc., 2014c). Patients at risk should be closely monitored. Finally, neurotoxicity may occur, usually grade 1 and sensory in nature. The overall incidence was 21.2% in clinical trials, while grade 3 or higher peripheral neuropathy occurred in 2.2% of patients (Genentech, Inc., 2014c; Verma et al., 2012).

Brentuximab vedotin is a chimeric IgG1 mAb directed against the CD30 antigen on Hodgkin and anaplastic lymphoma cells. The mAb is linked to auristatin E, a microtubular disrupting agent, and causes cell death when brought into the lymphoma cell. The drug is indicated for treatment of patients with (a) Hodgkin lymphoma after failure of autologous stem cell transplant (ASCT), or after failure of at least two prior multiagent chemotherapy regimens, in patients who are not ASCT candidates, or (b) systemic anaplastic large cell lymphoma, after failure of at least one prior multiagent chemotherapy regimen.

Brentuximab vedotin is administered as an IV infusion over 30 minutes every three weeks for a maximum of 16 cycles. Grade 1 or 2 infusion reactions occurred in 19% of patients in clinical trials (e.g., chills, nausea, dyspnea, pruritus, fever, cough). If this develops, patients should be premedicated prior to the next cycle with acetaminophen, an antihistamine, and a corticosteroid. For toxicity, the dose is modified for new or worsening grade 2 or 3 peripheral neuropathy and grade 3 or 4 neutropenia. Growth factor support should be considered for the next cycle in patients who develop grade 3 or 4 neutropenia. Because of additive pulmonary toxicity, the drug is contraindicated in combination with bleomycin. Patients with a high tumor burden are at risk for TLS (Seattle Genetics, Inc., 2014). Most common side effects related to brentuximab vedotin are bone marrow depression (e.g., neutropenia, thrombocytopenia, anemia), peripheral sensory neuropathy, fatigue, nausea and vomiting, upper respiratory tract infection, diarrhea, pyrexia, rash, and cough (Seattle Genetics, Inc., 2014). mAbs are large molecules and therefore must be administered parenterally, whereas kinase inhibitors are small molecules, permitting oral administration (Wilkes, 2011b).

An increased understanding of the role of the microenvironment in carcinogenesis has led to the development of drugs that modulate the immune system and interfere with angiogenesis, including thalidomide, lenalidomide, and the most recent, pomalidomide. In addition, vaccines continue to be studied, and FDA has approved one vaccine, sipuleucel-T. Immunomodulatory drugs, vaccines, and miscellaneous drugs, along with their potential side effects, are shown in Table 4-4.

Single-Targeted Tyrosine Kinase Inhibitors

Protein kinase inhibitors work within the cell and interrupt signaling pathways to stop uncontrolled cell signaling related to tumor mutations or epigenetic changes. Figure 4-5 depicts cellular signaling pathways.

EGFR inhibitors include both mAbs (discussed with cetuximab) and tyrosine kinase inhibitors (TKIs) (small molecules given orally). EGFR is a receptor tyrosine kinase that regulates cell growth and differentiation. When it is mutated or overexpressed, or when an overabundance of the ligand epidermal growth factor exists, EGFR leads to uncontrolled cell proliferation, angiogenesis, resistance to apoptosis, invasion, and metastasis. The aberrant signaling can be blocked at the extracellular domain by the mAbs cetuximab and panitumumab as previously discussed or by inhibiting the intracellular domain by TKIs. Normally, the message (cell signal) reaches the tyrosine kinase just inside the cell membrane. The tyrosine kinase phosphorylates, or adds a phosphate group from adenosine triphosphate (ATP), and this sends the message to the next signaling molecule in the pathway like a "bucket brigade" until it reaches

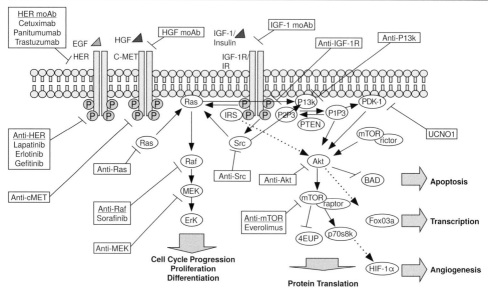

Depicted are the cellular signaling pathways involved in the proliferation, angiogenesis, and differentiation in neoplasms with the targets amenable to the therapeutic interventions in cancer therapy. Membrane-bound human epidermal growth factor receptors (HERs), c-MET, and insulin-like growth factor 1 receptor (IGF-1R) mediate mitogenic signals from extracellular ligands, such as epidermal growth factor (EGF), hepatocyte growth factor (HGF), and insulin growth factor (IGF), respectively. The Ras/Raf/MEK/Erk (mitogen-activated protein kinase, MAPK) and PI3k/Akt/mTOR pathways are major intracellular axes that regulate intracellular signaling traffic. The class and agents targeting the signaling proteins are indicated in boxes.

Figure 4-5. Cellular Signaling Pathways

Note. From "Targeted Therapy" (p. 563), by D. Wujcik in C.H. Yarbro, D. Wujcik, and B.H. Gobel (Eds.), *Cancer Nursing: Principles and Practice* (7th ed.), 2011, Burlington, MA: Jones & Bartlett Learning LLC. Copyright 2011 by Jones & Bartlett Learning LLC. Reprinted with permission.

the nucleus to bring about DNA transcription. This leads to protein synthesis, which directs cell growth and other functions. Protein kinases regulate cell signaling pathways in all cells and commonly are mutated in cancer (Weinberg, 2013). TKIs block the ATP binding domain so that phosphorylation, and hence signal transduction, cannot occur. Names of TKIs have the suffix of -inib. Compared to EGFR inhibitor mAbs, rash that occurs with TKIs is less severe in general and renal magnesium loss does not occur, but diarrhea tends to be more frequent and severe. These agents, side effects, and indications are shown in Table 4-5.

Erlotinib (Tarceva®) is indicated for the treatment of lung and pancreatic cancers. The bioavailability of erlotinib increases from 60% to about 100% when taken with food; therefore, the drug should be taken one hour before or two hours after a meal. The usual dose is 150 mg once a day. Studies showed no advantage when given together with chemotherapy (Astellas Pharma US, Inc., & Genentech, Inc., 2014). Like other TKIs, the drug is metabolized by the CYP3A4 microenzyme system in the liver and thus has potential drug interactions. Inducers increase metabolism (e.g., rifampin, phenytoin, phenobarbital, St. John's wort, carbamazepine, rifapentine, rifabutin); therefore, the dose may need to be increased. Inhibitors may decrease metabolism (e.g., ketoconazole, itraconazole, grapefruit or grapefruit juice, clarithromycin, metronidazole, isoniazid, telithromycin, voriconazole), and as such, the dose may need to be

Table 4-5. Molecular-Targeted Therapy: Small Molecules

Drug Class	Target	Drugs[a]	Side Effects[b]
Single-targeted kinase inhibitors	BRAF V600E	Dabrafenib (Tafinlar®) Indicated for treatment of patients with unresectable or metastatic melanoma with BRAF V600E mutation Drug should not be used in patients with BRAF wild-type gene, as melanoma may proliferate.	Most common are hyperkeratosis, headache, pyrexia, arthralgia, papilloma, alopecia, and palmar-plantar erythrodysesthesia syndrome (hand-foot syndrome). New cutaneous malignancies may develop; perform skin exam at baseline, every 2 months, and up to 6 months after therapy. Febrile drug reaction is possible; hold drug for fever ≥ 101.3°F (38.5°C). Hyperglycemia, uveitis, and iritis may occur. In patients with glucose-6-phosphate dehydrogenase deficiency: Monitor closely for hemolytic anemia. Avoid coadministration with strong CYP3A4 inhibitors and inducers, drugs that increase gastric pH, and others.
	BRAF V600E	Vemurafenib (Zelboraf®) Indicated for treatment of patients with unresectable or metastatic melanoma with BRAF V600E mutation Drug is not indicated for patients with melanoma who have the BRAF wild-type gene, as increased cell proliferation may occur (tumor promotion).	Most common are arthralgia, rash, alopecia, fatigue, photosensitivity reaction, nausea, pruritus, and skin papilloma. New primary cutaneous malignancies are possible; perform dermatologic evaluation at baseline and then every 2 months for up to 6 months after therapy ends. New cutaneous squamous cell cancers and serious hypersensitivity reactions may occur. QTc prolongation is possible: Monitor ECG and correct electrolyte imbalances (potassium, magnesium) before and during therapy; hold for QTc ≥ 500 ms. Hepatotoxicity is possible, as are uveitis and other serious ophthalmologic reactions.
	BTK, which signals messages through the BCR and cytokine receptor pathways. BCR regulates cell proliferation and survival and appears oncogenic in MCL and CLL.	Ibrutinib (Imbruvica®) Indicated for treatment of patients with • MCL who have received at least 1 prior therapy • CLL who have received at least 1 prior therapy • CLL with 17p deletion • Waldenström macroglobulinemia	Most common adverse effects are thrombocytopenia, neutropenia, diarrhea, anemia, fatigue, musculoskeletal pain, bruising, nausea, URI, and rash. Hemorrhage may occur; teach patient to report, and assess for during therapy. Infections: Teach patient to avoid infections and bleeding and to report fever, signs/ symptoms of infection, or bleeding right away. Monitor CBC at baseline and at least monthly. TLS may occur in patients who have a high tumor burden; prevent with prophylaxis. Occurrence of atrial fibrillation and development of secondary malignancy are rare. Teach women of reproductive potential to use effective contraception to avoid pregnancy.

(Continued on next page)

Table 4-5. Molecular-Targeted Therapy: Small Molecules *(Continued)*

Drug Class	Target	Drugs[a]	Side Effects[b]
Single-targeted kinase inhibitors *(cont.)*		Ibrutinib (Imbruvica®) *(cont.)*	Teach patient about drug interactions: Avoid strong and moderate CYP3A4 inhibitors and strong inducers. If a moderate CYP3A4 inhibitor is given in combination, reduce ibrutinib dose. Drug should not be administered to patients with moderate or severe baseline hepatic impairment; drug dose should be reduced in patients with mild hepatic impairment.
	CDK4, CDK6 CDKs advance cells through the cell cycle, leading to cell proliferation. Blocking this (preventing cells from going from G1 into S phase) prevents proliferation.	Palbociclib (Ibrance®) Indicated for treatment of postmenopausal women with ER+, HER2–negative advanced breast cancer, in combination with letrozole, as initial endocrine-based therapy	Most common are neutropenia, leukopenia, fatigue, anemia, URI, infection, nausea, stomatitis, alopecia, diarrhea, thrombocytopenia, decreased appetite, vomiting, asthenia, peripheral neuropathy, and epistaxis. Neutropenia: Monitor CBC/differential at baseline and at the beginning of each cycle, as well as on day 14 of the first 2 cycles, then as clinically indicated. Monitor patient for infections, and teach patient strategies to avoid infection and to report signs/symptoms of infection. Pulmonary embolism may occur (5% incidence). Teach women of reproductive potential to use effective contraception to avoid pregnancy, as drug is embryo-fetal toxic.
	EGFR1, including mutations in EGFR exon 19 deletion, or exon 212 (L858R) substitution	Afatinib (Gilotrif®) Indicated for the first-line treatment of patients with metastatic NSCLC whose tumors have EGFR exon 19 deletions or exon 21 (L858R) substitution mutations as detected by an FDA-approved test	Most common adverse effect are diarrhea, rash/dermatitis, rash/dermatitis acneform, stomatitis, paronychia, dry skin, decreased appetite, and pruritus. Diarrhea may be complicated by dehydration and renal failure; interrupt drug for severe and prolonged diarrhea that does not resolve with antidiarrheal therapy. Rarely, bullous and exfoliative skin reactions occur (e.g., blistering). Interrupt therapy if cutaneous reaction is severe and prolonged; discontinue drug if life threatening. ILD is a rare, potential class adverse effect of EGFRI therapy. Promptly evaluate acute-onset or worsening of pulmonary symptoms. If ILD is confirmed, discontinue drug. Hepatotoxicity may occur; monitor LFTs at baseline and periodically during therapy. Keratitis (e.g., acute or worsening eye inflammation, lacrimation, light sensitivity, blurred vision, eye pain, red eye) may rarely occur, with increased risk in patients wearing contact lenses or with a history of keratitis, ulcerative keratitis, or severe red eye. Interrupt drug if keratitis is suspected. If ulcerative keratitis is confirmed, consider drug discontinuation.

(Continued on next page)

Table 4-5. Molecular-Targeted Therapy: Small Molecules (*Continued*)

Drug Class	Target	Drugs[a]	Side Effects[b]
Single-targeted kinase inhibitors (*cont.*)		Afatinib (Gilotrif®) (*cont.*)	Drug should not be administered to patients with HER2-positive metastatic breast cancer receiving vinorelbine, as a study has shown increased patient mortality, higher rate of adverse effects, and higher rate of fatal events related to infection and cancer progression in those taking the combination.
	EGFR1, including mutations in EGFR exon 19 deletion, or exon 212 (L858R) substitution	Erlotinib (Tarceva®) Indicated for treatment of patients with • NSCLC – First-line, metastatic, tumors with exon 19 deletions or exon 21 substitution (L858R) mutations as detected by an FDA-approved test – Maintenance in locally advanced or metastatic, when disease has not progressed after 4 cycles of platinum first line – Locally advanced or metastatic after failure of at least one prior chemotherapy regimen • Pancreatic cancer: First-line treatment in locally advanced, unresectable or metastatic, in combination with gemcitabine	If increased toxicity, ensure patient is taking erlotinib on an **empty** stomach because food increases drug bioavailability. Most common adverse effects are rash, diarrhea, anorexia, fatigue, dyspnea, cough, nausea, and vomiting. In pancreatic carcinoma trial, rare MI, cerebrovascular accident, and microangiopathic hemolytic anemia with thrombocytopenia occurred. ILD is a rare, potential class adverse effect of EGFRI therapy. Promptly evaluate acute-onset or worsening of pulmonary symptoms, such as dyspnea, cough, and fever. If ILD is confirmed, discontinue drug. Renal failure has occurred; monitor renal function and electrolytes, especially in patients at risk for dehydration (e.g., older adults). Hepatotoxicity with or without impairment (e.g., hepatic failure) has been reported; monitor LFTs at baseline and periodically during therapy. Hold or discontinue drug if LFT abnormality is severe or worsening. GI perforations have been reported; discontinue drug if this occurs. Corneal perforation: Discontinue drug if perforation, ulceration, or persistent severe keratitis occurs. Patients taking warfarin or other coumarin-derivative anticoagulants are at risk for hemorrhage; monitor international normalized ratio regularly. Teach women of reproductive potential to use effective contraception to avoid pregnancy, as drug is embryo-fetal toxic. Avoid coadministration with strong CYP3A4 inhibitors or inducers (including smoking). Avoid drugs that affect gastric pH, as they decrease erlotinib plasma concentrations.

(Continued on next page)

Table 4-5. Molecular-Targeted Therapy: Small Molecules (Continued)

Drug Class	Target	Drugs[a]	Side Effects[b]
Single-targeted kinase inhibitors (cont.)	EGFR1, EGFR2	Lapatinib (Tykerb®) Indicated for treatment of patients with HER2-overexpressing breast cancer, in combination with • Capecitabine, in patients with advanced or metastatic disease, after prior therapy including an anthracycline, taxane, and trastuzumab • Letrozole, in patients with hormone receptor–positive, postmenopausal metastatic breast cancer	Most common, when given with capecitabine: Diarrhea, nausea, vomiting, fatigue, rash, and palmar-plantar erythrodysesthesia syndrome (hand-foot syndrome); when given with letrozole: Diarrhea, nausea, fatigue, and rash Rarely, decreased LVEF, hepatotoxicity, increased LFTs, ILD, pneumonitis, and prolonged QTc interval may result. • Confirm LVEF prior to starting drug and monitor during therapy. • Monitor LFTs at baseline, every 4–6 weeks during treatment, and as needed. • Consider ECG and electrolyte monitoring in patients at risk for QTc prolongation. Diarrhea may be severe and require antidiarrheal agents and fluid and electrolyte replacement. Monitor patients closely. Severe cutaneous reactions may occur; discontinue drug if life-threatening reaction suspected. Avoid coadministration with strong CYP3A4 inhibitors or inducers. Teach women of reproductive potential to use effective contraception to avoid pregnancy, as drug can cause fetal harm.
	MEK inhibitor (first in class), blocking cell proliferation MEK proteins regulate the ERK pathway, responsible for promoting cell proliferation.	Trametinib (Mekinist™) Indicated for treatment of patients with unresectable or metastatic melanoma with *BRAF V600E or BRAF V600K* mutations as detected by an FDA-approved test • As a single agent • In combination with dabrafenib	Most common are rash, diarrhea, and lymphedema. When combined with dabrafenib, pyrexia, chills, fatigue, rash, nausea, vomiting, diarrhea, abdominal pain, peripheral edema, cough, headache, arthralgia, night sweats, decreased appetite, constipation, and myalgia are most common. When drug is combined with dabrafenib, the following may occur: • New primary malignancies: Assess patients for new malignancies prior to starting therapy, during therapy, and after drug is discontinued. • Major hemorrhage: Teach patients to report bleeding, and monitor for signs/symptoms of bleeding and provide medical intervention. • Venous thromboembolism: DVT and PE • Serious febrile reactions: Hold dabrafenib for temperature ≥ 101.3°F; hold trametinib for temperature > 104°F. • Significant drug interactions (CYP3A4, CYP2C8). Cardiomyopathy: Obtain LVEF at baseline, after 1 month, and then every 2–3 months.

(Continued on next page)

Table 4-5. Molecular-Targeted Therapy: Small Molecules (Continued)

Drug Class	Target	Drugs[a]	Side Effects[b]
Single-targeted kinase inhibitors (cont.)		Trametinib (Mekinist™) (cont.)	Ocular toxicities: Retinal pigment epithelial detachment and retinal vein occlusion are possible. Perform ophthalmologic exam for any visual disturbance urgently (within 24 hours). ILD: Hold drug if patient develops new or progressive unexplained pulmonary symptoms; evaluate, and if ILD is diagnosed, discontinue drug. Serious skin toxicity: Monitor for skin toxicities and secondary skin infections; discontinue drug for intolerable grade 2, or grade 3–4 rash not improving in 3 weeks, despite dose interruption. Hyperglycemia: Monitor serum glucose in patients with existing diabetes mellitus or hyperglycemia. Teach women of reproductive potential to use effective contraception to avoid pregnancy, as drug is embryo-fetal toxic. Drug may impair fertility of men and women.
	mTOR (a serine-threonine kinase downstream of the PI3K/AKT pathway). Drug is a kinase inhibitor of mTOR. MTOR inhibitors bind to a protein, forming an inhibitory complex that blocks mTOR kinase from working. This blocks protein synthesis, expression of HIF-1 and reducing VEGF expression, thus turning off angiogenesis.	Everolimus (Afinitor®) Indicated for treatment of adult patients with • Postmenopausal advanced hormone receptor–positive, HER2-negative breast cancer in combination with exemestane recurring after letrozole or anastrozole failure • Progressive, unresectable, locally advanced or metastatic pNET • Advanced renal cell cancer after sorafenib or sunitinib failure, and other indications Aromatase inhibitors increase the antitumor activity of everolimus.	Most common are stomatitis, infection, fatigue, rash, diarrhea, edema, abdominal pain, nausea, fever, asthenia, cough, headache, and decreased appetite. Laboratory test alterations: Elevated serum creatinine, urinary protein, blood glucose, lipids; decreased hemoglobin, neutrophils, and platelets. Laboratory monitoring: Monitor renal function, blood glucose, lipids, and CBC/differential at baseline and periodically during treatment. Infections can be severe; monitor patients closely and treat promptly. Angioedema may occur in patients taking ACE inhibitor antihypertensive therapy. Oral ulceration is common (stomatitis, oral mucositis); teach patient oral self-assessment and systematic oral hygiene and to report ulcerations. Impaired wound healing and increased risk for wound-related complications may occur. Uncommon side effects include noninfectious pneumonitis and renal failure. Avoid live vaccinations and proximity to those who have received them. Teach women of reproductive potential to use effective contraception to avoid pregnancy, as drug is embryo-fetal toxic. Avoid coadministration with strong CYP3A4 inhibitors and inducers; if moderate CYP3A4 inhibitors must be used, reduce everolimus dose.

(Continued on next page)

Table 4-5. Molecular-Targeted Therapy: Small Molecules (Continued)

Drug Class	Target	Drugs[a]	Side Effects[b]
Single-targeted kinase inhibitors (cont.)		Temsirolimus (Torisel®) Indicated for treatment of patients with advanced RCC	Most common are rash, asthenia, mucositis, nausea, edema, and anorexia. Laboratory abnormalities: Monitor for anemia; hyperglycemia; hyperlipidemia; hypertriglyceridemia; elevated alkaline phosphatase, serum creatinine, AST; hypophosphatemia; thrombocytopenia; and leukopenia. Hypersensitivity/infusion reactions can occur with first infusion; monitor closely during infusion, stop infusion and treat with antihistamine if reaction occurs. Consider resuming at slower rate if not severe. Drug causes delayed wound healing; use cautiously if at all in perioperative period. Hepatotoxicity, rare ILD, bowel perforation, and renal failure may occur. Rarely, ILD, bowel perforation, and renal failure can occur. Evaluate urgently if patient has fever, abdominal pain, bloody stools, and/or acute abdomen to rule out bowel perforation. Older adult patients may have more severe diarrhea, edema, and pneumonia. Avoid coadministration with strong CYP3A4 inhibitors and inducers; if must coadminister, modify temsirolimus dose.
	PI3K-delta, which is found on normal and malignant B lymphocytes PI3K is key to cell growth, proliferation, motility, and survival.	Idelalisib (Zydelig®) Indicated for treatment of patients with • Relapsed CLL in combination with rituximab, when rituximab alone would be considered appropriate • Relapsed follicular B-cell NHL, after at least 2 prior systemic therapies • Relapsed small lymphocytic lymphoma, after at least 2 prior systemic therapies	Most common adverse effects include diarrhea, pyrexia, fatigue, nausea, cough, pneumonia, abdominal pain, chills, and rash. Drug is contraindicated in patients with a history of severe allergic reactions including anaphylaxis and toxic epidermal necrolysis. Teach patient that anaphylaxis may occur, and to call 911 if it occurs at home. Fatal and serious toxicities can occur. • Hepatotoxicity: Monitor LFTs at baseline and frequently (at least every 2 weeks during first 3 months of therapy); interrupt, dose reduce, or discontinue drug. • Diarrhea, colitis: Teach patient to report this right away, hold the drug, and to be evaluated right away. Drug dose should be reduced or discontinued once this resolves. • Pneumonitis: Monitor for pulmonary symptoms (e.g., cough, dyspnea, hypoxia, > 5% decrease in oxygen saturation). Teach patient to report new or worsening pulmonary symptoms right away. Assess x-ray for bilateral interstitial infiltrates, and interrupt or discontinue drug if confirmed.

(Continued on next page)

Table 4-5. Molecular-Targeted Therapy: Small Molecules (Continued)

Drug Class	Target	Drugs[a]	Side Effects[b]
Single-targeted kinase inhibitors (cont.)		Idelalisib (Zydelig®) (cont.)	• Intestinal perforation, which may occur during episodes of moderate to severe diarrhea: Teach patients to stop drug and to report right away any new or worsening abdominal pain, chills, fever, nausea, or vomiting. Drug should be discontinued if perforation occurs.
			Neutropenia: Grade 3–4 neutropenia occurred in 31% of patients in clinical trials. Monitor CBC/differential at least every 2 weeks for the first 3 months, then at least weekly when ANC is < 1,000/mm³.
			Teach female patients of reproductive potential to use effective contraception to avoid pregnancy, as drug is embryo-fetal toxic.
	26S proteasome Proteasomes degrade proteins no longer needed that are tagged with ubiquitin, thus regulating cellular contents of specific proteins, like those that move the cell cycle forward	Bortezomib (Velcade®) Indicated for treatment of patients with • Multiple myeloma • MCL and who have received 1 or more prior therapies	Most common are nausea, diarrhea, constipation, vomiting, anorexia, thrombocytopenia, neutropenia, anemia, lymphopenia, peripheral neuropathy, neuralgia, fatigue, pyrexia, and rash.
			Nausea, vomiting, and diarrhea may require antiemetic or antidiarrheal medications, as well as management with fluid replacement.
			Thrombocytopenia and neutropenia: Monitor CBC at baseline and regularly during therapy.
			Peripheral neuropathy is managed with dose reduction or discontinuance.
			Rarely, posterior reversible encephalopathy syndrome has occurred; evaluate MRI imaging if patient presents with new onset of visual or neurologic symptoms, and discontinue drug if diagnosis confirmed.
			Cardiac toxicity, manifested as worsening or development of cardiac failure, may occur; monitor patients with heart disease or risk factors closely.
			Acute respiratory syndromes have occurred. Monitor patient closely for signs/symptoms. TLS may develop in patients with high tumor burden.
			Hepatotoxicity is possible. Monitor at LFTs baseline and during therapy.
			Teach female patients of reproductive potential to use effective contraception to avoid pregnancy, as drug is embryo-fetal toxic.

(Continued on next page)

Table 4-5. Molecular-Targeted Therapy: Small Molecules (Continued)

Drug Class	Target	Drugs[a]	Side Effects[b]
Single-targeted kinase inhibitors (cont.)	20S proteasome; specifically, the core particle within the 26S proteasome, that breaks down proteins	Carfilzomib (Kyprolis®) Indicated for treatment of patients with multiple myeloma who progressed on at least 2 prior therapies, including bortezomib and an immunomodulatory agent, and progressed on or within 60 days of completion of last therapy	Most common are fatigue, anemia, nausea, thrombocytopenia, dyspnea, diarrhea, and pyrexia. Infusion reactions may develop: Hydrate patients prior to and after drug; premedicate with dexamethasone for cycle 1, first cycle of dose escalation, and if an infusion reaction develops or reappears. Teach patient to seek immediate medical care if symptoms develop. Cardiac problems, including heart failure and ischemia, have occurred. Assess for cardiac complications, use medical interventions to treat, and hold drug. Pulmonary hypertension may occur; hold drug if suspected. Pulmonary problems may arise; assess for and manage dyspnea urgently; interrupt drug until resolved. TLS may occur in patients with high tumor burden; hydrate for prevention, monitor patient closely, and treat if it occurs. Thrombocytopenia: Monitor platelet counts at baseline and regularly; reduce or interrupt drug as needed. Hepatic toxicity and hepatic failure have occurred; monitor LFTs at baseline and regularly; hold drug if suspected. Rarely, heart failure, ischemia, pulmonary HTN, hepatotoxicity, and liver failure occur. Teach female patients of reproductive potential to use effective contraception to avoid pregnancy, as drug is embryo-fetal toxic.
Multitargeted kinase inhibitors	Bcr-Abl, including multiple mutations, SRC family kinases	Bosutinib (Bosulif®) Indicated for treatment of adult patients with chronic-phase, accelerated-phase, or blast-crisis Ph+ CML with resistance or intolerance to prior therapy	Diarrhea, nausea, vomiting, abdominal pain, rash, pyrexia, anorexia, fatigue; neutropenia, thrombocytopenia, anemia; hepatotoxicity; and fluid retention (may be pleural, pericardial, pulmonary edema, or peripheral) may occur. Thrombocytopenia, neutropenia, anemia: Monitor CBC/differential weekly for the first month, then at least monthly thereafter. Manage diarrhea, nausea, and vomiting with antidiarrheals, antiemetics, and fluid replacement. Hepatotoxicity: Monitor AST and ALT monthly for the first three months of therapy, then as needed; if enzymes are elevated, monitor more frequently. Renal toxicity can occur; monitor renal function at baseline and during therapy, and more frequently in patients with preexisting renal impairment or risk factors. Modify dose if impairment is present at baseline or emerges during treatment.

(Continued on next page)

Table 4-5. Molecular-Targeted Therapy: Small Molecules *(Continued)*

Drug Class	Target	Drugs[a]	Side Effects[b]
Multitargeted kinase inhibitors *(cont.)*		Bosutinib (Bosulif®) *(cont.)*	Teach female patients of reproductive potential to use effective contraceptives to avoid pregnancy, as drug is embryo-fetal toxic. Avoid coadministration with strong and moderate CYP3A4 inhibitors and inducers; avoid proton pump inhibitors, and use short-acting antacids instead.
	Bcr-Abl, c-Kit, PDGFR-β	Dasatinib (Sprycel®) Indicated for treatment of newly diagnosed patients with chronic-phase Ph+ CML; patients with chronic-phase, accelerated-phase, or blast-crisis Ph+ CML; and patients with Ph+ ALL	Severe myelosuppression, fluid retention (including pleural and pericardial effusions), edema, nausea, vomiting, diarrhea, pain, headache, fatigue, arthralgia, and fatigue may occur. QTc interval prolongation is possible. Drug is teratogenic and embryo-fetal toxic. Patients should be taught to use effective contraception to avoid pregnancy.
	Bcr-Abl, c-Kit	Imatinib mesylate (Gleevec®) Multiple indications for patients with Ph+ CML (chronic phase, accelerated phase, and blast crisis), relapsed Ph+ ALL, newly diagnosed Ph+ ALL in children, adjuvant and treatment of unresectable GIST (Kit, CD117-positive) and others	Most common are edema, nausea, vomiting, muscle cramps, musculoskeletal pain, diarrhea, rash, fatigue, and abdominal pain. Edema and severe fluid retention may occur; weigh patients regularly, and interrupt drug to manage rapid weight gain, together with diuretics. Neutropenia, anemia, and thrombocytopenia may occur; monitor CBC/differential weekly for the first month, biweekly for the second month, then periodically after that. Severe CHF and left ventricular dysfunction have occurred, especially in patients with cardiac disease or risk factors. Monitor closely. Severe hepatotoxicity may occur; assess LFTs at baseline, then monthly. Bullous dermatologic reactions may develop. Drug is teratogenic (avoid pregnancy). Rare, severe hemorrhage in newly diagnosed patients may occur; GI perforation has been reported. Teach patients to avoid driving if dizzy, as motor vehicle accidents have occurred. If patient requires anticoagulation, low-molecular-weight or standard heparin should be given, not warfarin. Drug interactions with CYP3A4 inducers and inhibitors are possible.

(Continued on next page)

Table 4-5. Molecular-Targeted Therapy: Small Molecules (Continued)

Drug Class	Target	Drugs[a]	Side Effects[b]
Multitargeted kinase inhibitors (cont.)	Bcr-Abl kinase including those with multiple mutations, c-Kit, PDGFR, and others	Nilotinib (Tasigna®) Indicated for treatment of newly diagnosed patients with Ph+ CML in chronic phase; as well as adult patients in chronic or accelerated phase who are intolerant or resistant to prior therapy that included imatinib	Most common are rash, pruritus, headache, nausea, fatigue, myalgia, nasopharyngitis, constipation, diarrhea, abdominal pain, vomiting, arthralgia, pyrexia, URI, back pain, cough, and asthenia. Laboratory monitoring: Assess CBC every 2 weeks for 8 weeks, then monthly; chemistry panel including electrolytes, calcium, magnesium, LFTs, lipid profile, and glucose at baseline then periodically; ECG at baseline, 7 days after initiation, then periodically; and lipid profiles and glucose periodically, then at least yearly. If increased toxicity, ensure patient is taking medication on empty stomach. QTc prolongation with risk of sudden death may occur. Electrolyte abnormalities: Assess for hypophosphatemia, hyper- or hypokalemia, hypocalcemia, and hyponatremia; correct abnormalities prior to starting drug and periodically during therapy. Fluid retention, including pleural effusion, pericardial effusion, and ascites, may occur. Monitor patients closely for signs/symptoms. Pancreatitis and elevated serum lipase may develop. Cardiac and arterial vascular occlusive events: Teach patients to seek emergency care if signs/symptoms develop (ischemic heart disease or cerebrovascular events). Hepatotoxicity may develop; dose reduce initially if hepatic dysfunction is present. Tumor lysis syndrome (if high tumor burden) may occur. Avoid coadministration with strong inhibitors or inducers of CYP3A4; if a strong inhibitor must be coadministered, consider dose reduction of nilotinib and monitor QTc interval closely.
	Bcr-Abl kinase, including those with T315I mutation; also VEGFR, PDGFR, SRC family, c-Kit, and kinases	Ponatinib (Iclusig®) Indicated for treatment of adults with • Chronic-phase, accelerated-phase, or blast-crisis CML resistant or intolerant to prior TKIs • Ph+ ALL that is resistant to prior TKI therapy, or if the patient is intolerant to past TKIs	Common effects include HTN, rash, abdominal pain, headache, fatigue, dry skin, constipation, arthralgia, nausea, pyrexia, thrombocytopenia, neutropenia, and anemia. Serious side effects include arterial and venous thromboembolism; hepatotoxicity and liver failure; CHF; hypertensive crisis; pancreatitis; hemorrhage; cardiac arrhythmias (symptomatic bradycardia, supraventricular tachycardia); and grade 3–4 myelosuppression, which occurs in 48% of patients. Myelosuppression: Monitor complete blood count and differential every 2 weeks for 3 months, then monthly. Tumor lysis syndrome may occur in patients with high tumor burden.

(Continued on next page)

Table 4-5. Molecular-Targeted Therapy: Small Molecules (*Continued*)

Drug Class	Target	Drugs[a]	Side Effects[b]
Multitargeted kinase inhibitors (*cont.*)		Ponatinib (Iclusig®) (*cont.*)	Drug may cause decreased wound healing and GI perforation; interrupt drug at least 1 week before major surgery, and resume when wound has healed. Avoid coadministration with strong CYP3A4 inhibitors; if cannot avoid, reduce dose of ponatinib.
	ALK receptor tyrosine kinase, HGFR, c-Met, IGF-IR	Ceritinib (Zykadia®) Indicated for treatment of patients with ALK-positive metastatic NSCLC who have progressed on or are intolerant to crizotinib	Most common are diarrhea, nausea, elevated transaminases, vomiting, abdominal pain, fatigue, decreased appetite, and constipation. GI adverse effects can be severe and persistent; hold drug if unresponsive to antiemetics or antidiarrheals, then dose reduce once resolved. Hepatotoxicity: Monitor LFTs at baseline and then at least monthly. ILD/pneumonitis: If diagnosis is confirmed, discontinue drug. QTc interval prolongation: Monitor ECG and electrolytes in patients with CHF, bradyarrhythmias, and electrolyte abnormalities and in those taking medications that can prolong the QTc interval. Hyperglycemia: Monitor glucose and adjust antihyperglycemic medications. Bradycardia: Monitor heart rate and BP regularly. Avoid coadministration with strong CYP3A4 inhibitors and inducers. Teach women of reproductive potential to use effective contraception to avoid pregnancy, as drug is embryo-fetal toxic.
	ALK receptor tyrosine kinase, HGFR, c-Met, and others Mutation of the ALK gene forms an ALK fusion protein, which sends increased signals to increase tumor cell proliferation and survival	Crizotinib (Xalkori®) Indicated for patients with locally advanced or metastatic NSCLC having an ALK mutation as determined by an FDA-approved test	Most common are vision disorder, nausea, diarrhea, vomiting, edema, constipation, elevated transaminases, and fatigue. Hepatotoxicity and pneumonitis also may occur. Assess LFTs at baseline and monitor periodically during therapy. QTc prolongation: Monitor ECG in at-risk patients (e.g., those with history of or predisposition for QTc prolongation) at baseline and during therapy. Bradycardia: Do not use drug in combination with other agents that can cause bradycardia. Monitor BP and heart rate regularly. Drug dose is reduced in patients with severe renal failure. Teach women of reproductive potential to use effective contraception to avoid pregnancy, as drug is embryo-fetal toxic. Avoid coadministration with strong CYP3A4 inhibitors and inducers.

(Continued on next page)

Table 4-5. Molecular-Targeted Therapy: Small Molecules (Continued)

Drug Class	Target	Drugs[a]	Side Effects[b]
Angiogenesis inhibitors, multitargeted	VEGFR-1, VEGFR-2, VEGFR-3	Axitinib (Inlyta®) Indicated for treatment of patients with advanced RCC after failure of 1 prior systemic therapy	Most common adverse effects are diarrhea, HTN, fatigue, decreased appetite, dysphonia, palmar-plantar erythrodysesthesia (hand-foot) syndrome, weight loss, vomiting, asthenia, and constipation. Hemorrhagic events have occurred; drug is not recommended in patients with active GI bleeding or untreated brain metastases, as they have not been studied. Rare arterial and venous thrombosis and GI perforation or fistula may occur. Cardiac failure has been observed; patients should be monitored for signs or symptoms of cardiac failure during therapy. Stop drug prior to scheduled surgery because wound healing complications can occur. Proteinuria may occur; assess for urine protein before beginning drug and periodically during therapy; interrupt drug or reduce dose if moderate to severe proteinuria develops. Hypo- or hyperthyroidism may develop; monitor thyroid function studies at baseline and periodically during therapy; manage thyroid dysfunction if it develops. RPLS may rarely occur (seizure, headache, lethargy, confusion, blindness, other visual or neurological dysfunction) and may be accompanied by HTN; Evaluate by MRI and if RPLS confirmed, discontinue the drug. Hepatotoxicity may occur; monitor AST, ALT, and bilirubin at baseline and periodically during therapy. Drug dose should be reduced in patients with moderate hepatic impairment. Teach women of reproductive potential to use effective contraception to avoid pregnancy, as drug can cause fetal harm.
	VEGFR-1, VEGFR-2, VEGFR-3, c-Kit, FLT3, RET, MET, and others These receptor kinases control oncogenesis, tumor angiogenesis, tumor microenvironment maintenance, and metastasis.	Cabozantinib (Cometriq®) Indicated for treatment of patients with progressive, metastatic medullary thyroid cancer	Most common are diarrhea, stomatitis, palmar-plantar erythrodysesthesia syndrome (hand-foot syndrome), decreased weight and appetite, nausea, fatigue, oral pain, hair color changes, dysgeusia, HTN, and constipation. Most common lab abnormalities are increased AST, ALT, alkaline phosphatase, and bilirubin; decreased calcium and phosphate; and neutropenia and thrombocytopenia. Palmar-plantar erythrodysesthesia syndrome (hand-foot syndrome) occurs in 50% of patients and was severe in 13%. Thrombotic events, including MI and cerebral infarction, may occur. HTN: Monitor BP at baseline and regularly. Medically manage HTN. Wound complications: Hold drug for at least 28 days prior to scheduled surgery, and resume drug after adequate wound healing.

(Continued on next page)

Table 4-5. Molecular-Targeted Therapy: Small Molecules (Continued)

Drug Class	Target	Drugs[a]	Side Effects[b]
Angiogenesis inhibitors, multitargeted (cont.)		Cabozantinib (Cometriq®) (cont.)	Osteonecrosis of the jaw: Examine oral cavity and teeth prior to starting drug, and repeat regularly during therapy. If osteonecrosis occurs, discontinue drug. Hold drug for at least 28 days before invasive dental procedures. Teach patient oral hygiene practice. Proteinuria: Monitor urine protein at baseline and regularly during therapy. Uncommonly, GI fistula and GI perforation (3% incidence), proteinuria (2%), and RPLS (< 1%) may occur. Evaluate for RPLS if patient presents with seizures, headache, visual disturbances, confusion, or altered mental function. Drug should not be administered to patients with moderate or severe hepatic impairment. Avoid coadministration with strong CYP3A4 inhibitors or inducers. Teach women of reproductive potential to use effective contraception to avoid pregnancy, as drug can cause fetal harm.
	VEGFR-1, VEGFR-2, VEGFR-3, FGFR-1, FGFR-2, FGFR-3, FGFR-4, and others	Lenvatinib (Lenvima™) Indicated for treatment of patients with locally recurrent or metastatic, progressive, radioactive iodine-refractory differentiated thyroid cancer	Most common are HTN, fatigue, diarrhea, arthralgia/myalgia, decreased appetite, weight loss, nausea, stomatitis, headache, vomiting, proteinuria, palmar-plantar erythrodysesthesia syndrome, abdominal pain, and dysphonia. In clinical studies, 68% of patients required a dose reduction for adverse reactions. Dose reduce in patients with severe renal or hepatic impairment; hold drug for grade 3–4 renal failure/impairment. HTN is common; control before starting drug. Monitor BP after 1 week, then every 2 weeks for the first 2 months, and then at least monthly thereafter. The median time to onset or worsening of HTN was 16 days in clinical studies. Cardiac dysfunction (e.g., decreased left or right ventricular function, cardiac failure or pulmonary edema) may occur uncommonly. Monitor patients for signs/symptoms of cardiac decompensation. Arterial thromboembolic events are uncommon but may occur. Hepatotoxicity may occur; monitor LFTs at baseline, then every 2 weeks for the first 2 months, and at least monthly thereafter during treatment. Proteinuria occurs in about one-third of patients; assess urine dipstick prior to starting, then periodically during treatment. If dipstick is ≥ 2+, obtain 24-hour urine for protein. If protein excretion is ≥ 2 g/24 hours, hold drug, and resume at a reduced dose when urinary protein is < 2 g/24 hours.

(Continued on next page)

Table 4-5. Molecular-Targeted Therapy: Small Molecules (Continued)

Drug Class	Target	Drugs[a]	Side Effects[b]
Angiogenesis inhibitors, multitargeted (cont.)		Lenvatinib (Lenvima™) (cont.)	Drug impairs exogenous thyroid suppression; monitor TSH baseline and then monthly; adjust thyroid replacement medication as needed. Dehydration/hypovolemia related to diarrhea and vomiting may lead to severe renal impairment; monitor patients closely and control GI symptoms. Rarely, GI perforation and fistula. QTc interval prolongation, hypocalcemia, RPLS, and hemorrhagic events may occur. Monitor ECG at baseline and during therapy for patients with congenital long QT syndrome, CHF, bradyarrhythmias, or those taking drugs that prolong the QTc interval. Assess serum calcium at baseline and at least monthly and replete calcium as needed. Teach patients to report bleeding that does not stop (e.g., epistaxis).
	VEGFR-1, VEGFR-2, VEGFR-3, PDGFR-α, PDGFR-β, FGFR, c-Kit, and others	Pazopanib (Votrient®) Indicated for treatment of patients with • Advanced RCC • Advanced soft tissue sarcoma who have received prior chemotherapy • Efficacy not shown in treatment of adipocytic soft tissue sarcoma or GIST.	Most common are (a) RCC: diarrhea, HTN, hair color changes, nausea, anorexia, vomiting, fatigue, weight loss, decreased appetite, and vomiting; and (b) sarcoma: fatigue, diarrhea, nausea, vomiting, weight loss, HTN, decreased appetite, hair color changes, tumor pain, headache, dysgeusia, dyspnea, myalgia, GI pain, and musculoskeletal pain. Increased LFTs and severe hepatotoxicity may occur. Monitor LFTs at baseline and regularly during therapy. Prolonged QTc interval with torsades de pointes: Consider monitoring ECG and electrolytes. Cardiac dysfunction (e.g., CHF, decreased LVEF) has occurred. Monitor BP and control HTN before starting drug. Monitor BP within one week of starting drug, then frequently. Patients with cardiac risk should have LVEF assessed at baseline and periodically during therapy. Proteinuria: Monitor regularly; hold drug for 24-hour urine ≥ 3 g, then dose reduce. Interrupt therapy prior to surgery; resume after wound healing. Hypothyroidism may occur. Monitor TSH at baseline and repeat during therapy. Rarely, fatal hemorrhage has been reported. Use cautiously, if at all, in patients with hemoptysis or history of hemorrhage. Arterial and venous thrombotic events; GI perforation, fistula; RPLS; serious infection; and hypertensive crisis may occur. Avoid coadministration with strong CYP3A4 inhibitors or inducers. If must coadminister with a strong inhibitor, reduce pazopanib dose.

(Continued on next page)

Table 4-5. Molecular-Targeted Therapy: Small Molecules (*Continued*)

Drug Class	Target	Drugs[a]	Side Effects[b]
Angiogenesis inhibitors, multitargeted (*cont.*)		Pazopanib (Votrient®) (*cont.*)	Use together with simvastatin cautiously, as risk of ALT elevation is increased; monitor closely. Avoid concomitant administration with drugs that raise gastric pH (e.g., proton pump inhibitors, H_2 receptor antagonists) and use short-acting antacids instead. Separate dosing by several hours. Teach women of reproductive potential to use effective contraception to avoid pregnancy, as drug can cause fetal harm.
	VEGFR-1, VEGFR-2, VEGFR-3, c-Kit, PDGFR-α, PDGFR-β, *BRAF*, RET, and others	Regorafenib (Stivarga®) Indicated for treatment of patients with • *KRAS* wild-type mCRC after prior treatment with chemotherapy, anti-VEGF therapy, and anti-EGFR therapy • Locally advanced, unresectable, or metastatic GIST after prior treatment with imatinib and sunitinib	Most common are asthenia/fatigue, hand-foot skin reaction, diarrhea, decreased appetite, HTN, mucositis, dysphonia, infection, pain, weight loss, abdominal pain, fever, and nausea. Hepatotoxicity may be severe. Monitor LFTs at baseline and during drug therapy. Hold drug if elevated LFTs or hepatocellular necrosis occurs. Drug may decrease wound healing; stop drug before surgery, and discontinue if wound dehiscence occurs. Dermatologic toxicity may occur. Teach patient to administer with a low-fat breakfast. Rarely, hemorrhage, cardiac ischemia and infarction, RPLS, GI perforation, and fistula may occur. Avoid coadministration with strong CYP3A4 inhibitors or inducers. Teach women of reproductive potential to use effective contraception to avoid pregnancy as drug can cause fetal harm
	VEGFR-2, PDGFR-β, Raf kinase	Sorafenib (Nexavar®) Indicated for treatment of patients with • Unresectable hepatocellular carcinoma • Advanced renal cell carcinoma • Locally recurrent or metastatic, progressive, differentiated thyroid cancer refractory to radioactive iodine treatment	Most common are diarrhea, fatigue, infection, alopecia, hand-foot skin reaction, rash, weight loss, decreased appetite, nausea, GI and abdominal pain, HTN, and hemorrhage. HTN: Monitor BP weekly during the first 6 weeks and periodically thereafter. QTc prolongation: Monitor ECG and electrolytes in patients at increased risk for ventricular arrhythmias. Drug-induced hepatitis: Monitor LFTs baseline, then regularly during therapy; if transaminases become elevated without cause, discontinue drug. Cardiac ischemia and/or infarction may occur; temporarily or permanently discontinue drug. Bleeding: Teach patient to report this if it occurs.

(Continued on next page)

Table 4-5. Molecular-Targeted Therapy: Small Molecules *(Continued)*

Drug Class	Target	Drugs[a]	Side Effects[b]
Angiogenesis inhibitors, multitargeted *(cont.)*		Sorafenib (Nexavar®) *(cont.)*	Dermatologic toxicities: Interrupt or decrease dose; discontinue for severe or persistent reactions or if Stevens-Johnson syndrome or toxic epidermal necrolysis is suspected. Impairment of TSH suppression in differentiated thyroid cancer patients may occur; monitor TSH monthly and adjust thyroid replacement therapy as needed. Drug is teratogenic (avoid pregnancy). Avoid strong CYP3A4 inducers.
	VEGFR-1, VEGFR-2, VEGFR-3; PDGFR-α, PDGFR-β, FLT3, c-Kit, others	Sunitinib (Sutent®) Indicated for treatment of patients with • GIST after disease progression on or intolerance to imatinib mesylate • Advanced RCC • Progressive, well-differentiated pNET in patients with unresectable locally advanced or metastatic disease.	Most common are fatigue, asthenia, fever, diarrhea, nausea, mucositis/stomatitis, vomiting, dyspepsia, abdominal pain, constipation, HTN, peripheral edema, rash, hand-foot syndrome, skin discoloration, dry skin, hair color changes, altered taste, headache, back pain, arthralgia, extremity pain, cough, dyspnea, anorexia, and bleeding. Hepatotoxicity: Monitor LFTs baseline and during each treatment cycle. Cardiac toxicity, including decreased LVEF and cardiac failure: Monitor patients for signs and symptoms of CHF. QTc interval prolongation and torsades de pointes: Monitor ECG and electrolytes in patients at high risk. HTN may occur; monitor and treat. Hemorrhage, including tumor hemorrhage, has occurred; monitor serial CBC. Osteonecrosis of the jaw has been reported; encourage patient to have preventive dentistry prior to starting sunitinib, and avoid invasive procedures, especially if patient is also receiving IV bisphosphonate therapy. TLS, especially in patients with GIST and RCC with high tumor burden, may occur; monitor patients closely. Thyroid dysfunction: Assess for signs and symptoms of hypo- or hyperthyroidism, and monitor thyroid function. Hypoglycemia may occur; assess serum glucose at baseline and regularly during therapy. Modify antihyperglycemic medication as needed. Impaired wound healing occurs; interrupt drug prior to major surgical procedures. Proteinuria: Monitor urinalysis at baseline and during therapy, and 24-hour urine for protein; interrupt drug for protein ≥ 3 g/24 hours.

(Continued on next page)

Table 4-5. Molecular-Targeted Therapy: Small Molecules *(Continued)*

Drug Class	Target	Drugs[a]	Side Effects[b]
Angiogenesis inhibitors, multitargeted *(cont.)*		Sunitinib (Sutent®) *(cont.)*	Dermatologic toxicity: Discontinue drug if necrotizing fasciitis, erythema multiforme, Stevens-Johnson syndrome, or toxic epidermal necrosis occurs. Adrenal hemorrhage: Monitor adrenal function if surgery, trauma, or severe infection occurs. Drug interactions may occur with CYP3A4 inhibitors and inducers.
	VEGFR-1, VEGFR-2, VEGFR-3, EGFR family, Src, RET, and others	Vandetanib (Caprelsa®) Indicated for treatment of patients with unresectable, locally advanced or metastatic medullary thyroid cancer that is symptomatic or progressive	Drug is available through a restricted program, Caprelsa REMS® program, requiring prescriber, patient, and pharmacist education and commitment. Most common effects are diarrhea/colitis, rash, acneiform dermatitis, HTN, nausea, headache, URI, decreased appetite, and abdominal pain. Prolonged QTc, torsades de pointes, and sudden death may occur; monitor ECG, and keep serum levels of potassium, calcium, and magnesium within normal limits; monitor thyroid-stimulating hormone. Severe skin reaction (e.g., Stevens-Johnson syndrome) and ILD may occur. Rarely, Ischemic cerebrovascular events, heart failure, hemorrhage, and RPLS develop. Avoid coadministration with strong CYP3A4 inducers and drugs that prolong QTc interval. Drug is contraindicated in patients with congenital long QT syndrome.
	VEGF-A, VEGF-B Drug is the first in class VEGF TRAP, as it "traps" a soluble receptor that binds VEGF-A, preventing the blood vessel endothelial receptors from binding to the ligand VEGF.	Ziv-aflibercept (Zaltrap®) Indicated for treatment of patients with mCRC that is resistant to or has progressed after an oxaliplatin-containing regimen	Most common are leukopenia, diarrhea, neutropenia, proteinuria, increased ALT and AST, stomatitis, fatigue, thrombocytopenia, HTN, weight loss, decreased appetite, epistaxis, abdominal pain, dysphonia, increased serum creatinine, and headache. HTN: Monitor BP at baseline and control HTN before starting drug. Monitor BP through therapy. Diarrhea and increased risk of dehydration may occur; monitor older adult patients closely. Neutropenia: Monitor CBC/differential at baseline and prior to each treatment. Treat only if ANC ≥ 1.5 × 10⁹/L. Proteinuria: Monitor urine protein, and stop drug when proteinuria is ≥ 2 g/24 hours. Stop drug at least 4 weeks before major surgery, and do not resume for at least 4 weeks afterward, until wound is fully healed. Rarely, hemorrhage, GI perforation, fistula formation, arterial thrombotic events, and RPLS occur.

(Continued on next page)

Table 4-5. Molecular-Targeted Therapy: Small Molecules *(Continued)*

Drug Class	Target	Drugs[a]	Side Effects[b]
Angiogenesis inhibitors, multitargeted *(cont.)*		Ziv-aflibercept (Zaltrap®) *(cont.)*	Avoid strong CYP3A4 inducers and inhibitors. Teach male and female patients of reproductive potential to use highly effective contraception to avoid pregnancy during treatment and for at least 3 months after last dose.

[a] This table includes indications, but they change frequently. Please consult the manufacturer's product information as well as the FDA's Center for Drug Evaluation and Research website (www.accessdata.fda.gov/scripts/cder/drugsatfda/index.cfm), which offers an email service to alert subscribers when a new drug or new indication is approved by FDA, for updated information. Every effort has been made to ensure drug data are consistent with the most recent package insert, but typographical errors may occur, and drug information may be updated by the manufacturer. Please see drug package insert for complete prescribing information.

[b] All drugs are potentially fetotoxic, so women and men should be counseled use effective contraception to avoid pregnancy. In addition, most TKIs are metabolized by the CYP3A4 hepatic microenzyme system and require a review of the patient's medication profile for possible interactions.

ACE—angiotensin-converting enzyme; ALK—anaplastic lymphoma kinase; ALL—acute lymphoblastic leukemia; ALT—alanine aminotransferase; ANC—absolute neutrophil count; AST—aspartate transaminase; BCR—B-cell antigen receptor; BP—blood pressure; BTK—Bruton tyrosine kinase; CBC—complete blood count; CDK—cyclin-dependent kinase; CHF—congestive heart failure; CLL—chronic lymphocytic leukemia; CML—chronic myeloid leukemia; DVT—deep vein thrombosis; ECG—electrocardiogram; EGFR—epidermal growth factor receptor; EGFRI—epidermal growth factor receptor inhibitor; ER—estrogen receptor; ERK—extracellular signal-related kinase; FDA—U.S. Food and Drug Administration; FGFR—fibroblast growth factor receptor; GI—gastrointestinal; GIST—gastrointestinal stromal tumor; HGFR—hepatocyte growth factor receptor, also called Scatter factor, as involved in metastasis; HIF-1—hypoxia-inducible factor; HTN—hypertension; IGF-IR—insulin-like growth factor 1 receptor; ILD—interstitial lung disease; LFT—liver function test; LVEF—left ventricular ejection fraction; MCL—mantle cell lymphoma; mCRC—metastatic colorectal cancer; MI—myocardial infarction; MRI—magnetic resonance imaging; MEK—mitogen-activated extracellular signal regulated kinase 1 and 2, which regulate the ERK signaling pathway which promotes cell division; mCRC—metastatic colorectal cancer; MEK—mitogen-activated extracellular signal regulated kinase; MI—myocardial infarction; mTOR—mammalian target of rapamycin; NHL—non-Hodgkin lymphoma; NSCLC—non-small cell lung cancer; PDGFR—platelet-derived growth factor receptor; PE—pulmonary embolism; PI3K—phosphatidylinositol 3-kinase, expressed on normal and malignant B cells; pNET—pancreatic neuroendocrine tumor; RCC—renal cell cancer; RET—"rearranged during transfection" oncogene; RPLS—reversible posterior leukoencephalopathy syndrome; TKI—tyrosine kinase inhibitor; TLS—tumor lysis syndrome; TSH—thyroid-stimulating hormone; URI—upper respiratory tract infection; VEGF—vascular endothelial growth factor; VEGFR—vascular endothelial growth factor receptor

Note. Based on information from manufacturers' prescribing information.

decreased. Interaction with warfarin may increase international normalized ratio (INR), so this should be monitored closely.

As more is learned about EGFR mutations in NSCLC, new drugs that target specific mutations are being developed and FDA approved. Afatinib (Gilotrif®) is a TKI that binds to EGFR1, HER2, and HER4, inhibiting the kinase from turning itself on (autophosphorylation), so that EGFR signaling is downregulated. The drug is FDA-approved for first-line treatment of patients with metastatic NSCLC with EGFR exon 19 deletion or exon 21 L858R mutations. The drug should be taken on an empty stomach (at least one hour before or two hours after a meal), as the maximal concentration is reduced by 50%, and area under the curve (AUC, or bioavailability of the drug) is reduced by 39% when taken with a high-fat meal compared to fasting (Boehringer Ingelheim Pharmaceuticals, Inc., 2014). Diarrhea is the most common side effect and can be severe, resulting in dehydration and renal failure if not controlled. The drug should be held for refractory, prolonged diarrhea. Other side effects include rash/dermatitis acneform rash, stomatitis, paronychia, dry skin, decreased appetite, and pruritus. As with other EGFR inhibitors, the drug can rarely cause interstitial lung disease, so it should be held during the evaluation of patients with acute-onset or worsening pulmonary symptoms. Afatinib can cause hepatic toxicity, so baseline and periodic LFTs should be evaluated. The drug should be held or discontinued for severe or worsening LFTs. It can also rarely cause persistent keratitis (ulcerative), bullous or exfoliative skin disorders, and symptomatic left ventricular dysfunction; thus, it should be held or discontinued if these occur. The dose should be modified for grade 2 or higher diarrhea, grade 2 cutaneous reactions that are prolonged (more than seven days) or intolerable, and any grade 3 or higher toxicity. Coadministration of a P-glycoprotein (P-gp) inhibitor (e.g., ritonavir, cyclosporine A, ketoconazole, itraconazole, erythromycin, verapamil, quinidine, tacrolimus, nelfinavir, saquinavir, amiodarone) can increase afatinib exposure and toxicity. Coadministration with a P-gp inducer (e.g., rifampicin, carbamazepine, phenytoin, phenobarbital, St. John's wort) can decrease drug exposure. Avoid coadministration with both P-gp inducers and inhibitors; if this is not possible, the dose should be increased by 10 mg/day if given with an inducer or decreased by 10 mg/day if given with an inhibitor (Boehringer Ingelheim Pharmaceuticals, Inc., 2014). See Table 4-5 for a review of single-targeted and multitargeted kinase inhibitors.

Multitargeted Kinase Inhibitors

Many redundant cell signaling pathways exist, most of which are regulated by tyrosine kinases. Because multiple pathways are involved, multitargeted agents are needed. Several FDA-approved multitargeted TKIs are available. These are shown in Table 4-5. First-, second-, and third-generation Bcr-Abl TKIs for the treatment of Philadelphia chromosome–positive (Ph+) chronic myeloid leukemia (CML) now give options to develop a truly individualized therapeutic plan for patients with CML.

First-Generation Tyrosine Kinase Inhibitors Targeting Bcr-Abl

Imatinib mesylate (Gleevec®) was the first drug developed and is indicated for initial treatment of newly diagnosed patients with CML in chronic phase, as well as previously treated patients. Imatinib mesylate is a designer drug that inhibits Bcr-Abl tyrosine kinase, which is mutated in patients with Ph+ CML. In addition, the drug inhibits c-Kit, which is mutated in gastrointestinal stromal tumor (GIST), as well as tyrosine kinases for platelet-derived growth factor (PDGF) and stem cell factor (Novartis Pharmaceuticals Corp., 2015a).

Imatinib mesylate has a variety of doses for its many indications. It is metabolized by the cytochrome P450 microenzyme system, especially CYP3A4, and has a number of potential drug interactions. Drugs that may increase imatinib concentrations (substrates) are ketoconazole, itraconazole, erythromycin, and clarithromycin. Drugs that may decrease imatinib concentrations (inducers) are St. John's wort, dexamethasone, phenytoin, carbamazepine, rifampin, and phenobarbital. In addition, a number of drugs may have their plasma concentrations altered, including warfarin; if patients require anticoagulation, they should receive either low-molecular-weight heparin or unfractionated heparin (Novartis Pharmaceuticals Corp., 2015a).

Imatinib mesylate causes edema and potentially severe fluid retention, nausea, vomiting, diarrhea, muscle cramping, rash, and fatigue. Less common side effects are neutropenia, anemia, and thrombocytopenia; CHF in patients with cardiac risk factors; hepatotoxicity; hemorrhage; gastrointestinal perforation; severe skin manifestations (e.g., Stevens-Johnson syndrome); hypothyroidism in patients who have had thyroidectomy; and TLS. If patients continue to respond, treatment is lifelong, with potential risks to the liver, kidneys, and heart, as well as immunosuppression with resultant infection. Postmarketing data included reports of motor vehicle accidents in patients receiving imatinib, related to dizziness, blurred vision, or somnolence, so patient teaching should include using caution in operating motor vehicles or heavy machinery (Novartis Pharmaceuticals Corp., 2015a).

Second-Generation Tyrosine Kinase Inhibitors Targeting Bcr-Abl

Nilotinib (Tasigna®) is indicated for newly diagnosed patients with CML in chronic phase, or patients resistant or intolerant to other therapy, such as imatinib. Nilotinib is given orally, twice daily, 12 hours apart, but must be administered on an empty stomach (no food for two hours before or one hour after the dose) because the AUC is increased by 82% with food (Novartis Pharmaceuticals Corp., 2015b).

Nilotinib should be reduced in patients with hepatic dysfunction and in patients who develop neutropenia, thrombocytopenia, grade 3 toxicities or elevated laboratory values, or QTc greater than 480 msec. The drug can cause QTc prolongation, and sudden deaths have occurred. Hypokalemia and hypomagnesemia must be corrected before the drug is started and then must be monitored during therapy, keeping values in the high-normal range. Patients should be taught to avoid drugs prolonging QTc as well as strong CYP3A4 inhibitors, which can increase nilotinib serum levels (e.g., ketoconazole increases nilotinib AUC by threefold) and toxicity. If strong inhibitors (e.g., clarithromycin, itraconazole) must be given, nilotinib can be interrupted, but if the drug will be given long term, then nilotinib dose should be reduced. Nilotinib is metabolized by CYP3A4 microenzyme system in the liver. Inducers decrease nilotinib AUC (e.g., rifampicin decreases serum levels by 80%), so they should be avoided, including St. John's wort. In addition, nilotinib is an inhibitor or inducer of many microenzyme systems, so the patient's drug profile must be reviewed carefully. Common side effects are myelosuppression, rash, headache, fatigue, nausea, vomiting, myalgia, diarrhea or constipation, and asthenia. Other less common side effects include pancreatitis with elevated serum lipase and abdominal symptoms; hepatotoxicity with elevated LFTs; and electrolyte abnormalities (hypo- or hyperkalemia, hypocalcemia, hyponatremia, and hypophosphatemia) (Novartis Pharmaceuticals Corp., 2015b).

Dasatinib (Sprycel®) targets Bcr-Abl, c-Kit, and platelet-derived growth factor receptor (PDGFR)-beta. This drug is able to overcome imatinib resistance in most patients. Dasatinib is indicated for the treatment of adults with Ph+ CML in chronic phase (newly diagnosed), or with chronic-phase, accelerated-phase, or blast-crisis Ph+ CML resistant to prior therapy, or Ph+ acute lymphoblastic leukemia (ALL) resistant to prior therapy. The usual dose is 70 mg orally twice a day, taken in the morning and evening (Bristol-Myers Squibb Co., 2014b). It is metabolized in the liver by the CYP3A4 pathway and has potential drug interactions. CYP3A4 inducers are likely to decrease dasatinib plasma concentration and should be avoided (e.g., dexamethasone, phenytoin, carbamazepine, rifampin, pentobarbital). Substrates should be avoided as well (e.g., alfentanil, cisapride, cyclosporine, fentanyl, pimozide, quinidine, sirolimus, tacrolimus, ergotamine). Dasatinib solubility is pH dependent, so proton pump therapy should be replaced with antacids, which must be taken at least two hours before or after the dose. Patients should be instructed not to take St. John's wort and proton pump inhibitors.

Most common side effects related to dasatinib are myelosuppression, fluid retention, and diarrhea; headache, fatigue, dyspnea, and musculoskeletal pain also may occur. Neutropenia and thrombocytopenia may be severe, as may fluid retention. Ascites and pleural and pericardial effusions may be manifestations of fluid retention. QTc prolongation may occur, and dasatinib should be used cautiously, if at all, in patients with or having the potential to develop QTc prolongation. Dasatinib increases the risk for cardiac dysfunction and pulmonary artery hypertension (Bristol-Myers Squibb Co., 2014b).

Bosutinib (Bosulif®) is considered more potent than imatinib and can overcome mutations leading to resistance to imatinib (Cortes et al., 2011). However, the drug is resistant to the T315I point mutation, a common mutation for people who have been on these TKIs for a long time. Because it is very specific for *BCR-ABL* (the fusion gene, or Ph+ chromosome) and *SRC* (a proto-oncogene) mutations, it has less toxicity than other TKIs that are more multitargeted. It does not block growth factor receptors, like c-Kit and PDGFR, which spare normal hematopoietic cells (Cortes & Kantarjian, 2012). The incidence in clinical trials was neutropenia 16% (11% grade 3–4) and thrombocytopenia 40% (26% grade 3–4) (Pfizer Labs, 2014a). It also does not cause cardiotoxicity or pancreatitis. The most common side effect, affecting up to 80% of patients, is diarrhea, which is managed with standard care plans. Other side effects include nausea and vomiting, thrombocytopenia, anemia, abdominal pain, fatigue, rash, fever, and less commonly, hepatotoxicity and fluid retention. Bosutinib is given orally once daily with food, and the dose is adjusted for hepatic or renal impairment. The drug interacts with CYP3A4 inhibitors and inducers, so these should be avoided. In addition, proton pump inhibitor drugs may reduce bosutinib serum levels; short-acting antacids should be used instead (Pfizer Labs, 2014a).

Third-Generation Tyrosine Kinase Inhibitors Targeting Bcr-Abl

As patients live longer with CML, point mutations in the *BCR-ABL* oncogene are leading to resistance. Ponatinib (Iclusig®) was developed to address resistance, specifically T315I-positive and other mutations, and has been FDA-approved for treatment of adult patients with T315I-positive CML or Ph+ ALL, as well as for adult patients with CML or Ph+ ALL for whom other TKI therapy is not indicated (ARIAD Pharmaceuticals, Inc., 2014). Patients should be closely monitored for signs and symptoms of (a) thromboembolism and vascular occlusion, which occurred in at least 27% of patients; (b) cardiac dysfunction, as heart failure occurred in 8% of patients; and (c) hepatic dysfunction, as elevated aspartate aminotransferase (AST) and alanine aminotransferase (ALT) were elevated in 56% of patients (ARIAD Pharmaceuticals, Inc., 2014). Most common toxicities are (a) myelosuppression: thrombocytopenia, neutropenia, and anemia, which may require dose interruption and reduction; and (b) nonhematologic adverse reactions (20% or greater): hypertension, rash, abdominal pain, fatigue, headache, dry skin, constipation, arthralgia, nausea, and pyrexia. In addition, patients should be assessed and managed for hypertension, pancreatitis (monitor serum lipase monthly), neuropathy (cranial and peripheral), ocular toxicity (baseline and periodically during treatment), fluid retention, cardiac arrhythmias, myelosuppression, and TLS. Ponatinib should be interrupted for serious hemorrhage, as well as in patients undergoing major surgical procedures, because compromised wound healing and gastrointestinal perforation may occur. Finally, women of reproductive age should avoid pregnancy while taking ponatinib, and the drug should not be administered concomitantly with strong CYP3A4 inhibitors or inducers (ARIAD Pharmaceuticals, Inc., 2014). The Iclusig REMS program includes a letter and fact sheet advising prescribers of the revised drug indications, the risk of vascular occlusion, and new dosing considerations (ARIAD Pharmaceuticals, Inc., 2014).

Miscellaneous Drug Targeting Bcr-Abl

Omacetaxine (Synribo®) is an alkaloid translation inhibitor that has been approved for treatment of patients with CML with T315I mutations (Teva Pharmaceuticals USA, Inc., 2014). The drug requires subcutaneous administration. If a patient or family member is determined to be competent in administration, the educational plan should include administration technique, safe handling (PPE) and storage of syringes in the refrigerator, and disposal and cleanup of accidental spillage (with a spill kit sent home with the patient). The drug should be reconstituted and drawn in syringes by healthcare professionals. Most common adverse reactions are thrombocytopenia, anemia, neutropenia, diarrhea, nausea, fatigue, asthenia, injection-site reaction, pyrexia, infection and lymphopenia (Teva Pharmaceuticals USA, Inc., 2014) (see Table 4-4).

Angiogenesis Inhibitors

Tumors must make new blood vessels to deliver oxygen and nutrients and to remove waste products when they reach 1–2 mm in size (Folkman, 1971). Agents that can block either the ligand VEGF from binding to the VEGF receptor, or the receptor tyrosine kinase on the endothelial cell, can theoretically prevent tumor growth. The mAb bevacizumab was the first angiogenesis inhibitor to be approved (see Table 4-2). It has been followed by a number of multi-targeted kinase inhibitors: axitinib, cabozantinib, pazopanib, regorafenib, sorafenib, sunitinib, and ziv-aflibercept (see Table 4-5).

It is hypothesized that the improved response and patient survival rates with angiogenesis inhibitors when combined with chemotherapy are attributable to normalization of tumor vasculature, permitting entrance of chemotherapy into tumor cells (Chauhan et al., 2012; Jain, 2001). Tumor blood vessels have multiple structural and functional aberrations, making them leaky, with some vessels dilated and others constricted or even dead-ended, thus preventing distribution of chemotherapy into the tumor (Chauhan et al., 2012).

Hypertension is a class effect for this type of drug. Normal blood pressure depends upon nitric oxide for vasodilation, which depends upon VEGF. It is postulated that antiangiogenesis agents block nitric oxide, leading to vasoconstriction and hypertension (Horsley, Marti, & Jayson, 2012). In addition, angiogenesis is necessary for healing, so inhibition will lead to delayed wound healing. Finally, bleeding (i.e., epistaxis, but with risk of hemorrhage), possible gastrointestinal perforation, and proteinuria also are class effects. The drug should always be stopped prior to major surgery and resumed only after the wound has healed. Because angiogenesis is so important in the formation of the embryo, these drugs are fetotoxic. Women of childbearing age should use effective contraception to avoid pregnancy.

Sunitinib (Sutent®), an oral agent, targets multiple kinases and, similar to sorafenib, inhibits both angiogenesis and cell proliferation. Sunitinib is FDA-indicated for GIST after disease progression, advanced renal cell cancer, and progressive, well-differentiated pancreatic neuroendocrine tumors (pNETs) that are unresectable, locally advanced, or metastatic (Pfizer Labs, 2014c). Drug interactions are possible with CYP3A4 inhibitors (e.g., ketoconazole, itraconazole, clarithromycin, indinavir, telithromycin, voriconazole, grapefruit or grapefruit juice). These should not be coadministered, if possible; but if coadministration is necessary, sunitinib dose reduction should be considered. Similarly, coadministration with CYP3A4 inducers also should be avoided (e.g., rifampin, dexamethasone, phenytoin, phenobarbital, St. John's wort); if coadministration is necessary, sunitinib dose increase should be considered. The drug dose is 50 mg orally once a day for four weeks followed by two weeks off for GIST and advanced renal cell cancer, and 37.5 mg once daily continuously for pNET. Warnings include hepatotoxicity, including liver failure; cardiac toxicity with decrease in LVEF; prolonged QTc interval with torsades de pointes; osteonecrosis of the jaw; TLS; and thyroid dysfunction.

Sorafenib (Nexavar®), also an oral agent, targets VEGFR-1, VEGFR-2, and VEGFR-3 on the endothelial cell, as well as PDGFR (beta), FLT3, and c-Kit. It is both antiangiogenic and antiproliferative and is the first FDA-approved multikinase inhibitor. Drug interactions include CYP2C9 substrates (e.g., warfarin [monitor INR closely]), CYP3A4 inducers (e.g., rifampin, St. John's wort, phenytoin, phenobarbital, dexamethasone [expect decreased serum levels of sorafenib]), and antineoplastic agents (e.g., doxorubicin, irinotecan [do not coadminister]). Sorafenib is FDA-approved for the treatment of patients with unresectable hepatocellular carcinoma or advanced renal cell cancer. The usual dose is 400 mg orally twice a day, taken one hour before or two hours after eating. Warnings include cardiac ischemia or infarction, QTc prolongation, and drug-induced hepatitis; patients with risk factors require more intensive monitoring (Bayer Healthcare Pharmaceuticals Inc., 2013).

Axitinib (Inlyta®) is a multitargeted TKI of VEGFR-1, VEGFR-2, and VEGFR-3, blocking angiogenesis. It is approved for use after failure of one prior systemic therapy. Axitinib is started at 5 mg orally, twice daily, 12 hours apart. The dose should be decreased if given concurrently with a CYP3A4 or CYP3A5 inhibitor, or if the patient has moderate hepatic impairment. Strong CYP3A4 and CYP3A5 inducers should be avoided. Warnings include hypertension including hypertensive crisis; arterial and venous thrombotic events; hemorrhagic events, gastrointestinal perforation, and fistula formation; hypothyroidism; increased LFTs; and reversible posterior leukoencephalopathy syndrome. Patients should be monitored for proteinuria at baseline and periodically, and the drug should be interrupted for moderate to severe proteinuria. Axitinib should be stopped at least 24 hours before surgery (Pfizer Labs, 2014b).

Cabozantinib (Cometriq®) is a multitargeted TKI that inhibits the tyrosine kinase activity of VEGFR-1, VEGFR-2, VEGFR-3, c-Kit, FLT-3, and a number of others. It is FDA-approved for the treatment of patients with progressive, metastatic medullary thyroid cancer. The drug is given orally, once daily on an empty stomach (two hours before or at least one hour after a meal). The dose of cabozantinib is 140 mg. APNs should assess for possible drug interactions, as the drug is a CYP3A4 substrate. Strong CYP3A4 inhibitors can increase the drug's serum level, while strong CYP3A4 inducers can reduce serum levels; both should be avoided. Warnings include thrombotic events, wound complications, hypertension including hypertensive crisis, osteonecrosis of the jaw, palmar-plantar erythrodysesthesia syndrome, proteinuria, and reversible posterior leukoencephalopathy syndrome (Exelixis, Inc., 2012).

Pazopanib (Votrient®) is a multitargeted TKI, inhibiting the receptors for VEGFR-1, VEGFR-2, VEGFR-3, PDGFR (alpha and beta), c-Kit, and a number of others. The drug is approved for the treatment of patients with advanced renal cell cancer and those with advanced soft tissue sarcoma after prior chemotherapy. The dose is 800 mg orally, once daily without food (at least one hour before or two hours after a meal). The dose is reduced if patients have baseline moderate hepatic impairment, and the drug is not recommended for patients with severe hepatic dysfunction. As with other TKIs, coadministration with strong CYP3A4 inhibitors or inducers should be avoided. If coadministration with a strong CYP3A4 inhibitor is required, the pazopanib dose should be reduced. If patients are also taking simvastatin, the risk of elevated ALT is increased and they should be monitored closely (GlaxoSmithKline, 2014c). Warnings include hepatotoxicity, prolonged QTc interval with torsades de pointes, fatal hemorrhage, arterial and venous thrombotic events, gastrointestinal perforation, fistula, reversible posterior leukoencephalopathy syndrome, hypertension including hypertensive crisis, proteinuria, hypothyroidism, and serious infections. Severe and fatal hepatotoxicity may occur; LFTs should be monitored closely, and the drug interrupted, dose reduced, or discontinued as recommended in the manufacturer's prescribing information. Cardiac dysfunction (e.g., CHF) and decreased LVEF can occur; BP should be monitored closely and HTN managed promptly. In patients at risk for cardiac dysfunction, LVEF should be evaluated at baseline and periodically during therapy. APNs should monitor urine protein and perform a 24-hour urine for protein evaluation if present; if 3 g or higher, the drug should be interrupted, and dose reduced. If proteinuria continues despite dose reductions, the drug should be discontinued (GlaxoSmithKline, 2014c).

Regorafenib (Stivarga®) is a multitargeted inhibitor of VEGFR-1, VEGFR-2, VEGFR-3, c-Kit, PDGFR (alpha and beta), BRAF, BRAF V600E, and many others. It is FDA-approved for treatment of (a) patients with metastatic colorectal cancer previously treated with chemotherapy, an anti-VEGF agent, and, if *KRAS* wild-type, anti-EGFR therapy; and (b) patients with locally advanced, unresectable or metastatic GIST, previously treated with imatinib mesylate and sunitinib. The drug is given orally, once daily, for 21 days of a 28-day cycle, with a low-fat breakfast. Strong CYP3A4 inhibitors and inducers should be avoided. Warnings include hemorrhage, dermatologic toxicity, hypertension, cardiac ischemia and infarction, reversible posterior leukoencephalopathy syndrome, gastrointestinal perforation, fistula, and complications of wound healing (Bayer Healthcare Pharmaceuticals Inc., 2014).

Ziv-aflibercept (Zaltrap®) is indicated for the treatment of patients with metastatic colorectal cancer that is resistant to or has progressed following an oxaliplatin-containing regimen. Unlike the previous antiangiogenesis TKIs, aflibercept is administered by an IV infusion over one hour every two weeks, in combination with 5-FU, leucovorin, and irinotecan (FOLFIRI). Warnings include fistula formation, hypertension and hypertensive crisis, arterial thrombotic events, proteinuria, neutropenia and neutropenic complications, diarrhea with dehydration, and reversible posterior leukoencephalopathy syndrome (Sanofi-Aventis U.S. LLC & Regeneron Pharmaceuticals, Inc., 2014).

Other Classes of Targeted Agents

As more is learned about the specific mutations involved in malignant transformation and metastases, drugs are being developed to target the anomalies. These include inhibitors of Bruton kinase, BRAF kinase, PARP, MEK, PI3K, CDK, and Hedgehog pathway.

Bruton kinase inhibitor: The Bruton tyrosine kinase (BTK) helps pass the message through B-lymphocyte antigen receptor (BCR) and cytokine pathways, which are critical to B-cell trafficking, chemotaxis, and adhesion (Pharmacyclics, Inc., & Janssen Biotech, Inc., 2015). This results in inhibition of malignant B-cell proliferation, survival, migration, and adhesion. Ibrutinib (Imbruvica®) is a BTK inhibitor that is FDA-approved for treatment of patients with (a) mantle cell lymphoma who have received at least one prior therapy, (b) CLL who have received at least one prior therapy, and (c) Waldenström macroglobulinemia with 17p deletion. The most common adverse reactions include thrombocytopenia, neutropenia, diarrhea, anemia, fatigue, musculoskeletal pain, bruising, nausea, upper respiratory tract infection, and rash. The drug should not be given to patients with moderate or severe baseline hepatic impairment and should be dose reduced in patients with mild impairment (Pharmacyclics, Inc., & Janssen Biotech, Inc., 2015).

BRAF kinase inhibitors: About 50% of patients with malignant melanoma have a mutation in the BRAF gene (*BRAF V600E*), which makes a kinase that turns on the BRAF pathway, a part of the RAF pathway (Hodis et al., 2012) (see Figure 4-5). The mutated kinase sends messages that turn on the mitogen-activated protein kinase (MAPK) pathway when it should be off, called *constitutive activation* (Hodis et al., 2012). This contributes to cancer cell proliferation and survival. Drugs that inhibit BRAF kinase are vemurafenib (Zelboraf®) (Genentech, Inc., 2014d) and dabrafenib (Tafinlar®) (GlaxoSmithKline, 2014b), both FDA-approved for the treatment of patients with unresectable or metastatic melanoma and a *BRAF V600E* mutation. Dabrafenib is also approved in combination with trametinib (Mekinist®) (GlaxoSmithKline, 2014a), a reversible inhibitor of mitogen-activated extracellular signal-regulated kinase 1 and 2 activation and activity (MEK1 and MEK2). This combination targets two different tyrosine kinases and is FDA-approved for the treatment of patients with unresectable melanoma who have either a *BRAF V600E* or *V600K* mutation (GlaxoSmithKline, 2014a). While each drug has its specific potential adverse reactions, all of these agents may cause new primary cutaneous malignancies.

MEK inhibitor: MEK proteins are involved in the MAPK signaling cascade that regulates many cellular functions, including cellular proliferation and apoptosis. MEK1 and MEK 2 activate the extracellular signal-regulated kinase (ERK), one of the four MAPK pathways that regulate cell proliferation, differentiation, and survival (Roberts & Der, 2007). Trametinib is the first MEK-inhibitor and is approved for use in combination with dabrafenib, but only for patients who have not received prior BRAF-inhibitor therapy (GlaxoSmithKline, 2014a).

PARP inhibitor: Damage to DNA can be either singled or double stranded, and the cell has multiple repair mechanisms. Single strand breaks can be repaired by copying the intact strand (template) and removing the damaged base (called *base-excision repair*), using poly (ADP-ribose) polymerase (PARP) enzymes. If both strands are damaged, the DNA mistakes are repaired by homologous recombination. *BRCA1* and *BRCA2* are involved in repairing the double strand breaks. However, in *BRCA1*- or *BRCA2*-mutated breast or ovarian cancer, *BRCA* is unable to provide the repair. In this case, repair is attempted via PARP enzymes, and if these are inhibited, it results in cancer cell death (synthetic lethality) (Iglehart & Silver, 2009). Olaparib (Lynparza™) is a PARP inhibitor that is FDA-approved in patients with advanced ovarian cancer with germ-line mutation of the *BRCA* gene (actual or suspected) who have been treated with three or more prior lines of chemotherapy (AstraZeneca, 2014). The most common adverse reactions include anemia, nausea, fatigue, vomiting, diarrhea, dysgeusia, dyspepsia, headache, decreased appetite, arthralgia/musculoskeletal pain, myalgia, and dermatitis/rash. Laboratory abnormalities include increased creatinine, elevated mean corpuscular volume, decreased hemoglobin, decreased absolute neutrophil count, and decreased platelets (AstraZeneca, 2014).

PI3K inhibitor: Phosphoinositide-3-kinase (PI3K) mutation is involved with cancer development (Hemmings & Restuccia, 2012). PI3K-delta is found in normal and malignant B lymphocytes (B cells). Idelalisib (Zydelig®) (Gilead Sciences, Inc., 2014) is a PI3K-delta inhibitor that induces apoptosis and prevents cell proliferation in malignant B cells; it also inhibits other signaling pathways, including BCR signaling and others that help B cells to migrate to the lymph nodes and bone marrow so that chemotaxis and adhesion are lost and the malignant cell dies (Gilead Sciences, Inc., 2014). The drug is FDA-approved for treatment of patients with (a) relapsed CLL, in combination with rituximab, (b) relapsed follicular B-cell NHL who have had at least two systemic therapies, and (c) relapsed small lymphocytic lymphoma, who have received at least two systemic therapies. The most common adverse effects include diarrhea, pyrexia, fatigue, nausea, cough, pneumonia, chills, and rash. Laboratory abnormalities include neutropenia, hypertriglyceridemia, hyperglycemia, and increased AST and ALT.

Cyclin-dependent kinase (CDK) inhibitor: Palbociclib (Ibrance®) inhibits CDK4 and CDK6, which are responsible for pushing cell division forward, leading to cell proliferation. Almost all cancers involve abnormalities in the cell cycle. Palbociclib is FDA-approved in combination with letrozole for the treatment of postmenopausal women with estrogen receptor–positive, HER2-negative advanced breast cancer (Pfizer Labs, 2015). The most common adverse reactions include neutropenia, leukopenia, fatigue, anemia, upper respiratory tract infection, nausea, stomatitis, alopecia, diarrhea, thrombocytopenia, decreased appetite, vomiting, and peripheral neuropathy.

Hedgehog pathway inhibitor: This pathway is essential to the development and precise location of an embryo's organs and appendages but is largely turned off in adults (Wilkes, 2011b). Many basal cell cancers are associated with a mutation in a gene in this pathway, resulting in Hedgehog pathway activation. Vismodegib (Erivedge®) is a Hedgehog pathway inhibitor that shuts down the pathway; it is FDA-approved for the treatment of adults with metastatic basal cell carcinoma; those with locally advanced basal cell carcinoma that has recurred after surgery; or those who are not candidates for surgery or radiation therapy. Most common adverse effects are muscle spasms, alopecia, dysgeusia, weight loss, fatigue, nausea, vomiting, diarrhea, decreased appetite, constipation, arthralgias, and ageusia (Genentech, Inc., 2012). The drug can cause birth defects and embryo-fetal death, so men and women of reproductive potential should use effective contraception to prevent pregnancy while receiving the drug. In men, the drug is excreted in the sperm. Patients should be taught not to donate blood during and for seven months following cessation of the drug (Genentech, Inc., 2012).

Cytokines

Cytokines are substances released from activated lymphocytes that communicate between immune cells or affect the behavior of other immune cells. This group includes interleukins, interferons, tumor necrosis factor, and colony-stimulating factors. Interleukin-2 (Proleukin®) can cause a flu-like syndrome, as well as a more serious capillary leak syndrome (Prometheus Laboratories, Inc., 2012). The interferons also cause flu-like symptoms and may cause depression and suicidal ideation. Colony-stimulating factors such as erythropoietin are used to minimize the need for transfusions related to noncurative chemotherapy. These agents are summarized in Table 4-6.

Gene Therapy

As cancer is a disease of cellular mutations, gene therapy offers the promise of normalization of mutated oncogenes, tumor suppressor genes, and mismatch repair genes, as well as significant genes such as *TP53* and cell cycle genes. However, this work is still investigational (NCI, 2013).

Resources

The Oncology Nursing Society (ONS) has established standards for oncology nurses who are administering chemotherapy and biotherapy in the *Chemotherapy and Biotherapy Guidelines and Recommendations for Practice* (Polovich et al., 2014). This comprehensive resource should be used for principles of drug administration, specific chemotherapy and biotherapy drug toxicities, and assessment and management of patients receiving these agents. ONS also has developed a Putting Evidence Into Practice (PEP) initiative, which is a valuable resource in summarizing the evidence for several nursing-sensitive patient outcomes (see www.ons.org/practice-resources/pep). The American Society of Clinical Oncology (ASCO) and ONS published chemotherapy administration safety standards including standards for the safe administration and management of oral chemotherapy (www.ons.org/practice-resources/clinical-practice/ascoons-chemotherapy-administration-safety-standards). ASCO (www.asco.org) has also published practice guidelines (e.g., antiemetic use in oncology, use of white blood cell and erythropoietin growth factors, use of chemotherapy protectants) and quality care initiatives. NCCN (www.nccn.org) has consensus-developed evidence-based guidelines that include chemotherapy and biotherapy and each tumor type and location, as well as supportive care. These guidelines are frequently updated to reflect changing practice standards.

Table 4-6. Cytokines in Cancer Treatment

Drug Class	Mechanism of Action	Drug	Side Effects/Comments
Cytokines			
Interleukin-2	Produced by T cells after antibody-antigen reaction to amplify the immune response; induces killer cell activity, and gamma interferon	Aldesleukin (Proleukin®)	Flu-like symptoms (chills, rigors, fever, headache, myalgia, arthralgia, malaise, anorexia, asthenia); nausea, vomiting, diarrhea (which can be severe); hepatotoxicity; renal dysfunction; anemia, thrombocytopenia; rash Capillary leak syndrome with hypotension, arrhythmias Patients should have normal cardiac, pulmonary, hepatic, and CNS functioning to receive the drug; use extreme caution in patients with normal stress test and PFTs but have cardiac or pulmonary disease. Impaired neutrophil function with increased risk of disseminated infection
IFN alfa	IFN-α: Stimulated by viruses and tumor cells; has antiviral activity which is greater than its antiproliferative activity, which is greater than its immunomodulatory activity; at least 20 subtypes	IFN-α: IFN alfa-2a (Roferon®-A) IFN-α-2b (Intron® A) Pegylated IFN alfa-2b (Sylatron®)	Fever, chills, headache, myalgias, fatigue, nausea, vomiting, anorexia, diarrhea, depression, suicidal ideation, alopecia, blood disorders, increased LFTs; injection-site discomfort; retinopathy Pegylated IFN alfa-2b: Rare cardiovascular events, hepatic failure in patients with cirrhosis, endocrinopathies
IFN beta	IFN-ß: Stimulated by viruses; equal antiviral, antiproliferative, and immunomodulatory activity; 2 subtypes	IFN-ß-1a (Avonex®)	Flu-like symptoms (fever, chills, diaphoresis, myalgias, fatigue); depression, suicidal ideation, and psychotic disorder; hepatotoxicity; allergic reactions; CHF; decreased peripheral blood counts; autoimmune disorders
IFN gamma	IFN-γ: Produced by activated T cells and natural killer cells, involved in regulating immune and inflammatory response	IFN-γ-1b (Actimmune®)	Neutropenia, thrombocytopenia, hepatotoxicity, decreased mental status, unsteady gait, dizziness, flu-like symptoms, worsening of cardiac dysfunction

(Continued on next page)

Table 4-6. Cytokines in Cancer Treatment *(Continued)*

Drug Class	Mechanism of Action	Drug	Side Effects/Comments
Colony-Stimulating Factors (CSFs)			
Erythropoietin (ESAs)	Stimulate erythro-poiesis in the same way that endogenous erythropoietin does	Darbepoetin alfa (Aranesp®) Epoetin alfa (Procrit®)	Increased risk of tumor progression and death in some patients when hemo-globin > 12 g/dl; use only the lowest dose needed to prevent RBC trans-fusions. Prescribers and hospitals must enroll in and comply with ESA APPRISE Oncology Program to prescribe and dispense ESAs to patients with cancer (www.esa-apprise.com). ESAs are to be used only for anemia from myelosuppressive chemother-apy not intended for cure; discontinue drug after chemotherapy is completed. Drug is not approved for myeloid malignancies. Increased risk of thrombosis (MI, stroke) and mortality if hemoglobin > 11 g/dl; rare red cell aplasia
Granulocyte-CSFs Neutrophil cell line stim-ulation	Stimulates prolifera-tion, differentiation, end-cell activation of neutrophil cell line	Filgrastim (Neupogen®) Tbo-filgrastim (Granix®) Pegfilgrastim (Neulasta®)	Bone pain, rare allergic reaction, rare splenic rupture, rare ARDS in neutro-penic patients with sepsis
Myeloid pro-genitor Granulocyte macrophage–CSF	Stimulates produc-tion and differentiation of myeloid progenitor cells, including macro-phages and neutrophils	Sargramostim (Leukine®)	Flu-like syndrome, bone pain, rash, injection-site reaction; rare dyspnea, supraventricular arrhythmias, renal and hepatic dysfunction

ARDS—acute respiratory distress syndrome; CHF—congestive heart failure; CNS—central nervous system; ESA—erythropoietin-stimulating agent; IFN—interferon; LFTs—liver function tests; MI—myocardial infarction; PFTs—pulmo-nary function tests; RBC—red blood cell

Note. Based on information from manufacturers' prescribing information. This table does not review indications, as they change frequently. Please consult the manufacturer's product information, as well as the U.S. Food and Drug Adminis-tration's (FDA's) Center for Drug Evaluation and Research website (www.accessdata.fda.gov/scripts/cder/drugsatfda/index.cfm), which offers an email service to alert subscribers when a new drug or new indication is approved by the FDA, for updated information. Every effort has been made to ensure drug data are consistent with the most recent pack-age insert, but typographical errors may occur, and drug information may be updated by the manufacturer. Please see drug package insert for complete prescribing information.

In terms of personal protection in administering hazardous drugs, the following guides provide the national standard. The Occupational Safety and Health Administration's *OSHA Technical Manual*, Section VI, Chapter 2, "Controlling Occupational Exposure to Hazardous Drugs," identifies recommended personal protective safety guidelines and a list of some haz-ardous drugs. However, this list does not include any new, targeted therapies or most mAbs. ONS also publishes *Safe Handling of Hazardous Drugs* (Polovich, 2011). Finally, the National Institute for Occupational Safety and Health (www.cdc.gov/niosh) publishes updates to the appendices of its original publication *Preventing Occupational Exposure to Antineoplastic and Other Hazardous Drugs in Health Care Settings*.

Patient and Family Education

Chemotherapy has a very narrow therapeutic window. Therefore, toxicities are anticipated that would not be tolerated by patients receiving any other medications. As a result, oncology APNs have successfully developed patient and family education plans (and materials that can be individualized) for those receiving chemotherapy, as the evidence base for prevention and management of side effects has become clearer. These include self-assessment and self-care measures to minimize infection, bleeding, fatigue, nausea and vomiting, diarrhea, cognitive dysfunction, hand-foot syndrome, and injury from peripheral neuropathy, to name a few. In addition, APNs must ensure that patients have the knowledge required to make an informed decision to undergo therapy. Often, APNs, through knowledge of the science and clinical trial data, as well as the individual strengths of the patient, can best help patients to make a decision about which chemotherapy regimen to select when all other factors are equal, such as in patients with newly diagnosed advanced colorectal cancer. Other chapters within this book discuss in detail the patient teaching in each of these areas.

With the rapidly progressing evolution of targeted therapies, anecdotal reports form the basis for many patient and family education materials. Nurses need to work together to conduct prospective trials of potential prevention and intervention strategies to establish evidence-based practice. Skin rash and other skin complications from EGFR inhibitors are probably among the most challenging symptoms.

Implications for Oncology Advanced Practice Nurses

APNs are recognized by patients and families as key members of the healthcare team, advocating for patients and families and ensuring that they understand discussions with the physician about the disease, treatment, and care planning goals. APNs who are prescribing chemotherapy or managing patients receiving chemotherapy must understand the potential toxicities and preassessment criteria, such as baseline bone marrow, renal, hepatic, and, depending on the drug, cardiac and other organ functions. In addition, most patients receive chemotherapy in an ambulatory care setting, with most toxicities occurring while patients are at home. Patients must be able to self-assess and provide self-care or rely on a competent family member to do this. APNs must be able to use knowledge of differential diagnoses to evaluate patient complications between scheduled visits and work collaboratively with the triage nurse. As molecular-targeted treatments become more numerous, APNs will not only have to maintain a knowledge base of this rapidly exploding field but also must be able to simplify the mechanism of action, potential side effects, and self-care measures so that patients can make informed decisions about treatment choices and management. Complicating this is the rising cost of cancer therapy, as some targeted therapies cost in excess of $10,000 per month. APNs and physicians will need to ensure that patients know the cost, expected coverage, and co-pays when discussing treatment options. Ramsey et al. (2013) found that in the state of Washington, patients with cancer were 2.65 times more likely to become bankrupt than people without cancer.

APNs must be active in establishing the evidence base for interventions to prevent or minimize symptoms and provide structure and monitoring, as patients will be on these therapies for the rest of their lives. As these agents become FDA-approved and are more commonly used, new toxicities will emerge that perhaps were not recognized during clinical trials of patients with very good performance status. APNs must ensure that this information is communicated to the appropriate agencies and to oncology APN colleagues. The future has never been brighter in oncology care.

Conclusion

This chapter has reviewed principles of chemotherapy, biotherapy, and molecular therapy and general toxicities of agents. As the understanding of malignant transformation and molecular flaws in cell signaling and function develops, this new paradigm in cancer diagnosis and treatment will continue to change. Already, genetic fingerprints of different tumor types of breast cancer have been identified, leading to individualized or precision treatment planning. This has paved the way for similar study in lymphoma and colorectal, lung, and prostate cancers. Nanotechnology will allow precise, rapid diagnosis, real-time monitoring of response, and treatment. APNs must take steps to ensure knowledge and understanding of these developments in order to translate them to patients and their families and provide competent care. APNs also must take a leadership role in undertaking nursing research to provide the evidence base for new side effect prevention and management as new targeted agents are approved by FDA.

Case Study

J.C. is a 48-year-old patient with metastatic colorectal cancer who is coming in for her first cycle of infusional FOLFOX (5-FU, leucovorin, and oxaliplatin) and bevacizumab. She had a history of bright red blood per rectum for four months but thought it was related to hemorrhoids. When she started feeling tired and lost her appetite, she went to the emergency department for evaluation, as she had no primary care provider. Her computed tomography (CT) scan showed a questionable obstructing lesion in her ascending colon, along with liver and lung metastases. She underwent a hemicolectomy to prevent obstruction. Her laboratory values were within normal limits, except for carcinoembryonic antigen, which was 240 ng/dl preoperatively and 50 ng/dl postoperatively (normal is less than 5 ng/dl); alkaline phosphatase, which was slightly elevated at 300 U/L (normal is 70–230 U/L); and lactate dehydrogenase, which was 175 U/L (normal is 90–190 U/L). She has no known drug allergies.

J.C. is divorced, and her two children are married and live nearby. She works as a housekeeper for a family in the nearby city. She does not smoke. She has a past medical history of type II diabetes that is well controlled by metformin 1 g PO BID, exercises "in her work," and has a history of alcoholism. She goes to Alcoholics Anonymous regularly. She has a family history of cardiovascular disease but has no history of cancer in either her mother's or father's family.

On physical examination, the APN notes a young-appearing African American woman who is in no acute distress. Her blood pressure is 120/80 mm Hg. Her incision is well healed. She is appropriately sad about her diagnosis but hopeful that the treatment will "slow the cancer" so she can "live to see her grandchildren born."

J.C. has tolerated the treatment well, except for acute cold-induced neuropathy that has subsequently been prevented by calcium and magnesium infusions immediately before and after the oxaliplatin infusion. Her nadir blood counts are absolute neutrophil count of 1,200/

mm^3, platelet count of 100,000/mm^3, and hemoglobin of 12 g/dl. Her serum electrolytes, including magnesium and calcium, and renal and liver function tests are within normal limits. She has a urinalysis for protein every month, and today has trace protein in her urine. Her recent CT has shown a 50% reduction in measurable disease. She receives dexamethasone plus a serotonin antagonist to prevent nausea and vomiting. She has grade 0–1 persistent peripheral neuropathy characterized by paresthesias in her fingertips and toes.

J.C. experiences a hypersensitivity reaction to her FOLFOX. After she has been stabilized, she is admitted and observed overnight. The next day, the oxaliplatin is restarted to infuse over six hours following premedication with diphenhydramine, famotidine, and dexamethasone. She tolerates the infusion without further hypersensitivity reaction. She then continues to receive six more biweekly cycles of FOLFOX and then on follow-up CT shows disease progression. She is begun on FOLFIRI (5-FU, leucovorin, and irinotecan) for three cycles, but no interval improvement is shown on CT. Her chemotherapy regimen is changed to irinotecan plus cetuximab.

1. As the APN prepares to complete an assessment prior to the patient beginning FOLFOX chemotherapy, what are five key factors to assess?
   - She is receiving oxaliplatin, which has as a cumulative dose-limiting toxicity of peripheral neuropathy. It is very important, given her past history of alcoholism and type II diabetes, that the APN does a complete neurologic examination, paying close attention to sensory peripheral neuropathy, especially that of the large-fiber nerves, for position and vibration.
   - Bevacizumab can cause hypertension over time, so the APN would want to know her blood pressure status. She is normotensive, and the APN would monitor this before each treatment.
   - The clinician would assess her gastrointestinal status because she will be at risk for developing diarrhea from the 5-FU, leucovorin, and oxaliplatin. She is at risk for nausea and vomiting from the oxaliplatin, but the APN will use aggressive antiemetics to prevent this.
   - Because she is receiving bevacizumab and has a history of diabetes, she is at risk for proteinuria. Thus, the APN would want to check a baseline urinalysis for protein and monitor this at least monthly during her treatment.
   - The APN would want to do a baseline nasal septum evaluation because, rarely, bevacizumab can cause nasal septum perforation.
2. J.C. complains of a feeling of chest tightness during the oxaliplatin infusion, slight shortness of breath, and feeling very cold. Her blood pressure is 100/70 mm Hg (baseline 118/80), heart rate is 120 beats per minute (baseline 82), respiratory rate is 24 breaths per minute (baseline 13), and O$_2$ saturation is 92% (baseline 99%). What would the APN suspect, and how would he or she manage this?
   - Delayed hypersensitivity can occur with oxaliplatin, usually in about cycle 8–12. The APN would stop the drug, provide oxygen, and reassess. If it was severe, with symptomatic bronchospasm or severe hypotension, the APN would give epinephrine 1:1,000 intramuscularly, as well as IV saline for hypotension. The patient has already received dexamethasone, so the APN would also give her IV hydrocortisone. Patients have been successfully desensitized (Gammon, Bhargava, & McCormick, 2004), and given J.C.'s success with the current regimen, the APN would discuss this with her oncologist as well as the patient and family.
3. Prior to J.C.'s first cycle of FOLFIRI, the APN reviews the potential side effects of this regimen, including potential toxicity and self-care measures with irinotecan. What areas would he or she cover in teaching the patient about cetuximab?
   - The APN would teach her that although uncommon, hypersensitivity reaction may occur during the first infusion (3% incidence, and 90% occur during the first infusion). The APN reassures her that she will be closely monitored during the infusion. The APN also tells her about possible skin changes, including rash.

4. What specific teaching would the APN give her about skin changes?
   • The APN would teach her about skin changes, which include the following.
     – She may develop a sunburn-like skin effect initially, which she may not notice because she has dark skin. To manage this, she should use skin emollients to keep the skin moist and well hydrated.
     – The rash may get worse at about 15 days after the first treatment but will improve over time. It is very important for her not to scratch her face, as that may lead to infection. She should continue to use moisturizers and keep out of the sun, as sun exposure makes the rash worse. (She is African American and may or may not have the rash.) If she needs to go out in the sun, she should use a zinc-based sunscreen with SPF 30 or higher. She should call for anti-itch medication if an itch develops that cannot be controlled by a moisturizer.
     – The rash will crust over. She needs to assess her skin for the formation of blisters (vesicles), yellow crusting, or drainage. These should be reported immediately to the healthcare provider, as they may be an indication of infection. She may receive antibiotics (tetracycline-class antibiotic, topical and/or systemic depending upon the severity).
5. The APN also would teach her about changes in her hair and fingers. What specifically would the APN tell her?
   • The APN would teach her that she may develop hair changes, such as thinning of the hair, scalp dryness, and lengthening of her eyelashes. It is important that J.C. notify the healthcare provider if she develops conjunctivitis or eye irritation, and she will be referred to an ophthalmologist for evaluation.
   • Additionally, the APN teaches her that she may develop paronychia or fissures on her fingers. She should wear gloves when working around the house or doing dishes, and she needs to inform the healthcare provider if this occurs and is difficult to manage. The APN will then advise her about and may prescribe steroid tape if this becomes uncomfortable.

Key Points

• Advances in the development of chemotherapy include nanotechnology.
• Major advances have occurred in the understanding of cancer and biologic pathways, resulting in targeted agents that are changing the paradigm of cancer care.
• Chemotherapy most often interferes with frequently dividing normal cell populations, including bone marrow, gonads, hair follicles, and gastrointestinal mucosa, with resulting potential problems of myelosuppression, infertility, alopecia, and mucositis (including diarrhea).
• Biotherapy and targeted therapy require vigilance to prevent reactions or to intervene rapidly and efficiently if hypersensitivity reactions occur.
• Antiangiogenesis agents have class effects including hypertension and bleeding.
• EGFR inhibitors have class effects including sterile, inflammatory rash, diarrhea, hypomagnesemia (mAbs), and interstitial lung disease.
• Advances in targeted therapy are occurring frequently. APNs must understand cell physiology, cell signaling, angiogenesis, and other vital cell functions to be able to prepare patients for treatment.

Chemotherapy

• Drugs are classified as cell cycle specific (working in one specific phase of the cell cycle) or nonspecific (working throughout all phases of the cell cycle).
• Major class side effects are as follows.
  – Antimetabolites: Bone marrow depression, mucositis (stomatitis, diarrhea)

- – Alkylating agents: Bone marrow depression, damage to reproductive organs
- – Mitotic inhibitors: Neuropathy, many are vesicants
- – Antitumor antibiotics: Bone marrow depression, damage to cardiac myocytes, most are vesicants
- Nursing care focuses on teaching self-care measures to patients, as side effects often occur when patients are at home or outside the hospital.

Monoclonal Antibodies

- Monoclonal antibodies are unconjugated or conjugated
- They have two portions: The Fab portion, which binds to the antigen, and the Fc portion, which calls and binds immune effector cells to the antigen to kill it.
- Principal ways the immune cells kill antigen-containing cells are ADCC and CDC.

Tyrosine Kinase Inhibitors

- TKIs can have single or multiple targets. The more targets, the more side effects the drug has, as more signaling pathways are involved.
- Almost all TKIs are metabolized by the cytochrome P450 microenzyme system and thus have potential drug interactions.
- Side effects are class specific, as well as related to the individual drug.

Antiangiogenesis Agents

- Class effects of these drugs include hypertension, bleeding, proteinuria, rare arterial or venous embolism, gastrointestinal perforation, and fistula formation.
- Most drugs require assessment of urine protein prior to IV doses (e.g., bevacizumab) and periodically during therapy.
- Drug should be stopped prior to major surgery and resumed at some point afterward once the wound has healed (drug prescribing information may be specific as to number of days based on drug half-life).

Recommended Resources for Oncology Advanced Practice Nurses

Patient Teaching

- American Society of Clinical Oncology (www.cancer.net): The website offers publications and resources, with topics including coping and managing costs related to cancer.
- CancerCare offers many other self-empowering resources related to chemotherapy side effects at www.cancercare.org/patients_and_survivors.
- Fleishman, S.B., Fox, L.P., Garfield, D.H., Viele, C.S., & Messner, C. (2009). *Tips for managing treatment-related rash and dry skin.* Available from CancerCare at www.cancercare.org/pdf/booklets/ccc_managing_rash.pdf

Drug Information and Clinical Practice Guidelines

- American Society of Clinical Oncology (ASCO)

- ASCO and ONS published administration safety standards (www.ons.org/practice-resources/standards-reports/chemotherapy), including standards for the safe administration and management of oral chemotherapy.
    - ASCO Institute for Quality has also published practice guidelines (e.g., use of white blood cell and erythropoietin growth factors, as well as disease treatment), available at www.instituteforquality.org/practice-guidelines.
- FDA Center for Drug Evaluation and Research oncology tools: www.fda.gov/AboutFDA/CentersOffices/OfficeofMedicalProductsandTobacco/CDER/ucm091745.htm
- NCCN (www.nccn.org/professionals/physician_gls/f_guidelines.asp): NCCN publishes consensus-developed evidence-based guidelines that include chemotherapy and biotherapy and each tumor type and location, as well as supportive care. These guidelines are frequently updated to reflect changing practice standards.
- ONS
    - Polovich, M., Olsen, M., & LeFebvre, K.B. (Eds.). (2014). *Chemotherapy and biotherapy guidelines and recommendations for practice* (4th ed.). Pittsburgh, PA: Oncology Nursing Society. This resource covers principles of drug administration, specific chemotherapy and biotherapy drug toxicities, and assessment and management of patients receiving these agents.
    - Putting Evidence Into Practice resources (www.ons.org/practice-resources/pep): These resources summarize the evidence for several nursing-sensitive patient outcomes.

Personal Protection in Administering Hazardous Drugs

- National Institute for Occupational Safety and Health publishes updates to its appendices to the original 2004 publication *Preventing Occupational Exposure to Antineoplastic and Other Hazardous Drugs in Health Care Settings* (www.cdc.gov/niosh/docs/2004-165). The most recent update to the list of drugs considered hazardous was published in 2014.
- Occupational Safety and Health Administration identifies recommended personal protective safety guidelines and a list of some hazardous drugs in Section VI, Chapter 2: "Controlling Occupational Exposure to Hazardous Drugs" of the 1995 *OSHA Technical Manual* (www.osha.gov/dts/osta/otm/otm_vi/otm_vi_2.html). However, this list does not include any new, targeted therapies or most mAbs.
- Polovich, M. (Ed.). (2011). *Safe handling of hazardous drugs* (2nd ed.). Pittsburgh, PA: Oncology Nursing Society.

References

Adams, G.P., & Weiner, L.M. (2005). Monoclonal antibody therapy of cancer. *Nature Biotechnology, 23,* 1147–1153.

Alberta Health Services. (2012). *Prevention and treatment of rash in patients treated with EGFR inhibitor therapies.* Edmonton, Alberta, Canada: Author.

ARIAD Pharmaceuticals, Inc. (2014). *Iclusig® (ponatinib)* [Package insert]. Cambridge, MA: Author.

Astellas Pharma, Inc. (2014). *Xtandi® (enzalutamide)* [Package insert]. Northbrook, IL: Author.

Astellas Pharma US, Inc., & Genentech, Inc. (2014). *Tarceva® (erlotinib)* [Package insert]. Northbrook, IL, and South San Francisco, CA: Authors.

AstraZeneca. (2014). *Lynparza™ (olaparib)* [Package insert]. Wilmington, DE: Author.

Baird, R.D., & Caldas, C. (2013). Genetic heterogeneity in breast cancer: The road to personalized medicine? *BMC Medicine, 11,* 151. doi:10.1186/1741-7015-11-151

Balagula, Y., Garbe, C., Myskowski, P.L., Hauschild, A., Rapoport, B.L., Boers-Doets, C.B., & Lacouture, M.E. (2011). Clinical presentation and management of dermatological toxicities of epidermal growth factor receptor inhibitors. *International Journal of Dermatology, 50,* 129–146. doi:10.1111/j.1365-4632.2010.04791.x

Baselga, J., Perez, E.A., Pienkowski, T., & Bell, R. (2006). Adjuvant trastuzumab: A milestone in the treatment of HER-2-positive early breast cancer. *Oncologist, 11*(Suppl. 1), 4–12. doi:10.1634/theoncologist.11-90001-4

Bayer Healthcare Pharmaceuticals Inc. (2013). *Nexavar® (sorafenib)* [Package insert]. Whippany, NJ: Author.

Bayer Healthcare Pharmaceuticals Inc. (2014). *Stivarga® (regorafenib)* [Package insert]. Whippany, NJ: Author.

Biogen Idec, Inc., & Genentech, Inc. (2014). *Rituxan® (rituximab)* [Package insert]. South San Francisco, CA: Author.

Boehringer Ingelheim Pharmaceuticals, Inc. (2014). *Gilotrif® (afatinib)* [Package insert]. Ridgefield, CT: Author.

Borkar, D.S., Lacouture, M.E., & Basti, S. (2013). Spectrum of ocular toxicities from epidermal growth factor receptor inhibitors and their intermediate-term follow-up: A five-year review. *Supportive Care in Cancer, 21*, 1167–1174. doi:10.1007/s00520-012-1645-y

Bowles, E.J., Wellman, R., Feigelson, H.S., Onitilo, A.A., Freedman, A.N., Delate, T., … Pharmacovigilance Study Team. (2012). Risk of heart failure in breast cancer patients after anthracycline and trastuzumab treatment: A retrospective cohort study. *Journal of the National Cancer Institute, 104*, 1293–1305. doi:10.1093/jnci/djs317

Bristol-Myers Squibb Co. (2013). *Yervoy® (ipilimumab)* [Package insert]. Princeton, NJ: Author.

Bristol-Myers Squibb Co. (2014a). *Opdivo® (nivolumab)* [Package insert]. Princeton, NJ: Author.

Bristol-Myers Squibb Co. (2014b). *Sprycel® (dasatinib)* [Package insert]. Princeton, NJ: Author.

Celgene Corp. (2014). *Abraxane® (paclitaxel protein-bound particles for injectable suspension)* [Package insert]. Summit, NJ: Author.

Chauhan, V.P., Stylianopoulos, T., Martin, J.D., Popović, Z., Chen, O., Kamoun, W.S., … Jain, R.K. (2012). Normalization of tumour blood vessels improves the delivery of nanomedicines in a size-dependent manner. *Nature Nanotechnology, 7*, 383–388.

Chobanian, A.V., Bakris, G.L., Black, H.R., Cushman, W.C., Green, L.A., Izzo, J.L., Jr., … Roccella, E.J. (2003). The seventh report of the Joint National Committee on prevention, detection, evaluation, and treatment of high blood pressure: The JNC 7 report. *JAMA, 289*, 2560–2572. doi:10.1001/jama.289.19.2560

Chung, C.H., Mirakhur, B., Chan, E., Le, Q.T., Berlin, J., Morse, M., … Platts-Mills, T.A. (2008). Cetuximab-induced anaphylaxis and IgE specific for galactose-α-1, 3-galactose. *New England Journal of Medicine, 358*, 1109–1117. doi:10.1056/NEJMoa074943.

Citron, M.L., Berry, D.A., Cirrincione, C., Hudis, C., Winer, E.P., Gradishar, W.J., … Norton, L. (2003). Randomized trial of dose-dense versus conventionally scheduled and sequential versus concurrent combination chemotherapy as postoperative adjuvant treatment of node-positive primary breast cancer: First report of Intergroup Trial C9741/Cancer and Leukemia Group B Trial 9741. *Journal of Clinical Oncology, 21*, 1431–1439. doi:10.1200/JCO.2003.09.081

Clifford, D.B., Ances, B., Costello, C., Rosen-Schmidt, S., Andersson, M., Parks, D., … Tyler, K.L. (2011). Rituximab-associated progressive multifocal leukoencephalopathy in rheumatoid arthritis. *Archives of Neurology, 68*, 1156–1164. doi:10.1001/archneurol.2011.103

Cortes, J., & Kantarjian, H.M. (2012). How I treat newly diagnosed chronic phase CML. *Blood, 120*, 1390–1397. doi:10.1182/blood-2012-03-378919

Cortes, J.E., Kantarjian, H.M., Brümmendorf, T.H., Kim, D.W., Turkina, A.G., Shen, Z.X., … Gambacorti-Passerini, C. (2011). Safety and efficacy of bosutinib (SKI-606) in chronic phase Philadelphia chromosome-positive chronic myeloid leukemia patients with resistance or intolerance to imatinib. *Blood, 118*, 4567–4576. doi:10.1182/blood-2011-05-355594

Curtis, C., Shah, S.P., Chin, S.F., Turashvili, G., Rueda, O.M., Dunning, M.J., … Aparicio, S. (2012). The genomic and transcriptomic architecture of 2,000 breast tumours reveals novel subgroups. *Nature, 486*, 346–352.

Di Nicolantonio, F., Martini, M., Molinari, F., Sartore-Bianchi, A., Arena, S., Saletti, P., … Bardelli, A. (2008). Wild-type *BRAF* is required for response to panitumumab or cetuximab in metastatic colorectal cancer. *Journal of Clinical Oncology, 26*, 5705–5712. doi:10.1200/JCO.2008.18.0786

Eisai Inc. (2013). *Halaven® (eribulin mesylate)* [Package insert]. Woodcliff Lake, NJ: Author.

Eli Lilly and Co. (2014). *Gemzar® (gemcitabine for injection)* [Package insert]. Indianapolis, IN: Author.

Escalante, C.P., & Zalpour, A. (2011). Vascular endothelial growth factor inhibitor-induced hypertension: Basics for primary care providers. *Cardiology Research and Practice, 2011*, Article ID 816897. doi:10.4061/2011/816897

Ewer, M.S., & Ewer, S.M. (2010). Cardiotoxicity of anticancer treatments: What the cardiologist needs to know. *Nature Reviews Cardiology, 7*, 564–575.

Exelixis, Inc. (2012). *Cometriq® (cabozantinib)* [Package insert]. South San Francisco, CA: Author.

Fakih, M., & Vincent, M. (2010). Adverse events associated with anti-EGFR therapies for the treatment of metastatic colorectal cancer. *Current Oncology, 17*(Suppl. 1), S18–S30.

Fecher, L.A., Agarwala, S.S., Hodi, F.S., & Weber, J.S. (2013). Ipilimumab and its toxicities: A multidisciplinary approach. *Oncologist, 18*, 733–743. doi:10.1634/theoncologist.2012-0483

Fellner, C. (2012). Ipilimumab (Yervoy) prolongs survival in advanced melanoma: Serious side effects and a hefty price tag may limit its use. *Pharmacy and Therapeutics, 37*, 503–511, 530. Retrieved from http://www.ncbi.nlm.nih.gov/pmc/articles/PMC3462607/pdf/ptj3709503.pdf

Finigan, J.H., Downey, G.P., & Kern, J.A. (2012). Human epidermal growth factor receptor signaling in acute lung injury. *American Journal of Respiratory Cell and Molecular Biology, 47,* 395–404. doi:10.1165/rcmb.2012 -0100TR

Folkman, J. (1971). Tumor angiogenesis: Therapeutic implications. *New England Journal of Medicine, 285,* 1182–1186. doi:10.1056/NEJM197111182852108

Gammon, D., Bhargava, P., & McCormick, M.J. (2004). Hypersensitivity reactions to oxaliplatin and the application of a desensitization protocol. *Oncologist, 9,* 546–549. doi:10.1634/theoncologist.9-5-546

Genentech, Inc. (2012). *Erivedge® (vismodegib)* [Package insert]. South San Francisco, CA: Author.

Genentech, Inc. (2014a). *Avastin® (bevacizumab)* [Package insert]. South San Francisco, CA: Author.

Genentech, Inc. (2014b). *Herceptin® (trastuzumab)* [Package insert]. South San Francisco, CA: Author.

Genentech, Inc. (2014c). *Kadcyla® (ado-trastuzumab emtansine)* [Package insert]. South San Francisco, CA: Author.

Genentech, Inc. (2014d). *Zelboraf® (vemurafenib)* [Package insert]. South San Francisco, CA: Author.

Gilead Sciences, Inc. (2014). *Zydelig® (idelalisib)* [Package insert]. Foster City, CA: Author.

GlaxoSmithKline. (2014a). *Mekinist® (trametinib)* [Package insert]. Research Triangle Park, NC: Author.

GlaxoSmithKline. (2014b). *Tafinlar® (dabrafenib)* [Package insert]. Research Triangle Park, NC: Author.

GlaxoSmithKline. (2014c). *Votrient® (pazopanib)* [Package insert]. Research Triangle Park, NC: Author.

Gravalos, C., & Jimeno, A. (2008). HER2 in gastric cancer: A new prognostic factor and a novel therapeutic target. *Annals of Oncology, 19,* 1528–1529. doi:10.1093/annonc/mdn169

Haddadin, S., & Perry, M.C. (2012). Appendix I: Chemotherapeutic agents. In M.C. Perry, D.C. Doll, & C.E. Freter (Eds.), *Perry's the chemotherapy source book* (5th ed., p. 732). Philadelphia, PA: Wolters Kluwer Health/Lippincott Williams & Wilkins.

Hanahan, D., & Weinberg, R. (2011). Hallmarks of cancer: The next generation. *Cell, 144,* 646–674. doi:10.1016/j.cell .2011.02.013

Hansel, T.T., Kropshofer, H., Singer, T., Mitchell, J.A., & George, A.J. (2010). The safety and side effects of monoclonal antibodies. *Nature Reviews Drug Discovery, 9,* 325–338.

Hemmings, B.A., & Restuccia, D.F. (2012). PI3K-PKB/Akt pathway. *Cold Spring Harbor Perspectives in Biology, 4*(9), a011189. doi:10.1101/cshperspect.a011189

Hodis, E., Watson, I.R., Kryukov, G.V., Arold, S.T., Imielinski, M., Theurillat, J.-P., ... Chin, L. (2012). A landscape of driver mutations in melanoma. *Cell, 150,* 251–263. doi:10.1016/j.cell.2012.06.024

Hong, D.I., Bankova, L., Cahill, K.N., Kyin, T., & Castells, M.C. (2012). Allergy to monoclonal antibodies: Cutting edge desensitization methods for cutting-edge therapies. *Expert Review of Clinical Immunology, 8,* 43–54. doi:10.1586/eci .11.75

Horsley, L., Marti, K., & Jayson, G.C. (2012). Is the toxicity of anti-angiogenic drugs predictive of outcome? A review of hypertension and proteinuria as biomarkers of response to anti-angiogenic therapy. *Expert Opinion on Drug Metabolism and Toxicology, 8,* 289–293. doi:10.1517/17425255.2012.656845

Iglehart, J.D., & Silver, D.P. (2009). Synthetic lethality—A new direction in cancer-drug development. *New England Journal of Medicine, 361,* 189–191. doi:10.1056/NEJMe0903044

ImClone LLC & Bristol-Myers Squibb Co. (2013). *Erbitux® (cetuximab)* [Package insert]. Branchburg, NJ: ImClone LLC.

Jain, P.K. (2001). Normalizing tumor vasculature with antiangiogenic therapy: A new paradigm for combination therapy. *Nature Medicine, 7,* 987–989.

Janssen Products, LP. (2013). *Doxil® (doxorubicin hydrochloride liposome injection)* [Package insert]. Horsham, PA: Author.

Kazar, M.W., & Harmon, A.S. (2011). Prostate cancer. In C.H. Yarbro, D. Wujcik, & B.H. Gobel (Eds.), *Cancer nursing: Principles and practice* (7th ed., pp. 1609–1633). Burlington, MA: Jones & Bartlett Learning.

LabCorp. (2013). *HER2 by dual ISH.* Retrieved from http://labcorp.com

Lacouture, M.E., Anadkat, M.J., Bensadoun, R.-J., Bryce, J., Chan, A., Epstein, J.B., ... MASCC Skin Toxicity Study Group. (2011). Clinical practice guidelines for the prevention and treatment of EGFR inhibitor-associated dermatologic toxicities. *Supportive Care in Cancer, 19,* 1079–1095. doi:10.1007/s00520-011-1197-6

Lacouture, M.E., Mitchell, E.P., Piperdi, B., Pillai, M.V., Shearer, H., Iannotti, N., ... Yassine, M. (2010). Skin Toxicity Evaluation Protocol With Panitumumab (STEPP), a phase II, open-label, randomized trial evaluating the impact of a pre-emptive skin treatment regimen on skin toxicities and quality of life in patients with metastatic colorectal cancer. *Journal of Clinical Oncology, 28,* 1351–1357. doi:10.1200/JCO.2008.21.7828

Loprinzi, C.L., Qin, R., Dakhil, S.R., Fehrenbacher, L., Flynn, K.A., Atherton, P., ... Grothey, A. (2014). Phase III randomized, placebo-controlled, double-blind study of intravenous calcium and magnesium to prevent oxaliplatin-induced sensory neurotoxicity (N08CB/Alliance). *Journal of Clinical Oncology, 32,* 997–1005. doi:10.1200/JCO.2013.52.0536

Lum, D.W.K., Perel, P., Hingorani, A.D., & Holmes, M.V. (2013). *CYP2D6* genotypes and tamoxifen response for breast cancer: A systematic review and meta-analysis. *PLOS ONE, 8*(10), e76648. doi:10.1371/journal.pone.0076648

Luoh, S.-W., Ramsey, B., Newell, A.H., Troxell, M., Hu, Z., Chin, K., … Keenan, E. (2013). HER-2 gene amplification in human breast cancer without concurrent HER-2 over-expression. *Springerplus, 2,* 386. doi:10.1186/2193-1801-2-386

Lynch, T.J., Jr., Kim, E.S., Eaby, B., Garey, J., West, D.P., & Lacouture, M.E. (2007). Epidermal growth factor receptor inhibitor–associated cutaneous toxicities: An evolving paradigm in clinical management. *Oncologist, 12,* 610–621. doi:10.1634/theoncologist.12-5-610

Melosky, B., Burkes, R., Rayson, D., Alcindor, T., Shear, N., & Lacouture, M. (2009). Management of skin rash during EGFR-targeted monoclonal antibody treatment for gastrointestinal malignancies: Canadian recommendations. *Current Oncology, 16*(1), 16–26.

Merck & Co., Inc. (2015). *Keytruda® (pembrolizumab)* [Package insert]. Whitehouse Station, NJ: Author.

Merkle, C.J. (2011). Biology of cancer. In C.H. Yarbro, D. Wujcik, & B.H. Gobel (Eds.), *Cancer nursing: Principles and practice* (7th ed., pp. 3–22). Burlington, MA: Jones & Bartlett Learning.

Mould, D.R., Fleming, G.F., Darcy, K.M., & Spriggs, D. (2006). Population analysis of a 24-h paclitaxel infusion in advanced endometrial cancer: A gynaecological oncology group study. *British Journal of Clinical Pharmacology, 62,* 56–70. doi:10.1111/j.1365-2125.2006.02718.x

Naidoo, J., Page, D.B., & Wolchok, J.D. (2014). Immune modulation for cancer therapy. *British Journal of Cancer, 111,* 2214–2219. doi:10.1038/bjc.2014.348

National Cancer Institute. (2013). Biological therapies for cancer. Retrieved from http://www.cancer.gov/cancertopics/factsheet/Therapy/biological

National Comprehensive Cancer Network. (2015). *NCCN Clinical Practice Guidelines in Oncology (NCCN Guidelines®): Breast cancer* [v.2.2015]. Retrieved from http://www.nccn.org/professionals/physician_gls/PDF/breast.pdf

National Institutes of Health. (2006). *The NCI strategic plan for leading the nation to eliminate the suffering and death due to cancer* (NIH Publication No. 06-5773). Washington, DC: Author.

Noble, D.J., & Donaldson, L.J. (2010). The quest to eliminate intrathecal vincristine errors: A 40-year journey. *Quality and Safety in Health Care, 19,* 323–326. doi:10.1136/qshc.2008.030874

Norton, L., & Simon, R. (1977). Tumor size, sensitivity to therapy, and design of treatment schedules. *Cancer Treatment Reports, 61,* 1307–1317.

Novartis Pharmaceuticals Corp. (2015a). *Gleevec® (imatinib mesylate)* [Package insert]. East Hanover, NJ: Author.

Novartis Pharmaceuticals Corp. (2015b). *Tasigna® (nilotinib)* [Package insert]. East Hanover, NJ: Author.

Pardoll, D.M. (2012). The blockade of immune checkpoints in cancer immunotherapy. *Nature Reviews Cancer, 12,* 252–264.

Perez, E.A., Suman, V.J., Davidson, N.E., Sledge, G.W., Kaufman, P.A., Hudis, C.A., … Rodeheffer, R.J. (2008). Cardiac safety analysis of doxorubicin and cyclophosphamide followed by paclitaxel with or without trastuzumab in the North Central Cancer Treatment Group N9831 adjuvant breast cancer trial *Journal of Clinical Oncology, 26,* 1231–1238. doi:10.1200/JCO.2007

Pfizer Labs. (2014a). *Bosulif® (bosutinib)* [Package insert]. New York, NY: Author.

Pfizer Labs. (2014b). *Inlyta® (axitinib)* [Package insert]. New York, NY: Author.

Pfizer Labs. (2014c). *Sutent® (sunitinib)* [Package insert]. New York, NY: Author.

Pfizer Labs. (2015). *Ibrance® (palbociclib)* [Package insert]. New York, NY: Author.

Pharmacia & Upjohn Co. (2014). *Camptosar® (irinotecan)* [Package insert]. New York, NY: Author.

Pharmacyclics, Inc., & Janssen Biotech, Inc. (2015). *Imbruvica® (ibrutinib)* [Package insert]. Sunnyvale, CA, & Horsham, PA: Authors.

Polovich, M. (Ed.). (2011). *Safe handling of hazardous drugs* (2nd ed.). Pittsburgh, PA: Oncology Nursing Society.

Polovich, M., Olsen, M., & LeFebvre, K.B. (Eds.). (2014). *Chemotherapy and biotherapy guidelines and recommendations for practice* (4th ed.). Pittsburgh, PA: Oncology Nursing Society.

Prometheus Laboratories, Inc. (2012). *Proleukin® (aldesleukin)* [Package insert]. San Diego, CA: Author.

Ramsey, S., Blough, D., Kirchhoff, A., Kreizenbeck, K., Fedorenko, C., Snell, K., … Overstreet, K. (2013). Washington State cancer patients found to be at greater risk for bankruptcy than people without a cancer diagnosis. *Health Affairs, 32,* 1143–1152. doi:10.1377/hlthaff.2012.1263

Ricke, R.M., & van Deursen, J.M. (2011). Correction of microtubule-kinetochore attachment errors: Mechanisms and role in tumor suppression. *Seminars in Cell and Developmental Biology, 22,* 559–565. doi:10.1016/j.semcdb.2011.03.007

Roberts, P.J., & Der, C.J. (2007). Targeting the Raf-MEK-ERK mitogen-activated protein kinase cascade for the treatment of cancer. *Oncogene, 26,* 3291–3310. doi:10.1038/sj.onc.1210422

Romond, E.H., Perez, E.A., Bryant, J., Suman, V.J., Geyer, C.E., Jr., Davidson, N.E., … Wolmark, N. (2005). Trastuzumab plus adjuvant chemotherapy for operable HER2-positive breast cancer. *New England Journal of Medicine, 353,* 1673–1684. doi:10.1056/NEJMoa052122

Rowinsky, E.K., Gilbert, M.R., McGuire, W.P., Noe, D.A., Grochow, L.B., Forastiere, A.A., … Sartorius, S.E. (1991). Sequences of taxol and cisplatin: A phase I and pharmacologic study. *Journal of Clinical Oncology, 9,* 1692–1703.

Sanofi-Aventis U.S. LLC. (2014). *Eloxatin® (oxaliplatin)* [Package insert]. Bridgewater, NJ: Author.

Sanofi-Aventis U.S. LLC & Regeneron Pharmaceuticals, Inc. (2014). *Zaltrap® (ziv-aflibercept)* [Package insert]. Bridgewater, NJ: Author.

Scott, A.M., Wolchok, J.D., & Old, L.J. (2012). Antibody therapy of cancer. *Nature Reviews Cancer, 12,* 278–287.

Seattle Genetics, Inc. (2014). *Adcetris® (brentuximab vedotin)* [Package insert]. Bothell, WA: Author.

Singh, M.S., Francis, P.A., & Michael, M. (2011). Tamoxifen, cytochrome P450 genes and breast cancer clinical outcomes. *Breast, 20,* 111–118. doi:10.1016/j.breast.2010.11.003

Skipper, H.E. (1971). Kinetics of mammary tumor cell growth and implications for therapy. *Cancer, 28,* 1479–1499. doi:10.1002/1097-0142(197112)28:6<1479::AID-CNCR2820280622>3.0.CO;2-M

Slamon, D., Eiermann, W., Robert, N., Pienkowski, T., Martin, M., Press, M., … Crown, J. (2011). Adjuvant trastuzumab in HER2-positive breast cancer. *New England Journal of Medicine, 365,* 1273–1283. doi:10.1056/NEJMoa0910383

Slamon, D., Eiermann, W., Robert, N., Pienkowski, T., Martin, M., Rolski, J., … Crown, J. (2009). Phase III randomized trial comparing doxorubicin and cyclophosphamide followed by docetaxel (AC→T) with doxorubicin and cyclophosphamide followed by docetaxel and trastuzumab (AC→TH) with docetaxel, carboplatin and trastuzumab (TCH) in Her2neu positive early breast cancer patients: BCIRG 006 study. *Cancer Research, 69*(24, Suppl. 3), Abstract 62. doi:10.1158/0008-5472.SABCS-09-62

Sliwkowski, M.X., Lofgren, J.A., Lewis, G.D., Hotaling, T.E., Fendly, B.M., & Fox, J.A. (1999). Nonclinical studies addressing the mechanism of action of trastuzumab (Herceptin). *Seminars in Oncology, 26*(4, Suppl. 12), 60–70.

Sparreboom, A., van Zuylen, L., Brouwer, E., Loos, W.J., de Bruijn, P., Gelderblom, H., … Verweij, J. (1999). Cremophor EL-mediated alteration of paclitaxel distribution in human blood: Clinical pharmacokinetic implications. *Cancer Research, 59,* 1454–1457. Retrieved from http://cancerres.aacrjournals.org/content/59/7/1454.long

Suter, T.M., Procter, M., van Veldhuisen, D.J., Muscholl, M., Bergh, J., Carlomagno, C., … Piccart-Gebhart, M.J. (2007). Trastuzumab-associated cardiac adverse effects in the Herceptin Adjuvant trial. *Journal of Clinical Oncology, 25,* 3859–3865. doi:10.1200/JCO.2006.09.1611

Swain, S.M., Kim, S.B., Cortes, J., Ro, J., Semiglazov, V., Campone, M., … Baselga, J. (2013). Pertuzumab, trastuzumab and docetaxel for HER2-positive metastatic breast cancer (CLEOPATRA study): Overall survival results from a randomized, double-blind placebo-controlled, phase 3 study. *Lancet Oncology, 14,* 461–471. doi:10.1016/S1470-2045(13)70130-X

Tan-Chiu, E., Yothers, G., Romond, E., Geyer, C.E., Jr., Ewer, M., Keefe, D., … Bryant, J. (2005). Assessment of cardiac dysfunction in a randomized trial comparing doxorubicin and cyclophosphamide followed by paclitaxel, with or without trastuzumab as adjuvant therapy in node-positive, human epidermal growth factor receptor 2-overexpressing breast cancer: NSABP B-31. *Journal of Clinical Oncology, 23,* 7811–7819. doi:10.1200/JCO.2005.02.4091

Teva Pharmaceuticals USA, Inc. (2014). *Synribo® (omacetaxine mepesuccinate)* [Package insert]. North Wales, PA: Author.

Verma, S., Miles, D., Gianni, L., Krop, I.E., Welslau, M., Baselga, J., … Blackwell, K. (2012). Trastuzumab emtansine for HER2-positive advanced breast cancer. *New England Journal of Medicine, 367,* 1783–1791. doi:10.1056/NEJMoa1209124

Vogelstein, B., Sur, S., & Prives, C. (2010). p53: The most frequently altered gene in human cancers. *Nature Education, 3*(9), 6. Retrieved from http://www.nature.com/scitable/topicpage/p53-the-most-frequently-altered-gene-in-14192717

Von Eschenbach, A.C. (2006). Progress with a purpose: Eliminating suffering and death due to cancer. *Oncology, 20,* 1691–1696. Retrieved from http://www.cancernetwork.com/oncology-journal/progress-purpose-eliminating-suffering-and-death-due-cancer

Von Minckwitz, G., Zielinski, C., Maarteense, E., Vogel, P., Schmidt, M., Eidtmann, H., … Loibl, S. (2008). Capecitabine vs. capecitabine + trastuzumab in patients with HER2-positive metastatic breast cancer progressing during trastuzumab treatment: The TBP phase III study (GBG 26/BIG3-05). *Journal of Clinical Oncology, 26*(Suppl. 15), Abstract 1025. Retrieved from http://meeting.ascopubs.org/cgi/content/short/26/15_suppl/1025

Walko, C.M., & McLeod, H. (2009). Pharmacogenomic progress in individualized dosing of key drugs for cancer patients. *Nature Clinical Practice Oncology, 6,* 153–162. doi:10.1038/ncponc1303

Weinberg, R.A. (2013). *The biology of cancer* (2nd ed.). New York, NY: Garland Science/Taylor & Francis.

Wilkes, G.M. (2011a). Chemotherapy administration. In C.H. Yarbro, D. Wujcik, & B.H. Gobel (Eds.), *Cancer nursing: Principles and practice* (7th ed., pp. 390–458). Burlington, MA: Jones & Bartlett Learning.

Wilkes, G.M. (2011b). *Targeted cancer therapy: A handbook for nurses.* Burlington, MA: Jones & Bartlett Learning.

Woods, M.L., Lech, T., & Fadol, A.P. (2013). Hypertension in patients with cancer. In A.P. Fadol (Ed.), *Cardiac complications of cancer therapy* (pp. 95–107). Pittsburgh, PA: Oncology Nursing Society.

CHAPTER 5

Surgery

Joanne Lester, PhD, CNP, ANP-BC, AOCN®

Introduction

Surgical oncology is a branch of health care that deals with the management and eradication of malignant neoplasms. Surgery as an intervention is the oldest treatment modality for cancer and remains a primary intervention for patients with solid tumors. Adequate surgical resection of malignant tumors is an essential strategy in the treatment of cancer (Lochan, French, & Manas, 2011).

Surgical oncology involves the early detection and prevention of cancer occurrence, diagnosis of a primary or metastatic site, surgical resection as a primary or secondary treatment, postoperative care, surgical access for administration of therapy, rehabilitation with reconstructive procedures, surveillance for recurrence and second primaries, and palliation with symptom management. Oncologic emergencies also may necessitate a surgical procedure for resolution. Surgical oncology, medical and radiation oncology, and interventional radiology constitute the framework of the oncology healthcare team. Advanced practice nurses (APNs) are integral members of this team throughout the cancer trajectory and use evidence-based practice for nursing-sensitive patient outcomes in symptom management.

This chapter outlines current surgical oncology evidence-based interventions and the management of common cancers. It discusses innovative interventional radiology techniques and minimally invasive surgical procedures that provide the same level of surgical care as traditional open surgeries without large incisions, prolonged hospitalizations, and immobility.

Oncologic Surgical Strategies

Surgery is central to patient care and provides strategic interventions for cancer prevention, diagnosis, resection, postoperative care, access, rehabilitation, surveillance, and palliation (see Figure 5-1). The surgical healthcare team consists of physicians, APNs, RNs, ancillary staff, and support personnel. This team is a common thread throughout the cancer trajectory, offering expert assessment, psychosocial support, education, symptom management, and prevention of complications.

The *prevention* of cancer in high-risk patients results from improvements in the understanding of cancer biology with more effective risk assessments, early detection, screening, and potentially lifesaving interventions, including prophylactic surgical procedures. The sur-

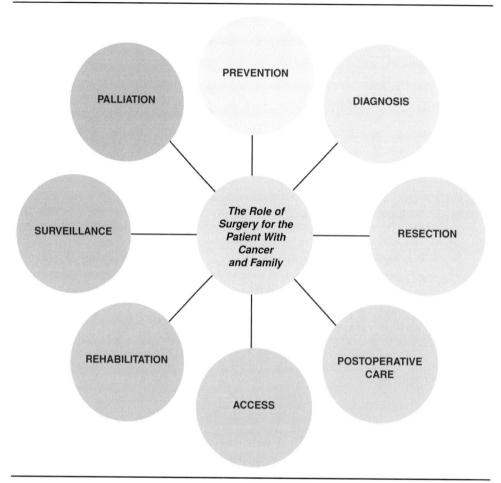

Figure 5-1. Surgical Interventions in Cancer Care

gical *diagnosis* of cancer employs innovative techniques that can identify early-stage cancers, which may improve the chances for cure. The surgical *resection* of cancer allows for removal of cancerous tissue and accurate pathologic staging of disease. Less-invasive surgical procedures are possible because of advances in bioengineering and biotechnology and use of interventional radiology techniques, laparoscopic approaches, and innovations such as robotic surgery.

Postoperative care involves maintenance or reestablishment of homeostasis, with prevention of complications related to surgical intervention. Surgically implanted *access* devices provide necessary routes for nutrition, medications, and chemotherapy while affording additional comfort to the patient. *Rehabilitation* after the cancer diagnosis employs surgical procedures that repair or reconstruct to enhance function and well-being. *Surveillance* of patients with cancer and their families provide screening and periodic observation to detect recurrent cancer, hereditary syndromes, or subsequent primary cancers. Finally, surgical *palliation* uses interventions in tumor control and symptom management for patients with recurrent or metastatic disease or in cancers that challenge a curative surgical approach.

This model of integrated surgical oncologic care, as illustrated in Figure 5-1, is an effective framework that promotes collaborative relationships between APNs and other members of the surgical oncology healthcare team (hereafter, *surgical team*). These strategies, as applied to the surgical trajectory, may undergo expansion, repetition, reversal, or omission based on individual characteristics of patients and families. APN interventions in colorectal cancer illustrate application of the model (see Table 5-1).

Prevention and Early Detection

The surgical team often is involved in the screening, early detection, and prevention of cancer. A thorough medical history is important to obtain information that can reduce or con-

Table 5-1. Advanced Practice Nursing Surgical Interventions in Colorectal Cancer

Cancer Trajectory	Education	Management
Prevention	Identification of risk factors and behaviors, family history, genetic risk, and screening practices	Evaluation of risk factors and behaviors, colonoscopy, genetic counseling, dietary interventions, and control of coexisting colorectal disease
Diagnosis	Ordering the required testing to obtain specimen; identification of location and extent of disease	Assessment of signs and symptoms of colorectal disease, appropriate workup with colonoscopy, and radiology studies and computed tomography to rule out metastatic disease
Resection	Determination of the extent of disease, surgical intervention for staging and resection, pain management, cardiac/pulmonary toilet, type of surgery, ostomy potential, postoperative care, home care, and adjuvant therapies	Preoperative assessment with surgical clearance, role of neoadjuvant therapy, perioperative management of body systems and homeostasis, postoperative management to prevent infection and maximize outcomes, consultation with dietitian and enterostomal therapist (if necessary), determination of disease stage, and adjuvant therapy
Access	Venous access for chemotherapy and/or gut access for nutrition	Assessment of venous access and options for therapy, and nutritional needs related to oral intake/gut absorption
Rehabilitation	Ostomy care and reversal, dietary habits, colon function, postchemotherapy/postradiation care	Assessment of current status, possible ostomy reversal, enterostomal and skin care, elimination patterns, and coping mechanisms
Surveillance	Lifetime recommendations, follow-up care, and family history implications	Appropriate screening and colonoscopy schedule, assessment of current status, symptoms, preventive healthcare maintenance, and screening of family members
Palliation	Diagnosis of recurrent disease, pain and symptom management, nutritional status, and end-of-life issues	Assessment of signs and symptoms of recurrent disease, and pain and symptom management

Note. Based on information from Lester, 2011.

trol comorbid conditions. An accurate personal and family history identifies patterns related to familial and genetic predispositions and may indicate the need for genetic counseling referrals. Information about health behaviors, risks, and personal habits can target behaviors that may affect cancer occurrence, such as smoking, alcohol intake, dietary patterns, and exercise habits. Discussion of risk-reduction strategies enables adjustment of behaviors to reduce the overall cancer risk (Liverani, 2013).

Routine screening practices potentially reduce the incidence, morbidity, and mortality of common cancers such as breast, cervical, colorectal, prostate, and skin. Primary or secondary investigation of the absence or presence of cancer can involve physical examination, radiographic and serum studies, screening interventions (such as colonoscopy), and tissue sampling (Green, 2013). Screening for asymptomatic or unrecognized cancers and subsequent evaluation of abnormal screening results often are responsibilities of the surgical team (Lambert, 2012). Surgeons frequently are the primary provider of health care, especially in otherwise healthy patients. As such, the APN can conduct these healthy surgical visits, with discussion about genetic risk factors and potential occurrence of related cancers.

Another fundamental responsibility of the surgical team is individual risk assessment with evaluation of patient eligibility for prophylactic surgical interventions. Patients identified as having a significantly increased risk of cancers such as testicular, colon, thyroid, breast, and ovarian may benefit from removal of the nonvital organ. In-depth discussion about the cancer risk and comparison to the risk and morbidity of surgery often arises (Borreani et al., 2014); the surgical oncology APN can be a vital link between the patient and surgeon during these difficult and prolonged discussions. Possible chemoprevention strategies also deserve exploration and discussion. The surgical team needs to remain current with the evidence about chemoprevention to help patients and families discern between proven interventions and those that require further study (Morris et al., 2013). These surgical and chemoprevention strategies must be tailored to the specific cancer and individual based on the patient's personal health history, risk profile, lifestyle, goals, and available options.

Early detection and prevention strategies provide unique opportunities for involvement of APNs in surgical oncology clinics. Discussion of personal risk profiles with avoidance of risky behaviors requires time, a reasonable plan of action, and subsequent evaluation. Detailed documentation of historical events is vital for accurate individual assessment of the relative and actual risks of cancer development (Brock, Wallace, Romagnuolo, & Hoffman, 2013). Often, repetitive and reframed questions are required to provide clarification. A prime example lies in patient descriptions of gynecologic cancers (e.g., confusion regarding the distinction between cervical intraepithelial neoplasia, cervical cancer, uterine cancer, and ovarian cancer). Obtaining a copy of the pathology reports for placement in the patient's medical record is ideal.

Diagnosis

A confirmatory diagnosis of cancer relies on tissue acquisition for pathologic, cytologic, and possibly histologic review. When a malignancy is suspected, consultation with the surgical team typically occurs. A potential cancer diagnosis must be distinguished from other diseases, with a systematic comparison of signs and symptoms. Information obtained from an individualized approach with review of documented history, physical examination, objective observation, radiology and laboratory review, and patient subjective interview is invaluable. This prediagnostic summary guides the development of the surgical plan for appropriate tissue acquisition.

Knowledge about the natural history of various cancers and their presentation is integral to the differential diagnosis process and appropriate workup (Bednar, Scheiman, McKenna, &

Simeone, 2013). After the initial consultation, the surgical team discusses the suspected cancer origin, appropriate type of biopsy, timing, and further staging. If another discipline, such as radiology, receives the diagnostic consult, clinicians must be sure to apply this same scrutiny to the overall diagnostic assessment. APNs are often the coordinators of care, providing continuity between services and relaying updates to patients and families.

A variety of biopsy techniques are available that can provide sufficient tissue for the pathologic and histologic diagnosis of a suspected cancer (see Table 5-2). The surgical team selects the appropriate tissue sampling technique based on information gained from the initial con-

Table 5-2. Biopsy Techniques

Biopsy Type	Advantages	Disadvantages	Common Cancer Use
Fine needle aspiration biopsy • Obtains cellular material with 20- or 21-gauge needle and syringe	Is easy for patients Can be performed in ambulatory setting/office Requires minimal preparation Is less invasive Is inexpensive Produces quick results Leaves no scar Can be done with ultrasound guidance Can be performed with local skin/tissue anesthesia Allows patients to resume activities immediately	Can be painful Requires experienced practitioners and pathologists Yields minimal pathologic information, as it is based on cellular material only Can cause development of problematic hematoma at biopsy site May still require core needle or open biopsy	Palpable masses Breast masses Skin lesions Palpable lymph nodes in neck, clavicle, and axillae Groin areas
Core needle biopsy • Obtains core(s) of tissue via spring-loaded device with 14- or 16-gauge core of tissue Stereotactic biopsy • Obtains core(s) of tissue using stereotactic machine via 12- or 14-gauge needle; usually vacuum-assisted Vacuum-assisted core needle biopsy • Uses suction through probe to draw multiple samples of tissue	Can be used on palpable masses Is somewhat easy for patients Can be performed in ambulatory setting/office Requires minimal preparation Is less invasive Is less expensive Leaves only a tiny nick/scar Retractable needle contains tissue fragments Can be performed by several disciplines Can be combined with radiographic guidance, including ultrasound, magnetic resonance imaging (MRI), computed tomography, or stereotactic imaging Provides pathologic and histologic information Can be performed with local skin/tissue anesthesia Allows patients to resume activities the next day	Can be painful Can be performed as a "procedure only" by other disciplines without evaluation or examination of patients Can cause development of problematic hematoma at biopsy site Requires removal of needle track if malignant May still require open biopsy Stereotactic biopsy of the breast requires prone position.	Palpable soft tissue masses Breast masses, microcalcifications Prostate masses Brain lesions Palpable lymph nodes

(Continued on next page)

Table 5-2. Biopsy Techniques *(Continued)*

Biopsy Type	Advantages	Disadvantages	Common Cancer Use
Mammotome® • Obtains core(s) of tissue using stereotactic guidance via vacuum-assisted device that rotates and cuts tissue	Is fairly easy for patients Can be performed in ambulatory setting/office Is less invasive Leaves a small scar with one or more sutures Needle contains tissue Can be performed by several disciplines Can be performed with ultrasound, mammography, or MRI Provides pathologic and histologic information Allows small lesions/nodules to be completely removed Can be performed with local skin/tissue anesthesia Allows patients to resume activities the next day	Can be painful Can be performed as a "procedure only" by other disciplines without evaluation or examination of patients Can cause development of problematic hematoma at biopsy site Requires removal of needle track if malignant May still require an open biopsy for margins Is an understudied procedure for breast cancer removal (i.e., without additional surgery)	Breast masses, microcalcifications
Incisional biopsy • Removes part of tumor mass via small skin incision	Can be performed on an outpatient basis or, less often, in the office Provides pathologic and histologic information Can be performed with local skin/tissue anesthesia Can be performed with flexible fiber-optic instrument	Is more involved for patients Can be painful Is more invasive Requires small incision/ leaves scar with sutures May require sedation or anesthesia Is not intended to obtain clean margin of tissue Will require further treatment if malignant May delay patients' return to daily activities	Any mass
Excisional biopsy • Removes all of tumor mass via small skin incision Needle localization • Uses tiny wire with hooked end to mark nonpalpable masses for open biopsy	Can be performed on an outpatient basis/same-day surgery Provides pathologic and histologic information Can be performed under local skin/tissue anesthesia Can be performed with flexible fiber-optic instrument	Is more involved for patients Can be painful Is more invasive Requires small incision/ leaves scar with sutures May require sedation or anesthesia Will require further treatment if malignant Is not intended to obtain clean margin of tissue May delay patients' return to daily activities	Any mass

Note. Based on information from Atkins et al., 2013; Bugalho et al., 2013; Chen, H.-J., et al., 2013; James et al., 2014; Jurado et al., 2013; Masroor et al., 2012; Tryggvason et al., 2013.

sultation. A fine needle aspiration (FNA) biopsy, using a 20-gauge needle and a 10 ml syringe, can obtain cells from a palpable mass for identification of the presence or absence of malignant cells in the sample. FNA does not indicate histologic differences necessary for treatment; therefore, patients typically require a more definitive tissue biopsy. Procurement of additional pathologic markers may be imperative, such as when neoadjuvant chemotherapy is under consideration, to obtain adequate information for cancer care throughout the trajectory. A larger-gauge core needle biopsy (CNB) may be an appropriate method to obtain additional tissue that provides a diagnosis with histologic detail. The benefits of needle biopsy include easy access, minimal or no scarring, and minimal discomfort. When performed by a skillful clinician, needle biopsies are reliable methods of obtaining tissue to begin the diagnostic process (James, Mace, Virnig, & Geller, 2012; Tryggvason et al., 2013).

All needle biopsies carry a word of caution: a negative biopsy reading obtained by FNA or CNB does not ensure a benign lesion. If a lesion is highly suspect for malignancy and a needle biopsy yields negative or inconclusive results, another technique or open biopsy is necessary to obtain enough tissue to verify a diagnosis (Bugalho et al., 2013). In the case of precursor neoplastic findings, as in lobular carcinoma in situ of the breast, a needle biopsy is insufficient for diagnosis and management. A follow-up surgical excision removes additional tissue for pathologic examination to exclude adjacent malignant cells (Atkins, Cohen, Nicholson, & Rao, 2013).

Intraluminal access to specific areas and tissues provides additional portals of entry to acquire tissue for biopsies and include the mouth, urethra, and anus. Sites accessible through the mouth include the posterior pharynx and larynx, bronchi, esophagus, stomach, and small intestine. Sites accessible through the anus include the prostate, colon, and rectum, whereas the urethra provides access to the bladder and ureters. These luminal openings are typically accessed by general or specialty surgeons with rigid or flexible thin tubes with lighted ends (Jurado et al., 2013; McWilliams, Shaipanich, & Lam, 2013; Siddiqui et al., 2013).

Open biopsies, otherwise known as incisional or excisional, are performed through a skin incision and are used in certain masses relative to size, location, and the suspected malignancy type. An incisional biopsy removes part of the visible mass for pathologic review, whereas an excisional biopsy removes visible components of the mass in its entirety. Imaging studies may be of benefit to localize lesions, especially in the case of nonpalpable lesions or areas of microcalcification in the breast (Gumus et al., 2013). Needle localization biopsy combines radiographic guidance with a small gauge and flexible wire to isolate the lesion or area of concern. Radiology guidance may be done through ultrasound, mammography, computed tomography, or magnetic resonance imaging, depending on the location of the suspect lesion, ease of access, and anticipated accuracy (Masroor, Afzal, Shafqat, & Rehman, 2012). Preoperative placement of a thin needle relative to the area of concern marks the site to be biopsied. As the placement needle is withdrawn, a fine wire with a hooked end remains to localize the area or mass of concern that requires tissue sampling. Wire removal occurs at the time of biopsy; the wire typically is attached to the biopsy specimen as it exits the body.

All tissue biopsies, whether performed by the surgical or interventional radiology teams, require adherence to the following principles in anticipation of identification of a malignancy: (a) mark a suitable anatomic plane and position for needle tracks and incisions before tissue removal, (b) avoid contamination of adjacent tissue planes, (c) avoid hematoma formation by providing adequate hemostasis, (d) meticulously mark the orientation of the specimen to ensure proper identification of tissue fragments, and (e) obtain adequate tissue for subsequent clinical or surgical decision making (Chen, H.-J., et al., 2013). Lack of attention to these details can be deleterious to the patient and can create situations that may compromise decision making throughout the cancer trajectory (James et al., 2012).

APNs, depending on the practice setting, may select the biopsy type and approach, arrange the procedure, and assist with the biopsy. They may even perform less-invasive biopsies such as FNA, CNB, and punch biopsy, depending on institutional and state regulatory guidelines (Schramp, Holtcamp, Phillips, Johnson, & Hoff, 2010). Prior to assuming this independent role, the nurse must meet core competencies, including performing an agreed-upon number of mentored procedures without complication. Communication between the surgical team and radiology is essential, along with possible concomitant radiology film review for clarification. Often, APNs bridge this gap with knowledge about the clinical and radiographic presentation of the patient.

Pathology and Staging

Correlation of the pathologic information obtained from the tissue biopsy with radiology studies, physical examination, and the patient's history is crucial to accurate identification of a malignancy. The surgical team often performs this critical role to establish an accurate, site-specific diagnosis. If further clarification is warranted, additional testing or tissue sampling may be necessary. APNs employ intuitive skills to assemble the diagnostic pieces of cancer presentations, such as in the preparation of clinically relevant cases for tumor board meetings (Lamb et al., 2013).

Clinical Stage

The healthcare team assesses the presenting clinical stage using professional judgment, physical examination and assessment, and radiologic reports to determine clinical evidence of malignancy at the primary or metastatic site(s) and estimate the size (Leibovici et al., 2013). All malignancies, regardless of planned surgical interventions, have an initial intuitive "clinical" estimation of stage. This clinical stage is particularly prudent when administration of neoadjuvant chemotherapy precedes definitive surgery. APNs, as clinical providers, often are responsible for accurate documentation of clinical stage prior to and throughout neoadjuvant therapy. (Chapter 3 provides in-depth staging information.)

Upon completion of neoadjuvant therapy, primary surgical removal of the tumor typically occurs with pathologic examination of excised tissue. If a complete remission has occurred (i.e., no pathologic evidence of malignancy exists in tissue removed from the primary and/or regional nodal surgical sites), the clinical stage may stand as the only means of documentation of the presenting cancer stage (Chen, K., et al., 2013). True pathologic staging cannot occur, as the specimen may show limited evidence of disease. An accurate clinical stage prior to and during neoadjuvant therapy is essential to provide the most accurate estimation of disease stage, as this often is the only accurate staging measurement (De Nardi & Carvello, 2013).

Surgical Staging

Surgical staging is an invasive assessment using laparoscopic or open surgical procedures that enable the surgeon to visualize structures, assess the visible extent of disease, and obtain necessary tissue for pathologic examination. The surgical team assesses the cancer from a surgical standpoint, noting tumor size, enlarged lymph nodes, and possible metastatic sites. All surgically removed tissue undergoes pathologic examination. Adequate tissue sampling must occur for the pathologist to derive the most accurate pathologic stage of the tumor. Surgical oncology APNs, armed with clinical and surgical staging assessments, must verify that the pathology team receives patients' identifying information and tissue.

Pathologic Staging

Pathologic staging derives its information from gross and microscopic examination of provided tissue. Pathologic staging defines a cancer as related to the organ or organs of origin, stating the tumor size, lymph node status, and metastatic sites. Additional histologic data, including differentiation, mitotic rate, receptors, and special stains, often are requisite to a better understanding of the biology of the specific cancer.

Ideally, surgical and pathologic staging correlate, thus validating that excision of all suspicious sites occurred with subsequent pathologic examination. The surgical team is responsible for marking tissue with regard to orientation and margins. At some institutions, the pathologist enters the operating room to view and receive the tissue specimens and to verify orientation of the specimen with the surgeon.

Ultimately, the site or origin of the malignancy and information derived from clinical, surgical, and pathologic staging provide the information needed to devise, or revise, the treatment plan (Poullis et al., 2012). Additional surgery may be necessary to secure clear tissue margins around the primary or metastatic site. Surgical oncology APNs must be familiar with cancer types and staging, including an understanding of tumor markers and characteristics as well as possible sites of metastasis. Identification of metastatic disease in another organ or distant organs may alter the treatment plan, but the malignancy retains the original pathologic diagnosis (Peck, Hitchcock, Maguire, Dickerson, & Bush, 2012). For example, lung cancer (that originates in the lung) is a "lung cancer." Lung cancer that metastasizes to the liver pathologically remains a "lung cancer"; it does not become "liver cancer." Therefore, pathologic examination of a cancerous lesion in the liver can essentially confirm a primary lung cancer diagnosis. This concept often is confusing to patients and families and requires explanation and education from the APN to avoid misinterpretation of information.

Oncogene Typing

Oncogene typing can provide adjunct information to the pathologic findings, thereby allowing for improved stratification of prognostic factors. This study of gene expression in combination with clinical markers and biomarkers can suggest potential target genes for treatment, as well as aid in the prediction of progression of the cancer and clinical outcomes. Subsequently, systemic treatments may be individually tailored, with avoidance of over- or undertreatment of patients (Litsas, 2013). Surgical APNs must be familiar with the basic concepts of the rapidly expanding field of oncogene typing, as this information may guide treatment decisions (Bardhan & Liu, 2013; Ghigna, Riva, & Biamonti, 2013; Lane, Segura-Cabrera, & Komurov, 2014; West et al., 2012).

Staging Systems

The tumor-node-metastasis (TNM) anatomic system from the American Joint Committee on Cancer and the Surveillance, Epidemiology, and End Results Program reports the pathologic staging of tumors based on tissue received by the pathologist. The TNM system divides cancers into stages with numeric markings of 0–IV. In this system, higher numbers indicate more disease. Unfortunately, no standardized system exists that includes all tumor characteristics such as histologic grade, estrogen and progesterone receptors, HER2/neu status, biologic markers, and molecular and genetic information, which are all inherent to definitive staging with accurate prognostic outcomes (Boyce, Fan, Watson, & Murphy, 2013; Smith, Nelson, & Schwarz, 2014). Astute clinicians must carefully combine all information to create a prognostic profile, as the TNM system cannot fulfill this requirement in current cancer care. Ongoing clinical trials will aid in the establishment of future staging systems (Schmitt, Brewer, Bordeaux, & Baum, 2014). Chapter 3 provides further information on diagnosis and staging.

Role of Advanced Practice Nurses

APNs often are the team members who explain these difficult concepts to surgical patients and their families to promote understanding of the disease process and treatment. The presumed tumor stage stated at the initial consultation may change based on final pathologic findings. Previously discussed treatment plans may be altered, resulting in confusion and frustration for patients and families. APNs provide continuity and reassurance throughout this difficult and stressful time.

Surgical APNs must be knowledgeable about related modalities of cancer therapy to teach and inform patients and families of all available treatment options that may, in turn, influence their decision-making processes. Certain cancer types have a planned trajectory with few options. Other cancer types, such as breast cancer, have multiple options that require continuing explanation to enable an informed patient choice (Gojon, Fawunmi, & Valachis, 2014). Treatment options may require modification for older adult patients (Palmeri, Berretta, & Palmeri, 2013).

Surgical APNs may facilitate interdisciplinary consultations or case conference discussions necessary for disease or health status evaluation. They often become an "interpreter" for both healthcare professionals and patients because they are frequently the closest provider to patients with biologic and psychosocial data. APNs are patient advocates and navigators who provide the continuity that patients and families seek as they strive to synthesize massive amounts of information resulting in difficult treatment decisions (Trossman, 2013).

The surgical treatment of cancer involves decision making on the part of the patient as well as the surgical team. Patients require information about cancer risk or a specific cancer, with the related treatment trajectory, anticipated outcome, and long-term prognosis. Involvement of the patient's family and support system is inherent to achieving successful outcomes, including discharge planning and short- and long-term care. Explanations about possible neoadjuvant or adjuvant therapies are important to patients, as they may be unaware of the concept of micrometastasis or the potential need for further surgery to determine the type or extent of systemic treatment (Gojon et al., 2014). APNs play vital roles as patient navigators, educators, and advocates during this difficult process in an effort to personalize the survivor's trajectory (Hoppo & Jobe, 2013; Trossman, 2013).

Preoperative Phase

Surgical resection is an integral part of solid tumor treatment. Additional modalities, such as radiation, chemotherapy, and biologic therapies, may be administered at the time of surgery to increase their individual and synergistic therapeutic effects (Shylasree, Bryant, & Athavale, 2013; Zaorsky, Trabulsi, Lin, & Den, 2013). The potential combinations of cancer modalities and their approach for each cancer type are too lengthy to list given the variability of host factors, tumor types, and tumor characteristics. These potential treatment combinations are specific to individual solid tumor types but share the same overall principles of surgical resection and local tumor control that are inherent in the treatment of solid tumors with systemic treatment (Shylasree et al., 2013). Marrow tumors, such as lymphoma and leukemia classifications, seldom use surgery as the primary interventional treatment because of the characteristics inherent to these tumor types. Nevertheless, a role for surgery does exist for marrow tumors, including access device placement and palliative surgical interventions for symptom management (Bagga, Yapa, Craven, Romanowski, & Jellinek, 2013).

The goals of cancer surgical therapy should be reviewed with patients and families. These goals include (a) maximizing potential for control or cure of cancer, (b) minimizing comorbidities, and (c) retaining active participation of patients and families (Rizk, 2013). A cancer diagnosis is challenging in itself, but the enormous amount of information given in a short time span by multiple providers can be even more difficult for patients and family members to manage as they prepare for surgical intervention. APNs play a pivotal role in maintaining the balance of these three goals and are the constant throughout the patient's disease course. Involvement of primary care providers is inherent to a coordinated approach (Hudson, 2013).

Preoperative Assessment

Preoperative assessment and evaluation are important for the safe completion of the surgical intervention and a decrease in postoperative complications. The surgical team determines the operative risk and weighs the potential benefits against the risks of cancer-related surgical interventions, with examination of past and current health history and current physical status. Surgery is demanding of the body's homeostatic mechanisms. Identification and resolution of problems that may increase morbidity and mortality risk are essential to optimal outcomes. Attention to concomitant diagnoses and comorbid conditions is an important component of efficient, effective surgical care. Consultations with other services, such as cardiology, pulmonology, or endocrinology, are best done in the preoperative phase, prior to the stress of surgery. If the benefits of surgery outweigh the identified risks, a thorough preoperative workup alerts the anesthesia and surgical teams to possible difficulties during the intra- and postoperative periods (Kwaan et al., 2013). Geriatric considerations include safety issues, functional status, frailty, medications, and comorbid conditions and must be assessed prior to surgery to enhance outcomes (Dale et al., 2014; Revenig et al., 2013). APNs play a critical role in patient evaluation as well as in communication within and between teams.

Attention to preexisting medical conditions with possible adverse outcomes is crucial in the preoperative evaluation. APNs are frequently participating members of the preoperative evaluation and must perform a thorough assessment that includes previous medical, surgical, and psychosocial histories; nutritional status; medications; laboratory and imaging studies; and teaching needs. Appropriate management of comorbid diseases, especially those related to mental health, endocrinology disease or diabetes, heart disease, or pulmonary, renal, and gastrointestinal function, as well as safety issues, must occur concomitantly with cancer care. The Surgical Care Improvement Project includes core measures with evidence-based surgical interventions monitored by the Joint Commission (2014): broad-spectrum prophylactic antibiotics within one hour of surgical incision and discontinuation within 24 hours following surgery; close glucose monitoring with 6 am sample on postoperative day 1; avoidance of preoperative hair removal with a razor; removal of urinary catheters on postoperative day 1 or 2 when able; maintenance of perioperative core temperature with warming blankets; administration of beta-blockers the morning of surgery and repeated in the perioperative phase; and implementation of venous thromboembolic prophylaxis measures with lower limb compression pumps and anticoagulant prophylaxis with heparin or low-molecular-weight blood thinners.

Statistics provide evidence that certain comorbid conditions may increase the risk of adverse events during the surgical procedure as well as during the postoperative period (Robinson et al., 2013). In general, a personal history of congestive heart failure leads to an increase in hospital stay, and a history of hypertension confers a twofold increase in the intraoperative risk of a cardiac event. A history of asthma is associated with a fivefold increase in the risk of respiratory events, such as bronchospasms, and smoking is responsible for a fourfold increase in postoperative respiratory difficulties. Obesity is responsible for a fourfold increase in intraoperative and postoperative respiratory events, and a history of uncontrolled reflux allows for an eightfold increase in intubation events, including aspiration (Amri, Bordeianou, Sylla, & Berger, 2014). APNs are responsible for obtaining a thorough history and physical and have the opportunity to improve a patient's outcome from surgery with consideration of the aforementioned criteria. Comorbid conditions must be medically controlled to prevent additional complications; if not, the surgery may be postponed until greater control is achieved.

Preoperative Assessment of Infection Risk

Surgical site infection (SSI) is a major cause of patient morbidity and mortality, as well as increased healthcare costs and length of hospital stay. Several factors create the infection matrix, including the patient's health status, the physical environment of the surgery, clinical risks, patient selection, preparation for surgery, antibiotic prophylaxis, hand hygiene of the surgical team, and the facility's use of universal precautions. Bacterial sources can be endogenous or exogenous, with a myriad of potential carriers. APNs are responsible for preemptively identifying infection risk factors and for preventing or eliminating as many of these factors as possible.

Critical examination of the clinical risks of infection relative to each patient is important to predict potential infection risk (Itatsu et al., 2014; Ortega-Deballon et al., 2014). Review of concomitant illnesses or diagnoses, age, preoperative nutritional status, and smoking habits provides baseline information that allows APNs to intervene. Suboptimal nutritional states increase the risk of infection (Hennessey et al., 2010). Nutritional supplements and possibly enteral feedings may be necessary to prepare the body for surgery and to improve nitrogen balance and protein stores. Patients suffering from significant malnutrition caused by a catabolic state or inability to ingest adequate nutrition may require parenteral feedings prior to a major surgery (Shinkawa et al., 2013). Control of metabolic disease, such as diabetes, is imperative in order to arm the body with necessary defenses (Schroeder, 2014). Tight control of serum blood sugars with sliding-scale insulin may improve the infection threshold (Kiran, Turina, Hammel, & Fazio, 2013). Attention to drug use, especially recent chemotherapy, chronic steroid use, and immunosuppressive drugs, may offer additional avenues for intervention (Schroeder, 2014). Although smoking cessation is desired, abstinence from smoking for as little as one week before surgery can make a positive impact on tissue oxygenation (Mills et al., 2011). Appropriate preoperative skin and bowel preparations reduce bacterial flora, especially endogenous bacteria. Avoidance of a preoperative admission may decrease nosocomial bacterial exposure, as the rate of nosocomial infections is reduced in same-day admissions versus preoperative admissions to the hospital unit (Kiran et al., 2013).

Review of the patient's health status and personal hygiene habits with a focus on potential acute and chronic infections may identify additional interventions. Appropriate antibiotic use preoperatively for acute infection can reduce bacterial load and potentially eliminate postoperative infection from host bacteria. Cultures of acute infection and serum titers of administered antibiotics may be helpful to target bacteria and ascertain systemic absorption of antibiotics. Culturing of chronic infection sites, such as skin ulcers, is not helpful, as normal skin flora and secondary organisms typically contaminate the specimen. Examination of body fluids, such as urine and sputum, may enable APNs to troubleshoot harboring bacteria that could cause a catheter-induced bladder infection or pneumonia (Anaya et al., 2012).

Unlike elective, planned surgeries, the timing of a cancer surgery often does not allow for correction of preexisting comorbidities. APNs should involve patients and families in recommended changes in the immediate pre- and postoperative periods, as well as long-term lifestyle changes. Modifications that can immediately affect surgical outcomes are smoking cessation, increase in dietary protein, control of serum glucose, and engagement in aerobic and pulmonary exercise with deep breathing (Hennessey et al., 2010; Itatsu et al., 2014; Kiran et al., 2013; Mills et al., 2011; Ortega-Deballon et al., 2014; Schroeder, 2014; Shinkawa et al., 2013). Patients and families are dealing with the cancer diagnosis itself, making it difficult to address poor personal habits and lifestyle choices.

Medications Affecting Surgery

Attention to preoperative drug dosing or discontinuation of certain medications is important to avoid anesthesia-related complications or excessive bleeding. Detailed personal or family history of difficulties with anesthesia is crucial information to obtain preoperatively, specifically in regard to anesthesia-induced hyperthermia. This condition, known as malignant hyperthermia (termed *malignant* but is unrelated to cancer), is a rare and often hereditary condition that occurs after exposure to certain anesthetic agents, such as volatile gases or muscle relaxants (Schuster, Johannsen, Schneiderbanger, & Roewer, 2013). Symptoms range from an increased fever and hypoxia to circulatory collapse and death. If the patient or family has a history of malignant hyperthermia, this information must be communicated to the anesthesia team. The anesthesia team will perform a more in-depth preoperative assessment and discuss a plan of care with the patient, family, and surgeon.

Avoidance of abrupt changes to the following medications is prudent in the preoperative period to avoid withdrawal or a rebound effect: beta-blockers, alpha-agonists, barbiturates, and opioids. Other medications that require adjustment, especially in the pre- and perioperative period, include oral hypoglycemics, insulin, corticosteroids, angiotensin-converting enzyme inhibitors, and calcium channel blockers. If possible, discontinuation of monoamine oxidase inhibitors should occur several days preoperatively. Table 5-3 lists some of the common medications that require discontinuation before surgery. Special attention to these medications may prevent patients with cancer from experiencing unnecessary side effects during the pre-, peri-, and postoperative periods. APNs are responsible for reviewing all medications, including over-the-counter drugs, for possible interaction or reaction with the cancer diagnosis and pending surgical procedure. Alterations in medication type, brand, or dosage optimally occur prior to the surgery to ascertain the patient's tolerance to the adjustment.

Drugs that alter platelet aggregation or prolong bleeding should be evaluated several weeks before surgery, if possible, to ensure proper dosage adjustments. These drugs include herbal remedies and antithrombolytic and antiplatelet agents. Discontinuation of these drugs may be required to avoid unnecessary bleeding, hemorrhage, or hematoma formation in the peri- or postoperative period (see Table 5-3). In the review of patient anticoagulant use, attention to underlying health conditions is necessary to investigate the clinical reason for anticoagulation (Savina & Couturaud, 2011), such as a history of hypercoagulable state, significant cardiac valvular disease, artificial cardiac valves, atrial fibrillation, and thrombotic events such as deep vein thrombosis or pulmonary embolism. In these serious hypercoagulable states, maintenance of anticoagulation with short-acting heparin may be implemented during the time the patient is unable to take routine anticoagulation medication. Hospital admission for this bridge therapy with heparin may be necessary to avoid thromboembolytic events (Lyman et al., 2013). APNs provide continuity among the primary care physician, the surgical team, and the house staff and often direct the stop of oral or subcutaneous anticoagulants, the start of IV heparin, the stop of heparin on the day of surgery, anticoagulant orders in the postoperative

Table 5-3. Drugs and Their Interfering Properties in the Preoperative Setting

Name of Drug	Interfering Properties	Preoperative (Preop) Discontinuation
Angiotensin-converting enzyme inhibitors	Intensify hypotension, effects of anesthesia	Individual consideration; 24 hours preop
Angiotensin receptor blockers	Intensify hypotension	Individual consideration; 24 hours preop
Calcium-channel blockers	Intensify hypotension, effects of anesthesia	Individual consideration; 24 hours preop
Aspirin Clopidogrel Eptifibatide Ticlopidine Tirofiban	Antiplatelet effect	7–10 days preop
Celecoxib Naproxen	Antiplatelet effect	72 hours preop
Ketorolac	Antiplatelet effect	24 hours preop
Fenoprofen	Antiplatelet effect	12 hours preop
Monoamine oxidase inhibitors	Fatal drug reaction with anesthetic agents	2 weeks preop
Tricyclic antidepressants	Cardiac arrhythmias, hypotension	Individual consideration; cessation probably not necessary; norepinephrine is drug of choice
Benzodiazepines Selective serotonin reuptake inhibitors	Withdrawal effects	Important not to alter preoperatively
Herbals: Garlic, ginseng, ginkgo, ginger, kava, valerian, St. John's wort	Antiplatelet, anticoagulation effect	2 weeks preop
Warfarin	Anticoagulation effect	Individual consideration; 3–5 days preop; may consider heparin bridge
Heparin	Anticoagulation effect	Just prior to surgery

Note. Based on information from Joint Commission, 2014; Kiran et al., 2013; Livingston, 2013; Lyman et al., 2013; Nicholson et al., 2013; Savina & Couturaud, 2011; Schroeder, 2014; Schuster et al., 2013.

phase, and the transition to oral and subcutaneous anticoagulation with serum monitoring in the home setting.

Perioperative Phase

The scope of this chapter does not allow for sufficient discussion of issues relevant to potential APN roles in the perioperative phase of cancer surgery. Intraoperative APNs, such as certified registered nurse anesthetists, receive certification by boards outside of oncology nursing and may not be the largest audience of this text. Nevertheless, the perioperative phase includes issues relevant to the APN and essential to surgery itself, for example, anesthesia, safety, blood products, fluid management, infection, electrolyte balance, cardiac hemostasis, pulmonary function, oxygenation, and positioning (Nicholson, Coldwell, Lewis, & Smith, 2013). Other chapters in this book include additional information about these topics. Information related to perioperative anesthesia, infection, and positioning follows.

Anesthesia

A variety of anesthesia approaches are used in cancer surgeries: general, regional, or local. The surgical team, anesthesiologist, and patient decide on the selection (MedlinePlus, 2013). General anesthesia induces a reversible state of loss of consciousness and provides the surgeon with a controlled, motionless operating field and a secure airway, with total unawareness for the patient. General anesthesia can produce analgesia, amnesia, muscle relaxation, unconsciousness, and inhibition of reflexes. IV agents such as ultrashort-acting barbiturates or tranquilizers frequently are used to obtain a rapid onset of unconsciousness. A number of inhaled anesthetic agents also can be used, which provide a safe form of anesthesia in combination with narcotics and muscle relaxants. Although these side effects may be desirable, general anesthesia carries risks, including the potential for cardiac dysfunction with myocardial infarction, arrhythmias, and cerebral vascular accident. Other negative side effects include nausea and vomiting, headache, blurred vision, disorientation, sore throat secondary to intubation, respiratory paralysis, muscle pain, a feeling of cold and shivering, dizziness, and drowsiness (MedlinePlus, 2013).

Local and regional anesthetic agents involve a reversible blockage of pain perception. Topical/skin anesthesia occurs after application of topical anesthetic agents to the skin or mucous membranes. Local anesthesia of a specific anatomic area occurs through injection of anesthetic agents directly into the operative field. These methods can involve short-acting or long-acting drugs, depending on the blockage time interval desired. Peripheral nerve blocks achieve pain blockage to a regional area of nerve trunks, thus providing anesthesia to an entire anatomic area, such as the arm or leg. These approaches are administered alone or in combination with general anesthesia (MedlinePlus, 2013).

Potential alternatives to general anesthesia include regional epidural or spinal anesthesia. These methods produce numbness of the area below the injected nerve roots. Epidural anesthesia, either short or long term, can be achieved by depositing analgesic or anesthetic drugs into the extradural space of the spinal canal using a spinal needle. A catheter may be left in place for continued, intermittent interjection of either set of drugs, even after the surgical procedure has been completed. Epidural anesthesia, in combination with general anesthesia, is a common approach for intensely painful surgeries, such as thoracic procedures. Drugs can be delivered directly to the injured nerves to optimize pain control and minimize systemic side effects. Spinal anesthesia is induced with an injection of local anesthetic agents into the cerebrospinal fluid after puncture of the dural sac between the L2 and L4 vertebrae. This provides anesthesia to the lower abdomen and extremities without the side effects of general anesthesia, thereby allowing the patient to remain in a semiconscious or awake state with spontaneous breathing (Narouze et al., 2012; Wuethrich, Thalmann, Studer, & Burkhard, 2013). Long-acting local skin anesthetic agents may be injected to relieve incisional pain, including the small incisions associated with laparoscopic surgery.

Preoperative oral analgesics and IV opioids prior to administration of general anesthesia may improve management and outcomes (Niwa, Rowbotham, Lambert, & Buggy, 2013). Regional anesthesia is frequently used with IV sedation, which may eliminate the need for general anesthesia (Narouze et al., 2012; Wuethrich et al., 2013).

APNs are responsible for ascertaining appropriate patient education for methods of anesthesia. In addition, APNs should share their assessment knowledge with staff RNs to enhance overall observation of patients and improve team surveillance.

Infection Risk

The risk of SSI is a systems issue requiring diligent attention to asepsis and infection control guidelines. To maintain the patient's host defense mechanisms, the physical environment of surgery is controlled. This includes preoperative surgical decisions, timing of surgery, surgical technique, use of blood products, control of blood loss, duration and extent of surgery, perioperative glucose control, adequate tissue oxygenation, normothermia, normovolemia, pain control, and sterility.

Preparation of the skin overlying the surgical site requires use of an antibacterial scrub and removal of body hair that is adjacent to the incision line (Zinn, Jenkins, Swofford, Harrelson, & McCarter, 2010). Clipping of the hair is preferred. If complete removal of body hair surrounding the surgical site is necessary, removal just prior to the skin incision in surgery is preferred rather than in the hours prior to surgery. This reduces potential areas of inflammation and subsequent superficial infection caused by trauma to the skin (Joint Commission, 2014). Use of depilatory products for surgical patients is not advisable because of the risk of skin inflammation.

The administration of preoperative and intraoperative antibiotics occurs depending on individual patient risk factors, type of surgery, anatomic location of surgery, and length of surgical time. The risk of infection increases as surgery time lengthens, although SSIs can establish several hours after exposure to an endogenous or exogenous pathogen. Administration of antibiotics before contamination reduces the risk of subsequent infection. Proper choice of an antimicrobial and timing of administration are crucial to effective prophylaxis.

Antibiotics are not indicated for patients undergoing short (less than two hours) surgical procedures in tissues outside of the alimentary tract (designated as "clean" cases). Exceptions to this guideline are surgeries in patients with a known infection, immunocompromised state, significant cardiac valvular disease, or artificial valves or joints, or if surgical time may extend beyond two hours. These cases may benefit from administration of an IV broad-spectrum antibiotic just prior to skin incision (Roos et al., 2013).

Cases involving the alimentary tract, including oral and digestive organs (designated as "dirty" cases), abscess drainage, or overt infections require preoperative and intraoperative administration of antibiotics. Surgical procedures involving the upper or lower digestive tracts (e.g., colon resection) also may require preoperative sterilization with multiple doses of oral agents (Roos et al., 2013). Surgical placement of vascular access devices requires prophylactic antibiotic administration just prior to the skin incision because of the possible introduction of skin flora into the circulatory system, as well as the placement of a foreign body that can trap organisms.

Positioning

Patient positioning during surgery is imperative to the prevention of postoperative complications related to muscular and neuropathic injury and compartmental syndromes (Valdivieso, Hueber, & Zorn, 2013). Attention to deficits from coexisting conditions, such as osteoarthritis, artificial joints, spinal disorders, and rheumatoid diseases, can potentially decrease postoperative discomfort and time to ambulation. Well-documented information on the surgical chart by the APN can alert surgical personnel to preexisting physical conditions. Care can include simple interventions such as ensuring proper alignment, placing pillows under the knees, avoiding abduction/adduction movements, taking special care during transfers, and using padding for lithotomy positioning. Avoidance of unnatural positioning can decrease unnecessary myalgias and avoid neuropathic injuries.

Of added importance are the gravitational effects of positioning on the circulatory and pulmonary systems. Supine positioning increases the cardiac output because of enhanced return of lower extremity venous blood to the heart. The supine lithotomy position can create an even greater cardiac return secondary to elevation of the lower extremities. Supine positioning can alternatively decrease functional lung capacity. Perfusion changes related to a decreased flow of blood to the lung bases can negatively affect oxygenation status. Trendelenburg positioning, as used in abdominal surgeries, can increase the pressure of abdominal contents on diaphragmatic movement and alter pulmonary expansion (Valdivieso et al., 2013).

Operative Procedure

The role of surgery in cancer treatment is dependent upon the presentation of the cancer and complications that can occur throughout the cancer trajectory. Knowledge of cancer development and progression is essential in understanding the disease and resulting surgical recommendations. Cancer-related characteristics drive the surgical approach; patients present with individual factors that likewise can direct surgical options. For example, a woman newly diagnosed with breast cancer with a previous history of upper chest wall radiation therapy for the treatment of Hodgkin lymphoma is unable to choose between the breast-conserving treatment option of a lumpectomy plus radiation versus a mastectomy, as she is unable to receive radiation therapy to the chest wall again. Therefore, she must have a total mastectomy to treat her breast cancer.

Minimally invasive approaches in cancer surgery can offer a significant reduction in surgical-related morbidities and postoperative recovery (Valdivieso et al., 2013). Advances in screening and early detection provide the ability to detect cancers in their earliest stage, with the accompanying benefit of less-invasive measures of resection. Unfortunately, not all cancers are amenable to these improved surgical approaches, nor are all cancers found in an early stage. Thus, the radical en bloc resection of a cancer and surrounding organs remains a discouraging reality with its associated disfigurement and morbidity.

Resection of Malignancy

Resection remains the primary therapy to eradicate solid tumors and involves removal of the tumor with adequate margins of normal tissue. The goals of every surgery are to remove the cancer while maintaining normal function of related organs and to remove tissue as necessary to avoid local recurrence. In most cancer surgeries, negative pathologic margins provide quantification of surgical clearance of local tumor evidence. Adequate margins vary from cancer to cancer; the important work of clinical trials serves to document what constitutes a "negative" or adequate margin with each individual cancer (Diaz et al., 2014; Thompson et al., 2014). Unfortunately, most cancers initiate their invasive growth many years before detection. As a result, micrometastatic disease is a possibility, indicating probable systemic disease that was not evident in the preoperative assessment. Therefore, the statement "We got it all" can only theoretically apply to local surgical therapy and seldom indicates a "cure" of the cancer.

Neoadjuvant chemotherapy and/or radiation therapy may precede surgery in an effort to decrease the overall size of the tumor and potentially allow a less-aggressive surgical approach (Larentzakis & Theodorou, 2014). In some examples of neoadjuvant chemotherapy, systemic treatment of the cancer may simultaneously provide treatment of micrometastasis. Intraoperative radiation therapy (i.e., administered during the surgical procedure) also may be a treatment option and involves application of concentrated doses of radiation directly to the tumor bed after the surgical team completes initial resection of visible disease (Azria & Lemanski, 2014). Consideration of these multimodality approaches optimally occurs prior to surgery, with involvement and education of patients and families.

Surgical intervention to debulk the tumor involves the surgical removal of visible or palpable tumor to decrease overall tumor burden in advanced presentations. The goal is not necessarily to achieve clean margins or remove all microscopic evidence of disease. Instead, debulking aims to improve quality of life and enhance the ability of systemic therapy to treat advanced cancer (Robinson & Cantillo, 2014).

Surgical resection of metastatic sites may be a strategy for patients with advanced cancer. This approach resects cancers confined to one metastatic organ, typically colorectal cancer with metastasis to the liver or osteogenic soft tissue sarcomas with metastasis to the lung. With respect to each individual case, surgical excision of these metastatic sites can improve five-year overall survival by 25%–40% (Gil-Gil et al., 2014; Moreno et al., 2013). Research is ongoing regarding the resection of metastatic cancer, although most cancer types are not amenable to this approach because of the malignant potential from systemic, micrometastatic disease.

Surgical Procedures

The surgical algorithm and subsequent interventions are dependent upon the specific cancer, presentation, symptoms, and individual host characteristics. The specific surgical approach varies according to the surgical team's skill level, the equipment available, and regional practices that affect decision making. The science of surgery originates from evidence-based practice, with the art of surgery arising from the skill and experience of the surgical team. Emerging innovations and advancements in technology and instrumentation have transformed operative procedures, with the surgical oncologist, interventional radiologist, and endoscopist often working in concert. At times, the roles blur, yet the goal is always to provide the highest level of care with the least invasive approach and side effect profile and optimized recovery. This multimodality approach and the potential combination of interventions enable creation and tailoring of the surgical approach to individuals with cancer (Sofocleous, Sideras, & Petre, 2013).

The surgical approach includes assessment and evaluation of the individual patient. Only then can surgical planning begin, with revision as needed. The surgical approach may be minimally invasive, traditional open, or combined (Altorki et al., 2014), depending on specific factors individual to each patient, disease presentation, and the surgical team.

Lymph Node Evaluation

Regional lymph nodes are the most common site of metastasis for the majority of solid tumors. Surgical resection of regional lymph nodes generally is part of the staging workup of the cancer, even if visible tumor is not evident in the lymph nodes (Lumachi, Basso, Santeufemia, Bonamini, & Chiara, 2013). If visible tumor is evident, or if intraoperative pathology verifies microscopic tumor, a lymph node dissection is performed to provide regional control of the cancer. In some cancers, it is uncertain whether a full lymph node dissection plays a role in eliminating future sites of systemic metastasis (Giuliano, Morrow, Duggal, & Julian, 2012). Elective lymph node resection (e.g., without evidence of disease or positive results with lymph node biopsy) bears skepticism, as aggressive removal of micrometastatic disease may not improve mortality rates although may increase morbidity (Giuliano et al., 2012). These concepts support the notion that many solid tumors undergo years of transformational growth with micrometastatic seeding via the lymphatic and hematologic pathways, which occurs many years before actual detection of the cancer. Treatments such as systemic chemotherapy, hormonal therapy, or biologic therapy may be sufficient to eradicate the disease in clinically benign lymph nodes without an extensive resection (Guiliano et al., 2012; Lumachi et al., 2013).

Sentinel lymph node biopsy (SLNB) is a surgical approach to evaluate regional lymph nodes in breast cancer and melanoma, although its use has been evaluated in multiple other cancer types. On the day of surgery, injections of a radioactive tracer and/or vital blue dye occur, directed at the tumor bed and lymph supply. These provide the surgeon with visible and radioactive maps to the first node or nodes that drain the tumor. After the visual identification of blue dye and measurement of in vivo gamma-ray counts, excision of the sentinel node (or nodes) occurs with intraoperative pathologic evaluation. If the lymph node is pathologically negative for tumor, often a node dissection is not performed, and the surgery proceeds to removal of the primary malignancy only (Guiliano et al., 2013). If the lymph node is pathologically positive, surgery often commences to remove regional lymph nodes along with the scar of the prior tumor. Clinical trials continue to validate the use of SLNB in various cancers and its overall reliability in identifying occult lymph node involvement (Yagata et al., 2013). The identification of micrometastasis in regional lymph nodes may be adequate to indicate the stage of disease and guide appropriate systemic treatment, with ultimate avoidance of lymph node dissection even if the sentinel node is positive.

Minimally Invasive Surgery

Minimally invasive surgery has been one of the most transforming areas in surgery over the past two decades, with multiple advances in techniques and instrumentation. In addition, the staff involved in minimally invasive surgery has expanded to include interventional radiologists and multidisciplinary teams that perform interrelated or tandem procedures with the surgical oncologist.

Minimally invasive surgery is performed with small incisions (less than 1 cm) and typically via laparoscopic access with specialized techniques and instruments. The type of minimally invasive surgery depends on which body part requires access (e.g., organ, body space, joint, bone). Instead of large incisions being used to access to the particular body part, small portholes provide access for the passage of laparoscopes. Visualization of the inside of the body is accomplished via inflation of the body cavity with carbon dioxide and insertion of laparoscopes that contain miniature cameras with microscopes, tiny fiber-optic flashlights, and high-definition monitors (Correa-Gallego et al., 2013; Wright et al., 2012). Instruments pass through the laparoscopes, which enable surgeons to perform a number of surgical techniques.

Generally, minimally invasive surgery is advantageous over an open procedure because of decreased trauma to the body, decreased blood loss, smaller surgical scars, less overall surgical pain, and decreased postoperative stay. Most patients who undergo minimally invasive surgery are able to leave the hospital sooner and with quicker return to normal activities compared to patients who undergo surgery with a conventional open incision.

One example of a minimally invasive surgery is an esophagectomy rather than an open procedure with transthoracic, right-side manipulation that mandates one-lung ventilation, postoperative chest tube, destruction of the thoracic wall and mediastinal pleura, and mechanical damage to the ventilated and collapsed lungs (Mori et al., 2013). The robotic-aided surgery is far less invasive than the open approach, although the patient essentially undergoes the same surgical procedure internally, with a modified external approach (e.g., the body must still heal) (Jacobs & Kamyab, 2013). APNs must often remind patients of this need to heal, as well as the realization of the side effects of prolonged anesthesia that results from longer procedures via the laparoscopic approach. Disadvantages for the surgeon related to minimally invasive surgery compared to traditional open surgery include decreased depth perception, lack of tactile feedback with the surgical field (although removed tissue can still be palpated once outside the body), and decreased intracavitary ease of suturing.

Minimally invasive surgery typically is reserved for early-stage cancer surgical procedures, although research continues to study its use in more advanced presentations. It is used widely in diagnostic and staging procedures (Hennon & Demmy, 2012), second-look procedures, diagnosis of recurrent disease, and palliative care. For example, in a woman who is clinically and radiographically diagnosed with stage II ovarian cancer, her surgical procedure may start with a diagnostic and exploratory laparoscopy. Tissue can be obtained for intraoperative confirmation of ovarian cancer, and the lower abdomen can be explored for evidence of disseminated disease, allowing an intraoperative decision as to the surgical approach.

Another example is in a patient with pancreatic cancer. If an exploratory laparoscopy reveals widespread disease, an en bloc procedure may be aborted, thus sparing the patient the morbidity and healing that accompany a large abdominal incision (Mori et al., 2013). The use of diagnostic laparoscopy in cancer surgery may prevent the traditional "open and close" approach or, more importantly, undesirable exenterative procedures. With laparoscopic surgeries, the opportunity to begin systemic treatment is not typically complicated by the delays related to surgical morbidity and healing. Another example of the benefits of laparoscopy surgery is the preservation of fertility in women with cervical cancer (Dursun, Caglar, Akilli, & Ayhan, 2013). The management of cancer continues to change with the emergence of new techniques that are safe and reasonable options in cancer care.

Video-Assisted Thoracoscopic Surgery

Video-assisted thoracoscopic surgery (VATS) is a minimally invasive approach that allows visualization of the chest and access for biopsies of the pleura, diaphragm, and pericardium. Pulmonary wedge resection using the VATS approach is a standard method of obtaining tissue for pathologic diagnosis of small, indeterminate pulmonary nodules. VATS also is useful for the diagnosis and treatment of pleural effusions, allowing for biopsies and pleurodesis. Robotic VATS can aid in mediastinal lymph node dissection, esophagectomy, and cardiac windows. VATS is not a minor surgery, but it is a minimally invasive approach to complex intrathoracic procedures (Hennon & Demmy, 2012; Swanson et al., 2014).

Robotic Surgery

Robotic surgery enables the surgeon to obtain three-dimensional access and vision using an intuitive robotic system, such as ZEUS® or, most recently, the da Vinci® Surgical System. The robot itself is a programmable and multifunctional machine that manipulates and performs a variety of tasks through the surgical team's guidance (Sooriakumaran et al., 2014). Robotic assistance in minimally invasive surgery bridges the gap between standard laparoscopic procedures and the traditional open approach, providing extensive manipulation, motion tracking, and three-dimensional imaging. This set of operative equipment includes the surgeon's console, a computerized control system, two instrument robotic arms, and a fiber-optic camera. The traditional laparoscope approach is used, and the robot "holds" the ports, with insertion of robotic instruments through the port openings. These instruments together provide controls for the surgeon to micromanipulate the robot, which in turn copies the movements made by the surgeon. This allows a full range of motion similar to the surgeon's hands and wrists beyond what is possible in standard laparoscopy. The pictures emitted on the screen are high definition and three-dimensional, unlike with traditional laparoscopic surgery, in which images are less distinct and two-dimensional. This method of computer-aided surgery can overcome some of the drawbacks of traditional minimally invasive laparoscopic surgery, allowing improved access and visualization and precise dissection, especially around arteries, veins, and nerves.

In a retrospective study of patients undergoing a radical prostatectomy, those patients who had robotic surgery or the laparoscopic (e.g., keyhole) approach were more likely to have negative tumor margins than those patients who underwent a traditional open technique. However, favorable margins were dependent on the center's volume of laparoscopic and robotic cases (Sooriakumaran et al., 2014).

As with traditional minimally invasive surgery, robotic surgery has the potential advantages of reduced pain and trauma, minimal blood loss, less postoperative pain, reduced infection risk, shorter hospital stay, improved recovery, and reduced scarring. Unfortunately, robotic-assisted laparoscopy surgery often can take 1.5 times longer than traditional open surgery (Lang, Wong, Tsang, Wong, & Wan, 2014). Appropriate patient selection is important to avoid additional surgical and anesthesia time. APNs play a pivotal role in identifying potentially eligible patients for robotic surgery with appropriate preoperative clearance. Additional education is necessary for patients and families, as well as staff members, related to new equipment, procedures, preoperative and postoperative patient care, and environmental and social issues that require attention for patients undergoing robotic surgery. This high-technologic approach may work for some cancer surgeries but not necessarily for all approaches, such as thyroidectomy, in which operating room time, hospital stay, and nerve injury rate were higher than with conventional open procedure (Lang et al., 2014).

Endoluminal Instrumentation

Endoluminal instrumentation is yet another form of minimally invasive surgery. This technique enables endoscopists to perform a variety of procedures, including suturing, dissecting, and ligating. This endoscopic approach can be more advantageous than laparoscopy, as procedures can be done with patients under conscious sedation, on an outpatient basis, and without abdominal wounds. These advantages result in less pain, improved cosmetic result, faster recuperation, and reduced costs. Examples of the endoluminal approach include a snare polypectomy (versus transabdominal colotomy for polypectomy); procedures performed to inject, cauterize, or clip lower or duodenal bleeding (versus transabdominal approach for duodenectomy); ligation and transjugular intrahepatic portosystemic shunting (versus transabdominal portal systemic shunt for variceal bleeding); percutaneous endoscopic gastrostomy (versus transabdominal approach for placement of a feeding tube); endoscopic retrograde cholangiopancreatography (versus transabdominal approach of common bile duct exploration); endoluminal suturing (versus Nissen fundoplication, a complex surgical procedure to treat intractable gastroesophageal reflux or hiatal hernia); and endoscopic mucosal resection (Chen, K., et al., 2013; Kim et al., 2012; Schurr et al., 2011).

Transluminal Endoscopic Surgery

Transluminal endoscopic surgery, or natural orifice transluminal endoscopic surgery (NOTES), is an emerging alternative to conventional surgery that combines minimally invasive endoscopic and laparoscopic techniques to diagnose and treat intra-abdominal disease. In this procedure, the surgeon inserts the endoscope through a natural orifice, such as the mouth, anus, urethra, or vagina, and enters the peritoneal cavity via a transvisceral incision. This potential means of access to the abdominal cavity from the lumen of hollow viscera can eliminate multiple laparoscopic or larger incisions that traverse through skin and muscle, thus reducing complications such as wound infection, hernia, pain, and adhesions (Emhoff, Lee, & Sylla, 2014).

Some of the more common uses of NOTES include the external insertion of percutaneous feeding tubes with endoscopic lighted access, sphincter access, and balloon dilation methods. Although these procedures are common, this passage from the lumen of hollow viscera into the abdominal cavity requires additional research with translation of animal to human studies and perfection of adequate closure of the viscerotomy (Emhoff et al., 2014).

Adjuncts to Surgical Resection

Radiofrequency Ablation

Radiofrequency ablation (RFA) is a method of tissue removal through the application of high-frequency radio waves that provide local destruction of tumor, either primary or metastatic. Uses of RFA for the primary treatment of cancers, such as breast cancer and hepatocellular carcinoma, continue to be under scientific investigation. Most often, RFA is used for control of metastatic liver disease, typically if conventional control of the disease has failed (Cabibbo et al., 2013). RFA employs percutaneous, laparoscopic, or open surgical access to tumors, with subsequent destruction of targeted tumor. Often, noninvasive surgical approaches are successful and cause minimal discomfort to patients.

Cryosurgery

Cryosurgery uses liquid nitrogen to destroy malignant tissue and provide local control of tumor growth. A variety of cryosurgical delivery methods exist to provide external or internal death of tissue, which may result in semipermanent or permanent cell death. Cryoablation and cryolocalization are methods undergoing study for use in the treatment and diagnosis of breast disease. Salvage cryosurgery for locally recurrent prostate cancer following radiation therapy may be an alternative to salvage radical prostatectomy (Cerruto, D'Elia, & Artibani, 2012).

Unlike RFA, as discussed earlier, patients potentially may better withstand cryoablation because cold is analgesic in nature, whereas heat can be more uncomfortable. Cryoablation, as a freezing technique, produces necrosis and local destruction of tissue. However, margins are difficult to ascertain; therefore, it remains most useful in benign disease such as fibroadenomas. Cryolocalization can create a well-delineated mass of frozen tissue around a tumor and may provide an alternative approach to needle localization for surgical removal of a breast mass. Additional research is necessary in the field of cryotechnology before it replaces surgical excision for removal of malignant tissue.

Radioimmunoguided Surgery

Radioimmunoguided surgery (RIGS) employs a radioactive tracer to identify possible malignant tissue. Intraoperatively, a neoprobe localizes radioactivity, guiding resection with the potential of identifying areas of malignancy distant from the main primary and reducing operating time. Examples include SLNB as previously described, radioguided parathyroidectomy, and radioimmunoguided intraoperative radiation therapy. Studies continue to identify labeled radiographic tracers specific for various cancer types and subtypes that successfully guide surgeons to malignant tissue (Tiernan et al., 2012).

Light Amplification by Stimulated Emission

Light amplification by stimulated emission of radiation (known as *laser*) employs an intense narrow beam, enabling precise surgery for removal of precancerous or cancerous lesions. Laser also can enable procedures that relieve symptoms of cancer. Different types of laser approaches and instrumentation exist that allow direct application of laser therapy through an open incision or endoscopic instruments. As with most minimally invasive techniques, the use of laser with endoscopic assistance results in less bleeding and damage than with other resection methods. Photodynamic therapy is another laser therapy technique that uses an injectable photosensitizing agent followed by targeted laser therapy to destroy malignant cells. Another laser modality, laser-induced interstitial thermotherapy, uses laser light to heat and kill malignant cells. This procedure may have more benefit if used in conjunction with arterial embolization, as in the case of liver metastases. These laser techniques offer additional approaches to destroy cancer cells, although the benefit does not typically persist (Rengan, Jagtap, De, Banerjee, & Srivastava, 2014).

Postoperative Care

Evaluation of patients with cancer and their family and caregivers during the preoperative phase of surgery minimizes the stress of the operative procedure and thus promotes a prompt return to a state of health during the postoperative phase. Criticism surrounds shorter lengths of hospital stays with concern that patients are not well enough to return home or have not remained in the hospital long enough to heal from their procedures. Shorter lengths of stay have led patients to be active sooner after surgery, leading to decreased levels of postoperative pain (Tighe, Harle, Boezaart, Aytug, & Fillingim, 2014), enhanced mobility and exercise capacity, and improved enteral intake soon after surgery. Body measurements, such as temperature, pulse, respiration, blood pressure, weight, and intake and output of fluids and urine, remain important indices upon which to measure postoperative stability and progress. Additionally, results of postoperative laboratory studies, specifically renal function, hematologic status, oxygenation, and electrolyte balance, enable APNs to augment surgical outcomes and minimize complications (Souza et al., 2014).

Preexisting comorbid conditions, such as cardiac, pulmonary, renal, and hepatic disease, present additional postoperative challenges in balancing metabolic disease with the stress of surgery. Appropriate volume resuscitation with isotonic fluids is required to maintain intravascular volume and adequate hydration (Hofer, Rex, & Ganter, 2014). Vital signs and urine output provide guides for adjustments in volume and fluid type. Control of peripheral capillary permeability prevents unwanted effects that lead to uncomfortable peripheral edema causing limited movement and ineffective ambulation. Patients with inadequate renal or cardiac function may require diuretics, but otherwise, a natural diuresis will occur postoperatively as fluid mobilizes from the periphery into vascular spaces. A variety of perioperative and postoperative symptoms can occur in patients, including electrolyte imbalances, anemia, mental status changes, and acid-base disorders. Various chapters throughout this text contain information regarding management of some of these conditions. In healthy surgical patients, pain, nausea and vomiting, and infection are the three largest threats to homeostasis and will be addressed here.

Pain

Postoperative pain is a constellation of unpleasant experiences precipitated by surgical injury that can be acute or chronic in nature. These sensory, emotional, and mental experiences are associated with autonomic, psychological, and behavioral responses. The control of postoperative pain aims to provide subjective comfort and inhibit blunt trauma–induced nociceptive impulses (Chiu et al., 2014). Management of these autonomic and somatic reflex responses to pain enables restoration of function with early ambulation accompanied by objective and subjective improvement. APNs have a compendium of analgesics to reduce or eliminate postoperative pain. In addition, nonpharmaceutical interventions with attention to mechanical positioning often are successful in reducing overall pain.

Special attention is required for patients with a history of chronic pain requiring management with narcotics for acute pain related to a surgical procedure. APNs are responsible for assessing patients' pain management strategies prior to surgery and the change in level of pain after surgery. In some cases, the surgical procedure actually may reduce pain that was caused by compression, thereby resulting in less overall pain for patients postoperatively (Nader et al., 2013). In other cases, incisional pain may increase overall pain needs, requiring narcotic dosages greater than patients' usual doses. APNs must ascertain that appropriate pain management techniques and dosages are in place, with frequent reassessment, and must educate those involved in the care of these compromised patients (Tighe et al., 2014).

Of all cancer surgeries, thoracotomy and major abdominal procedures are potentially the most painful. A combination approach to pain management is often required, with consideration of local anesthetics and opioids through an epidural catheter, systemic nonsteroidal anti-inflammatory drugs (NSAIDs) or cyclooxygenase-2 inhibitors, and systemic opioids (Yan, Butler, Kurowski, & Perloff, 2014). This combination of agents provides both synergistic and additive effects. Abdominal procedures also can present challenges related to decreased bowel motility and ileus. If possible, use of systemic opioids should be minimal until bowel motility returns as evidenced by flatus and passage of stool. Often, the addition of IV NSAIDs provides enhanced pain relief with smaller doses of narcotics compared to the use of narcotics alone. Use of patient-controlled analgesia is one method to monitor pain medication requirements if only the patient is requesting the medication through activation of the pump.

Epidural pain management can be effective for major mid-chest, abdominal, and lower extremity surgeries. Epidural medications are difficult to administer for head, neck, upper chest, and upper extremity surgeries, as the location of the epidural catheter with concomitant administration of pain medication may compromise respiratory function. Epidural pain management requires close monitoring of appropriate drug, dosage, and infusion rate because of the concentration of drug. Frequent assessment by the entire surgical team for bladder distension, lower extremity motor loss, and impaired skin integrity is essential, as patients are unlikely to accurately report these signs and symptoms because of a lack of sensation. APNs can be effective in optimizing pain management for patients undergoing these surgeries by including potential epidural pain management, as well as anesthesia when appropriate, in their discussion with the surgical team. APNs often are responsible for adequate postoperative pain management and must be prepared to alter the pain regimen as needed.

Nausea and Vomiting

Nausea and vomiting are common in postoperative patients and are responsible for unplanned hospital admission of ambulatory surgery patients, delay in discharge, significant discomfort, and patient dissatisfaction. Risk factors for postoperative nausea and vomiting include female sex, pediatric patient, prior history of nausea and vomiting with anesthesia, history of motion sickness, ingestion of food too quickly after surgery, side effects of pain medication, duration of surgery, and ear, nose, and throat and breast augmentation procedures (Sharma & Jamal, 2013). APNs often coordinate preoperative care and therefore are responsible for obtaining and synthesizing the history and a list of the patient's current medications, smoking history, and perceived barriers to nausea and vomiting management. With this information, the anesthesia team then may modify their management strategy and avoid the use of emesis-inducing agents such as fentanyl, nitrous oxide, and other volatile inhalational gases.

The receptor systems for nausea and vomiting in postoperative patients are similar to those related to chemotherapy (see Chapter 4 for further explanation). In most cases, stimulation of receptors in the brain from anesthetic agents induces nausea and vomiting, as opposed to chemical irritation of the stomach itself. Concomitantly, once vomiting begins, the epigastric muscles experience spasms that exacerbate symptoms. Therefore, interventions for both sources of nausea and vomiting often are necessary, with the use of a serotonin antagonist and a smooth muscle relaxant. Serotonin antagonists are effective and safe drugs with minimal side effects. Smooth muscle relaxants often cause somnolence but otherwise are well tolerated. An additional preventive approach can be used to decrease stimulation of histamine receptors in the brain with the application of a scopolamine patch several hours before surgery, especially in patients with a history of motion sickness. Control of postoperative nausea and vomiting begins in the operating room and includes a multimodal approach with serotonin antagonists and other antiemetic agents (Sharma & Jamal, 2013).

Fever and Infection

Fever in the postoperative setting is common and often is not associated with an infectious process. Typically, fever of noninfectious origin occurs early in the postoperative period and resolves, whereas fever related to an infection occurs days after surgery and persists. Fever generally increases in the evening and decreases in the morning. It is important to remember that the absence of fever does not rule out infection. This is especially true in immunocompromised patients, whose host defense mechanisms, including temperature response, are altered. Disease processes, including cancer, also can cause persistent temperatures. These are typically low grade in nature (less than 100.5°F [38°C]) but can exhibit fevers as high as 103°F (39.4°C) (Godfrey, Villa, Dawson, Swindells, & Schouten, 2013).

Physical examination is the most useful tool in the differential diagnosis of an infectious process. The most common sites of postoperative fever arise in the pulmonary system, urinary tract, or operative site and also can be related to medications or occur as a result of phlebitis. Bacterial infections in postoperative patients can be endogenous or exogenous and can originate from preexisting conditions, the surgical procedure, or nosocomial risk from rotating staff (Godfrey et al., 2013). In seriously ill individuals, one or more sources of infection can exist at the same time or secondarily as a result of stress on the immune system. Single-room occupancy is desirable, if possible, to reduce potential nosocomial infection through direct contact with other patients and family members. Infection surveillance is extremely important throughout the postoperative phase.

SSIs can occur in a variety of anatomic locations: superficial incision, deep incision, and organ space. An SSI occurs within the first 30 days after surgery. Infections occurring after 30 days are not termed SSIs and are not attributable to the surgical procedure or immediate postoperative phase. One exception is surgical implants; infections up to one year following the operation can be attributable to the surgical procedure. Superficial incision SSI occurs in the skin layers and subcutaneous tissues related to the incision. Deep incisional SSI involves the deep soft tissues. Organ space SSI occurs in adjacent organ space, regardless of whether the organ remains.

Surgical drain placement often is necessary for intracavitary drainage of the surgical bed to prevent pooling of bodily fluids that inadvertently delays wound healing, yet these drains also are a source of infection. The number of drains placed, the duration of placement, and the type of drainage apparatus are all factors related to possible SSI. Closed suction apparatus are preferred to minimize contamination from airborne sources. Prompt removal of drains is desirable to reduce the potential for surgical wound infections, although this cannot occur until intracavitary fluid accumulation slows (Ishizawa et al., 2014). Removal of drains can occur as early as two to three days after surgery, or they may remain in place for many weeks, pending decrease in accumulated fluid drainage. Any external tube is a portal for infection to the inside of the body. These tubes can colonize with bacteria, creating yet another source of infection.

Pneumonia can occur when normal host mechanisms of defense are unable to prevent pathogenic invasion. A number of factors are involved in the development of postoperative pneumonia, including the cancer diagnosis, intubation for general anesthesia, nosocomial exposure, inactivity, and other host risk factors. APNs must assess patient-specific risk factors, monitor clinical signs and symptoms, observe patient progress, and preemptively intervene as needed to maintain pulmonary health. Expedient recovery and prevention of additional infection-related complications rely on implementation of evidence-based nursing interventions relative to the care of patients with pneumonia as well as postoperative mobilization.

Additional Complications

A number of postoperative cardiac and pulmonary conditions can occur related to pre-existing conditions or resulting from the physical stress of surgery. Treatment of these conditions with evidence-based interventions specific to the cardiac or pulmonary event can prevent further serious adverse events. APNs can address these common adverse events in surgical patients to improve healing and avoid deleterious events. For example, postoperative hypertension commonly is caused by surgical pain or hypoxia; thus, adequate pain control and oxygenation are necessary. Use of various monitoring devices to measure oxygenation is warranted, as adequate oxygenation is necessary for tissue healing. Treatment of persistent hypertension is essential to prevent cardiac events, such as myocardial infarction, arrhythmias, and cerebral vascular accident. Respiratory complications, including atelectasis, aspiration, and pneumonia, often are preventable with therapeutic interventions, especially in high-risk patients. Upright positioning and early ambulation are essential to mobilization of secretions and prevention of pneumonia.

Diabetes mellitus is a preexisting chronic condition that can necessitate acute attention during the postoperative phase. Diabetic patients require close management with careful avoidance of hypoglycemia or hyperglycemia and associated complications of diabetic ketoacidosis and dehydration. Diabetes can have a significant negative impact on wound healing and may require tight control with sliding-scale insulin to maximize outcomes (Schroeder, 2014).

Thromboembolism, presenting as pulmonary embolism or deep vein thrombosis, is another serious potential side effect of surgery because of stasis of blood. Risk factors include age older than 40 years, obesity, immobilization, hypercoagulable states, Virchow triad (e.g., stasis, endothelial vessel injury, hypercoagulability), venous access devices, varicosities, pregnancy, history of malignancy, hormonal drugs, history of prior thromboembolism, and complicated, lengthy surgery. A variety of prophylactic measures are available, such as elevation of the legs with knee flexion, mobilization, pneumatic boots, leg exercises, elastic stockings, and anticoagulation with heparin (Livingston, 2013). Interventions by APNs must aim at prevention as well as primary and secondary treatment.

Access Devices

The infusion of chemotherapy and blood products often requires reliable and easy venous access, ensuring safety and maximum comfort for patients with cancer. Totally implantable access ports are widely used, with insertion by the surgical or interventional radiology team. Typically, either a cephalic vein cutdown or subclavian vein puncture technique is used. APNs are instrumental in identifying those patients who may benefit from the insertion of venous access devices, as well as in educating the healthcare team to anticipate this need for their patients.

Rehabilitation

Comprehensive rehabilitation of patients with cancer is a responsibility of all members of the oncology healthcare team, including surgical oncology. Rehabilitation begins in the hospital setting based on discussion with patients and families in the preoperative setting. Survival rates for most cancers continue to improve, yet life-altering treatments may be necessary to bring lifesaving results. The goals of cancer rehabilitation include improvements in quality of life and reduction in handicaps from cancer and its related treatments. All cancers share common rehabilitation goals, but each cancer brings its own set of challenges (Lester, 2011).

Wounds

Acute Wounds

Acute surgical wound management is the interaction of appropriate surgical closure, postoperative healing, and preexisting or acquired comorbid conditions. Initially, most cancer wounds are a result of mechanical trauma resulting from surgery. Primary closure of the wound occurs at the time of surgery; internal suturing and external suturing or staples create an incision line that heals as a scar (Shantz, Vernon, Leiter, Morshed, & Stranges, 2012). Secondary closure occurs if a surgical incision has opened or if the incision was intentionally left open at the time of surgery with healing by secondary intent (e.g., from the inside out). Tertiary closure involves mechanical or natural closure of the wound after a period of secondary healing. Wounds heal through an inflammatory response with immunomodulation of macrophages and monocytes in tissue repair (Mokarram & Bellamkonda, 2014). The proliferative phase occurs with fibroblasts and angiogenesis, formation of granulation tissue, epithelialization, with eventual wound contraction and healing. The goal of acute wound management is to facilitate healing and remodeling with minimal scarring. In marrow deficiencies, wound healing may be deterred secondary to macrophage production (Brown et al., 2012).

Cancer wounds can occur because of surgical intervention or from the cancer itself, with erosion of surrounding healthy tissue causing fistula formation, abscess, edema, or vascular changes. Superficial wounds involve the epidermis; partial-thickness wounds involve the dermis; and full-thickness wounds involve all layers of the skin, subcutaneous tissue, muscle, and/or bone. Treatment centers on the control or elimination of causative factors, as well as pressure, shearing force, friction, moisture, adequate circulation, and neuropathy. An understanding of the cellular response is essential to the healing of cancer-related wounds (Brown et al., 2012; Mokkaram & Bellamkonda, 2014).

In patients with comorbid conditions, additional interventions may be necessary to maximize wound healing and prevent skin breakdown. Assessment of factors revolving around nutritional status, preexisting cancer, diabetes, uremia, liver function or jaundice, advanced age, use of systemic corticosteroids, use of chemotherapy agents, previous radiation therapy, and alcoholism is imperative (Shalaby, Blume, & Sumpio, 2014). Prophylactic antibiotics are indicated for patients with contaminated wounds, patients who are immunocompromised or diabetic, patients with cardiac valvular disease, and patients with artificial prostheses, such as valve and joint replacements. Lymphedematous extremities are particularly prone to cellulitis and are of priority when performing surgery on these limbs. Patients who have stool-contaminated wounds or wounds that come into contact with gastrointestinal contents typically are treated with prophylactic antibiotics.

Smoking impairs tissue oxygenation, stimulates vasoconstriction, and contributes to factors of chronic atherosclerosis and vascular disease. All these conditions potentially can affect tissue and wound healing. Smoking cessation is ideal in the preoperative phase and imperative after surgery for maximal wound healing. Nutritional and fluid support is necessary, with a balanced diet and adequate hydration to provide the body with appropriate nutrients for healing. Attention to nitrogen and protein balance is essential to wound healing and often can be improved with dietary interventions. Frequently, patients with cancer require nutritional supplements, such as supplemental protein shakes, dietary supplements, and, in some cases, total parenteral nutrition, to boost the natural healing process.

The avoidance and prevention of surgical wound dehiscence is paramount in cancer surgical care. Recognition of risk factors is essential, and elimination of mechanical stress on the incision is necessary to prevent wound dehiscence. A dehisced wound may require immediate surgical intervention or may heal by secondary intent. APNs must recognize those patients who are at risk for wound dehiscence and provide added surveillance with the surgical team.

Soft tissue infections can involve the skin and underlying subcutaneous tissue, fascia, or muscle. These infections are divided into necrotizing and non-necrotizing categories: non-necrotizing infections are resolved primarily with antibiotic therapy, whereas necrotizing infections or skin or tissue death may also require operative debridement followed by antibiotics. Blood cultures rarely are positive and are only recommended when the patient exhibits concomitant high fever and chills. Other debridement techniques may be used instead of or after surgery, such as high-pressure, mechanical irrigation or wet-to-dry dressings. Vacuum-assisted closure therapy may be helpful in wound healing, especially for deep, chronic wounds of moderate to high exudate. This technique creates topical negative pressure with improved blood flow, decreased edema, and removal of excessive fluid from the wound bed. Improved tissue perfusion and oxygenation can result with increased tissue granulation and regeneration. Stem cell therapy may be effective in chronic ischemic wounds (e.g., diabetic foot) when vascularization is compromised (Shalaby et al., 2014). The hypoxic environment across the wound surface prevents survival of aerobic bacteria.

Chronic Wounds

Chronic wounds are distinguished from acute wounds by their healing characteristics and etiology and can persist for months or years. The most common chronic wound etiologies include changes related to burns, vasculitis, or dermatitis and complications related to delays in surgical wound healing, fistulas, manifestation of cancer in the skin, and tissue damage or death from radiation therapy. Although wound healing typically occurs in an orderly fashion, impediment of this process can occur in patients with cancer. Classification of chronic wounds related to etiology, wound depth, or degree of tissue damage is important, but accurate assessment of the wound and resulting healing is imperative to the plan of care (Shalaby et al., 2014).

Wound Assessment

Wound status must be assessed throughout the treatment period, which is a responsibility of APNs and the surgical team. Evidence-based scales and descriptors are helpful for quantitative assessment, with attention to anatomic characteristics of the wound: size, depth, edges, undermining, necrotic tissue type, necrotic tissue amount, exudate type, exudate amount, skin color surrounding the wound, peripheral tissue edema, peripheral tissue induration, granulation tissue, and epithelialization (García-Fernández, Pancorbo-Hidalgo, & Agreda, 2014). Education of staff members, patients, and families augments wound management and partnership in wound rehabilitation.

Risk assessment and prevention of pressure ulcers are essential in the care of patients with cancer. Conditions for skin breakdown are ideal because of the cancer itself, suboptimal nutrition, fatigue, and immunosuppression. Multiple comorbid risk factors also exist that contribute to development of pressure ulcers. Preventive measures with meticulous skin assessment are necessary, focusing on the individual patient's risk assessment, skin care, fluid balance, and nutrition. If a pressure wound develops, early intervention may avoid progression of tissue damage and ultimately surgical debridement.

Malignant Wounds

Malignant fungating wounds can present in advanced cancer as a result of local invasion by the primary tumor or metastatic disease. Unless treated, the tumor spreads and creates additional tissue destruction with resulting skin ulceration. Vascular and lymphatic supplies may change, leading to edema, exudates, bleeding, and tissue necrosis. The tumor mass may extend above the skin surface, presenting as an erosive and ulcerative lesion or a cauliflower-like growth. The wound bed typically consists of friable or necrotic tissue with fragile surrounding skin secondary to neoplastic ulceration (Sopata, Tomaszewska, Muszyński, Ciupińska, & Kotlińska-Lemieszek, 2013). Tissue necrosis and underlying infection are responsible for significant malodor. Management of odor occurs by decreasing local bacterial colonization, cleansing the wound, and debriding the wound. Dressing needs vary depending on the location of the wound, amount of exudates, and ability to secure the dressing to surrounding healthy skin. Adequate pain management is essential to maintaining patient comfort. Education and emotional support with attention to cosmesis and odor control potentially can improve quality of life for patients and caregivers.

Wound Care Management

Multiple (more than 800) wound care products are available to aid in preventing or treating delayed wound healing and fungating masses. These include but are not limited to hydrocolloids, impregnated gauze, hydrogels, alginates, film dressings, foam, hydrofibers, creams, ointments, sprays, enzymatic agents, powders, skin sealants, collagen matrix products, biologic or skin substitutes, and accessory products. Basic principles of wound assessment and management are essential to guide the treatment plan and dressing selection. APNs play an important role in wound management related to cancer therapy and may be consulted in the initial assessment phase. Enterostomal therapists are valuable resources for wound management and selection of wound care products specific to each patient (Hoedema & Suryadevara, 2010).

Stoma Care

A stoma is a mouth-like opening created surgically on the skin surface for access to underlying organs. Stoma openings are necessary in cancer surgery to divert normal internal lumens and to provide an alternative airway or method of elimination for urine or feces. The most common cancers requiring stoma are those related to the oropharynx and larynx, small and large bowel, and urinary system. The decision to create a stoma is based on the location and extent of a cancer along with concomitant issues such as infection or comorbid conditions (e.g., chronic obstructive pulmonary disease, scar tissue from previous surgeries).

Skin complications can occur as a result of irritation from surface contact with digestive fluids, poor skin integrity, excessive moisture, and restrictive appliances. External drainage apparatus containing bile or digestive products require attention to skin integrity maintenance, as degradation may occur in skin surfaces that are in frequent contact with digestive enzymes. Various products exist to improve stoma fit and to shield the skin from contact, thus preventing skin breakdown. Careful planning and education during the preoperative and postoperative phases are integral to successful adaptation of the body and the patient to a stoma. Enterostomal therapy nurses and wound, ostomy, and continence nurses are important resources for appliance fit and skin interventions (Hoedema & Suryadevara, 2010).

Skin Grafting

The extent of surgery, deformity, loss of function, and cosmetic results are factors to consider regarding skin grafting. If possible, skin grafting occurs at the time of tumor resection to maximize use of the anesthesia time and minimize postoperative colonization of endogenous and exogenous bacteria. Often, the decision of whether to graft is made at the time of surgery and can be difficult to predict because of potential unknown circulatory deficits (Actis & Actis, 2011). Assumed circulation to surrounding tissue and appropriate dressings may preclude the necessity of grafting, given adequate surface skin for closure. Delayed surgical graft placement can occur if healing does not progress, although closure of the wound by secondary intent or natural means often is preferred at this point. Skin grafting can be necessary in any surgery, as a result of the amount of removed subcutaneous tissue and skin, but the more common cancer types requiring grafting include head and neck cancer, melanoma, and cancer in a limb (i.e., amputation).

Skin graft healing is concomitant with wound healing, as the skin graft covers the wound with its own architecture. Skin graft revascularization occurs as blood and lymphatic vessels begin to grow from the surgical site into the graft and as preexisting vessels connect between the two sites. Blood and lymphatic flow to the graft approaches near-normal levels about seven days postoperatively. Maturity of the vascular supply continues and often is near normal by day 21 (Actis & Actis, 2011).

Reconstruction

Reconstruction of body parts altered by surgical treatment for cancer continues to evolve, with choices of immediate reconstruction (performed at the time of the cancer surgery) and delayed reconstruction (performed in a separate procedure after the cancer surgery). Reconstructive techniques include procedures such as tissue expansion, pedicled flaps, myocutaneous flaps, and free tissue transfer. The most common areas of reconstruction are the head and neck, breast, vagina, and extremities. The goal of reconstructive surgery in cancer is to eliminate suffering, decrease the deformity caused by cancer surgery, and restore wholeness (Alderman et al., 2011).

An increasing number of patients with breast cancer receive adjuvant radiation therapy after a mastectomy, with or without a reconstructed breast mound. Unsatisfactory results of conventional immediate reconstruction techniques when followed by radiation therapy have led to the formation of new algorithms. Questions remain as to the best method, timing, and outcomes for women undergoing immediate and delayed breast reconstruction without prior knowledge of the need for radiation therapy. Unfortunately, nodal status often is unknown during the decision-making phase for the type of breast surgery and possible type of reconstruction. The lack of this important information can lead to complications in the plastic surgery trajectory when postoperative radiation therapy is submitted for consideration after the definitive surgery has been performed (Eriksson et al., 2013).

The scope of this chapter does not permit detailed discussion of the various reconstructive procedures. APNs have a responsibility to identify patients who will have significant morbidity secondary to their cancer surgery and to tailor a personalized plan for their surgical care. Patients choose reconstruction to restore their removed body part and achieve symmetry, balance, weight replacement, and functionality. Reconstruction is an important component of restoring cosmesis and self-esteem. The plastic surgery team is responsible for restoring wholeness after the surgical team removes the cancer. Guiding patients and families through this trajectory can pose challenges that require ongoing revision for patients, both physically and psychologically.

Surveillance

All patients with cancer require ongoing surveillance for the unique medical needs related to their cancer diagnosis. Monitoring for possible local tumor recurrence, as well as disseminated disease, is necessary, including periodic interaction with patients and updated history information and physical examinations. Patients may be at risk for recurrence of their primary tumor, development of a second or related primary tumor because of genetic susceptibility, or development of a second primary tumor resulting from the cancer treatment. Unfortunately, in most cancers, extensive batteries of laboratory and imaging studies do not improve survival benefit. Surveillance tests designed for tumor-specific management provide long-term follow-up in this group of patients with diverse physical and psychosocial needs. (See Chapter 18 for more information on cancer surveillance following treatment.) The surgical team often maintains an ongoing relationship with patients with cancer and their families, thus assuming responsibility for appropriate surveillance testing with integral interventions.

APNs must take a leadership role in primary care of cancer survivors to promote effective cancer screening, healthy lifestyle choices, and continuing rehabilitation of the known cancer. Attention to the prevalence of multiple cancers is necessary, with review of genetic predisposition, environmental exposure, tobacco use, and aging. The spectrum of needs of cancer survivors and their families is extensive, requiring awareness of pertinent issues such as cancer-specific tumor biology, surveillance, genetic counseling and testing, second primaries, complications related to treatment, physiologic alterations, altered lifestyle, and psychosocial and caregiver challenges. APNs often fulfill the role of advocate, attending to the best interests of patients and families (Koch et al., 2014; Lester, 2011; Northouse, Williams, Given, & McCorkle, 2012).

Palliation

Palliation from a surgical perspective begins at the cancer diagnosis for all cancers. The goal is to maximize life and minimize side effects and disability, with the hope that the cancer will not recur locally or systemically. Although a few cancers can claim "cure" following a designated time period after surgery, the characteristics of most solid tumors do not avail a guarantee of cure with surgery alone. However, prolongation of life is not the only measure of success in cancer treatment. Palliation accomplished by surgical procedures is measured by disease-free intervals and the degrees of freedom from distress, rather than merely duration of life.

Each surgical intervention has risks and benefits. Surgical decisions, made together by the surgical team and patient, occur after thorough and thoughtful review of the patient's presentation, comorbid disease states, extent of disease, and wishes of the patient. Consideration of age alone as a factor is not relevant to decision making about palliative care, as older people are heterogeneous in terms of physical and psychological functioning. Discussion about goals, expectations, and physical cost of the intervention must be weighed against the potential negative side effects and complications, all in concert with personal belief systems, ethics, and end-of-life desires.

Surgical interventions to relieve symptom distress caused by side effects from metastatic cancer and to improve quality of life are becoming more common prior to the debilitating presence of life-threatening complications. Surgeons, endoscopists, interventional radiologists, anesthesiologists, and APNs all offer surgical expertise in controlling cancer-related symptoms. The rapid expansion of minimally invasive surgical approaches significantly decreases postoperative morbidity and hastens an improved outcome from the surgical intervention itself. Patient and procedure selection together require scrutiny in an effort to improve quality of life, sustain quantity of desired length of life, and maximize the side effect profile. And, as with all phases of medicine and the human body, no guarantees for outcome exist.

Conclusion

The role of surgery for patients with cancer and their families occurs throughout the cancer continuum, from prevention to diagnosis, from surgical resection through postoperative care, from access and rehabilitation to surveillance, and finally palliative care. Members of the surgical healthcare team, including APNs, play a vital role in the education, support, and care of patients with cancer and their families.

Case Study

J.L. is a 56-year-old Caucasian man who lives in an Appalachian county of southern Ohio. He recently saw a dentist for the first time in more than 15 years and noted that his "mouth is bleeding and hurts." His dentist noted several areas of leukoplakia on his tongue and an open friable lesion on his lower right posterior gum. J.L. was referred to an oral surgeon for evaluation of these findings.

1. How would the APN staffing this oral surgery clinic proceed?
   - The APN would interview the patient to obtain a complete history, including family history of cancer, personal cancer and health history, oral care history, smoking/tobacco use, alcohol use, drug use, and current medications. In addition, a full physical examination would be performed.
   - J.L.'s physical examination is consistent with the following.
     – Multiple areas of leukoplakia on superior and inferior surface of the tongue with lesions ranging from 0.3 to 1.5 cm, with the largest lesion noted on the right posterolateral edge of the tongue
     – One larger (approximately 1.5 cm), indurated, and friable lesion noted on the right posterolateral gum
     – A 3 cm firm, indurated, and friable lesion noted on the right lower posteromedial edge of the gum
     – Poor dentition with tobacco staining on remaining teeth
     – Clubbed fingers bilaterally with tobacco-stained nail beds and distal digits
     – Bilateral scattered rhonchi with decreased breath sounds in lower bases bilaterally.
     – J.L. admits to a 30+ pack-per-day smoking history. He occasionally smokes a pipe and also uses chewing tobacco on a daily basis. He drinks six to eight beers every evening and sometimes adds one to two hard-liquor drinks per night.
   - The oral surgeon reviews the physical examination information, examines the patient, and discusses the need for biopsies.

2. What would the surgeon and APN discuss next?
   - The surgeon and APN would
     – Arrange for scheduling of biopsies in the outpatient setting for the lesions on the tongue and gum
     – Order a chest x-ray, computed tomography scans, and general laboratories, as well as a complete preoperative examination
     – Discuss biopsies with patient
     – Discuss importance of smoking cessation and alcohol reduction, with referral of J.L. to smoking cessation clinic, and explain the importance of smoking cessation because of the tongue and gum lesions. (Note: These interventions must be in agreement with the patient's goals.)
   - The APN would discuss with J.L. the concern that these physical findings are highly suspicious for a locally advanced mouth cancer and need to be biopsied.

3. Following the biopsies, what will the surgeon and APN discuss?
   - The APN and surgeon discuss findings of the biopsies: squamous cell cancer of the tongue (multiple sites) and squamous cell cancer of mucosa of lower jaw.
   - The APN and surgeon discuss surgery to remove the lesions: removal of tongue, removal of lower jaw, SLNB/possible removal of cervical lymph nodes; followed by reconstruction of the jaw with bone and skin grafts

- The APN discusses the seriousness of these surgical procedures, including the necessary reconstructive procedures and grafts, with attention to emotional and decisional responses from patient and family.
- The APN discusses the impact of alcohol and tobacco use on surgical healing, especially skin and bone grafts. The patient and APN will create a care plan to successfully eliminate these behaviors. The surgery will be delayed until the patient has been tobacco free for two to four weeks, as the evidence supports improved healing of tissues. J.L. admits that he has not discontinued tobacco use, although has successfully weaned off alcohol because it burns his biopsy sites.
- The APN discusses the need for nutritional support after surgery and throughout postoperative radiation therapy. This will most likely consist of an oral feeding tube or external gastric or jejunostomy feeding tube. At this point, the patient decided he was not going to undergo any surgical interventions.
- The APN discusses the seriousness of J.L.'s diagnoses and the continued ulceration and skin erosion that will occur if no surgical interventions are performed. The APN was successful in helping J.L. to attain his recommended treatment. The APN, J.L., and J.L.'s family agree that additional counseling is needed before surgery in order to cope with these life-altering events.
- The APN discusses these issues with the surgeon and calls the psychologist for an emergency consult later in the day.
- The APN follows up with J.L. and his family to ensure appropriate emotional and physical support. Goals, objectives, and barriers will be communicated by the ambulatory clinic APN to the inpatient surgical team/APN to maximize patient outcomes.
- Postoperatively, the APN will be involved in J.L.'s rehabilitation and survivorship care, with awareness that multiple challenges await J.L.

Key Points

- Surgery is the oldest modality for cancer treatment and today is still the only means of cure in many cancers. It is used in every aspect of oncology care, including cancer prevention, diagnosis, resection, postoperative care, access, rehabilitation, surveillance, and palliation.
- Surgery involves removal of the tumor with adequate margins of normal tissue. Adequate margins vary from cancer to cancer.
- A diagnosis of cancer relies on tissue acquisition for pathologic, cytologic, and possibly histologic review. Information obtained from the history, physical examination, observation, and diagnostic testing guides the surgical plan for tissue acquisition. Correlation of pathologic information obtained from the tissue biopsy with radiology studies, physical examination, and the patient's history is necessary for accurate diagnosis.
- A negative needle biopsy (fine or core needle) does not ensure that a lesion is benign. If suspicion for malignancy is high and the needle biopsy is negative or inconclusive, an open biopsy is necessary to verify a diagnosis.
- Surgical APNs often serve as navigators or interpreters for patients and families by explaining available treatment options that may influence patients' decision-making processes, facilitating interdisciplinary consultations, and providing continuity of care during transition to other care settings.
- The goals of cancer surgical therapy are to (a) maximize potential for control or cure of cancer, (b) minimize comorbidities, and (c) retain active participation of patients and families.
- The preoperative assessment includes medical, surgical, and psychosocial history, nutritional status, medication review, laboratory and imaging studies, teaching needs, and risk of post-

surgical infection. Potential surgical benefits are weighed against the risks of the surgical interventions.

- Regional lymph nodes, the most frequent site of metastasis for most solid tumors, often are resected as part of the staging workup of the tumor even if visible tumor is not evident. If visible tumor is evident (or is confirmed by intraoperative pathology), then lymph node dissection is performed for regional control of the cancer.
- SLNB is a surgical approach to evaluate regional lymph nodes by using a radioactive tracer or dye directed at the tumor bed and lymph supply that enables the surgeon to visualize the first node or nodes draining the tumor. If the first lymph node is pathologically negative for tumor, node dissection often is not performed, thus saving the patient from unnecessary surgery.
- Surgical resection of metastatic sites removes cancers that are confined to one metastatic organ, improving overall five-year survival by 25%–40% (depending on the cancer and metastatic site). However, most cancer types are not amenable to this approach because of the malignant potential caused by systemic, micrometastatic disease.
- Minimally invasive surgery lessens the degree of trauma and blood loss and involves smaller surgical scars, less overall surgical pain, and decreased postoperative stays. It typically is reserved for early-stage cancer and is widely used in diagnostic and staging procedures, second-look procedures, diagnosis of recurrent disease, and palliative care.

Recommended Resources for Oncology Advanced Practice Nurses

- Davidson, G.W., Lester, J.L., & Routt, M. (Eds.). (2014). *Surgical oncology nursing*. Pittsburgh, PA: Oncology Nursing Society.
- InPractice for Nurses, Oncology Nursing (2014): http://inpractice.com
- Joint Commission Surgical Care Improvement Project (2014): www.jointcommission.org/surgical_care_improvement_project
- National Comprehensive Cancer Network Clinical Practice Guidelines in Oncology (NCCN Guidelines®): www.nccn.org
- Oncology Nursing Society's *Site-Specific Cancer Series* books

References

Actis, A.G., & Actis, G. (2011). Reconstruction of the upper eyelid with flaps and free grafts after excision of basal cell carcinoma. *Case Reports in Ophthalmology, 2,* 347–353. doi:10.1159/000334674

Alderman, A.K., Hawley, S.T., Morrow, M., Salem, B., Hamilton, A., Graff, J.J., & Katz, S. (2011). Receipt of delayed breast reconstruction after mastectomy: Do women revisit the decision? *Annals of Surgical Oncology, 18,* 1748–1755. doi:10.1245/s10434-010-1509-y

Altorki, N.K., Yip, R., Hanaoka, T., Bauer, T., Aye, R., Kohman, L., … Henschke, C.I. (2014). Sublobar resection is equivalent to lobectomy for clinical stage IA lung cancer in solid nodules. *Journal of Thoracic and Cardiovascular Surgery, 147,* 754–764. doi:10.1016/j.jtcvs.2013.09.065

Amri, R., Bordeianou, L.G., Sylla, P., & Berger, D.L. (2014). Obesity, outcomes and quality of care: Body mass index increased the risk of wound-related complications in colon cancer surgery. *American Journal of Surgery, 207,* 17–23. doi:10.1016/j.amjsurg.2013.05.016

Anaya, D.A., Cormier, J.N., Xing, Y., Koller, P., Gaido, L., Hadfield, D., … Feig, B.W. (2012). Development and validation of a novel stratification tool for identifying cancer patients at increased risk of surgical site infection. *Annals of Surgery, 255,* 134–139. doi:10.1097/SLA.0b013e31823dc107

Atkins, K.A., Cohen, M.A., Nicholson, B., & Rao, S. (2013). Atypical lobular hyperplasia and lobular carcinoma in situ at core breast biopsy: Use of careful radiologic-pathologic correlation to recommend excision or observation. *Radiology, 269,* 340–347. doi:10.1148/radiol.13121730

Azria, D., & Lemanski, C. (2014). Intraoperative radiotherapy for breast cancer. *Lancet, 383,* 578–581. doi:10.1016/S0140-6736(13)62304-1

Bagga, V., Yapa, S., Craven, I., Romanowski, C., & Jellinek, D. (2013). Lymphoblastic leukaemia presenting as a carotid-cavernous fistula. *Neuroradiology Journal, 26,* 94–96.

Bardhan, K., & Liu, K. (2013). Epigenetics and colorectal cancer pathogenesis. *Cancers, 5,* 676–713. doi:10.3390/cancers5020676

Bednar, R., Scheiman, J.M., McKenna, B.J., & Simeone, D.M. (2013). Breast cancer metastasis to the pancreas. *Journal of Gastrointestinal Surgery, 17,* 1826–1831. doi:10.1007/s11605-013-2291-5

Borreani, C., Manoukian, S., Bianchi, E., Brunelli, C., Peissel, B., Caruso, A., … Peirotti, M.A. (2014). The psychological impact of breast and ovarian cancer preventive options in *BRCA1* and *BRCA2* mutation carriers. *Clinical Genetics, 85,* 7–15. doi:10.1111/cge.12298

Boyce, S., Fan, Y., Watson, R.W., & Murphy, T.B. (2013). Evaluation of prediction models for the staging of prostate cancer. *BMC Medical Informatics and Decision Making, 13,* 126. doi:10.1186/1472-6947-13-126

Brock, A.S., Wallace, K., Romagnuolo, J., & Hoffman, B.J. (2013). Patients' short-term knowledge of personal polyp history inadequate despite systematic notification of results after polypectomy. *Southern Medical Journal, 106,* 285–289. doi:10.1097/SMJ.0b013e31828de5f6

Brown, B.N., Londono, R., Tottey, S., Zhang, L., Kukla, K.A., Wolf, M.T., … Badylak, S.F. (2012). Macrophage phenotype as a predictor of constructive remodeling following the implantation of biologically derived surgical mesh materials. *Acta Biomaterialia, 8,* 978–987. doi:10.1016/j.actbio.2011.11.031

Bugalho, A., Ferreira, D., Eberhardt, R., Dias, S.S., Videira, P.A., Herth, F.J., & Carreiro, L. (2013). Diagnostic value of endobronchial and endoscopic ultrasound-guided fine needle aspiration for accessible lung cancer lesions after non-diagnostic conventional techniques: A prospective study. *BMC Cancer, 13,* 130. doi:10.1186/1471-2407-13-130

Cabibbo, G., Maida, M., Genco, C., Alessi, N., Peralta, M., Butera, G., … Camma, C. (2013). Survival of patients with hepatocellular carcinoma (HCC) treated by percutaneous radio-frequency ablation (RFA) is affected by complete radiological response. *PLOS ONE, 8*(7), e70016. doi:10.1371/journal.pone.0070016

Cerruto, M.A., D'Elia, C., & Artibani, W. (2012). Focal salvage therapy for locally recurrent prostate: A review. *Urologia, 79,* 219–231 doi:10.5301/RU.2012.9908

Chen, H.-J., Yang, J.-J., Xu, C.-R., Lei, Y.-Y., Luo, D.-L., Yan, H.-H., & Wu, Y.-L. (2013). Principles of biopsy in suspected lung cancer: Priority still based on invasion in the era of targeted therapy? *Journal of Thoracic Disease, 5,* E93–E97. doi:10.3978/j.issn.2072-1439.2013.04.17

Chen, K., Xu, X.W., Zhang, R.C., Pan, Y., Wu, D., & Mou, Y.P. (2013). Systematic review and meta-analysis of laparoscopy-assisted and open gastrectomy for gastric cancer. *World Journal of Gastroenterology, 19,* 5365–5376. doi:10.3748/wjg.v19.i32.5365

Chiu, M., Bryson, G.L., Lui, A., Watters, J.M., Taljaard, M., & Nathan, H.J. (2014). Reducing persistent postoperative pain and disability 1 year after breast cancer surgery: A randomized, controlled trial comparing thoracic paravertebral block to local anesthetic infiltration. *Annals of Surgical Oncology, 21,* 795–801. doi:10.1245/s10434-013-3334-6

Correa-Gallego, C., Dinkelspiel, H.E., Sulimanoff, I., Fisher, S., Vinuela, E.F., Kingham, T.P., … Allen, P.J. (2013). Minimally-invasive vs. open pancreaticoduodenectomy: Systematic review and meta-analysis. *Journal of the American College of Surgeons, 218,* 129–139. doi:10.1016/j.jamcollsurg.2013.09.005

Dale, W., Hemmerich, J., Kamm, A., Posner, M.C., Matthews, J.B., Rothman, R., … Roggin, K.K., (2014). Geriatric assessment improves prediction of surgical outcomes in older adults undergoing pancreaticoduodenectomy: A prospective cohort study. *Annals of Surgery, 259,* 960–965. doi:10.1097/SLA.0000000000000226

De Nardi, P., & Carvello, M. (2013). How reliable is current imaging in restaging rectal cancer after neoadjuvant therapy? *World Journal of Gastroenterology, 19,* 5964–5972. doi:10.3748/wjg.v19.i36.5964

Diaz, E.S., Aoyama, C., Baquing, M.A., Beavis, A., Silva, E., Holschneider, C., & Cass, I. (2014). Predictors of residual carcinoma or carcinoma-in-situ at hysterectomy following cervical conization with position margins. *Gynecologic Oncology, 132,* 76–80. doi:10.1016/j.ygyno.2013.11.019

Dursun, P., Caglar, M., Akilli, H., & Ayhan, A. (2013). Large conization and laparoendoscopic single-port pelvic lymphadenectomy in early-stage cervical cancer for fertility preservation. *Case Reports in Surgery, 2013,* Article 207191. doi:10.1155/2013/207191

Emhoff, I.A., Lee, G.C., & Sylla, P. (2014). Transanal colorectal resection using natural orifice translumenal endoscopic surgery (NOTES). *Digestive Endoscopy, 26*(Suppl. 1), 29–42. doi:10.1111/den.12157

Eriksson, M., Anveden, L., Celebioglu, F., Dahlberg, K., Meldahl, I., Lagergren, J., … de Boniface, J. (2013). Radiotherapy in implant-based immediate breast reconstruction: Risk factors, surgical outcomes, and patient-reported outcome measures in a large Swedish multicenter cohort. *Breast Cancer Research and Treatment, 142,* 591–601. doi:10.1007/s10549-013-2770-0

García-Fernández, F.P., Pancorbo-Hidalgo, P.L., & Agreda, J.J.S. (2014). Predictive capacity of risk assessment scales and clinical judgment for pressure ulcers: A meta-analysis. *Journal of Wound, Ostomy, and Continence Nursing, 41,* 24–34. doi:10.1097/01.WON.0000438014.90734.a2

Ghigna, C., Riva, S., & Biamonti, G. (2013). Alternative splicing of tumor suppressors and oncogenes. *Cancer Treatment and Research, 158,* 95–117. doi:10.1007/978-3-642-31659-3_4

Gil-Gil, M.J., Martinez-Garcia, M., Sierra, A., Conesa, G., del Barco, S., González-Jimenez, S., & Villà, S. (2014). Breast cancer brain metastases: A review of the literature and a current multidisciplinary management guideline. *Clinical and Translational Oncology, 16,* 436–446. doi:10.1007/s12094-013-1110-5

Giuliano, A.E., Morrow, M., Duggal, S., & Julian, T.B. (2012). Should ACOSOG Z0011 change practice with respect to axillary lymph node dissection for a positive sentinel lymph node biopsy in breast cancer? *Clinical and Experimental Metastasis, 29,* 687–692. doi:10.1007/s10585-012-9515-z

Godfrey, C., Villa, C., Dawson, L., Swindells, S., & Schouten, J.T. (2013). Controlling healthcare-associated infections in the international research setting. *Journal of Acquired Immune Deficiency Syndromes, 62,* e115–118. doi:10.1097/QAI.0b013e3182845b95

Gojon, H., Fawunmi, D., & Valachis, A. (2014). Sentinel lymph node biopsy in patients with microinvasive breast cancer: A systematic review and meta-analysis. *European Journal of Surgical Oncology, 40,* 5–11. doi:10.1016/j.ejso.2013.10.020

Green, V.L. (2013). Breast cancer risk assessment, prevention, and the future. *Obstetrics and Gynecology Clinics of North America, 40,* 525–549. doi:10.1016/j.ogc.2013.05.003

Gumus, H., Mills, P., Fish, D., Gumus, M., Devalia, H., Jones, S.E., & Sever, A.R. (2013). Breast microcalcifications: Diagnostic value of calcified and non-calcified cores on specimen radiographs. *Breast Journal, 19,* 156–161. doi:10.1111/tbj.12069

Hennessey, D.B., Burke, J.P., Ni-Dhonochu, T., Sields, C., Winter, D.C., & Mealy, K. (2010). Preoperative hypoalbuminemia is an independent risk factor or the development of surgical site infection following gastrointestinal surgery: A multi-institutional study. *Annals of Surgery, 252,* 325–329. doi:10.1097/SLA.0b013d3183e9819a

Hennon, M.W., & Demmy, T.L. (2012). Video-assisted thoracoscopic surgery (VATS) for locally advanced lung cancer. *Annals of Cardiothoracic Surgery, 1,* 37–42. doi:10.3978/j.issn.2225-319X.2012.03.05

Hoedema, R.E., & Suryadevara, S. (2010). Enterostomal therapy and wound care of the enterocutaneous fistula patient. *Clinics in Colon and Rectal Surgery, 23,* 161–168. doi:10.1055/s-0030-1262983

Hofer, C.K., Rex, S., & Ganter, M.T. (2014). Update on minimally invasive hemodynamic monitoring in thoracic anesthesia. *Current Opinion in Anaesthesiology, 27,* 28–25. doi:10.1097/ACO.0000000000000034

Hoppo, T., & Jobe, B.A. (2013). Personalizing therapy for esophageal cancer patients. *Thoracic Surgery Clinics, 23,* 471–478. doi:10.1016/j.thorsurg.2013.07.001

Hudson, S.V. (2013). Continuous primary care is central to comprehensive cancer care: Are we ready to meet growing needs? *Journal of the American Board of Family Medicine, 26,* 623–625. doi:10.3122/jabfm.2013.06.130256

Ishizawa, T., Zuker, N.B., Conrad, C., Lei, H.-J., Ciacio, O., Kokudo, N., & Gayet, B. (2014). Using a 'no drain' policy in 342 laparoscopic hepatectomies: Which factors predict failure? *HPB, 16,* 494–499. doi:10.1111/hpb.12165

Itatsu, K., Sugawara, G., Kaneoka, Y., Kato, T., Takeuchi, E., Kanai, M., … Nagino, M. (2014). Risk factors for incisional surgical site infections in elective surgery for colorectal cancer: Focus on intraoperative meticulous wound management. *Surgery Today, 44,* 1242–1252. doi:10.1007/s00595-013-0677-3

Jacobs, M.J., & Kamyab, A. (2013). Total laparoscopic pancreaticoduodenectomy. *Journal of the Society of Laparoendoscopic Surgeons, 17,* 188–193. doi:10.4293/108680813X13654754534792

James, T.A., Mace, J.L., Virnig, B.A., & Geller, B.M. (2012). Preoperative needle biopsy improves the quality of breast cancer surgery. *Journal of the American College of Surgeons, 215,* 562–568. doi:10.1016/j.jamcollsurg.2012.05.022

Joint Commission. (2014, October 16). Surgical Care Improvement Project. Retrieved from http://www.jointcommission.org/surgical_care_improvement_project

Jurado, J., Saqi, A., Maxfield, R., Newmark, A., Lavelle, M., Bacchetta, M., … Bulman, W. (2013). The efficacy of EBUS-guided transbronchial needle aspiration for molecular testing in lung adenocarcinoma. *Annals of Thoracic Surgery, 96,* 1196–1202. doi:10.1016/j.athoracsur.2013.05.066

Kim, H.R., Lee, W.Y., Jung, K.U., Yun, H.-R., Cho, Y.B., Yun, S.H., … Chun, H.-K. (2012). Early surgical outcomes of NiTi endoluminal compression anastomotic clip (NiTi CAC 30) use in patients with gastrointestinal malignancy. *Journal of Laparoendoscopic and Advanced Surgical Techniques, 22,* 472–478. doi:10.1089/lap.2011.0406

Kiran, R.P., Turina, M., Hammel, J., & Fazio, V. (2013). The clinical significance of an elevated postoperative glucose value in nondiabetic patients after colorectal surgery: Evidence for the need for tight glucose control? *Annals of Surgery, 258,* 599–604. doi:10.1097/SLA.0b013e3182a501e3

Koch, L., Bertram, H., Eberle, A., Holleczek, B., Schmid-Höpfner, S., Waldmann, A., … Arndt, V. (2014). Fear of recurrence in long-term breast cancer survivors—Still an issue. Results on prevalence, determinants, and the association with quality of life and depression from the Cancer Survivorship—A multi-regional population-based study. *Psycho-Oncology, 23,* 547–554. doi:10.1002/pon.3452

Kwaan, M.R., Vogler, S.A., Sun, M.Y., Sirany, A.M.E., Melton, G.B., Madoff, R.D., & Rothenberger, D.A. (2013). Readmission after colorectal surgery is related to preoperative clinical conditions and major complications. *Diseases of the Colon and Rectum, 56,* 1087–1092. doi:10.1097/DCR.0b013e31829aa758

Lamb, B.W., Green, J.S.A., Benn, J., Brown, K.F., Vincent, C.A., & Sevdalis, N. (2013). Improving decision making in multidisciplinary tumor boards: Prospective longitudinal evaluation of a multi-component intervention for 1,421 patients. *Journal of the American College of Surgeons, 217,* 412–420. doi:10.1016/j.jamcollsurg.2013.04.035

Lambert, R. (2012). Endoscopy in screening for digestive cancer. *World Journal of Gastrointestinal Endoscopy, 16,* 518–525. doi:10.4253/wjge.v4.i12.518

Lane, A., Segura-Cabrera, A., & Komurov, K. (2014). A comparative survey of functional footprints of EGFR pathway mutations in human cancers. *Oncogene, 33,* 5078–5089.

Lang, B.H.-H., Wong, C.K.H., Tsang, J.S., Wong, K.P., & Wan, K.Y. (2014). A systematic review and meta-analysis comparing surgically-related complications between robotic-assisted thyroidectomy and conventional open thyroidectomy. *Annals of Surgical Oncology, 21,* 850–861. doi:10.1245/s10434-013-3406-7

Larentzakis, A., & Theodorou, D. (2014). A multicenter study of survival after neoadjuvant radiotherapy/chemotherapy and esophagectomy for ypT0N0K0R0 esophageal cancer. *Annals of Surgery, 259,* e67. doi:10.1097/SLA.0000000000000364

Leibovici, D., Shikanov, S., Gofrit, O.N., Zagaja, G.P., Shilo, Y., & Shalhav, A.L. (2013). How accurate is our clinical prediction of "minimal prostate cancer"? *Israel Medical Association Journal, 15,* 359–363. Retrieved from http://www.ima.org.il/FilesUpload/IMAJ/0/65/32860.pdf

Lester, J.L. (2011). Cancer survivorship care plans. In J.L. Lester & P. Schmitt (Eds.), *Cancer rehabilitation and survivorship: Transdisciplinary approaches to personalized care* (pp. 359–369). Pittsburgh, PA: Oncology Nursing Society.

Litsas, G. (2013). Individualizing care for women with early-stage breast cancer: The role of molecular assays. *Clinical Journal of Oncology Nursing, 17,* 332–334. doi:10.1188/13.CJON.332-334

Liverani, C.A. (2013). The four steps in the prevention of human papillomavirus-associated neoplasia: Considerations for preventive measures, screening, disease impact, and potential overtreatments in HPV-related pathology. *Archives of Gynecology and Obstetrics, 288,* 979–988. doi:10.1007/s00404-013-3011-9

Livingston, E.H. (2013). Postoperative venous thromboembolic disease: Prevention, public reporting, and patient protection. *JAMA, 310,* 1453–1454. doi:10.1001/jama.2013.280049

Lochan, R., French, J.J., & Manas, D.M. (2011). Surgery for retroperitoneal soft tissue sarcomas: Aggressive re-resection of recurrent disease is possible. *Annals of the Royal College of Surgeons of England, 93,* 39–43. doi:10.1308/003588410X12771863936729

Lumachi, F., Basso, S.M., Santeufemia, D.A., Bonamini, M., & Chiara, G.B. (2013). Ultrasonic dissection system technology in breast cancer: A case-control study in a large cohort of patients requiring axillary dissection. *Breast Cancer Research and Treatment, 142,* 399–404. doi:10.1007/s01549-013-2746-0

Lyman, G.H., Khorana, A.A., Kuderer, N.M., Lee, A.Y., Arcelus, J.I., Balaban, E.P., … Falanga, A. (2013). Venous thromboembolism prophylaxis and treatment in patients with cancer: American Society of Clinical Oncology clinical practice guideline update. *Journal of Clinical Oncology, 31,* 2189–2204. doi:10.1200/JCO.2013.49.1118

Masroor, I., Afzal, S., Shafqat, G., & Rehman, H. (2012). Usefulness of hook wire localization biopsy under imaging guidance for nonpalpable breast lesions detected radiologically. *International Journal of Women's Health, 4,* 445–449. doi:10.2147/IJWH.S35280

McWilliams, A., Shaipanich, T., & Lam, S. (2013). Fluorescence and navigational bronchoscopy. *Thoracic Surgery Clinics, 23,* 153–161. doi:10.1016/j.thorsurg.2013.01.008

MedlinePlus. (2013). Anesthesia. Retrieved from http://www.nlm.nih.gov/medlineplus/anesthesia.html

Mills, E., Eyawo, O., Lockhart, I., Kelly, S., Wu, P., & Ebbert, J.O. (2011). Smoking cessation reduces postoperative complications: A systematic review and meta-analysis. *American Journal of Medicine, 124,* 144–154.e8. doi:10.1016/j.amjmed.2010.09.013

Mokarram, N., & Bellamkonda, R.V. (2014). A perspective on immunomodulation and tissue repair. *Annals of Biomedical Engineering, 42,* 338–351. doi:10.1007/s10439-013-0941-0

Moreno, P., de la Quintana Basarrate, A., Musholt, T.J., Paunovic, I., Puccini, M., Vidal, O., … Ramia, J.M. (2013). Adrenalectomy for solid tumor metastases: Results of a multicenter European study. *Surgery, 154,* 1215–1223. doi:10.1016/j.surg.2013.06.021

Mori, K., Yamagata, Y., Wada, I., Shimizu, N., Nomura, S., & Seto, Y. (2013). Robotic-assisted totally transhiatal lymphadenectomy in the middle mediastinum for esophageal cancer. *Journal of Robotic Surgery, 7,* 385–387. doi:10.1007/s11701-013-0398-z

Morris, N.S., Field, T.S., Wagner, J.L., Cutrona, S.L., Roblin, D.W., Gaglio, B., … Mazor, K.M. (2013). The association between health literacy and cancer-related attitudes, behaviors, and knowledge. *Journal of Health Communication: International Perspectives, 18*(Suppl. 1), 223–241. doi:10.1080/10810730.2013.825667

Nader, A., Kendall, M.C., De Oliveira, G.S., Jr., Puri, L., Tureanu, L., Brodskaia, A., … McCarthy, R.J. (2013). A dose-ranging study of 0.5% bupivacaine or ropivacaine on the success and duration of the ultrasound-guided, nerve-stimulator-assisted sciatic nerve block: A double-blind, randomized clinical trial. *Regional Anesthesia and Pain Medicine, 38,* 492–502. doi:10.1097/AAP.0b013e3182a4bddf

Narouze, S.N., Provenzano, D., Peng, P., Eichenberger, U., Lee, S.C., Nicholls, B., & Moriggl, B. (2012). The American Society of Regional Anesthesia and Pain Medicine, the European Society of Regional Anesthesia and Pain Therapy, and the Asian Australasian Federation of Pain Societies Joint Committee recommendations for education and training in ultrasound-guided interventional pain procedures. *Regional Anesthesia and Pain Medicine, 37,* 657–664. doi:10.1097/AAP.0b013e318269c189

Nicholson, A., Coldwell, C.H., Lewis, S.R., & Smith, A.F. (2013). Nurse-led versus doctor-led preoperative assessment for elective surgical patients requiring regional or general anesthesia. *Cochrane Database of Systematic Reviews, 2013*(11). doi:10.1002/14651858.CD010160.pub2

Niwa, H., Rowbotham, D.J., Lambert, D.G., & Buggy, D.J. (2013). Can anesthetic techniques or drugs affect cancer recurrence in patients undergoing cancer surgery? *Journal of Anesthesia, 27,* 731–741. doi:10.1007/s00540-013-1615-7

Northouse, L., Williams, A.L., Given, B., & McCorkle, R. (2012). Psychosocial care for family caregivers of patients with cancer. *Journal of Clinical Oncology, 30,* 1227–1234. doi:10.1200/JCO.2011/39.576

Ortega-Deballon, P., Duvillard, L., Scherrer, M.-L., Deguelte-Lardière, S., Bourredjem, A., Petit, J.-M., & Bonithon-Kopp, C. (2014). Preoperative adipocytokines as a predictor of surgical infection after colorectal surgery: A prospective survey. *International Journal of Colorectal Disease, 29,* 23–29. doi:10.1007/s00384-013-1782-x

Palmeri, S., Berretta, M., & Palmeri, L. (2013). Medical treatment of elderly patients with breast cancer. *Anti-Cancer Agents and Medicinal Chemistry, 13,* 1325–1331. doi:10.2174/18715206113136660358

Peck, J.R., Hitchcock, C.L., Maguire, S., Dickerson, J., & Bush, C. (2012). Isolated cardiac metastasis from plasmacytoid urothelial carcinoma of the bladder. *Experimental Hematology and Oncology, 1*(1), 16. doi:10.1186/2162-3619-1-16

Poullis, M., McShane, J., Shaw, M., Woolley, S., Shackcloth, M., Page, R., & Mediratta, N. (2012). Lung cancer staging: A physiological update. *Interactive Cardiovascular and Thoracic Surgery, 14,* 743–749. doi:10.1093/icvts/ivr164

Rengan, A.K., Jagtap, M., De, A., Banerjee, R., & Srivastava, R. (2014). Multifunctional gold coated thermo-sensitive liposomes for multimodal imaging and photo-thermal therapy of breast cancer cells. *Nanoscale, 6,* 916–923. doi:10.1039/c3nr04448c

Revenig, L.M., Canter, D.J., Taylor, M.D., Tai, C., Sweeney, J.F., Sarmiento, J.M., … Ogan, K. (2013). Too frail for surgery? Initial results of a large multidisciplinary prospective study examining preoperative variables predictive of poor surgical outcomes. *Journal of the American College of Surgeons, 217,* 665–670.e1. doi:10.1016/j.jamcollsurg.2013.06.012

Rizk, N. (2013). Surgery for esophageal cancer: Goals of resection and optimizing outcomes. *Thoracic Surgery Clinics, 23,* 491–498. doi:10.1016/j.thorsurg.2013.07.009

Robinson, T.N., Wu, D.S., Pointer, L., Dunn, C.L., Cleveland, J.S., Jr., & Moss, M. (2013). Simple frailty score predicts postoperative complications across surgical specialties. *American Journal of Surgery, 206,* 544–550. doi:10.1016/j.amjsurg.2013.03.012

Robinson, W., & Cantillo, E. (2014). Debulking surgery and intraperitoneal chemotherapy are associated with decreased morbidity in women receiving neoadjuvant chemotherapy for ovarian cancer. *International Journal of Gynecological Cancer, 24,* 43–47. doi:10.1097/IGC.0000000000000009

Roos, D., Dijksman, L.M., Tijssen, J.G., Gouma, D.J., Gerhards, M.F., & Oudemans-van Straaten, H.M. (2013). Systematic review of perioperative selective decontamination of the digestive tract in elective gastrointestinal surgery. *British Journal of Surgery, 100,* 1579–1588. doi:10.1002/bjs.9254

Savina, E.N., & Couturaud, F. (2011). [Optimal duration of anticoagulation of venous thromboembolism]. *Journal des Maladies Vasculaires, 36*(Suppl. 1), S28–S32. doi:10.1016/S0398-0499(11)70005-1

Schmitt, A.R., Brewer, J.D., Bordeaux, J.S., & Baum, C.L. (2014). Staging for cutaneous squamous cell carcinoma as a predictor of sentinel lymph node biopsy results: Meta-analysis of American Joint Committee on Cancer criteria and a proposed alternative system. *JAMA Dermatology, 150,* 19–24. doi:10.1001/jamadermatol.2013.6675

Schramp, L.C., Holtcamp, M., Phillips, S.A., Johnson, T.P., & Hoff, J. (2010). Advanced practice nurses facilitating clinical translational research. *Clinical Medicine and Research, 8,* 131–134. doi:10.3121/cmr.2010.911

Schroeder, S.M. (2014). Perioperative management of the patient with diabetes mellitus: Update and overview. *Clinics in Podiatric Medicine and Surgery, 31,* 1–10. doi:10.1016/j.cpm.2013.10.002

Schurr, M.O., Baur, F., Ho, C.N., Anhoeck, G., Kratt, T., & Gottwald, T. (2011). Endoluminal full-thickness resection of GI lesions: A new device and technique. *Minimally Invasive Therapy and Allied Technologies, 20,* 189–192. doi:10.3109/136445706.2011.582119

Schuster, F., Johannsen, S., Schneiderbanger, D., & Roewer, N. (2013). Evaluation of suspected malignant hyperthermia events during anesthesia. *BMC Anesthesiology, 13*(1), 24. doi:10.1186/1471.2253–13-24

Shalaby, S.Y., Blume, P., & Sumpio, B.E. (2014). New modalities in the chronic ischemic diabetic foot management. *Clinics in Podiatric Medicine and Surgery, 31,* 27–42. doi:10.1015/j.cpm.2013.09.009

Shantz, J.A., Vernon, J., Leiter, J., Morshed, S., & Stranges, G. (2012). Sutures versus staples or wound closure in orthopaedic surgery: A randomized controlled trial. *BMC Musculoskeletal Disorders, 13,* 89. doi:10.1186/1471-2474-13-89

Sharma, A., & Jamal, M.M. (2013). Opioid induced bowel disease: A twenty-first century physicians' dilemma. *Current Gastroenterology Reports, 15,* 334. doi:10.1007/s11894-013-0334-4

Shinkawa, H., Takemura, S., Uenishi, T., Sakae, M., Ohata, K., Urta, Y., … Kubo, S. (2013). Nutritional risk index as an independent predictor factor for the development of surgical site infection after pancreaticoduodenectomy. *Surgery Today, 43,* 276–283. doi:10.1007/s00595-012-0350-2

Shylasree, T.S., Bryant, A., & Athavale, R. (2013). Chemotherapy and/or radiotherapy in combination with surgery for ovarian carcinosarcoma. *Cochrane Database of Systematic Reviews, 2013*(2). doi:10.1002/14651858.CD006246.pub2

Siddiqui, M.M., Rais-Bahrami, S., Truong, H., Stamatakis, L., Vourganti, S., Nix, J., … Pinto, P.A. (2013). Magnetic resonance imaging/ultrasound-fusion biopsy significantly upgrades prostate cancer versus systematic 12-core transrectal ultrasound biopsy. *European Urology, 64,* 713–719. doi:10.1016/j.eururo.2013.05.059

Smith, D.D., Nelson, R.A., & Schwarz, R.E. (2014). A comparison of five competing lymph node staging schemes in a cohort of resectable gastric cancer patients. *Annals of Surgical Oncology, 21,* 875–882. doi:10.1245/s10434-013-3356-0

Sofocleous, C.T., Sideras, P., & Petre, E.N. (2013). "How we do it"—A practical approach to hepatic metastases ablation techniques. *Technology in Vascular Interventional Radiology, 16,* 219–229. doi:10.1053/j.tvir.2013.08.005

Sooriakumaran, P., Srivastava, A., Shariat, S.F., Stricker, P.D., Ahlering, T., Eden, C.G., … Tewari, A.K. (2014). A multinational, multi-institutional study comparing positive surgical margin rates among 22393 open, laparoscopic, and robot-assisted radical prostatectomy patients. *European Urology, 66,* 450–456. doi:10.1016/j.eururo.2013.11.018

Sopata, M., Tomaszewska, E., Muszyński, Z., Ciupińska, M., & Kotlińska-Lemieszek, A. (2013). The pilot study assessing efficacy and versatility of novel therapy for neoplastic ulceration: Clinical and microbiological aspects. *Advances in Dermatology and Allergology, 30,* 237–245. doi:10.5114/pdia.2013.37034

Souza, P.S., Braga, A.C., Meira, C.A., Takahama, S.E., Seiko, K.C., Maidi, V.A.L., … Pereira, Y.W. (2014). Implementation of a guideline for physical therapy in the postoperative period of upper abdominal surgery reduces the incidence of atelectasis and length of hospital stay. *Revista Portuguesa de Pneumologia, 20,* 69–77. doi:10.1016/j.rppneu.2013.07.005

Swanson, S.J., Miller, D.L., McKenna, R.J., Jr., Howington, J., Marshall, M.B., Yoo, A.C., … Meyers, B.F. (2014). Comparing robot-assisted thoracic surgical lobectomy with conventional video-assisted thoracic surgical lobectomy and wedge resection: Results from a multihospital database (Premier). *Journal of Thoracic and Cardiovascular Surgery, 147,* 929–937. doi:10.1016/j.jtcvs.2013.09.046

Thompson, J.E., Egger, S., Böhm, M., Haynes, A.-M., Matthews, J., Rasiah, K., & Stricker, P.D. (2014). Superior quality of life and improved surgical margins are achievable with robotic radical prostatectomy after a long learning curve: A prospective single-surgeon study of 1552 consecutive cases. *European Urology, 65,* 521–531. doi:10.1016/j.eururo.2013.10.030

Tiernan, J.P., Ansari, I., Hirst, N.A., Millner, P.A., Hughes, T.A., & Jayne, D.G. (2012). Intra-operative tumour detection and staging in colorectal cancer surgery. *Colorectal Diseases, 14,* E510–E520. doi:10.1111/j.1463-1318.2012.03078.x

Tighe, P.J., Harle, C.A., Boezaart, A.P., Aytug, H., & Fillingim, R. (2014). Of rough starts and smooth finishes: Correlations between post-anesthesia care unit and postoperative days 1–5 pain scores. *Pain Medicine, 15,* 306–315. doi:10.1111/pme.12287

Trossman, S. (2013). Keeping patients on course: Nurse navigators help coordinate care all along the way. *American Nurse, 45*(1), 9.

Tryggvason, G., Gailey, P., Hultstein, S.L., Karnell, L.H., Hoffman, H.T., Funk, G.F., … Van Daele, D.J. (2013). Accuracy of fine-needle aspiration and imaging in the preoperative workup of salivary gland mass lesions treated surgically. *Laryngoscope, 123,* 158–163. doi:10.1002/lary.23613

Valdivieso, R.F., Hueber, P.A., & Zorn, K.C. (2013). Robot assisted radical prostatectomy: How I do it. Part I: Patient preparation and positioning. *Canadian Journal of Urology, 20,* 6957–6961. Retrieved from http://www.canjurol.com/html/free-articles/V20I5_17F_DrValdivieso.pdf

West, L., Vidwans, S.J., Campbell, N.P., Shrager, J., Simon, G.R., Bueno, R., … Salgia, R. (2012). A novel classification of lung cancer into molecular subtypes. *PLOS ONE, 7*(2), e31906. doi:10.1371/journal.pone.0031906

Wright, J.D., Burke, W.M., Wilde, E.T., Lewin, S.N., Charles, A.S., Kim, J.H., … Hershman, D.L. (2012). Comparative effectiveness of robotic versus laparoscopic hysterectomy for endometrial cancer. *Journal of Clinical Oncology, 30,* 783–791. doi:10.1200/JCO.2011.36.7508

Wuethrich, P.Y., Thalmann, G.N., Studer, U.E., & Burkhard, F.C. (2013). Epidural analgesia during open radical prostatectomy does not improve long-term cancer-related outcome: A retrospective study in patients with advanced prostate cancer. *PLOS ONE, 8*(8), e72873. doi:10.1371/journal.pone.0072873

Yagata, H., Yamauchi, H., Tsugawa, K., Hayashi, N., Yoshida, A., Kaijura, Y., … Nakamura, S. (2013). Sentinel node biopsy after neoadjuvant chemotherapy in cytologically proven node-positive breast cancer. *Clinical Breast Cancer, 13,* 471–477. doi:10.1016/j.cibc.2013.08.014

Yan, P.Z., Butler, P.M., Kurowski, D., & Perloff, M.D. (2014). Beyond neuropathic pain: Gabapentin use in cancer and perioperative pain. *Clinical Journal of Pain, 30,* 613–629. doi:10.1097/AJP.0000000000000014

Zaorsky, N.G., Trabulsi, E.J., Lin, J., & Den, R.B. (2013). Multimodality therapy for patients with high-risk prostate cancer: Current status and future directions. *Seminars in Oncology, 40,* 308–321. doi:10.1053/j.seminoncol.2013.04.006

Zinn, J., Jenkins, J.B., Swofford, V., Harrelson, B., & McCarter, S. (2010). Intraoperative patient skin prep agents: Is there a difference? *AORN Journal, 92,* 662–674. doi:10.1016/j.aorn.2010.07.016

CHAPTER 6

Radiation Therapy

Tracy K. Gosselin, PhD, RN, AOCN®

Introduction

Radiation therapy (RT) is an integral component of cancer treatment. This treatment modality has experienced advancement, refinement, and greater biologic understanding in the past 20 years. RT may be used alone or in combination with other therapies in the neo-adjuvant, adjuvant, and palliative care settings. Approximately 50% of patients with cancer will receive RT at some point in their disease trajectory (Delaney, Jacob, Featherstone, & Barton, 2005). What is unique about RT compared to other cancer treatments is the variety of treatments that can be offered as well as the population receiving treatment. In many RT centers, adult and pediatric patients receive treatment in the same facility, thus requiring healthcare providers to have additional knowledge and skills related to the care of all patient populations.

The advanced practice nurse (APN) role is a newer role in radiation oncology. Several publications in the 1980s and 1990s were related to the role of nursing in radiation oncology. Since 1999, descriptive studies also have included the role of the APN. Depending on the practice setting, APNs may have administrative, clerical, patient care, and research responsibilities. This chapter will provide an overview of RT for the APN, including indications for treatment, patient and family education, and implications for practice. A list of common terms used in RT can be found in Table 6-1, and the minimal and maximal tissue doses are noted in Table 6-2.

Indications

General

RT can be used for cure, control, palliation, and prophylaxis in a variety of disease sites (see Table 6-3). In the curative setting, RT commonly is used to treat skin cancer, prostate cancer, and early-stage Hodgkin lymphoma. This also is referred to as *definitive RT*. In this setting, the disease is confined to a particular area or organ. When the goal of treatment is that of control, patients typically present with advanced disease. The goal is to provide a symptom-free interval for patients. Palliative RT often is a shorter course of treatment that focuses on providing comfort when cure is not possible. Treatment also is given to minimize pain in patients

Table 6-1. Common Radiation Therapy Definitions

Term	Definition	Comments
Acute toxicity	This type of side effect arises during the course of radiation therapy (RT) and typically subsides within weeks once treatment is completed. Patients experience these effects at the treatment site but also may experience global symptoms such as fatigue. When the symptoms persist following treatment, they are referred to as *late effects*.	Common acute effects include nausea, diarrhea, mucositis, xerostomia, esophagitis, and skin reaction.
Boost	This term commonly is used to describe a smaller field within the larger field of radiation that typically is treated at the end of radiation.	Women who undergo a lumpectomy may receive external beam RT to the entire breast, followed by a boost to the surgical scar to minimize the risk of recurrence.
Brachytherapy	This therapy involves the use of radioactive seeds or liquids. Seeds may be placed on or near a tumor, whereas liquids may be given intravenously or orally. Treatment can be either high dose rate (HDR) or low dose rate (LDR). Sources may be left in place permanently (e.g., prostate LDR) or temporarily (e.g., cervix HDR, prostate HDR, sarcoma LDR, cervix LDR).	—
Chemoradiotherapy	Chemotherapy is given daily, weekly, or as a continuous infusion while the patient is undergoing RT for a synergistic effect.	Diseases treated with chemoradiotherapy include breast, lung, head and neck, gastrointestinal, and gynecologic cancers. This is based on pathology and staging of disease.
Dose-volume histogram (DVH)	A DVH is a graphical representation of the amount and percentage of RT that is given to the planned treatment volume and other surrounding anatomic structures.	—
Dosing	Dosing is broken down from a total dose (gray [Gy]) to individual doses (centigray [cGy]); this commonly is referred to as *fractionation*.	If the total dose is 54 Gy, this equals 5,400 cGy. If a patient is to receive 30 treatments, this becomes the denominator and divides into 5,400, giving a daily treatment dose of 1.8 Gy or 180 cGy.
Fractionation	The total dose of RT is divided into equal fractions. This is one of the most common methods of delivering RT, with treatments given once daily, Monday through Friday, for a prescribed number of weeks.	—

(Continued on next page)

Table 6-1. Common Radiation Therapy Definitions *(Continued)*

Term	Definition	Comments
GliaSite® Radiation Therapy System (Cytyc Corp.)	GliaSite is used in the treatment of malignant brain tumors. A balloon with a catheter is inserted into the resected tumor cavity, and iodine-125 is inserted into the catheter to give LDR RT over 3–7 days.	–
Hyperfractionation	When RT is given twice a day, separated by six hours, it is referred to as *hyperfractionation*. The total dose of treatment often is increased, while the dose per fraction is decreased.	Treatment may be given this way in certain cases of head and neck and pediatric cancers. This also may be used in breast brachytherapy, as well as in patients requiring total body irradiation for stem cell transplantation.
Hypofractionation	The dose of RT per fraction is increased, and the total dose and treatment time are decreased. This type of fractionation has changed how many patients with bone metastasis are treated, in that they receive a higher daily dose over a shorter amount of time.	–
Intensity-modulated radiation therapy (IMRT)	IMRT is an advanced form of RT whereby the intensity of the dose can be controlled within each treatment field by small beamlets. This allows the patient to receive more or less of a dose to a certain part of the treatment field based on tumor characteristics, anatomy, and physiology.	–
Late effects	These are side effects that persist months to years after treatment has been completed or effects that arise months to years later at the site of treatment.	Common late effects include fibrosis, enteritis, xerostomia, telangiectasia, and vaginal stenosis.
Particulate radiation	Particulate radiation consists of different particles that are used in different ways to treat cancer. • Alpha particles: Large, positively charged particles that have poor penetration and are emitted during the decay of radioactive sources • Beta particles: Electrons that are emitted during the decay of radioactive sources • Electrons: Small, negatively charged particles that are accelerated to high energies and do not penetrate deeply • Neutrons: Large, uncharged particles • Protons: Large, positively charged particles that penetrate deeply and have a stopping point	Electrons commonly are used to treat cutaneous T-cell lymphoma (mycosis fungoides) and also commonly are used during a boost treatment. Proton therapy is provided only at select centers across the United States because of the cost of equipment and facilities needed to operate. Brachytherapy and radioimmunotherapy are types of alpha, beta, and gamma rays.

(Continued on next page)

Table 6-1. Common Radiation Therapy Definitions *(Continued)*

Term	Definition	Comments
Radiobiology	This is the study of the effect of absorbed ionizing radiation on cells and comprises the four R's: repair, redistribution, repopulation, and reoxygenation. • Repair: This is key in normal cells and allows for the cells to repair themselves between doses of RT. Repair also may happen in tumor cells. • Redistribution: Cell kill increases as cells move through the cell cycle. As cells are delayed in each cycle, cell kill increases as DNA damage occurs. • Repopulation: This is key in normal cells to minimize acute and late effects. In cancer cells, repopulation rarely happens, as the cells attempt to divide because of the multiple RT treatments. • Reoxygenation: As the tumor shrinks, it becomes better oxygenated and more sensitive to the effects of RT.	–
Radiosensitivity	Radiosensitivity is concerned with how sensitive tumor cells and other structures and tissues respond to the radiation. It is an important consideration, as acute and late toxicities are related to this concept. Cells in the late G_2 and M phases are most sensitive to RT, whereas those in the S phase are more resistant.	–
Respiratory gating	A small, lightweight, reflective block is placed on the patient's chest that tracks to an infrared camera in the ceiling; this camera monitors the patient's breathing cycle and can turn the beam on and off based on the patient's breathing cycle. This technique assists in minimizing treatment to normal healthy tissue.	This may be used in patients with breast, thoracic, and abdominal malignancies.
Simulation	This is part of the treatment planning process and may take 1–2 hours depending on the patient. Fluoroscopy is used to visualize anatomy. Patients may or may not receive IV contrast, and a positioning device is typically made for treatment positioning.	This may take place on a conventional simulator or a computed tomography (CT)–based simulator. This is done prior to initiation of treatment.
Stereotactic radiosurgery	This type of treatment is used to treat tumors that are intracranial or extracranial and primary or metastatic in origin. It typically is one large dose of radiation that uses multiple arcs/beams to treat a focal area.	This treatment can be used in patients with metastatic disease to the brain, lung, and spinal cord and may be used as a primary treatment for prostate cancer using more than one treatment.

(Continued on next page)

Table 6-1. Common Radiation Therapy Definitions *(Continued)*

Term	Definition	Comments
Stereotactic radiotherapy	This type of treatment is used to treat intra-cranial lesions that may or may not be malignant. Treatments are fractionated and may use multiple arcs/beams.	–
Teletherapy	Teletherapy is also known as external beam RT; often the acronym EBRT is used. This treatment is given on a linear accelerator or with a cobalt unit.	–
Three-dimensional (3-D) confor-mal RT	This type of treatment uses computer-based treatment planning and CT during the planning process to develop a 3-D image of the tumor, which allows for a tighter margin around the tumor.	–
Tolerance dose	This is the dose of radiation that can be given that will still allow the tissue and/or organ to function (see Table 6-2).	–
Total body irra-diation	This is a type of photon treatment that is given to the whole body in patients undergoing stem cell transplantation.	–

Note. Based on information from Gosselin, 2011; Iwamoto et al., 2012.

with metastatic disease to the bone and to stop bleeding in patients whose tumors are friable. Furthermore, RT is used to treat structural oncologic emergencies (see Chapter 16), including increased intracranial pressure from brain metastases, spinal cord compression, and superior vena cava syndrome. Lastly, RT is used for prophylaxis in patients with small cell lung cancer who are at high risk for brain metastases. These patients receive prophylactic whole brain RT. The next section will focus on breast, colorectal, non-small cell lung, and prostate cancers and palliative radiation treatments, as these are some of the most common indications for RT.

Breast Cancer

Treatment of breast cancer with RT has undergone rapid evolution over the past 45 years. The studies conducted by the National Surgical Adjuvant Breast and Bowel Project (NSABP) have made breast-conserving treatment (BCT) a standard of care in the United States that provides patients with the option of breast preservation. Ongoing research continues to look at different types of treatment for breast cancer using RT.

Breast cancer is one of the most commonly treated diseases in RT departments; therefore, a comprehensive knowledge base about treatment options regarding this disease is critical. Radiation may be used after lumpectomy, after mastectomy, and in the setting of metastatic disease. Patients who present with large tumors also may undergo RT and/or chemotherapy prior to surgery (neoadjuvant therapy). Radiation usually is delivered via external beam or brachytherapy with the use of photons and electrons. Photons are administered the first four to five weeks of treatment, followed by electrons if the patient is to receive a boost treatment to the surgical scar. Photons penetrate the whole breast, whereas electrons are superficial.

Table 6-2. Minimal and Maximal Tissue Tolerance to Radiation Dose

Tissue	Dose-Related Injury	Minimal Tolerance Dose (TD) 5/5[a] (Gy)	Maximal TD 50/5[b] (Gy)	Amount of Tissue Treated (Field Size or Length)
Eye	Blindness			
	• Retina	55	70	Whole
	• Cornea	50	> 60	Whole
	• Lens	5.0	12	Whole
Bone marrow	Aplasia, pancytopenia	2.5	4.5	Whole
		30	40	Segmental
Liver	Acute and chronic hepatitis	25	40	Whole
		15	20	Whole (strip)
Stomach	Perforation, ulcer, hemorrhage	45	55	100 cm²
Intestine	Ulcer, perforation, hemorrhage	45	55	400 cm²
		50	65	100 cm²
Brain	Infarction, necrosis	60	70	Whole
Spinal cord	Infarction, necrosis	45	55	10 cm
Heart	Pericarditis, pancarditis	45	55	60%
		70	80	25%
Lung	Acute and chronic pneumonitis	30	35	100 cm²
		15	25	Whole
Kidney	Acute and chronic nephro-sclerosis	15	20	Whole (strip)
		20	25	Whole
Uterus	Necrosis, perforation	> 10	> 200	Whole
Vagina	Ulcer, fistula	90	> 100	Whole
Fetus	Death	2.0	4.0	Whole

[a] TD 5/5 = minimal tolerance dose; the dose, given to a population of patients under a standard set of treatment conditions, that will result in no more than a 5% rate of severe complications within five years after treatment.

[b] TD 50/5 = maximal tolerance dose; the dose, given to a population of patients under a standard set of treatment conditions, that will result in a 50% rate of severe complications within five years after treatment.

Note. Based on information from Bentel et al., 1989; Rubin et al., 1975.

From *Manual for Radiation Oncology Nursing Practice and Education* (4th ed., p. 25), by R.R. Iwamoto, M. Haas, and T.K. Gosselin (Eds.), 2012, Pittsburgh, PA: Oncology Nursing Society. Copyright 2012 by Oncology Nursing Society. Reprinted with permission.

Patients who receive BCT may have a diagnosis of ductal carcinoma in situ (DCIS) or invasive breast cancer. RT should only be given after a careful physical assessment has been completed and all laboratory results, pathologic reports, and radiologic studies have been reviewed (Senkus et al., 2013). Contraindications related to RT use in patients undergoing BCT are addressed in the National Comprehensive Cancer Network® (NCCN®) breast cancer treatment guidelines (NCCN, 2015c). In a comparison of four prospective trials, Solin (2010) found that women who underwent breast-conserving surgery and RT had a 42%–59% decrease in ipsilateral local recurrence compared to women who were treated with BCT alone. Treatment of DCIS with RT continues to be controversial, and factors that affect the decision to use RT include age at diagnosis, tumor grade, tumor size, and comedo histology. Women should be educated on their treatment options and factors that may increase the risk of recurrence.

The treatment planning process for the management of breast cancer includes computed tomography (CT) and simulation. These are used together to develop a three-dimensional treatment plan. A treatment-positioning device is made, with the patient's arm being raised above the head on the side that is being treated. During the treatment planning process, a dose-volume histogram (DVH) is constructed to show the dose to the breast and other anatomic structures. In patients with breast cancer, it is common to look at the dose to the head of the clavicle, heart, lung, and stomach because of anatomy and treatment beam arrangement. Surgical clips that are placed at the time of surgery also may assist in identifying the treatment area. If a patient is at risk for cardiac exposure, a heart block may be placed to minimize the RT dose. Intensity-modulated radiation therapy (IMRT) is not used as commonly as three-dimensional conformal RT in patients with breast cancer.

Table 6-3. Common Disease Sites/Diseases Treated With Radiation Therapy

Disease Site	Radiation Therapy Technique That May Be Used
Brain	External beam radiation therapy, stereotactic radiosurgery, stereotactic radiotherapy, GliaSite® Radiation Therapy System (Cytyc Corp.)
Head and neck	External beam radiation therapy, high-dose-rate brachytherapy, low-dose-rate brachytherapy
Breast	External beam radiation therapy, high-dose-rate brachytherapy
Lung	External beam radiation therapy, high-dose-rate brachytherapy, whole brain radiation therapy in small cell lung cancer
Gastrointestinal	External beam radiation therapy, intraoperative radiation therapy
Prostate	External beam radiation therapy, high-dose-rate brachytherapy, low-dose-rate brachytherapy
Gynecologic	External beam radiation therapy, high-dose-rate brachytherapy, low-dose-rate brachytherapy
Skin	External beam radiation therapy
Leukemia	Total body irradiation
Lymphoma	External beam radiation therapy
T-cell lymphoma	Total skin external beam therapy
Nonmalignant (keloids, heterotopic bone)	External beam radiation therapy
Metastatic disease to bone, brain, spinal column	External beam radiation therapy, stereotactic radiosurgery (for intracranial and extracranial metastasis)

Note. External beam radiation therapy includes the use of parallel fields, three-dimensional conformal therapy, and intensity-modulated radiation therapy.

Common RT treatment fields to the whole breast include tangential fields (medial and lateral fields that are directed obliquely at the breast) and a variety of additional fields if nodal involvement exists. These fields may include the axilla, intramammary, and supraclavicular nodal areas. It is critical that these fields do not overlap, as patients may be at higher risk in that area for acute and late effects. A small part of the lung volume also may be included, but efforts should be taken to minimize any potential heart exposure. For whole breast irradiation, patients typically are prescribed a dose of 45–50 gray (Gy) (Foxson, Lattimer, & Felder, 2011; NCCN, 2015c). This dose is then divided into daily doses of 1.8–2 Gy, which are administered five days a week over the course of five to six weeks. This dose range is similar for patients who require nodal irradiation.

Patients undergoing BCT commonly receive treatment to what is known as a *boost field*. This field usually is treated alone once the patient has completed treatment to the entire breast. This treatment field is around the surgical scar, and treatment is aimed at local tissues, as this area has a high chance of recurrence. Treatment is commonly given to women who are younger than age 50 and in those who have high-grade disease (NCCN, 2015c). It is commonly delivered with electrons as opposed to photons, which are used to treat the whole breast, and a patient typically receives 2 Gy a day for a total of six to eight treatments. Some institutions deliver the boost treatment via brachytherapy. Patients typically receive a total of 30–33 treatments inclusive of whole breast RT and the boost treatment. If treatment is delivered via brachytherapy, catheters are placed into the breast, and high-dose radiation is administered. Patients go home with the catheters in place until the treatment is complete.

Partial breast irradiation (PBI) commonly is referred to as *accelerated partial breast irradiation* and can be performed using the MammoSite® (Cytyc Corp.) treatment device (single catheter), on a linear accelerator, or via high-dose-rate (HDR) brachytherapy (multiple catheters). The MammoSite treatment device comes in either a spherical or an elliptical shape and can be placed into the lumpectomy cavity at the time of surgery or postoperatively with a trocar. Patients receive a total of 10 treatments over the course of five days. Each day, the patient typically receives two treatments separated by six hours. The catheter is attached to the HDR afterloader machine, and treatment is accomplished with iridium-192. This type of treatment decreases dosage to the heart and lung while giving the most dose to the area at greatest risk of recurrence. Small studies report a benefit with the use of MammoSite (Shah et al., 2013; Vargo et al., 2014). However, few studies have long-term follow-up (greater than five years) because this treatment is relatively new. In one study of 194 women, the five-year actuarial recurrence rate was 3.39% and the disease-free survival rate was 93.2% (Ferraro et al., 2012). The American Society of Breast Surgeons (2011) and the American Society for Radiation Oncology (Smith et al., 2009) have consensus statements that outline criteria for women who could possibly receive accelerated PBI. The total dose of PBI is 34 Gy with a daily dose of 3.4 Gy. Currently, NSABP and the Radiation Therapy Oncology Group are conducting a clinical trial to evaluate the feasibility of this type of treatment in select patients with breast cancer. NCCN (2015c) recommends that women who receive PBI should participate in a clinical trial.

Side effects related to the use of the MammoSite include fat necrosis, infection, seroma, skin retraction, and telangiectasias (Khan et al., 2012). Women also may experience pain related to the catheter site, as well as erythema related to the dose distribution. Late effects, including contralateral breast disease and local recurrence, are issues that APNs should be prepared to discuss with patients who are considering PBI. Until long-term follow-up studies are able to document the advantages and disadvantages as they have with BCT and whole breast RT, practitioners need to continue to be aware of the current treatment recommendations.

Patients who require RT after mastectomy typically have similar fields and treatment doses as those who elect to undergo BCT. Patients may require the use of bolus doses along the scar to provide enhanced dosing during part of the treatment. Photons and electrons also are used during this treatment.

Patients undergoing RT for breast cancer are at risk for developing a variety of acute and late effects. The two most common acute side effects related to RT for breast cancer are fatigue and skin reaction (dermatitis). It is estimated that approximately 63% of women with breast cancer have fatigue at the onset of chemotherapy (Liu et al., 2009), reaching up to 80% while receiving treatment (de M Alcântara-Silva, Freitas-Junior, Freitas, & Machado, 2013). The onset and duration of fatigue are different for each patient, and a baseline assessment prior to the initiation of RT is warranted. Patients who have received prior treatment (chemotherapy or surgery) and have not fully recovered may come into RT with a baseline measure of fatigue that is higher than a patient who has not had prior treatment. Both the Oncology Nursing Society (Mitchell et al., 2014) and NCCN (2015d) have evidence-based practice guidelines to support patient intervention.

Skin reactions are a common side effect of RT and are dependent on treatment site and dose. Typically, skin reaction occurs in the second week of treatment and is dose and time dependent. This side effect may initially start as a dry, flaky, pruritic rash that may then progress into erythema, dry desquamation, and lastly, moist desquamation. Hair loss within the treatment field may be noted, as well as skin pigmentation changes, depending on the individual's complexion. A variety of factors affect the development of an acute skin reaction, including total RT dose, fractionation (how many treatments, how many per day), type of energy (electrons are superficial and therefore more likely to cause a reaction), and total treatment time (Gosselin, Schneider, Plambeck, & Rowe, 2010). Additionally, individual factors such as age (older), breast size (larger breast size), and other comorbid conditions, such as collagen vascular disease and diabetes, affect patients' risk, as do lifestyle behaviors such as smoking. Patients receiving concurrent chemotherapy also may be at higher risk and potentially develop a skin reaction earlier in their course of treatment than those not receiving chemotherapy.

Standard management of these acute reactions often varies across settings. Many products used to treat these reactions can be purchased over the counter or have been approved by the U.S. Food and Drug Administration as a medical device, making the determination of the best product challenging for healthcare providers and patients. Patients should be encouraged to bathe as they normally would and to keep the skin clean and dry. An alcohol-free moisturizer can be used to minimize dryness and manage pruritus. A variety of ointments, creams, and gels are available, with many having been evaluated with mixed results. Women with large breasts and those receiving treatment to the axilla should be instructed to keep the area as dry as possible to minimize breakdown in the skin folds. Patients should avoid trauma and sun exposure to the treatment area. Skin products should be applied no sooner than four hours prior to treatment, although this varies from institution to institution. The concern is that certain skin products can create a bolus effect to the skin, resulting in administration of a higher dose of radiation.

Patients experiencing moist desquamation may benefit from the use of a hydrocolloid dressing to minimize the risk of infection, promote healing, and enhance comfort. Patients should be cautioned against the use of cornstarch to manage moisture, as once an area develops moist desquamation, this product can lead to a yeast infection. Evidence-based practice reviews have concluded that gentle skin washing and the use of antiperspirants are supported (Bolderston, Lloyd, Wong, Holden, & Robb-Blenderman, 2006; Gosselin et al., 2014; Wong et al., 2013). An alcohol-free, lanolin-free moisturizer can be used (Bolderston et al., 2006). Mometasone, a topical corticosteroid, may also be used to minimize pruritus (Wong et al., 2013).

Patients who have a MammoSite catheter or multiple brachytherapy catheters in place should be taught catheter care to minimize the risk of infection. Catheter care can be developed institutionally. Pain assessment and management are essential, as the catheters may cause some level of discomfort.

Late effects of RT to the skin include atrophy, scaling, fibrosis, telangiectasia, necrosis, and pigmentation changes (Archambeau, Pezner, & Wasserman, 1995; Davis et al., 2003; Harper, Franklin, Jenrette, & Aguero, 2004). These side effects arise months to years after treatment, typically are not reversible, and occur with dose ranges of 2.5–3 Gy/day. They affect the ultimate cosmetic outcome and should be discussed with patients prior to initiation of RT.

Follow-up care for each patient is individualized but should include physical examination, clinical breast examination, and mammograms based on recommended guidelines from NCCN (2015c). Practitioners also should closely examine the treated breast, as well as the scar, for changes related to RT. Women may verbalize changes they have noticed since treatment and should be encouraged to perform breast self-examinations, as their treated breast tissue will change over time. Patients receiving hormonal therapy should be evaluated regularly by a gynecologist.

Colorectal Cancer

Colorectal cancer (CRC) is divided into two treatment areas: the colon and the rectum, with the latter being more commonly treated with RT (Butler et al., 2013). RT typically is not used alone but rather is used in the neoadjuvant (preoperative) or adjuvant setting (postoperative or after the primary treatment) with chemotherapy. The goals of treatment in the neoadjuvant setting for CRC are to reduce tumor burden (generally done with rectal tumors), thus making the tumor more resectable and sparing healthy tissue at the time of resection, and to downstage the tumor (Garajová et al., 2011). In addition, sphincter preservation, pelvic disease control, and lower rates of acute and late side effects have been demonstrated in neoadjuvant studies (Czito & Willett, 2008). In the adjuvant setting, RT is used to minimize the risk of local recurrence.

Radiation can be delivered via external beam or with an intraoperative RT approach, which is given while patients are in the operating room. Therapy is given over the course of five to six weeks. A total dose of 45–50.4 Gy usually is prescribed and given as a daily dose of 1.8 Gy for a total of 25–28 treatments with photons (neoadjuvant or postoperative) (NCCN, 2015g). A treatment boost also may be given to the tumor bed, with the dose and number of fractions varying based on preoperative or postoperative status. A treatment boost typically is performed once patients reach 45 Gy and includes anywhere from three to five fractions (NCCN, 2015g). Patients with CRC typically have three to four treatment fields. A three-field treatment approach incorporates the use of posterior-anterior, right lateral, and left lateral fields. A four-field treatment approach uses all of the same fields as the three-field approach but has an anteroposterior field in addition, in which radiation is delivered from the front of the patient versus the back. IMRT should be used in a clinical trial or in a clinical case that may require reirradiation to the area (NCCN, 2015g), as it is often not covered by insurance because of insufficient data. Concurrent chemotherapy with a 5-fluorouracil (5-FU)-based agent should be used. Endocavitary RT also may be used in select patient populations (e.g., patients with small, mobile lesions) for sphincter preservation (Mendenhall et al., 2009).

Patients receiving RT need to undergo careful treatment planning to minimize the amount of small bowel in the treatment field, as this is the dose-limiting organ and can cause significant side effects. During simulation, a positioning device is made, and a rectal tube, vaginal marker, or BBs or wires (on the skin) may be used to outline the anatomy during the planning process. Some patients may be placed in the prone position on a belly board that allows for the bowel to fall away from the treatment field to minimize side effects during treatment. A DVH constructed during the planning phase will show doses to the planning target volume (PTV), including the femoral heads, bladder, and rectum. Treatment fields should include the tumor bed, a 2–5 cm margin, and the presacral and internal iliac nodes (NCCN, 2015g).

Intraoperative RT may be considered in patients with positive margins after resection (NCCN, 2015g) and also may be given in combination with external beam RT, with or without chemotherapy and surgical resection (Willett, Czito, & Tyler, 2007). This particular type of therapy can be performed by two different methods, depending on the treating facility. If performed in the operating suite, the room may have a linear accelerator in the suite, or an HDR unit may be brought to the suite to perform the treatment during the surgical procedure. The surgical room requires special shielding, and staff members need to be trained in radiation safety. The other option is for the patient to be transported to the radiation department during the operation to receive treatment. The latter option has multiple challenges related to patient transport and safety. During this treatment, the patient receives radiation to the surgical bed and surrounding areas that the surgical and radiation teams deem necessary.

Patients receiving RT for CRC are at risk for developing a variety of acute and late toxicities related to treatment (see Figure 6-1). Many of these side effects are RT specific, but many also can be attributed to the role that chemotherapy plays in treating this disease. For example, myelosuppression is not common in patients receiving RT alone but occurs more frequently in patients receiving RT plus chemotherapy. Many patients undergoing RT for CRC also receive concurrent 5-FU. Coordination of this therapy, including management of an ambulatory infusion pump and understanding of the side effects, is critical to patient care and compliance with treatment. Common side effects of RT alone and with chemotherapy for CRC include fatigue, nausea, diarrhea, and skin reactions.

APNs must assess for chemotherapy-related side effects in the RT setting with patients receiving combined-modality therapy. Complete blood cell counts should be evaluated throughout treatment. Nausea should be assessed, as this symptom is not common with RT but can develop with chemotherapy. The American Society of Clinical Oncology (Basch et al., 2011), the Multinational Association of Supportive Care in Cancer (Roila et al., 2010), and NCCN (2015b) have developed evidence-based guidelines for the management of nausea and vomiting in patients receiving chemotherapy and RT.

Diarrhea is a dose-limiting toxicity of 5-FU, and the small bowel is a dose-limiting factor in RT. Diarrhea occurs as a result of cell death in the crypt epithelium, which results in insufficient replacement of the crypt cells and atrophy of the villi with breakdown of the mucosal barrier (Hauer-Jensen, Wang, & Denham, 2003). This then results in a loss of absorptive function and diarrhea. Patients will need to be educated early in their treatment about this side effect and what to expect. Diarrhea typically occurs one to two weeks into treatment and can worsen with the administration of chemotherapy. The amount and dura-

Acute
- Allergic reaction
- Alopecia
- Anorexia
- Cholinergic syndrome
- Cystitis, dysuria, hematuria
- Diarrhea
- Fever
- Hand-foot syndrome
- Mucositis
- Myelosuppression
- Nausea, vomiting
- Peripheral neuropathy
- Proteinuria
- Skin erythema, desquamation
- Urgency, incontinence
- Vaginal dryness, dyspareunia, stenosis
- Vascular effects

Late
- Anorexia
- Diarrhea
- Enteritis
- Peripheral neuropathy
- Skin fibrosis
- Sterility
- Tenesmus
- Vaginal dryness, dyspareunia, stenosis

Figure 6-1. Common Acute and Late Toxicities of Colorectal Treatment With Radiation Therapy and Chemotherapy

Note. Based on information from Gosselin-Acomb, 2006.

tion of diarrhea are patient dependent and should be routinely assessed. Dietary modifications, such as a low-residue diet, and over-the-counter and prescription medications may be necessary, as well as IV fluids, depending on the patient's vital signs at the time of assessment. A dietitian may work with the team, particularly if probiotics are incorporated into the patient's diet (Delia et al., 2007; Visich & Yeo, 2010). Common medications used to manage diarrhea associated with RT to the small bowel include loperamide (Imodium® A-D) and diphenoxylate and atropine (Lomotil®). Some patients also may complain of rectal discharge or tenesmus (feeling of incomplete defecation), which usually results from inflammation or scarring of the bowel. APNs should recommend that patients use absorbent pads or briefs if this condition occurs.

Skin reactions typically arise in the perianal area about two to three weeks into treatment, depending on the location of the treatment field. The most common areas at risk for skin reactions are the gluteal folds and the perineal area. Patients initially present with erythema that can progress into dry and then moist desquamation over the course of treatment. Patients are instructed to use a mild skin cleanser and to apply a moisturizing protective cream. Haisfield-Wolfe and Rund (2000) developed a perineal-rectal skin care protocol (see Table 6-4) to be used in clinical practice to manage this uncomfortable side effect, which can be exacerbated by diarrhea. Good hygiene during this time is essential to alleviate and reduce the risk of infection and pain associated with skin reaction.

Late effects of RT in this population may include enteritis and sexuality issues. Enteritis is characterized by dysmotility (changes in movement through the bowel) and malabsorption that may need further diagnostic evaluation (Shadad, Sullivan, Martin, & Egan, 2013). These side effects take months to years to develop, and patients may experience adhesions, fibrosis, fistulas, and obstruction (Shadad et al., 2013). Mild cases of enteritis may require dietary modification with a low-residue diet, whereas more severe cases may require additional fiber to assist in stool formation and over-the-counter or prescription medications.

Sexuality issues related to dyspareunia, vaginal dryness, and vaginal stenosis may arise in women, and men may experience weakened orgasm and erectile dysfunction resulting from the effect of RT on the tissues. Patients must understand the risks of these symptoms along with the interventions that may be used to assist them in maintaining intimacy in their relationship. Interventions for women may include the use of vaginal dilators to keep the vagina open for sexual intercourse and for pelvic examinations (NCCN, 2015g). For men, pharmacologic and nonpharmacologic interventions may be used, including vasoactive agents and penile prostheses (Iwamoto, Haas, & Gosselin, 2012). The American Cancer Society has published two brochures, one for women and one for men, titled *Sexuality and Cancer* that can be provided and reviewed with patients. Female patients also may require education and instruction on the use of a vaginal dilator.

Follow-up care for each patient is individualized but should include physical examination, carcinogenic embryonic antigen monitoring, and colonoscopy. NCCN (2015g) recommends a physical examination and blood work every three to six months for two years and then every six months for a total of five years. Colonoscopy should be performed the first year after treatment and, if abnormal, repeated in a year. If no polyps are present, the test should be repeated in three years and then every five years (NCCN, 2015g).

Non-Small Cell Lung Cancer

RT can be used in the treatment of non-small cell lung cancer (NSCLC) in the curative or palliative treatment setting. The multidisciplinary team should evaluate patients and obtain appropriate imaging studies before developing final treatment plans. NCCN (2015e) recom-

Table 6-4. Perineal-Rectal Skin Care Protocol

Routine Care

During morning care and after each episode of urination or defecation, the patient will receive the following care.

- Gently cleanse skin with tepid water or a mild cleansing agent followed by gently patting areas dry **or** cleanse with tepid to cool sitz baths.
- If open lesions are present, cleanse with a wound cleanser or normal saline solution and treat.
- Apply a moisturizing cream.
- Recommend cotton undergarments; avoid restrictive clothing.
- Perform a full assessment of the perineal-rectal skin.
- Perform a nutrition assessment followed by nutrition consult, if needed.
- Consult an enterostomal therapy or wound-care nurse as needed.

Assessment	Recommendations for Care
Erythema signs and symptoms Pink Tenderness	Gently cleanse using a mild cleansing agent (perineal skin cleansers). Apply a moisturizing, protective cream. If cleanser is not accessible and soap must be used, use a soap without perfumes and thoroughly rinse all soap residues from the skin. Avoid lotions or creams containing perfume and talc (if receiving radiation therapy to area, avoid products containing metals or ointments or cleanse area prior to receiving radiation therapy). Frequency of skin care: Daily and after toileting
Dry desquamation signs and symptoms Scaling Flaking Pruritus Pain	Cleanse with tepid water or a wound cleanser. Apply a protective cream. Assess for pruritus. If present, • Apply topical antihistamine creams. • Take a cool shower or bath. • Consider analgesics or antihistamines. Assess for fungal infection. If present, • Treat with topical antifungal or systemic antifungal agent. Frequency of skin care: Twice a day/as needed after toileting
Moist desquamation signs and symptoms Pain Weeping Sloughing Abscess	Recommend sitz bath, shower, whirlpool as needed. Cleanse with a wound cleanser as needed. Apply a protective cream that will adhere to open skin. Apply an adhesive peripad or a pantyliner without deodorant to the undergarments. Assess need for analgesics, pain medications. If desquamation worsens, apply a wound hydrogel. Frequency of skin care: Twice a day/as needed after toileting
Possible complications of moist desquamation Vesicles Furuncle Carbuncles Abscess formation	Consult with physician or advanced practice nurse for treatment and systematic antibiotics. If vesicles are present, rule out herpes and treat appropriately.

(Continued on next page)

Table 6-4. Perineal-Rectal Skin Care Protocol *(Continued)*

Report to Physician	Documentation
Worsening of skin alteration Increase in inflammation Appearance of furuncle, carbuncles, abscess Appearance of vesicles Pain or increase in pain, change in character of pain	Anatomical area involved Size of involvement • Area may be difficult to measure because of the perineal-rectal anatomy. • Attempt to record in centimeters. • Measure from where the normal skin stops to where it begins again (use a disposable ruler). If open areas develop, measure width, length, and depth. • Record daily in acute care or weekly in home or long-term care. Changes in skin or wound conditions Colors of skin Drainage (i.e., amount, odor, color, consistency) Presence of sloughing or necrosis Presence and intensity of pain or pruritus Patient outcomes

Note. From "Nursing Protocol for the Management of Perineal-Rectal Skin Alterations," by M.E. Haisfield-Wolfe and C. Rund, *Clinical Journal of Oncology Nursing, 4,* p. 19. Copyright 2000 by Oncology Nursing Society. Reprinted with permission.

mends that RT or stereotactic body radiation therapy (SBRT) may be used in patients with stage I disease who are medically inoperable. For patients with stage II and III disease, chemotherapy and RT is often recommended after surgery (and sometimes before surgery). NCCN (2015e) provides recommendations as to whether patients should receive concurrent or sequential chemotherapy and RT; the decision depends on the results of surgery. For patients with advanced disease, RT is used for palliation of the symptoms associated with the primary tumor or sites of metastatic disease.

Treatment planning should include a CT scan and simulation; in some institutions, positron-emission tomography (PET) and CT scans will be done. Patients will have a treatment positioning device made to help position their arms above their head. Three-dimensional treatment planning then will take place, and a DVH will be constructed to identify doses to the PTV, including the lung, heart, and other tissues of concern. Planning the fields for this treatment often can be complex because of the anatomy of the chest, which includes the heart, stomach, and esophagus, and if nodal fields are involved, including the hilar, mediastinal, and supraclavicular areas. Multiple fields and oblique beams may be used to provide adequate dosing, as well as opposed fields (left and right laterals) in some cases. Total doses of RT may be 45–50 Gy in the preoperative setting, 50–70 Gy in the postoperative setting, and 60–74 Gy in the definitive setting (NCCN, 2015e). Dosing and fractionation may differ based on the treatment approach. Patients undergoing SBRT typically receive 3–5 fractions over 10–14 days (Kelsey & Salama, 2013). The Radiation Therapy Oncology Group (RTOG) currently is conducting a prospective study looking at dosing for NSCLC (RTOG, 2014). Daily doses for external beam RT usually are 1.8–2 Gy, and treatment typically is delivered over five to six weeks. Some patients may undergo respiratory gating (see Table 6-1) with each treatment, which requires additional time on the linear accelerator machine each day. IMRT as well as HDR brachytherapy may be used in select cases.

Acute side effects of RT for treatment of NSCLC include cough, fatigue, skin reactions, and esophagitis/pharyngitis. APNs need to obtain a baseline assessment of patients' symptoms before initiating RT. Patients may experience cough, dyspnea, anorexia, and weight loss related to the disease itself and not the treatment. If patients are receiving concurrent chemotherapy, assessment of the effects of combination therapy is important.

Esophagitis typically arises during the second or third week of therapy and is caused by the RT irritating the esophagus. This side effect may appear sooner if the patient is receiving concurrent chemotherapy. Patients may complain of dysphagia and the feeling of a lump in the throat. They also may report heartburn and occasional chest pain. Dietary modification should include eating soft, moist foods and consuming liquids with foods to make swallowing easier. Medications that coat the irritated area as well as pain medications may be beneficial. Use of the NCCN (2015a) guidelines for adult cancer pain may help as well. Providers also need to rule out an oral *Candida* infection, as this often can arise early in treatment and can be confused with esophagitis. *Candida* infection usually is treated with fluconazole. Some patients may require IV fluids if their vital signs and fluid status demonstrate dehydration.

A skin reaction will appear about two to three weeks into treatment and is characterized by pruritus, dry skin, and erythema. Patients also will experience temporary hair loss on the chest within the treatment field and should be encouraged to use an alcohol-free moisturizing lotion. Patients may have an additional area of pruritus at the exit site of the radiation beam, based on the beam arrangement. This occurs when the beam is exiting the body on the posterior side.

A cough can arise during treatment, which usually is caused by tissue irritation and typically subsides with the use of antitussive therapy with or without codeine. Fatigue is common in patients being treated for lung cancer. NCCN and ONS have guidelines that provide pharmacologic and nonpharmacologic recommendations for the management of fatigue (Mitchell et al., 2014; NCCN, 2015d). Pneumonitis can be both an acute and late side effect of RT and can be attributed to the total dose of radiation, volume of lung treated, fractionation schedule, and use of concomitant chemotherapy. Patients with pneumonitis usually present with shortness of breath with or without cough (Yirmibesoglu et al., 2012). Depending on the severity, patients may have a low-grade fever and the cough may be productive. Treatment generally includes the use of steroids (Yazbeck, Villaruz, Haley, & Socinski, 2013). Antibiotics typically are not used unless an associated infection is present. Fibrosis is a late effect of RT in which patients present with cough, dyspnea, and tachypnea. Management is similar to that of patients with pneumonitis.

Follow-up care for each patient is individualized but should include physical examination and diagnostic tests based on recommendations from NCCN (2015e). Patients should undergo a physical examination and a chest CT with contrast every 6–12 months for two years, and then a noncontrast-enhanced CT annually. Patients should be referred to smoking cessation programs as needed (NCCN, 2015e).

Prostate Cancer

Prostate cancer can be treated with a variety of RT approaches, as well as with watchful waiting, hormone therapy, surgery, and chemotherapy. Cryosurgery has seen recent improvements and also can be used to treat localized prostate cancer (Sverrisson, Jones, & Pow-Sang, 2013). Controversy still exists as to whether radical prostatectomy or radiation is superior, both as a treatment and in relation to acute or late effects that may arise. Initial treatment decisions should focus on the extent of the tumor; both surgery and RT can be used when the tumor is confined to the prostate. Other factors related to the initial treatment decision include the patient's age, general health status, and pretreatment bowel, bladder, and sexual function. Men who decide to undergo RT may receive external beam RT, brachytherapy, or a combination of the two.

Simulation for men undergoing external beam RT includes the development of a positioning device, the placement of rectal and urethral catheters, and the use of a penile clamp to stop the flow of contrast during the planning session. The urethral catheter is used to delineate the prostate base, whereas the rectal catheter shows the contour of the rectum. A planning CT also will be performed in patients who are to receive three-dimensional conformal or IMRT treatment. A variety of treatment techniques have been employed in treating prostate cancer. These include a four-field technique, a six-field approach (beams are coming in from six angles), three-dimensional conformal therapy, and IMRT, with the latter two being the more popular choices today because they minimize toxicity (NCCN, 2015f). Some patients may have fiducials or markers placed in the prostate to assist with treatment planning. The DVH would include the amount and percentage of radiation to the prostate, femoral heads, bladder, rectum, and seminal vesicles.

Based on NCCN (2015f) guidelines, patients with low-risk cancers should receive doses of 75.6–79.2 Gy given in 35–41 conventional fractions, whereas those with intermediate- or high-risk disease should receive doses up to 81 Gy. The risk categories (see Table 6-5) factor in staging, Gleason score, and prostate-specific antigen (PSA) level, which are used together to determine what type of treatment may be best for the patient. Daily doses typically are 1.8 Gy, and patients with intermediate- or high-risk disease also may receive treatment to the pelvic lymph nodes to a dose of 50 Gy. Men receiving IMRT will have more treatment fields and a tighter margin around the PTV to minimize side effects. HDR brachytherapy may be used in combination with external beam to provide a boost. The number of fractions varies depending on the total boost dose (NCCN, 2015f).

Brachytherapy can be used as a monotherapy or in addition to external beam treatment as a boost. As a monotherapy, it is used in patients with early-stage disease. Brachytherapy is used with other therapies for patients with high-grade tumors. Patient convenience, costs, and short recovery time factor into why men may choose brachytherapy over external beam therapy. Potential contraindications for brachytherapy include a large prostate, symptoms of bladder outlet obstruction (International Prostate Symptom Score greater than 15), or a previous transurethral resection of the prostate (NCCN, 2015f). This treatment can be given at a low dose rate (LDR) or HDR (see Table 6-1).

Treatment planning for LDR brachytherapy includes a CT scan one to two weeks before the implant. This scan assists physicians in determining optimum placement of the permanent seeds. LDR brachytherapy is accomplished while patients are receiving general or spinal anesthesia. While patients are in a lithotomy position, a perineal template and a transrectal ultrasound (TRUS) probe are placed. TRUS allows visualization of the needles and seeds as they are placed, and the template provides stabilization of the needles into the prostate. The seeds can be preloaded in the needle or inserted once the needles are in place. A total of 18–30 needles and 75–150 tiny seeds may be placed, depending on prostate volume. Once the seeds are

Table 6-5. Prostate Cancer Risk

Diagnosis Components	Low	Intermediate	High
Staging	T1–2a	T2b–T2c	T3a
Gleason score	2–6	7	8–10
Prostate-specific antigen	< 10 ng/ml	10–20 ng/ml	> 20 ng/ml

Note. Based on information from Carroll et al., 2005; National Comprehensive Cancer Network, 2015f.

deposited, the needles are removed and the patient is sent to the postoperative holding area. Because patients go home the same day, discharge teaching is a critical component of care. Discharge instructions should include contact numbers in the event of acute urinary retention, information about expected side effects (e.g., pain, seed migration, sexuality issues, skin and urinary changes), safety precautions related to the radioactive seeds, and follow-up appointments. Safety precautions include straining urine for seeds and using condoms during intercourse. Additionally, maximizing the distance between the patient and other individuals, particularly pregnant or possibly pregnant women and young children, also should be reviewed with the patient and family.

Iodine-125 and palladium-103 seeds commonly are used in LDR because they have a short range, slow dose rate, and low energy source; can give adequate dose levels to the prostate; and can avoid radiation to the bladder and rectum. However, side effects from LDR are more prolonged than those from HDR because of the half-life of the isotopes used.

In patients receiving HDR brachytherapy, the setup is the same as with LDR brachytherapy, except the perineal template is sutured into the perineum to secure it for placement of the needles. The needles or flexiguides are left in place because they will be attached to the afterloading machine for treatment. After CT-based treatment planning, several high-dose fractions are given. Iridium-192 is the source of radiation, and each treatment takes approximately 20–30 minutes (Waring & Gosselin, 2010). Patients will remain on bed rest until all fractions are given and will be transported to the radiation department for each fraction. Typically, two fractions are given each day, with six hours between fractions. Patients will have a urinary catheter in place and potentially could have a continuous bladder irrigation running to keep the urine clear. Patients also will be put on a clear liquid diet and will receive parenteral analgesics for pain and other supportive care medications. Antidiarrheals may be used so that patients do not have a bowel movement during this period of two to three days. Pain management is critical in these patients. After each treatment, the seeds are returned to the afterloader; therefore, patients are not radioactive between treatments or at the time of discharge. When the needles and template are removed, patients may experience perineal bleeding and swelling. A pressure dressing should be applied following treatment, and side effects, including perineal bleeding and swelling and urinary and bowel changes, should resolve in two to four weeks. Some patients may receive this treatment during external beam RT and may receive HDR brachytherapy more than once.

Acute and late toxicities of RT to the prostate include bowel and urinary changes, fatigue, sexual dysfunction, and skin reactions. APNs should conduct a baseline symptom assessment before the start of treatment so that they can document changes over time. Bowel changes are more prevalent in patients undergoing three-dimensional conformal treatment than those receiving IMRT. Diarrhea may develop a few weeks into treatment, which, for many patients, can be managed with a low-residue diet and Imodium A-D or Lomotil. Proctitis is another side effect that may occur. It is characterized by inflammation of the rectal lining and causes pain, bleeding, and a mucous or purulent discharge. This side effect can occur months to years after RT and may require laser treatment (Do, Nagle & Poylin, 2011).

Patients may experience perianal hair loss and skin changes from external beam RT. Men may experience mild erythema and desquamation, although desquamation is less common in these patients. For patients who experience skin breakdown, although uncommon, use of perianal skin care guidelines, such those in Table 6-4, would be beneficial.

Urinary side effects of RT to the prostate may include dysuria, frequency, hematuria, hesitancy, nocturia, and urgency. Patients must understand that these are expected side effects of treatment that result from the effects of radiation on the tissue and should be reported so that appropriate symptom management can be initiated. Ruling out bladder obstruction and infection is essential to the management of these symptoms. Patients should drink plenty of fluids throughout the day and decrease their intake in the evening. A variety of pharmacologic medications, including ibuprofen, oxybutynin chloride, phenazopyridine, tamsulosin hydrochloride, terazosin hydrochloride, and doxazosin, can be used to manage urinary symptoms (Iwamoto et al., 2012).

Sexual dysfunction is a common side effect of prostate cancer therapy. As with other side effects, APNs need to understand patients' pretreatment sexual function. Sexual dysfunction related to RT of the prostate includes impotence, premature ejaculation, and retrograde ejaculation. Treatment for dysfunction may include counseling and use of the American Cancer Society brochure *Sexuality for the Man With Cancer* (available at www.cancer.org/acs/groups/cid/documents/webcontent/002910-pdf.pdf). Medications such as vardenafil, tadalafil, and sildenafil may be used in men who are experiencing erectile dysfunction (Heidelbaugh, 2010). Vasoactive agents, such as intracavernosal injections and intraurethral suppositories, as well as vacuum devices and penile prostheses, may be beneficial for patients who cannot achieve or maintain an erection (Hogle, 2007).

Follow-up care for each patient is individualized but should include physical examination, digital rectal examination (DRE), and PSA monitoring based on recommended NCCN guidelines. The PSA test may be done as frequently as every three months, whereas DRE may be performed every year (NCCN, 2015f). Patients also should be evaluated for erectile dysfunction, as this is a common side effect of treatment (NCCN, 2015f).

Radiation Therapy With Palliative Intent

Patients with advanced disease often present with pain, bleeding, neurologic changes, and other symptoms that cause distress to patients and caregivers. Approximately half of the RT used in the United States is delivered with palliative intent (Murphy, Nelson, Chang, Mell, & Le, 2013). In patients with advanced disease, a prompt history and physical are essential, including attaining a thorough understanding of prior cancer therapies that patients have received. Prior RT treatment fields, dose, and volume treated are important in determining the potential for overlap of treatment fields, which may lead to unacceptable toxicities in patients with advanced disease. For example, a patient with NSCLC may complain of pain in the mid-back and undergo magnetic resonance imaging (MRI) that confirms spinal cord compression. The patient then would be started on steroids to reduce edema in the spinal cord and receive RT. The goal of therapy is not to cure but rather to palliate the symptom of pain and enhance patient comfort. The patient also may require pain medications. A course of palliative RT is much shorter than a curative course, usually by several weeks. NCCN treatment guidelines outline the management of patients with advance disease (NCCN, 2015c, 2015e, 2015f, 2015g). Pain assessment and management are critical during this time, and the APN should provide referral to palliative care or hospice if the patient is an appropriate candidate. Ongoing dialogue with caregivers also is important, as they may need to bring the patient back and forth to the center providing RT or may require the use of ambulance services.

Pediatric Considerations

Pediatric patients undergoing RT and their families often have unique treatment considerations. One of the primary concerns in the treatment of children is the ability of these patients to remain still during treatment. Typically, patients younger than three or four years old require sedation for simulation and treatment. This requires patients to be evaluated by the anesthesia staff. Consultation with child life experts to work with patients and families is critical in minimizing the use of sedation by doing play therapy with the positioning device, although cognitive impairment related to disease may affect patients' ability to forgo sedation. Parents need to be educated about dietary restrictions if their child is to undergo daily or hyperfractionated RT with anesthesia. Other potential areas of education include the use of growth hormone, fertility issues, and secondary malignancies (Iwamoto et al., 2012). Growth hormone deficiency is a common disorder in children who have received RT to the hypothalamus and can occur months to years after treatment. Fertility issues arise when the testes or ovaries receive RT, and an example of a secondary malignancy would be the development of breast cancer later in life in a woman who underwent RT for Hodgkin lymphoma as a teenager. It is important that as the child continues to grow and develop that the parents and child understand the need for lifelong follow-up and surveillance.

Geriatric Considerations

With approximately half of all cancers diagnosed in those older than age 65, this population is often predominant in RT centers. Caring for older patients who are receiving RT can potentially pose logistical issues, depending on their functional status and ability to perform activities of daily living. Patients with impaired vision may require a driver for their daily treatment appointments or request that their appointments be earlier in the day. Also, older adults are at an increased risk for skin reactions because of the natural aging and thinning of the skin. Care coordination with family and friends and appropriate assessment and intervention are critical when caring for this population (Iwamoto et al., 2012).

Standards

Standards of care and professional performance are outlined in the *Manual for Radiation Oncology Nursing Practice and Education* (Iwamoto et al., 2012). The standards of care pertain to interactions between the provider and patients and families, whereas standards of professional performance relate to how providers look to enhance their professional development and patient outcomes. Eight standards exist related to professional practice, and each will be interpreted in relation to the role of the APN in radiation oncology.

Quality of care: APNs should systematically evaluate and document the effectiveness of clinical care. This documentation includes completion and documentation of patients' history and physical examination, ordering of laboratory and radiology tests, performance of procedures, and documentation of weekly treatment and follow-up visits. APNs may prescribe supportive care medications (with appropriate prescriptive privileges) and should evaluate the medication's effectiveness in patient care. Additionally, APNs may review nursing practice and make recommendations regarding documentation tools, as well as serve on safety and quality committees. Furthermore, they may assume "on-call" responsibilities, evaluating patients in the emergency department or rounding on hospitalized patients on weekends and holidays (Carper & Haas, 2006).

Accountability: APNs will educate medical staff in defining the APN role, understanding the privileges that are set forth by the state, and establishing any competencies.

Education: APNs entering into the field of radiation oncology will need to evaluate their current level of RT knowledge in comparison to what is required on the job, as the role varies with practice setting. APNs will develop a self-education plan, as well as an education plan for other professionals in the department. They may facilitate education sessions and provide education to healthcare professionals outside of the department. APNs should review and develop patient education materials, as well as conduct support groups.

Leadership: APNs may serve as managers of nurses or other APNs in the department and therefore should serve as role models. This may require interviewing, hiring, performance management, budgetary functions, and oversight of staff and patient programs. APNs will be involved with both departmental and facility committees.

Ethics: APNs ensure that patient needs are met regardless of background and incorporate diversity and sensitivity into practice. APNs must be aware of role limitations. This also involves serving as a resource for staff members who are having difficulty managing a particular care situation.

Collaboration: APNs are part of the multidisciplinary team and assist in care coordination across the continuum. They develop symptom management plans and communicate significant findings and issues to others on the team. Barriers to practice may exist, and APNs may need to advocate for and educate colleagues and policy makers about their role in the delivery of quality cancer care.

Research: APNs translate research into practice but also are able to develop research studies to enhance patient care and outcomes. They may develop studies that are population or treatment based that investigate symptom management, patient education, palliative care, and acute and late side effects. APNs should look at the role of technology in care and how it can assist both patients and providers and should examine how the APN role can improve patient care and satisfaction.

Resource utilization: APNs understand the resource needs of both patients and the larger community. APNs will serve primarily in a clinical role and see patients in the inpatient and outpatient settings, as well as in multidisciplinary clinics.

Patient and Family Education

RT is a unique treatment, and most patients are unfamiliar with the planning process, technology, and highly technical aspects of care, thus making patient and family education a critical component of the APN role. APNs can assist in minimizing patients' and families' anxiety by providing education to meet their learning needs. In a 2003 survey, 93% of APN respondents indicated that they provided education related to expectations of RT and specific symptom management strategies (Moore-Higgs et al., 2003). A variety of materials are available for APNs to use in practice that can assist in supplementing verbal instruction regarding RT (see Table 6-6).

Patient education starts at the time of consultation, once it is determined that the patient will receive RT. APNs should educate the patient about the goals of treatment, the treatment planning process, treatments, and weekly treatment check, as well as acute and late side effects of treatment. This often is an overwhelming amount of information provided in one session, so CD-ROMs, DVDs, and written materials should be used to supplement the verbal instruction. Educational media also are helpful in educating patients who are not able to read. Written consent also may be appropriate at this time or when the patient returns for the simulation appointment. Ongoing education that reinforces self-care is important because side effects arise during treatment and typically subside one to two weeks after treatment.

Table 6-6. Sample of Available Patient Education Materials

Type of Education	Resources	Organization
General	*Radiation Therapy and You*	National Institutes of Health and National Cancer Institute
	Understanding Radiation Therapy: A Guide for Patients and Families	American Cancer Society
Population specific	*Caring for Adolescents and Young Adults*	National Comprehensive Cancer Network® (NCCN®)
Site specific	Breast, colorectal, lung, prostate, and 28 other disease-site booklets	National Cancer Institute
	Brochures on bladder, brain, breast, colorectal, gynecologic, head and neck, lung, prostate, and skin cancers and Hodgkin and non-Hodgkin lymphoma	American Society for Radiology Oncology
	Guidelines on breast, colon, lung, ovarian, and prostate cancers, and melanoma, among others	NCCN
Symptom management	*Sexuality for the Woman With Cancer Sexuality for the Man With Cancer*	American Cancer Society
	Patient and Caregiver Resources (Understanding a Diagnosis, Life With Cancer, and many others)	NCCN

Simulation and Treatment Planning

During most simulations, patients will be asked to wear a hospital gown, and they need to know that the area that is to receive treatment will be exposed. Patients must understand this prior to treatment, as it can cause emotional distress. It is important for patients to understand how long the procedure will take and that a body mold or mask may be made to assist in positioning and the reproducibility of the treatment field, as well as the need for them to remain still during this time. Certain patients may need placement of an IV for contrast administration or insertion of a urinary catheter, rectal tube, or vaginal marker. Simulation can be completed on a variety of different machines, such as a conventional simulator and a CT simulator. During this time, marks may be made on the patient's skin (using a marker) to outline the treatment area, and patients should not remove these until instructed to do so.

Patients also may be required to undergo additional tests, including PET scans, MRI, and CT scans, to provide an understanding of anatomic and physiologic information to be used for the development of the treatment plan. The treatment plan will then be developed, and in most cases where cure is the goal of therapy, it may take anywhere from one to two weeks before the patient starts treatment.

Treatment

Patients undergoing daily RT can expect to be in the RT department anywhere from 30–90 minutes. Conventional RT and three-dimensional conformal treatments typically take an average of 15–30 minutes of treatment time, whereas IMRT treatments can take up to 30–60 minutes. The addition of onboard imaging, which allows for visualization of the treatment site and ensures beam accuracy as well as respiratory gating, will require more time. Patients who are receiving hyperfractionated RT will need to come twice a day, and the feasibility of this schedule needs to be determined at the time of consultation/simulation. The radiation therapist will make permanent tattoos on the patient's skin once therapy has been initiated. Once these tattoos are made, the markings made during simulation can be removed.

The treatment team will evaluate the patient at least once a week. This will include checking the patient's weight and vital signs and providing an opportunity for the patient to address any concerns related to the care and treatment. The healthcare provider will review the treatment prescription, evaluate any expected and unexpected acute effects, and provide evidence-based symptom management strategies. Patients may be seen more frequently because of toxicity and placed on a treatment break if needed, although treatment breaks are not favored in RT because of cell repopulation.

Planning for Follow-Up

As patients are preparing to complete treatment, they must be educated on the follow-up plan of care, including the frequency of appointments, laboratory and radiology studies, and cancer screenings as defined by NCCN and American Cancer Society. Patients also should be educated about the resolution of their symptoms and what to expect over the next two to four weeks as their symptoms subside.

Implications for Oncology Advanced Practice Nurses

The American Society for Radiation Oncology (formerly the American Society for Therapeutic Radiology and Oncology) conducted a descriptive survey in 1997 on the role of nonphysician providers (Kelvin & Moore-Higgs, 1999). The survey received a total of 76 APN respondents (45 clinical nurse specialists [CNSs] and 31 nurse practitioners [NPs]). Based on the nurse's role, the researchers found that CNSs and NPs completed a patient history at the time of consultation (63% and 57% of the time, respectively), during treatment visits (67% and 80%), or during follow-up (62% and 58%). CNSs and NPs completed physical examinations at the time of consult (19% and 42%), during treatment (36% and 74%), and during follow-up (26% and 57%). They found that CNSs were more likely than NPs to develop patient education materials, lead patient education programs, and participate in planning new programs. NPs were found to be more involved with ordering laboratory studies and radiology studies and prescribing medications. Involvement with simulation also was reported, but not by practice role (Kelvin & Moore-Higgs, 1999).

In a survey of 1,000 APN members of ONS, only 6% of respondents listed RT as their primary specialty (Lynch, Cope, & Murphy-Ende, 2001). All respondents identified that patient care and education were the most common activities they performed in their role. Lastly, in a smaller sample of 28 NPs who work in RT, it was found that the top three activities performed by the respondents included providing symptom management, conducting weekly treatment visits, and seeing patients at follow-up visits (Carper & Haas, 2006).

In another study comparing the different roles of RT nurses (staff nurses, nurse managers, and APNs), it was found that APNs spent the majority of their time in direct patient care and education (Moore-Higgs et al., 2003). APNs also were involved with triage, research, and consultations. One interesting finding from this study was that all the roles studied reported involvement with patient education. The APN role is still in development in this specialty. APNs may see patients at the time of consultation, during weekly treatments for symptom management, or during follow-up care. Depending on the practice setting, APNs may obtain informed consent from patients, assist in treatment planning, and assist in the development of plans of care. Collaboration with the medical and surgical oncology teams is critical for APNs in RT because many patients are receiving combined-modality treatment and may require additional treatment following RT. Telephone triage and on-call responsibilities also may be part of the APN role (Carper & Haas, 2006). Furthermore, APNs may use other resources to improve the quality of care for patients receiving RT, such as dietitians, financial counselors, and social workers. Issues such as housing, transportation, out-of-pocket costs and insurance, child care, and support systems may all affect patients' adherence to the prescribed treatment.

APNs play a critical role in symptom assessment and management. Issues related to contrast reactions, allergies, pregnancy, and sexuality during treatment are all important topics that often may go unaddressed. APNs should be able to manage both acute and late effects of treatment. Collaboration with the team is essential when patients are experiencing significant side effects and are in need of a treatment break. In planning for discharge and follow-up, APNs may develop survivorship care plans and guidelines for routine screening and follow-up for patients.

Conclusion

The APN role in the radiation oncology setting is one of excitement and opportunity. APNs have tremendous opportunity in this field to showcase their knowledge and expertise to other healthcare providers, as well as to be a pivotal provider of patient care services. APNs should look to develop programs that improve patient outcomes and satisfaction with care. These types of programs may include development and coordination of a fast-track symptom management program, development of a survivorship clinic, or establishment of palliative care programs to support patients and families. The growing need to provide the right care at the right time is fundamental to the APN role in radiation oncology.

Case Study

H.B. is a 54-year-old postmenopausal woman diagnosed with a T1N0M0 breast cancer. In December, a screening mammogram showed an abnormality in the lateral left breast. A biopsy in February of the following year was positive for adenocarcinoma that was estrogen receptor and progesterone receptor positive, HER2 negative, and epidermal growth factor receptor negative. Surgery later that month revealed a 1.5 cm invasive ductal carcinoma. Surgical margins were negative, and one sentinel node was negative. She has recovered well from surgery and presents today for evaluation and discussion about her treatment options. Upon entry into the room, the APN notices that H.B. is anxious and alone. The nurse quickly assesses the situation and asks if anyone is with her. The nurse then explains to her the purpose of her visit today, and that based on her surgical report, she had clean margins. H.B. breathes a sigh of relief, and the nurse begins taking a history. The nurse notes that H.B. is a mother of two children, aged 16 and 18. The review of systems is negative, except for her breast scar, and H.B. reports that she has had sharp, shooting pains intermittently in her left lateral breast and axilla since surgery.

The APN makes an appointment for H.B. to return in three days for simulation and then reviews with her what simulation is and what will occur during this time. The APN then discusses treatment, weekly visits while under treatment, and the acute and late effects of RT.

On the day of her simulation, the therapist tells H.B., "We are going to remove the gown over your breast." H.B. states, "What do you mean?" The therapist tells her that she will need to be able to make appropriate marks on her skin and that no one else can see her except for them. H.B. takes a breath and closes her eyes. The therapists ask her if she would like to listen to some music. She responds yes. After the planning session, H.B. is given a tour of the department.

Treatment planning is completed, and H.B. starts treatment five days later. She is going to receive 23 treatments for a total dose of 46 Gy, with a boost to the surgical area for eight additional treatments at 200 centigray (cGy) a day, bringing her total dose to 62 Gy. Later that week, the APN sees her for her weekly treatment check. Her blood counts are normal, and she has no complaints.

The next two weeks are uneventful. She reports minor fatigue but attributes it to taking care of her kids and her home. At the end of week three, she reports that she has been experiencing some redness and itching of her breast. She says she just does not like the way she looks right now. The APN discusses her concerns with her and asks if there is anything else the healthcare team can do for her. H.B. says no and thanks the nurse for listening.

During the fourth week of treatment, H.B. has dry desquamation and asks for treatment recommendations. She says she has heard about a variety of different products from others who have gone through this treatment and shows the nurse a cream she has bought that has a floral scent. The nurse recommends a moisturizing product such as Aquaphor® and tells her not to use the product she bought because it contains alcohol.

The final two weeks of treatment are uneventful for H.B. She continues to use Aquaphor, and her fatigue continues to be low. On her final day before treatment, the nurse meets with her and reviews her discharge instructions and follow-up care. H.B. is told that her skin reaction will resolve within the next two to four weeks and that her fatigue also should improve.

1. At the time of the history taking, the patient asks the APN why she has to come back in before starting treatment. How would the APN respond?
   • A CT and simulation (treatment planning) are always performed prior to treatment to set up the precise treatment field that is required for RT.
2. The patient wants to know again the acute effects of radiation that she is going to experience from the treatment. What would the APN tell her?
   • Because RT is a local therapy, side effects generally will occur related to the areas of the body that have been treated. H.B. will likely experience fatigue and skin changes to the breast, including erythema and dry desquamation, which can lead to moist desquamation.
3. What is the purpose of a boost treatment?
   • A boost treatment is used to provide a "boost" of radiation to the surgical site at the completion of radiation to the entire breast. The treatment field includes the area around the surgical scar (as this area has a high chance of developing a recurrence).
4. Which recommendation should the APN provide to H.B. when she is experiencing dry desquamation?
   • No standard of care exists for the management of skin changes of the breast related to RT. Best practice dictates keeping the skin clean and dry along with using alcohol-free moisturizers. The patient also should be taught to avoid sun exposure to the site that has been irradiated.

Key Points

• Radiation oncology is a rapidly evolving field with new treatment modalities.

- Patient treatment is customized and requires careful planning to outline critical structures and anatomy.
- For the majority of patients, a curative course of RT is five to six weeks of treatment.
- Radiation side effects are treatment site dependent versus systemic.
- Acute and late effects of RT are influenced by the type of radiation used, the volume of tissue irradiated, the total dose and daily dose of radiation, the radiosensitivity of the organ or site, and the use of concurrent chemotherapy.
- Patients across all age groups are treated in RT departments; therefore, staff competencies and skill sets need to be current in relation to the diverse age groups.
- APNs should provide appropriate discharge instructions to patients outlining their required follow-up plans.
- The APN role in radiation oncology is evolving. APNs should look to develop programs to support patients throughout the care continuum.

Recommended Resources for Oncology Advanced Practice Nurses

- American Society for Radiation Oncology: www.astro.org
- Gunderson, L.L., & Tepper, J.E. (Eds.). (2012). *Clinical radiation oncology* (3rd ed.). Philadelphia, PA: Elsevier.
- Haas, M.L., Hogle, W.P., Moore-Higgs, G., & Gosselin-Acomb, T.K. (Eds.). (2007). *Radiation therapy: A guide to patient care.* St. Louis, MO: Elsevier Mosby.
- Iwamoto, R.R., Haas, M.L., & Gosselin, T.K. (Eds.). (2012). *Manual for radiation oncology nursing practice and education* (4th ed.). Pittsburgh, PA: Oncology Nursing Society.
- NCCN: www.nccn.org

References

American Society of Breast Surgeons. (2011). Consensus statement for accelerated partial breast irradiation. Retrieved from https://www.breastsurgeons.org/statements/PDF_Statements/APBI.pdf

Archambeau, J.O., Pezner, R., & Wasserman, T. (1995). Pathophysiology of irradiated skin. *International Journal of Radiation Oncology, Biology, Physics, 31,* 1171–1185. doi:10.1016/0360-3016(94)00423-I

Basch, E., Prestrud, A.A., Hesketh, P.J., Kris, M.G., Feyer, P.C., Somerfield, M.R., … Lyman, G.H. (2011). Antiemetics: American Society of Clinical Oncology clinical practice guideline update. *Journal of Clinical Oncology, 29,* 4189–4198. doi:10.1200/JCO.2010.34.4614

Bentel, G.C., Nelson, C.E., & Noell, K.T. (1989). *Treatment planning and dose calculation in radiation oncology* (4th ed.). Elmsford, NY: Pergamon Press.

Bolderston, A., Lloyd, N.S., Wong, R.K.S., Holden, L., & Robb-Blenderman, L. (2006). The prevention and management of acute skin reactions related to radiation therapy: A systematic review and practice guideline. *Supportive Care in Cancer, 14,* 802–817. doi:10.1007/s00520-006-0063-4

Butler, E.N., Chawla, N., Lund, J., Harlan, L.C., Warren, J.L., & Yabroff, K.R. (2013). Patterns of colorectal cancer care in the United States and Canada: A systematic review. *Journal of the National Cancer Institute Monographs, 2013*(46), 13–35. doi:10.1093/jncimonographs/lgt007

Carper, E., & Haas, M. (2006). Advanced practice nursing in radiation oncology. *Seminars in Oncology Nursing, 22,* 203–211. doi:10.1016/j.soncn.2006.07.003

Carroll, P.R., Carducci, M.A., Zietman, A.L., & Rothaermel, J.M. (2005). *Report to the nation on prostate cancer: A guide for men and their families.* Santa Monica, CA: Prostate Cancer Foundation.

Czito, B.G., & Willett, C.G. (2008). Thirty years of rectal cancer research: A brief history. *Oncology, 22,* 1441–1442.

Davis, A.M., Dische, S., Gerber, L., Saunders, M., Leung, S.F., & O'Sullivan, B. (2003). Measuring postirradiation sub-cutaneous soft-tissue fibrosis: State-of-the-art and future directions. *Seminars in Radiation Oncology, 13,* 203–213. doi:10.1016/S1053-4296(03)00022-5

Delaney, G., Jacob, S., Featherstone, C., & Barton, M. (2005). The role of radiotherapy in cancer treatment: Estimating optimal utilization from a review of evidence-based clinical guidelines. *Cancer, 104,* 1129–1137. doi:10.1002/cncr.21324

Delia, P., Sansotta, G., Donato, V., Frosina, P., Messina, G., De Renzis, C., & Famularo, G. (2007). Use of probiotics for prevention of radiation-induced diarrhea. *World Journal of Gastroenterology, 13,* 912–915. doi:10.3748/wjg.v13.i6.912

de M Alcântara-Silva, T.R., Freitas-Junior, R., Freitas, N.M.A., & Machado, G.D.P. (2013). Fatigue related to radio-therapy for breast and/or gynaecological cancer: A systematic review. *Journal of Clinical Nursing, 22,* 19–20. doi:10.1111/jocn.12236

Do, N.L., Nagle, D., & Poylin, V.Y. (2011). Radiation proctitis: Current strategies in management. *Gastroenterology Research and Practice, 2011,* Article 917941. doi:10.1155/2011/917941

Ferraro, D.J., Garsa, A.A., DeWees, T.A., Margenthaler, J.A., Naughton, M., Aft, R., ... Zoberi, I. (2012). Comparison of accelerated partial breast irradiation via multicatheter interstitial brachytherapy versus whole breast radiation. *Radiation Oncology, 7,* 53. doi:10.1186/1748-717X-7-53

Foxson, S.B., Lattimer, J.G., & Felder, B. (2011). Breast cancer. In C.H. Yarbro, D. Wujcik, & B.H. Gobel (Eds.), *Cancer nursing: Principles and practice* (7th ed., pp. 1091–1145). Burlington, MA: Jones & Bartlett Learning.

Garajová, I., Di Girolamo, S., de Rosa, F., Corbelli, J., Agostini, V., Biasco, G., & Brandi, G. (2011). Neoadjuvant treatment in rectal cancer: actual status. *Chemotherapy Research and Practice, 2011,* Article 839742. doi:10.1155/2011/839742

Gosselin, T.K. (2011). Principles of radiation therapy. In C.H. Yarbro, D. Wujcik, & B.H. Gobel (Eds.), *Cancer nursing: Principles and practice* (7th ed., pp. 249–268). Burlington, MA: Jones & Bartlett Learning.

Gosselin, T.K., McQuestion, M., Beamer, L., Feight, D., Merritt, C., Omabegho, M., & Shaftic, A. (2014). Putting evidence into practice: Radiodermatitis. Retrieved from https://www.ons.org/practice-resources/pep/radiodermatitis

Gosselin, T.K., Schneider, S.M., Plambeck, M.A., & Rowe, K. (2010). A prospective randomized, placebo-controlled skin care study in women diagnosed with breast cancer undergoing radiation therapy. *Oncology Nursing Forum, 37,* 619–626. doi:10.1188/10.ONF.619-626

Gosselin-Acomb, T.K. (2006). Colorectal cancer. In K.H. Dow (Ed.), *Nursing care of women with cancer* (pp. 139–165). St. Louis, MO: Elsevier Mosby.

Haisfield-Wolfe, M.E., & Rund, C. (2000). A nursing protocol for the management of perineal-rectal skin alterations. *Clinical Journal of Oncology Nursing, 4,* 15–21.

Harper, J.L., Franklin, L.E., Jenrette, J.M., & Aguero, E.G. (2004). Skin toxicity during breast irradiation: Pathophysiology and management. *Southern Medical Journal, 97,* 989–993. doi:10.1097/01.SMJ.0000140866.97278.87

Hauer-Jensen, M., Wang, J., & Denham, J.W. (2003). Bowel injury: Current and evolving management strategies. *Seminars in Radiation Oncology, 13,* 357–371. doi:10.1016/S1053-4296(03)00032-8

Heidelbaugh, J.J. (2010). Management of erectile dysfunction. *American Family Physician, 81,* 305–312. Retrieved from http://www.aafp.org/afp/2010/0201/p305.html

Hogle, W.P. (2007). Male genitourinary cancers. In M.L. Haas, W.P. Hogle, G.J. Moore-Higgs, & T.K. Gosselin-Acomb (Eds.), *Radiation therapy: A guide to patient care* (pp. 234–266). St. Louis, MO: Elsevier Mosby.

Iwamoto, R.R., Haas, M.L., & Gosselin, T.K. (Eds.). (2012). *Manual for radiation oncology nursing practice and education* (4th ed.). Pittsburgh, PA: Oncology Nursing Society.

Kelsey, C.R., & Salama, J.K. (2013). Stereotactic body radiation therapy for treatment of primary and metastatic pulmonary malignancies. *Surgical Oncology Clinics of North America, 22,* 463–481. doi:10.1016/j.soc.2013.02.011

Kelvin, J.F., & Moore-Higgs, G.J. (1999). Description of the role of nonphysician practitioners in radiation oncology. *International Journal of Radiation Oncology, Biology, Physics, 45,* 163–169. doi:10.1016/S0360-3016(99)00144-3

Khan, A.J., Vicini, F.A., Beitsch, P., Goyal, S., Kuerer, H.M., Keisch, M., ... Haffty, B.G. (2012). Local control, toxicity, and cosmesis in women > 70 years enrolled in the American Society of Breast Surgeons Accelerated Partial Breast Irradiation Registry Trial. *International Journal of Radiation Oncology, Biology, Physics, 84,* 323–330. doi:10.1016/j.ijrobp.2011.12.027

Liu, L., Fiorentino, L., Natarajan, L., Parker, B.A., Mills, P.J., Sadler, G.R., ... Ancoli-Israel, S. (2009). Pre-treatment symptom cluster in breast cancer patients is associated with worse sleep, fatigue and depression during chemotherapy. *Psycho-Oncology, 18,* 187–194. doi:10.1002/pon.1412

Lynch, M.P., Cope, D.G., & Murphy-Ende, K. (2001). Advanced practice issues: Results of the ONS Advanced Practice Nursing survey. *Oncology Nursing Forum, 28,* 1521–1530.

Mendenhall, W.M., Zlotecki, R.A., Snead, F.E., George, T.J., Jr., Marsh, R.D., Mendenhall, C.M., & Rout, W.R. (2009). Radiotherapy in the treatment of resectable rectal adenocarcinoma. *American Journal of Clinical Oncology, 32,* 629–638. doi:10.1097/COC.0b013e31817ff8e4

Mitchell, S.A., Clark, J.C., DeGennaro, R.M., Hoffman, A.J., Poirier, P., Robinson, C.B., … Weisbrod, B.M. (2014). Putting evidence into practice: Fatigue. Retrieved from https://www.ons.org/practice-resources/pep/fatigue

Moore-Higgs, G.J., Watkins-Bruner, D., Balmer, L., Johnson-Doneski, J., Komarny, P., Mautner, B., & Velji, K. (2003). The role of licensed nursing personnel in radiation oncology part A: Results of a descriptive study. *Oncology Nursing Forum, 30,* 51–58. doi:10.1188/03.ONF.51-58

Murphy, J.D., Nelson, L.M., Chang, D.T., Mell, L.K., & Le, Q.-T. (2013). Patterns of care in palliative radiotherapy: A population-based study. *Journal of Oncology Practice, 9,* e220–e227. doi:10.1200/JOP.2012.000835

National Comprehensive Cancer Network. (2015a). *NCCN Clinical Practice Guidelines in Oncology (NCCN Guidelines®): Adult cancer pain* [v.1.2015]. Retrieved from http://www.nccn.org/professionals/physician_gls/pdf/pain.pdf

National Comprehensive Cancer Network. (2015b). *NCCN Clinical Practice Guidelines in Oncology (NCCN Guidelines®): Antiemesis* [v.1.2015]. Retrieved from http://www.nccn.org/professionals/physician_gls/pdf/antiemesis.pdf

National Comprehensive Cancer Network. (2015c). *NCCN Clinical Practice Guidelines in Oncology (NCCN Guidelines®): Breast cancer* [v.2.2015]. Retrieved from http://www.nccn.org/professionals/physician_gls/pdf/breast.pdf

National Comprehensive Cancer Network. (2015d). *NCCN Clinical Practice Guidelines in Oncology (NCCN Guidelines®): Cancer-related fatigue* [v.2.2015]. Retrieved from http://www.nccn.org/professionals/physician_gls/pdf/fatigue.pdf

National Comprehensive Cancer Network. (2015e). *NCCN Clinical Practice Guidelines in Oncology (NCCN Guidelines®): Non-small cell lung cancer* [v.5.2015]. Retrieved from http://www.nccn.org/professionals/physician_gls/pdf/nscl.pdf

National Comprehensive Cancer Network. (2015f). *NCCN Clinical Practice Guidelines in Oncology (NCCN Guidelines®): Prostate cancer* [v.1.2015]. Retrieved from http://www.nccn.org/professionals/physician_gls/PDF/prostate.pdf

National Comprehensive Cancer Network. (2015g). *NCCN Clinical Practice Guidelines in Oncology (NCCN Guidelines®): Rectal cancer* [v.2.2015]. Retrieved from http://www.nccn.org/professionals/physician_gls/pdf/rectal.pdf

Radiation Therapy Oncology Group. (2014, March 9). RTOG 0813 protocol information. Retrieved from http://www.rtog.org/ClinicalTrials/ProtocolTable/StudyDetails.aspx?study=0813

Roila, F., Herrstedt, J., Aapro, M., Gralla, R.J., Einhorn, L.H., Ballatori, E., … Warr, D. (2010). Guideline update for MASCC and ESMO in the prevention of chemotherapy- and radiotherapy-induced nausea and vomiting: Results of the Perugia consensus conference. *Annals of Oncology, 21*(Suppl. 5), v232–v243. doi:10.1093/annonc/mdq194

Rubin, P., Cooper, R., & Phillips, T.L. (Eds.). (1975). *Radiation biology and radiation pathology syllabus (Set R.T.1: Radiation oncology).* Chicago, IL: American College of Radiology.

Senkus, E., Kyriakides, S., Penault-Llorca, F., Poortmans, P., Thompson, A., Zackrisson, S., & Cardoso, F. (2013). Primary breast cancer: ESMO clinical practice guidelines for diagnosis, treatment and follow-up. *Annals of Oncology, 0,* 1–17. doi:10.1093/annonc/mdt284

Shadad, A.K., Sullivan, F.J., Martin, J.D., & Egan, L.J. (2013). Gastrointestinal radiation injury: Symptoms, risk factors and mechanisms. *World Journal of Gastroenterology, 19,* 185–198. doi:10.3748/wjg.v19.i2.185

Shah, C., Badiyan, S., Wilkinson, J.B., Vicini, F., Beitsch, P., Keisch, M., … Lyden, M. (2013). Treatment efficacy with accelerated partial breast irradiation (APBI): Final analysis of the American Society of Breast Surgeons MammoSite breast brachytherapy registry trial. *Annals of Surgical Oncology, 10,* 3279–3285. doi:10.1245/s10434-013-3158-4

Smith, B.D., Arthur, D.W., Buchholz, T.A., Haffty, B.G., Hahn, C.A., Hardenbergh, P.H., … Harris, J.R. (2009). Accelerated partial breast irradiation consensus statement from the American Society for Radiation Oncology (ASTRO). *International Journal of Radiation Oncology, Biology, Physics, 74,* 987–1001. doi:10.1016/j.ijrobp.2009.02.031

Solin, L.J. (2010). The impact of adding radiation treatment after breast conservation surgery for ductal carcinoma in situ of the breast. *Journal of the National Cancer Institute Monographs, 2010*(41), 187–192. doi:10.1093/jncimonographs/lgq020

Sverrisson, E., Jones, J.S., & Pow-Sang, J.M. (2013). [Cryosurgery for prostate cancer: A comprehensive review]. *Archivos Españoles de Urología, 66,* 546–556. Retrieved from http://aeurologia.com/articulo_prod.php?id_art=2739529438606

Vargo, J.A., Verma, V., Kim, H., Kalash, R., Heron, D.E., Johnson, R., & Beriwal, S. (2014). Extended (5-year) outcomes of accelerated partial breast irradiation using MammoSite balloon brachytherapy: Patterns of failure, patient selection, and dosimetric correlates for late toxicity. *International Journal of Radiation Oncology, Biology, Physics, 88,* 285–291. doi:10.1016/j.ijrobp.2013.05.039

Visich, K.L., & Yeo, T.P. (2010). The prophylactic use of probiotics in the prevention of radiation therapy-induced diarrhea. *Clinical Journal of Oncology Nursing, 14,* 467–473. doi:10.1188/10.CJON.467-473

Waring, J., & Gosselin, T.K. (2010). Developing a high-dose rate brachytherapy program. *Clinical Journal of Oncology Nursing, 14,* 199–205. doi:10.1188/10.CJON.199-205

Willett, C.G., Czito, B.G., & Tyler, D.G. (2007). Intraoperative radiation therapy. *Journal of Clinical Oncology, 25,* 971–977. doi:10.1200/JCO.2006.10.0255

Wong, R.K.S., Bensadoun, R.-J., Boers-Doets, C.B., Bryce, J., Chan, A., Epstein, J.B., … Lacouture, M.E. (2013). Clinical practice guidelines for the prevention and treatment of acute and late radiation reactions from the MASCC Skin Toxicity Study Group. *Supportive Care in Cancer, 21,* 2933–2948. doi:10.1007/s00520-013-1896-2

Yazbeck, V.Y., Villaruz, L., Haley, M., & Socinski, M. (2013). Management of normal tissues toxicity associated with chemoradiation (primary skin, esophagus, and lung). *Cancer Journal, 19,* 231–237. doi:10.1097/PPO.0b013e31829453fb

Yirmibesoglu, E., Higginson, D.S., Fayda, M., Rivera, M.P., Halle, J., Rosenman, J., … Marks, L.B. (2012). Challenges scoring radiation pneumonitis in patients irradiated for lung cancer. *Lung Cancer, 76,* 350–353. doi:10.1016/j.lungcan.2011.11.025

CHAPTER 7

Blood and Marrow Stem Cell Transplantation

Hollie Devine, MSN, ANP-BC

Introduction

For approximately a century, physicians and scientists have collaborated, investigating the use of bone marrow to treat inherited diseases of immune function, marrow failure syndromes, and leukemia. The experiences of early studies were disappointing, and many were skeptical of its potential. Translating animal models to humans was met with many challenges, and its beginnings were cumbersome. A majority of these patients had refractory disease and were known to be the sickest of patients on the medical units. Death due to complications of primary disease, infections, and graft-versus-host disease (GVHD) characterized the outcomes of these patients. As a result of understanding immunologic processes, medical resiliency, and persistent fortitude, blood and marrow stem cell transplantation has become a therapeutic option for many malignant and nonmalignant diseases. Although much has been learned, new and improved strategies of blood and marrow stem cell transplantation continue to be discovered.

Knowledge of the historical background in blood and marrow transplantation can help to elucidate the use of this treatment today. In the discipline of blood and marrow stem cell transplantation, there has been a lack of worldwide scientific agreement on a single terminology used to describe this process. For example, terms such as *bone marrow*, *peripheral blood* (peripheral blood), and *hematopoietic stem cell* (HSC) transplant may be used interchangeably. To provide historical context, the derived stem cell source will be described. Thereafter, the term *hematopoietic stem cell transplantation* (HSCT) will be used throughout this chapter as a general term to cover transplantation of progenitor cells from any source (i.e., bone marrow, peripheral blood, umbilical cord blood).

History of Hematopoietic Stem Cell Transplantation

The scientific investigations and principles of HSCT commenced in animal models. In 1922, Fabricious-Moeller observed that when legs of guinea pigs were shielded during total body irradiation (TBI), cytopenias and bleeding were prevented (Kersey, 2004). This observation was overlooked until 1949 when Jacobson and colleagues rediscovered that mice exposed to doses of radiation experienced bone marrow aplasia, which could be prevented by shielding the spleen, a hematopoietic organ in mice (Kersey, 2004). Shortly thereafter, Lorenz, Uphoff, Reid, and Shelton (1951) demonstrated that lethally irradiated mice and guinea pigs could be protected by IV administration of syngeneic (identical twin) bone marrow. Using histochemical and genetic markers, scientists proved that protection from the lethal effects of TBI was due to the colonization of recipient donor cells.

In 1957, Barnes and Loutit reported survival differences of murine leukemia models that received supralethal radiation followed by either syngeneic or allogeneic (from a matched donor) cells (Kersey, 2004). Results demonstrated that syngeneic spleens provided bone marrow recovery and no further evidence of leukemia. However, 56% of mice infused with allogeneic splenic cells died prior to day 100. Other researchers were identifying similar findings in mice studies of allogeneic cell transplantation. Mice were dying because of severe diarrhea, weight loss, skin lesions, and hepatic necrosis. These observations provided the fundamental characteristics of GVHD, a potential complication of allogeneic HSCT. Although early animal studies were performed in the murine systems, a group of researchers in Seattle directed their efforts at identifying a more suitable preclinical animal model. Dogs were chosen because of their random-bred nature, large body habitus, longevity, and genetic diversity. Besides humans, they were the only other mammal species with these qualities. Thus, the canine model provided important information about bone marrow transplantation that was applicable to humans. Two salient findings included the predictive value of histocompatibility testing and its outcome on transplant, as well as being an effective model for evaluating diseases such as hemophilia, inherited metabolic disorders, and malignancies (Kersey, 2004).

In 1957, early attempts at HSCT demonstrated that large amounts of bone marrow could be safely infused intravenously followed by a transient engraftment (Thomas, Lochte, Lu, & Ferrebee, 1957). In 1959, Thomas and colleagues demonstrated the clinical use of syngeneic bone marrow infusions between sisters. One sister with end-stage leukemia received TBI to destroy the cancer, which was followed by an infusion of bone marrow from her healthy sister. The result was a three-month disease-free state of the recipient's leukemia (Thomas, Lochte, Cannon, Sahler, & Ferrebee, 1959).

In the following years, human leukocyte antigen (HLA) typing allowed physicians to find histocompatible donors for recipients (Kersey, 2004). In 1968, Mathé summarized his early experience of performing bone marrow transplants in 21 patients with leukemia. During this time, a majority of the patients were not HLA typed. Patients succumbed to graft failure, GVHD, recurrent leukemia, or infection (Kersey, 2004; Mathé, 1968). However, in 1968, Gatti and colleagues reported a successful allogeneic bone marrow transplant in three patients with severe combined immunologic deficiency (Gatti, Meuwissen, Allen, Hong, & Good, 1968). As of 1994, all three patients were alive and well (Thomas, 1999).

The 1970s proved that HSCT was becoming accepted as a treatment modality. In 1975, a review in the *New England Journal of Medicine* summarized the state of bone marrow transplant knowledge (Thomas et al., 1975). This article described 37 patients with aplastic anemia and 73 with advanced leukemia who failed conventional therapy and were then transplanted. Although engraftment was successful in some patients with aplastic anemia, few patients with leukemia survived. In 1977, 100 patients with advanced acute leukemia were given bone marrow from HLA-matched siblings. At the time of publication, 17 out of 100 patients were alive one to three years later (Thomas, Buckner, et al., 1977). Twenty-three years later, 8 of those 17 were long-term survivors (Thomas, 2000).

The 1980s and beyond demonstrated that HSCT was indeed a treatment option for those with malignant and nonmalignant diseases. This was evident by the increase in the number of transplants being performed. In the late 1980s, a volunteer registry was established, the National Marrow Donor Program (NMDP). In 1990, the Nobel Prize in Medicine was awarded to Dr. E. Donnell Thomas for his discoveries and contributions in the field of HSCT. In the late 1990s, CD34+ was recognized as a protein that identified hematopoietic progenitor cells, and isolation of hematopoietic progenitor cells from the peripheral blood would provide another stem cell source. With the introduction of cytokines, successful mobilization of CD34+ from the bone marrow into the peripheral circulation was achieved (de la Morena & Gatti, 2011). In addition, umbilical cord blood represented another alternative source of HSCs for both adults and children with hematopoietic disorders and malignancies (Gluckman et al., 1989, 1997). In 1998, cord blood programs were launched, and in 2001, NMDP built a donor repository that became one of the world's largest tissue sample storage facilities used for medical research and included donor access to stem cell sources that included bone marrow, peripheral blood, and umbilical cord blood.

In 2004, the research arm of NMDP partnered with the Autologous Blood and Marrow Transplant Registry of the Medical College of Wisconsin to create the Center for International Blood and Marrow Transplant Research (CIBMTR) (U.S. Department of Health and Human Services Health Resources and Services Administration, 2012). These organizations have more than 30 years of experience in collecting, managing, and analyzing data about various sources of HSCs. CIBMTR contributes to the scientific literature and encourages HSCT experts to use their data for research. They also work closely with federal agencies and international experts in hematology, oncology, transplantation, histocompatibility, biostatistics, bioinformatics, psychology, and health policy. Furthermore, CIBMTR continues to develop and maintain an electronic information system that collects and manages data about bone marrow and cord blood transplants and provides this information to interested individuals, organizations, and regulatory agencies. It is also experienced in creating and managing research sample repositories.

The number of autologous HSCTs in the United States continues to rise because of its treatment impact on those with plasma cell malignancies and lymphoproliferative disorders, as well as the increase in the number of patients older than age 60 receiving transplants. Since 2006, the number of allogeneic transplants from unrelated donors has exceeded those from related donors. Contributing factors to this trend include the growth of unrelated donor databases, improvements in unrelated donor transplants, and the increased numbers of allogeneic transplants for patients older than age 60 with reduced-intensity conditioning regimens (Pasquini & Zhu, 2014).

Basic Concepts of the Hematopoietic System

Hematopoiesis and immunology provide the foundation for oncology principles and are the scientific basis of HSCT. Hematopoiesis is a multistep process involving interactions between HSCs, the bone marrow microenvironment, cellular adhesion molecules, chemokines, and cytokines. The main objective of hematopoiesis is to maintain the peripheral blood with a constant level of different types of blood cells.

HSCs are cells that remain dormant in the bone marrow until activated. They express numerous proteins on the surface of their cell membrane. These surface proteins serve as "markers" that identify the type and function of the cell. The "cluster of differentiation" (CD) system is used to identify cell surface proteins. CD34+ is a marker of HSCs and is used to separate them from other populations of leukocytes. Immunophenotyping, or flow cytometry, is a laboratory methodology used to identify cell lineage, differentiation, and maturation. Once HSCs are activated, they rise to progenitor cells. Progenitor cells are more limited than HSCs in that once progenitor cells commit to a cell lineage, they are on a path to becoming a specific cell type. The two types of progenitor cell lineages are myeloid and lymphoid. The common myeloid progenitor cells give rise to red blood cells, white blood cells, and platelets. The lymphoid progenitor cells give rise to natural killer cells, T lymphocytes, and B lymphocytes (Manz, Akashi, & Weissman, 2004). As an HSC differentiates, it loses its CD34 status and acquires other markers specific to a cell lineage. For example, T cells will acquire CD4 or CD8 surface markers, and B cells will acquire surface immunoglobulin markers and antigen-specific receptors (Manz et al., 2004). Figure 7-1 demonstrates the evolution of the HSC, and Table 7-1 further outlines the different types and functions of blood cells that evolve as a result of hematopoiesis.

Given that the specialized cells of the immune system develop from HSCs, immune function is partially dependent on hematopoiesis. Problems arise within the immune system as a result of overwhelming infection, aging, medications, inherited genetic mutations, and acquired disorders (Hunt, Walsh, Voegeli, & Roberts, 2010). Furthermore, malignancies and therapies affecting cells originating from HSCs further contribute to immune malfunction.

Indications for Hematopoietic Stem Cell Transplantation

The clinical indications for use of HSCT as a treatment modality include both malignant and nonmalignant conditions. Examples of conditions treated with HSCT are listed in Table 7-2. The most common indications include leukemia, lymphoma, and multiple myeloma.

Types of Hematopoietic Stem Cell Transplantation

Autologous Transplantation

In autologous transplantation, the HSCs are collected from oneself. Bone marrow or peripheral blood is procured when the malignancy is in remission or in a state of minimal residual disease. Prior to myeloablative therapy, HSCs are mobilized (i.e., the process by which HSCs are released from the bone marrow into peripheral blood), collected, and cryopreserved. The rationale for administering myeloablative therapy is to give dose-intensive therapy to obliterate cancer cells. As a result of this therapy, patients may experience severe or complete depletion of bone marrow. Thus, to restore bone marrow functioning, autologous HSCs are reinfused, or transplanted back into the patient. To facilitate post-transplant hematopoiesis, cytokines are administered after the autologous infusion (Devine, Tierney, Schmit-Pokorny, & McDermott, 2010). The cytokine commonly used in HSCT is granulocyte–colony-stimulating factor (G-CSF).

Cytokines are intracellular signaling proteins that act by binding to a receptor on a target cell (Dinarello, 2007; Lee & Margolin, 2011). Cytokines have numerous functions and are involved with immune system regulation, inflammatory reactions, wound healing, cancer, and hematopoiesis (Dinarello, 2007; Shaikh, 2011). A variety of cytokines stimulate HSCs to proliferate and differentiate. Cytokines that induce proliferation and differentiation of the myeloid lineage include interleukin (IL)-1, IL-3, IL-6, erythropoietin, thrombopoietin, stem cell factor,

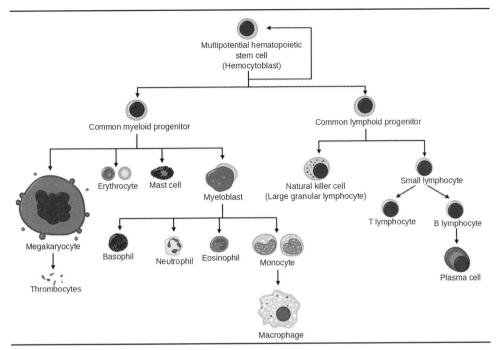

Figure 7-1. Hematopoiesis

Note. From Wikimedia Commons, http://en.wikipedia.org/wiki/File:Hematopoiesis_simple.svg; by Mikael Häggström (no attribution required), from original by A. Rad. Used under the Creative Commons Attribution-Share Alike 3.0 Unported license: http://creativecommons.org/licenses/by-sa/3.0/us/legalcode.

G-CSF, and granulocyte macrophage–colony-stimulating factor (GM-CSF) (Dinarello, 2007; Shaikh, 2011). Other cytokines in the bone marrow microenvironment that induce proliferation and differentiation of the lymphoid lineage include interferons, IL-1, IL-6, FMS-like tyrosine kinase 3 ligand (known as FLT-3 ligand), and tumor necrosis factor (Lee & Margolin, 2011; Shaikh, 2011).

Autologous HSCT may be considered part of the initial treatment plan, such as with multiple myeloma, or reserved for those with persistent disease or who have relapsed. Other diseases that are treated with autologous HSCT are listed in Table 7-2 and include non-Hodgkin lymphoma, Hodgkin lymphoma, and pediatric malignancies (e.g., germ cell tumors, sarcomas, neuroblastoma, Wilms tumor). An advantage of autologous HSCT includes ready access to HSCs and lack of GVHD risk. However, a disadvantage includes the risk of tumor contamination and the lack of graft-versus-tumor (GVT) effect.

Allogeneic Transplantation

Allogeneic transplantation is the use of HLA-matched related or unrelated donor HSCs to reconstitute hematopoiesis and immunity in recipients with hematologic malignancies or genetic or immunologic diseases. The goal of allogeneic HSCT is to generate long-term disease-free survival and cure the underlying condition (Spitzer, Dey, Chen, Attar, & Ballen, 2012). The donor T cells react against host antigens, providing the antitumor reaction known as the GVT effect (Spitzer et al., 2012; Zhang, Chen, & Chao, 2011). Stem cell sources include bone marrow, peripheral blood, and umbilical cord blood.

Table 7-1. Types and Functions of Blood Cells

Lineage	Role	Cell Type	Function
Lymphoid	Immune system cells that respond to foreign substances and are dependent upon the production of cytokines from antigen-presenting cells	Natural killer (NK) cells	Kill selected tumor cells without having to be activated or immunized against a tumor cell Participate early in host defenses against intracellular organisms and viral infections The difference between NK cells and killer T cells is that NK cells destroy their targets without a prior "conference" in the lymphoid organs.
		T lymphocytes	Are important in mediating an immune response Participate in delayed-type hypersensitivity Helper T (TH) cells secrete chemicals that recruit other immune cells and facilitate in coordinating their attack; express the CD4 protein on their cell surface. Cytotoxic T (TC) cells attack virally infected cells; express the CD8 protein on their cell surface. Regulatory T (Treg) cells suppress T-cell–mediated immunity toward the end of an immune reaction. Treg cells may have a crucial role in the generation and maintenance of immune tolerance. Treg cells express CD4, CD8, and CD25. Memory T cells are involved in secondary immune responses and long-term protection. Memory cells may be CD4+ or CD8+ and express CD45RO+.
		B lymphocytes	B lymphocytes or B cells have a receptor protein that allows the B cell to bind to a specific antigen. Principal function is to produce antibodies, known as immunoglobulins (Ig). Five known classes of these antigen-specific antibodies exist: • IgG: Are the major immunoglobulin in the blood; enter tissue spaces; coat microorganisms, speeding their destruction by other cells of the immune system • IgA: Guard the entrance to the body; concentrate in body fluids such as tears, saliva, and secretions of the respiratory and gastrointestinal tracts • IgM: Link together in the bloodstream to kill invaders • IgE: Participate in allergic reactions • IgD: Regulate cell activation in B-cell membranes
Myeloid	Respond early and nonspecifically to infection; includes monocytes, macrophages, and granulocytes (neutrophils)	Megakaryocytes	Known as platelets Fragments of cytoplasm that remain in the bone marrow to form platelets just before release into the circulation Assist with coagulation

(Continued on next page)

Table 7-1. Types and Functions of Blood Cells *(Continued)*

Lineage	Role	Cell Type	Function
Myeloid *(cont.)*		Erythrocytes	Known as red blood cells (RBCs) Provide tissue nourishment and transport oxygen throughout the body
		Myeloblasts	Produce granulocytes that are composed of neutrophils, basophils, and eosinophils Neutrophils are the first cells to arrive at the site of an infection or tissue damage and contribute to the acute inflammatory response Eosinophils attack parasites and secrete leukotrienes, prostaglandins, and other cytokines Basophils possess receptors for IgE; thus, when involved in allergic responses, inflammatory mediators such as histamine, prostaglandins, and serotonin are triggered Assist in the facilitation of monocytes leaving the blood and entering tissues, thus turning into macrophages or dendritic cells, depending on the signals they receive from T and B lymphocytes

Note. Based on information from Clayberger & Krensky, 2005; Delves & Roitt, 2000a, 2000b; Gutcher & Becher, 2007; Jiang & Chess, 2004; Parkin & Cohen, 2001; Sallusto et al., 1999, 2004; Ziegler-Heitbrock, 2007.

To identify a suitable donor, HLA typing must be performed on both the recipient and all potential donors. Determining the degree of HLA match is critical because it facilitates and predicts outcomes of cell, tissue, and organ transplantation. The major histocompatibility complex (MHC) also plays an integral role in transplant rejection. MHC molecules are located on the surface of nucleated cells and control immune responses by recognizing self from nonself. The MHC gene is located on the short arm of chromosome 6 and encodes the glycoprotein on the cell surface known as HLA (Ferrara, Levine, Reddy, & Holler, 2009; Mickelson & Petersdorf, 2009; Petersdorf, 2013). The HLA region is subdivided into three subgroups: class I, which is found on every cell in the body and presents antigens to cytotoxic T cells; class II, which is found on B cells, macrophages, and other antigen-presenting cells and presents antigens to helper T cells; and class III, which is involved in complement pathways and cytokines (Mickelson & Petersdorf, 2009). If individuals are HLA compatible, their tissues are immunologically compatible with one another. Thus, HLA typing and the degree of the match are critical in allogeneic HSCT, as studies have demonstrated that the accuracy of tissue typing for HSCT between the donor and recipient improves overall survival, reduces the incidence of acute and chronic GVHD, and improves rates of engraftment (Park & Seo, 2012; Petersdorf, 2013). For the purposes of allogeneic HSCT, the HLA-A, HLA-B, HLA-C, HLA-DRB1, and HLA-DQB1 antigens are the most important (Park & Seo, 2012; Petersdorf, 2013). HLA typing traditionally has been performed by serologic methods. However, medical technology is advancing to the point where HLA typing can initially be accomplished by obtaining cells from swabbing the buccal mucosa.

Each nucleated human cell has two HLA haplotypes, one inherited from the mother and the other inherited from the father. Because parental haplotypes can segregate in different combinations, there is a 25% chance that any one sibling would be identical to the other (see Figure 7-2). Aside from monozygotic twins, who share exactly the same HLA genotype, full siblings are most likely to share the same HLA haplotypes because they come from the same gene pool.

If a sibling is not an HLA match, unrelated donors or cord blood products may be identified through registries, such as NMDP. NMDP is the largest registry used in HSCT. Since 1986, NMDP has facilitated searches for unrelated donors worldwide and has coordinated the procurement and delivery of HSCs to transplant centers. The amount of time it takes to find an HLA-matched donor varies but may take four to six weeks or longer. Despite worldwide unrelated donor registries, finding a donor has been limited by finding a phenotypically matched unrelated donor. A phenotype is any observable characteristic of an organism and is determined by genes and environment (Lewontin, 2011). For example, the chance of finding a matched unrelated donor transplant is 60%–70% for Caucasians but less than 10% for ethnic minorities (Anasetti, Aversa, & Brunstein, 2012). Ethnic tendencies in HLA inheritance can make HLA matching with an unrelated donor difficult among members of ethnic minorities or people with mixed ethnic heritage (Bray et al., 2008). Thus, the use of HSCs from relatives who are partially HLA matched provides some advantages for patients lacking an HLA-matched sibling donor or fully matched unrelated donor. In such situations, a haploidentical transplant can be considered.

By definition, haploidentical donors are half matched, as genetic material comes from each parent. Virtually all patients have at least one partially HLA-matched family member who may

Table 7-2. Hematologic and Nonhematologic Conditions Treated With Blood and Marrow Stem Cell Transplantation

Type of Transplant	Malignant Conditions	Nonmalignant Conditions

Allogeneic	• Hematologic diseases
	  – Acute lymphocytic leukemia
	  – Acute myeloid leukemia
	  – Agnogenic myeloid metaplasia (myelofibrosis)
	  – Chronic lymphocytic leukemia
	  – Chronic myeloid leukemia
	  – Chronic myelomonocytic leukemia
	  – Hodgkin lymphoma
	  – Juvenile chronic myeloid leukemia
	  – Juvenile myelomonocytic leukemia
	  – Multiple myeloma
	  – Myelodysplastic syndrome
	  – Non-Hodgkin lymphoma
	  – Refractory anemia
		• Bone marrow failure syndromes
		  – Aplastic anemia
		  – Diamond-Blackfan anemia
		  – Fanconi anemia
		• Hemoglobinopathies
		  – Beta thalassemia major
		  – Chronic granulomatous disease
		  – Familial erythrophagocytic lymphohistiocytosis
		  – Kostmann syndrome
		  – Paroxysmal nocturnal hemoglobinuria
		  – Reticular dysgenesis
		  – Sickle-cell anemia
		• Inherited immune system disorders
		  – Chediak-Higashi syndrome
		  – Severe combined immunodeficiency
		  – Wiskott-Aldrich syndrome
		• Other: Osteopetrosis
		• Inherited metabolic disorders
		  – Adrenoleukodystrophy
		  – Gaucher disease
		  – Hunter syndrome
		  – Hurler syndrome
		  – Krabbe disease
		  – Maroteaux-Lamy syndrome (mucopolysaccharidosis type VI)
		  – Metachromatic leukodystrophy
		  – Sly syndrome

(Continued on next page)

Table 7-2. Hematologic and Nonhematologic Conditions Treated With Blood and Marrow Stem Cell Transplantation *(Continued)*

Type of Transplant	Malignant Conditions	Nonmalignant Conditions

Autologous	• Hematologic diseases
	  – Acute myeloid leukemia
	  – Hodgkin lymphoma
	  – Multiple myeloma
	  – Non-Hodgkin lymphoma
	• Solid tumors
	  – Astrocytomas
	  – Desmoplastic small round cell tumor
	  – Ewing sarcoma
	  – Germ cell tumors
	  – Hepatoblastoma
	  – Medulloblastoma
	  – Neuroblastoma
	  – Peripheral neuroectodermal tumor
	  – Retinoblastoma
	  – Rhabdomyosarcoma
	  – Sarcomas
	  – Wilms tumor
		• Amyloid light-chain amyloidosis
		• Autoimmune diseases (remains investigational)
		  – Multiple sclerosis
		  – Rheumatoid arthritis

Note. Based on information from Burt et al., 2008, 2015; Copelan, 2006; Gassas et al., 2015; Gratwohl et al., 2015; National Marrow Donor Program, n.d.; Pasquini & Zhu, 2014; Sureda et al., 2015.

be available to serve as a donor. Therefore, the donor can be a parent, sibling, or child. The availability of a haploidentical donor in most families is a potential advantage, both for avoiding the need to find an alternative unrelated donor and for the potentially greater GVT effect that can be induced. However, it is the donor T cells from the HSC graft that contribute to the increased risk of GVHD, as well as a decreased risk of relapsed disease (Raza & Vierling, 2014). Although the elimination of donor T cells, or the use of T cell–depleted grafts, may decrease the incidence of GVHD, the risk of infection and relapsed disease is increased (Ferrara et al., 2009). Thus, numerous challenges associated with haploidentical HSCT must be overcome.

Strategies to deplete T cells from stem cell grafts by various selection techniques include pharmacologic approaches and graft manipulation. Pharmacologic agents, such as calcineurin inhibitors, corticosteroids, and monoclonal antibodies (mAbs), are commonly managed by advanced practice nurses (APNs) in clinical practice. Pharmacologic approaches to prevent and treat GVHD are listed in Figure 7-3. Another strategy to deplete T cells is graft manipulation. This component of HSCT may go unrecognized, as this process occurs prior to the infusion of HSCs in a stem cell laboratory.

Graft manipulation can be divided into three main categories: physical, immunologic, and combined physical and immunologic separation methods (Daniele et al., 2012). Physical separation methods such as soybean agglutinin/T-cell rosetting, elutriation, and specific mAb (i.e., anti-CD8) depletion are some examples of T cell–depletion methods that have been used for the acute leukemias and lymphomas. However, relapse is still problematic in recipients with chronic myeloid leukemia, myelodysplastic syndrome, and multiple myeloma (Daniele et al., 2012). Therefore, other approaches, such as immunologic techniques, have been used.

Prior to HSCT, mAbs in combination with rabbit complement factors are directed against T cells. This method has been improved with cell-sorting devices that use antibodies in combi-

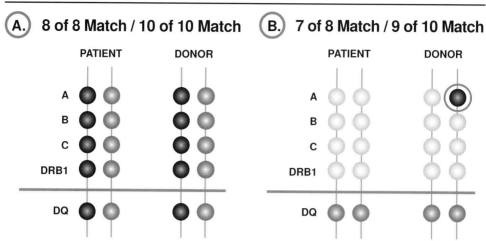

Example A shows that the patient's markers match the donor's. When HLA markers A, B, C, and DRB1 from the patient and the donor match, it is called an 8 of 8 match. When A, B, C, DRB1, and DQ markers all match, it's called a 10 of 10 match.

Example B shows that one of the patient's A markers does not match one of the donor's A markers. Therefore, this is a 7 of 8 match or, if the DQ marker matches, a 9 of 10 match.

Figure 7-2. Example of Human Leukocyte Antigen (HLA) Typing and Matching of Siblings

Note. From "HLA Matching," by Be The Match, 2015. Retrieved from http://bethematch.org/for-patients-and-families/ finding-a-donor. Copyright 2015 by National Marrow Donor Program® (NMDP). Reprinted with permission.

nation with immune-magnetic beads. These approaches are the combined physical and immunologic methods. Antibodies are coated with magnetic beads that bind to antigens present on the surface of cells. The cells of interest, which in this case are the T cells, are captured. As a result, there is an increased concentration of bead-attached T cells. A magnetic wash then occurs within the cell-sorting device. The final product is a graft that has been depleted of T cells. The two common cell-sorting devices used in HSCT are the Isolex® 300i Magnetic Cell Selection System and the CliniMACS® device. The Isolex 300i device is indicated for processing autologous HSC graft products to obtain a CD34+ cell–enriched population intended for hematopoietic reconstitution after myeloablative therapy in patients with CD34– tumors. However, this device has been evaluated in haploidentical donors (Daniele et al., 2012). The CliniMACS device efficiently removes donor T cells from the graft prior to transplantation by enriching CD34+ stem cells (Devine et al., 2011; Pasquini et al., 2012). The approval was based on data from a phase II, single-arm, multicenter study (Devine et al., 2011). The trial demonstrated that following intensive myeloablative conditioning, HSCT from an HLA-matched sibling donor graft processed using the CliniMACS device as the sole means of GVHD prophylaxis led to a low incidence of chronic GVHD (19% at two years after transplantation) without negatively affecting relapse, engraftment, overall survival, or disease-free survival (Pasquini et al., 2012). Thus, T-cell depletion offers the possibility of preventing GVHD and reducing transplant-related morbidity and mortality, thereby contributing to a better quality of life.

Allogeneic donor selection is critical and may influence the success of HSCT. In addition to HLA type and stem cell source, other factors such as age, gender, parity, and infectious disease serologies warrant further consideration (Erkurt, Berber, Kuku, Kaya, & Nizam, 2014). Age is the only donor-related factor that affects overall and disease-free survival. Although older age does not preclude one from being a donor, younger donors, ages 18–55, are preferred (Nannya et al., 2011). Mobilization failure rates and increased incidence of acute and chronic GVHD have been associated with older donors, thus affecting survival (Erkurt et al., 2014). Irrespective of recipient gender, female donors with a history of previous pregnancies increases the risk of GVHD. This

---

Systemic Immunosuppression
- Calcineurin inhibitors: Cyclosporine and tacrolimus
- Corticosteroids
- Folate antagonist: Methotrexate
- Mammalian target of rapamycin inhibitor: Sirolimus
- Mycophenolate mofetil
- Purine analog: Azathioprine

Monoclonal Antibody–Based Therapies
- Alemtuzumab
- Antilymphocyte globulin
- Antithymocyte globulin
- Basiliximab
- Daclizumab
- Denileukin diftitox
- Etanercept
- Infliximab
- Milatuzumab (investigational)
- Pentostatin (investigational)
- Rituximab

Other Systemic Therapies
- Bortezomib (investigational)
- Hydroxychloroquine
- Maraviroc (investigational)
- Rapamycin
- Repifermin (investigational)
- Retinoids (investigational)
- Thalidomide

Phototherapy
- 8-Methoxypsoralen plus ultraviolet A irradiation (PUVA)
- Extracorporeal photopheresis
- Ultraviolet B phototherapy

Local and Topical Therapy
- Corticosteroid mouthwash
- Intralesional steroid injections (mouth only)
- Ophthalmic cyclosporine
- Prosthetic replacement of the ocular surface ecosystem (known as PROSE)
- Topical corticosteroids
- Topical tacrolimus
- Vaginal cyclosporine or tacrolimus ointment/gel

Cell-Sorting Devices
- CliniMACS®
- Isolex® 300i

Figure 7-3. Options for Graft-Versus-Host Disease Prevention and Treatment

Note. Based on information from Ferrara et al., 2009; Johnson, 2013; Mohty & Mohty, 2011; Pavletic & Fowler, 2012; Pavletic et al., 2006; Raza & Vierling, 2014; Reshef et al., 2012; Rogosheske et al., 2014; Spitzer et al., 2012.

is a result of alloreactive immunogenicity in males created by minor histocompatibility antigens coded on the Y chromosome (Erkurt et al., 2014). In the event of multiple donors, male donors are preferable to female counterparts. If only female donors are identified, those without a history of delivery are preferable to those with previous histories of deliveries. In addition, allogeneic HSCT donors are excluded if they have an active cancer or cancer history or test positive for hepatitis C or HIV. Hepatitis B surface antigen–positive recipients usually are excluded. However, if an infected donor is the only option or the recipient is also positive, a hepatitis B–infected donor may be considered. Furthermore, the donor should begin anti-hepatitis B therapy as soon as possible to decrease the risk of disease transmission (Liang, 2009). Cytomegalovirus (CMV) positivity should also be considered in allogeneic donors. If multiple donors are available, CMV-seronegative donors are preferred, especially if the recipient is also CMV seronegative. Any blood products needed should also be CMV seronegative. Even if the recipient is CMV-seropositive, CMV-seronegative donors are preferred over CMV-seropositive donors (Schmidt-Hieber et al., 2013). Blood group typing does not interfere with allogeneic HSCT (Kanda et al., 2009). Although Rh mismatch between the donor and recipient is not an adverse risk factor in allogeneic HSCT, there is an increased risk of hemolytic anemia (Erkurt et al., 2014).

Syngeneic Transplantation

Syngeneic transplantation is a type of allogeneic transplant in which HSCs from an identical twin are transfused into the other twin following myeloablative therapy. Although the patient is at risk for conditioning regimen–related toxicities, theoretically, the recipient is not at risk for GVHD because the donor is considered to be genetically identical to the recipient. However, Fouillard et al. (2008) reported a large series of 116 adult patients who underwent syngeneic HSCT for acute myeloid leukemia or acute lymphoid leukemia. Nineteen patients developed acute GVHD, of which eight patients received GVHD prophylaxis and still developed acute GVHD. One patient died of acute GVHD. Three patients developed chronic GVHD. At one year after transplant, the leukemia-free survival was approximately 41% in both types of leukemia. Thus, GVHD may be observed after syngeneic HSCT, indicating that a syngeneic graft-versus-leukemia effect exists.

Sources of Stem Cells

HSCs are primitive blood cells that reside in the bone marrow. HSCs are capable of self-renewal and give rise to progenitor cells, which are multipotent cells that differentiate and proliferate into the mature cells of the blood and immune system (see Figure 7-1) (Devine, 2013). The quantity of HSCs differs depending on the source. For example, in the bone marrow, the steady state of HSCs is 1.1%, whereas in the peripheral circulation, it is 0.06% (Körbling & Anderlini, 2001). Three main sources of HSC are used for HSCT: bone marrow, peripheral blood, and umbilical cord blood.

Bone Marrow

Bone marrow cells were the first source of HSCs used in transplantation. This method of stem cell collection involves a sterile surgical procedure performed in the operating room under general anesthesia. With the individual lying on his or her abdomen, multiple needle aspirations are collected from the posterior iliac crest. The aspirated marrow is mixed with anticoagulants in a sterile bag system and then filtered to remove fat or particles of bone. The bone marrow dose needed depends on the recipient's body weight as well as the HSCT center. However, a standard total nucleated cell dose of 2–4×10^8 cells/kg is usually the target goal during the harvest procedure (Fagioli et al., 2014). The bone marrow cells are then taken to the laboratory for further processing. An advantage of bone marrow collection is that it is well tolerated and can be performed on an outpatient basis or require 24-hour observation. However, disadvantages of bone marrow harvests are complications associated with anesthesia, bleeding, bone pain, and infection.

Peripheral Blood

Peripheral blood remains the most common source of stem cells requested and used for blood and marrow transplantation. Because a majority of HSC resides in the bone marrow, methods to mobilize HSCs into the peripheral blood must be used. When to commence peripheral blood stem cell collection varies depending on the strategy used in the mobilization process, as well as the transplant center's criteria. This may include the total white blood cell count, the absolute neutrophil count, the number of days of cytokine administration, or the number of HSCs circulating in the peripheral blood (Devine et al., 2010). In the peripheral blood, HSCs are measured by CD34. CD34 is an antigen that can be used to quantify HSCs after mobilization and to determine the cell dose needed for transplantation. Peripheral blood CD34+ cell counts may be monitored to determine when apheresis should commence (Sorasio et al., 2014). Thresholds of CD34+ cell counts vary according to institutional practice and research protocols. Irrespective of the varying collection goals and criteria for the initiation of apheresis, the collection goal often cited in the literature is 2–4×10^6 CD34+ cells/kg of body weight (Chepovetsky et al., 2013; D'Rozario, Parisotto, Stapleton, Gidley, & Owen, 2014). Although it has been purported that higher numbers of CD34+ cells collected are associated with a more robust engraftment of neutrophils and platelets, no strong evidence supports that CD34+ cell doses above 2×10^6 cells/kg are associated with any substantial clinical benefits. Furthermore, data regarding survival advantage with higher CD34+ cell doses and any other advantages, such as early discharge after transplant or decreased transfusion requirements, are insignificant (DiPersio, Micallef, et al., 2009; DiPersio, Stadtmauer, et al., 2009).

The procedure used to collect peripheral blood stem cells is known as apheresis. Apheresis involves the removal of large volumes of whole blood through a device that simultaneously collects, separates, and returns blood components. These components are red blood cells, which are the densest, and plasma, white blood cells, and platelets, which are the least dense (Devine et al., 2010). HSCs circulate in the buffy coat, the layer between red and white blood cells. The buffy layer is collected, and the remaining cells are returned to the individual. The length of time an individual is on the apheresis machine ranges from four to six hours and varies based on the collection goal, size of the recipient, total blood volume, blood flow rate, and tolerance to the procedure (Devine et al., 2010).

For collection of peripheral blood stem cells, placement of large bore needles in the antecubital veins is required. If peripheral access is inadequate, a large-bore, dual-lumen external central venous catheter may be surgically placed. Once peripheral blood stem cells are collected, the cells are taken to the laboratory for further processing. If the recipient is undergoing an allogeneic HSCT, the cells are infused within hours after collection. If the recipient is undergoing an autologous HSCT, the cells are cryopreserved, or frozen until ready for use.

Advantages of using peripheral blood stem cells include faster marrow reconstitution compared to bone marrow–derived stem cells and shorter durations of neutropenia and thrombocytopenia. Thus, there is potential decrease in antibiotic use, risk of infections, use of blood and platelet products, and inpatient hospitalization, which may result in lower healthcare costs.

Potential complications of peripheral blood stem cell collection may be due to the approach used for mobilization, as well as complications that may occur during the apheresis procedure. Apheresis complications may include hypocalcemia, hypovolemia, thrombocytopenia, issues related to placement of a central venous catheter, and chilling. Donors undergoing apheresis generally do not experience pain related to the apheresis procedure. However, they may experience side effects from the cytokines.

Mobilization of stem cells consists of causing the stem cell to move from the bone marrow to the peripheral blood for collection. In the setting of autologous donors, successful mobilization of CD34+ stem cells has been accomplished through the administration of cytokines alone, cytokines with chemokine antagonists, or cytokines combined with chemotherapy. Cytokines used for stem cell mobilization include G-CSF (filgrastim) and GM-CSF (sargramostim). The most commonly used cytokine for stem cell mobilization is G-CSF (Bensinger, DiPersio, & McCarty, 2009). G-CSF is administered as a subcutaneous injection, which can be self-administered. When mobilization is initiated with cytokines alone, apheresis usually begins on the fourth or fifth day of administration. G-CSF is well tolerated; however, some common side effects include bone pain, gastrointestinal (GI) symptoms, skin reactions or bruising at the injection sites, headache or flu-like symptoms, or elevations in liver function tests (Amgen Inc., 2013). G-CSF is also the most commonly used cytokine in allogeneic and unrelated donor peripheral blood HSC mobilization.

Plerixafor is a chemokine antagonist that has been shown to efficiently mobilize HSCs into the peripheral circulation (Devine et al., 2010). Two multicenter phase III studies compared the use of plerixafor and G-CSF versus placebo and G-CSF to mobilize autologous HSC (DiPersio, Micallef, et al., 2009; DiPersio, Stadtmauer, et al., 2009). Those who received plerixafor and G-CSF collected more HSCs than those who had received G-CSF alone. Plerixafor is a stem cell mobilizer that is indicated in combination with G-CSF to mobilize HSCs to the peripheral blood for collection and subsequent autologous transplantation in patients with multiple myeloma and non-Hodgkin lymphoma. It is administered as a subcutaneous injection after the autologous donor has received G-CSF for four days. In addition, plerixafor is administered 11 hours prior to apheresis. Common side effects of plerixafor include diarrhea, nausea, injection-site reactions, headache, arthralgia, orthostatic hypotension, and thrombocytopenia (Genzyme Corp., 2013). Optimal mobilization requires approximately four to six days of G-CSF administration.

Allogeneic donors may experience significant inconvenience, including bone pain and absence from work during the mobilization process. A pilot trial was conducted from HLA-matched sibling donors (N = 25) who were mobilized and collected using only plerixafor (Devine et al., 2008). Plerixafor was administered by subcutaneous injection, and apheresis was then initiated four hours later. Two-thirds of the donors collected an allograft with a CD34+ cell dose sufficient for transplantation after one dose of plerixafor. No donor experienced more than a grade 1 toxicity, defined as mild symptoms requiring no intervention (National Cancer Institute Cancer Therapy Evaluation Program, 2010). The most common side effects attributed to plerixafor were GI symptoms (e.g., upset stomach, flatulence), injection-site erythema, and paresthesias. After a myeloablative regimen, 20 patients with hematologic malignancies received allografts collected with plerixafor-mobilized HSCs. At 277 days after transplant (range = 139–964 days), 14 allogeneic recipients were surviving, in remission, had robust trilineage hematopoiesis, and were transfusion free. Plerixafor may provide a more rapid and possibly less toxic and cumbersome alternative to traditional G-CSF–based mobilization strategies in healthy donors. Phase II studies in HLA-matched sibling donors are ongoing.

Following chemotherapy plus G-CSF, collection of HSCs occurs approximately 17 days after chemotherapy administration. This usually occurs around the time when white blood cell counts begin to recover. Many chemotherapy regimens have been used to mobilize HSCs and include cyclophosphamide, etoposide, paclitaxel, and cytarabine (Bensinger et al., 2009). For patients with lymphoma, disease-specific chemotherapy regimens and cytokines may be used. Benefits of combination chemotherapy and cytokines include a reduced number of apheresis procedures and rapid engraftment due to a greater number of CD34+ cells collected. Several disadvantages include the need for hospitalization to administer chemotherapy, exposure to side effects and toxicities associated with chemotherapy, the risk of neutropenia and infection, the need for blood and platelet transfusions, and the variability in time for the recovery of white blood cells, which can make scheduling apheresis difficult.

Umbilical Cord Blood

Umbilical cord blood represents another source of HSCs for allogeneic transplant when an HLA-matched sibling and unrelated donor are unavailable. Thus, umbilical cord blood transplants have become a standard option for children and adults with hematopoietic disorders and malignancies (de la Morena & Gatti, 2011). Immediately after a baby is delivered, cord blood can be collected from the placenta and umbilical cord. A syringe is inserted in the umbilical vein to collect blood. The whole procedure takes less than 10 minutes, and about 75 ml of cord blood is used for storing. The collected blood is then sent to the cord blood bank for HLA typing and is cryopreserved, or frozen, for future use.

The advantages of using HSCs from umbilical cord blood over bone marrow or peripheral blood include the low rate of viral contamination, lower rates of GVHD, and ready availability of units (Rocha & Gluckman, 2009). Disadvantages of using umbilical cord blood include delayed engraftment and immune reconstitution and an increase in opportunistic infections. While this may be a consequence of the low cell doses in single umbilical cord blood grafts, it also reflects the relative immaturity of cellular immunity within cord blood (Danby & Rocha, 2014). In an effort to improve engraftment, decrease the period of aplasia, and improve survival after umbilical cord blood transplants, many approaches have been investigated, such as the use of double-unit umbilical cord blood transplants (Barker et al., 2005; Brunstein et al., 2007; Oran & Shpall, 2012). Umbilical cord blood banks have been established worldwide as a result of international registries. These banks share registries and collect clinical and long-term follow-up data on transplanted patients.

Conditioning Regimens in Hematopoietic Stem Cell Transplantation

The preparative or conditioning regimen is a critical part of the HSCT process. Based on the expected duration and reversibility of cytopenias after HSCT, conditioning regimens can be classified as myeloablative, reduced-intensity, or nonmyeloablative (Bacigalupo et al., 2009; Shi, Li, & Ikehara, 2013). The purpose of the preparative regimen is to provide adequate immunosuppression to prevent rejection of the transplanted graft and eradicate the disease for which the transplant is being performed.

Myeloablative Regimens

Myeloablative regimens consist of a combination of agents given at maximally tolerated doses expected to eradicate HSCs in the bone marrow and result in profound pancytopenia within one to three weeks from the time of administration. The resulting pancytopenia is long-lasting, usually irreversible, and, in most instances, fatal unless hematopoiesis is restored by infusion of HSCs (Bacigalupo et al., 2009; Shi et al., 2013). Examples of myeloablative regimens are listed in Table 7-3 and include TBI, cyclophosphamide, busulfan, thiotepa, melphalan, and etoposide. Myeloablative regimens are most commonly used for refractory hematologic malignancies and autologous transplantation.

Nonmyeloablative Regimens

Treatment-related mortality increases with age; thus, the aim of developing nonmyeloablative regimens was to reduce treatment side effects. These regimens result in minimal cytopenias and are also immunoablative (Bacigalupo et al., 2009; Shi et al., 2013). The potential to promote a cure in patients undergoing a nonmyeloablative preparative regimen relates to the development of a GVT effect. Examples of nonmyeloablative regimens include fludarabine, cyclophosphamide, antithymocyte globulin, and TBI $\leq$ 2 Gy (see Table 7-3).

Reduced-Intensity Conditioning

Reduced-intensity conditioning regimens are an intermediate category of regimens that do not fit the definition of myeloablative or nonmyeloablative (Bacigalupo et al., 2009; Shi et al., 2013). Such regimens cause cytopenias, which may be prolonged and result in significant morbidity and mortality, thus requiring HSC support. These regimens differ from myeloablative regimens in that the dose of alkylating agents and TBI is reduced by 30%. Examples of reduced-intensity conditioning regimens include fludarabine-based conditioning regimens combined with busulfan, cyclophosphamide, melphalan, or TBI (Bacigalupo et al., 2009; Shi et al., 2013).

Chimerism and Donor Lymphocyte Infusions

Two main types of conditioning regimens previously described include myeloablative and nonmyeloablative. Myeloablative preparative regimens in allogeneic HSCT are designed to eradicate the lymphohematopoietic system of the recipient, which is subsequently replaced by donor cells. Conversely, nonmyeloablative regimens provide sufficient immunosuppression to prevent rejection of donor cells and facilitate engraftment. As a result, donor immune cells eliminate both normal and malignant host hematopoiesis. These regimens were designed to treat hematologic disorders in older adult recipients or those with comorbidities who otherwise would not be considered for intensive therapies.

Chimerism is the coexistence of donor and host lymphohematopoietic cells and can be further characterized as full, mixed, or split chimerism (Antin et al., 2001). Recipients who demonstrate no evidence of host DNA at any time during the post-transplant follow-up are considered to be fully chimeric, meaning that 100% of donor cells are detected. Recipients with full donor chimerisms are associated with a low risk of relapse and better prognosis. Recipients with both donor and recipient DNA are defined as having mixed chimerism. Split chimerism is when one or more whole lineages are host and one or more lineages are donor. Following HSCT, chimerism status can be monitored in the recipient's peripheral blood or bone marrow by using various laboratory methods, for example, analysis of short tandem repeats or variable number tandem repeats, polymerase chain reaction, or fluorescent in situ hybridization (FISH). If the transplant is a sex-mismatched HSCT, evaluations for XX/XY can be performed by FISH or standard cytogenetic testing.

Table 7-3. Common Conditioning Regimens Used in Hematopoietic Stem Cell Transplantation*

Abbreviation	Regimen/Agents	Indications/Disease
Cy/TBI	Cyclophosphamide and total body irradiation	AML, ALL, CLL, CML, HL, MDS, MM, NHL, myeloablative
TBI/VP	Total body irradiation and etoposide	AML, ALL, NHL, HL, myeloablative
Bu/Cy	Busulfan and cyclophosphamide	AML, ALL, CLL, CML, HL, MDS, MM, NHL, myeloablative
Bu/Cy/VP	Busulfan, cyclophosphamide, and etoposide	AML, ALL, CLL, CML, HL, MDS, MM, NHL, myeloablative
Cy/ATG	Cyclophosphamide and antithymocyte globulin	Severe aplastic anemia, myeloablative
TBI/Mel	Total body irradiation and melphalan	MM, myeloablative
Mel	Melphalan	MM, myeloablative
CEC	Cyclophosphamide, etoposide, and carboplatin	Germ cell tumors, myeloablative
CBV	Cyclophosphamide, carmustine, and etoposide	NHL, HL, myeloablative
BEAM	Carmustine, etoposide, cytarabine, and melphalan	NHL, HL, myeloablative
TBI	Total body irradiation	Nonmyeloablative
Fludara/Bu/ATG	Fludarabine/busulfan/antithymocyte globulin	Nonmyeloablative
Fludara/Cy	Fludarabine and cyclophosphamide	Nonmyeloablative/RIC
Fludara/Cy/ATG	Fludarabine, cyclophosphamide, and antithymocyte globulin	Nonmyeloablative/RIC
Fludara/Mel	Fludarabine and melphalan	Nonmyeloablative/RIC

* This list is not all-inclusive and serves only to provide examples of preparative regimens.

ALL—acute lymphocytic leukemia; AML—acute myeloid leukemia; CLL—chronic lymphocytic leukemia; CML—chronic myeloid leukemia; HL—Hodgkin lymphoma; MDS—myelodysplastic syndrome; MM—multiple myeloma; NHL—non-Hodgkin lymphoma; RIC—reduced-intensity conditioning

Note. Based on information from Bacigalupo et al., 2009; Shi et al., 2013.

Consensus from a collaborative meeting of HSCT experts sponsored by NMDP and the International Bone Marrow Transplant Registry (IBMTR) regarding chimerism analysis monitoring after allogeneic HSCT revealed it was unnecessary to obtain these tests in recipients of myeloablative regimens unless there was a change in the recipient's clinical status (Antin et al., 2001). However, in recipients of nonmyeloablative regimens, post-transplant surveillance was standard, and evaluations at 1, 3, 6, and 12 months after HSCT were recommended. However, in a study comparing donor chimerism following myeloablative and nonmyeloablative allogeneic HSCT, permanent eradication of the recipient lymphohematopoietic system does not always occur following myeloablative regimens, and more frequent monitoring may be necessary (Mickelson et al., 2011). Thus, patterns of chimerism analysis can be used to identify recipients at risk for graft rejection, relapse, and acute and chronic GVHD, as well as the need for donor lymphocyte infusions (DLIs).

DLIs facilitate donor cell conversion to achieve a GVT effect. The dose of DLIs varies according to institutional guidelines or clinical trial protocols. DLIs may be administered prophylactically in patients with high-risk disease, such as acute myeloid leukemia (Liu, 2013). In some cases, additional lymphocytes are obtained at the time of initial HSC collection and cryopreserved for infusion at a later time after HSCT to trigger an immune response, resulting in a GVT effect. Related or unrelated donors may be asked to donate additional lymphocytes. The effectiveness of DLI in promoting antitumor activity has been described to be greatest for the treatment of persistent chronic myeloid and lymphoid leukemias, acute myeloid and lymphoid leukemias, and lymphomas following HSCT (Liu, 2013).

Pre-Hematopoietic Stem Cell Transplantation Evaluation

The treatment trajectory of HSCT patients is multidisciplinary and includes a team of physicians, scientists, cellular therapy laboratory technicians, transfusion medicine physicians, apheresis nurses, APNs, physician assistants, ambulatory and hospital-based nurses, pharmacists, dietitians, research personnel, transplant coordinators, social workers, and other support staff. Although patients may only see staff members who are at the forefront of patient care, many healthcare professionals collaborate in navigating the complexities of HSCT recipients.

Factors considered in determining if the patient is eligible for HSCT include age, whether the disease is chemosensitive, disease status, comorbidities, performance status, identification of the type and source of HSCT, and treatment compliance. In 1996, the Foundation for the Accreditation of Cellular Therapy (FACT) was formed to standardize as well as promote quality medical practices. Centers that meet rigorous standards of quality medical and cellular therapy laboratory practices are recognized with certificates of accreditation (FACT, 2012).

FACT recommends that clinical evaluations of autologous donors include documenting the history of present illness; past medical, surgical, and family history; allergies and medications; if female, a gynecologic history; vaccinations; history of blood transfusions; travel history; and psychosocial assessment. A psychosocial assessment of autologous donors and their families should be obtained prior to HSCT to identify family, social, and financial concerns, as well as spiritual issues. If the donor is a child, neuropsychological testing should be performed for baseline measures. Furthermore, a complete physical examination should be performed, including laboratory and diagnostic tests to evaluate baseline organ function and infectious disease markers. Figure 7-4 further outlines evaluations needed prior to continuing with the HSCT process. Finally, consent to collect HSCs must be obtained prior to the mobilization phase of transplant. If the donor is a minor, the parent or guardian must consent. However, if the child is younger than 18 years old and understands and expresses willingness to participate, the child may sign an assent form (FACT, 2012).

Allogeneic donors must also go through a thorough clinical evaluation and psychosocial assessment as previously described. The medical history should address whether the potential donor is at high risk for transmission of communicable diseases, inherited conditions, or hematologic or immunologic diseases, as well as a past history of malignant diseases. Similar to autologous donors, allogeneic donors must undergo a complete physical examination including basic laboratory and infectious disease evaluations.

Laboratory Evaluations
- Complete blood count with differential
- Chemistry profile, including liver and renal function tests
- Electrolytes, magnesium, calcium, and phosphorus
- Blood grouping and Rh typing
- Human leukocyte antigen typing
- Prothrombin time, partial thromboplastin time, and international normalized ratio
- Pregnancy test
- Creatinine clearance
- Blood urea nitrogen and creatinine
- Chest x-ray

Infectious Disease Titers
- Cytomegalovirus
- Epstein-Barr virus
- Hepatitis B virus (surface antigen, core antigen)
- Hepatitis C virus (antibody)
- Herpes simplex virus
- Human immunodeficiency virus types 1 and 2
- Human T-cell lymphotropic virus types 1 and 2
- *Treponema pallidum* (syphilis)
- West Nile virus
- *Trypanosoma cruzi* (Chagas disease)

Organ Function Testing
- Dental examination
- Pulmonary function test
- 12-Lead electrocardiogram
- Multigated acquisition scan/echocardiogram

Disease Evaluation
- Bone marrow biopsy and aspiration
- Computed tomography scans
- Lumbar puncture
- Magnetic resonance imaging
- Myeloma blood and urine studies: Serum protein electrophoresis, urine protein electrophoresis, serum light chains, 24-hour urine protein, creatinine
- Myeloma skeletal survey
- Positron-emission tomography or gallium scan
- Positron-emission tomography scans

Figure 7-4. Clinical Evaluations for Hematopoietic Stem Cell Transplantation

Note. Based on information from Foundation for the Accreditation of Cellular Therapy, 2012.

Infusion of Hematopoietic Stem Cells

On a designated day following completion of the conditioning regimen, the recipient is scheduled on "day 0" for the infusion of HSCs. Autologous and umbilical cord blood HSCT recipients are transplanted with HSCs that have been cryopreserved. Cryopreservatives are additives that protect the HSCs from the freezing and thawing process. These cryoprotectants inhibit the formation of intra- and extracellular crystals and prevent cell death in these living cells (Berz, McCormack, Winer, Colvin, & Quesenberry, 2007; Cox, Kastrup, & Hrubiško, 2012). The standard cryoprotectant used in HSCT is dimethyl sulfoxide (DMSO), which has been established to be safe and nontoxic to stem cells (Berz et al., 2007; Cox et al., 2012). However, DMSO has been associated with clinically significant side effects that include fevers, chills, cough, nausea, vomiting, diarrhea, dyspnea, tachypnea, abdominal cramps, facial flushing, hypertension, cardiac arrhythmias, chest tightness, and hemoglobinuria (Berz et al., 2007; Cox et al., 2012). Because DMSO penetrates the skin, the unusual property that many HSCT recipients may perceive is a garlic-like taste in the mouth after contact with DMSO. Others may note an abnormal breath and body odor as the DMSO is released through carbon dioxide and the pores of the skin. These symptoms usually resolve within 24–48 hours. Prior to receiving HSC products that contain DMSO, recipients may be given IV hydration to promote renal perfusion and minimize hemolysis. Symptomatic treatment of adverse effects usually is effective, but occasionally the stem cell infusion may need to be slowed or briefly stopped. Premedications prior to the infusion may include an antiemetic, acetaminophen, and diphenhydramine. For additional safety purposes, emergency equipment, including oxygen and cardiac monitoring, should be readily available (AABB, American Red Cross, America's Blood Centers, & Armed Services Blood Program, 2013).

Allogeneic HSCs are usually infused within hours of procurement; thus, recipients experience fewer side effects. Adverse effects may occur and are similar to complications that can occur with blood transfusions. These include hives, chills, rash, fever, nausea, vomiting, flushing, shortness of breath, hypotension or hypertension, tachycardia, chest pain or tightness, or anaphylaxis. If the donor and recipient are ABO mismatched, an immediate or delayed immune hemolysis may occur (AABB et al., 2013). Because the life span of red blood cells is approximately 120 days, recipients should be monitored for approximately four months following HSCT. Additionally, an immune hemolysis, or passenger lymphocyte syndrome (PLS), may occur as a result of ABO incompatibly. PLS is caused by the production of donor B lymphocytes against recipient red blood cell antigens (Reed, Yearsley, Krugh, & Kennedy, 2003). Management of PLS may include transfusion of ABO-compatible red blood cells, use of corticosteroids, exchange transfusion, and maintenance of renal perfusion. Over time, the recipient's blood type converts to that of the donor's, and the risk of hemolysis resolves. Blood evaluations, including recipient ABO titers, are monitored to detect when the transition to donor blood type occurs. During this time, patients receive type O blood products to minimize the risk of transfusion-related hemolysis (AABB et al., 2013).

Engraftment and Recovery

Engraftment refers to the hematopoietic and immunologic recovery that occurs after HSCT. Factors that affect the rate of engraftment include the source of stems cells used, the type of transplant, the conditioning regimen, the use of cytokines during peripheral blood HSC mobilization, the use of cytokines after HSCT, and the occurrence of infection or GVHD. Approximately five to seven days after the HSCT, the nadir of blood counts may occur as a result of the conditioning regimen. Engraftment may be delayed in patients who develop GVHD or infections, particularly viral infections.

In autologous HSCT, engraftment using cytokine-mobilized HSCs derived from the peripheral blood occurs approximately one week earlier than with stem cells collected from the bone marrow (Körbling & Anderlini, 2001). Engraftment is accelerated by the use of cytokines during peripheral blood HSC mobilization and collection, as well as its use post-HSCT to facilitate in engraftment.

Engraftment after a myeloablative allogeneic HSCT is variable but has been demonstrated to occur earlier with HSCs derived from peripheral blood compared to bone marrow. Bensinger et al. (2001) described recovery of blood counts following allogeneic peripheral blood HSCT as a neutrophil count greater than 500/mm³ at day 16 and platelet count greater than 20,000/mm³ at day 13. Engraftment with bone marrow–derived HSCs occurred more slowly and was reported as a neutrophil count greater than 500/mm³ at day 21 and platelet count greater than 20,000/mm³ at day 19 post-transplant.

Following nonmyeloablative HSCT, the duration of myelosuppression is diminished because the conditioning regimen is myelosuppressive rather than myeloablative. White blood cell recovery is faster, and transfusion of red blood cells and platelets may be avoided. Engraftment after umbilical cord blood HSCT is slower compared to HSCT using cells derived from peripheral blood or bone marrow. Although a high concentration of HSCs are present in umbilical cord blood, blood count recovery occurs at approximately day 28 for neutrophils and day 60 for platelets. In some cases, the number of CD34+ cells collected may not be sufficient for an adult recipient (Barker et al., 2005; Brunstein et al., 2007; Oran & Shpall, 2012).

Post-Hematopoietic Stem Cell Transplantation Care

Historically, the process of HSCT has occurred in the hospital milieu. However, transplant centers have expanded their facilities and resources for HSCT recipients to receive their conditioning regimen, infusion of HSCs, and post-transplant care in the ambulatory setting. Preparation of the transplant center to successfully coordinate care in this setting involves many factors, including the availability of lodging, homecare resources, outpatient care facilities, and nursing and pharmacy staff members. Caregivers are trained to assist HSCT recipients with activities of daily living, hygiene, maintaining nutrition, medication administration, central venous catheter care, and transportation to outpatient appointments. Autologous HSCT recipients are referred back to their primary oncologist after they have engrafted and recovered for treatment-related toxicities. However, allogeneic recipients are observed closely by HSCT staff for monitoring of infections, management of immunosuppressive drugs, and performance of physical examinations to identify symptoms of GVHD.

Post-transplant follow-up focuses on adherence to standard guidelines for routine care and disease monitoring, tapering of immunosuppressive medications, and observance of clinical trial protocols. Comprehensive published guidelines for infection control in the hospital and home setting, safe living after HSCT (i.e., food, water, and sexual practice safety), and infectious disease monitoring are available (Tomblyn et al., 2009). Table 7-4 outlines the most recent vaccination schedule for both autologous and allogeneic HSCT recipients.

Immune reconstitution after HSCT consists of two distinct phases: numeric recovery from bone marrow cells (i.e., white blood cells, red blood cells, and platelets) and functional recovery of cellular interactions (i.e., B cells, T cells, and NK cells) (Storek et al., 2008). Numerous factors can affect post-transplant immune reconstitution. As previously described, this includes the type of HSCT (i.e., autologous versus allogeneic; myeloablative versus reduced-intensity versus T-cell depletion), source of stem cells (i.e., bone marrow, peripheral blood, or umbilical cord blood), recipient age, underlying malignancy and the treatment regimen, donor immunity, histocompatibility, immunosuppressive medications, donor age and gender, GVHD status, and presence of graft rejection (Bernstein, Boyd, & van den Brink, 2008; Erkurt et al., 2014; Jiménez, Ercilla, & Martínez, 2007; Kollman et al., 2001; Loren et al., 2006; Nannya et al., 2011). Strategies to enhance post-HSCT immune reconstitution are emerging and remain under clinical investigation. This includes medications that inhibit sex steroids (e.g., gonadotropin-releasing hormone agonist treatment), growth factor therapies (e.g., G-CSF, GM-CSF), cytokine therapies (e.g., IL-7), and cellular therapies (e.g., T-cell administration) to

Table 7-4. Vaccination Recommendations for Autologous and Allogeneic Hematopoietic Stem Cell Transplant (HSCT) Recipients

Vaccine	Recommended for Use After HSCT	Time Post-HSCT to Initiate Vaccine	Number of Doses
Tetanus, diphtheria, acellular pertussis toxoid[ab]	Yes	6–12 months	3
Haemophilus influenzae, type b conjugate	Yes	6–12 months	3
Hepatitis B series[c]	Follow country recommendations for general population.	6–12 months	3
Pneumococcal conjugate vaccine (PCV)[d] 23-Valent pneumococcal polysaccharide (PPSV23)	Yes	3–6 months	3–4
Inactivated influenza[e]	Yes	Starting 4–6 months, then annually	1–2
Inactivated polio	Yes	6–12 months	3
Meningococcal conjugate	Follow country recommendations for general population.	6–12 months	1
Measles-mumps-rubella[f]	Yes	24 months	1–2

[a] DTaP is preferred, but not licensed for adults. If only Tdap available, administer.

[b] Should continue to be revaccinated every 10 years as recommended for all adults

[c] Initial dose, then dose two 3–4 weeks later, and third dose 3–6 months thereafter. Serum titer should be checked 1–2 months after third dose. If antibody is not present, series of three vaccinations should be repeated. Vaccination is recommended for HBsAg- or HBcAb-positive patients because vaccination can reduce the risk for reverse seroconversion.

[d] When given during the first year after transplantation, PPSV23 elicits inadequate responses; thus, PCV is the preferred vaccine.

[e] For children younger than 9 years of age, two doses are recommended annually and up to age 9.

[f] Live attenuated vaccine—administer only to patients assumed to be immunocompetent. In children, two doses are favored.

Note. From "Guidelines for Preventing Infectious Complications Among Hematopoietic Cell Transplantation Recipients: A Global Perspective," by M. Tomblyn, T. Chiller, H. Einsele, R. Gress, K. Sepkowitz, J. Storek, ... M.J. Boeckh, 2009, *Biology of Blood and Marrow Transplantation, 15,* p. 1173. doi:10.1016/j.bbmt.2009.06.019. Copyright 2009 by American Society for Blood and Marrow Transplantation. Adapted with permission.

enhance malignancy/viral specific immunity (Bernstein et al., 2008; Zakrzewski, Holland, & van den Brink, 2007).

A potential sequela of immunosuppressive therapy is the development of opportunistic infections. Quantitative recovery of immunity does not always correlate with qualitative cellular function. Therefore, an important consideration for oncology APNs is to educate other nurses and patients that normal laboratory parameters do not eliminate the HSCT recipient's risk of infection. In determining the patient's risk for infection, obtaining or having knowledge of the patient's history is critical. In addition to a thorough history and physical examination, laboratory investigations to assess immune reconstitution may further assist in determining the duration of prophylactic antimicrobials. These tests include T-cell analysis by immuno-phenotyping (T-cell subsets), B-cell analysis (i.e., quantitative and immunoglobulin G subclass analysis), NK cell reconstitution, dendritic cell, and chimerism analysis. Additionally, disease-specific tests, as well as infection surveillance or detection strategies (such as blood cultures and polymerase chain reaction), can further assist with identifying infections and commencing treatment.

Complications of Hematopoietic Stem Cell Transplantation

Graft-Versus-Host Disease

GVHD is a complication of allogeneic HSCT that may occur in 40%–60% of cases and, if severe, can lead to a 50% mortality rate (Ferrara et al., 2009; Spitzer et al., 2012). GVHD has been reported to occur less frequently with the use of umbilical cord blood HSCT because of the lower number of T cells. A randomized multicenter trial of 172 patients who underwent bone marrow or peripheral blood HSCT demonstrated a faster recovery of neutrophils and platelets in recipients who received peripheral blood–derived HSCs compared to bone marrow–derived HSCs (Bensinger et al., 2001). However, no significant difference was noted between peripheral blood and bone marrow as the source of stem cells in the cumulative incidence of grades 2–4 acute GVHD (discussed below) at 100 days after transplant. There was also no significant difference between peripheral blood and bone marrow HSCTs in the cumulative incidence of chronic GVHD at two years after transplant, although a trend favored fewer cases of chronic GVHD with bone marrow HSCT. The overall estimated two-year probability and rate of post-transplant disease-free survival was better in patients who received peripheral blood–derived HSCs. Although much progress has occurred in the understanding of GVHD, including prophylaxis and management, it remains a complex complication of allogeneic HSCT that remains challenging.

Pathophysiology

GVHD is an immune reaction that occurs between recipient cells and the immunologically competent donor T lymphocytes. It is an immune-mediated process that consists of several steps involving the MHC and T-cell activation (Ferrara et al., 2009; Raza & Vierling, 2014). The HLA antigens or genes that currently determine tissue typing include the class I antigens (HLA-A, HLA-B, and HLA-C) and class II antigens (HLA-DR, HLA-DP, and HLA-DQ). Class I HLA-C antigen matching decreases the incidence of GVHD in unrelated transplants (Ferrara et al., 2009). Matching of HLA antigens of the recipient and donor decreases the risk of developing GVHD, whereas the risk increases if the donor and recipient are HLA mismatched. In addition, minor histoincompatible differences may exist despite HLA typing, which can also lead to the development of GVHD.

The immune system of the allogeneic recipient must be incompetent so that the recipient cells do not recognize donor cells as foreign. Conversely, the donor T lymphocytes must be immunologically competent to recognize and attack the defined target organs of the recipient. Induction of acute GVHD begins by administration of myeloablative conditioning regimens. This results in ablating the recipient's immune system, contributing to tissue and organ system damage. As a result of cytokine release, organs such as the skin, GI tract, and liver are affected. Donor T lymphocytes proliferate, recognize, and destroy target organs of the recipient. Additional cytokines are released as tissue damage continues to perpetuate the clinical sequelae of GVHD (Ferrara et al., 2009).

The pathophysiology of chronic GVHD has been described but is not well understood. It is purported that an alloreactivity of T cells (defined as strong primary T-cell response to the minor histocompatibility antigens) and dysfunctional immune recovery occur (Ferrara et al., 2009; Raza & Vierling, 2014). The clinical manifestations of chronic GVHD appear similar to autoimmune disorders. For example, skin changes are comparable to scleroderma features and the sicca complex of Sjögren syndrome (Ferrara et al., 2009; Pavletic & Fowler, 2012; Spitzer et al., 2012).

The benefits of GVHD following allogeneic HSCT are related to the immune response of donor T lymphocytes toward residual tumor cells. A GVT effect is considered beneficial following nonmyeloablative transplant. Maintaining post-transplant remission or disease control due to the occurrence of GVHD resulting in a GVT effect has been reported. Post-transplant DLIs may be given to trigger a GVT effect in patients who have relapsed or who have persistent mixed chimerism (donor and recipient cells). Conversion to full donor chimerism (donor cells) and occurrence of GVHD are predictive of reaching a complete remission.

Risk Factors

Many risk factors have been identified in the development of GVHD. These include histo-incompatibilities, HLA disparities, unrelated allogeneic transplant, cumulative blood transfusions, increasing age, and multiparous donor (Erkurt et al., 2014; Spitzer et al., 2012). The existence of acute GVHD increases the risk for development of chronic GVHD.

Clinical Manifestations

Acute GVHD is defined as occurring before day 100 after allogeneic HSCT, whereas chronic GVHD is defined as occurring after day 100 (Ferrara et al., 2009; Pavletic & Fowler, 2012; Raza & Vierling, 2014; Spitzer et al., 2012). Clinical manifestations of acute GVHD involve the skin, upper and lower GI tract, and liver. Figure 7-5 highlights the clinical manifestations of GVHD, including diagnostic evaluations. The diagnosis of acute GVHD is made by clinical evaluation; however, biopsies of the skin, GI tract, or liver assist in ruling out other etiologies of abnormal findings identified on physical examination or by laboratory investigations.

The staging and grading of acute GVHD has been described by Glucksberg et al. (1974), Thomas et al. (1975), and IBMTR (Przepiorka et al., 1995) as involving three organ systems: skin, liver, and GI tract. Cahn et al. (2005) evaluated the use of the Glucksberg and IBMTR grading systems in 607 patients to compare scoring systems for acute GVHD. Both scoring systems were found to be similar in predicting long-term survival outcomes based on the maximum grade of acute GVHD. The Rule of Nines (see Figure 7-6) is used to describe the extent of skin involvement that correlates with the stage of cutaneous involvement. The Glucksberg et al. and IBMTR staging and grading systems for acute GVHD are described in Tables 7-5 and 7-6.

Chronic GVHD has been described as a multiorgan condition involving the mouth, eyes, skin, liver, lungs, GI tract, and hematopoietic system (Ferrara et al., 2009; Mohty & Mohty, 2011; Pavletic & Fowler, 2012; Pavletic, Lee, Socie, & Vogelsang, 2006; Raza & Vierling, 2014; Spitzer et al., 2012). Clinical manifestations and diagnostic evaluations related to organ systems involved in chronic GVHD are further described in Figure 7-5.

Limited and *extensive* have been used to describe chronic GVHD based on the extent of organ involvement. These descriptions of chronic GVHD have limited usefulness in describing the full spectrum of its clinical sequelae. The National Institutes of Health consensus criteria for diagnosis and severity grading of chronic GVHD categorized chronic GVHD as classic chronic GVHD (without features or characteristics of acute GVHD) and an overlap syndrome

Clinical Manifestations
- Acute GVHD
  - Gastrointestinal: Nausea, vomiting, diarrhea, oral lesions
  - Liver: Elevated liver enzymes, hyperbilirubinemia
  - Mouth: Erythema, lesions
  - Skin: Maculopapular rash
- Chronic GVHD
  - Gastrointestinal: Nausea, vomiting, diarrhea, malabsorption, esophageal strictures
  - Hematologic: Cytopenias, autoimmune, eosinophilia, decreased platelet count
  - Liver: Elevated alkaline phosphatase, hyperbilirubinemia, cholestasis
  - Mouth: Erythema, lichen-type hyperkeratosis, ulcerations, xerostomia, sensitivities, leukoplakia, lichenoid appearance, dry mouth
  - Neuromuscular: Joint motion affected in patients with scleroderma; muscle cramping, fasciitis, joint stiffness
  - Ocular: Dry eyes, reduced tear flow
  - Pulmonary: Bronchiolitis obliterans
  - Reproductive: Lichen planus, dry skin–type features; women may have inflammation, mucosal dryness, adhesions, vaginal stenosis; men may have impotence, erectile dysfunction
  - Skin: Macular, erythematous eruption; thickened, tight, sclerotic patches; lichen planus–type features

Diagnostic Evaluation
- Skin biopsy
- Schirmer test
- Open lung biopsy
- Endoscopy with biopsy
- Colonoscopy with biopsy
- Pulmonary function tests
- High-resolution computed tomography of the chest

Figure 7-5. Clinical Manifestations and Diagnostic Evaluation of Graft-Versus-Host Disease (GVHD)

Note. Based on information from Ferrara et al., 2009; Mohty & Mohty, 2011; Raza & Vierling, 2014.

in which diagnostic or distinctive features of chronic and acute GVHD appear together. The clinical scoring system for chronic GVHD is based on a scale of 0–3 (see Table 7-7) and allows providers to evaluate the involvement of individual organs and sites. Systemic therapy should be considered for patients who meet criteria for moderate to severe global severity (Filipovich et al., 2005). These criteria were recently validated but had limited significance in predicting outcomes (Aisa et al., 2013). Guidelines for treatment suggest that local therapies may be indicated for mild chronic GVHD, and systemic therapy is recommended if three or more organs are involved or if a score of 2 or higher is present in any organ system (Filipovich et al., 2005).

Prophylaxis and Management

Pharmacologic approaches to prevent acute GVHD include administration of a combination of systemic immunosuppressive medications (see Table 7-3). The folate antagonist methotrexate, cyclosporine (CSA), and calcineurin inhibitors (e.g., tacrolimus), as well as mycophenolate mofetil, antithymocyte globulin, and mammalian target of rapamycin inhibitors (e.g., sirolimus), are pharmacologic therapies commonly initiated prior to HSCT (Pavletic & Fowler, 2012). Other medications that are being evaluated for GVHD prophylaxis include the proteasome inhibitor bortezomib in combination with tacrolimus and methotrexate (Reshef et al., 2012).

Monitoring of drug levels and side effects of these drugs is necessary to anticipate potential toxicities. Although serum drug levels vary according to institutional practices or research protocols, suggested therapeutic ranges are 200–400 mcg/ml for CSA and 5–15 mcg/ml for tacrolimus (Rogosheske et al., 2014). Numerous drug interactions may occur that increase or decrease serum CSA or tacrolimus levels. Some drugs that may alter calcineurin inhibitor or CSA levels include calcium channel blockers, antifungal agents, antibiotics, prokinetic agents, and anticonvulsants (Ferrara et al., 2009; Raza & Vierling, 2014). Common adverse effects related to these immunosuppressive medications include renal, metabolic, neurologic, GI, cardiovascular, hematologic, cutaneous, and infusion-related toxicities. Renal insufficiency and electrolyte abnormalities may occur, including increased creatinine, hyperglycemia, hypomagnesemia, and hyperkalemia. Seizure activity and change in mental status have been reported

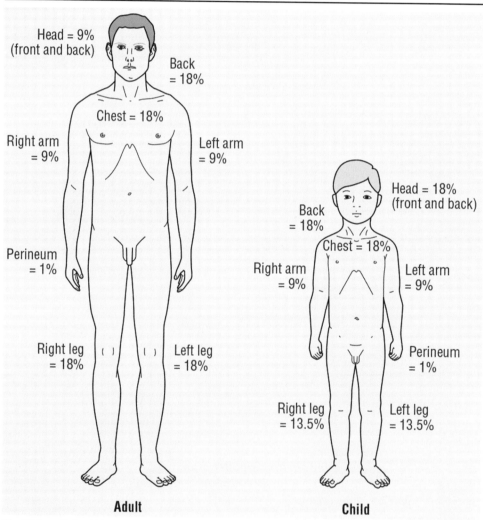

The Wallace Rule of Nines can be used to determine the percentage of body surface area involved with cutaneous graft-versus-host disease.

Figure 7-6. Rule of Nines

Note. From "Initial Management of a Major Burn: II—Assessment and Resuscitation," by S. Hettiaratchy and R. Papini, 2004, *BMJ, 328,* p. 101. doi:10.1136/bmj.329.7457.101. Copyright 2004 by BMJ Publishing Group Ltd. Reprinted with permission.

Table 7-5. Staging and Grading Systems for Acute Graft-Versus-Host Disease (GVHD)

Clinical Staging and Grading of Acute GVHD

Organ	Stage	Description
Skin	+1	Maculopapular eruption over < 25% of body area
	+2	Maculopapular eruption over 25%–50% of body area
	+3	Generalized erythroderma
	+4	Generalized erythroderma with bullous formation and often with desquamation
Liver	+1	Bilirubin 2–3 mg/dl
	+2	Bilirubin 3.1–6 mg/dl
	+3	Bilirubin 6.1–15 mg/dl
	+4	Bilirubin > 15 mg/dl
Gut	+1	Diarrhea > 500 ml/day or > 30 ml/kg
	+2	Diarrhea > 1,000 ml/day or > 60 ml/kg
	+3	Diarrhea > 1,500 ml/day or > 90 ml/kg
	+4	Severe abdominal pain with or without ileus

Overall Grade

Grade	Skin	Liver	Gut	Performance Status
I	+1 to +2	0	0	No decrease
II	+1 to +3	+1	and/or +1	Mild decrease
III	+2 to +3	+2 to +3	and/or +2 to +3	Marked decrease
IV	+2 to +4	+2 to +4	and/or +2 to +4	Extreme decrease

Note. Based on information from Glucksberg et al., 1974; Thomas et al., 1975.

with calcineurin inhibitors, and nausea, vomiting, hirsutism, hypertension, and gum hypertrophy have been described with CSA (Ferrara et al., 2009; Raza & Vierling, 2014). Immunosuppressive medications are tapered gradually over a few months after the transplant according to institutional guidelines or research protocols.

Other pharmacologic agents used to prevent or treat GVHD include steroids, IL-2 targeting agents (e.g., basiliximab, daclizumab, denileukin diftitox), alemtuzumab, etanercept, infliximab, and pentostatin (Martin et al., 2012). Research is ongoing to determine the most effective method to prevent and treat GVHD. Nonpharmacologic approaches used to prevent acute GVHD include extracorporeal photopheresis, phototherapy, T-cell or lymphocyte depletion of HSCs pretransplant, or total lymphoid irradiation. Figure 7-3 lists options for the prevention and treatment of GVHD.

Table 7-6. Criteria for the International Bone Marrow Transplant Registry Severity Index for Acute Graft-Versus-Host Disease

Index*	Skin Involvement			Liver Involvement			Gastrointestinal (GI) Involvement		
	Stage (max.)	Extent of Rash		Stage (max.)	Total Bilirubin (µmol/L)		Stage (max.)	Volume of Diarrhea (ml/d)
A	1	< 25%		0	< 34		0	< 500
B	2	25%–50%	or	1–2	34–102	or	1–2	550–1,500
C	3	> 50%	or	3	103–255	or	3	> 1,500
D	4	Bullae	or	4	> 255	or	4	Severe pain and ileus

* Assign index based on maximum involvement in an individual organ system.

Note. From "IBMTR Severity Index for Grading Acute Graft-Versus-Host Disease: Retrospective Comparison With Glucksberg Grade," by P.A. Rowlings, D. Przepiorka, J.P. Klein, R.P. Gale, J.R. Passweg, P.J. Henslee-Downey, ... M.M. Horowitz, 1997, *British Journal of Haematology, 97,* p. 859. doi:10.1046/j.1365-2141.1997.1112925.x. Copyright 1997 by Blackwell Science Ltd. Reprinted with permission.

Hematologic Complications

In addition to GVHD, additional complications may occur with HSCT. These are further described in Table 7-8. Profound pancytopenia and immune suppression following HSCT result from the effects of the conditioning regimen and the immunosuppressive agents used in allogeneic transplant to prevent GVHD. Myeloablative conditioning regimens eradicate hematopoietic function, thus resulting in severe anemia, neutropenia, and thrombocytopenia. Most patients require red blood cell and platelet transfusions during the post-transplant course if their hemoglobin is less than 7 g/dl and platelet count is less than 10,000/mm³ (Carson et al., 2012; Wandt et al., 2012). Diagnostic studies used to assess bleeding may include guaiac of stool and emesis, urinalysis, and a computed tomography (CT) scan of the head to evaluate for intracranial hemorrhage. Because nonmyeloablative conditioning regimens are less toxic, suppression of blood counts may not be as severe and blood counts may recover more quickly, thus minimizing the need for transfusions. Furthermore, the duration of neutropenia is dependent on the stem cell source, type of transplant, and cytokine used for stem cell mobilization and during the post-transplant course. Chronic GVHD is commonly associated with chronic cytopenias and eosinophilia (Ferrara et al., 2009). Recipients with thrombocytopenia in association with GVHD have a poor prognosis (Kuzmina et al., 2012).

Infections

The risk of infection related to HSCT exists throughout the transplant trajectory. Supportive care is essential for patients with both acute and chronic GVHD. Viral, bacterial, fungal, and protozoan infections occur at various time points after transplantation as described in Figure 7-7 and Table 7-9.

Various measures can reduce the risk of infection, including protective isolation, positive air pressure rooms, air filtration systems such as high-efficiency particulate air filtration, hand washing, limited visitation, and other institution-specific guidelines (FACT, 2012). Despite a variety of preventive measures used, hand washing is the most effective practice to minimize

Table 7-7. National Institutes of Health Consensus Development of Chronic Graft-Versus-Host Disease Staging

Organ/Site	Score 0	Score 1	Score 2	Score 3
Performance Score: ☐ **KPS ECOG LPS**	☐ Asymptomatic and fully active (ECOG 0; KPS or LPS 100%)	☐ Symptomatic, fully ambulatory, restricted only in physically strenuous activity (ECOG 1; KPS or LPS 80%–90%)	☐ Symptomatic, ambulatory, capable of self-care, > 50% of waking hours out of bed (ECOG 2; KPS or LPS 60%–70%)	☐ Symptomatic, limited self-care, > 50% of waking hours in bed (ECOG 3–4; KPS or LPS < 60%)
Skin _Clinical features:_ ☐ Maculopapular rash ☐ Lichen planus–like features ☐ Papulosquamous lesions or ichthyosis ☐ Hyperpigmentation ☐ Hypopigmentation ☐ Keratosis pilaris ☐ Erythema ☐ Erythroderma ☐ Poikiloderma ☐ Sclerotic features ☐ Pruritus ☐ Hair involvement ☐ Nail involvement **% BSA involved**	☐ No symptoms	☐ < 18% BSA with disease signs but **NO** sclerotic features	☐ 19%–50% BSA **OR** involvement with superficial sclerotic features "not hidebound" (able to pinch)	☐ > 50% BSA **OR** deep sclerotic features "hidebound" (unable to pinch) **OR** impaired mobility, ulceration or severe pruritus
Mouth	☐ No symptoms	☐ Mild symptoms with disease signs but not limiting oral intake significantly	☐ Moderate symptoms with disease signs **with** partial limitation of oral intake	☐ Severe symptoms with disease signs on examination **with** major limitation of oral intake
Eyes	☐ No symptoms	☐ Mild dry eye symptoms not affecting ADL (requiring eye drops ≤ 3 × per day) **OR** asymptomatic signs of keratoconjunctivitis sicca	☐ Moderate dry eye symptoms partially affecting ADL (requiring drops > 3 × per day or punctal plugs) **WITHOUT** vision impairment	☐ Severe dry eye symptoms significantly affecting ADL (special eyewear to relieve pain) **OR** unable to work because of ocular symptoms **OR** loss of vision caused by keratoconjunctivitis sicca

(Continued on next page)

Table 7-7. National Institutes of Health Consensus Development of Chronic Graft-Versus-Host Disease Staging *(Continued)*

Organ/Site	Score 0	Score 1	Score 2	Score 3
GI tract	☐ No symptoms	☐ Symptoms such as dysphagia, anorexia, nausea, vomiting, abdominal pain or diarrhea without significant weight loss (< 5%)	☐ Symptoms associated with mild to moderate weight loss (5%–15%)	☐ Symptoms associated with significant weight loss > 15%, requires nutritional supplement for most calorie needs **OR** esophageal dilation
Liver	☐ Normal LFT	☐ Elevated bilirubin, AP[a], AST or ALT < 2 × ULN	☐ Bilirubin > 3 mg/dl or bilirubin enzymes 2–5 × ULN	☐ Bilirubin or enzymes > 5 × ULN
Lungs[b]	☐ No symptoms	☐ Mild symptoms (shortness of breath after climbing one flight of steps)	☐ Moderate symptoms (shortness of breath after walking on flat ground)	☐ Severe symptoms (shortness of breath at rest; requiring O_2)
FEV$_1$ [ ] DLCO [ ]	☐ FEV$_1$ > 80% **OR** LFS = 2	☐ FEV$_1$ 60%–79% **OR** LFS = 3–5	☐ FEV$_1$ 40%–59% **OR** LFS = 6–9	☐ FEV$_1$ ≤ 39% **OR** LFS = 10–12
Joints and fascia	☐ No symptoms	☐ Mild tightness of arms or legs, normal or mild decreased range of motion (ROM) **AND** not affecting ADL	☐ Tightness of arms or legs **OR** joint contractures, erythema thought due to fasciitis, moderate decrease in ROM **AND** mild to moderate limitation of ADL	☐ Contractures **WITH** significant decrease of ROM **AND** significant limitation of ADL (unable to tie shoes, button shirts, dress self, etc.)
Genital tract	☐ No symptoms	☐ Symptomatic with mild signs on exam **AND** no effect on coitus and minimal discomfort with gynecologic exam	☐ Symptomatic with moderate signs on exam **AND** with mild dyspareunia or discomfort on gynecologic exam	☐ Symptomatic **WITH** advanced signs (stricture, labial agglutination or severe ulceration) **AND** severe pain with coitus or inability to insert vaginal speculum

(Continued on next page)

Table 7-7. National Institutes of Health Consensus Development of Chronic Graft-Versus-Host Disease Staging *(Continued)*

Other indicators, clinical manifestations or complications related to chronic GVHD (check all that apply and assign a score to its severity [0–3] based on its functional impact where applicable [none – 0, mild – 1, moderate – 2, severe – 3])

Esophageal stricture or web__	Pericardial effusion__	Pleural effusion(s)__
Ascites (serositis)__	Nephrotic syndrome__	Peripheral neuropathy__
Myasthenia gravis__	Cardiomyopathy__	Eosinophilia > 500µl__
Polymyositis__	Cardiac conduction defects__	Coronary artery involvement__
Platelets < 100,000/µl__	Progressive onset__	

Others: Specify:_____

[a] AP may be elevated in growing children and not reflective of liver dysfunction.

[b] Pulmonary scoring should be performed using both the symptom and pulmonary function testing (PFT) scale whenever possible. When discrepancy exists between pulmonary symptom or PFT scores the higher value should be used for final scoring. Scoring using the Lung Function Score (LFS) is preferred, but if DLCO is not available, grading using FEV₁ should be used. The LFS is a global assessment of lung function after the diagnosis of bronchiolitis obliterans has already been established. The percent predicted FEV₁ and DLCO (adjusted for hematocrit but not alveolar volume) should be converted to a numeric score as follows: > 80% = 1; 70%–79% = 2; 60%–69% = 3; 50%–59% = 4; 40%–49% = 5; < 40% = 6. The LFS = FEV_1 score + DLCO score, with a possible range of 2–12.

ADL—activities of daily living; ALT—alanine aminotransferase; AP—alkaline phosphatase; AST—aspartate aminotransferase; BSA—body surface area; ECOG—Eastern Cooperative Oncology Group; GVHD—graft-versus-host disease; KPS—Karnofsky Performance Status; LFTs—liver function tests; LPS—Lansky Performance Status; ULN—upper limit of normal

Note. From "National Institutes of Health Consensus Development Project on Criteria for Clinical Trials in Chronic Graft-Versus-Host Disease: I. Diagnosis and Staging Working Group Report," by A.H. Filipovich, D. Weisdorf, S. Pavletic, G. Socie, J.R. Wingard, S.J. Lee, … M.E.D. Flowers, 2005, *Biology of Blood and Marrow Transplantation, 11,* pp. 952–953. doi:10.1016/j.bbmt.2005.09.004. Copyright 2005 by American Society for Blood and Marrow Transplantation. Reprinted with permission.

the risk of infection (FACT, 2012; Tomblyn et al., 2009). The risk of infection in allogeneic transplantation is complex because of the profound immunosuppression induced by both the conditioning regimen and the medications used to prevent or treat GVHD. Risk of infection after allogeneic transplant is greatest during the early postengraftment phase but also may occur in later months following transplant as a result of prolonged immunosuppression (see Figure 7-7 and Table 7-9).

Following autologous HSCT, the risk of infection is greatest during the early postengraftment period because of neutropenia. Both autologous and allogeneic transplant recipients are at greatest risk for the development of infection while neutropenic, with an absolute neutrophil count less than 500/mm³. Neutrophil engraftment is described as a neutrophil count greater than 500/mm³ (Tomblyn et al., 2009). Medications recommended for post-transplant infection prophylaxis include antibacterial, antiviral, and antifungal agents (see Table 7-10).

Risk factors for the development of bacterial infections in transplant recipients include central venous catheters, altered oral mucosa, and altered GI tract because of bacterial translocation. Bacterial infections following HSCT are caused by gram-positive organisms such as *Staphylococcus aureus, Staphylococcus epidermidis,* and *Streptococcus viridans* (Kedia et al., 2013). Forty percent of bacterial infections are from gram-negative organisms such as *Escherichia coli, Kleb-*

Table 7-8. Complications of Hematopoietic Stem Cell Transplantation

Complication	Risk Factors/Causes	Clinical Sequelae	Diagnostic Findings
Bleeding	Anemia Thrombocytopenia Altered coagulation factors Altered mucosal barriers Sinusoidal obstructive syndrome Failed or delayed engraftment ABO-incompatible transplant	Petechiae, ecchymosis, easy bruising Hematuria, menorrhagia Bloody stool or emesis Epistaxis, hemoptysis Headache, change in pupil response or mental status	Platelet count < 10,000–20,000/mm^3 Hemoglobin < 8 g/dl Elevated prothrombin time, international normalized ratio, partial thromboplastin time Blood revealed on chemstick Guaiac-positive stool, emesis Computed tomography (CT) of the head—intracranial bleed
Cardiac	Cardiomyopathy—previous exposure to anthracyclines; administration of cyclophosphamide; total body irradiation (TBI)	Pulmonary edema, poor peripheral perfusion, systemic edema	Electrocardiogram (ECG)—decreased voltage Echocardiogram—cardiomegaly, decreased ejection fraction
	Cardiac arrhythmias	Palpitations, chest discomfort, anxiety, abnormal heart sounds, hypotension	ECG findings specific to type of arrhythmia
	Cardiac infections—endocarditis related to bacteremia	Nonspecific symptoms of fever, chills, malaise, night sweats Arrhythmias	ECG conduction or rhythm disturbances Echocardiogram—valvular vegetations, decreased ventricular function
Pulmonary	Idiopathic pneumonia syndrome (IPS)—TBI used in preparative regimen, graft-versus-host disease (GVHD), methotrexate for GVHD prophylaxis	IPS—fever, dyspnea, nonproductive cough, hypoxemia, respiratory failure	IPS—chest radiograph (CXR) and CT diffuse or multilobular interstitial or alveolar infiltrates, thickened deep and superficial interlobular septa, nodules of varying sizes
	Diffuse alveolar hemorrhage (DAH)—radiation prior to transplantation, age > 40, solid tumors, severe mucositis, granulocyte recovery, fever, renal insufficiency, acute GVHD	DAH—dyspnea, cough, hemoptysis, hypoxemia, respiratory failure	DAH—CXR unilateral or bilateral infiltrates, diffuse alveolar pattern; bronchial alveolar lavage bloody fluid and hemosiderin-laden macrophages, diffuse alveolar damage
Renal insufficiency	Hypovolemia Dehydration Septic shock Nephrotoxic drugs Prolonged ischemia Hemorrhagic cystitis Tumor lysis syndrome Acute tubular necrosis Congestive heart failure	Doubling of baseline creatinine Oliguria Fluid and electrolyte imbalance Pulmonary edema Cardiac compromise Multiple organ failure	Urinalysis Fluid balance Blood chemistries

(Continued on next page)

Table 7-8. Complications of Hematopoietic Stem Cell Transplantation *(Continued)*

Complication	Risk Factors/Causes	Clinical Sequelae	Diagnostic Findings
Sinusoidal obstruction syndrome	Hepatitis prior to transplant Repeated courses and higher doses of chemotherapy Hepatotoxic radiation therapy Immunosuppressive agents Elevated liver function tests prior to transplant Infection/sepsis Estrogen or progesterone therapy	Azotemia Ascites Weight gain Hepatomegaly Encephalopathy Fluid balance intake greater than output	Hyperbilirubinemia Elevated alkaline phosphatase Elevated serum aspartate aminotransferase and alanine aminotransferase Elevated prothrombin time Liver biopsy

Note. Based on information from AABB et al., 2013; Carson et al., 2012; del Campo et al., 2014; Kedia et al., 2013; Kimura et al., 2008; Mohty & Mohty, 2011; Nishiguchi et al., 2009; O'Donghaile et al., 2012; Raza & Vierling, 2014; Rubio-Augusti & Bataller, 2012; Savani et al., 2011; Sengsayadeth et al., 2012; Singh et al., 2013; Tomblyn et al., 2009; Wandt et al., 2012.

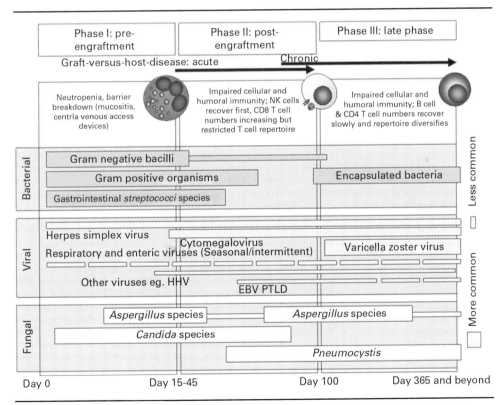

Figure 7-7. Phases of Opportunistic Infections Among Allogeneic Hematopoietic Stem Cell Transplant Recipients

EBV—Epstein-Barr virus; HHV—human herpesvirus 6; PTLD—post-transplant lymphoproliferative disorder

Note. From "Background to Hematopoietic Cell Transplantation, Including Post Transplant Immune Recovery," by C. Mackall, T. Fry, R. Gress, K. Peggs, J. Storek, and A. Toubert, 2009, *Bone Marrow Transplantation, 44,* p. 461. doi:10.1038/bmt.2009.255. Copyright 2009 by Macmillan Publishers Limited. Reprinted with permission.

Table 7-9. Infectious Complications and Occurrence in Blood and Marrow Stem Cell Transplantation Recipients

Organism	Common Sites	Treatment
First Month Post-Transplant		
Viral		
Herpes simplex virus	Oral, esophageal, skin, gastrointestinal (GI) tract, genital	Acyclovir, valacyclovir, famciclovir
Respiratory syncytial virus (RSV)	Sinopulmonary	Aerosolized ribavirin
Epstein-Barr virus	Oral, esophageal, skin, GI tract	Treatment usually is not indicated.
Bacterial		
Gram positive (*Staphylococcus epidermidis, Staphylococcus aureus, Streptococci*)	Skin, blood, sinopulmonary	Third- and fourth-generation cephalosporins, quinolones, aminoglycosides, vancomycin
Gram negative (*Escherichia coli, Pseudomonas aeruginosa, Klebsiella*)	GI, blood, oral, perirectal	Fluoroquinolone with antipseudomonal activity. Important to check institution's epidemiologic data regarding resistant patterns
Fungal		
Candida species (*C. albicans, C. glabrata, C. krusei*)	Oral, esophageal, skin	Fluconazole, voriconazole, itraconazole, amphotericin B, liposomal amphotericin
Aspergillus (*fumigatus, flavus*)	Sinopulmonary	Aerosolized liposomal amphotericin B, voriconazole
1–4 Months Post-Transplant		
Viral		
Cytomegalovirus (CMV)	Pulmonary, hepatic, GI	Ganciclovir, foscarnet, valacyclovir, acyclovir
Enteric viruses (rotavirus, Coxsackievirus, adenovirus)	Pulmonary, urinary, GI, hepatic	No specific treatment
RSV	Sinopulmonary	Aerosolized ribavirin
Parainfluenza	Pulmonary	Possibly ribavirin, but no standard treatment
Bacterial		
Gram positive	Sinopulmonary	Third- and fourth-generation cephalosporins, quinolones, aminoglycosides, vancomycin
Fungal		
Candida species	Oral, hepatosplenic, integument	Fluconazole, voriconazole, itraconazole, amphotericin B, liposomal amphotericin. posaconazole, micafungin

(Continued on next page)

Table 7-9. Infectious Complications and Occurrence in Blood and Marrow Stem Cell Transplantation Recipients *(Continued)*

Organism	Common Sites	Treatment
Aspergillus species	Sinopulmonary, central nervous system (CNS)	Fluconazole, voriconazole, itraconazole, amphotericin B, liposomal amphotericin. posaconazole, micafungin
Mucormycosis	Sinopulmonary	Liposomal formulations of amphotericin B
Coccidioidomycosis	Sinopulmonary	Amphotericin B
Cryptococcus neoformans	Pulmonary, CNS	Liposomal formulations of amphotericin B
Protozoan		
Pneumocystis jiroveci	Pulmonary	Standard is trimethoprim-sulfamethoxazole (TMP-SMZ). Pentamidine, atovaquone may be used if allergic to sulfa.
Toxoplasma gondii	Pulmonary, CNS	Pyrimethamine and sulfonamides may be combined with clindamycin and spiramycin, especially if sulfa allergy.
4–12 Months Post-Transplant		
Viral		
CMV, echoviruses, RSV, varicella-zoster virus (VZV)	Integument, pulmonary, hepatic	CMV—ganciclovir, foscarnet, valacyclovir, acyclovir RSV—aerosolized ribavirin VZV—acyclovir, valacyclovir, famciclovir Echoviruses—no specific treatment, IVIG
Bacterial		
Gram positive (*S. pneumoniae, Haemophilus influenzae, Pneumococci*)	Sinopulmonary, blood	Third- and fourth-generation cephalosporins, quinolones, aminoglycosides, vancomycin
Fungal		
Aspergillus	Sinopulmonary	Fluconazole, voriconazole, itraconazole, amphotericin B, liposomal amphotericin
Coccidioidomycosis	Sinopulmonary	Amphotericin B
Protozoan		
Pneumocystis jiroveci	Pulmonary	Standard is TMP-SMZ. Pentamidine, atovaquone may be used if allergic to sulfa.
Toxoplasma gondii	Pulmonary, CNS	Pyrimethamine and sulfonamides may be combined with clindamycin and spiramycin, especially if sulfa allergy.

(Continued on next page)

Table 7-9. Infectious Complications and Occurrence in Blood and Marrow Stem Cell Transplantation Recipients *(Continued)*

Organism	Common Sites	Treatment
Greater Than 12 Months Post-Transplant		
Viral		
VZV	Integument	Acyclovir, valacyclovir, famciclovir
Bacterial		
Gram positive (*Streptococci, Haemophilus influenzae,* encapsulated bacteria)	Sinopulmonary, blood	Third- and fourth-generation cephalosporins, quinolones, aminoglycosides, vancomycin

Note. Based on information from Foundation for the Accreditation of Cellular Therapy, 2012; Kedia et al., 2013; Liu et al., 2013; Tomblyn et al., 2009.

siella pneumoniae, Enterobacter, and *Pseudomonas aeruginosa* (Kedia et al., 2013; Tomblyn et al., 2009). The Centers for Disease Control and Prevention does not recommend specific guidelines for antibacterial prophylaxis for afebrile transplant recipients (Tomblyn et al., 2009). Institutional guidelines for antibacterial prophylaxis are based on commonly occurring infections, resistant organisms, and antibiotic susceptibilities. Antibiotic regimens for the empiric treatment of neutropenic or febrile HSCT recipients may include third- and fourth-generation cephalosporins, quinolones, aminoglycosides, and vancomycin. If cultures remain negative, vancomycin should be discontinued because of the risk of vancomycin-resistant enterococci (Tomblyn et al., 2009).

Common viral infections that may reactivate during the early post-transplant period include herpes simplex virus (HSV) types I and II, human herpesvirus 6 (HHV-6), and cytomegalovirus (CMV) (Kedia et al., 2013; Liu et al., 2013). Pretransplant viral serologic testing is performed to determine past exposure to viral infections of the transplant recipient and donor. Prophylactic use of antiviral medications such as acyclovir, valacyclovir, or famciclovir is common during the HSCT process. HSV most commonly is associated with oral mucositis. Risk factors for the development of CMV infections include CMV seropositivity prior to transplant, infusion of CMV-seropositive blood products to CMV-seronegative patients, GVHD, and the use of immunosuppressive agents. Another measure for the prevention of viral infections includes the use of leukocyte filters for blood product transfusions (Tomblyn et al., 2009). Antigen detection techniques to test for CMV and Epstein-Barr virus (EBV) should be performed on allogeneic HSCT recipients because patients are at risk for developing EBV infections due to the profound immunosuppression after allogeneic transplant. Local or disseminated varicella-zoster virus infections may occur as a result of prolonged immunosuppression at 4–12 months or later after transplant and require treatment with high-dose acyclovir or valacyclovir (Kedia et al., 2013).

Fungal infections may occur during the post-transplant period and commonly include *Candida* species or *Aspergillus*. Prophylactic antifungal agents may include fluconazole, itraconazole, or voriconazole. Oral antifungal agents may be used to prevent oral candidiasis caused by mucositis. Invasive fungal infections have been reported including *Aspergillus, Fusarium,* and *Mucor*. Prolonged antifungal therapy may be necessary with amphotericin, caspofungin, itraconazole, voriconazole, or posaconazole (Kedia et al., 2013; Tomblyn et al., 2009).

Many other infections may occur following transplant. These include pneumocystis pneumonia (PCP), *Toxoplasma gondii,* and *Clostridium difficile*. The use of prophylactic sulfonamides to prevent PCP has nearly eliminated this post-transplant infectious complication (Kedia et al., 2013; Tomblyn et al., 2009). Toxoplasmosis infections have occurred in transplant recipients because of profound immunosuppression. The most effective treatment for toxoplasmosis infections is the use of combination therapy including pyrimethamine and sulfonamides (Tomblyn et al., 2009). *Clostridium difficile* infection may develop post-transplant in patients who are treated with antibiotics allowing for GI overgrowth of other organisms. GI symptoms that are associated with colitis, such as diarrhea, nausea, and vomiting, usually are present. Treatment with oral vancomycin, metronidazole, or fidaxomicin is preferred to allow for GI absorption of the medications.

Bleeding

Thrombocytopenia and anemia commonly occur post-transplant as a result of the profound myelosuppressive effects of the conditioning regimen. Institutional guidelines for transfusion of blood products should be used to develop a standard of practice. Transfusion needs must be individualized for each patient based on signs and symptoms of bleeding, presence of red blood cell or platelet antibodies, response to transfusions, and the presence of refractoriness to blood products. Current evidence suggests that red blood cell transfusions should be considered at a hemoglobin concentration of 8 g/dl or less or for symptoms (Carson et al., 2012). In critically ill patients, a hemoglobin level of 7–8 g/dl should be maintained (Carson et al., 2012). Routine prophylactic platelet transfusions are recommended if platelets are less than 10,000/mm^3 (Wandt et al., 2012). In a study that compared prophylactic platelet transfusions at

Table 7-10. Centers for Disease Control and Prevention Recommendations for Infection Prophylaxis

Pathogen	Recommendations
Pneumocystis	Alternative therapy includes dapsone, pentamidine, or atovaquone.
Toxoplasma gondii	Trimethoprim-sulfamethoxazole double strength, 1 pill three times per week Alternative therapy includes clindamycin plus pyrimethamine, plus leucovorin. Begin therapy after engraftment and continue until 6 months after hematopoietic stem cell transplant (HSCT) and patient is off immunosuppressive medications.
Herpes simplex virus	Acyclovir 200 mg PO three times a day or 250 mg/m^2/dose every 12 hours from beginning of conditioning regimen until engraftment or mucositis resolves Alternative therapy: Valacyclovir 500 mg PO daily Prophylaxis for seropositive allogeneic HSCT recipients
Cytomegalovirus	Ganciclovir 5 mg/kg/dose IV twice daily for 5–7 days, then daily until day 100 post-HSCT Alternative therapy includes foscarnet.
Fungal—*Candida* species	Fluconazole 400 mg PO or IV daily Alternative therapy includes itraconazole solution 200 mg orally twice a day; micafungin 50 mg IV daily; voriconazole 200 mg orally twice a day; or posaconazole 200 mg orally three times a day. Begin at the day of transplant and continue until engraftment or until 7 days after the absolute neutrophil count > 1,000 cells/mm^3.
Molds or fluconazole-resistant *Candida* species	Micafungin 50 mg IV daily; posaconazole 200 mg orally three times a day Alternative therapy: Voriconazole 200 mg orally twice a day

Note. Based on information from Tomblyn et al., 2009.

10×10^9 versus 30×10^9 cells/kg, the number of platelet transfusions and cost associated with transfusions were reduced using the lower platelet threshold. The risk of bleeding or significant bleeding events was not increased by giving prophylactic platelet transfusion for a level of 10 $\times 10^9$ (AABB et al., 2013; Wandt et al., 2012). Platelet transfusions may be necessary at higher levels if signs of bleeding, coagulation abnormalities, rapidly falling platelet count, or invasive procedures are involved. Fresh frozen plasma and cryoprecipitate may be given for coagulation abnormalities as needed. In ABO-mismatched allogeneic HSCT, the ABO type of the recipient will change to the ABO type of the donor in approximately three to four months. The ABO titer of the recipient must be monitored to detect when this change occurs so that blood transfusions can be adjusted appropriately. Type O blood products usually are used for transfusion until the recipient's blood type completely changes to the donor ABO type (Kimura et al., 2008; O'Donghaile, Kelley, Klein, & Flegel, 2012).

Gastrointestinal Complications

GI complications after autologous and allogeneic transplant may occur as a result of the conditioning regimen, infections, or GVHD. Post-transplant GI complications include the upper and lower GI systems. Upper GI symptoms may include nausea, vomiting, oral mucositis, pharyngitis, xerostomia, dysphagia, and dysgeusia. For prevention of oral mucositis as a sequela of myeloablative regimens, palifermin may be considered (Tomblyn et al., 2009). Use of antiemetics and analgesics can manage symptoms. Daily weight, calorie counts, and intake and output measurements are helpful to monitor nutritional and fluid status. A dietary consultation may be needed to assist with nutritional support. As a result of mucosal injury, translocation and colonization of bacteria (e.g., *Streptococcus viridans, Staphylococcus aureus*) can occur, especially during the neutropenic phase of transplant (Kedia et al., 2013; Tomblyn et al., 2009). Oral hygiene should be maintained with sterile water, normal saline, or sodium bicarbonate at least four to six times a day. In addition, tooth brushing two to three times a day should occur; however, toothpaste is optional (Tomblyn et al., 2009). Invasive fungal infections can occur from endogenous *Candida* species in the GI tract. Topical antifungal drugs may decrease superficial colonization but not invasive fungal infections. Fluconazole is commonly used for prophylaxis, but it does not cover *Candida krusei* or *Candida glabrata* (Kedia et al., 2013; Tomblyn et al., 2009).

Lower GI symptoms affect more than 80% of HSCT recipients and usually are the result of hepatobiliary symptoms, acute GVHD, and pseudomembranous and neutropenic colitis (del Campo, León, Palacios, Lagana, & Tagarro, 2014). In cases of colitis, patients may complain of right lower quadrant pain and bloody or watery diarrhea. Obtaining CT scans may assist in determining a diagnosis, and obtaining a stool sample for detection of *Clostridium difficile* may be sufficient for diagnosis (del Campo et al., 2014). Prophylaxis with metronidazole may reduce anaerobic bacteria in the GI tract; however, the data are insufficient to recommend it for gut decontamination in the HSCT setting (Tomblyn et al., 2009). Encouraging perineal hygiene is important because the perirectal area is another site that can be an entry portal for infections. Assessing for abscess formation may facilitate early detection and prevention of surgical interventions, such as incision and drainage, as well as wound care.

Hepatic Complications

The etiology of hepatic manifestations following HSCT may initially present as hyperbilirubinemia, increased serum alkaline phosphatase and aminotransferase levels, and coagulopathies. Liver damage may occur after transplant for many reasons, including sinusoidal obstructive syndrome, hepatitis B infection, hepatitis C infection, iron overload, cholangitis, and drug toxicity (Raza & Vierling, 2014; Savani, Griffith, Jagasia, & Lee, 2011). Multiorgan system consequences may occur as a result of liver dysfunction and can include ascites, hypotension, coagulopathies, hyponatremia, hypoalbuminemia, encephalopathy, renal insufficiency, fluid overload, pleural effusion, and pulmonary edema (Raza & Vierling, 2014). Management of sinusoidal obstructive syndrome involves adjusting dosages of medications that are metabolized by the liver and symptomatically treating the organ dysfunction that results from the liver insufficiency.

Pulmonary Complications

Lung injury is a frequent complication after HSCT that may account for post-transplant morbidity and mortality (Savani et al., 2011; Sengsayadeth, Srivastava, Jagasia, & Savani, 2012). Delayed pulmonary injury can occur as a result of the conditioning regimen. Thus, the risk of pulmonary complications in long-term allogeneic HSCT survivors is 30%–60% (Sengsayadeth et al., 2012). Restrictive changes may be the result of muscle weakness from prolonged steroid use, pulmonary fibrosis, or sclerotic chronic GVHD involving the thorax (Savani et al., 2011).

Bronchiolitis obliterans syndrome is a unique pulmonary complication of allogeneic HSCT and is associated with chronic GVHD. Data suggest that viral infections, gastroesophageal reflux disease, and chemotherapy and radiation conditioning regimens may be contributing factors (Savani et al., 2011). Progressive shortness of breath results from obstructive airway disease causing occlusion of the bronchioles. Histologic confirmation is invasive; therefore, a diagnosis is made based on diagnostic tests including pulmonary function tests and chest imaging. Treatment consists of corticosteroids, immunosuppressive therapies, and macrolide antibiotics (Sengsayadeth et al., 2012).

Numerous pulmonary infections can develop following transplantation, including bacterial, viral, fungal, protozoan, and parasitic infections. Bacterial pneumonia may be caused by both gram-positive and gram-negative organisms. The most common gram-positive organisms responsible for pulmonary infections include *Staphylococcus aureus*, *Staphylococcus epidermidis*, and *Streptococcus pneumoniae*. Gram-negative organisms may include *Klebsiella* and *Pseudomonas* species (Tomblyn et al., 2009). Prolonged immunosuppression caused by chronic GVHD may be a risk factor for pneumococcal pneumonia.

Post-transplant viral pneumonia most commonly is caused by CMV (Liu et al., 2013). The most significant risk factors for CMV pneumonia include prior CMV exposure and the immunosuppressive therapies used during the transplant process. Respiratory syncytial virus (RSV) may also result in pneumonia and is very contagious. Protective precautions are necessary to avoid the spread of RSV to other patients. Additional viruses reported to cause pneumonia in transplant recipients include adenovirus, parainfluenza virus, influenza virus, and HHV-6. Parasitic infections such as PCP also may lead to pneumonia in transplant recipients. Trimethoprim-sulfamethoxazole often is given after allogeneic HSCT following engraftment for prophylaxis against PCP and is continued until immunosuppression therapy is stopped (Savani et al., 2011). Several fungal infections have been reported in transplant recipients, including *Aspergillus*, *Candida*, *Cryptococcus neoformans*, *Fusarium*, *Penicillium*, and *Mucor*. Fungal prophylaxis for pneumonia may include fluconazole, itraconazole, voriconazole, and posaconazole (Tomblyn et al., 2009).

Cardiac Complications

Cardiac complications following HSCT are uncommon and occur because of the cardiotoxic effects of chemotherapy and radiation therapy given prior to transplant or as part of the conditioning regimen. Chemotherapeutic agents with well-described cardiac toxicity include anthracyclines and cyclophosphamide, both of which may cause cardiomyopathy (Savani et al., 2011). TBI and total lymphoid irradiation have been reported to cause cardiac toxicity in rare cases. Cardiac arrhythmias have been reported during the transplant course. Cardiac infections are rare but most commonly are associated with endocarditis in the presence of bacteremia. Fungal organisms, such as *Aspergillus*, also have been found to be associated with the development of endocarditis (Tomblyn et al., 2009).

Renal Complications

Older age, hypertension, poor renal function prior to transplant, drug-induced toxicity, and infection account for the etiology of renal insufficiency in HSCT recipients (Mohty & Mohty, 2011). Acute kidney injury affects 15%–60% of HSCT recipients, has a higher incidence in the allogeneic compared to autologous transplant population, and is associated with a high mortality rate (Singh et al., 2013). Furthermore, if hemodialysis is indicated, the mortality rate may be greater than 70%. Causes of acute kidney injury following HSCT can be prerenal (e.g., dehydration, sepsis, drugs, sinusoidal obstructive syndrome, decreased cardiac output), intrinsic renal (e.g., acute tubular necrosis, infection, vascular), and postrenal (e.g., tumor lysis syndrome, drug precipitation, hemorrhagic cystitis) (Singh et al., 2013). Administration of medications such as calcineurin inhibitors, nonsteroidal anti-inflammatory drugs, chemotherapy, and antibiotics is challenging because of their potential renal toxicity. Management of acute kidney injury depends on the etiology and ranges from administration of IV fluid to removal of the offending agent. Chronic kidney disease develops in 15%–20% of recipients and is defined as a slow yet steady rise in the creatinine along with progressive hypertension and anemia (Singh et al., 2013). Three common causes of chronic kidney disease include chronic calcineurin inhibitor nephrotoxicity, chronic GVHD–associated glomerulonephritis, and HSCT-associated thrombotic microangiopathy. A renal biopsy is a useful diagnostic tool in chronic calcineurin inhibitor nephrotoxicity and chronic GVHD–associated glomerulonephritis. However, in HSCT-associated thrombotic microangiopathy, the diagnosis is based on clinical characteristics such as rising serum creatinine levels, anemia, thrombocytopenia, presence of schistocytes, elevated lactate dehydrogenase, low serum haptoglobin, and hypertension (Singh et al., 2013). Treatment of chronic kidney disease involves medical management and discontinuation or dose adjustment of the instigating agent.

Neurologic Complications

The incidence of post-HSCT neurologic complications ranges from 8% to 42% (Rubio-Augusti & Bataller, 2012). Central nervous system (CNS) complications in the HSCT setting depend on the degree and duration of myelosuppression, immunosuppression, and GVHD (Nishiguchi et al., 2009). Figure 7-8 provides an overview of neurologic complications observed in HSCT recipients. Viral encephalitis from reactivation of latent herpesviruses, EBV, and varicella-zoster virus is common. Symptoms such as acute-onset mental alterations, drowsiness, and short-term memory loss are clinical manifestations (Nishiguchi et al., 2009; Rubio-Augusti & Bataller, 2012). Vascular complications (e.g., intracranial hemorrhage, thrombotic and embolic events in the cerebrovascular system) usually are related to chronic GVHD or tumor relapse. Therapies that contribute to CNS complications include high-dose chemotherapy, radiation therapy, immunosuppressive agents, infections, and metabolic disturbances. Cyclosporine and tacrolimus have been associated with posterior reversible encephalopathy syndrome. Risk factors for this include sepsis, shock associated with multiorgan fail-

- Chemotherapy agents
  - Busulfan
  - Carmustine
  - Cisplatin
  - Cytarabine
  - Etoposide
  - Ifosfamide
  - Methotrexate
  - Paclitaxel
- Total body irradiation
- Immunosuppressive agents
  - Cyclosporine
  - Steroids
  - Tacrolimus
- Anti-infective agents
  - Acyclovir
  - Aminoglycosides
  - Cephalosporins
  - Ganciclovir
  - Imipenem
- Central nervous system (CNS) infections
  - Bacterial—*Streptococcus epidermidis*, *Staphylococcus aureus*, *Pseudomonas aeruginosa*, *Haemophilus influenzae*, pneumococcus
  - Fungal—*Aspergillus*, *Candida*
  - Protozoan—toxoplasmosis
  - Viral—human herpesvirus 6, cytomegalovirus, Epstein-Barr virus, varicella-zoster virus
- CNS hemorrhage or stroke
- Encephalopathy
  - Leukoencephalopathy
  - Metabolic encephalopathy
- Immune-mediated toxicities
  - Inflammatory demyelinating polyneuropathy
  - Myasthenia gravis
  - Polymyositis

Figure 7-8. Common Etiologies of Neurologic Complications

Note. Based on information from Nishiguchi et al., 2009; Rubio-Augusti & Bataller, 2012.

ure, chemotherapy, and GVHD, as well as cyclosporine or tacrolimus toxicity (Nishiguchi et al., 2009; Rubio-Augusti & Bataller, 2012). Sudden mental status alterations, headaches, psychosis, unconsciousness, and convulsions are initial clinical manifestations. No correlation exists between serum drug levels and severity of toxicity; however, neurologic improvement has been observed with withdrawal of these agents (Nishiguchi et al., 2009). CT scans and magnetic resonance imaging may demonstrate CNS lesions and assist in obtaining the correct diagnosis so that treatment can commence.

Late Effects After Hematopoietic Stem Cell Transplantation

Many late effects following HSCT are associated with delayed toxicities of the preparative regimen, the occurrence of GVHD, or the administration of steroids. Careful and diligent evaluation for late effects is essential to the overall well-being and recovery of patients after transplant. Figure 7-9 further describes late effects of HSCT. In addition to what has been described in this section thus far, diabetes may develop as a result of prolonged steroid therapy used for the treatment of GVHD. Monitoring hemoglobin A1c levels with a goal of less than 7%, as well as encouraging a healthy diet and exercise, should be considered. Furthermore, diabetes has implications for ocular, renal, peripheral vascular, and cardiovascular diseases (Savani et al., 2011). Dyslipidemia may occur as a result of steroids, sirolimus, and calcineurin inhibitors. As a result, APNs should assess fasting lipid levels annually in patients with GVHD and treat with statins if clinically indicated (Savani et al., 2011). Fasting lipid panels should be evaluated every three months to assess effectiveness of interventions (Savani et al., 2011). Infertility, hypogonadism, thyroid dysfunction, and growth hormone deficiency are the most common endocrine late effects that may occur. Late renal dysfunction is not well understood but may be related to the effects of the preparative regimen and other nephrotoxic agents used during the transplant process. The most common musculoskeletal disorders following HSCT include avascular necrosis, diminished bone density, and vitamin D deficiency. Vitamin D and bisphosphonates should be considered, and bone density evaluations should be performed

Cardiac
- Conduction abnormalities
- Hypertension
- Left ventricular dysfunction

Endocrine
- Dyslipidemia
- Gonadal dysfunction
- Growth hormone deficiency
- Infertility
- Primary ovarian insufficiency
- Thyroid dysfunction

Gastrointestinal
- Cytomegalovirus
- Gallstones
- Gastritis/esophagitis
- Graft-versus-host disease
- Hepatitis
- Iron overload
- Oral health impairment

Immune Reconstitution
- Late infections
- Returned by one year after transplant or longer

Integument
- Hyperpigmentation
- Hypopigmentation
- Nail loss
- Thinning hair

Musculoskeletal
- Avascular necrosis
- Contractures
- Diminished bone density
- Myositis
- Osteochondromas
- Polymyositis

Neurocognitive
- Cognitive function abnormalities
- Psychological function abnormalities

Ophthalmologic
- Blepharitis
- Cataracts
- Photophobia
- Sicca syndrome

Pulmonary
- Bronchiolitis obliterans
- Chronic bronchitis
- Hepatopulmonary syndrome
- Idiopathic pneumonia syndrome
- Pulmonary fibrosis

Renal
- Chronic kidney disease

Secondary Malignancy
- Acute myeloid leukemia
- Epithelial cancers
- Myelodysplasia
- Post-transplant lymphoproliferative disorders

Figure 7-9. Late Effects of Blood and Marrow Transplantation

Note. Based on information from Mohty & Mohty, 2011; Savani et al., 2011.

at least every two years. Use of steroids for the treatment of GVHD predisposes individuals to develop avascular necrosis, which may necessitate a surgical joint replacement. The mean time to developing this is one to two years after transplant (Savani et al., 2011). Pain and limited activity are the first signs of this disabling complication. Immune function recovery may be delayed for a year or longer with prolonged use of immunosuppressive medications and can increase the risk of developing late infections. Cognitive and psychological effects of cancer therapy have been described in both adults and children and require ongoing assessment.

Late Secondary Malignancies After Allogeneic Hematopoietic Stem Cell Transplantation

As the age and life expectancy of HSCT survivors increase, so do the risks of secondary malignancies. The cumulative incidence of secondary malignancies ranges from 2% to 6% at 10 years after HSCT (Savani et al., 2011). Post-transplant lymphoproliferative disorders (PTLDs), late relapse of primary disease, squamous cell skin and oral cancers, myelodysplastic syndrome, and acute myeloid leukemia have been described.

PTLD risk factors include HLA-mismatched transplant, positive EBV serology, and splenectomy prior to transplant. PTLDs also have been reported to occur in solid organ transplant. Presence of EBV, proliferation of B lymphocytes, and clinical features of lymphadenopathy are common findings associated with PTLDs. The mortality rate of PTLDs is high, and treatment options include rituximab, an anti-B-lymphocyte antibody (Savani et al., 2011). Strategies to predict the risk of PTLDs and careful monitoring of EBV after transplant are important considerations.

It is recommended that HSCT survivors adhere to the cancer screening guidelines for the general population. Furthermore, patients should be counseled about their higher risk for secondary malignancies (Savani et al., 2011).

Standards of Care

Several organizations have developed standards of care for HSCT programs. National and international organizations have developed guidelines for various aspects of transplant program development and the clinical care of transplant recipients. In the 1970s, IBMTR was formed to serve as a site to collect and analyze data from all participating transplant centers. The Autologous Blood and Marrow Transplant Registry (ABMTR) was formed in 1990 to accomplish similar goals in the autologous transplant setting. CIBMTR was formed to unite IBMTR, ABMTR, and NMDP. The purpose of CIBMTR is to design and conduct clinical research to promote clinical expertise in the field of transplantation. In 1996, FACT formed to promote quality medical and laboratory practice related to HSCT. Many transplant centers seek FACT accreditation. FACT standards have been developed for all aspects of the HSCT clinical program, including hematopoietic progenitor cell collection and processing, as well as the acute transplant phase of HSCT (FACT, 2012).

Implications for Oncology Advanced Practice Nurses

As scientific and clinical advancements in the field of blood and marrow transplantation continue, advancements in patient care will evolve. Over the years, the role of APNs working with HSCT recipients also has evolved. In many settings, APNs have taken on more clinical and direct patient care responsibilities that traditionally were performed by physicians, including residents and interns. The daily assessment and management of patients during the inpatient hospital stay and at outpatient visits often are coordinated by APNs. Patient continuity also is important, not only for the physical clinical outcomes and quality care but also for patients' and families' psychosocial well-being. It is critical that patients participate in medical and nursing studies. By doing so, improvement can continue in all domains of patient care that will greatly influence patient outcomes and quality of life.

Conclusion

Much advancement has occurred in the field of HSCT as a treatment for malignant and nonmalignant diseases. Although much has been learned and has positively affected both medical and nursing practice, the basic concepts of transplantation have remained the same over the years. Myeloablative and nonmyeloablative preparative regimens are used to treat a variety of diseases. Nonmyeloablative regimens offer less toxicity and mortality, thus enabling older patients and patients with some comorbid conditions to undergo transplantation. Ongoing research continues on strategies for mobilization of stem cells, use of immunosuppressive agents, prophylactic anti-infective medications, DLIs, and treatment of GVHD. Nursing management of transplant recipients remains complex and challenging. The multidisciplinary transplant team must work together to provide education to physicians, APNs, staff nurses, and other staff members to keep up to date on changes in practice related to transplantation.

Case Study

B.J. is a 44-year-old Caucasian man with a history of acute lymphocytic leukemia who is 196 days post a one-antigen–mismatched allogeneic HSCT from a sex- and ABO-mismatched graft. His conditioning regimen included TBI and etoposide. B.J.'s post-transplant course was uneventful, and he has not experienced any complications.

B.J. presents to the outpatient clinic for his scheduled every-other-month routine history and physical examination. As B.J. approaches, the APN notices he is dyspneic. After B.J. is questioned about his symptoms, he states that for approximately a month, he has experienced shortness of breath with stair climbing and walking long distances. B.J. also admits to having oral mucosa, ocular, and cutaneous dryness. Physical examination findings are significant for dry mucous membranes and skin, bilateral conjunctivitis, diminished skin turgor, and scleroderma changes of his arms bilaterally and his posterior thorax. His breath sounds are diminished, and his inspiratory effort is poor. Vital signs are as follows: temperature = 97.8°F (36.6°C), heart rate = 104 beats per minute, respiratory rate = 32 breaths per minute, blood pressure = 140/82 mm Hg, and oxygen saturation = 89% on room air. B.J. has been off his immunosuppressant medications for two months and is currently on no medications. Diagnostic studies based on his symptoms demonstrate the following: white blood cell count = 4,200/mm^3, hemoglobin = 12.6 g/dl, platelets = 148,000/mm^3, absolute neutrophil count = 3,200/mm^3, eosinophils = 18%, and chest x-ray = normal. Results of pulmonary function tests show diffusing capacity of the lung for carbon monoxide (DCLO) = 48%, forced expiratory volume in one second (FEV$_1$) = 46%, and a pattern of obstructive ventilatory defect.

1.   What differential diagnoses in this patient should the APN consider?
   • Pneumonia, because he is short of breath and has diminished breath sounds and a poor inspiratory effort; and his respiratory rate is 32 and oxygen saturation is 89%.

- Pulmonary embolism, because he complains of shortness of breath, diminished breath sounds, and poor inspiratory effort, and his respiratory rate is 32 and oxygen saturation is 89%.
- Chronic GVHD, because he is 196 days post allogeneic HSCT and complains of shortness of breath. Examination demonstrates diminished breath sounds; poor inspiratory effort; respiratory rate of 32; oxygen saturation of 89%; dry mouth, eyes, and skin; loss of skin turgor and scleroderma changes of arms and back; DLCO of 48%; FEV_1 of 46%; and pattern of obstructive ventilatory defect.
2. What other diagnostic studies could be ordered to further evaluate the patient's pulmonary condition?
   - CT of the chest
   - Arterial blood gases
   - Open lung biopsy
3. What treatment options would be initiated for chronic GVHD of the lungs, skin, mouth, and eyes?
   - Initiate immunosuppressive therapy with corticosteroids or other immunosuppressive agents.
   - Perform a skin biopsy to confirm chronic GVHD of the skin.
   - Apply steroid skin cream (i.e., triamcinolone cream).
   - Refer the patient for an ophthalmology consult.
   - Apply eye drops/ointment.
   - Provide supportive care as needed, such as home oxygen.

Key Points

- The types of transplants discussed in the chapter include autologous, allogeneic, and syngeneic HSCT.
- Types of allogeneic HSCT include sibling donor, haploidentical donor, and unrelated donor, as well as myeloablative and nonmyeloablative transplant.
- The three sources of stem cells used in HSCT are the bone marrow, peripheral blood, and umbilical cord blood.
- Malignant diseases (e.g., leukemia, lymphoma, multiple myeloma) and nonmalignant diseases are treated with HSCT.
- The process of peripheral blood stem cell mobilization and collection was described, including combinations of chemotherapy and cytokines, cytokines alone, and cytokines and chemokine antagonists.
- The steps of HSC infusion and potential side effects were discussed.
  - Autologous HSCs are cryopreserved and stored prior to transplant.
    * Adverse effects of autologous HSC infusion are related to the preservative DMSO, red blood cell contamination, or the volume of cells infused.
    * Common side effects of autologous HSCT are related to DMSO and include fever, chills, cough, nausea, vomiting, diarrhea, dyspnea, tachypnea, abdominal cramps, facial flushing, hypertension, cardiac arrhythmias, chest tightness, hemoglobinuria, and garlic-like taste in recipient's mouth.
  - Allogeneic stem cells generally are reinfused fresh.
    * Adverse effects include hives, fever, chills, rash, nausea, vomiting, flushing, shortness of breath, hypotension, hypertension, tachycardia, chest pain or tightness, and anaphylaxis.
    * Emergency equipment, including oxygen and cardiac monitoring equipment, should be readily available during infusion of HSCs.

- The day of infusion is day 0.
- Complications of HSCT include GVHD, infection, bleeding, organ toxicities (GI, hepatic, pulmonary, cardiac, renal, neurologic), late effects, and secondary malignancies.
- Clinical manifestations, prevention, and treatment of acute and chronic GVHD were described.
  - GVHD is an immune reaction that occurs between the recipient cells and immunologically competent donor T lymphocytes.
  - Acute GVHD can occur from time of engraftment until approximately day 100 post-transplant. It primarily affects the skin, liver, and upper and lower GI tract.
  - Pharmacologic approaches to prevent acute GVHD include combinations of systemic immunosuppressive medications.
  - Chronic GVHD can occur after day 100 post-transplant. It affects multiple organ systems and involves the mouth, eyes, skin, GI tract, liver, lungs, and hematopoietic system.
  - Pharmacologic (as used for acute GVHD) and nonpharmacologic approaches are used to treat chronic GVHD.
- DLIs may be given to promote conversion of recipient cells to donor cells and to achieve a GVT effect. DLI cell dose varies according to institutional practice or research protocols.
- Chimerism studies often are performed following allogeneic HSCT to determine conversion to donor cells.
  - Stem cell transplant recipients are considered to have converted to full chimerism if all of their HSCs and lymphoid cells are derived from the allogeneic donor.
  - Full chimerism is a good prognostic sign in patients who have undergone allogeneic HSCT.

Recommended Resources for Oncology Advanced Practice Nurses

A plethora of guidelines are available regarding numerous aspects related to HSCT. The following resources contain evidence-based information that is readily available and can be used in the clinical setting.
- AABB: www.aabb.org
- American Society for Blood and Marrow Transplantation: www.asbmt.org
- Centers for Disease Control and Prevention: www.cdc.gov
- CIBMTR: www.cibmtr.org
- FACT: www.factwebsite.org
- National Comprehensive Cancer Network®: www.nccn.org
- NMDP/Be The Match: www.nmdp.org; https://bethematchclinical.org

The author would like to acknowledge Susan A. Ezzone, MS, RN, CNP, AOCNP®, for her contribution to this chapter that remains unchanged from the first edition of this book.

References

AABB, American Red Cross, America's Blood Centers, & Armed Services Blood Program. (2013). *Circular of information for the use of human blood and blood components.* Retrieved from http://www.aabb.org/resources/bct/Documents/coi0413.pdf

Aisa, Y., Mori, T., Kato, J., Yamane, A., Kohashi, S., Kikuchi, T., & Okamoto, S. (2013). Validation of NIH consensus criteria for diagnosis and severity-grading of chronic graft-versus-host disease. *International Journal of Hematology, 97,* 263–271. doi:10.1007/s12185-013-1268-1

Amgen Inc. (2013). *Neupogen® (filgrastim)* [Package insert]. Thousand Oaks, CA: Author.

Anasetti, C., Aversa, F., & Brunstein, C.G. (2012). Back to the future: Mismatched unrelated donor, haploidentical related donor, or unrelated umbilical cord blood transplantation? *Biology of Blood and Marrow Transplantation, 18*(Suppl. 1), S161–S165. doi:10.1016/j.bbmt.2011.11.004

Antin, J.H., Childs, R., Filipovich, A.H., Giralt, S., Mackinnon, S., Spitzer, T., & Weisdorf, D. (2001). Establishment of complete and mixed donor chimerism after allogeneic lymphohematopoietic transplantation: Recommendations from a workshop at the 2001 Tandem Meetings. *Biology of Blood and Marrow Transplantation, 7,* 473–485. doi:10.1053/bbmt.2001.v7.pm11669214

Bacigalupo, A., Ballen, K., Rizzo, D., Giralt, S., Lazarus, H., Ho, V., … Horowitz, M. (2009). Defining the intensity of conditioning regimens: Working definitions. *Biology of Blood and Marrow Transplantation, 15,* 1628–1633. doi:10.1016/j.bbmt.2009.07.004

Barker, J.N., Weisdorf, D.J., DeFor, T.E., Blazar, B.R., McGlave, P.B., Miller, J.S., … Wagner, J.E. (2005). Transplantation of 2 partially HLA-matched umbilical cord blood units to enhance engraftment in adults with hematologic malignancy. *Blood, 105,* 1343–1347. doi:10.1182/blood-2004-07-2717

Barnes, D.W.H., & Loutit, J.F. (1957). Treatment of murine leukaemia with X-rays and homologous bone marrow: II. *British Journal of Haematology, 3,* 241–252. doi:10.1111/j.1365-2141.1957.tb05793.x

Bensinger, W.I., DiPersio, J.F., & McCarty, J.M. (2009). Improving stem cell mobilization strategies: Future directions. *Bone Marrow Transplantation, 43,* 181–195. doi:10.1038/bmt.2008.410

Bensinger, W.I., Martin, P.J., Storer, B., Clift, R., Forman, S.J., Negrin, R., … Appelbaum, F.R. (2001). Transplantation of bone marrow as compared with peripheral-blood cells from HLA-identical relatives in patients with hematologic cancers. *New England Journal of Medicine, 344,* 175–181. doi:10.1056/NEJM200101183440303

Bernstein, I.D., Boyd, R.L., & van den Brink, M.R.M. (2008). Clinical strategies to enhance post-transplant immune reconstitution. *Biology of Blood and Marrow Transplantation, 14*(Suppl. 1), 94–99. doi:10.1016/j.bbmt.2007.10.003

Berz, D., McCormack, E.M., Winer, E.S., Colvin, G.A., & Quesenberry, P.J. (2007). Cryopreservation of hematopoietic stem cells. *American Journal of Hematology, 82,* 463–472. doi:10.1002/ajh.20707

Bray, R.A., Hurley, C.K., Kamani, N.R., Woolfrey, A., Müller, C., Spellman, S., … Confer, D.L. (2008). National Marrow Donor Program HLA matching guidelines for unrelated adult donor hematopoietic cell transplants. *Biology of Blood and Marrow Transplantation, 14*(Suppl. 9), 45–53. doi:10.1016/j.bbmt.2008.06.014

Brunstein, C.G., Barker, J.N., Weisdorf, D.J., DeFor, T.E., Miller, J.S., Blazar, B.R., … Wagner, J.E. (2007). Umbilical cord blood transplantation after nonmyeloablative conditioning: Impact on transplantation outcomes in 110 adults with hematologic disease. *Blood, 110,* 3064–3070. doi:10.1182/blood-2007-04-067215

Burt, R.K., Balabanov, R., Han, X., Sharrack, B., Morgan, A., Quigley, K., … Burman, J. (2015). Association of nonmyeloablative hematopoietic stem cell transplantation with neurological disability in patients with relapsing-remitting multiple sclerosis. *JAMA, 313,* 275–284. doi:10.1001/jama.2014.17986

Burt, R.K., Testori, A., Craig, R., Cohen, B., Suffit, R., & Barr, W. (2008). Hematopoietic stem cell transplantation for autoimmune diseases: What have we learned? *Journal of Autoimmunity, 30,* 116–120. doi:10.1016/j.jaut.2007.12.010

Cahn, J.-Y., Klein, J.P., Lee, S.J., Milpied, N., Blaise, D., Antin, J.H., … Socié, G. (2005). Prospective evaluation of 2 acute graft-versus-host (GVHD) grading systems: A joint Société Française de Greffe de Moëlle et Thérapie Cellulaire (SFGM-TC), Dana Farber Cancer Institute (DFCI), and International Bone Marrow Transplant Registry (IBMTR) prospective study. *Blood, 106,* 1495–1500. doi:10.1182/blood-2004-11-4557

Carson, J.L., Grossman, B.J., Kleinman, S., Tinmouth, A.T., Marques, M.B., Fung, M.K., … Djulbegovic, B. (2012). Red blood cell transfusion: A clinical practice guideline from the AABB. *Annals of Internal Medicine, 157,* 49–58. doi:10.7326/0003-4819-157-1-201206190-00429

Chepovetsky, J., Yoon, S.C., Blouin, A.G., Tindle, S., Bertinelli, A., Nash, E., & Wu, D.W. (2013). Roles of peripheral blood CD34+ cell count and midpoint collection CD34+ cell yield for peripheral blood stem cell collections from autologous patients mobilized by G-CSF and plerixafor. *North American Journal of Medicine and Science, 6*(2), 63–70. Retrieved from http://najms.net/v06i02p063a

Clayberger, C., & Krensky, A.M. (2005). T-cell and NK cell immunity. In R. Hoffman, E.J. Benz Jr., S.J. Shattil, B. Furie, H.J. Cohen, L.E. Silberstein, & P. McGlave (Eds.), *Hematology: Basic principles and practice* (4th ed., pp. 135–149). Philadelphia, PA: Elsevier Churchill Livingstone.

Copelan, E.A. (2006). Hematopoietic stem-cell transplantation. *New England Journal of Medicine, 354,* 1813–1826. doi:10.1056/NEJMra052638

Cox, M.A., Kastrup, J., & Hrubiško, M. (2012). Historical perspectives and the future of adverse reactions associated with haemopoietic stem cells cryopreserved with dimethyl sulfoxide. *Cell and Tissue Banking, 13,* 203–215. doi:10.1007/s10561-011-9248-2

Danby, R., & Rocha, V. (2014). Improving engraftment and immune reconstitution in umbilical cord blood transplantation. *Frontiers in Immunology, 5,* 68. doi:10.3389/fimmu.2014.00068

Daniele, N., Scerpa, M.C., Caniglia, M., Ciammetti, C., Rossi, C., Bernardo, M.E., … Zinno, F. (2012). Overview of T-cell depletion in haploidentical stem cell transplantation. *Blood Transfusion, 10,* 264–272. doi:10.2450/2012.0106-11

de la Morena, M.T., & Gatti, R.A. (2011). A history of bone marrow transplantation. *Hematology/Oncology Clinics of North America, 25,* 1–15. doi:10.1016/j.hoc.2010.11.001

del Campo, L.D., León, N.G., Palacios, D.C., Lagana, C., & Tagarro, D. (2014). Abdominal complications following hematopoietic stem cell transplantation. *RadioGraphics, 34,* 396–412. doi:10.1148/rg.342135046

Delves, P.J., & Roitt, I.M. (2000a). The immune system, part 1. *New England Journal of Medicine, 343,* 37–49. doi:10.1056/NEJM200007063430107

Delves, P.J., & Roitt, I.M. (2000b). The immune system, part 2. *New England Journal of Medicine, 343,* 108–117. doi:10.1056/NEJM200007133430207

Devine, H. (2013). Overview of hematopoiesis and immunology: Implications for hematopoietic stem cell transplantation In S.A. Ezzone (Ed.), *Hematopoietic stem cell transplantation: A manual for nursing practice* (2nd ed., pp. 1–11). Pittsburgh, PA: Oncology Nursing Society.

Devine, H., Tierney, D.K., Schmit-Pokorny, K., & McDermott, K. (2010). Mobilization of hematopoietic stem cells for use in autologous transplantation. *Clinical Journal of Oncology Nursing, 14,* 212–222. doi:10.1188/10.CJON.212-222

Devine, S.M., Carter, S., Soiffer, R.J., Pasquini, M.C., Hari, P.N., Stein, A., … O'Reilly, R.J. (2011). Low risk of chronic graft-versus-host disease and relapse associated with T cell–depleted peripheral blood stem cell transplantation for acute myelogenous leukemia in first remission: Results of the Blood and Marrow Transplant Clinical Trials Network Protocol 0303. *Biology of Blood and Marrow Transplantation, 17,* 1343–1351. doi:10.1016/j.bbmt.2011.02.002

Devine, S.M., Vij, R., Rettig, M., Todt, L., McGlauchlen, K., Fisher, N., … DiPersio, J.F. (2008). Rapid mobilization of functional donor hematopoietic cells without G-CSF using AMD3100, an antagonist of the CXCR4/SDF-1 interaction. *Blood, 112,* 990–998. doi:10.1182/blood-2007-12-130179

Dinarello, C.A. (2007). Historical insights into cytokines. *European Journal of Immunology, 37*(Suppl. 1), S34–S45. doi:10.1002/eji.200737772

DiPersio, J.F., Micallef, I.N., Stiff, P.J., Bolwell, B.J., Maziarz, R.T., Jacobsen, E., … Calandra, G. (2009). Phase III prospective randomized double-blind placebo-controlled trial of plerixafor plus granulocyte colony-stimulating factor compared with placebo plus granulocyte colony-stimulating factor for autologous stem-cell mobilization and transplantation for patients with non-Hodgkin's lymphoma. *Journal of Clinical Oncology, 27,* 4767–4773. doi:10.1200/JCO.2008.20.7209

DiPersio, J.F., Stadtmauer, E.A., Nademanee, A., Micallef, I.N., Stiff, P.J., Kaufman, J.L., … Calandra, G. (2009). Plerixafor and G-CSF versus placebo and G-CSF to mobilize hematopoietic stem cells for autologous stem cell transplantation in patients with multiple myeloma. *Blood, 113,* 5720–5726. doi:10.1182/blood-2008-08-174946

D'Rozario, J., Parisotto, R., Stapleton, J., Gidley, A., & Owen, D. (2014). Pre infusion, post thaw CD34+ peripheral blood stem cell enumeration as a predictor of haematopoietic engraftment in autologous haematopoietic cell transplantation. *Transfusion and Apheresis Science, 50,* 443–450. doi:10.1016/j.transci.2014.02.021

Erkurt, M.A., Berber, I., Kuku, I., Kaya, E., & Nizam, I. (2014). Donor selection in allogeneic stem cell transplantation. *American Journal of Clinical Medicine Research, 2,* 32–35. doi:10.12691/ajcmr-2-1-8. doi:10.12691/ajcmr-2-1-8

Fabricious-Moeller, J. (1922). *Experimental studies of hemorrhagic diathesis from X-ray sickness.* Copenhagen, Denmark: Levin and Munksgaard.

Fagioli, F., Quarello, P., Pollichieni, S., Lamparelli, T., Berger, M., Benedetti, F., … Sacchi, N. (2014). Quality of harvest and role of cell dose in unrelated bone marrow transplantation: An Italian Bone Marrow Donor Registry–Gruppo Italiano Trapianto di Midollo Osseo Study. *Hematology, 19,* 1–9. doi:10.1179/1607845413Y.0000000086

Ferrara, J.L., Levine, J.E., Reddy, P., & Holler, E. (2009). Graft-versus-host disease. *Lancet, 373,* 1550–1561. doi:10.1016/S0140-6736(09)60237-3

Filipovich, A.H., Weisdorf, D., Pavletic, S., Socie, G., Wingard, J.R., Lee, S.J., … Flowers, M.E.D. (2005). National Institutes of Health consensus development project on criteria for clinical trials in chronic graft-versus-host disease: I. Diagnosis and Staging Working Group report. *Biology of Blood and Marrow Transplantation, 11,* 945–956. doi:10.1016/j.bbmt.2005.09.004

Fouillard, L., Labopin, M., Gratwohl, A., Gluckman, E., Frassoni, F., Beelen, D.W., … Rocha, V. (2008). Results of syngeneic hematopoietic stem cell transplantation for acute leukemia: Risk factors for outcomes of adults transplanted in first complete remission. *Haematologica, 93,* 834–841. doi:10.3324/haematol.11277

Foundation for the Accreditation of Cellular Therapy. (2012). *FACT-JACIE international standards for cellular therapy product collection, processing and administration* (5th ed.). Omaha, NE: Author.

Gassas, A., Ashraf, K., Zaidman, I., Ali, M., Krueger, J., Doyle, J., … Leucht, S. (2015). Hematopoietic stem cell transplantation in infants. *Pediatric Blood and Cancer, 62,* 517–521. doi:10.1002/pbc.25333

Gatti, R.A., Meuwissen, H.J., Allen, H.D., Hong, R., & Good, R.A. (1968). Immunological reconstitution of sex-linked lymphopenic immunological deficiency. *Lancet, 292,* 1366–1369. doi:10.1016/S0140-6736(68)92673-1

Genzyme Corp. (2013). *Mozobil® (plerixafor)* [Package insert]. Cambridge, MA: Author.

Gluckman, E., Broxmeyer, H.E., Auerbach, A.D., Friedman, H.S., Douglas, G.W., Devergie, A., … Boyse, E.A. (1989). Hematopoietic reconstitution in a patient with Fanconi's anemia by means of umbilical-cord blood from an HLA-identical sibling. *New England Journal of Medicine, 321,* 1174–1178. doi:10.1056/NEJM198910263211707

Gluckman, E., Rocha, V., Boyer-Chammard, A., Locatelli, F., Arcese, W., Pasquini, R., … Chastang, C. (1997). Outcome of cord-blood transplantation from related and unrelated donors. Eurocord Transplant Group and the European Blood and Marrow Transplantation Group. *New England Journal of Medicine, 337,* 373–381. doi:10.1056/NEJM199708073370602

Glucksberg, H., Storb, R., Fefer, A., Buckner, C.D., Neiman, P.E., Clift, R.A., … Thomas, E.D. (1974). Clinical manifestations of graft-versus-host disease in human recipients of marrow from HL-A-matched sibling donors. *Transplantation, 18,* 295–304. doi:10.1097/00007890-197410000-00001

Gratwohl, A., Pasquini, M.C., Aljurf, M., Atsuta, Y., Baldomero, H., Foeken, L., … Niederwieser, D. (2015). One million haemopoietic stem-cell transplants: A retrospective observational study. *Lancet Haematology, 2,* e91–e100. doi:10.1016/S2352-3026(15)00028-9

Gutcher, I., & Becher, B. (2007). APC-derived cytokines and T cell polarization in autoimmune inflammation. *Journal of Clinical Investigation, 117,* 1119–1127. doi:10.1172/JCI31720

Hunt, K.J., Walsh, B.M., Voegeli, D., & Roberts, H.C. (2010). Inflammation in aging, part I: Physiological and immunological mechanisms. *Biological Research for Nursing, 11,* 245–252. doi:10.1177/1099800409352237

Jiang, H., & Chess, L. (2004). An integrated view of suppressor T cell subsets in immunoregulation. *Journal of Clinical Investigation, 114,* 1198–1208. doi:10.1172/JCI200423411

Jiménez, M., Ercilla, G., & Martínez, C. (2007). Immune reconstitution after allogeneic stem cell transplantation with reduced-intensity conditioning regimens. *Leukemia, 21,* 1628–1637. doi:10.1038/sj.leu.2404681

Johnson, N.L. (2013). Ocular graft-versus-host disease after allogeneic transplantation. *Clinical Journal of Oncology Nursing, 17,* 621–626. doi:10.1188/13.CJON.621-626

Kanda, J., Ichinohe, T., Matsuo, K., Benjamin, R.J., Klumpp, T.R., Rozman, P., … Uchiyama, T. (2009). Impact of ABO mismatching on the outcomes of allogeneic related and unrelated blood and marrow stem cell transplantations for hematologic malignancies: IPD based meta-analysis of cohort studies. *Transfusion, 49,* 624–635. doi:10.1111/j.1537-2995.2008.02043.x

Kedia, S., Acharya, P.S., Mohammad, F., Nguyen, H., Asti, D., Mehta, S., … Mobarakai, N. (2013). Infectious complications of hematopoietic stem cell transplantation. *Journal of Stem Cell Research and Therapy.* doi:10.4172/2157-7633.S3-002

Kersey, J.H. (2004). Historical background to hematopoietic stem cell transplantation. In K. Atkinson, R. Champlin, J. Ritz, P.W.E. Fibble, P. Ljungman, & M. Brenner (Eds.), *Clinical bone marrow and blood cell transplantation* (3rd ed., pp. 1–10). Cambridge, United Kingdom: Cambridge University Press.

Kimura, F., Sato, K., Kobayashi, S., Ikeda, T., Sao, H., Okamoto, S., … Ashida, H. (2008). Stem cell transplantation-impact of ABO-blood group incompatibility on the outcome of recipients of bone marrow transplants from unrelated donors in the Japan Marrow Donor Program. *Haematologica, 93,* 1686–1693. doi:10.3324/haematol.12933

Kollman, C., Howe, C.W., Anasetti, C., Antin, J.H., Davies, S.M., Filipovich, A.H., … Confer, D.L. (2001). Donor characteristics as risk factors in recipients after transplantation of bone marrow from unrelated donors: The effect of donor age. *Blood, 98,* 2043–2051. doi:10.1182/blood.V98.7.2043

Körbling, M., & Anderlini, P. (2001). Peripheral blood stem cell versus bone marrow allotransplantation: Does the source of hematopoietic stem cells matter? *Blood, 98,* 2900–2908. doi:10.1182/blood.V98.10.2900

Kuzmina, Z., Eder, S., Böhm, A., Pernicka, E., Vormittag, L., Kalhs, P., … Greinix, H.T. (2012). Significantly worse survival of patients with NIH-defined chronic graft-versus-host disease and thrombocytopenia or progressive onset type: Results of a prospective study. *Leukemia, 26,* 746–756. doi:10.1038/leu.2011.257

Lee, S., & Margolin, K. (2011). Cytokines in cancer immunotherapy. *Cancers, 3,* 3856–3893. doi:10.3390/cancers3043856

Lewontin, R. (2011). The genotype/phenotype distinction. In *The Stanford encyclopedia of philosophy.* Retrieved from http://plato.stanford.edu/archives/sum2011/entries/genotype-phenotype

Liang, R. (2009). How I treat and monitor viral hepatitis B infection in patients receiving intensive immunosuppressive therapies or undergoing hematopoietic stem cell transplantation. *Blood, 113,* 3147–3153. doi:10.1182/blood-2008-10-163493

Liu, H. (2013). Prophylactic donor lymphocyte infusion to prevent relapse after allogeneic stem cell transplantation. *Journal of Clinical and Medical Case Reports, 1*(1), 3. Retrieved from http://fulltextarticles.avensonline.org/jcmcr-2332-4120-01-0002.html

Liu, Q., Lin, R., Liu, C., Wu, M., Xuan, L., Jiang, X., … Sun, J. (2013, December). Epstein-Barr virus infection in recipient of allogeneic hematopoietic stem cell transplantation: The role of cytomegalovirus (Abstract No. 4555). Abstract presented at the 55th ASH Annual Meeting and Exposition, New Orleans, LA. Retrieved from https://ash.confex.com/ash/2013/webprogram/Paper60324.html

Loren, A.W., Bunin, G.R., Boudreau, C., Champlin, R.E., Cnaan, A., Horowitz, M.M., … Porter, D.L. (2006). Impact of donor and recipient sex and parity on outcomes of HLA-identical sibling allogeneic hematopoietic stem cell transplantation. *Biology of Blood and Marrow Transplantation, 12,* 758–769. doi:10.1016/j.bbmt.2006.03.015

Lorenz, E., Uphoff, D.E., Reid, T.R., & Shelton, E. (1951). Modification of irradiation injury in mice and guinea pigs by bone marrow injections. *Journal of the National Cancer Institute, 12,* 197–201.

Manz, M.G., Akashi, K., & Weissman, I.L. (2004). Biology of hematopoietic stem and progenitor cells. In K.G. Blume, S.J. Forman, & F.R. Appelbaum (Eds.), *Thomas' hematopoietic cell transplantation* (3rd ed., pp. 69–95). Malden, MA: Blackwell.

Martin, P.J., Rizzo, J.D., Wingard, J.R., Ballen, K., Curtin, P.T., Cutler, C., … Carpenter, P.A. (2012). First- and second-line systemic treatment of acute graft-versus-host disease: Recommendations of the American Society of Blood and Marrow Transplantation. *Biology of Blood and Marrow Transplantation, 18,* 1150–1163. doi:10.1016/j.bbmt.2012.04.005

Mathé, G. (1968). Bone marrow transplantation. In F.T. Rappaport & J. Dausset (Eds.), *Human transplantation* (pp. 284–303). New York, NY: Grune and Stratton.

Mickelson, D.M., Sproat, L., Dean, R., Sobecks, R., Rybicki, L., Kalaycio, M., … Copelan, E.A. (2011). Comparison of donor chimerism following myeloablative and nonmyeloablative allogeneic hematopoietic SCT. *Bone Marrow Transplantation, 46,* 84–89. doi:10.1038/bmt.2010.55

Mickelson, E., & Petersdorf, E.W. (2009). Histocompatibility. In F.R. Appelbaum, S.J. Forman, R.S. Negrin, & K.G. Blume (Eds.), *Thomas' hematopoietic cell transplantation: Stem cell transplantation* (4th ed., pp. 145–162). Oxford, United Kingdom: Wiley-Blackwell.

Mohty, B., & Mohty, M. (2011). Long-term complications and side effects after allogeneic hematopoietic stem cell transplantation: An update. *Blood Cancer Journal, 1,* e16. doi:10.1038/bcj.2011.14

Nannya, Y., Kataoka, K., Hangaishi, A., Imai, Y., Takahashi, T., & Kurokawa, M. (2011). The negative impact of female donor/male recipient combination in allogeneic hematopoietic stem cell transplantation depends on disease risk. *Transplant International, 24,* 469–476. doi:10.1111/j.1432-2277.2011.01229.x

National Cancer Institute Cancer Therapy Evaluation Program. (2010). *Common terminology criteria for adverse events* [v.4.03]. Retrieved from http://ctep.cancer.gov/protocolDevelopment/electronic_applications/ctc.htm

National Marrow Donor Program. (n.d.). Disease-specific HCT indications and outcomes data. Retrieved from https://bethematchclinical.org/transplant-indications-and-outcomes/disease-specific-indications-and-outcomes

Nishiguchi, T., Mochizuki, K., Shakudo, M., Takeshita, T., Hino, M., & Inoue, Y. (2009). CNS complications of hematopoietic stem cell transplantation. *American Journal of Roentgenology, 192,* 1003–1011. doi:10.2214/AJR.08.1787

O'Donghaile, D., Kelley, W., Klein, H.G., & Flegel, W.A. (2012). Recommendations for transfusion in ABO-incompatible hematopoietic stem cell transplantation. *Transfusion, 52,* 456–458. doi:10.1111/j.1537-2995.2011.03465.x

Oran, B., & Shpall, E. (2012). Umbilical cord blood transplantation: A maturing technology. *Hematology: American Society of Hematology Education Program Book, 2012,* 215–222. doi:10.1182/asheducation-2012.1.215

Park, M., & Seo, J.J. (2012). Role of HLA in hematopoietic stem cell transplantation. *Bone Marrow Research, 2012,* Article ID 680841. doi:10.1155/2012/680841

Parkin, J., & Cohen, B. (2001). An overview of the immune system. *Lancet, 357,* 1777–1789. doi:10.1016/S0140-6736(00)04904-7

Pasquini, M.C., Devine, S., Mendizabal, A., Baden, L.R., Wingard, J.R., Lazarus, H.M., … Soiffer, R.J. (2012). Comparative outcomes of donor graft CD34+ selection and immune suppressive therapy as graft-versus-host disease prophylaxis for patients with acute myeloid leukemia in complete remission undergoing HLA-matched sibling allogeneic hematopoietic cell transplantation. *Journal of Clinical Oncology, 30,* 3194–3201. doi:10.1200/JCO.2012.41.7071

Pasquini, M.C., & Zhu, X. (2014). Current uses and outcomes of hematopoietic stem cell transplantation: 2014 CIBMTR summary slides. Retrieved from http://www.cibmtr.org/ReferenceCenter/SlidesReports/SummarySlides/Pages/index.aspx

Pavletic, S.Z., & Fowler, D.H. (2012). Are we making progress in GVHD prophylaxis and treatment? *Hematology: American Society of Hematology Education Program Book, 2012,* 251–264. doi:10.1182/asheducation-2012.1.251

Pavletic, S.Z., Lee, S.J., Socie, G., & Vogelsang, G. (2006). Chronic graft-versus-host disease: Implications of the National Institutes of Health consensus development project on criteria for clinical trials. *Bone Marrow Transplantation, 38,* 645–651. doi:10.1038/sj.bmt.1705490

Petersdorf, E.W. (2013). Genetics of graft-versus-host disease: The major histocompatibility complex. *Blood Reviews, 27,* 1–12. doi:10.1016/j.blre.2012.10.001

Przepiorka, D., Weisdorf, D., Martin, P., Klingemann, H.G., Beatty, P., Hows, J., & Thomas, E.D. (1995). 1994 Consensus Conference on Acute GVHD Grading. *Bone Marrow Transplantation, 15,* 825–828.

Raza, A., & Vierling, J.M. (2014). Graft-versus-host disease. In M.E. Gershwin, J.M. Vierling, & M.P. Manns (Eds.), *Liver immunology: Principles and practice* (2nd ed., pp. 425–441). doi:10.1007/978-3-319-02096-9_29

Reed, M., Yearsley, M., Krugh, D., & Kennedy, M. (2003). Severe hemolysis due to passenger lymphocyte syndrome after hematopoietic stem cell transplantation from an HLA-matched related donor. *Archives of Pathology and Laboratory Medicine, 127,* 1366–1368. Retrieved from http://www.archivesofpathology.org/doi/full/10.1043/1543-2165(2003)127%3C1366:SHDTPL%3E2.0.CO;2

Reshef, R., Luger, S.M., Hexner, E.O., Loren, A.W., Frey, N.V., Nasta, S.D., … Porter, D.L. (2012). Blockade of lymphocyte chemotaxis in visceral graft-versus-host disease. *New England Journal of Medicine, 367,* 135–145. doi:10.1056/NEJMoa1201248

Rocha, V., & Gluckman, E. (2009). Improving outcomes of cord blood transplantation: HLA matching, cell dose and other graft-and transplantation-related factors. *British Journal of Haematology, 147,* 262–274. doi:10.1111/j.1365-2141.2009.07883.x

Rogosheske, J.R., Fargen, A.D., DeFor, T.E., Warlick, E., Arora, M., Blazar, B.R., … Brunstein, C.G. (2014). Higher therapeutic CsA levels early post transplantation reduce risk of acute GVHD and improves survival. *Bone Marrow Transplantation, 49,* 122–125. doi:10.1038/bmt.2013.139

Rubio-Augusti, I., & Bataller, L. (2012). Neurologic complications of hematopoietic stem cell transplantation. *European Association of NeuroOncology Magazine, 2,* 78–83.

Sallusto, F., Geginat, J., & Lanzavecchia, A. (2004). Central memory and effector memory T cell subsets: Function, generation, and maintenance. *Annual Review of Immunology, 22,* 745–763. doi:10.1146/annurev.immunol.22.012703.104702

Sallusto, F., Lenig, D., Förster, R., Lipp, M., & Lanzavecchia, A. (1999). Two subsets of memory T lymphocytes with distinct homing potentials and effector functions. *Nature, 401,* 708–712. doi:10.1038/44385

Savani, B.N., Griffith, M.L., Jagasia, S., & Lee, S.J. (2011). How I treat late effects in adults after allogeneic stem cell transplantation. *Blood, 117,* 3002–3009. doi:10.1182/blood-2010-10-263095

Schmidt-Hieber, M., Labopin, M., Beelen, D., Volin, L., Ehninger, G., Finke, J., … Mohty, M. (2013). CMV serostatus still has an important prognostic impact in de novo acute leukemia patients after allogeneic stem cell transplantation: A report from the Acute Leukemia Working Party of EBMT. *Blood, 122,* 3359–3364. doi:10.1182/blood-2013-05-499830

Sengsayadeth, S.M., Srivastava, S., Jagasia, M., & Savani, B.N. (2012). Time to explore preventive and novel therapies for bronchiolitis obliterans syndrome after allogeneic hematopoietic stem cell transplantation. *Biology of Blood and Marrow Transplantation, 18,* 1479–1487. doi:10.1016/j.bbmt.2012.03.008

Shaikh, P.Z. (2011). Cytokines and their physiologic and pharmacologic functions in inflammation: A review. *International Journal of Pharmacy and Life Sciences, 2,* 1247–1263. Retrieved from http://www.ijplsjournal.com/issues%20PDF%20files/nov2011/11.pdf

Shi, M., Li, M., & Ikehara, S. (2013). Novel conditioning regimens for bone marrow transplantation. *Blood and Lymphatic Cancer: Targets and Therapy, 3,* 1–9. doi:10.2147/BLCTT.S26390

Singh, N., McNeely, J., Parikh, S., Bhinder, A., Rovin, B.H., & Shidham, G. (2013). Kidney complications of hematopoietic stem cell transplantation. *American Journal of Kidney Diseases, 61,* 809–821. doi:10.1053/j.ajkd.2012.09.020

Sorasio, R., Bonferroni, M., Grasso, M., Strola, G., Rapezzi, D., Marenchino, D., … Gallamini, A. (2014). Peripheral blood CD34+ percentage at hematological recovery after chemotherapy is a good early predictor of harvest: A single-center experience. *Biology of Blood and Marrow Transplantation, 20,* 717–723. doi:10.1016/j.bbmt.2014.02.002

Spitzer, T.R., Dey, B.R., Chen, Y.-B., Attar, E., & Ballen, K.K. (2012). The expanding frontier of hematopoietic cell transplantation. *Cytometry, 82B,* 271–279. doi:10.1002/cyto.b.21034

Storek, J., Geddes, M., Khan, F., Huard, B., Helg, C., Chalandon, Y., … Roosnek, E. (2008). Reconstitution of the immune system after hematopoietic stem cell transplantation in humans. *Seminars in Immunopathology, 30,* 425–437. doi:10.1007/s00281-008-0132-5

Sureda, A., Bader, P., Cesaro, S., Dreger, P., Duarte, R.F., Dufour, C., … Madrigal, A. (2015). Indications for allo- and auto-SCT for haematological diseases, solid tumours and immune disorders: Current practice in Europe, 2015. *Bone Marrow Transplantation.* Advance online publication. doi:10.1038/bmt.2015.6

Thomas, E.D. (1999). Bone marrow transplantation: A review. *Seminars in Hematology, 36*(Suppl. 7), 95–103.

Thomas, E.D. (2000). Bone marrow transplantation: A historical review. *Medicina, 33,* 209–218.

Thomas, E.D., Buckner, C.D., Banaji, M., Clift, R.A., Fefer, A., Flournoy, N., … Weiden, P.L. (1977). One hundred patients with acute leukemia treated by chemotherapy, total body irradiation, and allogeneic marrow transplantation. *Blood, 49,* 511–533. Retrieved from http://www.bloodjournal.org/content/49/4/511.long

Thomas, E.D., Flournoy, N., Buckner, C.D., Clift, R.A., Fefer, A., Neiman, P.E., & Storb, R. (1977). Cure of leukemia by marrow transplantation. *Leukemia Research, 1,* 67–70. doi:10.1016/0145-2126(77)90065-0

Thomas, E.D., Lochte, H.L., Jr., Cannon, J.H., Sahler, O.D., & Ferrebee, J.W. (1959). Supralethal whole body irradiation and isologous marrow transplantation in man. *Journal of Clinical Investigation, 38,* 1709–1716. doi:10.1172/JCI103949

Thomas, E.D., Lochte, H.L., Jr., Lu, W.C., & Ferrebee, J.W. (1957). Intravenous infusion of bone marrow in patients receiving radiation and chemotherapy. *New England Journal of Medicine, 257,* 491–496. doi:10.1056/NEJM195709122571102

Thomas, E.D., Storb, R., Clift, R.A., Fefer, A., Johnson, F.L., Neiman, P.E., ... Buckner, C.D. (1975). Bone-marrow transplantation. *New England Journal of Medicine, 292,* 895–902. doi:10.1056/NEJM197504242921706

Tomblyn, M., Chiller, T., Einsele, H., Gress, R., Sepkowitz, K., Storek, J., ... Boeckh, M.J. (2009). Guidelines for preventing infectious complications among hematopoietic cell transplantation recipients: A global perspective. *Biology of Blood and Marrow Transplantation, 15,* 1143–1238. doi:10.1016/j.bbmt.2009.06.019

U.S. Department of Health and Human Services Health Resources and Services Administration. (2012). Bone marrow and cord blood donation and transplantation. Retrieved from http://bloodcell.transplant.hrsa.gov/index.html

Wandt, H., Schaefer-Eckart, K., Wendelin, K., Pilz, B., Wilhelm, M., Thalheimer, M., ... Ehninger, G. (2012). Therapeutic platelet transfusion versus routine prophylactic transfusion in patients with haematological malignancies: An open-label, multicentre, randomised study. *Lancet, 380,* 1309–1316. doi:10.1016/S0140-6736(12)60689-8

Zakrzewski, J.L., Holland, A.M., & van den Brink, M.R.M. (2007). Adoptive precursor cell therapy to enhance immune reconstitution after hematopoietic stem cell transplantation. *Journal of Molecular Medicine, 85,* 837–843. doi:10.1007/s00109-007-0175-4

Zhang, P., Chen, B.J., & Chao, N.J. (2011). Prevention of GVHD without losing GVL effect: Windows of opportunity. *Immunologic Research, 49,* 49–55. doi:10.1007/s12026-010-8193-7

Ziegler-Heitbrock, L. (2007). The CD14+ CD16+ blood monocytes: Their role in infection and inflammation. *Journal of Leukocyte Biology, 81,* 584–592. doi:10.1189/jlb.0806510

CHAPTER 8

Complementary and Integrative Therapies

Colleen O. Lee, MS, ANP-BC, AOCN®, CLNC

Introduction

Many definitions abound in the growing health trend of complementary and integrative therapies. Complementary and alternative medicine (CAM) is a broad domain of resources that surrounds the modalities, practices, and health belief systems and their associated theories that differ from those of the surrounding society or culture within a historical period of time (Institute of Medicine Committee on the Use of Complementary and Alternative Medicine by the American Public, 2005). *Complementary* medicine modalities are used alongside conventional medicine, whereas *alternative* medicine modalities are used instead of conventional medicine. Some modalities are considered both complementary and alternative. *Conventional medicine* is medicine that is practiced by medical doctors, osteopaths, and allied health professionals and also is termed *allopathic* or *Western* medicine. Conventional approaches, known as *standard*, *traditional*, or *biomedical* approaches, are those that historically have seen broad application in the United States since the 1800s.

Integrative medicine (IM), or *integrative health care*, is the combination of complementary and conventional approaches (National Center for Complementary and Integrative Health [NCCIH], 2014). IM emphasizes the therapeutic relationship, and neither rejects conventional medicine nor accepts alternative therapies without critical consideration (Weil, 2014b). Increased public acceptance of IM is attributed to its focus on health promotion versus disease prevention, as well as access to lower-cost, evidence-based therapies believed to be as good as or better than conventional approaches (Weil, 2014a).

Integrative oncology (IO) is possibly a "next step" in the evolution of cancer care. IO incorporates the successful outcomes of conventional approaches that maintain an evidence base and expands the focus of cancer care in several ways (Mumber, 2006a). IO (a) considers body, mind, soul, and spirit within cultural groups, (b) renews the focus of medicine back to its foundational guiding principles, (c) expands the goal of intervention to include translational, preventive, and supportive medicine, and (d) includes the development of recommendations based on therapy goals and individual risk-benefit analyses (Mumber, 2006b). As a discipline that seeks to blend conventional and complementary care, its goal is to increase the efficacy of conventional cancer treatment programs, reduce symptoms, and improve quality of life for patients with cancer. Although a formal definition has not been established, CAM practitioners generally are thought to be individuals who deliver CAM modalities as part of or all of their practice. They may hold state, national, or certifying body licensure and may practice across multiple settings. CAM researchers, likewise, generally are thought to be individuals who embrace an interest in developing theoretical frameworks and sound methodology for the investigation of CAM modalities in preclinical and clinical settings as part of or all of their research endeavors.

The main categories of CAM therapies are (a) alternative medical systems, (b) energy therapies, (c) exercise therapies, (d) manipulative and body-based methods, (e) mind-body interventions, (f) nutritional therapeutics, (g) pharmacologic and biologic treatments, and (h) spiritual therapies (National Cancer Institute [NCI] Office of Cancer Complementary and Alternative Medicine, 2012). Definitions and examples of CAM modalities, as well as those currently being evaluated in clinical trials, are listed in Table 8-1.

Use of Complementary and Integrative Therapies in the United States

The use of CAM has been steadily increasing in recent decades in the United States, as have surveys measuring its use. Topics significant in understanding CAM use are prevalence (the frequency with which use occurs), motive (the reasons for using CAM), and patient characteristics (the people who use it). Data from the 2007 National Center for Health Statistics (NCHS)/NCCIH survey indicated that 38% of adults in the United States had used some form of CAM therapy during the previous 12 months (Barnes, Bloom, & Nahin, 2008). This survey compared results to the 2002 published survey (Barnes, Powell-Griner, McFann, & Nahin, 2004).

Back or neck pain, joint pain and stiffness, and arthritis were the most common conditions for which adults sought CAM therapies. The most commonly used CAM therapies were non-vitamin, non-mineral natural products, deep breathing exercises, meditation, chiropractic or osteopathic manipulation, massage, and yoga (in descending order by percentage). CAM therapies for which use increased between 2002 and 2007 were mind-body therapies (deep breathing exercises, meditation, yoga), acupuncture, massage therapy, and naturopathy.

A number of secondary analyses of the 2002 and 2007 NCHS/NCCIH data have been published in recent years. For example, one secondary analysis of the 2002 NCHS data exploring the type and amount of CAM use in 218 men with a history of prostate cancer revealed that more than 90% of the men reported using CAM, specifically biologically based and mind-body therapies (Ross et al., 2012). Another secondary analysis of complementary therapy use in the cancer and noncancer populations in the 2007 survey data revealed similar patterns of use between cancer survivors and the general population, although a greater percentage of cancer survivors used CAM therapies. The five most common complementary practices and products used by individuals with cancer were supplements (including vitamins and minerals), prayer for self, intercessory prayer, manipulation therapies (including chiropractic and osteopathic approaches), and herbal therapies (Anderson & Taylor, 2012).

Surveys of general CAM use solely in adult patients with cancer in the past five years (2008–2013) are not as plentiful as earlier surveys between 2002 and 2008, as researchers have opted

Table 8-1. Complementary and Alternative Medicine Modalities in Clinical Trials

Domain	Definition	Examples	Examples of Modalities Studied in Clinical Trials
Alternative medical systems	Systems built on theory and practices that preceded conventional systems	Acupuncture, Ayurveda, homeopathy, naturopathy, Tibetan medicine, traditional Chinese medicine	Acupuncture, acupressure, homeopathy, traditional Chinese medicine
Energy therapies	Therapies using energy fields, some still scientifically unproven	Qigong, Reiki, therapeutic touch	Reiki, Qigong
Exercise therapies	Modalities used to improve patterns of bodily movement	Tai Chi, Feldenkrais, hatha yoga, Alexander technique, dance therapy, Rolfing structural integration, Trager psychophysical integration, applied kinesiology	Exercise, yoga, tai chi, kinesiology
Manipulative and body-based methods	Based on manipulation and/or movement of one or more parts of the body	Chiropractic, therapeutic massage, osteopathy, reflexology	Massage, reflexology, chiropractic, osteopathy
Mind-body interventions	Techniques designed to enhance the mind's capacity to affect bodily function and symptoms	Meditation, hypnosis, art therapy, biofeedback, imagery, relaxation therapy, support groups, music therapy, cognitive behavioral therapy, aromatherapy, animal-assisted therapy	Biofeedback, hypnosis, mindfulness relaxation
Nutritional therapeutics	Assortment of nutrients, food components, and/or special diets as cancer prevention or treatment strategies	Macrobiotics, Gerson therapy, Kelley-Gonzalez regimen, vitamins, dietary macronutrients, supplements, antioxidants, melatonin, selenium, coenzyme Q10	Omega-3 fatty acids, glutamine, soy protein isolate, *Antrodia cinnamomea*, selenium, selected vegetable and herb mix, curcumin
Pharmacologic and biologic treatments	Drugs, complex natural products, vaccines, and other biologic interventions not yet accepted in mainstream medicine; off-label use of prescription drugs	Antineoplastons, 714-X, low-dose naltrexone, Met-enkephalin, immunoaugmentive therapy, Laetrile, hydrazine sulfate, Newcastle virus, ozone therapy, thymus therapy, enzyme therapy, high-dose vitamin C	Antineoplastons, ascorbic acid (high-dose ascorbate), ozone therapy
Complex natural products	Pharmacologic and biologic treatments including plant samples, extracts of crude natural substances, and extracts from marine organisms	Herbs and herbal extracts, tea polyphenols, shark cartilage, mistletoe	*Astragalus*-based formula, silymarin, green tea, green tea polyphenol E

(Continued on next page)

Table 8-1. Complementary and Alternative Medicine Modalities in Clinical Trials
(Continued)

Domain	Definition	Examples	Examples of Modalities Studied in Clinical Trials
Spiritual therapies	Interventions geared to beliefs and feelings, including sense of peace and connectedness	Intercessory prayer, spiritual healing	Intercessory prayer, distance healing

Note. Based on information from National Cancer Institute, n.d.-a; National Cancer Institute Office of Cancer Complementary and Alternative Medicine, 2012; National Center for Complementary and Integrative Health, 2014.

From "Clinical Trials in Cancer Part I: Biomedical, Complementary, and Alternative Medicine: Finding Active Trials and Results of Closed Trials," by C.O. Lee, 2004, *Clinical Journal of Oncology Nursing, 8,* p. 534. Copyright 2004 by Oncology Nursing Society. Adapted with permission.

to perform secondary analyses on previously published large-scale data, such as the NCHS data, or develop a subfocus on CAM use in specific populations, such as men with prostate cancer (Butler et al., 2011; Philippou, Hadjipavlou, Khan, & Rane, 2013; Ross et al., 2012) and women with breast cancer (Carpenter, Ganz, & Bernstein, 2009; Saquib et al., 2012; Wyatt, Sikorskii, Wills, & Su, 2010).

CAM use in the cancer survivor population has gained increasing research interest. A survey of 614 cancer survivors revealed that CAM use appeared to be associated with positive changes and increased spiritual importance (Mao, Palmer, Healy, Desai, & Amsterdam, 2011). Additionally, a secondary analysis examined the relationships among gender and symptoms (depression, fatigue, insomnia, and pain) and the use of specific CAM therapies among cancer survivors (Fouladbakhsh & Stommel, 2010). Researchers noted that CAM therapy use was more common among middle-aged, well-educated Caucasian females. Specific symptoms such as depression, insomnia, and pain were strong predictors of use, with differences noted by gender and the type of CAM therapy.

Despite the increasing number of surveys, comparatively little is known about what patients expect from CAM therapy versus what is experienced, characteristics differentiating the use of one versus more than one therapy, the relationship between health status and CAM use, patterns of use over time, reasons for participating in clinical trials involving CAM, reasons for referral (or lack of referral), and more specific use among patients with cancer. Recent inquiry is attempting to address some of these areas (Ge et al., 2013; Ramsey et al., 2012).

Regulation, Monitoring, and Guidelines

Dietary Supplement Health and Education Act of 1994

CAM's influence on individuals, the public, hospitals, managed care plans, schools of nursing and medicine, and pharmacies is considerable. However, much remains unknown in terms of the safety and efficacy of most therapies. For those therapies that are not provider-based, such as nutritional therapies or dietary supplements, the U.S. Food and Drug Administration (FDA) provides oversight through the Dietary Supplement Health and Education Act (DSHEA) of 1994 (U.S. FDA, 2014). According to DSHEA, a dietary supplement is a product taken by mouth that contains a "dietary ingredient" intended to supplement the diet and may

be found in various forms such as tablets, capsules, softgels, gel caps, liquids, powders, or bars. Examples include
- Vitamins
- Minerals
- Herbs or other botanicals
- Amino acids and substances such as enzymes and metabolites
- Extracts or concentrates.

Whatever their form may be, DSHEA places dietary supplements in a special category under the general umbrella of "foods," not drugs, and requires that every supplement be labeled as a dietary supplement. DSHEA allows manufacturers to use various statements on a product label that do not need preapproval, but claims must not be made about the diagnosis, prevention, treatment, or cure for a specific disease. Manufacturers are responsible for ensuring that the dietary supplement is safe prior to marketing it. FDA may take action against any dietary supplement product that is unsafe; however, FDA at present does not have the authority to regulate supplements prior to marketing. DSHEA also resulted in creation of the National Institutes of Health Office of Dietary Supplements to promote, collect, and compile research and maintain a database on supplements and individual nutrients.

MedWatch

MedWatch is the main avenue in which the FDA's safety information and adverse event reporting program is publically visible (U.S. FDA, n.d.-b). This program provides important and timely product information and includes prescription and over-the-counter drugs, biologics, medical devices, and nutritional products. Healthcare professionals (HCPs) and consumers report problems they experience that are related or suspected to be related to certain FDA-regulated products. The total annual recalls of drug products, medical devices, biologic products, and dietary supplements has generally been rising, with 132 drug/biologic/device recalls in 2008 and 177 in 2012, and 2 dietary supplement recalls in 2008 to 24 in 2012 (U.S. FDA, n.d.-a). Common reasons for supplement recalls were undeclared drug ingredients, health problems associated with use, possible bacterial contamination, and misleading packaging or labeling. Examples of undeclared ingredients were detected presence of analogs of the drug sildenafil and hazardous amounts of minerals such as chromium or selenium (U.S. FDA, n.d.-a).

Guiding Principles and Model Guidelines

National Guidelines

The White House Commission on Complementary and Alternative Medicine Policy (WHCCAMP) guiding principles (U.S. Department of Health and Human Services, 2002) and the Institute of Medicine model guidelines (Institute of Medicine Committee on the Use of Complementary and Alternative Medicine by the American Public, 2005) remain the only existing framework for CAM use on a national level and have not been revised in more than a decade. In 2000, WHCCAMP was assembled at the request of the president and Congress to explore scientific policy and practice questions regarding CAM use. The commission proposed the following principles: (a) deliver high-quality health care of the whole person, (b) use science to generate evidence that protects and promotes public health, (c) support the right of patients to choose freely among safe and effective approaches and qualified practitioners,

(d) promote partnerships and teamwork in integrated health care among patients, HCPs, and researchers committed to creating healing environments and respecting diversity of healthcare traditions, (e) disseminate comprehensive, timely evidence about CAM systems, practices, and products, and (f) obtain input from informed consumers for incorporation in proposing priorities for healthcare, research, and policy decisions (U.S. Department of Health and Human Services, 2002).

In April 2002, the Special Committee for the Study of Unconventional Health Care Practices of the Federation of State Medical Boards approved the Model Guidelines for the Use of Complementary and Alternative Therapies in Medical Practice (Institute of Medicine Committee on the Use of Complementary and Alternative Medicine by the American Public, 2005). This model is used in educating and regulating physicians and those who co-manage patients, such as advanced practice nurses (APNs), who use CAM in their practices but may not be currently licensed by a governing body with licensed or state-regulated CAM providers. The guidelines affirm that all HCPs have a duty to avoid harm and to act in patients' best interests. The initiative encourages the medical community to adopt clinically responsible and ethically appropriate standards that promote public safety while at the same time educating HCPs on safeguards to ensure that services are provided within professional practice boundaries. The seven central areas are patient evaluation, treatment planning, consultation and/or referral to licensed or state-regulated HCPs, medical records documentation, education, selling of health-related products, and conformance to ethical standards when conducting clinical investigations. The ultimate emphasis is on balancing evidence-based practice while remaining compassionate and respectful of patient autonomy and dignity (Institute of Medicine Committee on the Use of Complementary and Alternative Medicine by the American Public, 2005).

Academic Initiatives

The Academic Consortium for Integrative Medicine and Health (formerly the Consortium of Academic Health Centers for Integrative Medicine), first established in 2004, has grown to include 60 academic medical centers and affiliate institutions in the United States and Canada. Its mission is to advance academic centers' principles and practices of integrative health care by developing curricula, supporting research initiatives, and informing healthcare policy (Academic Consortium for Integrative Medicine and Health, n.d.). Member centers of the consortium have emerged as some of the premier, well-regarded integrative medicine programs in the United States. Direct collaboration between these integrative medicine programs and the cancer centers associated within their university structure provides an opportunity for enhancement in the care of patients with cancer and integrative oncology research as a whole. In 2010, NCI's Office of Cancer Complementary and Alternative Medicine and NCI's Office of Communications and Public Liaison conducted a brief but comprehensive survey and inventory of integrative medicine programs offered by NCI cancer centers and other academic institution–based health centers in the United States, with 66 NCI-designated cancer centers of the Cancer Center Program and 41 integrative medicine programs eligible to participate. Although the inventory revealed that additional inquiry is needed, collaborative activities involving cancer care and CAM modalities between cancer centers and integrative medicine programs are ongoing (Mikhail et al., 2012).

Professional Societies

The professional association solely dedicated to the integration of CAM practice, education, and research into cancer care is the Society for Integrative Oncology (SIO), a nonprofit, multidisciplinary organization founded in 2003. SIO's mission is to promote and advance evidence-based integrative care to improve the lives of those affected by cancer (SIO, n.d.). As a landmark contribution to the field, SIO published its first iteration of evidence-based clinical practice guidelines for integrative oncology in 2007, which were later amended and made public in 2009 (Deng et al., 2009). The guidelines (available at www.integrativeonc.org/index.php/docguide) are for clinicians to use when making clinical choices for their patients. They may also be a source document for quality assurance and multidisciplinary care.

Although the documents from the WHCCAMP and Institute of Medicine provide a framework for a societal, academic, and healthcare approach to CAM use, they are void of specific recommendations for nursing. During 2000–2010, the American Holistic Nurses Association (AHNA) and the Oncology Nursing Society (ONS) developed position statements that provided guidance and minimal competency expectations for nurses at all levels of practice. AHNA published *Position on the Role of Nurses in the Practice of Complementary and Alternative Therapies* (AHNA, n.d.), and ONS's position (now retired) was titled *The Use of Complementary, Alternative, and Integrative Therapies in Cancer Care* (ONS, 2009).

Several state boards of nursing have addressed the use of CAM and offered guidance to nurses, such as California (www.rn.ca.gov/pdfs/regulations/npr-b-53.pdf), New York, and Oregon (www.oregon.gov/OSBN/pdfs/policies/complementary-alternative_modalities .pdf).

Complementary and Integrative Therapy Modalities in Cancer Treatment

Surveys, secondary analyses, systematic reviews, and studies support that CAM use is pervasive in all areas of oncology care, including prevention, supportive care (symptom management, palliative care, and end-of-life care), and treatment. Use, however, does not signify efficacy or safety. Applying CAM modalities to any of the areas of cancer care ultimately is a patient's choice, and the patient may or may not involve an oncology APN in the decision process. The prevention and conventional treatment of cancer are complex disciplines and characteristically involve a multimodality approach. Some CAM modalities can be safely and effectively used and have sufficient clinical research findings to support evidence-based recommendations, although for the most part, they remain under study. Table 8-2 lists examples of efficacy and safety of CAM therapies by modality.

Complementary and Integrative Therapy Modalities in Symptom Management

Symptom management spans the cancer spectrum from before diagnosis to survivorship. Tremendous advances have occurred in offering relief from symptoms associated with the disease process, its treatment, and the possible physical, emotional, spiritual, and psychological long-term consequences. The popularity and availability of CAM therapies have enhanced conventional approaches to symptom management in the past several years. Recent evidence-based reviews of both conventional and CAM modalities for common symptoms associated with cancer and its treatment are available for HCPs (Decker & Lee, 2010) and consumers (Lee & Decker, 2012).

Knowledge of symptom clusters better assists APNs in targeting individual symptoms, as well as how the symptom interacts with other symptoms within the cluster. Symptom clusters are two, three, or more coexisting symptoms that are related but may be of differing etiologies and of varying time lengths (Esper & Heidrich, 2005; Kim, McGuire, Tulman, & Barsevick, 2005). Untreated or poorly treated symptom clusters may unfavorably affect patient outcomes and contribute to overall patient morbidity. Examples of possible evidence-based CAM modalities for common cancer-related symptoms appear in Table 8-3.

Complementary and Integrative Therapy Practice

Licensure and Credentialing

Licensure refers to the laws that regulate a given occupation and has two functions: (a) to protect the title by preventing unqualified practitioners from using the title and (b) to define the scope of practice in delineating specific responsibilities that form that practice. Licensure occurs at the state level, and the scope of practice may be different from state to state. In most states, CAM providers who do not possess a license may be regarded as diagnosing and treating patients and as practicing medicine without a license. *Certification* is the process by which an individual accrediting body awards acknowledgments to a practitioner for meeting predetermined qualifications (e.g., didactic learning, practice hours, and/or examination). National certification ensures that a professional's credentials are recognized in every state and that the scope of practice is the same across states. Examples of CAM practices with educational preparation, licensure, and credentialing criteria are listed in Table 8-4.

Certification and Reimbursement for Nurses and Advanced Practice Nurses

Specifically for nurses, the American Holistic Nurses Credentialing Corporation (www.ahncc.org) is the sole nursing body that offers an inclusive CAM certification. Many nurses choose to undergo training in specific areas of CAM, such as Reiki, bodywork, aromatherapy, or homeopathy, and can then bill for these services separately. The International Classification of Diseases, Ninth Revision, Clinical Modification (ICD-9-CM) for coding conventional and integrative services has been extended for the 10th edition (ICD-10-CM) (see www.who.int/classifications/icd/en).

Core Competencies

A principal question arises as to what degree oncology APNs are responsible and accountable for baseline knowledge of CAM when patients choose to integrate conventional medicine with CAM. Compelling reasons exist to develop baseline knowledge. First, patients use CAM, often without provider knowledge; thus, the topic must be addressed in the provider-patient relationship. Second, safe and effective CAM modalities exist for some common conditions. Oncology APNs need to be familiar with these modalities so that they can suggest options for a comprehensive approach to clinical problems. Third, known or suspected interactions may occur between some CAM modalities and conventional care. Therefore, APNs need to be able to prevent and recognize these interactions in a timely manner.

The development of clinical core competencies and curricula to teach core competencies is a sequential progression for oncology APNs in the attainment of baseline knowledge in CAM.

Table 8-2. Examples of Efficacy and Safety of Complementary and Alternative Medicine Therapies by Modality

Therapy	Description	Evidence	Side Effects	Cautions/ Contraindications
		Alternative Medical Systems		
Homeopathy Also known as homeopathic, homeopathic medicine, homeopathic remedies	Whole system of medicine that uses highly diluted substances to induce the body's self-healing mechanisms to bring about symptom or disease resolution (Jonas & Jacobs, 1996).	NM: Insufficient reliable evidence to rate. No RCTs show the effectiveness of homeopathic medicine as a whole. PDQ: No PDQ summary is available for this therapy.	NM: Homeopathic preparations contain little or no active ingredients and are unlikely to have any beneficial or adverse effects. There are no published reports of serious adverse effects. PDQ: N/A	NM: No known interactions with herbs, supplements, foods, lab tests, or disease conditions. PDQ: N/A
Naturopathy Also known as naturopath, naturopathic, naturopathic doctor, naturopathic medical doctor, naturopathic medicine, ND.	Combines conventional medical understanding of human physiology and disease with alternative therapies aimed at stimulating the body's own ability over drugs and surgery. These therapies may include herbal and nutritional therapies, acupuncture, bodywork and body movement, hydrotherapy, meditation, and counseling.	NM: Insufficient reliable evidence to rate. No RCTs show the effectiveness of naturopathic medicine as a whole. PDQ: No PDQ summary is available for this therapy.	NM: There are no published reports of serious adverse effects. PDQ: N/A	NM: No known interactions with herbs, supplements, foods, lab tests, or disease conditions. PDQ: N/A

(Continued on next page)

Table 8-2. Examples of Efficacy and Safety of Complementary and Alternative Medicine Therapies by Modality *(Continued)*

Therapy	Description	Evidence	Side Effects	Cautions/ Contraindications
Traditional Chinese medicine (TCM) with a focus on acupuncture Also known as Chinese medicine, Oriental medicine, TAM, TCM, traditional Asian medicine	TCM is an ancient system of medicine that uses a variety of treatments, including herbs and specific combinations of herbal ingredients. One of the more common TCM methods is acupuncture. Acupuncture is a family of procedures involving the stimulation of anatomic points (acupoints) with a needle or pressure thought to stimulate the body to correct energy flow and balance.	NM: Possibly effective for back pain, chemotherapy-induced nausea and vomiting, labor pain, and osteoarthritis. Insufficient reliable evidence to rate for cancer pain, cocaine dependence, depression, enuresis, shoulder pain, smoking cessation, or stroke recovery. PDQ: Effect of acupuncture has been studied on immune function, nausea and vomiting, vasomotor symptoms, fatigue, and xerostomia, among others. Four RCTs, a nonrandomized clinical study, and two case series found that acupuncture enhanced or regulated immune function. Seven clinical studies of acupuncture on cancer pain showed effectiveness, but the findings have limited significance due to small sample sizes, varied regimens, and absence of blinding. A systematic review of the effect of acupuncture on nausea and vomiting described five clinical trials with consistent results showing that acupuncture is useful for treating chemotherapy-induced nausea and vomiting. Acupuncture point stimulation for chemotherapy-induced nausea and vomiting is more effective for acute vomiting than for acute or chronic nausea.	NM: Acupuncture is generally well tolerated. Side effects can occur but are rare. They can include dizziness, nausea and vomiting, pain, fainting, and infection of the needle insertion points. PDQ: Serious adverse effects of acupuncture are rare. Minor adverse effects are pain at needle insertion sites, hematoma, light-headedness, drowsiness, and localized skin irritation.	NM: No known interactions with drugs, herbs, supplements, foods, lab tests, or disease conditions. PDQ: None stated.

(Continued on next page)

Table 8-2. Examples of Efficacy and Safety of Complementary and Alternative Medicine Therapies by Modality (*Continued*)

Therapy	Description	Evidence	Side Effects	Cautions/ Contraindications
Energy Therapies				
Qigong Also known as Qi Gong, Chi Kung, energy healing, energy health, energy medicine, energy therapy, energy work, EQT, external Qi Gong therapy, Qigong healer, Qigong therapy	A traditional Chinese therapy that can be a self-trained exercise or applied by a qigong practitioner incorporating moderate intensity exercise, movements, posture, meditation, and breathing. The several varieties of qigong include tai chi, meditation, yoga, and Reiki.	NM: Possibly effective for hypertension. Insufficient reliable evidence to rate for atrial fibrillation, depression, diabetes, fibromyalgia, menopausal symptoms, osteoarthritis, osteoporosis, pain, and stress. PDQ: No PDQ summary is available for this therapy.	NM: There are no published reports of serious adverse effects. PDQ: N/A	NM: No known interactions with drugs, herbs, supplements, foods, lab tests, or disease conditions. PDQ: N/A
Reiki Also known as bioenergy therapy, biofield energy therapy, energy medicine, energy work, healing touch, Japanese Reiki, Reiki touch therapy	*Rei* means universal spirit and *ki* means life energy; Reiki therefore means "universal life energy." Considered an energy therapy and a touch therapy. The Reiki practitioner is the conduit for the transmission or transfer of energy.	NM: Insufficient reliable evidence to rate for Alzheimer disease, cancer-related fatigue, cancer-related pain, post-hysterectomy pain, stress, or stroke. PDQ: No PDQ summary is available for this therapy.	NM: Reiki therapy has been safely used in several small, preliminary clinical studies. There are no published reports of serious adverse effects. PDQ: N/A	NM: No known interactions with drugs, herbs, supplements, foods, lab tests, or disease conditions. PDQ: N/A

(Continued on next page)

Table 8-2. Examples of Efficacy and Safety of Complementary and Alternative Medicine Therapies by Modality (Continued)

Therapy	Description	Evidence	Side Effects	Cautions/ Contraindications
Exercise Therapies				
Tai chi Also known as moving meditation, Tai-Chi, Tai Chi Chih, Tai Chi martial arts	System of movements and positions that address the mind to reduce stress and increase memory and for the body to improve posture and strength. The five major styles are Chen, Yang, Wu/Hao, Wu, and Sun.	NM: Insufficient reliable evidence to rate for fall prevention, insomnia, or Parkinson disease. PDQ: No PDQ summary is available for this therapy.	NM: Tai chi has been safely used in clinical trials without any evidence of adverse outcomes. There are no published reports of serious adverse effects. PDQ: N/A	NM: No known interactions with drugs, herbs, supplements, foods, lab tests, or disease conditions. PDQ: N/A
Yoga Also known as hatha yoga, relaxing yoga, Tibetan yoga	Ancient system of relaxation, exercise, and healing aimed to achieve fitness and a healthy lifestyle. Schools of practice include hatha, karma, bhakti, and raja. The Eight Limbs are pranayama (breathing exercises), asana (physical postures), yama (moral behavior), niyama (healthy habit), dharana (concentration), pratyahara (sense withdrawal), dhyana (contemplation), and samadhi (higher consciousness).	NM: Possibly effective for back pain, depression, pregnancy, and tuberculosis. Insufficient reliable evidence to rate for anxiety, quality of life in patients with breast cancer, bronchitis, carpal tunnel syndrome, chemotherapy-induced nausea and vomiting, cognitive function, coronary artery disease, diabetes, epilepsy, fibromyalgia, hemodialysis, hypertension, or insomnia. PDQ: No PDQ summary is available for this therapy.	NM: Yoga has been safely used in several clinical trials. Reports of serious adverse events have occurred in people using the pranayama and kapalabhati pranayama techniques. PDQ: N/A	NM: No known interactions with drugs, herbs, supplements, foods, or lab tests. There is concern that some aggressive breathing techniques, such as kapalabhati pranayama, might place excessive pressure on the abdomen or increase blood pressure. PDQ: N/A

(Continued on next page)

Table 8-2. Examples of Efficacy and Safety of Complementary and Alternative Medicine Therapies by Modality *(Continued)*

Therapy	Description	Evidence	Side Effects	Cautions/ Contraindications
Manipulative and Body-Based Methods				
Massage (Swedish [most common], bodywork, Rolfing® [Rolf Institute of Structural Integration], shiatsu) Also known as aromatherapy massage, chair massage, classical massage, deep-tissue massage, foot reflexion massage, hand massage, hot stone massage, ice massage, myofascial release, neuromuscular massage, therapeutic massage, trigger point massage, tui na	*Massage* is a broad term encompassing a variety of approaches to the manipulation of soft tissue to achieve health benefits. Practitioners primarily use their hands but may also use their forearms, elbows, or even their feet. Lubricants often are added to reduce friction and discomfort. Massage is increasingly combined with other modalities in the development of integrative treatment programs for chronic or degenerative illness such as cancer.	NM: Likely effective for cancer-related pain. Possibly effective for back pain, labor pain, low birth weight, postpartum depression, stress, and surgical recovery. Insufficient reliable evidence to rate for anxiety, asthma, burns, chemotherapy-induced nausea and vomiting, constipation, fibromyalgia, headache, muscle strength, myofascial pain, neck pain, or shoulder pain. PDQ: No PDQ summary is available for this therapy.	NM: Massage therapy is not associated with major side effects. Likely safe when used in most stress-related and chronic pain conditions. About 10% of individuals may experience musculoskeletal discomfort following massage. PDQ: N/A	NM: No known interactions with drugs, herbs, supplements, or foods. Preliminary research suggests that a targeted 5-minute massage after dye injection in a sentinel lymph node biopsy may enhance the spread of injected dye through the tissues being examined. PDQ: N/A

(Continued on next page)

Table 8-2. Examples of Efficacy and Safety of Complementary and Alternative Medicine Therapies by Modality (Continued)

Therapy	Description	Evidence	Side Effects	Cautions/ Contraindications
Reflexology (auricular reflexology, body reflexology, chakra energy reflexology, foot acupressure, macroreflexology [ear-foot-hand], zone therapy, lymphatic reflexology)

Also known as bodywork therapy, ear reflexology, energy medicine, energy work, foot reflexology, foot therapy, hand reflexology, lymphatic reflexology, zone therapy | Reflexology is based on the concept that areas of the feet correspond to other body parts, and stimulation of these areas on the feet can affect the associated body part. Some practitioners perform reflexology of the ears and hands. | NM: Possibly effective for cancer-related pain. Possibly ineffective for menopausal symptoms. Insufficient reliable evidence to rate for quality of life for individuals receiving chemotherapy or those with migraine headache, overactive bladder, or tension headache.
PDQ: No PDQ summary is available for this therapy. | NM: Some individuals can experience symptoms of malaise, fatigue, nausea, or flulike symptoms after reflexology. These potential side effects are believed to be due to the body releasing toxins. There is no reliable scientific evidence to support this belief.
PDQ: N/A | NM: No known interactions with drugs, herbs, supplements, foods, lab tests, or disease conditions.
PDQ: N/A |

(Continued on next page)

Table 8-2. Examples of Efficacy and Safety of Complementary and Alternative Medicine Therapies by Modality *(Continued)*

Therapy	Description	Evidence	Side Effects	Cautions/ Contraindications
Mind-Body Intervention				
Aromatherapy Also known as aroma, aroma therapy, aroma treatment, aromatic oils, aromatic therapy, essential oils	Refers to several modalities that deliver essential oils to the body. Essential oils are mixed with a carrier oil or diluted in alcohol before being applied to the skin, sprayed in the air, or inhaled. Massage is a common means of delivering oils into the body through the skin.	NM: Possibly effective for alopecia areata. Insufficient reliable evidence to rate for agitation, anxiety, chemotherapy-induced nausea and vomiting, depression, insomnia, migraine headache, postoperative nausea and vomiting, or psychological well-being. PDQ: Twelve clinical trials using either lavender, rosewood, rose, or valerian showed mixed results: Seven studies showed improvement in quality of life, anxiety, pain, or mobility. Five studies showed no effect on mood, pain, or anxiety.	NM: By inhalation, aromatherapy is usually well tolerated. Topically, essential oils may cause skin irritation, especially if the oils are not diluted. Ingestion of undiluted oils may result in significant adverse events, including seizures and kidney failure. PDQ: Safety testing on essential oils has shown minimal adverse effects, although ingestion of large amounts is not recommended. May cause contact dermatitis with prolonged skin contact.	NM: No known interactions with herbs, supplements, foods, lab tests, or disease conditions. Moderate caution is required with the use of lavender and medications because it may cause drowsiness. Use of essential oils topically or via inhalation might enhance the therapeutic and adverse effects of CNS depressants. PDQ: Theoretical concern for women with estrogen-dependent tumors when using lavender and tea tree oils because of possible weak estrogenic and antiandrogenic effects.

(Continued on next page)

Table 8-2. Examples of Efficacy and Safety of Complementary and Alternative Medicine Therapies by Modality (Continued)

Therapy	Description	Evidence	Side Effects	Cautions/ Contraindications
Mindfulness meditation Also known as concentrative meditation, mindfulness, mindfulness training, TM, transcendental meditation	A practice used to free the mind of cluttered thoughts and focus on a relaxed mental and physical state. Types of meditation include concentrative mindfulness and transcendental mindfulness. Mindfulness meditation allows the mind to experience extraneous stimuli, but there is no reaction to the stimuli.	NM: Possibly effective for stress. Insufficient reliable evidence to rate for anxiety disorder, back pain, or fibromyalgia. PDQ: No PDQ summary is available for this therapy.	NM: Meditation has been safely used in clinical trials without any evidence of adverse outcomes. There are no published reports of serious adverse effects. PDQ: N/A	NM: No known interactions with drugs, herbs, supplements, foods, lab tests, or disease conditions. PDQ: N/A
Nutritional Therapeutics: Macrobiotics				
Macrobiotics Also known as macrobiotism or Zen macrobiotics	An approach to life rather than a diet, but diet is predominantly vegetarian, with emphasis on vegetables, fruits, legumes, seaweeds, with small amount white meat or fish once or twice per week. The three types are Zen, American, and integrative. Followers believe that food and food quality powerfully affect health, well-being, and happiness.	NM: Possibly safe in a diet containing dairy, fish, or nutritional supplementation. Clinical studies have shown that the macrobiotic diet may increase the risk for various nutrient deficiencies. Possibly unsafe in infants, children, and adolescents without supplementation with vitamin B_{12} and iron. Insufficient reliable evident to rate for cognitive function, hyperlipidemia, or obesity. PDQ: No PDQ summary is available for this therapy.	NM: May be associated with an increased risk of rickets and osteoporosis, as well as deficiencies in calcium, iron, vitamin B_2 (riboflavin), vitamin B_{12} (cobalamin), and vitamin D. PDQ: N/A	NM: No known interactions with drugs, herbs, supplements, foods, lab tests, or disease conditions. PDQ: N/A

(Continued on next page)

Table 8-2. Examples of Efficacy and Safety of Complementary and Alternative Medicine Therapies by Modality (Continued)

Therapy	Description	Evidence	Side Effects	Cautions/ Contraindications
Pharmacologic and Biologic Treatments/Complex Natural Products				
Melatonin Also known as 5-methoxy-n-acetyltryptamine, MEL, MLT, pineal hormone	Hormone synthesized endogenously in the pineal gland from the amino acid tryptophan. Primary role seems to be regulation of the body's circadian rhythm, endocrine secretions, and sleep patterns. Levels of melatonin in the blood are highest prior to bedtime.	NM: Likely effective for circadian rhythm sleep disorders and sleep-wake cycle disturbances. Possibly effective for benzodiazepine withdrawal, hypertension, insomnia, jet lag, preoperative anxiety and sedation. Possibly ineffective for exercise performance and shift work disorder. Likely ineffective for depression. Insufficient reliable evidence to rate for beta-blocker–induced insomnia, fibromyalgia, or migraine headache. PDQ: No PDQ summary is available for this therapy.	NM: Likely safe when used orally or parenterally short term. Possibly safe when used orally long term in adults but not in children or pregnant women. PDQ: N/A	NM: Drug interactions include anticoagulants, anticonvulsants, antidiabetics, antihypertensives, benzodiazepines, caffeine, CNS depressants, contraceptives, cytochrome P450 1A2 and 2C19 substrates, flumazenil, fluvoxamine, immunosuppressants, methamphetamine, nifedipine, and verapamil. No known interactions with foods. Known interactions with lab tests: bleeding time, temperature, and heart rate. PDQ: N/A

(Continued on next page)

Table 8-2. Examples of Efficacy and Safety of Complementary and Alternative Medicine Therapies by Modality (Continued)

Therapy	Description	Evidence	Cautions/ Contraindications
European mistletoe (*Viscum album*, *Iscador*, *Helixor*, *Eurixor*, *Isorel*)	One of the most widely studied CAM therapies for cancer. European mistletoe has been used in Europe in the treatment of cancer since the 1920s. Avoid confusing with American mistletoe and mistletoe from Australia, Korea, New Zealand, and others.	NM: Possibly ineffective for head and neck or pancreatic cancer. Insufficient reliable evidence to rate for bladder, breast, colorectal, gastric, liver, lung, and uterine cancers, leukemia, or melanoma. PDQ: Mistletoe is a widely studied CAM therapy for cancer. In some European countries, preparations made from European mistletoe (*Viscum album L.*) are among the most prescribed drugs offered to patients with cancer. Improvements in survival, quality of life, and/or stimulation of the immune system are reported with mistletoe extract. Most clinical studies conducted have had major weaknesses that raise doubts about the reliability of the findings. No evidence exists to support that stimulation of the immune system by mistletoe leads to improved ability to fight cancer.	NM: Possibly safe when used orally or subcutaneously; no more than three mistletoe berries or two leaves are recommended at any one time. Likely unsafe when used orally in high doses. More than three berries or two leaves can cause seizures, slow heart rate, low blood pressure, and death in some patients. PDQ: Soreness and inflammation at injection site, headache, fever, and chills; reports of severe allergic reactions, anaphylaxis.	NM: Drug interactions include antihypertensives, hepatotoxic drugs, and immunosuppressants. No known interactions with food. Laboratory interactions with eosinophilia and liver function tests. Disease interactions include autoimmune diseases such as multiple sclerosis and lupus, leukemia, organ transplant, and liver disease. PDQ: None reported.

(Continued on next page)

Table 8-2. Examples of Efficacy and Safety of Complementary and Alternative Medicine Therapies by Modality *(Continued)*

Therapy	Description	Evidence	Side Effects	Cautions/ Contraindications
Green tea Also known as *Camellia sinensis*; synonyms: *Camellia thea, Camellia theifera, Thea bohea, Thea sinensis, Thea viridis*	Tea from the *Camellia sinensis* plant that may be green, black, and oolong. Fresh leaves from the *Camellia sinensis* plant are steamed to produce green tea. Green tea and green tea extracts, such as its component EGCG, have been used to prevent and treat a variety of cancers. Usually brewed and drunk as a beverage; tea extracts can be taken in capsules and are sometimes used in skin products.	NM: Likely effective for mental alertness and hyperlipidemia. Possibly effective for cervical dysplasia, coronary artery disease, endometrial cancer, oral leukoplakia, ovarian cancer. Insufficient reliable evidence to rate for amyloidosis or bladder, esophageal, colorectal, gastric, oral, lung, prostate, breast, or pancreatic cancer. PDQ: No PDQ summary is available for this therapy. A fact sheet describing the strengths and limitations of tea and cancer prevention is available at www.cancer.gov/cancertopics/causes-prevention/risk/diet/tea-fact-sheet.	NM: Likely safe when consumed as a beverage in moderate amounts. Possibly unsafe when used orally long term in high doses. PDQ: N/A	NM: Long-term use of caffeine, especially in large amounts, may produce tolerance, habituation, and psychological dependence. Abrupt discontinuation of caffeine may result in physical withdrawal symptoms, including headache, irritation, nervousness, anxiety, and dizziness. Drug interactions include adenosine, alcohol, amphetamines, anticoagulants, antidiabetics, beta-adrenergic agonists, bortezomib, cimetidine, clozapine, cytochrome P450 3A4 substrates, and estrogens, among others. Food interactions include iron and milk. Laboratory interactions include most chemistry tests and bleeding time. PDQ: N/A

(Continued on next page)

Table 8-2. Examples of Efficacy and Safety of Complementary and Alternative Medicine Therapies by Modality *(Continued)*

Therapy	Description	Evidence	Side Effects	Cautions/ Contraindications
Spiritual Therapies				
Spiritual therapies Also known as distant healing, faith healing, faith therapy, intentional prayer healing, intentional religion, intercessory prayer, prayer healing, remote intercessory prayer, remote prayer	Spiritual therapies include different approaches that can use prayer to treat or prevent illness. May include distance healing and other techniques provided in a hospice setting, at home, in a medical facility, in a residential facility, and more recently, over the Internet.	NM: Insufficient reliable evidence to rate for leukemia, coronary heart disease, or alcoholism. PDQ: Research confirms both patients and family caregivers commonly rely on spirituality and religion to help them deal with serious physical illnesses, expressing a desire to have specific spiritual and religious needs and concerns acknowledged or addressed by medical staff. Additionally, spirituality has multiple expressed forms between and within cultural and religious traditions.	NM: Spiritual healing has been safely used in clinical studies. PDQ: None reported.	NM: No known interactions with drugs, herbs, supplements, foods, lab tests, or disease conditions. PDQ: None reported.

CNS—central nervous system; N/A—not applicable; NM—Natural Medicines; PDQ—Physician Data Query; RCTs—randomized controlled trials (double-blinded, nonblinded)

Note. Based on information from National Cancer Institute, n.d.-b; Natural Medicines, n.d.

From *Handbook of Integrative Oncology Nursing: Evidence-Based Practice* (pp. 25–42), by G.M. Decker and C.O. Lee, 2010, Pittsburgh, PA: Oncology Nursing Society. Copyright 2010 by Oncology Nursing Society. Adapted with permission.

This knowledge could be achieved through the completion of a smaller curriculum program or a larger fellowship program that teaches the established core competencies. Oncology APNs could then increase baseline knowledge and obtain nationally recognized certification. Ideally, the development of baseline knowledge could be potentially augmented and simplified with national adoption of the SIO clinical practice guidelines in conjunction with the WHH-CAMP guiding principles. To date, it is difficult to determine to what degree these guidelines and guiding principles are modeled and implemented across all oncology practice settings.

CAM core competencies are fundamental skills, abilities, and expertise in the area of CAM and integrated medicine as applied to clinical scenarios versus the skills and abilities to deliver CAM interventions. Decker and Lee (2011) offered the following endpoints for nurses in cancer CAM.

- Expand baseline knowledge.
- Provide high-quality education regarding safety and efficacy.
- Facilitate partnerships between patients, HCPs, and CAM providers.
- Seek proper training and credentials if practicing a CAM therapy.
- Require informed consent if delivering a CAM therapy.
- Guarantee credentialing of a provider if referring a patient.
- Establish standards of practice for the use of CAM within specified patient groups.
- Document consent procedures and response to therapy.
- Assist in the design or maintenance of any preexisting integrated program.
- Develop a working knowledge of cost issues and reimbursement.
- Assist in the design of methodologically sound, rigorous research.
- Contribute to the body of knowledge through publications and presentations.

Implications for Oncology Advanced Practice Nurses

Knowledge Expansion

Many patients want to be directly involved in the diagnosis, planning, and delivery of their own health care, and they are seeking information from various sources and investing significant out-of-pocket dollars in health and wellness. While in essence, self-motivated health behavior is beneficial for individuals and society, patients sometimes are seeking interventions without consultation with oncology APNs. Engaging in an open dialogue and offering positive direction in acquiring reliable information can assist patients in being fully informed to make critical healthcare decisions. APNs can direct patients to safe and reliable sources of information to facilitate decision making. It also is imperative that oncology APNs use evidence-based CAM resources to assess patient situations that are affected by or likely to be affected by integrative therapies. Such resources contribute to accurate assessments and preventive approaches.

Numerous opportunities exist for APNs to access resources and expand knowledge in the area of CAM therapies. Some include assessing patients' CAM knowledge and use; conducting integrative assessments; advising patients across the cancer spectrum from early detection to survivorship; and sharing evidence-based materials with colleagues across practice areas and consumers in the community.

Assessing Complementary and Alternative Medicine Knowledge

Many patients with cancer use CAM therapies without essential knowledge to inform their decisions. Wyatt, Sikorskii, and Wills (2013) developed a 13-item CAM knowledge instrument

Table 8-3. Examples of Possible Evidence-Based Complementary and Alternative Medicine Modalities for Common Cancer-Related Symptoms

Symptom/Condition	National Center for Complementary and Integrative Health	Natural Medicines
Anxiety	Transcendental meditation, chamomile capsules, acupuncture for post-traumatic stress, self-hypnosis, omega-3	Possible: Tryptophan, St. John's wort, S-adenosyl-L-methionine
Cognitive decline or impairment	Soy protein, sage	None at this time
Constipation	Flaxseed, flaxseed oil, aloe vera	Psyllium, magnesium, cascara, glycerol, senna
Depression	St. John's wort for mild depression, S-adenosyl-L-methionine, yoga	St. John's wort for mild depression, s-adenosyl-L-methionine, yoga
Diarrhea	Probiotics, stress management techniques (cognitive behavioral therapy, exercise), acupuncture, peppermint oil	Lactobacillus, zinc, bifidobacteria, psyllium
Fatigue	Yoga	Magnesium
Mucositis	Chamomile	Hyaluronic acid, chamomile, glutamine
Nausea or vomiting	Ginger	Acupuncture, ginger
Pain	Acupuncture, spinal manipulation, massage therapy	Camphor, capsicum, acupuncture, balneotherapy
Sleep disorders	Valerian, tai chi, relaxation techniques	Melatonin, valerian
Taste changes	None at this time	Zinc
Xerostomia	None at this time	None at this time

Note. Based on information from National Center for Complementary and Integrative Health, n.d.; Natural Medicines, n.d.

and initially validated the instrument in 800 breast cancer survivors. This instrument can be used, or one or both of the subsets can be used, for a more detailed examination of patients' knowledge.

A survey examining conversations between patients and their physicians regarding CAM use revealed that despite the high known use of CAM among people age 50 or older, 69% of those individuals do not talk to their physicians about it (AARP & NCCIH, 2007). According to a telephone survey of 1,559 respondents, patients did not discuss their CAM use with their physicians because the providers never asked (42%); the patients did not know that they should discuss it (30%); or patients did not have enough time during the office visit to discuss it (19%). Personal responsibility for one's health and obtaining health care has led patients to seek interventions, including CAM. Patients may consider CAM to be beneficial to maintaining wellness, treating symptoms, or perhaps even treating an acute or chronic disease state. In many settings, such as managed care, consumerism is encouraged, with the intended outcome that adopting wellness behaviors or more consistent symptomatic relief may decrease overall healthcare costs for insurers and the insured (Rizzo & Xie, 2006).

Table 8-4. Examples* of Complementary and Alternative Medicine Practices With Educational Preparation, Licensure, and Credentialing Criteria

Practice	Acronym	Certification or Licensing Body	Educational Preparation	Related Links
Acupuncture	LAc (licensed acupuncturist)	National Certification Commission for Acupuncture and Oriental Medicine (NCCAOM) training and certification resulting in the title Diplomate of Acupuncture or Diplomate of Oriental Medicine. The designation LAc is the state licensure to practice the discipline.	NCCAOM certification is a nationally recognized certification available to practitioners of acupuncture and Oriental medicine. NCCAOM certification is a requirement for licensure in most states.	NCCAOM www.nccaom.org
Animal-assisted activity or animal-assisted therapy	AAA or AAT	No formal credentialing or licensure process; many trained therapists (e.g., physical, occupational) can incorporate AAA or AAT into their practice. Pet Partners® therapy animal teams may be registered in the state in which they reside.	Pet Partners offers a comprehensive therapy animal program either in person on online.	Pet Partners www.petpartners.org
Aromatherapy	RA (registered aromatherapist)	No formal credentialing or licensure process exists at this time. Many trained practitioners incorporate essential oils into their practice.	The National Association for Holistic Aromatherapy (NAHA) approves aromatherapy courses according to their education standards. The Aromatherapy Registration Council Examination (ARC™) in Aromatherapy is open to anyone who has completed a minimum of a one-year level 2 program in aromatherapy from an NAHA-compliant college or school or Alliance of International Aromatherapists Educational Guidelines or anyone who could provide evidence of equivalent training.	NAHA www.naha.org Aromatherapy Registration Council http://aromatherapycouncil.org Alliance of International Aromatherapists www.alliance-aromatherapists.org

(Continued on next page)

Table 8-4. Examples* of Complementary and Alternative Medicine Practices With Educational Preparation, Licensure, and Credentialing Criteria *(Continued)*

Practice	Acronym	Certification or Licensing Body	Educational Preparation	Related Links
Art therapy	ATR-BC (art therapist, board certified)	Certification is offered through the Art Therapy Credentials Board (ATCB). In some states, a passing score on the ATCB exam is a condition for licensure. State approval is required in order to take the exam for state licensure in select states. Many trained practitioners incorporate art therapy into their practice.	Minimum educational and professional standards are established by the American Art Therapy Association, a membership and advocacy organization.	ATCB www.atcb.org
Ayurveda	BAMS (bachelor of Ayurvedic medicine and surgery) DAMS (doctor of Ayurvedic medicine and surgery)	No formal licensure or certification process exists in the United States. Many trained practitioners incorporate Ayurvedic medicine into their practice.	Ayurvedic training in India is obtained with either a bachelor's degree or doctorate degree. Several states in the United States have approved Ayurvedic schools encouraging up to 500 hours of clinical practice. Professional scopes of practice are available describing the roles of Ayurvedic Health Counselor, Ayurvedic Practitioner, and Ayurvedic Doctor.	National Ayurvedic Medical Association www.ayurvedanama.org
Chiropractic medicine	DC (doctor of chiropractic medicine)	Licensure in 50 states and in Washington, DC, following a national board examination. Practitioners are required to pass a series of four national board exams and be state licensed. Doctors of chiropractic (DCs) are designated as physician-level providers in the vast majority of states and federal Medicare program.	The curriculum includes a minimum of 4,200 hours of classroom, laboratory, and clinical experience.	American Chiropractic Association www.acatoday.org

(Continued on next page)

Table 8-4. Examples* of Complementary and Alternative Medicine Practices With Educational Preparation, Licensure, and Credentialing Criteria *(Continued)*

Practice	Acronym	Certification or Licensing Body	Educational Preparation	Related Links
Healing touch	HTCP (healing touch certified practitioner) or CHTP (certified healing touch practitioner)	Certification is offered through two organizations: Healing Touch Program™ and Healing Touch International, Inc. (dba) Healing Beyond Borders. No formal licensure process is available. Many trained practitioners incorporate healing touch into their practice.	The Healing Touch Certificate (HTCP) Program is endorsed by American Nurses' Credentialing Center and the National Certification Board for Therapeutic Massage and Bodywork. The Certified Healing Touch Practitioner program is endorsed by the American Holistic Nurses Association. It is sequenced through multiple levels of didactic and experiential learning.	Healing Touch Program™ www.healingtouchprogram.com Healing Beyond Borders Educating and Certifying the Health Touch™ http://healingbeyondborders.org
Homeopathy	Hom (homeopathic physician)	Certification is available through the Council for Homeopathic Certification. Effective in January 2018, the Council for Homeopathic Certification will require candidates to attend programs that are approved or fully accredited by the Accreditation Commission for Homeopathic Education in North America (ACHENA). No formal licensure process is available. Many trained practitioners incorporate homeopathy into their practice.	Several homeopathic programs in the United States offer a range of 10-week to 4-year curriculums. The American Medical College of Homeopathy Homeopathic Practitioner Program is an accredited program through ACHENA and is licensed through the State of Arizona Private Postsecondary Board of Education. This program is open to non-medically licensed practitioners as well as licensed practitioners.	Council for Homeopathic Certification www.homeopathicdirectory.com American Medical College of Homeopathy www.amcofh.org

(Continued on next page)

Table 8-4. Examples* of Complementary and Alternative Medicine Practices With Educational Preparation, Licensure, and Credentialing Criteria *(Continued)*

Practice	Acronym	Certification or Licensing Body	Educational Preparation	Related Links
Macrobiotics	None at this time	A Macrobiotics Counselor Training Program is offered through Macrobiotics America. A Macrobiotics Leadership Certificate Program is offered through the Kushi Institute. Many trained practitioners incorporate macrobiotics into their practice.	Several macrobiotic training programs in the United States involve online study and in-person training. The Macrobiotics Counselor training program requires one year of learning with focus on caregiver cooking, healthy lifestyle cooking, or teaching. The Macrobiotics Leadership Certificate requires 12 weeks of online study and in-person training.	Macrobiotics America www.macroamerica.com Kushi Institute www.kushiinstitute.org
Massage therapy	CMT-BC (certified massage therapist, board certified)	The Board Certification credential is offered through the National Certification Board for Therapeutic Massage and Bodywork (NCBTMB). Until 2013, the National Certification was offered. As of December 2016, all practitioners who had obtained National Certification will need to transition to Board Certification or the credential is invalid.	The Board Certification requires 750 hours of instruction and 250 hours of hands-on experience. Therapists must demonstrate mastery of core skills and pass a standardized NCBTMB exam. NCBTMB programs are accredited by the National Commission for Certifying Agencies.	NCBTMB www.ncbtmb.org
Music therapy	MT-BC (music therapist, board certified)	Certification is available through the Certification Board for Music Therapists (CBMT). No formal licensure process is available. Many trained practitioners incorporate music therapy into their practice.	Certification requires the completion of an academic and clinical training program approved by the American Music Therapy Association and completion of a written examination. CBMT programs are accredited by the National Commission for Certifying Agencies.	CBMT www.cbmt.org

(Continued on next page)

Table 8-4. Examples* of Complementary and Alternative Medicine Practices With Educational Preparation, Licensure, and Credentialing Criteria *(Continued)*

Practice	Acronym	Certification or Licensing Body	Educational Preparation	Related Links
Naturopathy	ND (doctor of naturopathy)	Certification can be obtained through the Naturopathic Physicians Licensing Examination Board and the North American Board of Naturopathic Examiners. 17 states, the District of Columbia, Puerto Rico, and the U.S. Virgin Islands have licensing laws for naturopathic doctors. In these states, naturopathic doctors are required to graduate from an accredited four-year residential naturopathic medical school and pass a postdoctoral board exam to receive a license.	Each of the six schools in North America is either accredited or is a candidate for accreditation by an agency of the U.S. Department of Education.	American Association of Naturopathic Physicians www.naturopathic.org Federation of Naturopathic Medicine Regulatory Authorities www.fnmra.org
Osteopathy	DO (doctor of osteopathy) C-NMM/OMM, FAAO (certified neuromusculoskeletal medicine and osteopathic manipulative medicine, fellow in the American Academy of Osteopathy)	The American Osteopathic Association has 18 certifying bodies. The two levels of certification are general certification in neuromusculoskeletal medicine and osteopathic manipulative medicine (C-NMM/OMM) and fellowship in the American Academy of Osteopathy (FAAO).	A number of osteopathic medical schools operate in the United States. Three specialty training programs exist: (1) two-year program in NMM/OMM; (2) one-year program in NMM and OMM followed by completion of an American Osteopathic Association–approved residency in another discipline, and (3) integrated three-year program in family practice and NMM and OMM.	American Academy of Osteopathy www.academyofosteopathy.org American Association of Colleges of Osteopathic Medicine www.aacom.org/home

(Continued on next page)

Table 8-4. Examples* of Complementary and Alternative Medicine Practices With Educational Preparation, Licensure, and Credentialing Criteria *(Continued)*

Practice	Acronym	Certification or Licensing Body	Educational Preparation	Related Links
Reflexology	None at this time	Certification is available through the American Reflexology Certification Board (ARCB). ARCB does not accredit schools, instructors, or curricula. Many trained practitioners incorporate reflexology into their practice.	A number of reflexology programs are available in the United States. Educational programs recognized by the ARCB possess a minimum of 100 hours of classroom study with 200 hours of clinical experience.	ARCB http://arcb.net Reflexology Association of America http://reflexology-usa.org
Reiki	RP (Reiki practitioner) RMT (registered massage therapist)	Certification is available through several groups. No formal licensure process exists. Many trained practitioners incorporate Reiki into their practice.	Training in traditional Reiki has three levels: First and second levels can be given in 8–12-hour classes over two weekends. Third-level training to become a Reiki master may be completed in a few weeks to years.	International Association of Reiki Professionals www.iarp.org Reiki License Commission for Reiki Masters and Healers http://reikilicense.com
Yoga	None at this time	Certification is available through the Yoga Alliance. No formal licensure process exists. Many trained practitioners incorporate yoga into their practice.	Yoga schools train individuals to become instructors with 200, 300, and 500 hours of training programs, enabling different entry levels into the field.	Yoga Alliance www.yogaalliance.org

* This is not a definitive guide to complementary and alternative medicine certification bodies, licensing laws, and education preparation of these providers. The information presented here is current at the time of printing and serves as examples only. Refer to state licensing boards or professional associations for more information.

Note. From *Handbook of Integrative Oncology Nursing: Evidence-Based Practice* (pp. 18–23), by G.M. Decker and C.O. Lee, 2010, Pittsburgh, PA: Oncology Nursing Society. Copyright 2010 by Oncology Nursing Society. Adapted with permission.

A cross-sectional survey of 305 patients receiving radiation therapy in an urban cancer center revealed that 43% (n = 133 patients) reported using CAM and 12% (n = 37) discussed CAM therapies with their radiation oncologist (Ge et al., 2013). Female patients, in particular, and patients who were employed full-time were less likely to discuss CAM with their radiation oncologists.

Conducting an Integrative Assessment

Integrative assessments conducted by oncology APNs can elicit pertinent information regarding patients' past and current use of CAM, as well as assess their potential for future use of CAM for cancer-related symptoms or treatment. By performing an integrative assessment, APNs can communicate an openness to learn the value and significance of CAM to patients. This, in turn, allows patients to express their willingness and desire to be involved in decision processes or to "take the lead" in affecting their care. An open dialogue can lead to an increased level of confidence on the part of patients in knowing that oncology APNs are interested in their viewpoints and concerns; identification of safe and effective modalities for specific symptoms; education regarding unsafe and ineffective modalities; and recognition of potential interactions between conventional and CAM modalities as care continues. Decker and Lee (2010) developed a standard integrative assessment tool that consists of the following.

- Health history basics: Demographics (including insurance), chief complaint, history of present illness, past medical history, medications (including adherence), allergies, social history, immunizations and travel, family history, review of systems, laboratory values, diagnostics
- Integrative assessment basics: Comprehensive medication assessment (as published in Decker & Lee, 2010), previous and current CAM therapies (use, duration, reason, benefit, provider, cost, location, side effects), general well-being, nutrition, physical activity/exercise, stress management, spirituality, personal image, view toward illness state and recommended conventional therapies, anticipated CAM use (or desire for more information)
- Treatment plan basics: Is a safe and effective conventional therapy available? Is receiving a conventional therapy desirable to the patient? Is a safe and effective CAM therapy available? Is the population studied similar to the patient? Does the patient or APN have a strong belief in the rationale of the CAM therapy? Is there agreement in the rationale of the CAM therapy between the APN and patient? Is the CAM therapy affordable? Can the patient be monitored during the treatment period? Are interactions between the conventional and CAM therapies a risk? Has a plan for consistent follow-up been established?

Advising Patients' Needs Across the Cancer Spectrum

A comprehensive guide to decision making in integrative oncology for nurses has not yet been developed, although many APNs are functioning daily in conducting assessments as described previously, advising patients about CAM, and developing integrative plans for cancer care. APNs who are in a position to refer or who are functioning in roles that facilitate integrative care are cognizant of the challenges posed by risk management assessment, referral practices, billing audits, and required medical record documentation, all while overseeing the safe and effective delivery of both conventional and CAM practices. Attention to detail in proper communication and documentation of interactions among APNs is critical to this aspect of practice.

A discussion on advising patients in selecting CAM therapies would be remiss without addressing the need to recognize and communicate potential drug interactions between herbal products and cytotoxic drugs. When herbs and cytotoxic drugs are taken simultaneously, the pharmacologic dynamics are not well understood and may not be realized in the short term. Overdosing or underdosing of cytotoxic agents can greatly affect a patient's course of care. APNs can perform an evaluation of interactions with the assistance of a pharmacist and known drug databases and can communicate potential concerns with the patient and other HCPs (Andersen et al., 2013; Lee, 2005). For patients who are receiving radiation therapy, widespread inquiry into the pharmacologic dynamics between simultaneous radiation therapy and herbal drug usage is currently underdeveloped, as many studies are in the bench phase of translational medicine in the conduct of smaller-scale, preclinical studies, leaving more unknown than known (Jia et al., 2013). For this reason, it is best to advise patients who are receiving radiation therapy to disclose all over-the-counter products taken while receiving treatment.

Ultimately, clinicians and patients should incorporate discussions of CAM to guide its appropriate use and to maximize possible benefit while minimizing potential harm.

Conclusion

Complementary and integrative therapies are common in the oncology population, where they are used for cancer prevention, cancer treatment, and management of symptoms caused by the disease and treatment. Knowledge of specific characteristics of people who use CAM can assist oncology APNs in detecting CAM users who may not disclose that information readily. Access to and proper interpretation of evidence-based resources is crucial to people with cancer and oncology APNs. Many current evidence-based resources are available. CAM is becoming a specialized area of nursing with opportunities for additional education for oncology APNs. However, many issues are left to be resolved with respect to curriculum development for certification, reimbursement for services, and improvement of patient communication with oncology APNs about the use of CAM.

Case Study

L.L. is a 32-year-old Caucasian man with progressive Ewing sarcoma diagnosed 15 months ago. He is now one-year post–nonmyeloablative stem cell transplant and graft-versus-host disease. Recently, he was treated with levofloxacin 500 mg daily for two weeks for pneumonia followed by diarrhea, which was positive for *Clostridium difficile* and treated with metronidazole 250 mg every eight hours for two weeks with resolution. He returned to the clinic for a scheduled chest computed tomography (CT) last month, which showed disease progression. He and his wife recently returned from a one-week cruise, which he enjoyed and tolerated well. Because of disease progression, he began radiation therapy to the chest wall for five days starting the same day as the CT documenting progression, per radiation oncology. He is seen today in the clinic following an aerosolized pentamidine treatment and is found to be febrile and tachypneic, with an oxygen saturation of 91%. He complains of auditory wheezing and intermittent nonproductive cough. His right lateral chest wall pain is controlled with oral opioids.

L.L.'s past medical history consists of
- Ewing sarcoma diagnosed 15 months ago
- Pneumonia one month ago
- Pulmonary emboli 15 months ago—currently on enoxaparin.

Current medications are
- Oxycodone controlled-release 10 mg every 12 hours
- Oxycodone 5 mg every 4 hours PRN
- Enoxaparin 80 mg every 12 hours
- Pentamidine monthly
- Valacyclovir 500 mg every day
- Clotrimazole troches 10 mg every 6 hours
- Docusate sodium 100 mg every 12 hours
- Penicillin V potassium 500 mg every 12 hours
- Diazepam 5 mg every 6 hours PRN.

He has no known drug allergies. He is married, does not use tobacco or alcohol, operates a part-time business, and lives in a rural area. His family history is noncontributory.

Temperature is 102°F (38.9°C), pulse is 120 bpm, and respirations are 24 breaths per minute. He is a well-developed, alert male in no acute distress. Pupils are equal and react to light and accommodation, extraocular muscles are intact, and no nystagmus is present. No oral ulcers or candidiasis is present, nor is any lymphadenopathy. He has expiratory wheezes bilaterally in all lobes and decreased breath sounds in the right posterior lobes. The apical pulse is 130 bpm, regular rate and rhythm, no murmur, rub, or gallop, S3 or S4; and no jugular vein distension or carotid bruits are found. The abdomen is soft and non-tender with positive bowel sounds. No hepatosplenomegaly or costovertebral angle tenderness is present. Pedal pulses are 2+; no edema. Skin is warm and dry. Healing bruises are present on the abdomen from subcutaneous injections; the right lateral chest wall has radiation therapy markings; and the patient has a healing anterior right chest wall chest tube site.

The patient is alert and oriented. The cranial nerves 2–12 are intact. Deep tendon reflexes are 1+ upper and lower extremities. Strength is 5/5. Gait is normal. Patient has full range of motion in the neck and all extremities.

- White blood cells = 24.8/mm^3
- Red blood cells (RBCs) = 3.12 × 10^6/mm^3
- Hemoglobin = 10.2 g/dl
- Hematocrit = 32.4%
- Mean corpuscular volume = 100.4 fL
- RBC distribution width = 18.7
- Platelets = 283 × 10^3/mm^3
- Neutrophils = 79.0%
- Lymphocytes = 50.0%
- Monocytes = 15%
- Eosinophils = 1.0%
- Basophils = 1.0%
- Blood cultures and sputum cultures are pending.

This is a 32-year-old man with stage IV progressive Ewing sarcoma who presents with fever, recurrent dyspnea, and desaturation. No obvious source of infection is noted on examination. Chest x-ray demonstrates an obstructive component. Recommendations include levofloxacin 500 mg once a day for two weeks, metronidazole 750 mg once a day for four weeks, and then metronidazole 250 mg every eight hours for four weeks. Additional recommendations were for the patient to continue radiation therapy per radiation oncology and to return to the clinic in two weeks for follow-up.

The goals of therapy are to (a) treat obstructive pneumonia, (b) complete radiation therapy (two days remaining), and (c) promote comfort and quality of life. L.L. and his wife are aware of the grave prognosis and completed a home hospice referral prior to the cruise. They are interested in combining complementary approaches for pain management, intermittent nausea, occasional constipation (and possible diarrhea while on an extended course of antibiotics), and dyspnea.

L.L. reports that his spirits are good and that he and his wife are adjusting to his prognosis. He would like to spend as much of his time at home helping his wife with the business, maximize his energy, and minimize his symptoms. His nutritional status is good, and he is able to eat a variety of foods and maintain his weight. For management of the symptoms L.L. reports, the APN explains that no modality has been tested sufficiently yet to determine whether strong evidence of efficacy exists. Good evidence exists for the use of massage therapy for pain management (see Table 8-3). They ask about acupuncture and whether it would be contraindicated because he is taking enoxaparin. The APN explains that there may be some concern about using acupuncture needles for the pain because he is on a low-molecular-weight heparin, but acupuncture-related interventions such as acupressure and acustimulation wrist bands are noninvasive and may be helpful for nausea. For occasional constipation (and also for the possible diarrhea while L.L. is on an extended course of antibiotics), the APN explains that good evidence exists that probiotics and psyllium are effective and are available over the counter. For dyspnea, the evidence is conflicting, but many patients enjoy the benefits of yoga and find that it eases breathing. L.L. and his wife decide that they would like to see an acupuncturist, and the APN provides a referral for a licensed provider in addition to the name of the yoga instructor in the cancer center. The APN cannot assure them that these services will be covered under their current insurance and explains this to the patient and his wife, and they verbalize understanding. The APN provides an opportunity for questions, documents the discussion in the progress note, and schedules a follow-up appointment for two weeks.

The APN has suggested a conservative integrated treatment plan that has no known interactions with L.L.'s current medications. The nurse also provided the opportunity for questions and open discussion. Following the visit, the APN initiates a phone consultation with the acupuncturist, discusses the referral, and requests a summary letter for the patient's file after the first and subsequent visits for other HCPs on L.L.'s team to review.

What would be the APN's assessment questions and the rationale?
1. Has a comprehensive medication assessment been conducted?
    • Rationale: A complete medication assessment includes prescription and over-the-counter medications along with products that may not come to mind as quickly, such as aerosols, topical creams, dietary supplements, enhanced sports drinks, or protein bars.
2. Is there a history of previous and current CAM therapies? (If so, what kind? Duration? Reason? Did it help? Who provided it? Was it costly?)
    • Rationale: Symptom management in cancer care may involve CAM modalities such as acupuncture, aromatherapy, cognitive behavioral therapy, exercise, massage, reflexology, and yoga, to name a few. Documenting the patient's experience with any modality, its impact on the patient's symptoms, and cost/benefit analysis is advantageous when creating an integrative plan of care.
3. How is L.L.'s overall well-being and endurance? Nutritional status? Stress level and management? View toward the status of his illness?
    • Rationale: Knowing the overall well-being of the patient physically, emotionally, and spiritually is important for the APN, as it assists in effective treatment planning. For example, if a patient is not able to eat solids, is he or she receiving adequate caloric intake to provide energy for daily activities? Or is the patient experiencing hopelessness that may affect his or her outlook and relationships with family members?
4. Does the treatment plan include any additional chemotherapy or surgery? Is continuing the radiation desirable to the patient? Are safe and effective CAM therapies available for his symptoms? What might be the APN's thoughts about L.L. integrating CAM therapies at this time? Do he and his wife have some therapies in mind? Do they anticipate a cost, and can they pay if insurance does not cover it? Does L.L. need to be monitored for particular side effects or interactions? Is there a plan for consistent follow-up?
    • Rationale: Participation in healthcare decision making is desirable for many patients, and treatment planning should reflect their input along with a method of evaluation. The

benefits and drawbacks of any intervention should be explained well. Many patients would like to try CAM therapies outside of conventional interventions. This patient is experiencing pain, nausea, constipation, and dyspnea. He may be interested in meeting with an acupuncturist to discuss the benefits, risks, and cost of a series of treatments for his pain. For the nausea, the APN may suggest drinking a cup of ginger tea. Psyllium often is used in conventional approaches for the relief of constipation but also is considered to be CAM. Some patients with dyspnea benefit from relaxation and special breathing techniques taught in yoga classes. The patient or family member can keep a log of what works and what does not and how the intervention was tolerated. As a provider, the APN can review the possible interventions, check for potential interactions, and make a plan for follow-up evaluation in several weeks.

Key Points

- Many patients are directly involved in the diagnosis, planning, and delivery of their care.
- Patients seek information from various sources and are investing out-of-pocket dollars in health and wellness.
- Many patients with cancer use CAM without the knowledge of APNs.
- Safe and effective CAM therapies exist for some cancer-related symptoms.
- CAM research must urgently fill the gaps between what is used by patients daily and what is proved to be safe and reliable in well-controlled studies.
- APNs must know how to access safe and reliable sources of CAM information, maintain knowledge about CAM, and assess for CAM use among patients.
- CAM licensure and credentialing is governed by state bodies, and requirements vary by state.
- Informed consent is suggested for patients using CAM services within an inpatient or outpatient setting.
- APNs can serve as facilitators in maintaining an open dialogue between patients and the oncology care team.

Recommended Resources for Oncology Advanced Practice Nurses

For Patients/Consumers

- NCCIH published an indispensable guide for pertinent questions to consider prior to considering adding complementary medicine into an individual's current medical treatment plan. The guide, titled *Are You Considering Complementary Health Approaches?*, identifies these key questions and provides suggestions for thorough review and is available at http://nccam.nih.gov/health/decisions/consideringcam.htm.
- Consumers are encouraged to review the NCCIH, FDA, National Institutes of Health, and Federal Trade Commission websites and contact the NCCIH Clearinghouse (https://nccih.nih.gov/health/clearinghouse) for available evidence-based materials.
- A joint publication sponsored by NCCIH and NCI, titled *Talking About Complementary and Alternative Medicine With Health Care Providers: A Workbook and Tips*, is available for free download at http://cam.cancer.gov/talking_about_cam.html.

For Colleagues/Healthcare Providers

Organizations and Government Agencies

- American Botanical Council
  - Commission E Monographs: http://cms.herbalgram.org/commissione/index.html
  - HerbClip™ Online: http://cms.herbalgram.org/herbclip/index.html
- American Cancer Society
  - Complementary and Alternative Medicine: www.cancer.org/treatment/treatmentsand sideeffects/complementaryandalternativemedicine/index
  - Complementary and Alternative Methods and Cancer: www.cancer.org/treatment/treatmentsandsideeffects/complementaryandalternativemedicine/complementaryand alternativemethodsandcancer/index
- Cochrane Library: www.cochranelibrary.com/home/topic-and-review-group-list.html?page =topic
- Select cancer centers with integrative medicine programs
  - Academic Consortium for Integrative Medicine and Health: www.imconsortium.org
  - Via NCI: http://cam.cancer.gov/health_programs.html
- FDA
  - Consumer Updates: http://www.fda.gov/ForConsumers/ConsumerUpdates/default.htm
  - Dietary Supplements: www.fda.gov/Food/DietarySupplements/default.htm
  - Protecting Yourself (information on buying medicines and medical products online): www.fda.gov/ForConsumers/ProtectYourSelf/default.htm
- U.S. Government Accountability Office
  - *Herbal Dietary Supplements: Examples of Deceptive or Questionable Marketing Practices and Potentially Dangerous Advice*: www.gao.gov/products/GAO-10-662T
- U.S. National Institutes of Health
  - MedlinePlus
    * Herbs and Supplements: www.nlm.nih.gov/medlineplus/druginformation.html
    * Complementary and Alternative Medicine: www.nlm.nih.gov/medlineplus/complementaryandalternativemedicine.html
  - National Library of Medicine: www.nlm.nih.gov
    * CAM on PubMed®: http://nccam.nih.gov/research/camonpubmed
    * Dietary Supplement Label Database: http://www.dsld.nlm.nih.gov/dsld
  - NCCIH: https://nccih.nih.gov/health
    * Clinical Practice Guidelines: https://nccih.nih.gov/health/providers/clinicalpractice.htm
    * Health Topics A–Z: https://nccih.nih.gov/health/atoz.htm
    * Herbs at a Glance (https://nccih.nih.gov/health/herbsataglance.htm)—complete list may be downloaded as a free e-book
  - NCI: www.cancer.gov
    * PDQ® Cancer Information Summaries: Complementary and Alternative Medicine: www .cancer.gov/cancertopics/pdq/cam
    * PDQ Cancer Information Summaries: Supportive and Palliative Care: www.cancer.gov/cancertopics/pdq/supportivecare
  - Office of Dietary Supplements Fact Sheets: http://ods.od.nih.gov/factsheets/list-all

Select Peer-Reviewed Journals

- *Alternative Therapies in Health and Medicine* (www.alternative-therapies.com)
- *Integrative Cancer Therapies* (http://ict.sagepub.com)

- *Journal of Alternative and Complementary Medicine* (www.liebertpub.com/overview/journal
  -of-alternative-and-complementary-medicine-the/26)
- *Journal of Holistic Nursing* (http://jhn.sagepub.com)

References

AARP & National Center for Complementary and Integrative Health. (2007). *Complementary and alternative medicine: What people 50 and older are using and discussing with their physicians.* Retrieved from http://assets.aarp.org/rgcenter/health/cam_2007.pdf

Academic Consortium for Integrative Medicine and Health. (n.d.). Consortium of Academic Health Centers for Integrative Medicine. Retrieved from http://www.imconsortium.org/about/home.cfm

American Holistic Nurses Association. (n.d.). Position on the role of nurses in the practice of complementary and alternative therapies. Retrieved from http://www.ahna.org/Resources/Publications/PositionStatements/tabid/1926/Default.aspx

Andersen, M.R., Sweet, E., Lowe, K.A., Standish, L.J., Drescher, C.W., & Goff, B. (2013). Dangerous combinations: Ingestible CAM supplement use during chemotherapy in patients with ovarian cancer. *Journal of Alternative and Complementary Medicine, 19,* 714–720. doi:10.1089/acm.2012.0295

Anderson, J.G., & Taylor, A.G. (2012). Use of complementary therapies for cancer symptom management: Results of the 2007 National Health Interview Survey. *Journal of Alternative and Complementary Medicine, 18,* 235–241. doi:10.1089/acm.2011.0022

Barnes, P.M., Bloom, B., & Nahin, R.L. (2008). *Complementary and alternative medicine use among adults and children: United States, 2007* (National Health Statistics Reports; No. 12). Retrieved from http://www.cdc.gov/nchs/data/nhsr/nhsr012.pdf

Barnes, P.M., Powell-Griner, E., McFann, K., & Nahin, R.L. (2004). *Complementary and alternative medicine use among adults: United States, 2002* (Advance Data From Vital And Health Statistics Reports; No. 343). Retrieved from http://www.cdc.gov/nchs/data/ad/ad343.pdf

Butler, S., Owen-Smith, A., DiIorio, C., Goodman, M., Liff, J., & Steenland, K. (2011). Use of complementary and alternative medicine among men with prostate cancer in a rural setting. *Journal of Community Health, 36,* 1004–1010. doi:10.1007/s10900-011-9402-6

Carpenter, C.L., Ganz, P.A., & Bernstein, L. (2009). Complementary and alternative therapies among very long-term breast cancer survivors. *Breast Cancer Research and Treatment, 116,* 387–396. doi:10.1007/s10549-008-0158-3

Decker, G.M., & Lee, C.O. (2010). *Handbook of integrative oncology nursing: Evidence-based practice.* Pittsburgh, PA: Oncology Nursing Society.

Decker, G., & Lee, C.O. (2011). Complementary and alternative medicine (CAM) therapies in integrative oncology. In C.H. Yarbro, D. Wujcik, & B.H. Gobel (Eds.), *Cancer nursing: Principles and practice* (7th ed., pp. 626–654). Burlington, MA: Jones & Bartlett Learning.

Deng, G.E., Frenkel, M., Cohen, L., Cassileth, B.R., Abrams, D.I., Capodice, J.L., … Sagar, S. (2009). Evidence-based clinical practice guidelines for integrative oncology: Complementary therapies and botanicals. *Journal of the Society for Integrative Oncology, 7,* 85–120.

Esper, P., & Heidrich, D. (2005). Symptom clusters in advanced illness. *Seminars in Oncology Nursing, 21,* 20–28. doi:10.1053/j.soncn.2004.10.004

Fouladbakhsh, J.M., & Stommel, M. (2010). Gender, symptom experience, and use of complementary and alternative medicine practices among cancer survivors in the U.S. cancer population [Online exclusive]. *Oncology Nursing Forum, 37,* E7–E15. doi:10.1188/10.ONF.E7-E15

Ge, J., Fishman, J., Vapiwala, N., Li, S.Q., Desai, K., Xie, S.X., & Mao, J.J. (2013). Patient-physician communication about complementary and alternative medicine in a radiation oncology setting. *International Journal of Radiation Oncology, Biology, Physics, 85,* e1–e6. doi:10.1016/j.ijrobp.2012.08.018

Institute of Medicine Committee on the Use of Complementary and Alternative Medicine by the American Public. (2005). *Complementary and alternative medicine in the United States.* Retrieved from http://www.nap.edu/catalog/11182.html

Jia, L., Ma, S., Hou, X., Wang, X., Qased, A.B.L., Sun, X., … Fan, F. (2013). The synergistic effects of traditional Chinese herbs and radiotherapy for cancer treatment. *Oncology Letters, 5,* 1439–1447. doi:10.3892/ol.2013.1245

Jonas, W.B., & Jacobs, J. (1996). *Healing with homeopathy: The complete guide.* New York: Warner Books.

Kim, H.-J., McGuire, D.B., Tulman, L., & Barsevick, A.M. (2005). Symptom clusters: Concept analysis and clinical implications for cancer nursing. *Cancer Nursing, 28,* 270–282. doi:10.1097/00002820-200507000-00005

Lee, C.O. (2005). Herbs and cytotoxic drugs: Recognizing and communicating potentially relevant interactions. *Clinical Journal of Oncology Nursing, 9,* 481–487. doi:10.1188/05.CJON.481-487

Lee, C.O., & Decker, G.M. (2012). *Cancer and complementary medicine: Your guide to smart choices in symptom management*. Pittsburgh, PA: Hygeia Media.

Mao, J.J., Palmer, C.S., Healy, K.E., Desai, K., & Amsterdam, J. (2011). Complementary and alternative medicine use among cancer survivors: A population-based study. *Journal of Cancer Survivorship, 5*, 8–17. doi:10.1007/s11764-010-0153-7

Mikhail, I., Austin, E., Buckman, S., Lee, C., Goodman, N., & White, J. (2012). P03.14. Cancer complementary and alternative medicine research among NCI's cancer centers program and the integrative medicine programs: An inventory [Poster presentation]. *BMC Complementary and Alternative Medicine, 12*(Suppl. 1), P267 doi:10.1186/1472-6882-12-S1-P267

Mumber, M.P. (2006a). Clinical decision analysis. In M.P. Mumber (Ed.), *Integrative oncology: Principles and practice* (pp. 145–164). New York, NY: Taylor & Francis.

Mumber, M.P. (2006b). Principles of integrative oncology. In M.P. Mumber (Ed.), *Integrative oncology: Principles and practice* (pp. 3–15). New York, NY: Taylor & Francis.

National Cancer Institute. (n.d.-a). Clinical trials search results [Treatment/Intervention: Complementary or alternative medicine procedure; Trial Status: Active]. Retrieved from http://www.cancer.gov/clinicaltrials/search/results?protocolsearchid=6462148

National Cancer Institute. (n.d.-b). PDQ®—NCI's comprehensive database. Retrieved from http://www.cancer.gov/cancertopics/pdq

National Cancer Institute Office of Cancer Complementary and Alternative Medicine. (2012). Categories of CAM therapies. Retrieved from http://cam.cancer.gov/health_categories.html

National Center for Complementary and Integrative Health. (n.d.). Health topics A–Z. Retrieved from http://nccam.nih.gov/health/atoz.htm

National Center for Complementary and Integrative Health. (2014). Complementary, alternative, or integrative health: What's in a name? Retrieved from http://nccam.nih.gov/health/whatiscam

Natural Medicines. (n.d.). Natural Medicine (formerly Natural Standard and Natural Medicine Comprehensive Database). Retrieved from https://naturalmedicines.therapeuticresearch.com

Oncology Nursing Society. (2009). The use of complementary, alternative, and integrative therapies in cancer care [Position statement; retired in 2012]. Pittsburgh, PA: Author.

Philippou, Y., Hadjipavlou, M., Khan, S., & Rane, A. (2013). Complementary and alternative medicine (CAM) in prostate and bladder cancer. *BJU International, 112*, 1073–1079. doi:10.1111/bju.12062

Ramsey, S.D., Zeliadt, S.B., Blough, D.K., Fedorenko, C.R., Fairweather, M.E., McDermott, C.L., … Arora, N.K. (2012). Complementary and alternative medicine use, patient-reported outcomes, and treatment satisfaction among men with localized prostate cancer. *Urology, 79*, 1034–1041. doi:10.1016/j.urology.2012.01.023

Rizzo, J.A., & Xie, Y. (2006). Managed care, consumerism, preventive medicine: Does a causal connection exist? *Managed Care Interface, 19*(7), 46–50.

Ross, L.E., Fletcher, A., Anderson, M.C., Meade, S.A., Powe, B.D., & Howard, D. (2012). Complementary and alternative medicine (CAM) use among men with a history of prostate cancer. *Journal of Cultural Diversity, 19*, 143–150.

Saquib, J., Parker, B.A., Natarajan, L., Madlensky, L., Saquib, N., Patterson, R.E., … Pierce, J.P. (2012). Prognosis following the use of complementary and alternative medicine in women diagnosed with breast cancer. *Complementary Therapies in Medicine, 20*, 283–290. doi:10.1016/j.ctim.2012.04.002

Society for Integrative Oncology. (n.d.). SIO mission. Retrieved from http://www.integrativeonc.org/index.php/about

U.S. Department of Health and Human Services. (2002). *White House Commission on Complementary and Alternative Medicine Policy: Final report* [NIH Publication No. 03-5411]. Retrieved from http://www.whccamp.hhs.gov

U.S. Food and Drug Administration. (n.d.-a). MedWatch safety alerts for human medical products. Retrieved from http://www.fda.gov/Safety/MedWatch/SafetyInformation/SafetyAlertsforHumanMedicalProducts/default.htm

U.S. Food and Drug Administration. (n.d.-b). MedWatch: The FDA safety information and adverse event reporting program. Retrieved from http://www.fda.gov/Safety/MedWatch/default.htm

U.S. Food and Drug Administration. (2014). Q&A on dietary supplements. Retrieved from http://www.fda.gov/Food/DietarySupplements/QADietarySupplements/default.htm

Weil, A. (2014a). Preface to the series. In D.I. Abrams & A.T. Weil (Eds.), *Integrative oncology* (2nd ed., pp. v–vii). New York, NY: Oxford University Press.

Weil, A. (2014b). Why integrative oncology? In D.I. Abrams & A.T. Weil (Eds.), *Integrative oncology* (2nd ed., pp. 1–12). New York, NY: Oxford University Press.

Wyatt, G., Sikorskii, A., & Wills, C.E. (2013). Development and initial validation of a complementary and alternative medicine (CAM) knowledge instrument. *Journal of Nursing Measurement, 21*, 55–63. doi:10.1891/1061-3749.21.1.55

Wyatt, G., Sikorskii, A., Wills, C.E., & Su, H.A. (2010). Complementary and alternative medicine use, spending, and quality of life in early stage breast cancer. *Nursing Research, 59*, 58–66. doi:10.1097/NNR.0b013e3181c3bd26

CHAPTER 9

Clinical Research

Lisa Aiello-Laws, MSN, RN, AOCNS®

Introduction

Clinical research is the systematic investigation of human biology, health, or illness that contributes to generalizable knowledge and provides evidence to support clinical practice (Polit & Beck, 2014). Oncology advanced practice nurses (APNs) have a multitude of roles related to clinical research: (a) translating research into practice, (b) educating nurses regarding evidence-based practice and new research findings, (c) critiquing and evaluating research studies, (d) developing and carrying out research as an investigator, (e) evaluating the feasibility of research, (f) being a member of an institutional review board (IRB), (g) advising staff on clinical research, (h) taking part in clinical trials as a research nurse or staff nurse, or (i) managing a clinical research program.

As the role of the APN is further defined through the doctorate of nursing practice (DNP), research responsibilities may increase. In nursing, a long-standing gap has existed between research and practice. The proposed collaborative relationships between PhD-prepared (academic) nurses and DNP-prepared (practice doctorate nurses) nurses include DNP-prepared nurses performing clinical research at the point of care and translating new research findings into practice. The PhD-prepared nurses will collaborate with DNP-prepared nurses and continue to perform rigorous scientific research, yet will remain more academic focused (Edwardson, 2010; Rolfe & Davies, 2009; Vincent, Johnson, Velasquez, & Rigney, 2010).

Types of Research

Two main types of research exist: quantitative and qualitative (Polit & Beck, 2014). *Quantitative* research usually involves introducing an intervention and/or observing. Data are collected, and statistical evaluation is completed. *Qualitative* research typically involves observing and describing the lived experiences of a group, such as quality of life. Medical research tends to be more quantitative, whereas nursing research tends to be more qualitative. This is understandable, given nursing's strong focus on holistic care and quality of life.

Research can be further classified by the profession performing the research. One type is medical research, where the physician is the principal investigator and the scientific process is used. Commonly, medical research in oncology is treatment focused. Chemotherapy trials typically test new agents, or they test approved agents for different diagnoses. These research trials are called clinical trials (National Cancer Institute [NCI], 2013). Clinical trials may be supported by the pharmaceutical company related to the study drug or by a cooperative group. Cooperative groups work with NCI and include researchers and clinicians in the United States, Canada, and Europe, thus allowing research studies to be performed at multiple centers, improving enrollment and generalizability of results. Cooperative groups are more regulated and must meet federal standards. Based on recommendation from the Institute of Medicine (2013), NCI consolidated its cooperative group program into the National Clinical Trials Network. This network centralizes the functions of the cooperative groups. Many former cooperative groups merged to form larger network groups. See Table 9-1 for a complete list of network groups.

Nursing research typically evaluates nursing-sensitive patient outcomes, interventions, symptom management, and education. It usually occurs at the point of care and focuses on "biobehavioral research with a primary focus on health promotion, symptom management, quality of care, and quality of life" (National Institute of Nursing Research, 2011, p. 1). The results of nursing research provide evidence to support nursing practice, add to the science of nursing, shape health policy, and influence the health of people worldwide (American Association of Colleges of Nursing, 2006). In nursing research, nurses are the principal investigators, and research also may be sponsored by pharmaceutical or cooperative groups. Many NCI-sponsored cooperative group trials are led by nurse scientists (Bruner & O'Mara, 2014). The focus of these nurse-led trials is commonly quality of life but also can include prevention, symptom management, treatment, patient-reported outcomes, and the evaluation of effectiveness and cancer care delivery. See Table 9-2 for milestones in nursing research, with emphasis on oncology nursing.

Table 9-1. National Cancer Institute National Clinical Trials Network

Network	Cooperative Groups Included/ Comments	Website
NRG Oncology	The National Surgical Adjuvant Breast and Bowel Project (NSABP), the Radiation Therapy Oncology Group (RTOG), and the Gynecologic Oncology Group (GOG)	www.nrgoncology.org
Alliance for Clinical Trials in Oncology	The American College of Surgeons Oncology Group (ACOSOG), Cancer and Leukemia Group B (CALGB), and North Central Cancer Treatment Group (NCCTG)	www.allianceforclinicaltrials inoncology.org
Children's Oncology Group (COG)	–	www.childrensoncologygroup .org
ECOG-ACRIN Cancer Research Group	The Eastern Cooperative Oncology Group (ECOG) and the American College of Radiology Imaging Network (ACRIN)	http://ecog-acrin.org
SWOG	Formerly the Southwest Oncology Group	www.swog.org
Canadian Cancer Clinical Trials Network (3CTN)	–	http://3ctn.ca

Note. Based on information from National Cancer Institute, 2015.

Table 9-2. Historical Nursing Research Milestones, With Emphasis on Oncology Nursing

Year	Event
1859	Florence Nightingale's *Notes on Nursing* is published.
1900	The American Nurses Association publishes first nursing journal, *American Journal of Nursing*.
1952	First nursing research journal, *Nursing Research*, is published.
1955	American Nurses Foundation developed as the research, education, and charitable affiliate of the American Nurses Association.
1963	Seminal research article is published by oncology nurse scientist Jeanne Quint Benoliel.
1973	American Cancer Society publishes *Proceedings of the National Conference on Cancer Nursing*.
1973	Oncology Nursing Society (ONS) publishes *Cancer Nursing Newsletter* (forerunner to the *Oncology Nursing Newsletter*, and then the *Oncology Nursing Forum*).
1978	ONS publishes first oncology nursing journal, *Oncology Nursing Forum*.
1981	ONS creates the Oncology Nursing Foundation, a source for research funding, later renamed to ONS Foundation.
1986	National Institutes of Health establishes the National Center for Nursing Research (NCNR), source for research funding.
1993	NCNR becomes the National Institute of Nursing Research.
2001	First ONS Research Agenda published.
2006	First ONS Putting Evidence Into Practice resources released.
2008	ONS publishes the second edition of the *Manual for Clinical Trials Nursing*.
2010	ONS publishes the *Oncology Clinical Trials Nurse Competencies*.
2013	ONS receives a grant from the Agency for Healthcare Research and Quality to test new strategies for improving the quality of cancer care.

Note. Based on information from American Nurses Foundation, n.d.; Lubejko et al., 2011; Mayer, 2000; Oncology Nursing Society, n.d., 2010; Penn Nursing Science, n.d.; Polit & Beck, 2014.

Medical research and nursing research are not dichotomous. Nurses, physicians, and other disciplines frequently collaborate on research and, at times, include each profession's hypotheses within the same study.

Evaluating Strength of Research Studies

Before the APN translates research into practice or educates other oncology nurses about the integration of new evidence, it is important to first identify the strength of the evidence. One of the initial evaluation methods includes assessing the level of evidence. Many scales are available that define the levels and strength of evidence (American Nurses Association, 2012). APNs needs to identify the scale being used in the clinical trial and its associated definitions. See Figure 20-7 in Chapter 20 for an explanation of the hierarchy of the levels of evidence.

Ethical Issues

Unfortunately, there is a worldwide history of mistreatment of participants in research studies (Polit & Beck, 2014). Today, these investigators would be guilty of ethical misconduct, although at that time, no guidelines or protections existed. For example, the Nazis performed experiments on prisoners of war in the 1930s and 1940s. The Tuskegee Syphilis Study in the United States investigated the effects of syphilis by withholding medical treatment to 400 African American men. In 1951, cell lines were made from the cervical cancer cells of Henrietta Lacks, a poor African American tobacco farmer in Virginia (Skloot, 2011). These cells, called HeLa cells, played a large role in medical progress, including development of the polio vaccine, cloning, gene mapping, and in vitro fertilization. However, Henrietta did not know her cells were collected. Despite years of contributions to scientific discovery resulting from these cells, her descendants then and today cannot afford health insurance. In all of these examples, the participants did not give informed consent.

As a result of ethical misconduct, many groups developed codes of ethics (Polit & Beck, 2014). Globally, the Nuremberg Code (U.S. Department of Health and Human Services Office for Human Research Protections, 2005) was developed in 1949 as a result of the Nazi human rights violations. The World Medical Association developed the Declaration of Helsinki in 1964, which was recently updated in 2008 (World Medical Association, 2008). The International Council of Nurses (ICN) developed the *ICN Code of Ethics for Nurses*, which was last revised in 2012 (ICN, 2012). The American Nurses Association (ANA) has developed many ethical guidelines for nurses, including *Ethical Guidelines in the Conduct, Dissemination, and Implementation of Nursing Research* in 1995 (Silva, 1995) and the *Code of Ethics With Interpretive Statements*, recently updated in 2015 (ANA, 2015). The National Commission for the Protection of Human Subjects of Biomedical and Behavioral Research issued the Belmont Report in 1979. This document has served as the basis for many guidelines and governmental regulations in the United States. Clinical trials have been regulated since the 1970s by the U.S. Food and Drug Administration (FDA). FDA ensures that researchers follow the guidelines of good clinical practice (GCP), which were developed by the International Conference on Harmonisation of Technical Requirements for Registration of Pharmaceuticals for Human Use (ICH) (Emanuel, Wendler, & Grady, 2008; ICH, 1996; U.S. FDA, 2014a). GCP includes guidelines related to informed consent, protection of children, financial disclosure by investigators, IRB rules, and investigational new drug applications. It is the responsibility of APNs to become familiar with these documents and regulations and to ensure adherence by nursing and/or research staff. See Table 9-3 for a timeline of the development of regulations.

Protection of Human Participants

As a result of the aforementioned ethical misconduct, the protection of human participants has become paramount. The researcher designing a study needs to compare the potential risks of participation to the potential benefits to participants (Polit & Beck, 2014). Benefits to participants may include access to investigational drugs that may provide benefit, the satisfaction of helping future generations, intensive observation and oversight by the medical team, and

Table 9-3. Documents for Protection of Human Subjects

Originally Published	Title	Purpose
1949	Nuremberg Code www.hhs.gov/ohrp/archive/nurcode.html	Established voluntary consent and justification for the research
1953	Guidelines for the Conduct of Research Involving Human Subjects at the National Institutes of Health http://grants.nih.gov/grants/policy/hs/hs_policies.htm	Required medical review of research at the National Institutes of Health Clinical Center
1962	Kefauver-Harris amendments to the Federal Food, Drug, and Cosmetic Act www.fda.gov/ForConsumers/ConsumerUpdates/ucm322856.htm	Mandated consent for drug testing
1964	Declaration of Helsinki www.wma.net/en/30publications/10policies/b3/17c.pdf	Declared that potential benefits must outweigh potential risks
1979	Belmont Report www.hhs.gov/ohrp/humansubjects/guidance/belmont.html	Defined principles of respect for persons, beneficence, and justice
1991	Code of Federal Regulations, Title 45, Part 46: Protection of Human Subjects; also known as the "Common Rule" www.hhs.gov/ohrp/humansubjects/guidance/45cfr46.html	Established role of the institutional review board to protect human subjects

Note. Based on information from Emanuel et al., 2008.

stipends or incentives. Risks may include untoward side effects, emotional distress, and monetary costs (e.g., transportation, missed time from work). Untoward side effects are reviewed regularly by the institution approving the clinical research at the site.

Informed Consent

The informed consent process provides participants with a clear explanation of the potential risks and benefits. This process protects the rights of participants and is highly regulated (Wilkinson, 2012). Many guidelines exist that define what must be included in informed consent documents. NCI (2011), U.S. FDA (2014c), and the U.S. Department of Health and Human Services Office for Human Research Protections (2014) developed recommendations for cancer clinical trial informed consent documents. A checklist to assist in the development of easy-to-read informed consent documents is available at https://accrualnet.cancer.gov/literature/checklist_easy_to_read_informed_consent#.VRBHE-F5_wA. The research team must be aware of the regulating bodies involved with specific research studies.

The informed consent document should clarify to participants that their participation is voluntary and that they can withdraw at any time. Updated consent forms must be developed for a study if findings or toxicities are released, further clarifying the risks and benefits. All participants already on the study must sign the new consent form. Informed consent documents must go through the IRB approval process to ensure inclusion of all required elements before they can be used. It typically is the responsibility of the clinical trial nurse (CTN) to prepare edited documents, submit them to the IRB for approval, and contact all current participants on the trial to obtain updated consent. See Table 9-4 for a list of the required elements of informed consent.

Confidentiality

It also is the responsibility of the research team to follow strict procedures to ensure confidentiality of any patient data (Polit & Beck, 2014). This may include a separate locked office or file cabinet, anonymity, or use of individual numbers, instead of protected health information (PHI), to identify participants. Only the research team should have the ability to decipher the identification numbers.

Vulnerable Populations

Specific vulnerable groups may need additional protections because they may be unable to give informed consent, may be at higher risk for side effects, or may feel obligated to participate because of their relationship with the researcher (Polit & Beck, 2014). These groups include children, pregnant women, and mentally ill, emotionally disabled, severely ill, ter-

Table 9-4. Required Elements of Informed Consent

Factor	Details
General requirements	• Consent must be obtained from the participant or participant's legal representative. • Process must allow sufficient opportunity for the patient to consider whether to participate. • Process must minimize the possibility of coercion or undue influence. • Language of consent must be understandable to the participant or representative. • Agreement must not release or appear to release the investigator, sponsor, institution, or its agents from liability for negligence.
Basic elements	• States that the study involves research • Describes purpose, expected duration, and procedures • Describes foreseeable risks and benefits • Discloses alternatives • Describes how confidentiality will be maintained • Explains what compensation or treatments are available if injury occurs • Defines whom to contact for questions about the research, the participant's rights, and research-related injury • Includes statements such as participation is voluntary, refusal to participate will not result in any penalty or loss of benefits, and participant may withdraw at any time without penalty or loss of benefits
Additional elements that could possibly be included	• Reasons participation may be stopped by the investigator without the participant's consent • Additional costs for participation • Consequences of participant's withdrawal and procedures for orderly termination • Notice that if significant new findings occur that relate to the study product, this information will be provided to the participant • Approximate number of participants to be enrolled

Note. Based on information from U.S. Department of Health and Human Services Office for Human Research Protections, 2014; U.S. Food and Drug Administration, 2014a.

minally ill, disabled, and institutionalized (i.e., patients, inmates) people. Additional safe-guards must be implemented when working with any of these populations.

Role of the Advanced Practice Nurse in Research

Whether the APN is involved in medical or nursing research, or is a clinical trials nurse, many of the roles and responsibilities may be the same. These responsibilities may include recruitment, informed consent, preparing for audits by sponsoring agencies (pharmaceutical and cooperative groups), assessing insurance coverage, evaluating appropriateness of research for a facility or employer, and managing clinical trial data, data entry, and paperwork. Other roles external to being a part of the research team include being a member of an IRB, managing a research team or department, interpreting research findings, educating staff about research and evidence-based practice, critiquing research, and translating research findings into practice (Catania et al., 2012).

Recruitment

An ever-present challenge facing researchers and the research team is the recruitment of research participants. Many obstacles to patient recruitment have been reported, including those that are physician related, patient related, and protocol related. However, a recurring obstacle is patients not being informed about trials or not offered participation. Only an estimated 3%–5% of people with cancer participate in a cancer clinical trial (Penberthy, Dahman, Petkov, & DeShazo, 2012). The suspected reasons vary for this discouraging low enrollment rate, but participation in cancer clinical research cannot increase without effective recruitment. Oncology APNs, because of their in-depth knowledge of the science that supports clinical research endeavors and oncology care, as well as their educational and communication skills, are the ideal practitioners to recruit research participants.

Recruitment involves the identification of eligible patients and enrollment of patients (Tramm, Daws, & Schadewaldt, 2013). Those who choose to participate usually report doing so to obtain access to newer treatments or out of altruism for future generations. Those who refuse participation may be concerned about privacy and confidentiality and may have mistrust for the medical establishment. The recruitment process is typically a challenge to researchers. Approximately 85% of patients with cancer report they were unaware of or were not offered participation in clinical trials (Penberthy et al., 2012; Stiles et al., 2011). However, minorities, those living in rural areas, and marginalized patients participate even less. This makes research findings less generalizable.

Historical mistreatment of minorities in research studies has led to mistrust among many marginalized groups. Women and minorities have reported specific barriers to trial participation, such as fear, mistrust, and the burden of participation (Schmotzer, 2012). Specific facilitators to participation were reported to be physician enthusiasm and good communication skills, a good provider-patient relationship, having a perceived benefit, and altruism. Ethnicity and culture must be considered when developing recruitment materials and training staff. It is important to develop relationships with patients and their community. It also is important to be sincere and to not just recruit with the primary focus of obtaining participants.

A common method of recruiting research participants is to deliver a message directly to the targeted sample. Direct advertisement may take many forms, including mailings, fliers, brochures, web postings, phone calls, magazine and newspaper postings, and radio or television announcements. All recruitment materials must be approved by the IRB prior to their use because advertisement for clinical research is considered part of the informed consent process. The first information that people receive about the research needs to be clear, concise, and free of misleading text. When research is conducted at multiple clinical sites, effective communication and a designated point person may enhance clinical trial participation (Tramm et al., 2012). When reviewing a prospective advertisement, the IRB ensures that the material states information clearly, discloses that this is clinical research, refers to possible risks, and is consistent with the actual study and consent form (Miller, 2008). It should not contain potential areas of misinterpretation, coercion, bias, or discrimination.

Another method of recruiting participants is through screening of current patients. If a nurse works for a practice, as an employee, the nurse can review patient records to identify those who may be eligible to participate. Then, typically, information about the study is left in the record for the provider to share with patients on their next visit. Because of Health Insurance Portability and Accountability Act regulations, researchers outside of the practice cannot review charts and access PHI without signing a confidentiality agreement. Screening for eligibility also can be addressed when the patient completes the initial paperwork required for a standard patient. The patient can then indicate whether he or she would be open to further conversation or a phone call to discuss possible research participation.

Great variability exists in the financial and time requirements of recruitment strategies. Consideration of successful strategies used to target similar sample populations and to establish community commitment may be beneficial. Consulting with clinical research colleagues, healthcare providers, and patients within the targeted community may lead to valuable recruitment initiatives.

Clinical Trial Nurse

Historically, the role of the CTN has not been well defined. It has been suggested that CTNs need to receive formal education with clearer career progression (Scott, White, & Roydhouse, 2013). A few master's degree programs in clinical trial nursing exist, although CTNs may be licensed practical nurses or RNs or may not be nurses at all (e.g., clinical research associates). Oncology CTNs typically receive extensive training on the regulations and management of a clinical trial by the sponsoring agency. The Oncology Nursing Society (ONS) provides educational support to CTNs via access to the Clinical Trial Nurses Special Interest Group (http://clinicaltrial.vc.ons.org) and development of core competencies for the novice CTN (Lubejko et al., 2011). Clinical trials may involve testing new drugs or treatments, evaluating prevention strategies, or testing other types of treatments, such as radiation, surgery, or symptom management. In addition to the responsibilities already discussed, CTNs are likely to be responsible for protocol implementation, participant visits, data collection and data entry, trial management, patient follow-up, and preparation and submission of documents to the IRB or sponsoring agency. They may be responsible for continual renewal of studies until completed, submission of case report forms, and patient advocacy. Other responsibilities include maintaining the study binder, data and document tracking, and individual participant research charts; providing a reference manual for staff, reporting patients' responses to the intervention, including adverse events; attending educational sessions provided by the sponsoring agency or research site; and being a liaison to the sponsoring agency. Collaboration with ancillary departments, such as pharmacy and laboratory, may be necessary, as well as educating the billing staff, securing document storage, managing the study budget, and ensuring that staff take part in mandatory ethics training (Poston & Buescher, 2010). CTNs are responsible for all of this management in addition to being prepared for audits of the aforementioned information by the endorsing agency or cooperative group.

Publishing Research Data

The International Committee of Medical Journal Editors (ICMJE) recommends that for a manuscript to be published in an ICMJE journal, the clinical trial must be registered before enrolling the first human subject (ICMJE, 2014). Currently, only 14 journals are official members of the ICMJE, although a large number of peer-reviewed journals follow these recommendations. The rationale for the ICMJE's recommendations is to establish a standardized approach for the preparation of research manuscripts. It is important for APNs to be aware of this requirement prior to initiating enrollment.

Phases of Clinical Trials

Clinical trials are defined by phase, which occur in a stepwise fashion (NCI, 2013). The steps are clarified by phase number. Phase 0 trials are the earliest step in testing treatments in humans. It is the first time a drug is given, in very small doses, to see how it is processed. Investigators are primarily looking at the pharmacokinetics and pharmacodynamics (or metabolism) of the drug. Only a small number of participants are needed (10–15 people), and these participants usually have advanced disease without any further treatment options.

Phase I trials are focused on the safety of the drug (NCI, 2013). The drug dosage is slowly titrated up to identify the maximum tolerated dose and harmful side effects. Effectiveness of the drug is also assessed. Phase I trials usually have 15–30 or more participants who also have advanced disease with no further treatment options.

Phase II trials are based on the findings of phase I trials (NCI, 2013). Once the maximum tolerated dose is identified, the drug is tested among a specific population with a specific disease. Efficacy is the main outcome assessed. These trials usually have fewer than 100 participants.

Phase III trials compare the treatment used in phase II studies against the current standard of care (NCI, 2013). Effectiveness and tolerability of side effects are evaluated. Phase III trials usually are randomized controlled trials, where each participant is randomized to either the control arm (standard treatment) or experimental arm (drug being tested). *Randomization* means that each participant is randomly assigned to one of the arms of the study without any input by the participant, clinician, or researcher. The number of participants can range from 100 to thousands.

Phase IV trials occur after the drug receives FDA approval for the proposed indication. These trials are frequently called *postmarketing surveillance trials*. Drug companies usually sponsor these programs to assess effectiveness and long-term effects. However, the ethics of these trials have come under recent scrutiny (Institute of Medicine, 2013; Mello & Goodman, 2012). When the risk-benefit ratio of an approved drug is in question, FDA needs to balance protecting the public's health versus protecting the research participants before requiring postmarketing research.

See Figure 9-1 for a summary of the phases of clinical trials.

Searching for Clinical Trials

As of March 23, 2015, more than 12,000 open trials and 25,000 closed trials were posted to the NCI database (available at www.cancer.gov/clinicaltrials/search) (NCI, n.d.). Although it initially may seem odd that the database includes clinical trials that are closed, there is a good

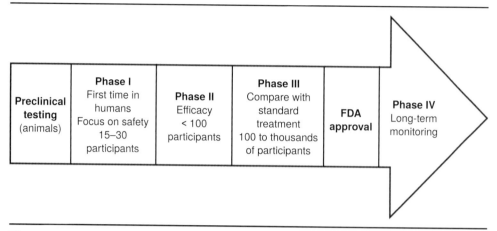

Figure 9-1. Phases of Clinical Trials

rationale. The World Health Organization (n.d.) fueled the momentum that prompted the current clinical trial registry mandate. Registering all clinical trials prior to knowing the success of the research and providing a summary of their results promotes the public's trust in how research is conducted and removes some of the mystery surrounding research. It also allows standardization of findings and avoids unnecessary duplication of research. Scientific and ethical integrity of clinical research is enhanced by the use of a universal system to register clinical trials.

Both clinicians and patients can search for clinical trials that would be appropriate for a patient. Many search engines exist, such as the following.
• CenterWatch Clinical Trials Listing Service™: www.centerwatch.com/clinical-trials/post
• ClinicalTrials.gov registry and results database of clinical studies of human participants conducted around the world: https://clinicaltrials.gov
• National Comprehensive Cancer Network® oncology clinical trial information for patients and caregivers: www.nccn.org/patients/resources/clinical_trials/default.aspx
• NCI clinical trials information: www.cancer.gov/clinicaltrials

Institutional Review Board

Before the first research participant is enrolled in a clinical research study, the study must receive certain approvals. All clinical research must be reviewed by the IRB. The IRB is the regulatory body authorized to review, approve, and regulate research. An IRB may be part of an academic or healthcare institution or an independent entity. The IRB's purposes include (a) protecting the rights and welfare of research participants, (b) determining that the potential benefits are greater than the risks, (c) ensuring that research participant recruitment is equitable, and (d) ensuring that appropriate consent is obtained and documented (U.S. FDA, 2014b). The IRB also reviews and approves the informed consent form for the clinical research study. The IRB, not the researchers, determines whether a study may be exempt from review. IRBs are federally regulated and monitored for compliance by the Office for Human Research Protections and FDA (Speers, 2008). Depending on the investigational product, approval by other regulatory bodies in addition to the IRB may be required. This regulatory body may be either internal or external to the institution. If the APN is a manager or program director, he or she may have to evaluate the feasibility of taking part in a research study at the clinical site. The feasibility assessment includes assessing cost to the facility or practice; staff requirements, including training and competency assessment; implications of regulations; and possible outside funding. Research studies and clinical trials typically cover procedures and testing that are performed that are not the standard of care and would not have been performed if the patient was not participating in research. However, each patient's individual health insurance policy may have stipulations regarding participation in clinical trials. Typically, investigational drugs or drugs used for investigational purposes (even if they are approved for another purpose) are not covered by insurance companies, but approved drugs that are considered standard care would be covered. However, it is always important to check the patient's individual plan.

Conclusion

Opportunities for oncology APNs to become involved with clinical research are diverse. APNs may refer patients for research; design the protocol; consent, screen, examine, and evaluate research participants; manage regulatory affairs; be a principal investigator or co- or subinvestigator; analyze the data; disseminate research findings; serve as a consultant to clinical researchers to identify and manage complications; or serve on a committee or board that provides scientific, regulatory, or ethical review. Many APNs are active in more than one of these clinical research roles.

Case Study

C.S. is a 54-year-old woman with advanced pancreatic cancer who wants to participate in a phase I clinical trial that was featured on the news two weeks ago. She made a consultation appointment with the oncology APN at the closest facility that is conducting the research. Unfortunately, C.S. has a five-hour drive to reach this facility. When C.S. first meets the oncology APN, she tells the nurse that since hearing the news that "a cure for pancreatic cancer has been found," she could hardly wait to get started. The APN notes that her handshake is weak and she appears frail. Her family reports that she did not eat any breakfast that morning because she is so nervous. C.S. shares that her appetite has not been good for the past few days because of the anxiety of waiting for this first consultation. She has been traveling with her family since before dawn to arrive for this early afternoon appointment. Her partner, her two adult children, and her father accompany her and appear very distressed over C.S.'s current condition. C.S. is extremely fatigued and was transported from the car to the office via a wheelchair. Her family indicates that she usually is more energetic and is "sleepy" now only because they all needed to wake up so early to arrive in time for the appointment. Her family believes that her fatigue and anorexia are related to this visit.

The plan of care was to obtain an informed consent at this visit for the cancer clinical trial and to initiate screening to determine eligibility.

1. After introductions are made and comfort measures are provided for the patient and her family, how should the oncology APN begin the consenting process?
    *   The oncology APN could begin the consenting process by discussing the research history of the new investigational product. During the initial greeting, C.S. shared information about how she learned about the cancer clinical trial. Earlier that week on the local evening news, a report indicated that the phase I study was going to start for a

new investigational product that cured mice of advanced pancreatic cancer. The oncology APN could briefly explain the phases of research, including the preclinical phase, in which animals (in this case, mice) are treated with the investigational product (see Figure 9-1). The APN would note that the successful results seen in mice do not always happen in humans. C.S. and her family need to know that the purpose of the phase I research study is to find out if the new investigational product can be given safely to humans and to determine the best dose. Phase I research studies are not designed to offer a therapeutic benefit. The APN's goal would be to deliver information that could balance a sense of hope with realism.

- C.S. and the family are puzzled now. They thought they had heard reliable news that reported the existence of a cure for pancreatic cancer. C.S.'s partner said, "You are just saying that to keep the publicity and malpractice claims under control. We know that you have the cure. Your lawyers are probably telling you to say that, right?" The oncology APN assures C.S. and her family that because this is the first time the investigational product will be given to humans, the effects are unknown. The drug may help, but it also may be harmful. The APN explains that this is a phase I, dose-escalating study and that even if the investigational product is found to be helpful, neither C.S. nor the healthcare providers will know if she will be receiving the optimal dose. And, in a phase I study, finding optimal dosing is the main objective.

2. After the oncology APN provides an overview of the essential elements of the informed consent, C.S. asks, "Can I sign the papers now?" Her partner states, "She's ready to sign up. Just tell her where to sign and let's be on with it." How should the oncology APN respond?

- The oncology APN knows that ensuring an adequate informed consent benefits the research participant and the cancer clinical trial. By knowing as much as possible about the cancer clinical trial, the research participant can be a partner in research. Having research participants understand their essential role in the cancer clinical trial can affect retention. The APN anticipated that C.S. would bring family and friends with her and provides extra copies of the informed consent document. Each person receives a copy of the consent and is asked to read the document thoroughly. The APN encourages them to mark the areas of the consent that they find to be unclear or have questions about. After they have read the consent, the oncology APN will return to answer their questions.

- Twenty minutes later, the family indicates that they have read the consent, and the nurse finds C.S. in a deep sleep. She arouses but is having difficulty staying awake. The family suggests that they allow C.S. to sleep, as she has already signed the informed consent document. They ask if she needs to be awake to receive the treatment.

3. What about this situation would cause concern to the APN?

- A few events could cause the oncology APN to become concerned. The oncology APN knows that the informed consent form needs to be signed in her presence. The nurse tells the family the consent needs to be reviewed with C.S. to determine *her* understanding of the content of the document. The oncology APN explains to the family that part of the routine consenting process includes validation from the research participant about what information is contained in the document that is being signed. This includes having the patient explain the purpose and process of the cancer clinical trial in her own words. The oncology APN also needs to assess her understanding of the time commitment required to be a research participant. Because C.S. is not mentally alert enough to continue with the consenting process, the oncology APN suggests they return another day to continue. The family indicates that they were planning to drive back home today and that these long drives are taking a toll on C.S. They ask if their local APN can sign the consent form with C.S. tomorrow.

4. Can the oncology APN arrange this for C.S.'s convenience?

• No, this is not an option. The oncology APN explains why C.S. will need to return to the clinical site to continue the consenting process. The oncology APN knows that only certain investigators who have received training about the study and have adequate education and experience are allowed to obtain informed consent. Also, for each study, investigators are selected by the principal investigator and approved by the IRB. The cancer clinical trial's regulatory records include the oncology APN's signed and dated curriculum vitae, APN license, and financial disclosure form. Another healthcare provider would not have approval by the IRB or the training to perform this function.

The oncology APN is sensitive to the family's desire to help their loved one and shares information about the signs and symptoms of advanced pancreatic cancer. The nurse acknowledges that while the long drive and the excitement of today's visit probably affected C.S.'s energy level, the decreasing performance status actually may reflect advancing disease. C.S.'s inability to eat also may be reflective of the anorexia that accompanies advanced pancreatic cancer. The APN encourages the family to call her tomorrow when C.S. is more alert. They do have a speaker phone at home, and all who are present today plan to talk tomorrow on the call. The oncology APN provides the family with several educational materials. The topics include dealing with advanced cancer, pancreatic cancer, hospice care, clinical trial information, and a list of Internet resources. The APN also plans to discuss with C.S.'s oncology healthcare provider that C.S. may not be a good candidate for the cancer clinical trial.

Key Points

• Clinical research is the systematic investigation of human biology, health, or illness that contributes to generalizable knowledge.
• General requirements of informed consent include the following.
    – Consent must be obtained from the participant or the participant's legal representative.
    – The process must allow sufficient opportunity for patients to consider whether to participate.
    – The process must minimize the possibility of coercion or undue influence.
    – The language of consent must be understandable to the participant or the participant's representative.
    – The consent must not release or appear to release the investigator, sponsor, institution, or its agents from liability for negligence.
• Only an estimated 3%–5% of people with cancer participate in a cancer clinical trial; thus, recruitment of participants to oncology trials must be a priority for oncology APNs.
• Oncology APNs have diverse roles in clinical research and may
    – Refer patients for research
    – Design the protocol
    – Consent, screen, examine, and evaluate research participants
    – Manage regulatory affairs
    – Be a co- or subinvestigator
    – Be a principal investigator
    – Analyze the data
    – Disseminate research findings
    – Serve as a consultant to clinical researchers to identify and manage complications
    – Serve on a committee or board that provides scientific, regulatory, or ethical review.

Recommended Resources for Oncology Advanced Practice Nurses

Education

- American Association of Colleges of Nursing Position Statement on Nursing Research: www.aacn.nche.edu/publications/position/NsgResearch.pdf
- ANA's Research Toolkit: www.nursingworld.org/Research-Toolkit
- National Institute of Nursing Research Strategic Plan: www.ninr.nih.gov/files/ninr-strategic-plan-2011.pdf
- ONS Resources for Researchers: www.ons.org/practice-resources/researchers
  - ONS Research Agenda
  - ONS Research Priorities Survey
  - ONS *Oncology Clinical Trials Nurse Competencies*: www.ons.org/sites/default/files/ctncompetencies.pdf

Training

- Health Resources and Services Administration—Protecting Human Subjects Training: www.hrsa.gov/publichealth/clinical/humansubjects
- National Institute of Nursing Research Nurse Scientists Training: www.ninr.nih.gov/training#.VRBgeOF5_wA
- National Institutes of Health—Human Subjects Protections Training: http://grants.nih.gov/grants/policy/hs/training.htm

Funding

- Agency for Healthcare Research and Quality: www.ahrq.gov/funding/index.html
- American Cancer Society Research Programs and Funding: www.cancer.org/research/researchprogramsfunding/index
- American Nurses Foundation: www.anfonline.org/MainCategory/NursingResearchGrant.aspx
- ONS Foundation: www.onsfoundation.org
- Sigma Theta Tau International Nursing Research Grants: www.nursingsociety.org/Research/Grants/Pages/Grantsbydate.aspx

The author would like to acknowledge Barbara A. Biedrzycki, RN, MSN, CRNP, AOCNP®, for her contribution to this chapter that remains unchanged from the first edition of this book.

References

American Association of Colleges of Nursing. (2006). AACN position statement on nursing research. Retrieved from http://www.aacn.nche.edu/publications/position/NsgResearch.pdf

American Nurses Association. (2012). Appraising the evidence. Research toolkit. Retrieved from http://nursingworld.org/MainMenuCategories/ThePracticeofProfessionalNursing/Improving-Your-Practice/Research-Toolkit/Appraising-the-Evidence

American Nurses Association. (2015). *Code of ethics for nurses.* Silver Spring, MD: American Nurses Publishing.

American Nurses Foundation. (n.d.). History of the American Nurses Foundation. Retrieved from http://www.anfonline.org/Main/AboutANF/History

Bruner, D.W., & O'Mara, A. (2014). Nurse scientists in cancer cooperative groups. *Seminars in Oncology Nursing, 30,* 4–10. doi:10.1016/j.soncn.2013.12.002

Catania, K., Askew, T., Brikhimer, D., Courtney, L., Hanes, D., Lamprecht, M., … Vendlinski, S. (2012). From unit based to population focused: Transforming the role of oncology clinical nurse specialists. *Clinical Nurse Specialist, 26,* 103–106. doi:10.1097/NUR.0b013e31824590d0

Edwardson, S.R. (2010). Doctor of philosophy and doctor of nursing practice as complementary degrees. *Journal of Professional Nursing, 26,* 137–140. doi:10.1016/j.profnurs.2009.08.004

Emanuel, E.J., Wendler, D., & Grady, C. (2008). An ethical framework for biomedical research. In E.J. Emanuel, C. Grady, R.A. Crouch, R.K. Lie, F.G. Miller, & D. Wendler (Eds.), *The Oxford textbook of clinical research ethics* (pp. 123–135). New York, NY: Oxford University Press.

Institute of Medicine. (2013). *Implementing a national cancer clinical trials system for the 21st century: Second workshop summary.* Washington, DC: National Academies Press.

International Committee of Medical Journal Editors. (2014, December). Recommendations for the conduct, reporting, editing, and publication of scholarly work in medical journals. Retrieved from http://www.icmje.org/icmje-recommendations.pdf

International Conference on Harmonisation of Technical Requirements for Registration of Pharmaceuticals for Human Use. (1996). Guideline for good clinical practice E6(R1). Retrieved from http://www.ich.org/fileadmin/Public_Web_Site/ICH_Products/Guidelines/Efficacy/E6/E6_R1_Guideline.pdf

International Council of Nurses. (2012). *The ICN code of ethics for nurses.* Retrieved from http://www.icn.ch/images/stories/documents/about/icncode_english.pdf

Lubejko, B., Good, M., Weiss, P., Schmieder, L., Leos, D., & Daugherty, P. (2011). Oncology clinical trials nursing: Developing competencies for the novice. *Clinical Journal of Oncology Nursing, 15,* 637–643. doi:10.1188/11.CJON.637-643

Mayer, D.K. (Ed.). (2000). Celebrating our past, creating our future [Special issue]. *Oncology Nursing Forum, 27*(Suppl.).

Mello, M.M., & Goodman, S.N. (2012). Ethical considerations in studying drug safety—The Institute of Medicine report. *New England Journal of Medicine, 367,* 959–964. doi:10.1056/NEJMhle1207160

Miller, F.G. (2008). Recruiting research participants. In E.J. Emanuel, C. Grady, R.A. Crouch, R.K. Lie, F.G. Miller, & D. Wendler (Eds.), *The Oxford textbook of clinical research ethics* (pp. 397–403). New York, NY: Oxford University Press.

National Cancer Institute. (n.d.). Search for clinical trials. Retrieved from http://www.cancer.gov/clinicaltrials/search

National Cancer Institute. (2011). Checklist for easy-to-read informed consent. AccrualNet. Retrieved from https://accrualnet.cancer.gov/literature/checklist_easy_to_read_informed_consent#.VRBll-F5_wB

National Cancer Institute. (2013). What are clinical trials? Retrieved from http://www.cancer.gov/clinicaltrials/learningabout/what-are-clinical-trials

National Cancer Institute. (2015). An overview of NCI's National Clinical Trials Network. Retrieved from http://www.cancer.gov/clinicaltrials/nctn

National Commission for the Protection of Human Subjects of Biomedical and Behavioral Research. (1979). The Belmont report. Retrieved from http://www.hhs.gov/ohrp/humansubjects/guidance/belmont.html

National Institute of Nursing Research. (2011). Bringing science to life: NINR strategic plan. Retrieved from https://www.ninr.nih.gov/sites/www.ninr.nih.gov/files/ninr-strategic-plan-2011.pdf

Oncology Nursing Society. (n.d.). ONS history. Retrieved from https://www.ons.org/about/history

Oncology Nursing Society. (2010). *Oncology clinical trials nurse competencies.* Retrieved from https://www.ons.org/sites/default/files/ctncompetencies.pdf

Penberthy, L.T., Dahman, B.A., Petkov, V.I., & DeShazo, J.P. (2012). Effort required in eligibility screening for clinical trials. *Journal of Oncology Practice, 8,* 365–370. doi:10.1200/JOP.2012.000646

Penn Nursing Science. (n.d.). Nursing, history and health care. Retrieved from http://www.nursing.upenn.edu/nhhc/Pages/Welcome.aspx

Polit, D.F., & Beck, C.T. (2014). *Essentials of nursing research: Appraising evidence for nursing practice* (8th ed.). Philadelphia, PA: Wolters Kluwer Health/Lippincott Williams & Wilkins.

Poston, R.D., & Buescher, C.R. (2010). The essential role of the clinical research nurse (CRN). *Urologic Nursing, 30,* 55–63, 77.

Rolfe, G., & Davies, R. (2009). Second generation professional doctorates in nursing. *International Journal of Nursing Studies, 46,* 1265–1273. doi:10.1016/j.ijnurstu.2009.04.002

Schmotzer, G.L. (2012). Barriers and facilitators to participation of minorities in clinical trials. *Ethnicity and Disease, 22,* 226–230.

Scott, K., White, K., & Roydhouse, J.K. (2013). Advancing the educational and career pathway for clinical trials nurses. *Journal of Continuing Education in Nursing, 44,* 165–170. doi:10.3928/00220124-20121217-38

Silva, M. (1995). *Ethical guidelines in the conduct, dissemination, and implementation of nursing research.* Silver Spring, MD: American Nurses Association.

Skloot, R. (2011). *The immortal life of Henrietta Lacks.* New York, NY: Broadway Books.

Speers, M.A. (2008). Evaluating the effectiveness of institutional review boards. In E.J. Emanuel, C. Grady, R.A. Crouch, R.K. Lie, F.G. Miller, & D. Wendler (Eds.), *The Oxford textbook of clinical research ethics* (pp. 560–568). New York, NY: Oxford University Press.

Stiles, C.R., Johnson, L., Whyte, D., Nergaard, T.H., Gardner, J., & Wu, J. (2011). Does increased patient awareness improve accrual into cancer-related clinical trials? *Cancer Nursing, 34*(5), E13–E19. doi:10.1097/NCC.0b013e31820254db

Tramm, R., Daws, K., & Schadewaldt, V. (2013). Clinical trial recruitment—A complex intervention? *Journal of Clinical Nursing, 22,* 2436–2443. doi:10.1111/jocn.12145

U.S. Department of Health and Human Services Office for Human Research Protections. (2005). The Nuremberg Code. Retrieved from http://www.hhs.gov/ohrp/archive/nurcode.html

U.S. Department of Health and Human Services Office for Human Research Protections. (2014). § 46.116 Informed consent checklist: Basic and additional elements. Retrieved from http://www.hhs.gov/ohrp/policy/consentckls.html

U.S. Food and Drug Administration. (2014a). Title 21: Food and drugs; Chapter I: Food and Drug Administration Department of Health and Human Services; Subchapter A: General; Part 50: Protection of human subjects. Retrieved from http://www.accessdata.fda.gov/scripts/cdrh/cfdocs/cfcfr/CFRSearch.cfm?fr=50.25

U.S. Food and Drug Administration. (2014b). Title 21: Food and drugs; Chapter I: Food and Drug Administration Department of Health and Human Services; Subchapter A: General; Part 56: Institutional review boards. Retrieved from http://www.accessdata.fda.gov/scripts/cdrh/cfdocs/cfcfr/CFRSearch.cfm?CFRPart=56

U.S. Food and Drug Administration. (2014c). A guide to informed consent—Information sheet. Retrieved from http://www.fda.gov/RegulatoryInformation/Guidances/ucm126431.htm

Vincent, D., Johnson, C., Velasquez, D., & Rigney, T. (2010). DNP-prepared nurses as practitioner-researchers: Closing the gap between research and practice. *American Journal for Nurse Practitioners, 14*(11/12), 28–34.

Wilkinson, K. (2012). Informed consent and patients with cancer: Role of the nurse as advocate. *Clinical Journal of Oncology Nursing, 16,* 348–350. doi:10.1188/12.CJON.348-350

World Health Organization. (n.d.). International Clinical Trials Registry Platform (ICTRP). Retrieved from http://www.who.int/ictrp/network/trds/en

World Medical Association. (2008). World Medical Association Declaration of Helsinki: Ethical principles for medical research involving human subjects. Retrieved from http://www.wma.net/en/30publications/10policies/b3/17c.pdf

CHAPTER 10

Pain, Fatigue, and Cognitive Impairment

Kimberly Noonan, RN, ANP-BC, AOCN®

Introduction

Pain, fatigue, and cognitive impairment are common problems encountered by advanced practice nurses (APNs) in oncology practice. Each of these factors may have a profound effect on patient quality of life and daily function. Assessment, diagnosis, and management of each will be addressed in this chapter.

Pain

Introduction

Pain is one of the most feared and prevalent symptoms associated with cancer and cancer treatments. Pain can severely affect the quality of life of patients with cancer; therefore, it is imperative that pain is managed to reduce physical and emotional distress (Mesgarpour et al., 2014). The European Society for Medical Oncology (ESMO) reported that more than 80% of patients with advanced metastatic disease will experience pain (Ripamonti, Santini, Maranzano, Berti, & Roila, 2012). Cancer pain can be caused by the infiltration of tumor; injury to nerves, bone, or soft tissue as a result of chemotherapy, radiation therapy, or surgery; or radiation-induced vascular occlusion (McMenamin, 2011; Portenoy, 2011). In 1996, the World Health Organization (WHO) estimated that about one-third of patients receiving cancer treatments and 60%–90% of patients with metastatic disease experience moderate to severe pain (WHO, 1996). Unfortunately, the epidemiology of cancer pain has remained consistent over the past 20 years, with numerous studies continuing to report that cancer pain remains under-treated (Miaskowski, 2010a). Pooled data from 52 articles reported pain in 64% of patients with advanced-stage cancer, 59% of patients receiving therapy, and 33% of patients receiving curative treatment (van den Beuken-van Everdingen et al., 2007). More than one-third of the patients rated their pain as moderate or severe. Actual pain incidence rates vary depending on the extent of disease, the type of cancer, the definition of pain, and the measurement methods used (Ripamonti et al., 2012). Because of the growing number of cancer survivors, the incidence of chronic pain following successful cancer treatment is increasing as well. Factors influencing chronic pain in cancer survivors following cancer treatment include chemotherapy-induced peripheral neuropathy, radiation-induced brachial plexopathy, postsurgical pain (such as postmastectomy or post-thoracotomy pain), and pelvic pain secondary to radiation (Ripamonti et al., 2012).

Several professional societies have position statements recommending specific treatment of for cancer pain. Some of these include Oncology Nursing Society (ONS, 2014), the American Society for Pain Management Nursing (Cooney et al., 2013; Reynolds, Drew, & Dunwoody, 2013), the American Academy of Pain Medicine (2013), and the American Association of Nurse Anesthetists (2010), among others. Several organizations also have published recommendation guidelines or standards of care for cancer pain treatment, such as the National Comprehensive Cancer Network® (NCCN®, 2015a), the American Pain Society (Chou et al., 2009), the Agency for Healthcare Research and Quality (2013), WHO (1996), and the American Society of Anesthesiologists (1996, 2010). Patient advocacy groups and professional organizations have emphasized routine pain assessment for well over a decade. Since 1999, many healthcare organizations have mandated assessment of pain as the "fifth vital sign" (Lorenz et al., 2009). Although effective pain management interventions are readily available for up to 80%–90% of patients experiencing pain, undertreatment is well documented and occurs in close to 50% of patients (Higginson & Gao, 2012). Barriers that may play a role in the undertreatment of cancer pain are complicated and involve the healthcare system, healthcare providers, patients, and family members (Mercadante, 2012; Ripamonti et al., 2012). The most common error in the treatment of cancer pain is inadequate assessment and failure to act upon that assessment by treating adequately or underdosing (Bennett et al., 2012). The optimal management of cancer pain is one of the most important tasks of oncology APNs and is accomplished through a multidisciplinary approach: blending various skills, knowledge, tools, therapies, policies, and beliefs of each member of the healthcare team, including the patient (NCCN, 2015a).

Definitions and Incidence

The concept of pain is complex, varying by individual and culture. The International Association for the Study of Pain (2011) defines pain as an unpleasant sensory and emotional experience related to actual or potential tissue damage. Pain can be acute or chronic. Acute pain is of shorter, limited duration, has an identifiable cause, and functions to warn and protect from tissue damage. Acute pain may be caused by diagnostic procedures, treatment, or surgical interventions. In most clinical situations, acute pain will improve over time. Chronic pain continues well past the expected recovery time following injury to the body. In general, chronic pain continues for longer than one to six months or recurs at various intervals. It can occur from sites of metastatic disease but also may develop because of preexisting conditions (such as diabetic peripheral neuropathy, osteoarthritis, and lower back pain) (Miaskowski, 2010a). Cancer pain may be acute or chronic, or both, as both types can occur simultaneously depending on the disease state, diagnostic procedure, or treatment.

Pain can be described as nociceptive when caused by ongoing tissue injury. The two types of nociceptive pain include somatic and visceral pain. Neuropathic pain is another type of pain that is caused by an abnormal somatosensory processing in the peripheral or central nervous system (Dworkin et al., 2010). It is important to recognize that patients with cancer may have one or a combination of the three mechanisms of pain (Bennett et al., 2012). For these reasons, it is essential that oncology practitioners are accurate in their assessment, treatment, and evaluation of patients experiencing pain.

Controlled-release opioids are prescribed for patients with cancer experiencing persistent moderate to severe chronic pain. Controlled-release opioids are administered around the clock and on a fixed schedule. Extended-release or long-acting medications include oxycodone, methadone, oxymorphone, hydromorphone, and transdermal fentanyl and buprenorphine.

Breakthrough pain is defined as transitory pain that occurs in the setting of adequately controlled pain by an opioid regimen. Breakthrough pain may be somatic, visceral, neuropathic, or a combination of these. Breakthrough pain medication is also known as "rescue" medication. Short-acting opioids are used to control breakthrough pain and include oxycodone, morphine, hydromorphone, and oxymorphone. Newer breakthrough pain medications include transmucosal fentanyl (NCCN, 2015a). Breakthrough pain can occur without stimulus or as a result of certain activities or biologic events and is associated with decreased quality of life and increased cost and hospitalizations (Wengström et al., 2014). The incidence of breakthrough pain is difficult to quantify. A prospective study of 63 patients with cancer pain reported that 64% had breakthrough pain of severe or excruciating intensity (Portenoy & Hagen, 1990). In this study, 29% of the cases of breakthrough pain were related to fixed opioid dosing, occurring at the end of the dosing interval. In 55% of the cases, the breakthrough pain was precipitated by some activity. Less than one-third were considered idiopathic and not under voluntary control (such as pain occurring with flatulence or coughing). Other studies have reported similar findings, with the prevalence of breakthrough pain ranging from 19% to 95% (Greco et al., 2011). Breakthrough pain is also costly: related hospitalizations, emergency department visits, and clinic or office visits in patients experiencing breakthrough pain was estimated at $12,000 per patient per year compared to $2,400 in patients without breakthrough pain (Wengström et al., 2014).

Optimal pain management requires understanding of addiction, physical dependence, and tolerance. *Addiction* is a disease with strong genetic, psychosocial, and environmental influences. Opioid addiction is uncommon among patients with cancer (Anghelescu, Ehrentraut, & Faughnan, 2013). The American Society for Pain Management Nursing defines *addiction* as a chronic, relapsing, treatable disease of the brain characterized by craving, dysfunctional behaviors, and an inability to control impulses regarding consumption of a substance with compulsive use despite harmful consequences (Oliver et al., 2012). Pseudoaddiction occurs because of inadequate pain management and often is interpreted as drug seeking (Anghelescu et al., 2013; Bell & Salmon, 2009). Pseudoaddictive behaviors are pain-relief–seeking behaviors that occur when a patient's pain is unrelieved and healthcare clinicians view the patient's request for more pain medication as addictive behavior. This is more likely to occur when the patient is undermedicated, requiring an adjustment in the current pain management strategy (Anghelescu et al., 2013).

Opioid dependence involves physical symptoms, including tolerance of opioid medication and symptoms of withdrawal when the opioids are withheld (Garland, Froeliger, Zeidan, Partin, & Howard, 2013). This is an anticipated response to ongoing opioid therapy and should not be confused with addiction. Physical dependence may occur within a few days, although it varies among patients. Physical dependence may be seen as a withdrawal syndrome if the drug is abruptly stopped, if the dose is rapidly reduced, or if an antagonist is administered. Withdrawal symptoms can be avoided by tapering the narcotic over a period of time (Anghelescu et al., 2013).

Tolerance is the need to increase the dosage of drug or the frequency of use to achieve the same level of pain relief and results from chronic administration (Garland et al., 2013). When tolerance occurs, the frequency of dosing should be increased or another opioid could be prescribed.

Etiology and Pathology

Nociceptors are specialized receptors (sensory neurons) located throughout the body (skin, viscera, and musculoskeletal tissues) that respond to painful stimuli. When nociceptors are activated by either mechanical or chemical stimuli, nociceptive information is sent along A-delta and C fibers to the brain, and the individual then experiences somatic and/or visceral pain. Non-nociceptive information (caused by damage to the nervous system) is conveyed by A-beta fibers, and when the brain receives them, neuropathic pain results (Fornasari, 2012). A-delta fibers are small, thinly myelinated fibers that are activated by stimuli such as pinpricks. C fibers are thin and unmyelinated and are activated by tissue damage. Tissue damage causes C fibers to release chemical metabolites called *transducers*, such as epinephrine, prostaglandins, leukotrienes, serotonin, bradykinin, and substance P, that sensitize the area of damage (causing inflammation) and activate nociceptors, thus causing pain. A-beta axons are larger and more heavily myelinated and are activated by light touch, therefore transmitting information much more rapidly than the A-delta or C fibers. Pain information enters the spinal cord via the dorsal root synapse, and transmission is mediated by excitatory amino acids, mainly glutamate but also aspartate, substance P, and calcitonin gene-related peptide. The pain information then crosses to the spinothalamic tracts and is transmitted to the thalamus and cortex. From there, the sensory cortex, frontal lobe, and reticular formation process the information, resulting in the perception of pain (Fornasari, 2012; Walker, 2010). Opioid receptors are located on ascending and descending pain pathways and will produce the analgesic effects of opioid pharmaceuticals. More opioid receptors are located in certain parts of the brain and spinal cord.

Understanding of the neurotransmitters involved in pain transmission has led researchers to explore targeted strategies for cancer pain management (Chou et al., 2009). Strategies include blocking pain at the periphery (as with nonsteroidal anti-inflammatory drugs [NSAIDs] and anesthetics), activating inhibitory processes in the spinal cord and brain (as with opioid treatments), and interfering with the perception of pain (as with relaxation therapy).

Somatic pain originates from skin, bone, muscle, blood vessels, subcutaneous tissue, and connective tissue. It is well localized when cutaneous but more diffuse when originating deeper. Patients may describe somatic pain as dull, constant, or aching. An example of somatic pain in oncology is bone metastases or postsurgical incision pain. Approximately one-third of all cancer pain is somatic (Miaskowski, 2010a).

The etiology of visceral pain may be caused by organ obstruction (e.g., bowel, pancreatic duct, ureteral) or injury to another pain-sensitive visceral structure such as the pleura, hepatic capsule, or peritoneum. It is important to determine the etiology of visceral pain and establish whether the pain is due to compression, infiltration, or distension of viscera when considering management strategies to control visceral pain. This type of pain occurs in patients with gastrointestinal and gynecologic malignancies (McMenamin, 2011). It usually is poorly localized in nature and may be described as deep, squeezing, cramping, splitting, or pressure-like. Visceral pain can occur when metastasis to an organ occurs. It is often referred to areas away from the actual site of disease. Causes include the tumor itself or injury resulting from chemotherapy, radiation therapy, or surgery.

Neuropathic pain is poorly localized and may be described as sharp, strange, shooting, hot or burning, electric shock–like, vise-like, or "painfully numb." If localized, it usually occurs at the site of injury, and this area may be hypersensitive to other stimuli. Neuropathic pain may be delayed in onset, occurring days to years after the nerve-damaging event. Several causes of neuropathic pain syndromes exist. Neoplastic invasion to the spinal cord, nerve roots, plexuses, or peripheral nerves is a common cause. Surgical procedures such as radical neck dissection, mastectomy, thoracotomy, nephrectomy, and limb amputation are another reason for the development of neuropathic pain syndromes. Chemotherapy toxicity from agents such as taxanes, cisplatin, bortezomib, and vinca alkaloids is also known to cause neuropathic pain. Infection also can be considered when patients report neuropathic pain symptoms (Miaskowski, 2010a).

The prevalence of neuropathic pain is estimated to occur in 18%–21% of patients with cancer (Bennett et al., 2012). It is interesting that when mixed pain is reported, neuropathic pain was reported more frequently and estimated to occur 19%–39% of the time (Bennett et al., 2012).

Several pain syndromes commonly appear in patients with cancer (see Table 10-1). A cancer pain syndrome is described as a constellation of meaningful signs and symptoms in a patient with cancer (Portenoy, 2011). Approximately 75% of patients with cancer with chronic pain have nociceptive or neuropathic pain that is directly related to the individual malignancy (Portenoy, 2011). Patients often experience mixed types of pain. For example, patients with bone metastasis (somatic pain) also may experience a component of neuropathic pain. Other causes of chronic pain occur as a result of antineoplastic treatments and disorders that are

Table 10-1. Common Oncologic Pain Syndromes

Pain Syndrome	Description
Bone metastasis pain	Form of nociceptive pain Sensitive to nonsteroidal and anti-inflammatory drugs Localized, sharp, aching, deep pain that may worsen with activity Most common site of metastases are the vertebrae, pelvis, hip, femur, and skull
Brachial plexopathy	Often occurs following radiation for lymphoma, breast cancer, and lung cancer Incidence up to 9% Onset varies from 6 months to 20 years after cancer treatment Dysesthesia, pain, weakness, flaccid arm, loss of hand function
Herpetic neuralgia	Painful paresthesia and dysesthesia, burning, aching, shock-like pain Risk factors: Increasing age, immunosuppression
Inflammatory pain	Caused by tissue damage leading to inflammation (migration of white blood cells to site releasing cytokines, prostaglandins, and bradykinin, thus activating nociceptors) Common causes: Tumor mass effect, treatment-induced gout, abscesses
Osteonecrosis (avascular necrosis)	Often caused by long-term corticosteroid use, usually within 3 years, most often in the femoral head Osteonecrosis of the jaw as rare result of bisphosphonate therapy Focal necrosis from radiation, bisphosphonate therapy, or chemotherapy Decreased range of motion, pain with activity, arthritis
Peripheral neuropathy	Painful paresthesias and dysesthesias, hyporeflexia Could lead to motor and sensory loss, including autonomic dysfunction May be chemotherapy induced Incidence and severity potentially increased by preexisting nerve damage

(Continued on next page)

Table 10-1. Common Oncologic Pain Syndromes *(Continued)*

Pain Syndrome	Description
Postamputation "phantom" pain	Prevalence rates up to 95% Phantom sensations, phantom pain, stump pain, burning dysesthesias Pain possibly exacerbated by movement Risk factors: Preamputation pain, female sex, severe postoperative pain, poorly fitted prosthesis, more proximal amputation, chemotherapy treatment
Postmastectomy pain syndrome	Tight, burning pain in mastectomy site, axilla, and back of arm; paresthesia, dysesthesia, allodynia, hyperalgesia, or loss of shoulder function; neuroma pain (scar pain); phantom breast pain Caused by intercostobrachial neuralgia and/or other nerve injuries Worse with arm movement Prevalence rates are approximately 25%–60% Risk factors: Postoperative radiation therapy, extent of axillary dissection, negative psychological states
Postnephrectomy pain syndrome	Dysesthesias; fullness and heaviness in flank, abdomen, or groin
Postradiation pain syndrome (radiation-induced plexopathy)	Radiation-induced neural damage, as well as compression causing radiation-induced fibrosis May have late onset (even up to 20 years) after treatment
Postradiation pelvic pain syndromes	Etiology: Pelvic insufficiency fracture, enteritis, visceral dysfunction, neural damage, prostate brachytherapy Often underreported
Post–radical neck dissection	Tight, burning pain in surgical site Dysesthesias, shock-like pains Incidence of neck pain approximately 33%; shoulder pain, 37%; myofascial pain, 47%; loss of sensation, 65% Possible pain years after treatment as result of radiation-induced neural damage
Post-thoracotomy pain syndrome	Aching, sharp pain in incision site, more intense at medial and apical points of incision Prevalence rates approximately 50%, with half of these reporting moderate to severe pain Etiology: Intercostal nerve injury and continuous chest wall movement
Radiation myelopathy	Injury to spinal cord by radiation Paresthesia, thermesthesia, algesthesia, muscle weakness, gait disturbance, hemiplegia Pain or dysesthesia at or below level of injury
Skeletal fractures	Pain that increases in severity; severe pain; reports of a "cracking" sound May exacerbate with activity
Tumor infiltration of peripheral nerve	Dysesthesia; localized, constant burning pain Radiating pain
Visceral pain	Most often found in abdominal cancers Associated with distension Dull, cramping pain, difficult to localize

Note. Based on information from Burton et al., 2007; Chang et al., 2006; Ephraim et al., 2005; Fallon, 2013; Khadilkar & Khade, 2013; McMenamin, 2011; National Comprehensive Cancer Network, 2015a; Portenoy, 2011; Schreiber et al., 2013; Sepsas et al., 2013.

unrelated to the disease (Bennett et al., 2012). Bone metastasis is a pain syndrome that is one of the most prevalent causes of chronic cancer pain (Falk & Dickenson, 2014).

Bone metastasis may be caused by direct tumor invasion, damage to adjacent structures, or a secondary pathologic fracture. The pain is often described as severe and localized. The exact mechanism of action is not known, but it is known that during this process, normal bone remodeling is disrupted. Bone metastasis may be associated with direct nociceptor activation by tumor, mechanical microfracture distortion, or the release of growth factors and chemical mediators (Monczewski, 2013; Portenoy, 2011). The most common sites of metastasis include the spine, pelvis, hip, femur, and skull. APNs need to monitor for specific complications of bone metastasis, which include cord compression, fracture, and hypercalcemia.

Many pain syndromes are treatment related, such as chemotherapy-induced peripheral neuropathy caused by an agent or combination of agents such as vincristine, thalidomide, bortezomib, platinum compounds, and taxanes (Ferrier, Pereira, Busserolles, Authier, & Balayssac, 2013). Even years after radiation therapy, patients may experience the onset of pain from neural damage.

The etiology of breakthrough pain in patients with cancer is not always clear (Greco et al., 2011). It can occur spontaneously or be precipitated by an activity such as walking, turning, or standing (volitional pain). Breakthrough pain may be nonvolitional, such as with abdominal distension or coughing, or incidental, such as pain related to a procedure or a therapeutic intervention. Breakthrough pain also may result from "end-of-dose failure" caused by declining analgesic levels—that is, pain occurring before the next scheduled dose of pain medication. The pathophysiology of breakthrough pain is believed to be consistent with the mechanisms outlined previously. However, hyperexcitability in the central nervous system or periphery may play a role as well (Hogan, Baker, Morón, & Carlton, 2013). Mechanical stimuli, nerve injuries, changes in the chemical environment of nociceptors, and the release of tumor growth factors may cause sensitization, and thus breakthrough pain may be evoked by stimuli that normally are minimally painful (i.e., hyperalgesia) or not painful (i.e., allodynia) (Portenoy, 2011).

Leptomeningeal metastasis is another example of a pain syndrome. This can be caused by any solid or hematologic malignancy but is more common in breast and lung cancer, as well as lymphoma and leukemia (Le Rhun, Taillibert, & Chamberlain, 2013). Patients may report headache; back pain, which may be accompanied by seizures; cognitive impairment; hemiparesis; neuropathy; or radiculopathy. Cranial neuralgias can develop from metastases involving the base of the skull or leptomeninges arising from the head, neck, or sinuses. Radiculopathies, or pain radiating from the spine, can be caused by compressed or inflamed nerve roots.

Plexopathies also may cause neuropathic pain. Tumor-related plexopathies can involve the cervical, brachial, or lumbosacral plexus. Cervical plexopathies may be due to a head and neck tumor or involved cervical lymph nodes. Brachial plexopathy may cause shoulder, arm, or hand pain. The underlying malignancies associated with brachial plexopathies include lung cancer, breast cancer, and lymphoma.

It is estimated that 20%–40% of patients receiving neurotoxic chemotherapy will develop painful peripheral neuropathy (McMenamin, 2011). Painful chemotherapy-induced neuropathy can persist for years after chemotherapy administration, significantly affecting the quality of life for patients with cancer (Smith et al., 2013).

Risk Factors

Many factors potentially increase the risk of cancer pain. Advanced disease increases the risk of pain. Additionally, the type of metastases may increase risk (Portenoy, 2011). The location of the cancer is another consideration. Studies show that psychosocial factors, such as depression, anxiety, and feelings of isolation, influence pain reports (Ripamonti et al., 2012). Patients with inadequate acute pain management during treatment are more likely to have subsequent chronic pain (Burton, Fanciullo, Beasley, & Fisch, 2007; Burton, Fine, & Passik, 2012). Data have suggested that preoperative patients with cancer with an increase in distress-related psychosocial factors, such as anxiety, somatization, catastrophizing, or depression, may be at risk for developing prolonged pain (Lautenbacher et al., 2011; Schreiber et al., 2013).

Factors also exist that increase the risk of inadequate pain management. These include age (older than 70 or younger than 3 years old), female sex, cognitive impairment, a history of substance abuse, and minority races (McMenamin, 2011; Walker, 2010). Pain management in the older adult population can be complicated, and pain often is undertreated (Curtiss, 2010; Miaskowski, 2010b). A recent literature review of 17 publications suggested the need for future research that would better define the complexity and nature of pain in older adult patients with cancer (Dunham, Ingleton, Ryan, & Gott, 2013).

Literature has suggested inadequate pain management in minority populations (Campbell & Edwards, 2012; Shavers, Bakos, & Sheppard, 2010). In a study conducted by Merry et al. (2011), researchers evaluated 155 patients participating in a multidisciplinary pain treatment program. Patients participating in this trial were African American or Caucasian, and the primary outcome variables included pain-related interference, pain severity, and depressive symptoms. A reduction in pain-related interference and depressive symptoms was noted for each group. However, patients in the Caucasian group also reported a reduction in pain severity, whereas the African American group did not. Another study conducted by Fisch et al. (2012) reported that minority patients were twice as likely to experience uncontrolled pain when compared to nonminority patients.

Signs and Symptoms

Acute, chronic, and neuropathic pain will have varying clinical signs and symptoms (see Figure 10-1). Autonomic signs (such as tachycardia or increased blood pressure) are present in acute pain but may be absent in chronic pain. The absence of autonomic signs does not necessarily indicate absence of pain. Neuropathic pain presents unique symptoms, such as hyperesthesia or dysesthesia. Assessment in nonverbal or cognitively impaired patients may be more difficult because of an absence of a self-report or an unreliable pain report. In such patients, cli-

Acute	Chronic	Neuropathic
• Autonomic signs*	• Autonomic signs absent	• Allodynia
– Diaphoresis	• Constipation	• Dysesthesias
– Elevated blood pressure	• Decreased appetite	• Hyperalgesia
– Pallor	• Decreased libido	• Hyperesthesia
– Tachycardia	• Depression	• Hyperpathia
	• Fatigue	• May follow neural pathway
	• Insomnia	
	• Social withdrawal	

Figure 10-1. Clinical Signs and Symptoms of Pain

* Autonomic signs are not sensitive in differentiating pain from other sources of distress. Absence of autonomic signs does not indicate absence of pain.

Note. Based on information from Kendall et al., 2013; Miaskowski, 2010a; National Comprehensive Cancer Network, 2015a; Portenoy, 2011; Ripamonti et al., 2012.

nicians should use a comprehensive approach to assess pain. A comprehensive approach may include metrics such as physical and emotional functional status, as well as overall improvement in quality of life (Miaskowski, 2010b).

Assessment

Cancer pain is a multidimensional experience. Pain assessment is a continuous process that often begins when vital signs are obtained and patients are asked to respond to the numeric rating scale (NRS) of 0–10. The assessment quantifies and qualifies pain but also considers the impact on physical and emotional functioning, previous interventions, success of interventions, and effects of symptoms or adverse events produced by the treatment (Miaskowski, 2010a). A comprehensive pain assessment is completed following any pain report. Failure to perform an adequate pain assessment is one of the most common causes of inadequate pain management (Miaskowski, 2010a; NCCN, 2015a).

The initial step in assessing pain is the patient's self-report. The specific site of pain, as well as the description, intensity, duration, etiology, and characteristics, should be discussed. Aggravating and alleviating factors also should be assessed. Interventions, such as medications, rest, activities, heat, or cold compresses, that have and have not controlled the pain should be considered (McMenamin, 2011; Miaskowski, 2010a; NCCN, 2015a). The psychosocial impact of pain should be considered during the process of a pain assessment. Patients should be questioned about the impact of pain, specifically, functional status and interference with activities of daily living. Other considerations regarding pain are past coping strategies, the economic impact of pain, and concerns about the use of opioids to manage pain (Greco et al., 2011; Ripamonti et al., 2012). A comprehensive pain assessment includes four important components. Obtaining a detailed history of pain is the initial step in assessing pain. Second, a psychosocial assessment should be considered. Third, examining the site of pain and determining the physical impact of pain is critical when assessing pain. Finally, following the history and physical examination, a diagnostic evaluation of the pain, the potential pain syndromes, and the effect on the patient's quality of life and overall function are determined (Miaskowski, 2010a; NCCN, 2015a; Tracy & Morrison, 2013).

Breakthrough pain assessment should be considered, and the location, intensity, and timing of breakthrough pain should be determined. Temporal patterns, precipitating or exacerbating factors, relieving factors, and response to interventions are part of a thorough assessment. The number of pain episodes per day should be documented. The relationship of breakthrough pain to the overall clinical status requires careful examination as well (Greco et al., 2011; NCCN, 2015a).

Rating pain is often subjective. Pain assessment tools or rating scales can be an effective way of quantifying and qualifying pain symptoms. Pain scales can be unidimensional or multidimensional. Unidimensional tools measure one pain component, while multidimensional scales are more comprehensive in the approach of identifying the meaning of pain (McMenamin, 2011). The appropriate pain rating scale depends on the patient population, a patient's preferences and abilities, an individual's past experiences, and the documentation system within the healthcare setting (Curtiss, 2010). When using a pain tool, it is important to consider barriers in communication, including language differences, cognitive difficulties, and hearing or vision impairment (Dunham et al., 2013).

Pain is assessed at regular intervals and when a change occurs in the patient's pain or when the patient has a new pain (NCCN, 2015a; Portenoy, 2011). Many assessment tools exist, with various strengths and weaknesses. In general, the baseline assessment is more comprehensive, whereas ongoing reassessment tools are more succinct. Table 10-2 lists common cancer pain

Table 10-2. Pain Assessment Tools

Tool	Description	Advantages/Disadvantages
Numeric Rating Scale (McCaffery & Pasero, 1999)	0–10 scale where 0 = no pain and 10 = worst pain imaginable	Rapid, good for assessment of intervention efficacy
Breakthrough Pain Questionnaire (Portenoy et al., 1999)	Structured interview	Designed to characterize breakthrough pain
Checklist of Nonverbal Pain Indicators (Feldt, 2000)	Six-item checklist rated by observer where 0 = behavior not observed and 1 = behavior observed	For patients who are cognitively impaired or otherwise unable to verbally rate pain presence or intensity
Edmonton Symptom Assessment Scale (Bruera et al., 1991)	Nine-item visual analog scale for symptoms in patients receiving palliative care	Gives a numeric score; higher scores reflect greater severity of patient condition; easy to perform
Memorial Symptom Assessment Scale (Fishman et al., 1987)	Assesses 32 symptoms in three dimensions: intensity, frequency, and distress	Broader range of information, more time consuming; two abbreviated forms available that assess 32 or 14 symptoms in one dimension; valid in patients with or without cancer
Wong-Baker FACES Pain Rating Scale (Wong & Baker, 1988)	Six faces that vary from smiling (0 and no pain) to crying (10 and worst pain)	Recommended for people age 3 or older; useful in patients with language barriers
McGill Pain Questionnaire (MPQ) (Melzack, 1987)	Three major classes of word descriptors—sensory, affective, and evaluative—used by patients to describe subjective pain experience; also has intensity scale	Qualitative and quantitative information; originally developed for nonmalignant pain, but valid in cancer populations as well
Multidimensional Affect and Pain Survey (Knotkova et al., 2006)	101 descriptors rated by patients as to closeness to their own feelings, emotions, and experiences	Similar to MPQ; takes no more than 15 minutes to complete; assesses somatosensory and emotional experiences and feelings of well-being
Brief Pain Inventory (Cleeland & Ryan, 1994; Tittle et al., 2003)	Measures pain by severity and interference with function	Developed for use in patients with cancer; validated across cultures and various languages; validated in surgical patients with cancer and chronic nonmalignant pain; time intensive

assessment tools. The use of validated pain assessment tools may improve pain intervention outcomes (Tracy & Morrison, 2013). Pain assessment tools can be tailored to meet an individual's needs. For example, the Wong-Baker FACES® Pain Rating Scale may be useful in children, patients who are cognitively impaired, or patients with a language barrier. Visual analog scales are widely used to measure pain and are well validated (McMenamin, 2011). Although no universal standard pain assessment tool exists, it is recommended that every cancer care setting adopt at least one standard tool for the assessment of pain.

Reassessment is performed following any intervention and uses patients' self-reports and the initial assessment tools. Reassessment includes assessment of intervention side effects, adverse events, and effects on quality of life (Apolone et al., 2009; Miaskowski, 2010a). Having patients use a pain management diary may help in assessing the efficacy of treatment strategies. This may give patients an enhanced awareness of pain and its contributing factors, as well as an increased sense of control over pain.

The patient report will guide the physical examination. Physical examination is an essential component of the assessment. The site of pain is examined for any physical changes, such as redness, bruising, edema, or tenderness. Activities, movements, or positions that reproduce the pain are evaluated. Diagnostic studies are ordered based on findings from the physical examination and patient report, as well as the medical history. Chapter 3 gives more information on diagnostic studies that may be appropriate for patients with cancer who are experiencing pain.

Differential Diagnosis

The differential diagnosis of pain may be related to its etiology and pathophysiology. Pain may be a result of a nonmalignant issue, such as peripheral neuropathy caused by diabetes, osteoarthritis, or chronic fatigue syndrome. Clinicians should consider the patient's past medical history when assessing and treating cancer pain, although the distinction often is unclear (Portenoy, 2011). Potential specific cancer pain syndromes, such as post-thoracotomy pain syndrome (see Table 10-1), and potential oncologic emergencies, such as spinal cord compression or hypercalcemia, should be considered in the differential (see Chapters 15 and 16 on oncologic emergencies).

Treatment of Cancer Pain

An individualized, multidisciplinary, and multimodal pain management approach that considers physical, mental, psychological, cultural, and social factors will provide an optimal outcome for patients with cancer (Miaskowski, 2010a; Ripamonti et al., 2012). An essential component of successful pain management is the oncology advanced practitioner's ability to work with the patient and the patient's caregivers and communicate the treatment plan. Treatment interventions are initiated based on the assessment, and treatment plans are evaluated on a continual basis. Changes are made based on the clinical situation (Miaskowski, 2010a). Clinicians should initiate pain treatment promptly while awaiting workup for specific etiology of the pain (Portenoy, 2011). Interventions include pharmacologic and nonpharmacologic strategies to control pain.

Pharmacologic Treatment

Initial pharmacologic intervention is based on the patient's report of pain severity. Pain rated 1–4 using the NRS is considered mild and may require nonopioid interventions. Moderate pain is usually described as 5 or 6, whereas severe pain is rated 7–10. Severe pain is considered a pain emergency requiring immediate interventions (Miaskowski, 2010a). Pharmacologic interventions include nonopioids, opioids, and coanalgesics. The most appropriate medication is based on the cause and severity of pain.

NCCN (2015a), ESMO (Ripamonti et al., 2012), and the American Pain Society (Chou et al., 2009) have established clinical practice guidelines for cancer pain management based on the WHO (1996) three-step analgesic ladder. Clinical practice guidelines provide evidence-based information to reduce variation in the clinical management of cancer pain and improve patient outcomes. Figure 10-2 defines some of the key concepts of cancer pain management based on these guidelines and the current literature. A crucial concept when treating cancer pain is that the assessment of pain is subjective and individualized, and treatment is based on the patient's pain intensity, comorbidities, and current medications (McMenamin, 2011; NCCN, 2015a).

Nonopioid analgesics: Following a comprehensive pain assessment, if the patient has a pain intensity of 1–3, a nonopioid analgesic agent such as an NSAID or acetaminophen may be administered, or a short-acting opioid can be considered. Any NSAID, including one that the patient has used successfully in the past, can be considered (NCCN, 2015a). Commonly used NSAIDs in the management of cancer pain include aspirin, salicylate, ibuprofen, acetaminophen, naproxen, and selective cyclooxygenase-2 inhibitors. NSAIDs have a ceiling effect and do not produce tolerance, dependence, or addiction. Common side effects associated with NSAIDs include dyspepsia, gastrointestinal bleeding, and renal insufficiency. NSAIDs inhibit the enzyme cyclooxygenase, which catalyzes the synthesis of endoperoxides from arachidonic acid. This, in turn, inhibits the cyclooxygenase pathway, reducing prostaglandin production (McMenamin, 2011; Portenoy, 2011). Acetaminophen appears to have fewer side effects. Daily acetaminophen dosing of greater than 4 g is not recommended because of the increased risk of hepatic toxicity that can occur, which is more likely in alcoholic individuals and those with liver disease (Miaskowski, 2010a). NSAIDs are used cautiously in patients at risk for gastrointestinal or renal toxicities. If two different NSAIDs are prescribed without successful control of pain, another strategy should be considered.

Opioid analgesics: Opioids are the principal analgesics to treat moderate to severe pain based on the WHO analgesic ladder (WHO, 1996). Opioids bind with mu opioid receptors within and outside the central nervous system (Miaskowski, 2010a). Morphine continues to be the opioid of choice for management of moderate to severe cancer pain. Although no controlled trials

---

- Pain is what the patient says it is.
- Use the oral route whenever possible; avoid intramuscular route.
- Scheduled dosing is preferable to episodic dosing.
- Opioid prescribing
  - Pain intensity 1–3: Increase dose by 25%.
  - Pain intensity 4–6: Increase dose by 25%–50%.
  - Pain intensity 7–10: Increase dose by 50%–100%.
  - Pain intensity < 4 and unmanageable side effects: Consider dose reduction of 25% and reassess.
  - Rescue doses of the short-acting form of the sustained-release medication at 10%–20% of the 24-hour dose should be given every hour as needed.
  - Patients on pure agonists should not be switched to either mixed agonist-antagonists or partial agonists, as the antagonistic element may precipitate withdrawal.
  - When acetaminophen dose of fixed combination opioid is > 4 g/day, switch to single-entity opioid.
  - Convert from short-acting to long-acting opioid when total 24-hour opioid dose is providing adequate pain control.
  - Adjuvant pharmacologic agents (non-narcotic) may be required.
  - Consider opioid rotation (switching) if more than two side effects (not including constipation) are present or if pain is not managed with increasing doses.
  - Opioid-induced side effects must be monitored and managed (e.g., a bowel regimen should begin when the patient begins an opioid intervention).
  - Meperidine, mixed agonist-antagonists, partial agonists, placebos, and propoxyphene are not recommended for treatment of adult cancer pain.

Figure 10-2. Key Concepts of Cancer Pain Management

Note. Based on information from Coyle & Layman-Goldstein, 2007; Grossman et al., 2006; National Comprehensive Cancer Network, 2015a.

have demonstrated its superiority over other agents, it is easily available, is relatively inexpensive, and has multiple routes of administration (McMenamin, 2011). Before an opioid is prescribed, nurses, providers, and pharmacists should have an understanding of the medication's mechanism of action, common starting doses, equivalence to other opioids, duration of effect, half-life, available routes, and associated adverse effects. Initial opioid titration for opioid-naïve patients is done at a slower pace than in opioid-tolerant patients (NCCN, 2015a).

Opioids that are prescribed for chronic pain should be administered on a regular basis. As previously discussed, long-acting pain medication or extended-release opioids provide a consistent release of analgesia. An oral or transdermal route of administration is preferred. Extended-release or long-acting pain medications (e.g., morphine, oxycodone, fentanyl patch) should be given along with medication that is administered for breakthrough pain. When long-acting opioids do not adequately control pain, a short-acting or breakthrough medication should be prescribed. Breakthrough pain medication may be needed at the end of the extended-release medication schedule or with increased activity during the day. Breakthrough pain medications include morphine, oxycodone, and hydromorphone. Other rapid-onset opioids include fentanyl transmucosal or fentanyl buccal tablets (McMenamin, 2011; Miaskowski, 2010a; NCCN, 2015a).

The only absolute contraindication to opioid use is hypersensitivity (Coyle & Layman-Goldstein, 2007). Opioid analgesics may be compounded with a nonopioid such as acetaminophen, which confers a ceiling dose because of the nonopioid component. Table 10-3 lists opioid classifications and agents, as well specific information about these drugs. Opioid use has the potential for addiction, yet this potential must not compromise appropriate pain manage-

Table 10-3. Opioid Classification and Dosing

Opioid Class	Class Effects	Agents

Pure opioid agonists	Increasing dose increases effectiveness but with no ceiling effect. Will not reverse or decrease effects of other pure opioid agonists if given together. Caution with impaired breathing, bronchial asthma, increased intracranial pressure, or liver failure	Morphine
		• Opioid of choice for cancer pain
		• Standard of comparison for opioids
		• IV
		• Oral
		  – Immediate release
		  – Extended release
		
		Hydromorphone
		• Synthetic opioid with short half-life
		• Useful in those intolerant of morphine
		• More potent than morphine
		• Peak effect slightly more rapid than morphine but with slightly shorter duration of action
		• May cause less nausea and hallucinations than morphine
		• IV
		• Oral
		
		Oxycodone
		• Synthetic opioid, better oral absorption than morphine
		• May cause less nausea and hallucinations than morphine but more constipation
		• No parenteral route, oral only

(Continued on next page)

Table 10-3. Opioid Classification and Dosing *(Continued)*

Opioid Class	Class Effects	Agents

Pure opioid agonists *(cont.)*		Fentanyl
		• Opioid with short half-life
		• Much more rapid onset of action but effect of shorter duration
		• Transdermal and transmucosal routes
		• May be less constipating than morphine
		• When given transdermally, the drug is stored in subcutaneous fat, and serum concentration may take several hours to decline.
		• IV
		• Transdermal
		• Transmucosal
		
		Methadone
		• Excellent oral and rectal absorption, long duration of action, low cost, and no known active metabolites
		• Used in severe pain situations such as neuropathic pain
		• Accumulates with repetitive dosing
		• After a few days, the interval of administration can be increased while maintaining analgesic effects.
		• For use by experienced prescribers
		• Careful titration and follow-up
		• IV
		• Oral
		
		Oxymorphone
		• Short half-life and more potent than morphine and an active metabolite of oxycodone
		• IV
		• Oral
		  – Immediate release
		  – Extended release
		
		Hydrocodone
		• Considered a weaker opioid than oxycodone agents
		• Often used in antitussive agents
		
		Propoxyphene
		• Not often used in treating cancer pain

Partial agonists	Less effect at the opioid receptor than full agonists	Buprenorphine • This class of opioids is not recommended for the treatment of cancer pain. • Ceiling effects • May precipitate withdrawal in patients on pure opioid
Mixed agonist-antagonists	Block or are neutral at one receptor but activate another; contraindicated in patients receiving an opioid agonist	Butorphanol, nalbuphine, and pentazocine • This class of opioids is not recommended for the treatment of cancer pain. • Ceiling effects • Risk of psychotomimetic effects such as dysphoria, delusions, and hallucinations

Note. Based on information from Coyle & Layman-Goldstein, 2007; Fallon, 2013; McMenamin, 2011; Miaskowski, 2010a; National Comprehensive Cancer Network, 2015a; Ripamonti et al., 2012; Vallejo et al., 2011.

ment. Pure opioid agonists (e.g., morphine, hydromorphone) are the most common opioids used in cancer pain management. The dose of opioids should be increased slowly based on the report of pain. In the clinical setting, when slowly increasing opioids based on the patient's report of pain, opioids do not have a ceiling dose.

Morphine is a potent analgesic with a strong affinity for the mu receptor in the brain and spinal cord. IV morphine is three times more potent than oral morphine and often is considered the first-line treatment for cancer pain. As with most opioids, morphine is metabolized by the liver. Morphine-3-glucuronide (M3G) and morphine-6-glucuronide (M6G) are two metabolites of morphine that have been identified. M6G is twice as potent as morphine and is excreted by the kidneys. Although M3G does not bind to opioid receptors, it may be responsible for some of the toxicities associated with morphine. Morphine is available as an IV and oral medication (McMenamin, 2011). Oral medication is available as extended-release or immediate-acting medications. Morphine also is available for rectal, intraspinal, epidural, or subarachnoid administration (McMenamin, 2011; NCCN, 2015a).

Hydromorphone is a semisynthetic morphine analog. It is five to eight times more potent than morphine. IV hydromorphone is five times more potent than oral hydromorphone (McMenamin, 2011). The metabolite, hydromorphone-3-glucuronide, is excreted by the kidney and has been identified to cause neuroexcitation at higher doses. Hydromorphone can be administered as IV, oral, rectal, and spinal formulations (McMenamin, 2011; Walker, 2010).

Oxycodone is a semisynthetic opioid derived from morphine. It is available as an oral medication as an extended-release or immediate-release formulation. The active metabolite of oxycodone is oxymorphone, which is a very potent analgesic.

Fentanyl is a potent lipophilic opioid that is 75–100 times more potent than morphine (McMenamin, 2011). Fentanyl is poorly absorbed in the gastrointestinal tract but well absorbed via the buccal mucosa, skin, and blood-brain barrier. Fentanyl patches are commonly used to control cancer pain and are recommended for opioid-tolerant patients currently on stable opioid medications. The absorption of transdermal fentanyl can be altered if patients are diaphoretic, febrile, or dehydrated. Transmucosal fentanyl citrate and fentanyl buccal tablets are rapid-onset opioid preparations that require enrollment into the risk evaluation and mitigation strategies program (McMenamin, 2011; Miaskowski, 2010a; NCCN, 2015a).

Methadone is a potent mu opioid and should be prescribed by providers with experience and understanding of methadone's unique pharmacologic characteristics. Methadone is metabolized by the P450 cytochrome system, and a large portion is excreted in the feces. Plasma concentrations of methadone increase slowly (up to one week); therefore, titration should take place slowly. The steady state of methadone is achieved after four to five half-lives (Aiello-Laws et al., 2009; Miaskowski, 2010a; NCCN, 2015a).

Partial agonists (e.g., buprenorphine) have little use in cancer pain because of their ceiling effects and their ability to precipitate withdrawal syndrome in patients on pure agonist agents (NCCN, 2015a). Patients receiving mixed agonist-antagonist agents (e.g., butorphanol, nalbuphine, pentazocine) may have more side effects, such as agitation, dysphoria, and confusion, than with pure opioid agonists. These agents are not recommended for cancer pain treatment.

If the patient's pain intensity is rated 4 or greater, a short-acting opioid is ordered and titrated to adequate analgesic effect (NCCN, 2015a). Adjuvant analgesics are given as indicated by assessment and response to initial opioid treatment. A pain reassessment is completed within 24 hours of treatment initiation. Upon reassessment, if the patient's pain is rated 1–3, then conversion to a sustained-release agent is recommended (see example in Figure 10-3). If pain continues to be rated 1–3, then the patient may be assessed weekly until comfortable, and then at each healthcare visit. However, if upon reassessment the patient's pain intensity is 4 or greater, opioid titration should continue.

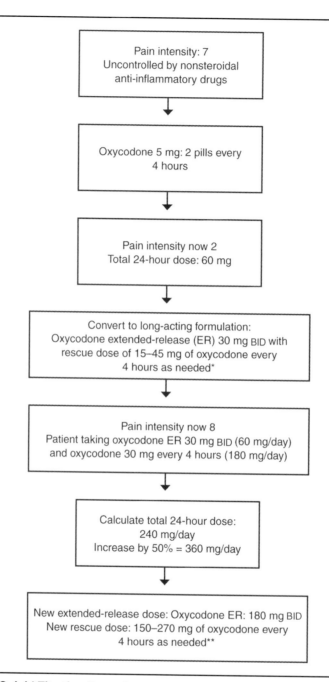

Figure 10-3. Opioid Titration Example

* Rescue dose calculated by multiplying total 24-hour dose by 10%–20% to be given every hour (60 mg × 10%–20% = 6–12 mg every hour). Given in 4-hour intervals: 24–48 mg every 4 hours PRN. Oxycodone tablets come in 5, 15, and 30 mg tablets; therefore, 15–45 mg every 4 hours is appropriate for breakthrough dose.

** Rescue dose calculated by multiplying 24-hour dose by 10%–20% as above (360 × 10%–20% = 36–72 mg every hour). Given in 4-hour intervals: 144–288 mg every 4 hours PRN; therefore, using oxycodone 30 mg tablets, dose is 5–9 pills (150–270 mg).

Note. Based on information from National Comprehensive Cancer Network, 2015a; Ripamonti et al., 2012.

Short-acting opioids have a peak effect at 60 minutes if given orally and 15 minutes if given intravenously. Generally, when clinicians are prescribing opioids, the dose is increased by 25% for pain intensity of 1–3; 25%–50% for pain intensity of 4–6; and 50%–100% for pain intensity of 7–10 (NCCN, 2015a). For the example in Figure 10-3, a patient is currently taking opioids but now reports pain rated at 8, and the total 24-hour dose (including the breakthrough doses) is calculated. The new scheduled dose is determined by the previous total 24-hour dose and increased by 50%. The new breakthrough dose is calculated at 10%–20% of this new 24-hour dose and is given every hour as needed. The most appropriate dose for any patient with cancer pain is whatever dose it takes to relieve the individual's pain.

Patient-controlled analgesia (PCA) is useful when a patient has uncontrolled pain or requires quick relief, or when the clinician is trying to determine the required opioid dose for adequate pain relief. This method allows patients to self-administer a preset dose of an analgesic within a prescribed time period (usually every 15–30 minutes), enabling timely and highly individualized management. A maximum dose is set as well (usually prescribed in 1–4-hour dose limits). An effective safeguard of PCA is that excessively sedated patients will not be able to activate the dosing button, thereby preventing delivery of further opioid. A continuous infusion may be prescribed along with patient-administered bolus doses. Once pain is controlled, the IV pharmacologic agent can be converted to an equianalgesic oral dose. PCA management is a poor choice of pain management for cognitively impaired patients. Caution is vital in prescribing and managing opioid-naïve patients with PCA (NCCN, 2015a). An American Society for Pain Management Nursing position paper (Cooney et al., 2013) cautioned that PCA by proxy (i.e., someone other than the patient activates the bolus dose delivery) is considered an unsafe practice. APNs must be familiar with concepts of narcotic equianalgesia and dosage conversions from one drug to another and also from one route to another. Conversions to a different opioid or route may be required because of inadequate analgesia, intolerable side effects, inability to use the oral route, insurance coverage, or formulary coverage. This information is found in many pain management references, including the NCCN (2015a) and ESMO (Ripamonti et al., 2012) guidelines on adult cancer pain. Doses of various opioid analgesics are compared to the equivalent of 10 mg of parenteral morphine (and 30 mg of oral morphine). It is imperative that clinicians maintain a consistent method of conversion using the same equianalgesic chart or program to promote safety. In most cases, the equianalgesic dose is reduced by 25%–50% to account for incomplete cross-tolerance and titrated liberally to gain adequate analgesic effect (NCCN, 2015a). When a dose needs to be rounded, rounding downward is preferred. The clinician also must prescribe an adequate breakthrough dose of the new medication and assess analgesia within 24 hours.

Breakthrough pain is anticipated in patients with cancer, and medication should be available as needed to control pain. Consideration of the etiology is critical (Greco et al., 2011). If the breakthrough pain is of neuropathic etiology, it may be beneficial to add an antidepressant, anticonvulsant, or other neuropathic agent. If the etiology is bone-related, then an NSAID or corticosteroid might be beneficial. Pretreatment for events expected to cause pain should be considered (NCCN, 2015a). For breakthrough pain caused by end-of-dose failure, increasing the dosage or frequency of the regular analgesic can improve pain control.

Treatment for breakthrough pain should have a rapid onset and short half-life. Adjustments in regularly scheduled analgesic dosing are considered if frequent episodes of breakthrough pain are reported (NCCN, 2015a; Portenoy, 2011). The rescue dose should reflect the amount of the regularly scheduled medication. Usually this dose is 10%–20% of the total daily opioid dose and may be given every hour as needed (Ripamonti et al., 2012); however, this can vary greatly among patients (NCCN, 2015a). Titration of the dose to patient response is necessary to adequately manage pain and to balance untoward side effects.

When adequate pain control is not achieved or if patients are experiencing intolerable opioid side effects, opioid rotation may be considered. Opioid rotation is defined as substituting one opioid with another using equianalgesic ratios. In one study, opioid rotation was conducted in 31% of outpatients with cancer with a 65% success rate (Reddy et al., 2013). When converting or rotating from one opioid to another, the first step is to determine the amount of the current opioid taken in a 24-hour period. When switching to any opioid (other than methadone or transdermal fentanyl), clinicians use the equianalgesic chart to calculate the new opioid dose. If the pain is controlled, the dose of the new medication should be reduced by 25%–50% to allow for the incomplete cross-tolerance between the two opioids. If the previous dose was ineffective, the dose of the new medication can be prescribed at 100%–125% of the equianalgesic dose (Fine & Portenoy, 2009; NCCN, 2015a; Ripamonti et al., 2012). If switching to methadone, the dose should be 75%–90% lower than the calculated equianalgesic dose. When changing from an opioid to transdermal patch, clinicians should obtain the package insert for accurate information regarding the titration procedure (Fine & Portenoy, 2009; NCCN, 2015a).

Management of Treatment Side Effects

Pharmacologic intervention for pain, particularly opioids, may produce a variety of side effects, many occurring as a result of the effects on the gastrointestinal system. The most common side effects of opioids are constipation, cognitive impairment, sedation, somnolence, nausea and vomiting, reduced libido, and delirium. Constipation, the one side effect that does not improve with routine opioid use, is best treated prophylactically. Initiation of a bowel regimen including a stimulant laxative such as polyethylene glycol, senna, bisacodyl, and a stool softener (docusate) and titrated to effect is critical when patients are started on opioid therapy (McMenamin, 2011; Mesgarpour et al., 2014; NCCN, 2015a).

Respiratory depression is one of the most feared toxicities of opioids. It occurs when there is decreased sensitivity of the medulla to rising carbon dioxide levels that normally create spontaneous respirations. Respiratory depression usually is not an issue for patients with cancer who are prescribed opioids for chronic pain. Patients with pulmonary conditions may be at risk for developing opioid-related respiratory depression. If respiratory depression occurs, it can be managed with naloxone (0.4 mg in 10 ml of normal saline) administered at 0.5 ml every two minutes to avoid abrupt withdrawal symptoms and severe pain as well as seizures (Miaskowski, 2010a; NCCN, 2015a). Methylphenidate, dextroamphetamine, or modafinil may be appropriate for the treatment of persistent opioid-induced sedation (Portenoy, 2011). Research suggests that psychomotor and cognitive functioning usually is not affected after stable doses of opioids are attained. Gaertner et al. (2006) found that the use of long-term (at least four weeks) controlled-release oxycodone did not prohibit driving, but they emphasized that individual assessment is vital and patients should be educated about the potential risks of driving after taking pain medication. Treatment of many common pain management side effects is discussed in other chapters of this book.

Coanalgesics

Coanalgesics often are used in conjunction with opioids or NSAIDs to treat neuropathic pain. Coanalgesic medications include antidepressants, anticonvulsants, corticosteroids, and topical agents such as capsaicin or local anesthetics (Fallon, 2013). Coanalgesics or adjuvant analgesics are medications that have pain-relieving properties in specific clinical situations; however, the primary indication of coanalgesics are not for the treatment of pain. Common coanalgesic medications include tricyclic antidepressants (such as nortriptyline), anticonvulsant medications (such as gabapentin), topical agents (such as capsaicin or lidocaine), and opioids (such as methadone). The Neuropathic Pain Special Interest Group of the International Association for the Study of Pain developed evidence-based guidelines for the treatment of neuropathic pain (Dworkin et al., 2010). Tricyclic antidepressants (nortriptyline or venlafaxine), calcium channel ligands (gabapentin or pregabalin), and topical lidocaine were recommended as first-line treatment interventions (Dworkin et al., 2010). Anticonvulsants often are used for pain related to peripheral neuropathy. Tricyclic antidepressants are effective and inexpensive medications used to treat neuropathic pain; however, patients should be monitored for cardiotoxicity, urinary retention, orthostatic hypotension, constipation, and drowsiness. Secondary amine tricyclic antidepressants such as nortriptyline or desipramine are preferred over tertiary amine tricyclic antidepressants (e.g., amitriptyline, imipramine) because they are better tolerated. Coanalgesic medications such as anticonvulsants and antidepressants should be increased slowly to avoid toxicities (Aiello-Laws et al., 2009; NCCN, 2015a).

Treatment of metastatic bone pain requires not only NSAIDs and opioids but also bisphosphonate therapy, which currently is accepted to provide moderate analgesic effects (Gralow et al., 2013; NCCN, 2015a). Local treatments such as external beam radiation therapy, radiofrequency ablation, and surgical interventions (e.g., bone stabilization procedures) also may be used. Strontium-89 and samarium-153 may be employed for widespread bone metastases. Chapter 6 provides more information on radiologic interventions.

Interventional Strategies

Although opioids are the foundation of pain management, it is estimated that 10%–20% of patients with cancer may require a combination of treatment interventions (Hanks et al., 2001; Mercadante, 2014). In this clinical situation, alternative methods of pain control should be considered. Interventional therapies are considered for a variety of reasons. Interventional strategies may be considered if adequate oral pain management has produced intolerable side effects or if pain is more likely to be controlled with a nerve block, as in the case of a celiac plexus block for uncontrolled pancreatic pain. Interventional approaches may include nerve blocks (temporary or permanent), neurostimulation, neuraxial analgesic infusion, neuroablation, and surgical intervention (McMenamin, 2011; NCCN, 2015a; Walker, 2010). Common procedures for neuraxial infusions include an epidural or intrathecal infusion of opioids, local anesthetic, or other analgesics to diffuse into the dorsal lamina and affect nociception (McMenamin, 2011). Neuroablative procedures such as brachial plexus neurolysis or cordotomy may be considered for well-localized pain syndromes. Neurostimulation procedures such as transcutaneous electrical nerve stimulation (TENS) modulate the pain stimulus transmission, thereby relieving pain (Walker, 2010). Surgical interventions such as a vertebroplasty or kyphoplasty also may be considered. Vertebroplasty involves injection of orthopedic cement into fractured vertebrae. Kyphoplasty is a procedure that involves the insertion of a vertebral catheter and then inflation of a "balloon" tamp to restore the height of the vertebrae before injecting orthopedic cement. Other surgeries for pain management might include amputation, tumor debulking, organ excision, or skeletal fixation (McMenamin, 2011).

Nonpharmacologic Treatment

Nonpharmacologic or integrative interventions often are used in conjunction with pharmacologic approaches for cancer-related pain. Cognitive and physical interventions are used to enhance a patient's ability to control pain (NCCN, 2015a). Cognitive interventions include imagery/hypnosis, distraction, relaxation, graded task assignments, cognitive behavioral training, or active coping training. Examples of physical nonpharmacologic interventions include physical therapy, energy conservation, massage, application of heat or ice, TENS, acupuncture, ultrasonic stimulation, or bed, bath, and walking supports (NCCN, 2015a; Running & Turnbeaugh, 2011). Integrative therapy is discussed in further detail in Chapter 8. Rehabilitative interventions, such as physical therapy, may improve range of motion, strength and endurance, and neuromuscular control, thus helping to relieve cancer pain. Massage, TENS, ultrasonic stimulation, and other modalities also may be appropriate to manage pain (NCCN, 2015a; Walker, 2010). Applications of heat or cold may be beneficial in certain types of pain, particularly postsurgical pain (NCCN, 2015a). Patients must be warned about the potential for burns, especially if neuropathy or other disorders are present that would disrupt their perception of pain or temperature.

Psychiatric symptoms, including anxiety and depression, in patients with cancer pain should first be considered to be a result of uncontrolled pain and then reassessed after pain is controlled. Patients with pain that interferes with their daily activities express more anxiety, which compounds intolerance of daily activities (Running & Turnbeaugh, 2011). Psychosocial support is vital, and patients and families should understand that emotional reactions to pain are normal and should be treated as part of the pain management plan (NCCN, 2015a). Reinforcing positive coping skills, enhancing personal control, and focusing on optimal quality of life are all part of psychosocial support to patients and families or support systems.

Complementary and Alternative Treatments

The treatment of pain with complementary or alternative medicine (CAM) is an evidence-based science. In a study reported by Templeton et al. (2013) of 342 patients with early-stage breast cancer, nearly half (46%) used at least one CAM treatment. Complementary and alternative methods used included vitamins (38%), teas (29%), homeopathy (19%), herbal medicine (19%), and mistletoe (16%). In a recent study, Ndao et al. (2013) reported that CAM therapies are used by 31%–84% of children with cancer, both within and outside of clinical trials. A wide variety of CAM pain interventions exist, including yoga, Qigong, Reiki, Shiatsu, hypnosis, imagery, massage, nutrition, meditation, acupuncture, acupressure, aromatherapy, magnet therapy, mind-body medicine, reflexology, spiritual cures, therapeutic touch, and traditional Chinese medicine (Running & Turnbeaugh, 2011). Patients with cancer use CAM for many reasons, but a common one is unrelieved pain (Running & Seright, 2012). Chapter 8 provides more detailed information about CAM. Cognitive behavioral interventions, such as keeping a pain diary or a journal about thoughts and emotions surrounding the pain experience, may promote feelings of control over the pain (NCCN, 2015a; Running & Turnbeaugh, 2011).

Perceived control over pain is an influential aspect of pain response (Templeton et al., 2013). Behavioral interventions examine behaviors that influence the pain experience. Biofeedback, hypnosis, music and art therapy, distraction training, systematic desensitization, and relaxation therapy are examples of behavioral interventions. Evidence suggests that cognitive behavioral interventions are effective in providing immediate but not long-term pain relief (Running & Turnbeaugh, 2011). Randomized controlled clinical trials are needed to evaluate CAM interventions in the management of cancer pain.

Treatment of Patients With Substance Abuse

Treatment of cancer pain in people with a history of substance abuse is an issue that oncology APNs should be prepared to encounter. While maintaining a respect for the potential for abuse of controlled substances such as opioid analgesics, one must understand that these medications are the most effective way to treat cancer pain. Patients with a known substance abuse history often are undermedicated (McMenamin, 2011; Modesto-Lowe, Girard, & Chaplin, 2012). Several organizations (including ONS and the American Cancer Society) and the

U.S. Drug Enforcement Administration have issued a joint statement titled *Promoting Pain Relief and Preventing Abuse of Pain Medications: A Critical Balancing Act* (U.S. Drug Enforcement Administration, 2002). This statement reinforces the need to prevent abuse of prescription pain medications while still ensuring availability for those who need them. The American Society for Pain Management Nursing stated that patients with addictive disease and cancer pain have the right to be treated with dignity, respect, and the same quality of pain management (Oliver et al., 2012). The management of pain in patients with addictive disease requires a nonjudgmental approach and assumes that patients' self-report is true. Higher doses may be required because patients may have developed a tolerance to some medications or increased sensitivity to pain because of drug use. A pain contract that includes clear, written patient expectations and responsibilities with nonnegotiable limits will help to deter aberrant behavior. A pain contract clearly outlines patient and clinician responsibilities, patient expectations, and consequences of aberrant behavior and sets clear, nonnegotiable limits. Patients should be monitored with periodic pill counts and drug screens. Careful documentation of pain etiology, assessment, education, prescription, management, and follow-up will protect clinicians while providing rationale for proper management (McMenamin, 2011; NCCN, 2015a; Oliver et al., 2012).

Patient and Family Education

A vital part of pain management plans is patient and family education. Lack of knowledge and incorrect beliefs about pain are barriers to optimal pain relief (Vallerand, Musto, & Polomano, 2011; Wengström et al., 2013). Research shows improvements in cancer pain management when patients and families are taught about their pain and its management (Vallerand et al., 2011). Individualized education may reduce the disparity in cancer pain management among minorities (Vallerand, Pieper, Crawley, Nordstrom, & Dinardo, 2013).

Evaluation of Outcomes

Following reassessment of cancer pain after therapeutic intervention, if pain control appears to be inadequate, oncology APNs should assess patients for factors that impede pain relief. Numerous studies have identified a range of barriers to optimal cancer pain management. Figure 10-4 is a nonexhaustive list of barriers to adequate pain management. Successful outcomes of pain interventions include not only a decrease in pain intensity but also an increase in functional abilities and improved quality of life. Reassessment should include patients' continued ability to obtain and afford medications or treatment (NCCN, 2015a). Documentation of outcomes is essential for continuity of care and for legal obligations. Compliance with the therapeutic regimen and follow-up also must be documented.

Ongoing continuous quality improvement is vital to improve the quality of cancer pain management, as well as to evaluate evidence-based practice (Vallerand et al., 2011). Continuing education of physicians, nurses, and ancillary staff improves the quality of pain management (Walker, 2010). Ideally, all practice settings should have a formal process for evaluation and improvement of cancer pain management (NCCN, 2015a). All healthcare providers must follow evidence-based standards of care. When patients transition from one healthcare setting to another (such as from the hospital to home), care must be taken to maintain optimal pain management.

Oncology nurses play a vital role in assessing and managing pain in patients with cancer. It is essential that oncology advanced practitioners assess pain on a consistent basis and manipulate treatment plans to optimize patients' quality of life. It also is important to educate patients

- Stoicism
- Fear of addiction
- Language barriers
- Healthcare staff turnover
- Desire to be a "good patient"
- Poor access to pain specialists
- Cost of medications/procedures
- Patients' lack of support people
- Misconceptions about cancer pain
- Lack of national policies on pain relief
- Healthcare providers' resistance to change
- Lack of consistent use of assessment tools
- Low expectations that pain can be relieved
- Inadequate dosing of pharmacologic agents
- Fear of side effects of pharmacologic agents
- Legal concerns on part of healthcare providers
- Inadequate time on part of healthcare providers
- Incomplete effectiveness of some interventions
- Inadequate reimbursement for healthcare providers
- Inadequate knowledge about cancer pain etiology and control
- Organizational factors (e.g., increasing paperwork, documentation)
- Varying rules and regulations on controlled substances state to state
- Nurses' or support people's reluctance to administer opioids
- Inadequate knowledge about cultural variations regarding pain responses
- Unmanaged negative psychosocial factors (such as depression and anxiety)
- Reluctance to report pain because of fear that pain stems from progressive or recurrent disease
- Shortages of healthcare providers, particularly those specializing in cancer pain management
- Poor recognition of importance of pain control or low priority of pain control in optimal cancer treatment and care
- Disagreement between patient and support system or patient and provider on presence and severity of pain
- Fear of tolerance (i.e., that cancer pain will worsen toward death and interventions will then be ineffective)
- Poor communication (e.g., between healthcare provider and patient; provider and provider; provider and support systems; patient and support systems)

Figure 10-4. Barriers to Optimal Cancer Pain Management

Note. Based on information from Miaskowski, 2010a; National Comprehensive Cancer Network, 2015a; Portenoy, 2011; Ripamonti et al., 2012.

and families about medication titration to achieve quality pain control. Nurses need to continually broaden their knowledge of pain management to provide continuous, safe, and excellent care to patients with cancer.

Fatigue

Introduction

Fatigue is a distressing and pervasive problem for patients receiving cancer treatment, cancer survivors, and patients with cancer who are at the end of their lives (Horneber, Fischer, Dimeo, Rüffer, & Weis, 2012; Weis, 2012). Cancer-related fatigue (CRF) is one of the most frequently recurring symptoms confronting oncology nurses. It is a nearly universal side effect of cancer and cancer treatment, affecting physical, psychological, and social functioning and causing significant distress for patients and caregivers (NCCN, 2015b). It often is underrecognized and undertreated and has a strong relationship with quality of life (Cleeland et al., 2013; Mitchell, 2011). Fatigue is subjective and multidimensional and often is reported as the most distressing symptom associated with cancer and its treatment, causing the most interference with daily life (NCCN, 2015b).

Definitions and Incidence

Fatigue often occurs as one element in a cluster of symptoms such as depression, pain, sleep disturbance, and menopausal symptoms but also may occur as an isolated symptom (Laird et al., 2011; Mitchell, 2010; Mortimer et al., 2010; Yennurajalingam, Palmer, Zhang, Poulter, & Bruera, 2008). CRF is defined by NCCN (2015b) as a distressing, persistent subjective sense of tiredness or exhaustion related to cancer or cancer treatment that is not proportional to recent activity and interferes with usual functioning. Compared to fatigue in healthy individuals, CRF is more severe, more distressing, and less likely to be relieved by rest (NCCN, 2015b). Fatigue is a subjective symptom, and the report of fatigue differs among individuals. Some patients may report fatigue as mental fogginess, inertia, or loss of efficiency, whereas others may describe it as an excessive need to rest, the inability to recover promptly from exertion, or muscle heaviness and weakness (Mitchell, 2011). More research is needed to better define and potentially standardize symptoms of fatigue. Disruptive symptoms of chronic fatigue are reported to persist for months to years after completion of cancer therapy (NCCN, 2015b).

A survey of more than 100 clinicians and 500 patients reported that regardless of cancer type, fatigue was ranked as the most distressing symptom (Butt et al., 2008). It is estimated that fatigue will occur throughout the cancer experience in 25%–99% of patients with cancer (Mitchell, 2011). Fatigue is an anticipated side effect of treatment. Although there are data describing CRF occurrence and severity based on treatment type, tumor stage, time from treatment completion, and demographic information, it is difficult to draw conclusions because of the variability factors. Studies have suggested that patients experience fatigue 40%–90% of the time while receiving chemotherapy or radiation therapy (Campos, Hassan, Riechelmann, & Del Giglio, 2011; Mitchell, 2010).

The prevalence of CRF in men with prostate cancer receiving long-term androgen deprivation therapy was estimated at greater than 40%, and the prevalence of fatigue in patients with breast cancer was estimated to be 30%–70% (de M Alcântara-Silva, Freitas-Junior, Freitas, & Machado, 2013; Storey et al., 2011). In a published literature review, Minton and Stone (2008) reported that there is an increase in fatigue in the breast cancer population when compared to a healthy population. Fatigue in patients with breast cancer occurred up to five years after completion of adjuvant therapy. The prevalence of post-treatment fatigue in Hodgkin lymphoma survivors was 11%–76% compared to a prevalence of 10% in the general population (Daniels, Oerlemans, Krol, van de Poll-Franse, & Creutzberg, 2013). Severe fatigue is reported in up to 78% of patients receiving palliative care (Stone & Minton, 2008).

Etiology and Pathophysiology

The primary mechanism of CRF is unclear and poorly understood and may involve several mechanisms. Various causative factors and multiple confounding factors exist to explain the etiology of fatigue. Although the precise etiology is unclear, many experts think that fatigue occurs as a side effect of treatment as well as a biologic effect of the disease itself (Campos et al., 2011; Horneber et al., 2012).

The etiology of CRF is multifactorial and includes various types of chemotherapy or radiation therapy that may cause bone marrow suppression and disrupt erythrocyte production, causing anemia. Anemia is common when individuals report fatigue. Although data support an improvement in fatigue symptoms when anemia is treated, the overall effects appear to be small (Mitchell, 2010). Other causes of CRF include psychological distress, generalized deconditioning, and insomnia (Stone & Minton, 2008), as well as myeloid suppression and concurrent symptoms such as pain and depression (Laird et al., 2011). Other possible explanations for CRF include infection, malnutrition, cachexia, and medications. Preexisting health issues, such as hypothyroidism and cardiac, pulmonary, hepatic, and renal impairments, can cause significant symptoms of fatigue, and these symptoms will increase in the setting of cancer-related treatment (Mitchell, 2011).

Several models have been proposed to explain CRF. These include energy balance/energy analysis models, fatigue as a stress response model, neuroendocrine-based regulatory fatigue models, and hybrid models (Mitchell, 2011). The energy balance/energy analysis model is an imbalance of intake, metabolism, and expenditure of energy that produces symptoms of fatigue. Several fatigue models exist that describe dysregulation in neuroendocrine-based regulatory systems. Some of these regulatory systems include the hypothalamic-pituitary-adrenal axis (HPA), neuroimmune system transmitter secretion, and circadian rhythms (Mitchell, 2010, 2011; Stone & Minton, 2008). All of these models could be helpful in identifying appropriate treatment strategies.

Proposed mechanisms of CRF include abnormal accumulation of metabolites, proinflammatory cytokine effects, changes in neuromuscular function, abnormalities in adenosine triphosphate synthesis, serotonin dysregulation, and vagal afferent activation (Horneber et al., 2012; Mitchell, 2010). Abnormalities in energy metabolism related to increased requirements because of tumor growth, infection, fever, or surgery also may cause fatigue (Mitchell, 2011).

Aberrant cytokine production (such as interleukin-1, interleukin-6, and tumor necrosis factor-alpha), as noted in post-treatment breast cancer survivors, may be associated with persistent fatigue (Minton et al., 2013). Some cytokines may be produced by tumors and directly cause fatigue. Abnormal cytokine production also is linked to cancer treatments (Bower et al., 2011; Horneber et al., 2012; Miaskowski & Aouizerat, 2012). They may contribute indirectly to fatigue by promoting cachexia and muscle wasting (Mitchell, 2010). Hyperglycemia also may contribute to CRF. Patients who are insulin resistant may experience an abnormal glucose uptake in the muscle, as well as an increase in body fat, causing an increase in fatigue (Berger, Gerber, & Mayer, 2012).

Risk Factors

NCCN (2015b) identified several contributing factors of CRF. Some of these factors include adverse side effects of medications, pain, emotional distress (e.g., depression, anxiety), sleep disturbances, nutritional imbalances, anemia, decrease in functional status (deconditioning, decreased activity level), and comorbidities. Patient demographic information, such as sex, age, marital status, and employment status, are not consistently identified as factors adding to CRF (Dhruva et al., 2010; Mitchell, 2010). Medical diagnoses that may contribute to CRF include electrolyte disturbances (e.g., hypercalcemia, hypomagnesemia), end-organ dysfunction (cardiac, pulmonary, hepatic, or renal), hypothyroidism, hypogonadism, adrenal insufficiency, infection, and dehydration (de M Alcântara-Silva et al., 2013; Mitchell, 2010).

At baseline, patients with certain preexisting conditions may be at increased risk for development of or increased level of fatigue. Individuals who have had a stroke or congestive heart failure have decreased reserves and may develop fatigue more easily (Giacalone et al., 2013).

Sleep disturbances, including hypersomnia, insomnia, or sleep apnea, contribute to fatigue. Physiologic stress may be a contributing factor. Paraneoplastic syndromes, such as syndrome of inappropriate antidiuretic hormone secretion and hypercalcemia, cause fatigue (Mitchell, 2011). Tissue injury and stress response attributable to surgery may result in fatigue that lasts six months or longer (Baumann, Zopf, & Bloch, 2012). People taking medications such as opioids, hypnotics, anxiolytics, antihistamines, antiemetics, anticonvulsants, or antihypertensives may experience medication-related fatigue (Mitchell, 2010). Immobility can result in deconditioning and muscle wasting, thereby causing fatigue (Mitchell, 2011).

Signs and Symptoms

Fatigue is multidimensional, including mental, physical, and emotional components (Horneber et al., 2012; Mitchell, 2011; Stone & Minton, 2008). Significant changes in behavioral patterns of sleep quality, stamina, cognition, and emotional reactivity are early indicators of impending fatigue. Eventually, body processes and social interactions are affected if behavioral patterns do not improve.

At least two dimensions of fatigue have been described: mental fatigue and physical fatigue. Mental fatigue symptoms include difficulties with cognition, concentration, and speed of information processing. Patients with fatigue may have difficulty understanding simple instructions or trying to complete a to-do list. They may complain of forgetfulness and miss appointments, omit medications, or have difficulty in communications with healthcare providers (Horneber et al., 2012). Patients may describe negative or unpleasant emotions, mental exhaustion, and impaired concentration and memory (Mitchell, 2010). Symptoms of mental fatigue may be difficult to differentiate from cancer-related cognitive impairment, which will be discussed later in this chapter.

Examples of physical fatigue symptoms include exhaustion, weakness, and tiredness (Horneber et al., 2012). Patients may describe feeling weary, sluggish, or dragged-out, having heavy limbs, or feeling slow and unable to carry out activities of daily living. Patients commonly report limited energy and an inability to complete routine tasks such as housecleaning or cooking or recreational hobbies. Even routine activities, such as getting dressed, require more effort than customary. Mental and physical fatigue may prevent individuals from participating in relationships and limit socialization, leading to isolation and loneliness (Horneber et al., 2012; NCCN, 2014, 2015b).

Patients may find that their ability to fulfill various roles is altered. They may describe changing roles within the family dynamics, and interactions with others may change because of patients' inability to carry out their normal routine and usual responsibilities. Patients may cease volunteerism in their community, school, or social groups. It is suggested that CRF can have an effect on employment status. Many people are forced to change their current employment status, causing a significant financial burden (Horneber et al., 2012).

Assessment

NCCN (2015b) guidelines recommend that every patient be screened for fatigue as a vital sign at regular intervals. Following a thorough history and physical examination, certain diagnostic tools may be necessary to form the diagnosis of CRF. However, consideration is given to the time required to complete the testing: it should not take so long that it causes fatigue (NCCN, 2014).

Data suggest that healthcare professionals may not appreciate the scope of the problem related to CRF (Mortimer et al., 2010). Communication barriers exist between patients and clinicians about the report of fatigue. Reasons for this miscommunication or failure to communicate are a lack of viable interventions by providers, lack of patient awareness of CRF treatment, reluctance of patients to use medication to improve CRF, and unwillingness of patients to report CRF because they did not want to complain (Mitchell, 2010; Quinten et al., 2011).

Assessment of CRF is subjective, relying on patient report, and is considered suboptimal partly due to the lack of consensus in the identification of a consistent method of measuring fatigue, as well as the frequency of measurement. CRF assessments include routine screening and rescreening of CRF and its impact on quality of life, characteristics of CRF, and potential contributing factors (Mitchell, 2010). Several CRF instruments have been validated and widely used. Single-item measures are used as a quick assessment but are not comprehensive in identifying the many dimensions of CRF. Other types of assessment tools, including self-report measures, multi-item unidimensional scales, and multidimensional tools, are used to assess CRF.

A single 11-item (0–10) NRS is commonly used to identify patients with CRF (NCCN, 2014). This is a quick, simple method of identifying patients who may benefit from CRF interventions. However, this assessment tool does not capture many important factors of fatigue. The NCCN guidelines recommend that all patients be screened at diagnosis, with each chemotherapy visit, and when there is a clinical change. Patients with a score of 0–3 are considered to have low to mild fatigue. Patients with scores of 4 or higher are considered to have moderate (4–6) to severe fatigue (7–10) (Campos et al., 2011; NCCN, 2015b).

In addition to the NRS, questions are posed about day-to-day functioning, such as the ability to work and engage in routine activities. The PQRST assessment tool refers to **P**rovocation, **Q**uality, **R**egion, **S**everity, and **T**iming of cancer symptoms. This assessment tool provides information regarding the onset, pattern, and duration of fatigue, changes over time, and associated or alleviating factors. Disease status, type and length of treatment, and the patients' response to treatment are documented. Comorbidities and contributing factors, such as pain, anemia, depression, altered nutritional status, medications, and sleep disturbances, are identified (Campos et al., 2011; NCCN, 2015b).

Multiple other instruments are available to evaluate fatigue. Three commonly referenced tools specific to CRF are the Piper Fatigue Scale (Piper et al., 1998; Reeve et al., 2012), the Brief Fatigue Inventory (Mendoza et al., 1999), and the Functional Assessment of Chronic Illness Therapy–Fatigue (FACIT-F) assessment tool (Yellen, Cella, Webster, Blendowski, & Kaplan, 1997).

A thorough list of patients' medications is an important consideration in the assessment of CRF. Patients' past medical history and comorbidities will influence the diagnosis and interventions of CRF and were previously discussed in this chapter. Concurrent symptoms are equally important when assessing fatigue. Symptoms such as depression, pain, shortness of breath, nausea and vomiting, and diarrhea are a few of many concurrent symptoms that may be present.

Physical Examination

Physical examination may provide clues to the causes of fatigue and identification of contributing factors (Mitchell, 2011; NCCN, 2015b). For example, constitutional signs might identify nutritional deficiencies, and vital signs might indicate the presence of infection. Assessment of general appearance, mood, and manner may reveal anxiety or depression. Assessment of the musculoskeletal system might reveal focal or generalized weakness, muscle mass loss, joint pain, warm or edematous joints, muscle pain, muscle twitching, limitations in range of motion, or bone pain. Abnormal skin turgor could indicate that dehydration might be contributing to fatigue. Decreased or adventitious lung sounds might indicate pulmonary edema, chronic obstructive pulmonary disease, or pneumonia that is affecting activity tolerance. Abnormal heart sounds and jugular venous distension might indicate that congestive heart failure is causing fatigue.

Diagnostic Testing

Diagnostic testing for fatigue may be problematic. No identified diagnostic tests exist for fatigue specifically. However, tests are available that assist in determining the cause or causes of fatigue and ruling out other potential diagnoses. Table 10-4 gives a nonexhaustive list of diagnostic tests to consider in the workup of patients with fatigue.

Differential Diagnosis

The differential diagnosis for CRF are vast and may include causes or contributing factors. These may potentially be treatable or reversible, such as pain, emotional distress, sleep disturbances, anemia, hypothyroidism, and hypercalcemia (Mitchell, 2011). Comorbidities such as infection or cardiac, pulmonary, renal, hepatic, neurologic, or endocrine dysfunction also may be part of the differential. CRF is now included as a diagnosis in the 10th revision of the International Classification of Diseases.

Treatment of Cancer-Related Fatigue

The treatment of CRF is individualized and tailored based on a comprehensive assessment and the etiology of fatigue. Communication between patients, family members, and the healthcare team regarding the plan of care should occur. It is essential that all involved in the care understand the scope of the problem and the relationship to other symptoms that patients are experiencing. Educating patients regarding fatigue before or soon after the onset can prompt early intervention before CRF becomes debilitating.

Prevention

The optimal intervention for CRF is prevention. Because there are so many potential contributing factors related to CRF, attention should focus on identifying correctable conditions. Clinical issues such as nutritional deficiencies, anemia, pain, emotional distress, and sleep disturbances should be evaluated and addressed to avoid the concomitant effects of CRF (Campos et al., 2011; Mortimer et al., 2010; NCCN, 2014, 2015b).

Table 10-4. Diagnostic Tests* to Consider in the Workup of Fatigue

Test	Rationale
Complete blood count and differential	Rule out anemia and infection.
Thyroid-stimulating hormone and T4 level	Evaluate thyroid function.
Electrolyte levels	Evaluate nutritional status, and rule out electrolyte imbalance.
Blood urea nitrogen and creatinine	Evaluate renal function as a potential factor in fatigue.
Liver function tests (aspartate aminotransferase, alanine aminotransferase, alkaline phosphatase, and bilirubin)	Rule out liver dysfunction or metastatic disease as a potential cause of fatigue.
Bone scan, computed tomography scans, or other diagnostic imaging tests	Rule out metastatic disease causing pain that in turn causes fatigue.

* Nonexhaustive listing

Pharmacologic Interventions

Although several medications are available that may improve fatigue (e.g., methylphenidate, donepezil, paroxetine, modafinil, bupropion), limited data exist to support the effectiveness in CRF. It is also important to recognize the side effects of these medications. No medications specifically for fatigue currently are approved by the U.S. Food and Drug Administration (FDA); however, certain drugs are approved to treat possible concomitant, contributing disease states that affect fatigue (Minton et al., 2013).

Psychostimulants such as methylphenidate, caffeine, and modafinil may be effective in decreasing fatigue and depression; however, the evidence is not yet sufficient to support a recommendation for routine use (Minton, Richardson, Sharpe, Hotopf, & Stone, 2011; Moraska et al., 2010; NCCN, 2015b; Stone, 2013). Adverse effects associated with psychostimulants include anorexia, insomnia, tremulousness, anxiety, delirium, and tachycardia (Minton et al., 2011).

The antidepressant paroxetine has been examined during and after chemotherapy treatment. Paroxetine is a selective serotonin reuptake inhibitor (SSRI). Although paroxetine has been shown to improve depression and mood, its effects on CRF are mixed. Other antidepressants such as bupropion, sertraline, and venlafaxine have been studied to evaluate the effectiveness in controlling CRF, also with mixed results (Mitchell, 2010).

Donepezil is a centrally acting reversible acetylcholinesterase inhibitor used to treat Alzheimer disease. In a double-blind randomized trial, fatigue was not significantly different in the treatment group compared to the control group (Bruera et al., 2007).

The use of erythropoiesis-stimulating agents (ESAs) has generated practice changes over the past several years. Seven meta-analyses concluded that although ESAs may improve CRF in patients with a hemoglobin of less than 10 g/dl, the effects are small (Mitchell, 2010). Data also suggest that ESA products are associated with significant risks consisting of hypertension and thrombosis and may have a negative impact on disease control and overall survival (Mitchell, 2011; NCCN, 2015b). Treatment of anemia may ameliorate fatigue and significantly improve quality of life. Transfusion may be necessary in some cases.

Evidence exists to suggest that dexamethasone may improve CRF symptoms. In a study by Yennurajalingam et al. (2013), 84 patients were randomized to receive dexamethasone or placebo to control CRF symptoms. The dose of dexamethasone was 4 mg twice per day for 14 days. The FACIT-F was used to measure the fatigue level of patients enrolled in the study. The study reported a significant improvement in the FACIT-F scores of the dexamethasone group at day 15 when compared to the placebo group. The improvement in total quality of life using FACIT-F scores also was significantly higher in the dexamethasone group at day 15. Dexamethasone is associated with side effects such as hyperglycemia, avascular necrosis, muscle weakness, emotional lability, inattention/hyperactivity, mania, psychosis, and altered sleep patterns. The adverse side effects should be considered when prescribing steroids to control fatigue (Vallance et al., 2010).

Nonpharmacologic Interventions

The management of fatigue positively affects physical, psychological, social, and vocational functioning and improves overall quality of life. However, as causes of CRF are poorly understood and are influenced by concomitant diseases and their various treatments, few specific and effective treatments exist (Campos et al., 2011). One important goal of fatigue intervention is to focus on eliminating stressors and increasing patients' resistance to stressors. Nonpharmacologic interventions include activity enhancement such as exercise, psychosocial interventions, integrative therapies, nutritional support, sleep therapy, and energy conservation (Campos et al., 2011; Mitchell, 2010; Mortimer et al., 2010; Mustian, Sprod, Janelsins, Peppone, & Mohile, 2012).

Whenever possible, the underlying cause of fatigue should be eliminated or treated. Managing pain, depression, infection, dehydration, hypoxia, insomnia, anemia, nutritional deficiencies, and electrolyte imbalances may improve fatigue and eliminate other symptoms as well (Campos et al., 2011; Irwin, Poirier, & Mitchell, 2014; NCCN, 2015b). Table 10-5 lists potential interventions that can be used to treat fatigue. Some of these interventions can also be used for prevention.

A meta-analysis of exercise in the setting of CRF reported an overall benefit of exercise during and following cancer treatment in breast cancer (Carayol et al., 2013). Encouraging activity and establishing a regular exercise program may prevent as well as treat fatigue (NCCN, 2014). A Cochrane review by Cramp and Byron-Daniel (2012) of 56 studies reported that aerobic exercise may be beneficial for patients who experience CRF during and after cancer therapy. This was especially true in the solid tumor population. ONS's Putting Evidence Into Practice (PEP) resource for fatigue lists exercise as recommended for practice in controlling CRF (Irwin et al., 2014).

Despite its recommendation as an intervention for fatigue, exercise has not been documented as a consistent intervention to improve fatigue, suggesting that more research is needed (Chiffelle & Kenny, 2013; Mishra et al., 2012; Mitchell, 2011; Mortimer et al., 2010). A Cochrane analysis published in 2012 concluded that exercise decreased fatigue levels from baseline at a 12-week follow-up (Mishra et al., 2012). While it is reasonable to encourage patients to con-

Table 10-5. Fatigue Interventions in Patients With Cancer

Category/Intervention	Comments/Examples
Nonpharmacologic	
Exercise	• No specific type of exercise is superior to another. • Activity enhancement is the primary goal. • Walking, jogging, swimming, and resistance exercises, such as lifting light weights, are common activities that should be considered. • Some contraindications to activity enhancement include bone metastases, thrombocytopenia, infection, and anemia.
Psychosocial therapies	• Cognitive behavioral therapy • Supportive-expressive therapies • Individual counseling • Stress reduction with relaxation training • Fatigue education • Psychoeducational therapies/educational therapies
Sleep patterns	• Sleep hygiene programs • Introduction of different bedtime practices • Sleep restrictions during the day • Falling asleep and waking up at the same time each day • Limiting caffeine or eating several hours before bedtime

Complementary and alternative medicine (CAM) therapies	• CAM is not well established for the treatment of fatigue.
	• Interventions include
	  – Acupuncture/acupressure
	  – Massage therapy
	  – Relaxation techniques
	  – Melatonin.

(Continued on next page)

Table 10-5. Fatigue Interventions in Patients With Cancer *(Continued)*

Category/Intervention	Comments/Examples
Pharmacologic	
Psychostimulants	• Methylphenidate* • Modafinil* • Corticosteroids*

Treatment of other causes of fatigue	• Treat secondary causes of fatigue such as anxiety, depression, or pain.
	• Classes of drugs include
	  – Benzodiazepines*
	  – Antidepressants*
	  – Nonsteroidal anti-inflammatory drugs for mild pain or bone pain*
	  – Opioids.*
	• Consider and treat comorbidities that may affect fatigue and interfere with the patient's ability to sleep, such as cardiac or pulmonary problems.

Sleep medications	• Consider sleep medication if the patient is having difficulty falling asleep or maintaining sleep.
	• Medications to be considered include
	  – Temazepam*
	  – Zolpidem*
	  – Zaleplon*
	  – Eszopiclone*
	  – Diphenhydramine*
	  – Doxepin.*

* These medications do not have U.S. Food and Drug Administration–approved indications for the treatment of cancer-related fatigue.

Note. Based on information from Berger et al., 2012; Campos et al., 2011; Horneber et al., 2012; National Comprehensive Cancer Network, 2015a, 2015b; Neefjes et al., 2013; Thorpy & Roth, 2013.

tinue or increase physical activity, no data exist to recommend a specific amount or type of physical activity. Referral to other expert practitioners, such as physical therapists, social services, or nutritionists, may be necessary (NCCN, 2015b). Oncology APNs are instrumental in coordinating these referrals.

Anxiety and depression can increase symptoms of fatigue. Psychological support can play an important role in managing patients with fatigue. A meta-analysis reported that behavioral interventions, including cognitive therapy, relaxation techniques, counseling, social support, hypnosis, and biofeedback, were beneficial in improving fatigue among patients with breast cancer during and after treatment (Duijts, Farber, Oldenburg, van Beurden, & Aaronson, 2011).

Changes in sleep patterns could easily cause or aggravate CRF. Symptoms of insomnia and hypersomnia may disrupt sleep. Nonpharmacologic interventions to improve sleep include cognitive behavioral, complementary, psychoeducation/information, and exercise therapies. Cognitive behavioral techniques include sleep restriction, sleep hygiene, and stimulus control. Stimulus control includes going to bed and waking up at the same time each day. Stimulus control also includes getting out of bed after 20 minutes if unable to fall asleep. Sleep restriction in the form of avoiding long or late afternoon naps, as well as limiting total time spent sleeping, also is considered an important strategy in managing fatigue. Sleep hygiene involves altering basic lifestyle habits that influence sleep. An example of lifestyle changes include limiting caffeine, alcohol, and smoking; relaxing before bedtime; taking warm baths; and getting adequate exercise during the day (Berger et al., 2012; Mitchell, 2011).

Cognitive behavioral techniques include interventions to relax patients before going to bed. These interventions include complementary therapies, breathing control, progressive muscle relaxation, and guided imagery techniques. Complementary therapies include massage therapy, yoga, and stress reduction using mindfulness (Berger et al., 2012; NCCN, 2015b).

Strategies for energy conservation may be helpful (Berger et al., 2012). NCCN (2015b) defines energy conservation as "deliberately planned management of one's personal energy resources to prevent their depletion" (p. MS-9). The goal of energy conservation is to maintain a balance between rest and activity so that valued activities may be completed.

Attention-restoring therapy may improve the capacity to concentrate or direct attention during times of stress. Enjoyment of natural environments improves cognitive ability and decreases attentional fatigue (NCCN, 2015b). Maintaining an active mind, even when the body is fatigued, improves the ability to concentrate (Mitchell, 2010). Psychosocial interventions also have a strong evidence base for treating fatigue and include education, support groups, individual counseling, stress management training, and tailored behavioral interventions to decrease anxiety, depression, and fatigue (Mitchell, 2011).

Nutritional consultation may be helpful in managing deficiencies caused by anorexia, diarrhea, nausea, and vomiting. Proper nutrition is thought to provide adequate fuel for the body to function (Mitchell, 2011). Hydration and replacement of deficient electrolytes, such as iron and folic acid, may prevent or treat fatigue (NCCN, 2015b).

Complementary and Alternative Therapies

Preliminary studies have noted massage therapy, acupuncture, expressive writing, yoga, muscle relaxation, healing touch, and mindfulness-based stress reduction as being effective in reducing fatigue in patients with cancer; however, further study is warranted (Berger et al., 2012; Mitchell, 2011; NCCN, 2014, 2015b). Chapter 8 provides more information about alternative therapies.

Evaluation of Outcomes

Assessment and evaluation of fatigue are essential at each clinic visit. APNs evaluate effectiveness of interventions and, if strategies are ineffective, consider alternatives. Assessment for the presence of several known treatable factors (e.g., medications, pain, emotional distress, sleep disturbances, anemia, alteration in nutrition, deconditioning, comorbidities) is ongoing. Fatigue occurs in the context of multiple symptoms, and these symptoms may act synergistically to worsen the overall symptom experience (NCCN, 2014, 2015a, 2015b). Multiple concurrent interventions may be required. Cause-specific interventions are indicated, but if no cause is identified, nonpharmacologic and pharmacologic treatments are implemented (NCCN, 2014).

Cancer-Related Cognitive Impairment

Introduction

As the diagnosis and treatment of cancer become more sophisticated and successful, more individuals will live longer as survivors. As this occurs, the long-term sequelae of systemic treatments will become more apparent. A long-term effect of cancer and cancer treatments being increasingly recognized by healthcare professionals is cancer-related cognitive impairment (CRCI), often called *chemobrain* by laypeople. CRCI is often a complex and distressing symptom (Von Ah, Jansen, Allen, Schiavone, & Wulff, 2011). The common presentation of CRCI is a decline in memory, concentration, and multitasking functions that may occur during or after treatment for cancer (Mulrooney, 2010). Quality of life is altered, as cancer survivors report that they are not confident to return to work because of a change in cognition and also describe significant changes in interpersonal relationships (Fardell, Vardy, Johnston, & Winocur, 2011).

Definitions and Incidence

Cognitive function is the ability to handle the informational aspects of human behavior. The multidimensional concept of cognitive function includes the domains of attention and concentration, executive function (including planning and problem solving), information processing speed, language, visuospatial skill, psychomotor ability, learning, and memory (Jansen, 2010; Von Ah et al., 2011). It is important for APNs to recognize the impact of CRCI on quality of life by assessing patients' economic, emotional, and intrapersonal lives (Boykoff, Moieni, & Subramanian, 2009).

Many patients report a subtle and intermittent decline in cognitive function after chemotherapy, making it difficult to obtain objective evidence of CRCI (Hermelink et al., 2010; O'Farrell, MacKenzie, & Collins, 2013). Initially, the focus of CRCI research was centered on children with cancer and women with breast cancer. In more recent times, more investigation has been undertaken involving patients with prostate, lung, colorectal, and hematologic malignancies. Generalizing the results of CRCI research has been difficult because of small sample sizes and inconsistent methods of testing cognitive function. The prevalence of CRCI varies, and an accurate incidence is unknown. CRCI occurs in patients prior to the initiation of therapy, and the prevalence is estimated to be 11%–35% in patients with breast cancer, 40% in people with leukemia, 46% in patients with testicular cancer, 50%–80% in people with brain tumors, and 70%–80% in patients with lung cancer (Boykoff et al., 2009; Mulrooney, 2010; Von Ah et al., 2011).

Approximately 15%–50% of patients were found to have mild to moderate cognitive changes on standardized neuropsychological assessments (Fardell et al., 2011). Ahles et al. (2002) reviewed patients with breast cancer and lymphoma who had been treated with chemotherapy in the past 10 years. Results demonstrated that cognitive deficits were present up to a decade after treatment.

Brezden, Phillips, Abdolell, Bunston, and Tannock (2000) surveyed women with breast cancer. They found that women who were previously treated or currently in treatment had measurable cognitive impairment when compared to the healthy control arm. The investigators concluded that more research was needed and that information about the potential for cognitive impairment should be included in the consenting process.

In another study, interviews were conducted to assess cognitive function in men receiving androgen deprivation therapy (Wu, Diefenbach, Gordon, Cantor, & Cherrier, 2012). Eight of the 11 men interviewed reported impairments in cognitive and neurobehavioral functions that affected their work and daily lives.

Ahles et al. (2010) examined the impact of age and cognitive reserve on cognitive function in patients with breast cancer undergoing adjuvant treatment by evaluating neuropsychological and psychological test results before treatment and after treatment at 1, 6, and 18 months. The data suggested that age and pretreatment cognitive reserve were related to post-treatment changes in processing speed. Chemotherapy was associated with a negative short-term impact on verbal ability. Although chemotherapy was associated with cognitive impairment in this study, it was not the only variable.

In a study by Jansen, Cooper, Dodd, and Miaskowski (2011), cognitive impairment was reported in 23% of patients with breast cancer before chemotherapy administration. Women who received chemotherapy developed a decrease in the cognitive domains of visuospatial skills, attention, delayed memory, and motor function. These deficits significantly improved six months after chemotherapy.

Determining actual incidence is difficult. Existing studies measure varying domains of cognitive function, use varying control groups for comparison, examine different points in time relative to administration of treatment, do not account for confounding factors, lack pre-treatment assessment for comparison, and lack consistency in many aspects of methodology (Fardell et al., 2011; Hermelink et al., 2010).

As previously discussed, studies have suggested subtle declines in cognitive function in approximately 23%–33% patients before the start of chemotherapy treatment (Ahles et al., 2010; Joly, Rigal, Noal, & Giffard, 2011). Although a definitive cause has not been identified, it is hypothesized that this may be the result of patient characteristics such as nutritional, hormonal, genetic, or immune factors; disease characteristics such as cytokines produced by the tumor; or the influence of the psychological impact of a cancer diagnosis (Fardell et al., 2011; Joly et al., 2011).

Etiology and Pathophysiology

Several mechanisms are hypothesized to contribute to the development of cognitive impairment, and it is likely multifactorial. Some likely responsible factors include endogenous hormones, genetic predisposition, depression, anxiety, fatigue, cytokines, cancer treatment, and thrombus in small blood vessels (Fardell et al., 2011; Hermelink et al., 2010; Von Ah et al., 2011).

Cognitive impairment is often described after chemotherapy. Common chemotherapy agents known to affect the nervous system include 5-fluorouracil (5-FU), nitrosoureas (carmustine, lomustine), methotrexate, cisplatin, ifosfamide, cytarabine, vinca alkaloids, and taxanes. Studies describe a higher incidence of CRCI when methotrexate and 5-FU are given at higher doses (Gehring, Roukema, & Sitskoorn, 2012; Myers, Pierce, & Pazdernik, 2008).

Several hypotheses exist regarding the cause of cognitive difficulties. Chemotherapy may damage blood vessels in the brain and cause ischemia or an infarction (Gehring et al., 2012). Yet another theory to explain CRCI involves chemotherapy drugs coming into direct contact with brain tissue when passing through the blood-brain barrier to the central nervous system, damaging nerve cells and potentially causing demyelination (Wefel & Schagen, 2012). Neurotransmitter levels also may be altered, potentially affecting cognition (Mulrooney, 2010). Other causes of CRCI include microvascular impairment, cytokine-induced inflammatory reaction, and hormonal changes (Joly et al., 2011; Myers, 2009). Radiation therapy of the brain is known to cause leukoencephalopathy caused by damage of the myelin found in the white matter of the brain. This can occur 6–24 months following whole brain irradiation and potentially affect cognition (Wefel & Schagen, 2012).

Cytokines may play a role in the development of CRCI. Specifically, interleukins and interferons are naturally occurring cytokines that are administered to treat cancer. It is postulated that cytokines can cross the blood-brain barrier, travel to the brain, and cause behavioral changes (Fardell et al., 2011).

A genetic predisposition may be associated with chemotherapy-induced cognitive impairment. Apolipoprotein E (APOE) is a glycolipo-protein that enables lipid uptake and transports and distributes ion lipids, as well as aiding in neuronal repair and plasticity after injury (Ahles & Saykin, 2007). Ahles and Saykin (2007) reported an association between the E4 allele of APOE and a diminished cognitive performance in breast cancer and lymphoma survivors (Mulrooney, 2010).

Symptoms such as depression, fatigue, and anxiety play a significant role in diminished cognition. While some research is supportive of these symptoms affecting cognition, other studies have found no association between these symptoms and cognitive impairment (Mulrooney, 2010). A relationship appears to exist between hormone therapy and cognition. Women prescribed anastrozole, an aromatase inhibitor for breast cancer, scored lower on tests of verbal and visual learning and memory than women who were prescribed tamoxifen (Bender et al., 2007). As previously discussed, men who were treated with androgen deprivation therapy compared to healthy men reported a decline in certain cognitive function over time (Wu et al., 2012), whereas another study found no significant differences (Joly et al., 2006).

Tumor location can have an obvious effect on cognition. Patients diagnosed with primary and metastatic brain tumors often present with cognitive impairment. The size, location, tumor histology, and treatment regimen will factor into the severity of CRCI. Patient age and related symptoms (such as pain, fatigue, and depression) also may play a role in cognitive impairment in patients with brain tumors (Gehring, Aaronson, Taphoorn, & Sitskoorn, 2010; Mulrooney, 2010).

Medications that are prescribed along with chemotherapy, such as antiemetics, steroids, sedatives, and antihistamines, may induce a short-term effect on cognitive ability. For example, steroids can have adverse effects on mental and emotional functioning, thus intensifying anxiety, depression, restlessness, and insomnia. Antiepileptic medications can cause sedation, distractibility, somnolence, dizziness, and impairment of attention and memory (Fardell et al., 2011; Gehring et al., 2010). Effects of hormonal changes associated with menopause, whether naturally occurring or induced by chemotherapy treatment, are hypothesized to influence cognitive function. Estrogen receptors are present in areas of the brain associated with attention, memory, and learning. Estrogen may have a neuroprotective effect and support the maintenance of cognitive function (Janelsins et al., 2011; O'Farrell et al., 2013). However, despite subjective reports, research has not proved a difference in cognitive function attributable to menopausal or hormonal changes (Mulrooney, 2010). Studies vary on the influence of additional psychological factors, such as anxiety, depression, and fatigue, on cognitive function. Heflin et al. (2005) concluded that cancer and chemotherapy treatment decrease cognitive reserve, and over time, survivors have a higher risk of reaching the threshold for measurable cognitive impairment.

Risk Factors

The Theory of Unpleasant Symptoms (TUS) and the Conceptual Model of Chemotherapy-Related Changes in Cognitive Function are models that may help to explain potential risk factors associated with CRCI (Myers, 2009). TUS was first described by Elizabeth Lenz in 1995. The model recognizes three factors that play a role in cognitive impairment: physiologic, psychological, and situational. The TUS model could be used to identify at-risk patients by identifying certain symptoms. Physiologic factors such as cardiovascular disease, infection, or nutritional problems could potentially place patients at risk for CRCI. Psychological factors such as depression, anxiety, or isolation could potentially confer a risk of developing CRCI as well. Situational factors such as family supports and employment or financial issues could also be identified as potential CRCI risk factors.

The conceptual model of Chemotherapy-Related Changes in Cognitive Function (Hess & Insel, 2007) defines cognitive function and the relationship to certain identified domains (executive function, attention, concentration, intelligence, memory/recall, psychomotor ability, processing, verbal ability, vigilance, and visuospatial and visuomotor ability). Cancer treatments are listed as antecedents. Mediators can be identified as risk factors, for example, physiologic factors, chemotherapy agents, radiation therapy, treatment dose, duration, concomitant medications, and psychosocial factors such as stress, depression, anxiety, and distress. Moderators in the model include age, education, intelligence, genetic factors, and coexisting neurocognitive disorders (Myers, 2009).

Not all patients receiving chemotherapy develop cognitive changes. Several studies have reported that cognitive impairment appears to affect a subset of patients, with the underlying risk or causative factors unknown and the severity of impairment varying among individuals (Brezden et al., 2000; Joly et al., 2011). No significant differences have been identified in sociodemographic characteristics, such as age, sex, employment status, IQ level, or education, or clinical characteristics, such as diagnosis. Studies controlling for confounding or associated factors show that certain risk factors such as age, education level, menopausal status, mood, fatigue, anxiety, and depression have not had a significant impact on results. The disparity in cognitive risk factor studies is thought to be due to the lack of standardized neuropsychological testing and the lack of available longitudinal studies (Freedman et al., 2013; Wefel, Vardy, Ahles, & Schagen, 2011).

Patients receiving high-dose chemotherapy regimens are at an increased risk for cognitive impairment before and after stem cell transplantation. Scherwath et al. (2013) found that the pretreatment regimen, graft-versus-host disease, total body irradiation, and conditioning regimen were not associated with CRCI. However, age and baseline intelligence were associated with changes in cognition (Scherwath et al., 2013).

The specific chemotherapy agents received may increase the risk for cognitive impairment. Most chemotherapy agents do not cross the blood-brain barrier, with the exception of methotrexate and 5-FU (Ahles, Root, & Ryan, 2012; Mulrooney, 2010). Data also suggest that many chemotherapy agents can potentially cause central nervous system toxicities, including encephalopathy, leukoencephalopathy, ototoxicity, and cerebellar symptoms. Although central nervous system toxicities are uncommon, detectable levels of radiolabeled cisplatin, carmustine, and paclitaxel have been detected in the brain after administration (Verstappen, Heimans, Hoekman, & Postma, 2003). The effect is seen as deterioration over time occurring in a subset of patients and is not consistently seen with a particular agent or combination of agents (Avisar et al., 2012; Joly et al., 2011).

Certain psychological complaints may increase the risk of developing cognitive impairment. Wefel et al. (2004) found that a significant number of patients with breast cancer reporting cognitive impairment also reported symptoms of anxiety, depression, and significant affective distress. Vearncombe et al. (2009) reported that patients experiencing anxiety were at risk for developing cognitive impairment. Schagen et al. (2008) reported no significant difference in objective cognitive testing; however, self-reports of cognitive impairment were associated with emotional distress and fatigue.

Anemia may contribute to cognitive impairment, thereby increasing risk. It can occur as a result of the treatment effect on stem cells, secretion of anemia-inducing factors by some types of tumors, or other conditions such as blood loss, B_{12} or folate deficiency, or renal disease. Symptoms of decreased mental alertness, poor concentration, and memory problems are associated with decreased hemoglobin concentration (Fardell et al., 2011; NCCN, 2014).

Signs and Symptoms

Patients frequently report mild cognitive impairment, including having mildly affected thinking ability but still being able to maintain adequate functioning. Difficulty with memory is reported, such as trouble remembering names, trouble remembering the flow of a conversation, and a tendency to misplace things. Mild cognitive impairment differs from dementia. In dementia, memory loss has progressed to such a point that normal independent function is impossible, and individuals can no longer successfully manage their finances or provide for their own basic needs.

Subtle changes in memory, concentration, language, visual-motor, and executive function are observed and negatively affect quality of life (Gehring et al., 2012; Von Ah et al., 2011). Many individuals report difficulty maintaining ability to work, continuing education, or fulfilling social responsibilities (Boykoff et al., 2009; Joly et al., 2011). A study by Jansen et al. (2011) reported a decrease in several cognitive measurements after chemotherapy administration in patients with breast cancer. While improvement in several domains (such as visuospatial skill, attention, motor skills, and delayed memory) were seen after six months, other domain measurements (immediate memory, language and executive function) did not change over time. Symptoms of cognitive impairment may persist for years following the completion of treatment. Patients usually will report these symptoms when their activities of daily living are adversely affected.

Over the past several years, neuroimaging has provided evidence of structural and functional differences following chemotherapy. A study using magnetic resonance imaging in patients with breast cancer found significant decreases in gray matter density bilaterally in the frontal, temporal, and cerebellar regions and the right thalamus shortly following completion of chemotherapy that were not evident in a disease or healthy control group (McDonald, Conroy, Ahles, West, & Saykin, 2010). Another study in patients with breast cancer performed positive-emission tomography along with neuropsychological testing in women who received treatment for breast cancer 5–10 years previously. It was found that during short-term recall tasks, modulation of cerebral blood flow in the frontal cortex and cerebellum was altered in chemotherapy-treated women when compared to untreated women (Silverman et al., 2007).

Assessment

Cognition is complex thought processes involving four components: receptive functions, memory and learning, thought processes, and expressive functions (Fardell et al., 2011; Jansen, 2010). As previously mentioned in this chapter, seven domains of cognitive functioning and neuropsychological testing exist. These cognitive processes include attention and concentration, executive function, information processing speed, language, visual-spatial skill, psychomotor ability, learning, and memory (Jansen, 2010; Mulrooney, 2010). These cognitive processes are interrelated, and when difficulty occurs in one area, disruption may occur in another (Von Ah et al., 2011). Neuropsychological testing is performed to measure the function of each cognition component. Neuropsychological testing is a long, involved process and can take up to eight hours to complete. Patients with cancer may find this difficult to complete. Several quick neuropsychological tests can be used; however, at present, accurate neuropsychological testing may not be possible for patients with cancer (Mulrooney, 2010). No validated practical and simple tests are available to measure cognitive impairment. This further limits the development of standardized guidelines to aid in the assessment and interventions of patients with cancer with cognitive impairment (Joly et al., 2011).

Patients who report subjective symptoms of cognitive impairment may not show impairment on neuropsychological testing. Changes in cognitive function often are mild but concerning to patients. While assessment may show decline from baseline after initiation of treatment, results of neuropsychological testing frequently remain within the normal range (Kanaskie,

2012). This discrepancy may occur because tests are not measuring the correct construct or may be insufficiently sensitive to detect mild deficits (Holmes, 2013).

Diagnostic Tests and Tools

Multiple measures are available to test various aspects of identified cognitive domains, but no valid and reliable clinical tool exists to evaluate the frequently subtle changes associated with cancer treatment (Jansen, 2010; Mulrooney, 2010; O'Farrell et al., 2013; Von Ah et al., 2011). Referral of patients for specific neuropsychological evaluation may be indicated if symptoms are severe. Administration and interpretation of these tests by a healthcare professional with training in neuropsychology is recommended (Hermelink et al., 2010; Kanaskie, 2012).

Physical Examination

Clinical observation is the most useful way to assess for cognitive changes (Boykoff et al., 2009). Individuals are assessed for changes in attention or concentration and their ability to perform routine tasks and are questioned regarding subjective signs of impairment. Asking directed questions may initiate discussion regarding problems with role function or quality-of-life issues. A physical examination is useful to rule out other causes of cognitive impairment, such as metastatic disease, electrolyte imbalance, or side effects of medications. Assessment may require laboratory tests, such as a complete blood count, metabolic panel, liver function tests, or imaging scans, as indicated (Mulrooney, 2010).

Symptom Rating Scale

A relationship appears to exist between subjective cognitive problems and psychological distress (O'Farrell et al., 2013). The NCCN (2014) guidelines for distress management suggest that clinicians assess the level and nature of the distress by asking patients to quantify the impact of CRCI on their life by rating their level of distress on a scale of 0–10 (where 0 indicates no distress, and 10 indicates extreme distress). A rating of 4 or higher indicates moderate to severe distress, and intervention should be planned. Patients are reevaluated on an ongoing basis to determine the effectiveness of interventions.

Differential Diagnosis

Mild cognitive changes may be attributed to fatigue, anxiety, depression, mood imbalances, or hormonal changes; therefore, the differential diagnosis may include psychological disorders. Potentially reversible causes, such as endocrine or metabolic dysfunction, must be ruled out (Von Ah et al., 2011). Infection, fever, nutritional deficits, sleep disorders, and advancing age may be indirect factors accounting for mild cognitive impairment and are included in the differential (Myers, 2009). Figure 10-5 is a nonexhaustive list of the differential diagnosis of

Psychological	Physiologic	Pharmacologic
• Anxiety	• Anemia	• Antidepressants
• Depression	• Fever	• Antiemetics
• Fatigue	• Hormonal changes	• Antiepileptics
• Insomnia/sleep disorder	• Infection	• Opioids
• Mood imbalance	• Nutritional deficits	• Sedatives
		• Steroids

Figure 10-5. Differential Diagnosis for Cognitive Impairment

cognitive impairment. Potential diagnoses could be psychological, physiologic, or pharmacologic in nature.

Treatment of Cancer-Related Cognitive Impairment

No treatment is currently FDA-approved to prevent or decrease any of the cognitive symptoms associated with chemotherapy (Mulrooney, 2010; Von Ah et al., 2011). In 2008, the International Cognition and Cancer Task Force convened and identified an urgent need for validated treatments and interventions for patients with cancer experiencing cognitive impairment (Fardell et al., 2011). Various treatments were proposed and are under study (see Figure 10-6). The passage of time may improve cognitive impairment (Ahles et al., 2010; Jansen et al., 2011; O'Farrell et al., 2013). Informing patients of this may be reassuring. It is important to first treat concomitant problems, such as anxiety, depression, pain, and fatigue, and maintain good nutrition, as well as to expertly manage comorbid diseases.

Pharmacologic Interventions

Hormonal strategies, antioxidants, monoamine oxidase inhibitors, growth factors, dopamine agonists, cholinesterase inhibitors, anti-inflammatory agents, thiamine, and steroids all

---

Pharmacologic Interventions (not yet supported by research study, and use may be limited by side effects)
• Methylphenidate (Ritalin®)
• Dexmethylphenidate (Focalin®)
• Modafinil (Provigil®)
• Cholinesterase inhibitors (Aricept®, Exelon®, Razadyne®)
• Erythropoietin

Nonpharmacologic Interventions
• Simplification
  – Limit/eliminate distraction.
  – Reduce background noise.
  – Clear clutter.
• Memory aids
  – Use calendars/lists.
  – Establish routines.
• Cognitive behavioral therapy
• Restorative natural environment
• Physical/mental exercise

Complementary and Alternative Interventions
• Herbs
  – Thiamine
  – Vitamins C and E
  – Ginkgo biloba
• Body awareness and movement
  – Yoga
  – Tai chi
• Aromatherapy
• Meditation

Figure 10-6. Treatment for Mild Cognitive Impairment

Note. Based on information from Cephalon, Inc., 2010; Eisai Inc., 2013; Fardell et al., 2011; Jotoi et al., 2005; Mulrooney, 2010; Novartis Pharmaceuticals Corp., 2013a, 2013b; Von Ah et al., 2011; Wefel et al., 2015.

have been noted to improve cognition in various clinical situations, but studies proving effectiveness and safety in patients with cancer are lacking (Fardell et al., 2011; Mulrooney, 2010; Von Ah et al., 2011).

Methylphenidate and dexmethylphenidate are psychostimulants that improve concentration, psychomotor slowing, fatigue, and attention. Methylphenidate is FDA-approved for attention-deficit/hyperactivity disorder but is not approved for use in patients experiencing CRCI (Von Ah et al., 2011). Methylphenidate acts by modulating catecholaminergic tone in the prefrontal cortex and by increasing extracellular dopamine levels and possibly noradrenergic and serotonergic neurotransmitter systems (Fardell et al., 2011; Mulrooney, 2010). Evidence to support the use of methylphenidate is conflicting. Gagnon, Low, and Schreier (2005) reported that the daily administration methylphenidate improved language, psychomotor function and attention deficit in patients with advanced cancer, whereas other studies report no significant impact on cognitive impairment in patients taking methylphenidate (Lower et al., 2009; Mar Fan et al., 2008). Psychostimulants increase tissue perfusion, vascular dilation, and cerebral blood flow. Side effects usually are mild and easily reversed with drug discontinuation. Adverse effects include headache, nausea, nervousness, insomnia, and cardiovascular symptoms (Von Ah et al., 2011). Contraindications include prior sensitivity to stimulants, glaucoma, symptomatic cardiovascular disease, and hyperthyroidism (Novartis Pharmaceuticals Corp., 2013a, 2013b).

Modafinil is a psychostimulant medication used for wakefulness and narcolepsy. It also has been used for patients with cancer experiencing fatigue. One small sample study reported an improvement in memory speed and quality of episodic memory and mean continuity of attention compared to the placebo group (Kohli et al., 2009; Von Ah et al., 2011). Modafinil is not approved for use in patients experiencing CRCI. Currently, it is under study in phase II and III trials for CRCI.

Donepezil is a cholinesterase inhibitor used for the treatment of Alzheimer disease and vascular dementia. Donepezil may stabilize memory capacity and improve cognitive function by selectively inhibiting acetylcholinesterase (Eisai Inc., 2013). One study reported that patients with brain tumors experienced an improvement in cognitive functioning and mood in the setting of treatment-related responsive disease (Shaw et al., 2006). Side effects include nausea, diarrhea, weight loss, asthenia, arthralgias, and, in rare cases, syncope and mild pancreatitis (Eisai Inc., 2013). Donepezil is not approved for CRCI; however, ongoing studies continue to evaluate its use in various oncology populations.

Although anemia may be a possible cause of CRCI, inadequate data exist to support the use of ESAs as a strategy to improve cognition. Studies examining the use of ESAs have been inconclusive (Fardell et al., 2011; Mar Fan et al., 2009; Von Ah et al., 2011).

Nonpharmacologic Interventions

Cognitive rehabilitation and training approaches may significantly improve cognitive function. A variety of methods are used in cognitive training programs and include group sessions with trained personnel, computer training programs, and individual sessions with all participants offered psychoeducational training sessions. The goal of psychoeducational training is to incorporate compensatory interventions into daily function (Von Ah et al., 2011). While some studies reported improvement in cognitive function (Gehring, Aaronson, Taphoorn, & Sitskoorn, 2011), other studies did not report an improvement in cognition when compared control group (Poppelreuter, Weis, & Bartsch, 2009), suggesting that more research is needed to identify specific cognitive training interventions.

Evidence suggests that exercise may improve CRCI (Fardell et al., 2011; Mustian et al., 2012; Myers, 2012). One study evaluated the effects of a 12-week combined psychoeducational and rehabilitation program. The exercise regimen consisted of two-hour sessions twice a week. The psychoeducational intervention included 7 two-hour sessions focused on coping with cancer. Improvement in global cognitive function was reported (Korstjens, Mesters, van der Peet, Gijsen, & van den Borne, 2006).

Myers (2012) conducted a qualitative descriptive study in 18 breast cancer survivors. Participants described several cognitive deficits, including inability to focus, difficulty driving, difficulty reading, short-term memory problems, and issues with word-finding. Other cognitive problems included fatigue, difficulty sleeping, neuropathy, and difficulty with balance and coordination. Women reported that exercise, adequate rest, and mind stimulation were important strategies that improved their symptoms. Although 11 of the 18 women interviewed reported that exercise was an important intervention, only 5 women were able to exercise during treatment. Schwartz, Thompson, and Masood (2002) evaluated visual attention, motor speed, and cognitive flexibility in combination with an aerobic exercise program four days per week that also included daily methylphenidate. Participants in this study showed an improvement in cognitive function, specifically visual attention, motor speed, and cognitive flexibility.

Simplifying tasks, commitments, and the environment reduces the stress caused by changes in memory, concentration, and the ability to multitask. Reducing work or dividing projects into manageable small steps, establishing a routine, decreasing work hours or academic credits, and avoiding performance of concurrent tasks may help to reduce stress. Limiting or eliminating distractions, such as background noise and clutter, makes the environment less stressful (Joly et al., 2011; Myers, 2012). Keeping lists of tasks or important items to remember and using a calendar to keep track of important dates and appointments will provide prompts rather than individuals having to rely on memory.

Memory and attention adaptation training (MAAT) is a cognitive behavioral treatment intervention that has been studied in cancer survivors. It has five cognitive-behavioral components: education about memory and attention; training about self-awareness; self-regulation using relaxation training; activity scheduling and pacing; and cognitive compensatory strategies training. Compensatory strategies of MAAT include self-instructional training, verbal rehearsal of auditory information, schedule making, external cueing, and outlining written material. In a small one-arm pilot study, MAAT interventions were implemented in patients with stage I or stage II breast cancer. The study reported an improvement in the self-report of cognitive function, quality of life, and standard neuropsychological test performance observed at post-treatment, two-month, and six-month follow-up. Participants also reported improvement in the ability to compensate for memory problems (Ferguson et al., 2007).

Ferguson et al. (2012) used the MAAT behavioral treatment intervention in a randomized trial in patients with breast cancer. Patients were evaluated by self-reported daily cognitive failures; quality of life; and neuropsychological performance. Findings noted significant improvements that persisted in areas of attention and concentration, spatial memory, verbal memory, and language. Use of electronic devices, such as an electronic calendar with an alarm, is helpful if short-term memory is affected, and a word-based direction finder or GPS can assist patients whose visuospatial memory is decreased. Mental exercise can improve cognition and slow mental decline. This could include working on crossword or math puzzles, participating in a book club, or taking a class. Use of mnemonic devices, such as a formula or rhyme, may aid patients in remembering information.

Complementary and Alternative Therapies

Herbs used to enhance mental alertness and memory include blessed thistle, blue cohosh, and ginkgo biloba and are controversial (Avisar et al., 2012; Fardell et al., 2011; Joly et al.,

2011). Ginkgo biloba may have antioxidant, membrane-stabilizing, and neuroprotective effects. It may inhibit loss of cholinergic receptors. Studies in healthy volunteers and older adults with Alzheimer disease and dementia suggest that ginkgo biloba may improve symptoms (van Dongen, van Rossum, Kessels, Sielhorst, & Knipschild, 2003), but studies in individuals with cancer are lacking (Fardell et al., 2011; Joly et al., 2011). Because of an antiplatelet effect, ginkgo may potentiate anticoagulants and antiplatelet drugs and should not be used in conjunction with these agents (Avisar et al., 2012).

Barton et al. (2013) conducted a two-arm randomized, placebo-controlled, double-blind, phase III clinical trial to evaluate the use of ginkgo biloba in the prevention of chemotherapy-related cognitive impairment. The trial enrolled 166 women, and the ginkgo biloba dose was 60 mg twice daily. The results of the trial did not support the use of gingko biloba in the prevention of chemotherapy-related cognitive impairment. Thus, it is difficult to recommend ginkgo biloba for CRCI.

Vitamin E or alpha-tocopherol is a fat-soluble antioxidant that may prevent the production of reactive oxygen. In a study assessing the effect of vitamin E on cognitive function, Chan, Cheung, Law, and Chan (2004) reported improvements in executive function, verbal memory, and visual memory in patients with brain and nasopharyngeal cancer who developed temporal lobe radionecrosis receiving 1,000 international units of vitamin E twice daily for more than one year.

Body awareness and movement, artwork, spiritual exploration, psychotherapy groups, supportive-expressive groups, yoga, and tai chi are interventions that can improve psychological outcomes (Avisar et al., 2012). Rigorous study of these techniques, however, is lacking. Interventions such as aromatherapy and meditation also may prove to be helpful.

Evaluation of Outcomes

Approximately 50% of patients who complain of cognitive impairment during chemotherapy demonstrate improvement 12–18 months after completion of treatment, and patients report improvement in ability to perform work-related activities one to two years following chemotherapy (Ahles et al., 2010; Fardell et al., 2011; Joly et al., 2011). The expectation is that most cancer survivors return to normal activity and function once treatment is completed, unless overt physical limitations exist. Most survivors "look normal"; therefore, subtle changes affecting their function and quality of life may persist without others appreciating the patients' concerns. Reinforcing, strengthening, or reestablishing previously effective mechanisms or patterns of cognitive activity that compensate for impaired processes is helpful. Quantifying changes over time to determine the benefit of various strategies used is an important aspect of rehabilitation. Screening patients for CRCI is critical, and when cognitive impairment is diagnosed, providing patients with education, support, reassurance, and information regarding management strategies is essential to potentially optimize patients' quality of life (O'Farrell et al., 2013).

Implications for Oncology Advanced Practice Nurses

Oncology nurses play an important role in the assessment, diagnosis, and treatment of cancer pain, fatigue, and CRCI. These symptoms often are seen in the cancer treatment setting and have a huge impact on the quality of life of patients with cancer. Understanding the pathophysiology of these toxicities and the elements of comprehensive assessment will enable APNs to successfully create an individualized, evidence-based management plan for each patient and adjust the plan as needed. Education about these toxicities is an essential part of initial training and ongoing continuing education programs for all cancer care providers.

Oncology APNs should be alert to vulnerable populations who are at risk for undertreatment of cancer pain and the barriers that exist to optimal pain management. Familiarity with myths surrounding cancer pain and its management will help APNs to disabuse patients, caregivers, and other healthcare professionals of these beliefs. Knowledge regarding the differences among addiction, tolerance, physical dependence, and pseudoaddiction will lead to optimal pain management, even in patients with a history of substance abuse.

Oncology APNs can reassure patients with cancer that fatigue is a common effect of cancer and its treatment and that fatigue does not necessarily indicate progressive disease. Management of fatigue is an integral part of the care of patients with cancer (NCCN, 2015b). Comorbidities or contributing factors are assessed and treated as part of the fatigue management plan.

Long-term cognitive impairment, even when relatively subtle, can have a profound influence on the daily lives of individuals with cancer (Joly et al., 2011). Concerns regarding subjective symptoms of cognitive impairment must not be minimized or ignored. When educating patients, clinicians ideally should support verbal information with written material to compensate for memory and processing problems (O'Farrell et al., 2013). Patients need to receive information on coping methods and how to compensate for changes in cognition and must be reassured that symptoms may decline over time. When considering CRCI, implications exist for informed consent and identification of treatment-related toxicities (Holmes, 2013). In order to make informed decisions regarding risks and benefits of proposed treatments, patients require accurate information regarding cognitive impairment as a potential side effect (Boykoff et al., 2009).

Oncology APNs have a multifaceted role in the management of patients with cancer- or cancer treatment–related toxicities. This includes participation in ongoing research to support effective, evidence-based intervention strategies. A particular need exists for continued research in cancer pain management (Hughes, Wu, Carducci, & Snyder, 2012). Recruitment of patients, especially older adults, women, and minorities, to clinical trials is critical. According to NCCN (2014, 2015b) guidelines, toxicities, such as CRF, are a vital part of studies of clinical health outcomes in patients with cancer.

Patient advocacy through legislative activities will broaden public understanding and awareness of cancer and increase funding for oncology research.

Conclusion

Patients who are experiencing pain, fatigue, or cognitive impairment are common in oncology practices. These toxicities may be related to the cancer or its treatment. Astute and timely assessment enables oncology APNs to accurately diagnose these toxicities. Advanced nursing knowledge allows oncology APNs to expertly manage pain, fatigue, and cognitive impairment, thus enhancing the quality of life and outcomes of patients with cancer.

Case Study

M.H. is a 43-year-old man diagnosed with non-Hodgkin lymphoma. He has received aggressive chemotherapy followed by stem cell transplantation. Now he returns to the ambulatory treatment unit for weekly follow-up appointments and blood work. He volunteers to the APN that he had to stop twice on the way in from the parking lot to rest, and earlier today he had to stop and rest while just walking to the refrigerator to get milk. He states that he feels exhausted but is unable to sleep soundly. He has difficulty concentrating and almost got lost coming to the clinic, even though he has been coming by the same route every week. He admits that his relationship with his wife is suffering because of his fatigue, as he does not have the energy to do things socially with her, and he feels emotionally numb.

1. What interventions would the oncology APN recommend for M.H.?
   - Although exercise is the only intervention proved to be effective, M.H. is too exhausted to begin with an activity intervention initially. The APN suggests that he keep a journal of activities with exacerbating and alleviating factors of his exhaustion. Methods to conserve energy were recommended, and concrete ways he could pace essential activities throughout the day, alternating with periods of rest, were planned. Sleep hygiene recommendations also were discussed.
   - Later in his disease trajectory, M.H. experiences recurrence of his disease. He relates to the oncology APN that his back and lower abdominal pain are no longer controlled by his current analgesic regimen of extended-release morphine sulfate 15 mg twice a day and short-acting morphine sulfate 15 mg every four hours. He rates his pain as 5 on a scale of 1–10. He feels that this pain is affecting his ability to go to his son's ball games and also is waking him from sleep at night.

2. How should the APN adjust M.H.'s pain medication to improve his pain relief?
   - The total previous 24-hour dose of morphine should first be calculated. He has been taking 30 mg of extended-release morphine plus 90 mg of short-acting morphine for a total of 120 mg of morphine in 24 hours. The APN decides to increase the scheduling dose by 50% of his previous 24-hour dose per NCCN (2015a) guidelines. The APN multiplies 150% by the total 24-hour dose of 120 mg and notes that this is 180 mg. Extended-release morphine is dosed in 30 mg and 60 mg release capsules. The APN writes a new prescription for extended-release morphine sulfate 60 mg TID. The APN also calculates a new breakthrough dose by multiplying the total new 24-hour dose by 10% (180 mg × 10% = 18 mg) and knows that 10%–20% of the total 24-hour dose may be given every hour as needed for breakthrough pain (18–36 mg). She writes a prescription for breakthrough pain as morphine sulfate 30 mg two to four tablets every four hours as needed for breakthrough pain. She advises him to expect an increase in constipation whenever pain medication is increased and instructs him in a bowel regimen to prevent this.
   - M.H.'s pain is now under control. He is receiving chemotherapy and biotherapy, and his last diagnostic scans show improvement. He reports experiencing memory changes over the past couple of months, which he has noticed since his initial diagnosis, but they now seem worse with the resumption of chemotherapy. He relates having difficulty in following television shows and has given up reading, one of his favorite pastimes, because of difficulty concentrating. He also has forgotten to take his oral medications several times and missed one healthcare appointment. He asks the APN if he might have "chemobrain" and what can be done about it. After ruling out other etiologies of cognitive impairment, such as metastatic disease, depression, and uncontrolled symptoms such as pain or sleep disorders, the oncology APN diagnoses cognitive impairment secondary to chemotherapy.

3. What interventions might the oncology APN suggest?
   - No medications are FDA-approved for cognitive impairment. The APN realizes that depression can cause or contribute to cognitive impairment, but the patient is currently on an antidepressant (an SSRI), and his depression is well controlled. She discusses the recent literature about central nervous system stimulants, such as methylphenidate, that currently are undergoing study in patients with cancer and cognitive impairment. However, M.H. is not interested in taking another medication. Therefore, the APN recommends behavioral interventions such as list-making and using an alarm for medication and appointment reminders. She encourages him to try some relaxation techniques, such as meditation and progressive muscle relaxation, at least once a day. The APN also assures him that the passage of time often relieves cognitive impairment.

Key Points

Pain

- Many barriers exist to optimal pain management that must be assessed.
- The pathophysiology of pain drives treatment management.
- Common oncologic pain syndromes exist that have specific treatments.
- A comprehensive pain assessment includes past and present physical, emotional, mental, and educational history.
- Certain populations are at risk for inadequate pain management, including young, older adult, cognitively impaired, and minority patients.

Fatigue

- CRF, one of the most common symptoms experienced by patients with cancer, is a distressing, persistent, subjective sense of tiredness or exhaustion related to cancer or cancer treatment that is not proportional to recent activity and interferes with usual functioning.
- Although CRF is widely prevalent, exact mechanisms of its pathophysiology are largely unknown.
- Seven treatable factors are known to contribute to fatigue: pain, emotional distress, sleep disturbances, anemia, alteration in nutrition, deconditioning, and comorbidities.
- Because the mechanisms causing fatigue are poorly understood, few effective treatments are available. Exercise is the only intervention proved by evidence-based research to effectively reduce fatigue.

Cognitive Impairment

- A subset of individuals treated for cancer will have difficulty with memory, concentration, executive function, and/or motor function.
- The subjective complaint of cognitive impairment associated with chemotherapy does not necessarily correlate with objective performance on neuropsychological testing.
- CRCI is multifactorial and possibly related to direct effects of drugs or cytokines on the brain, genetic predisposition, and factors such as anxiety, depression, and fatigue.
- No current pharmacologic therapy is approved for the treatment of mild cognitive impairment associated with chemotherapy, although behavioral interventions and cognitive therapy show some benefit in improving cognitive function.

Recommended Resources for Oncology Advanced Practice Nurses

Pain

- City of Hope Pain and Palliative Care Resource Center website (http://prc.coh.org): Information on pain and pain management, including clinical guidelines, information, assessment tools, resources, continuing education, patient education (including slide presentations, handouts, and outlines), staff education, and research tools
- National Cancer Institute Physician Data Query (PDQ®) information summary on pain (www.cancer.gov/cancertopics/pdq/supportivecare/pain/HealthProfessional): Information for providers about pain and pain management

- National Institutes of Health National Institute on Drug Abuse (www.drugabuse.gov): Information and continuing education on drug abuse; patient screening and resource tools; patient information; treatment information
- ONS PEP (www.ons.org/practice-resources/pep/pain): Evidence-based information about pain that can be used in the oncology setting
- StopPain.org (www.stoppain.org): Mount Sinai Beth Israel's Department of Pain Medicine and Palliative Care website that provides continuing online education on pain management

Fatigue

- National Cancer Institute PDQ summary on fatigue (www.cancer.gov/cancertopics/pdq/supportivecare/fatigue/HealthProfessional): Information about fatigue in cancer and its management
- ONS PEP resource on fatigue (www.ons.org/practice-resources/pep/fatigue): Evidence-based information on cancer fatigue and its management

Cognitive Impairment

- National Cancer Institute PDQ summary on delirium (www.cancer.gov/cancertopics/pdq/supportivecare/delirium/HealthProfessional): Comprehensive information about delirium and its management
- ONS PEP resource on cognitive impairment (www.ons.org/practice-resources/pep/cognitive-impairment): Evidence-based information on cognitive impairment

The author would like to acknowledge Wendy H. Vogel, MSN, FNP, AOCNP®, and Jean M. Rosiak, RN, MSN, ANP-BC, AOCNP®, for their contributions to this chapter that remain unchanged from the first edition of this book.

References

Agency for Healthcare Research and Quality. (2013). *Pain management guideline.* Rockville, MD: Author.

Ahles, T.A., Root, J.C., & Ryan, E.L. (2012). Cancer- and cancer treatment–associated cognitive change: An update on the state of the science. *Journal of Clinical Oncology, 30,* 3675–3686. doi:10.1200/JCO.2012.43.0116

Ahles, T.A., & Saykin, A.J. (2007). Candidate mechanisms for chemotherapy-induced cognitive changes. *Nature Reviews Cancer, 7,* 192–201.

Ahles, T.A., Saykin, A.J., Furstenberg, C.T., Cole, B., Mott, L.A., Skalla, K., … Silberfarb, P.M. (2002). Neuropsychologic impact of standard-dose systemic chemotherapy in long-term survivors of breast cancer and lymphoma. *Journal of Clinical Oncology, 20,* 485–493. doi:10.1200/JCO.20.2.485

Ahles, T.A., Saykin, A.J., McDonald, B.C., Li, Y., Furstenberg, C.T., Hanscom, B.S., … Kaufman, P.A. (2010). Longitudinal assessment of cognitive changes associated with adjuvant treatment for breast cancer: Impact of age and cognitive reserve. *Journal of Clinical Oncology, 28,* 4434–4440. doi:10.1200/JCO.2009.27.0827

Aiello-Laws, L., Reynolds, J., Deizer, N., Peterson, M., Ameringer, S., & Bakitas, M. (2009). Putting evidence into practice: What are the pharmacologic interventions for nociceptive and neuropathic cancer pain in adults? *Clinical Journal of Oncology Nursing, 13,* 649–655. doi:10.1188/09.CJON.649-655

American Academy of Pain Medicine. (2013). Use of opioids for the treatment of chronic pain [Position statement]. Retrieved from http://www.painmed.org/files/use-of-opioids-for-the-treatment-of-chronic-pain.pdf

American Association of Nurse Anesthetists. (2010). *Pain management.* Park Ridge, IL: Author.

American Society of Anesthesiologists. (1996). A report by the American Society of Anesthesiologists Task Force on Pain Management, Cancer Pain Section. *Anesthesiology, 84,* 1243–1257. doi:10.1097/00000542-199605000-00029

American Society of Anesthesiologists. (2010). Practice guidelines for chronic pain management: An updated report by the American Society of Anesthesiologists Task Force on Chronic Pain Management and the American Society of Regional Anesthesia and Pain Medicine. *Anesthesiology, 112,* 810–833. doi:10.1097/ALN.0b013e3181c43103

Anghelescu, D.L., Ehrentraut, J.H., & Faughnan, L.G. (2013). Opioid misuse and abuse: Risk assessment and management in patients with cancer pain. *Journal of the National Comprehensive Cancer Network, 11,* 1023–1031.

Apolone, G., Corli, O., Caraceni, A., Negri, E., Deandrea, S., Montanari, M., & Greco, M.T. (2009). Pattern and quality of care of cancer pain management: Results from the Cancer Pain Outcome Research Study Group. *British Journal of Cancer, 100,* 1566–1574. doi:10.1038/sj.bjc.6605053

Avisar, A., River, Y., Schiff, E., Bar-Sela, G., Steiner, M., & Ben-Arye, E. (2012). Chemotherapy-related cognitive impairment: Does integrating complementary medicine have something to add? Review of the literature. *Breast Cancer Research and Treatment, 136,* 1–7. doi:10.1007/s10549-012-2211-5

Barton, D.L., Burger, K., Novotny, P.J., Fitch, T.R., Kohli, S., Soori, G., … Loprinzi, C.L. (2013). The use of *Ginkgo biloba* for the prevention of chemotherapy-related cognitive dysfunction in women receiving adjuvant treatment for breast cancer, N00C9. *Supportive Care in Cancer, 21,* 1185–1192. doi:10.1007/s00520-012-1647-9

Baumann, F.T., Zopf, E.M., & Bloch, W. (2012). Clinical exercise interventions in prostate cancer patients—A systematic review of randomized controlled trials. *Supportive Care in Cancer, 20,* 221–233. doi:10.1007/s00520-011-1271-0

Bell, K., & Salmon, A. (2009). Pain, physical dependency and pseudoaddiction: Redefining addiction for nice people. *International Journal of Drug Policy, 20,* 170–178. doi:10.1016/j.drugpo.2008.06.002

Bender, C., Sereika, S., Brufsky, A., Ryan, C., Vogel, V., Rastogi, P., … Berga, S.L. (2007). Memory impairments with adjuvant anastrozole versus tamoxifen in women with early stage breast cancer. *Menopause, 14,* 995–998. doi:10.1097/gme.0b013e318148b28b

Bennett, M.I., Rayment, C., Hjermstad, M., Aass, N., Caraceni, A., & Kaasa, S. (2012). Prevalence and aetiology of neuropathic pain in cancer patients: A systematic approach. *Pain, 153,* 359–365. doi:10.1016/j.pain.2011.10.028

Berger, A., Gerber, L., & Mayer, D. (2012). Cancer-related fatigue. *Cancer, 118,* 2261–2269. doi:10.1002/cncr.27475

Bower, J., Ganz, P., Irwin, M., Kwan, L., Breen, E., & Cole, S. (2011). Inflammation and behavioral symptoms after breast cancer treatment: Do fatigue, depression, and sleep disturbance share a common underlying mechanism? *Journal of Clinical Oncology, 29,* 3517–3522. doi:10.1200/JCO.2011.36.1154

Boykoff, N., Moieni, M., & Subramanian, S.K. (2009). Confronting chemobrain: An in-depth look at survivors' report of impact on work, social networks, and health care response. *Journal of Cancer Survivorship, 3,* 223–232. doi:10.1007/s11764-009-0098-x

Brezden, C.B., Phillips, K., Abdolell, M., Bunston, T., & Tannock, I. (2000). Cognitive function in breast cancer patients receiving adjuvant chemotherapy. *Journal of Clinical Oncology, 18,* 2695–2701.

Bruera, E., El Osta, B., Valero, V., Driver, L.C., Pei, B.L., Shen, L., … Palmer, J.L. (2007). Donepezil for cancer fatigue: A double blind, randomized, placebo-controlled trial. *Journal of Clinical Oncology, 25,* 3475–3481. doi:10.1200/JCO.2007.10.9231

Bruera, E., Kuehn, N., Miller, M.J., Selmser, P., & Macmillan, K. (1991). The Edmonton Symptom Assessment System (ESAS): A simple method for the assessment of palliative care patients. *Journal of Palliative Care, 7*(2), 6–9.

Burton, A., Fanciullo, G., Beasley, R., & Fisch, M. (2007). Chronic pain in the cancer survivor: A new frontier. *Pain Medicine, 8,* 189–198. doi:10.1111/j.1526-4637.2006.00220.x

Burton, A.W., Fine, P.G., & Passik, S.D. (2012). Transformation of acute cancer pain to chronic cancer pain syndromes. *Journal of Supportive Oncology, 10,* 89–95. doi:10.1016/j.suponc.2011.08.004

Butt, Z., Rosenbloom, S., Abernethy, A., Beuamont, J., Paul, D., Hampton, D., & Cella, D. (2008). Fatigue is the most important symptom for advanced cancer patients who have had chemotherapy. *Journal of National Comprehensive Cancer Network, 6,* 448–455.

Campbell, C.M., & Edwards, R. (2012). Ethnic differences in pain and pain management. *Pain Management, 2,* 219–230. doi:10.2217/pmt.12.7

Campos, M.P.O., Hassan, B.J., Riechelmann, R., & Del Giglio, A. (2011). Cancer-related fatigue: A practical review. *Annals of Oncology, 22,* 1273–1279. doi:10.1093/annonc/mdq458

Carayol, M., Bernard, P., Boiché, J., Riou, F., Mercier, B., Cousson-Gélie, F., … Ninot, G. (2013). Psychological effect of exercise in women with breast cancer receiving adjuvant therapy: What is the optimal dose needed? *Annals of Oncology, 24,* 291–300. doi:10.1093/annonc/mds342

Cephalon, Inc. (2010). *Provigil® (modafinil)* [Package insert]. Frazer, PA: Author.

Chan, A., Cheung, M., Law, S., & Chan, J. (2004). Phase II study of alpha-tocopherol in improving the cognitive function of patients with temporal lobe radionecrosis. *Cancer, 100,* 398–401. doi:10.1002/cncr.11885

Chang, V., Janjan, N., Jain, S., & Chau, C. (2006). Regional cancer pain syndromes. *Journal of Palliative Medicine, 9,* 1435–1453. doi:10.1089/jpm.2006.9.1435

Chiffelle, R., & Kenny, K. (2013). Exercise for fatigue in hematopoietic stem cell transplantation recipients. *Clinical Journal of Oncology Nursing, 17,* 241–244. doi:10.1188/13.CJON.241-244

Chou, R., Fanciullo, J., Fine, P.G., Adler, J.A., Ballantyne, J.C., Davies, P., … Miaskowski, C. (2009). Clinical guidelines for the use of chronic opioid therapy in chronic noncancer pain. *Journal of Pain, 10,* 113–130. doi:10.1016/j.jpain.2008.10.008

Cleeland, C.S., & Ryan, K.M. (1994). Pain assessment: Global use of the Brief Pain Inventory. *Annals of the Academy of Medicine, Singapore, 23,* 129–138.

Cleeland, C.S., Zhao, F., Chang, V.T., Sloan, J.A., O'Mara, A.M., Gilman, P.B., … Fisch, M.J. (2013). The symptom burden of cancer: Evidence for a core set of cancer-related and treatment-related symptoms from the Eastern Cooperative Oncology Group Symptom Outcomes and Practice Patterns study. *Cancer, 119,* 4333–4340. doi:10.1002/cncr.28376

Cooney, M., Czarnecki, M., Dunwoody, C., Eksterowicz, N., Merkel, S., Oakes, L., & Wuhrman, E. (2013). American Society for Pain Management Nursing position statement with clinical practice guidelines: Authorized agent controlled analgesia. Retrieved from http://www.aspmn.org/documents/AuthorizedAgentControlledAnalgesia_PMN_August2013.pdf

Coyle, N., & Layman-Goldstein, M. (2007). Pharmacologic management of adult cancer pain. *Oncology, 21*(2, Suppl. Nurse Ed.), 10–22.

Cramp, F., & Byron-Daniel, J. (2012). Exercise for the management of cancer-related fatigue in adults. *Cochrane Database of Systematic Reviews, 2012*(11). doi:10.1002/14651858.CD006145.pub3

Curtiss, C.P. (2010). Challenges in pain assessment in cognitively intact and cognitively impaired older adults with cancer. *Oncology Nursing Forum, 37*(Suppl. 5), 7–16. doi:10.1188/10.ONF.S1.7-16

Daniels, L., Oerlemans, S., Krol, A., van de Poll-Franse, L., & Creutzberg, C. (2013). Persisting fatigue in Hodgkin lymphoma survivors: A systematic review. *Annals of Hematology, 92,* 1023–1032. doi:10.1007/s00277-013-1793-2

de M Alcântara-Silva, T.R., Freitas-Junior, R., Freitas, N.M., & Machado, G.D. (2013). Fatigue related to radiotherapy for breast and/or gynaecological cancer: A systematic review. *Journal of Clinical Nursing, 22,* 2679–2686. doi:10.1111/jocn.12236

Dhruva, A., Dodd, M., Paul, S.M., Cooper, B.A., Lee, K., West, C., … Miaskowski, C. (2010). Trajectories of fatigue in patients with breast cancer before, during, and after radiation therapy. *Cancer Nursing, 33,* 201–212. doi:10.1097/NCC.0b013e3181c75f2a

Duijts, S., Faber, M., Oldenburg, H., van Beurden, M., & Aaronson, N. (2011). Effectiveness of behavioral techniques and physical exercise on psychosocial functioning and health-related quality of life in breast cancer patients and survivors—A meta-analysis. *Psycho-Oncology, 20,* 115–126. doi:10.1002/pon.1728

Dunham, M., Ingleton, C., Ryan, T., & Gott, M. (2013). A narrative literature review of older people's cancer pain experience. *Journal of Clinical Nursing, 22,* 2100–2113. doi:10.1111/jocn.12106

Dworkin, R.H., O'Connor, A.B., Audette, J., Baron, R., Gorlay, G.K., Haanpaa, M.L., … Wells, C.D. (2010). Recommendations for the pharmacological management of neuropathic pain: An overview and literature update. *Mayo Clinic Proceedings, 85*(Suppl. 3), 3–14. doi:10.4065/mcp.2009.0649

Eisai Inc. (2013). *Aricept® (donepezil hydrochloride)* [Package insert]. Retrieved from http://labeling.pfizer.com/ShowLabeling.aspx?id=510

Ephraim, P.L., Wegener, S.T., MacKenzie, E.J., Dillingham, T.R., & Pezzin, L.E. (2005). Phantom pain, residual limb pain, and back pain in amputees: Results of a national survey. *Archives of Physical Medicine and Rehabilitation, 86,* 1910–1919. doi:10.1016/j.apmr.2005.03.031

Falk, S., & Dickenson, A.H. (2014). Pain and nociception: Mechanisms of cancer-induced bone pain. *Journal of Clinical Oncology, 32,* 1647–1657. doi:10.1200/JCO.2013.51.7219

Fallon, M.T. (2013). Neuropathic pain in cancer. *British Journal of Anaesthesia, 111,* 105–111. doi:10.1093/bja/aet208

Fardell, J., Vardy, J., Johnston, I., & Winocur, G. (2011). Chemotherapy and cognitive impairment: Treatment options. *Clinical Pharmacology and Therapeutics, 90,* 366–376. doi:10.1038/clpt.2011.112

Feldt, K.S. (2000). The Checklist of Nonverbal Pain Indicators (CNPI). *Pain Management Nursing, 1,* 13–21. doi:10.1053/jpmn.2000.5831

Ferguson, R.J., Ahles, T.A., Saykin, A.J., McDonald, B.C., Furstenberg, C.T., Cole, B.F., & Mott, L.A. (2007). Cognitive-behavioral management of chemotherapy-related cognitive change. *Psycho-Oncology, 16,* 772–777. doi:10.1002/pon.1133

Ferguson, R.J., McDonald, B.C., Rocque, M.A., Furstenberg, C.T., Horrigan, S., Ahles, T.A., & Saykin, A.J. (2012). Development of CBT for chemotherapy-related cognitive change: Results of a waitlist control trial. *Psycho-Oncology, 21,* 176–186. doi:10.1002/pon.1878

Ferrier, J., Pereira, V., Busserolles, J., Authier, N., & Balayssac, D. (2013). Emerging trends in understanding chemotherapy-induced peripheral neuropathy. *Current Pain and Headache Reports, 17,* 364. doi:10.1007/s11916-013-0364-5

Fine, P.G., & Portenoy, R.K. (2009). Establishing "Best Practices" for opioid rotation: Conclusions of an expert panel. *Journal of Pain and Symptom Management, 38,* 418–425. doi:10.1016/j.jpainsymman

Fisch, M.M., Lee, J.W., Weis, M., Wagner, L.I., Chang, V., Cella, D., … Cleeland, C.S. (2012). Prospective, observational study of pain and analgesic prescribing in medical oncology outpatients with breast, colorectal, lung or prostate cancer. *Journal of Clinical Oncology, 30,* 1980–1988. doi:10.1200/JCO.2011.39.2381

Fishman, B., Pasternak, S., Wallenstein, S., Houde, R., Holland, J., & Foley, K. (1987). The Memorial Pain Assessment Card: A valid instrument for the evaluation of cancer pain. *Cancer, 60,* 1151–1158. doi:10.1002/1097 -0142(19870901)60:5<1151::AID-CNCR2820600538>3.0.CO;2-G

Fornasari, D. (2012). Pain mechanisms in patients with chronic pain. *Clinical Drug Investigation, 32*(Suppl. 1), 45–52. doi:10.2165/11630070-000000000-00000

Freedman, R., Pitcher, B., Keating, N.L., Ballman, K.V., Mandelblatt, J., Kornblith, A.B., … Muss, H.B. (2013). Cognitive function in older women with breast cancer treated with standard chemotherapy and capecitabine on Cancer and Leukemia Group B 49907. *Breast Cancer Research and Treatment, 139,* 607–616. doi:10.1007/s10549-013-2562-6

Gaertner, J., Radbruch, L., Giesecke, T., Gerbershagen, H., Petzke, F., Ostgathe, C., … Sabatowski, R. (2006). Assessing cognition and psychomotor function under long-term treatment with controlled release oxycodone in non-cancer pain patients. *Acta Anaesthesiologica Scandinavica, 50,* 664–672. doi:10.1111/j.1399-6576.2006.01027.x

Gagnon, B., Low, G., & Schreier, G. (2005). Methylphenidate hydrochloride improves cognitive function in patients with advanced cancer and hypoactive delirium: A prospective clinical study. *Journal of Psychiatry and Neuroscience, 30,* 100–107. Retrieved from http://jpn.ca/vol30-issue2/30-2-100

Garland, E.L., Froeliger, B., Zeidan, F., Partin, K., & Howard, M.O. (2013). The downward spiral of chronic pain, prescription opioid misuse, and addiction: Cognitive, affective, and neuropsychopharmacologic pathways. *Neuroscience and Biobehavioral Reviews, 37,* 2597–2607. doi:10.1016/j.neubiorev.2013.08.006

Gehring, K., Aaronson, N.K., Taphoorn, M.J.B., & Sitskoorn, M.M. (2010). Interventions for cognitive deficits in patients with a brain tumor: An update. *Expert Review of Anticancer Therapy, 10,* 1779–1795. doi:10.1586/era.10.163

Gehring, K., Aaronson, N.K., Taphoorn, M.J.B., & Sitskoorn, M.M. (2011). A description of a cognitive rehabilitation programme evaluated in brain tumour patients with mild to moderate cognitive deficits. *Clinical Rehabilitation, 25,* 675–692. doi:10.1177/0269215510395791

Gehring, K., Roukema, J., & Sitskoorn, M. (2012). Review of recent studies on interventions for cognitive deficits in patients with cancer. *Expert Review of Anticancer Therapy, 12,* 255–269. doi:10.1586/era.11.202

Giacalone, A., Quitadamo, D., Zanet, E., Berretta, M., Spina, M., & Tirelli, U. (2013). Cancer-related fatigue in the elderly. *Supportive Care in Cancer, 21,* 2899–2911. doi:10.1007/s00520-013-1897-1

Gralow, J.R., Biermann, J.S., Farooki, A., Fornier, M.N., Gagel, R.F., Kumar, R., … Van Poznak, C.H. (2013). NCCN Task Force report: Bone health in cancer care. *Journal of the National Comprehensive Cancer Network, 11*(Suppl. 3), S1–S50. Retrieved from http://www.jnccn.org/content/11/suppl_3/S-1.long

Greco, M.T., Corli, O., Montanari, M., Deandrea, S., Zagonel, V., & Apolone, G. (2011). Epidemiology and pattern of care of breakthrough cancer pain in longitudinal sample of cancer patients: Results from the Cancer Pain Outcome Research Study Group. *Clinical Journal of Pain, 27,* 9–18. doi:10.1097/AJP.0b013e3181edc250

Grossman, S.A., Dunbar, E.M., & Nesbit, S.A. (2006). Cancer pain management in the 21st century. *Oncology, 20,* 1333–1339. Retrieved from http://www.cancernetwork.com/oncology-journal/cancer-pain-management-21st-century

Hanks, G.W., de Conno, F., Cherny, N., Hanna, M., Kalso, E., McQuay, H.J., … Ventafridda, V. (2001). Morphine and alternative opioids in cancer pain: The EAPC recommendations. *British Journal of Cancer, 84,* 587–593. Retrieved from http://www.ncbi.nlm.nih.gov/pmc/articles/PMC2363790/pdf/84-6691680a.pdf

Heflin, L., Meyerowitz, B., Hall, P., Lichtenstein, P., Johansson, B., Pedersen, N., & Gatz, M. (2005). Cancer as a risk factor for long-term cognitive deficits and dementia. *Journal of the National Cancer Institute, 97,* 854–856. doi:10.1093/jnci/dji137

Hermelink, K., Kuchenhoff, H., Untch, M., Bauerfeind, I., Lux, M., Buhner, M., … Munzel, K. (2010). Two different sides of 'chemobrain': Determinants and nondeterminants of self-perceived cognitive dysfunction in a prospective, randomized, multicenter study. *Psycho-Oncology, 19,* 1321–1328. doi:10.1002/pon.1695

Hess, L., & Insel, K. (2007). Chemotherapy-related change in cognitive function: A conceptual model. *Oncology Nursing Forum, 34,* 981–994. doi:10.1188/07.ONF.981-994

Higginson, I.J., & Gao, W. (2012). Opioid prescribing for cancer pain during the last 3 months of life: Associated factors and 9-year trends in a nationwide United Kingdom cohort study. *Journal of Clinical Oncology, 30,* 4373–4379. doi:10.1200/JCO.2012.42.0919

Hogan, D., Baker, A.L., Morón, J.A., & Carlton, S.M. (2013). Systemic morphine treatment induces changes in firing patterns and responses of nociceptive afferent fibers in mouse glabrous skin. *Pain, 154,* 2297–2309. doi:10.1016/j.pain.2013.05.033

Holmes, D. (2013). Trying to unravel the mysteries of chemobrain. *Lancet Neurology, 12,* 533–534. doi:10.1016/S1474-4422(13)70087-5

Horneber, M., Fischer, I., Dimeo, F., Rüffer, J.U., & Weis, J. (2012). Cancer-related fatigue: Epidemiology, pathogenesis, diagnosis, and treatment. *Deutsches Ärzteblatt International, 109,* 161–172. doi:10.3238/arztebl.2012.0161

Hughes, E., Wu, A., Carducci, M., & Snyder, C. (2012). What can I do? Recommendations for responding to issues identified by patient-reported outcomes assessments used in clinical practice. *Journal of Supportive Oncology, 10,* 143–148. doi:10.1016/j.suponc.2012.02.002

International Association for the Study of Pain. (2011). IASP taxonomy. Retrieved from http://www.iasp-pain.org/Taxonomy

Irwin, M., Poirier, P., & Mitchell, S.A. (2014). Fatigue. In M. Irwin & L.A. Johnson (Eds.), *Putting evidence into practice: A pocket guide to cancer symptom management* (pp. 111–132). Pittsburgh, PA: Oncology Nursing Society.

Janelsins, M.C., Kohli, S., Mohile, S.G., Usuki, K., Ahles, T.A., & Morrow, G.R. (2011). An update on cancer- and chemotherapy-related cognitive dysfunction: Current status. *Seminars in Oncology, 38*(3), 431–438. doi:10.1053/j.seminoncol.2011.03.014

Jansen, C. (2010). Cognitive changes. In J. Eggert (Ed.), *Cancer basics* (pp. 361–366). Pittsburgh, PA: Oncology Nursing Society.

Jansen, C., Cooper, B., Dodd, M., & Miaskowski, C. (2011). A prospective longitudinal study of chemotherapy-induced cognitive changes in breast cancer patients. *Supportive Care in Cancer, 19,* 1647–1656. doi:10.1007/s00520-010-0997-4

Joly, F., Alibhai, S., Galica, J., Park, A., Yi, Q., Wagner, L., & Tannock, I. (2006). Impact of androgen deprivation therapy on physical and cognitive function as well as quality of life of patients with nonmetastatic prostate cancer. *Journal of Urology, 176,* 2243–2247. doi:10.1016/j.juro.2006.07.151

Joly, F., Rigal, O., Noal, S., & Giffard, B. (2011). Cognitive dysfunction and cancer: Which consequences in terms of disease management? *Psycho-Oncology, 20,* 1251–1258. doi:10.1002/pon.1903

Jotoi, A., Kahanic, S., Frytak, S., Schaefer, P., Foote, R., Sloan, J., & Peterson, R. (2005). Donepezil and vitamin E for preventing cognitive dysfunction in small cell lung cancer patients: Preliminary results and suggestions for future study designs. *Supportive Care in Cancer, 13,* 66–69. doi:10.1007/s00520-004-0696-0

Kanaskie, M. (2012). Chemotherapy-related cognitive change: A principle-based concept analysis [Online exclusive]. *Oncology Nursing Forum, 39,* E241–E248. doi:10.1188/12.ONF.E241-E248

Kendall, S., Holm, N., Hojsted, J., Frich, L., Nielsen, P.R., Jensen, N., & Sjogren, P. (2013). Chronic pain and the development of a symptom checklist: A pilot study. *Acta Anaesthesiologica Scandinavica, 57,* 920–928. doi:10.1111/aas.12137

Khadilkar, S.V., & Khade, S.S. (2013). Brachial plexopathy. *Annals of Indian Academy of Neurology, 16,* 12–18. doi:10.4103/0972-2327.107675

Knotkova, H., Clark, W., Keohan, M., Kuhl, J., Winer, R., & Wharton, R. (2006). Validation of the multidimensional affect and pain survey (MAPS). *Journal of Pain, 7,* 161–169. doi:10.1016/j.jpain.2005.10.002

Kohli, S., Fisher, S., Tra, Y., Adams, M., Mapstone, M., Wesnes, K., … Morrow, G.R. (2009). The effect of modafinil on cognitive function in breast cancer survivors. *Cancer, 115,* 2605–2616. doi:10.1002/cncr.24287

Korstjens, I., Mesters, I., van der Peet, E., Gijsen, B., & van den Borne, B. (2006). Quality of life of cancer survivors after physical and psychosocial rehabilitation. *European Journal of Cancer Prevention, 15,* 541–547. doi:10.1097/01.cej.0000220625.77857.95

Laird, B.J.A., Scott, A.C., Colvin, L.A., McKeon, A.-L., Murray, G.D., Fearon, K.C.H., & Fallon, M.T. (2011). Pain, depression, and fatigue as a symptom cluster in advanced cancer. *Journal of Pain and Symptom Management, 42,* 1–11. doi:10.1016/j.jpainsymman.2010.10.261

Lautenbacher, S., Huber, C., Baum, C., Rossaint, R., Hochrein, S., & Heesen, M. (2011). Attentional avoidance of negative experiences as predictor of postoperative pain ratings and consumption of analgesics: Comparison with other psychological predictors. *Pain Medicine, 12,* 645–653. doi:10.1111/j.1526-4637.2011.01076.x

Le Rhun, E., Taillibert, S., & Chamberlain, M.C. (2013). Carcinomatous meningitis: Leptomeningeal metastases in solid tumors. *Surgical Neurology International, 4*(Suppl. 4), S265–S288. Retrieved from http://www.surgicalneurologyint.com/text.asp?2013/4/5/265/111304

Lorenz, K.A., Sherbourne, C.D., Shugarman, L.R., Rubenstein, L.V., Wen, L., Cohen, A., … Asch, S.M. (2009). How reliable is pain as the fifth vital sign? *Journal of the American Board of Family Medicine, 22,* 291–298. doi:10.3122/jabfm.2009.03.080162

Lower, E., Fleishman, S., Cooper, A., Zeldis, J., Faleck, H., Yu, Z., & Manning, D. (2009). Efficacy of dexmethylphenidate for the treatment of fatigue after cancer chemotherapy: A randomized clinical trial. *Journal of Pain and Symptom Management, 38,* 650–662. doi:10.1016/j.jpainsymman.2009.03.011

Mar Fan, H.G., Clemons, M., Xu, W., Chemerynsky, I., Breunis, H., Braganza, S., & Tannock, I.F. (2008). A randomised, placebo-controlled, double-blind trial of the effects of d-methylphenidate on fatigue and cognitive dysfunction in women undergoing adjuvant chemotherapy for breast cancer. *Supportive Care in Cancer, 16,* 577–583. doi:10.1007/s00520-007-0341-9

Mar Fan, H.G., Park, A., Xu, W., Yi, Q.-L., Braganza, S., Chang, J., … Tannock, I.F. (2009). The influence of erythropoietin on cognitive function in women following chemotherapy for breast cancer. *Psycho-Oncology, 18,* 156–161. doi:10.1002/pon.1372

McCaffery, M., & Pasero, C. (1999). Teaching patients to use a numerical pain-rating scale. *American Journal of Nursing, 99*(12), 22.

McDonald, B., Conroy, S., Ahles, T., West, J., & Saykin, A. (2010). Gray matter reduction associated with systemic chemotherapy for breast cancer: A prospective MRI study. *Breast Cancer Research and Treatment, 123,* 819–828. doi:10.1007/s10549-010-1088-4

McMenamin, E. (2011). Cancer pain management. In C.H. Yarbro, D. Wujcik, & B.H. Gobel (Eds.), *Cancer nursing: Principles and practice* (7th ed., pp. 685–712). Burlington, MA: Jones & Bartlett Learning.

Melzack, R. (1987). The short-form McGill Pain Questionnaire. *Pain, 30,* 191–197. doi:10.1016/0304-3959(87)91074-8

Mendoza, T.R., Wang, X.S., Cleeland, C.S., Morrissey, M., Johnson, B.A., Wendt, J.K., & Huber, S.L. (1999). The rapid assessment of fatigue severity in cancer patients: Use of the Brief Fatigue Inventory. *Cancer, 85,* 1186–1196. doi:10.1002/(SICI)1097-0142(19990301)85:5<1186::AID-CNCR24>3.0.CO;2-N

Mercadante, S. (2012). Cancer pain undertreatment and prognostic factors. *Pain, 153,* 1769–1771. doi:10.1016/j.pain.2012.03.032

Mercadante, S. (2014). Managing difficult pain conditions in the cancer patient. *Current Pain and Headache Reports, 18,* 395–402. doi:10.1007/s11916-013-0395-y

Merry, B., Edwards, R.R., Buenaver, L.F., McGuire, L., Haythornthwaite, J.A., Doleys, D.M., & Campbell, C.M. (2011). Ethnic group differences in the outcomes of multidisciplinary pain treatment. *Journal of Musculoskeletal Pain, 19,* 24–30. doi:10.3109/10582452.2010.538821

Mesgarpour, B., Griebler, U., Glechner, A., Kien, C., Strobelberger, M., Van Noord, M.G., & Michalek-Sauberer, A. (2014). Extended-release opioids in the management of cancer pain: A systematic review of efficacy and safety. *European Journal of Pain, 18,* 605–616. doi:10.1002/j.1532-2149.2013.00401.x

Miaskowski, C. (2010a). Cancer pain. In C.G. Brown (Ed.), *A guide to oncology symptom management* (pp. 369–403). Pittsburgh, PA: Oncology Nursing Society.

Miaskowski, C. (2010b). Outcome measures to evaluate the effectiveness of pain management in older adults with cancer. *Oncology Nursing Forum, 37*(Suppl. 5), 27–32. doi:10.1188/10.ONF.S1.27-32

Miaskowski, C., & Aouizerat, B. (2012). Biomarkers: Symptoms, survivorship and quality of life. *Seminars in Oncology Nursing, 28,* 129–138. doi:10.1016/j.soncn.2012.03.008

Minton, O., Berger, A., Barsevick, A., Cramp, F., Goedendorp, M., Mitchell, S., & Stone, P. (2013). Cancer-related fatigue and its impact on functioning. *Cancer, 119,* 2124–2130. doi:10.1002/cncr.28058

Minton, O., Richardson, A., Sharpe, M., Hotopf, M., & Stone, P.C. (2011). Psychostimulants for the management of cancer-related fatigue: A systematic review and meta-analysis. *Journal of Pain and Symptom Management, 41,* 761–767. doi:10.1016/j.jpainsymman.2010.06.020

Minton, O., & Stone, P. (2008). How common is fatigue in disease free breast cancer survivors? A systematic review of the literature. *Breast Cancer Research and Treatment, 112,* 5–13. doi:10.1007/s10549-007-9831-1

Mishra, S.I., Scherer, R.W., Snyder, C., Geigle, P.M., Berlanstein, D.R., & Topaloglu, O. (2012). Exercise interventions on health-related quality of life for people with cancer during active treatment. *Cochrane Database of Systematic Reviews, 2012*(8). doi:10.1002/14651858.CD008465.pub2

Mitchell, S. (2010). Cancer-related fatigue. In C.G. Brown (Ed.), *A guide to oncology symptom management* (pp. 271–297). Pittsburgh, PA: Oncology Nursing Society.

Mitchell, S. (2011). Cancer-related fatigue. In C.H. Yarbro, D. Wujcik, & B.H. Gobel (Eds.), *Cancer nursing: Principles and practice* (7th ed., pp. 772–791). Burlington, MA: Jones & Bartlett Learning.

Modesto-Lowe, V., Girard, L., & Chaplin, M. (2012). Cancer pain in the opioid-addicted patient: Can we treat it right? *Journal of Opioid Management, 8,* 167–175. doi:10.5055/jom.2012.0113

Monczewski, L. (2013). Managing bone metastasis in the patient with advanced cancer. *Orthopaedic Nursing, 32,* 209–214. doi:10.1097/NOR.0b013e31829a4da3

Moraska, A.R., Sood, A., Dakhil, S.R., Sloan, J.A., Barton, D., Atherton, P.J., … Loprinzi, C.L. (2010). Phase III, randomized, double-blind, placebo-controlled study of long-acting methylphenidate for cancer-related fatigue: North Central Cancer Treatment Group NCCTG-N05C7 trial. *Journal of Clinical Oncology, 28,* 3673–3679. doi:10.1200/JCO.2010.28.1444

Mortimer, J.E., Barsevick, A.M., Bennett, C.L., Berger, A.M., Cleeland, C., DeVader, S.R., … Rugo, H.S. (2010). Studying cancer-related fatigue: Report of the NCCN scientific research committee. *Journal of the National Comprehensive Cancer Network, 8,* 1331–1339.

Mulrooney, T. (2010). Cognitive impairment. In C.G. Brown (Ed.), *A guide to oncology symptom management* (pp. 123–137). Pittsburgh, PA: Oncology Nursing Society.

Mustian, K.M., Sprod, L.K., Janelsins, M., Peppone, L.J., & Mohile, S. (2012). Exercise recommendations for cancer-related fatigue, cognitive impairment, sleep problems, depression, pain, anxiety, and physical dysfunction: A review. *Oncology and Hematology Review, 8,* 81–88. Retrieved from http://www.ncbi.nlm.nih.gov/pmc/articles/PMC3647480

Myers, J.S. (2009). A comparison of the theory of unpleasant symptoms and the conceptual model of chemotherapy-related changes in cognitive function [Online exclusive]. *Oncology Nursing Forum, 36,* E1–E10. doi:10.1188/09.ONF.E1-E10

Myers, J.S. (2012). Chemotherapy-related cognitive impairment: The breast cancer experience [Online exclusive]. *Oncology Nursing Forum, 39*, E31–E40. doi:10.1188/12.ONF.E31-E40

Myers, J.S., Pierce, J., & Pazdernik, T. (2008). Neurotoxicology of chemotherapy in relation to cytokine release, the blood-brain barrier, and cognitive impairment. *Oncology Nursing Forum, 35*, 916–920. doi:10.1188/08.ONF.916-920

National Comprehensive Cancer Network. (2014). *NCCN Clinical Practice Guidelines in Oncology (NCCN Guidelines®): Distress management* [v.2.2014]. Retrieved from http://www.nccn.org/professionals/physician_gls/pdf/distress.pdf

National Comprehensive Cancer Network. (2015a). *NCCN Clinical Practice Guidelines in Oncology (NCCN Guidelines®): Adult cancer pain* [v.2.2015]. Retrieved from http://www.nccn.org/professionals/physician_gls/pdf/pain.pdf

National Comprehensive Cancer Network. (2015b). *NCCN Clinical Practice Guidelines in Oncology (NCCN Guidelines®): Cancer-related fatigue* [v.2.2015]. Retrieved from http://www.nccn.org/professionals/physician_gls/pdf/fatigue.pdf

Ndao, D.H., Ladas, E.J., Bao, Y., Cheng, B., Nees, S.N., Levine, J.M., & Kelly, K.M. (2013). Use of complementary and alternative medicine among children, adolescent, and young adult cancer survivors: A survey study. *Journal of Pediatric Hematology/Oncology, 35*, 281–288. doi:10.1097/MPH.0b013e318290c5d6

Neefjes, E., van der Vorst, M., Blauwhoff-Buskermolen, S., & Verheul, H. (2013). Aiming for a better understanding and management of cancer-related fatigue. *Oncologist, 18*, 1135–1143. doi:10.1634/theoncologist.2013-0076

Novartis Pharmaceuticals Corp. (2013a). Focalin: Highlights of prescribing information. Retrieved from http://www.pharma.us.novartis.com/product/pi/pdf/focalinXR.pdf

Novartis Pharmaceuticals Corp. (2013b). Ritalin: Highlights of prescribing information. Retrieved from http://www.pharma.us.novartis.com/product/pi/pdf/ritalin_ritalin-sr.pdf

O'Farrell, E., MacKenzie, J., & Collins, B. (2013). Clearing the air: A review of our current understanding of "chemo fog." *Current Oncology Reports, 15*, 260–269. doi:10.1007/s11912-013-0307-7

Oliver, J., Coggins, C., Compton, P., Hagan, S., Matteliano, D., Stanton, M., … Turner, H.N. (2012). American society for Pain Management Nursing position statement: Pain management in patients with substance use disorders. *Pain Management Nursing, 13*, 169–183. doi:10.1097/JAN.0b013e318271c123

Oncology Nursing Society. (2014). Cancer pain management [Position statement]. Retrieved from https://www.ons.org/advocacy-policy/positions/practice/pain-management

Piper, B.F., Dibble, S.L., Dodd, M.J., Weiss, M.C., Slaughter, R.E., & Paul, S.M. (1998). The revised Piper fatigue scale: Psychometric evaluation in women with breast cancer. *Oncology Nursing Forum, 25*, 677–684.

Poppelreuter, M., Weis, J., & Bartsch, H. (2009). Effects of specific neuropsychological training programs for breast cancer patients after adjuvant chemotherapy. *Journal of Psychosocial Oncology, 27*, 274–296. doi:10.1080/07347330902776044

Portenoy, R.K. (2011). Treatment of cancer pain. *Lancet, 377*, 2236–2242. doi:10.1016/S0140-6736(11)60236-5

Portenoy, R.K., & Hagen, N.A. (1990). Breakthrough pain: Definition, prevalence and characteristics. *Pain, 41*, 273–281. doi:10.1016/0304-3959(90)90004-W

Portenoy, R., Payne, D., & Jacobsen, P. (1999). Breakthrough pain: Characteristics and impact in patients with cancer pain. *Pain, 81*, 129–134. doi:10.1016/S0304-3959(99)00006-8

Quinten, C., Maringwa, J., Gotay, C., Martinelli, F., Coens, C., Reeve, B., … Bottomley, A. (2011). Patient self-reports of symptoms and clinician ratings as predictors of overall cancer survival. *Journal of the National Cancer Institute, 103*, 1851–1858. doi:10.1093/jnci/djr485

Reddy, A., Yennurajalingam, S., Pulivarthi, K., Palla, S.L., Wang, X., Kwon, J.H., … Bruera, E. (2013). Frequency, outcome, and predictors of success within 6 weeks of an opioid rotation among outpatients with cancer receiving strong opioids. *Oncologist, 18*, 212–220. doi:10.1634/theoncologist.2012-0269

Reeve, B.B., Stover, A.M., Alfano, C.M., Smith, A.W., Ballard-Barbash, R., Bernstein, L., … Piper, B.F. (2012). The Piper Fatigue Scale-12 (PFS-12). Psychometric findings and item reduction in a cohort of breast cancer survivors. *Breast Cancer Research and Treatment, 136*, 9–20. doi:10.1007/s10549-012-2212-4

Reynolds, J., Drew, D., & Dunwoody, C. (2013). American Society for Pain Management Nursing position statement: Pain management at the end of life. Retrieved from http://www.aspmn.org/documents/PainManagementattheEndofLife_August2013.pdf

Ripamonti, C.I., Santini, D., Maranzano, E., Berti, M., & Roila, F. (2012). Management of cancer pain: ESMO clinical practice guidelines. *Annals of Oncology, 23*(Suppl. 7), vii139–vii154. doi:10.1093/annonc/mds233

Running, A., & Seright, T. (2012). Integrative oncology: Managing cancer pain with complementary and alternative therapies. *Current Pain and Headache Reports, 16*, 325–331. doi:10.1007/s11916-012-0275-x

Running, A., & Turnbeaugh, E. (2011). Oncology pain and complementary therapy: A review of the literature. *Clinical Journal of Oncology Nursing, 15*, 374–379. doi:10.1188/11.CJON.374-379

Schagen, S.B., Boogerd, W., Muller, M.J., Huinink, W.T.B., Moonen, L., Meinhardt, W., & Van Dam, F.S. (2008). Cognitive complaints and cognitive impairment following BEP chemotherapy in patients with testicular cancer. *Acta Oncologica, 47*, 63–70. doi:10.1080/02841860701518058

Scherwath, A., Schirmer, L., Kruse, M., Ernst, G., Eder, M., Dinkel, A., … Mehnert, A. (2013). Cognitive functioning in allogeneic hematopoietic stem cell transplantation recipients and its medical correlates: A prospective multicenter study. *Psycho-Oncology, 22*, 1509–1516. doi:10.1002/pon.3159

Schreiber, K.L., Martel, M.O., Shnol, H., Shaffer, J.R., Greco, C., Viray, N., … Belfer, I. (2013). Persistent pain in postmastectomy patients: Comparison of psychophysical, medical, surgical, and psychosocial characteristics between patients with and without pain. *Pain, 154*, 660–668. doi:10.1016/j.pain.2012.11.015

Schwartz, A.L., Thompson, J.A., & Masood, N. (2002). Interferon induced fatigue with melanoma: A pilot study of exercise and methylphenidate [Online exclusive]. *Oncology Nursing Forum, 29*, E85–E90. doi:10.1188/02.ONF.E85-E90

Sepsas, E., Misthos, P., Anagnostopulu, M., Toparlaki, O., Voyagis, G., & Kakaris, S. (2013). The role of intercostal cryoanalgesia in post-thoracotomy analgesia. *Interactive Cardiovascular Thoracic Surgery, 16*, 814–818. doi:10.1093/icvts/ivs516

Shavers, V.L., Bakos, A., & Sheppard, V.B. (2010). Race, ethnicity, and pain among the U.S. adult population. *Journal of Health Care for the Poor and Underserved, 21*, 177–220. doi:10.1353/hpu.0.0255

Shaw, E.G., Rosdhal, R., D'Agostino, R.B., Jr., Lovato, J., Naughton, M.J., Robbins, M.E., & Rapp, S.R. (2006). Phase II study of donepezil in irradiated brain tumor patients: Effect on cognitive function, mood, and quality of life. *Journal of Clinical Oncology, 24*, 1415–1420. doi:10.1200/JCO.2005.03.3001

Silverman, D.H.S., Dy, C.J., Castellon, S.A., Lai, J., Pio, B.S., Abraham, L., … Ganz, P.A. (2007). Altered frontocortical, cerebellar, and basal ganglia activity in adjuvant-treated breast cancer survivors 5–10 years after chemotherapy. *Breast Cancer Research and Treatment, 103*, 303–311. doi:10.1007/s10549-006-9380-z

Smith, E.M.L., Pang, H., Cirrincione, C., Fleishman, S., Paskett, E.D., Ahles, T., … Shapiro, C.L. (2013). Effect of duloxetine on pain, function, and quality of life among patients with chemotherapy-induced painful peripheral neuropathy: A randomized clinical trial. *JAMA, 309*, 1359–1367. doi:10.1001/jama.2013.2813

Stone, P.C. (2013). Methylphenidate in the management of cancer-related fatigue. *Journal of Clinical Oncology, 31*, 2372–2373. doi:10.1200/JCO.2013.50.0181

Stone, P.C., & Minton, O. (2008). Cancer-related fatigue. *European Journal of Cancer, 44*, 1097–1104. doi:10.1016/j.ejca.2008.02.037

Storey, D.J., McLaren, D.B., Atkinson, M.A., Butcher, I., Frew, L.C., Smythe, J., & Sharpe, M. (2011). Clinically relevant fatigue in men with hormone-sensitive prostate cancer on long-term androgen deprivation therapy. *Annals of Oncology, 23*, 1542–1549. doi:10.1093/annonc/mdr447

Templeton, A.J., Thürlimann, B., Baumann, M., Mark, M., Stoll, S., Schwizer, M., … Ruhstaller, T. (2013). Cross-sectional study of self-reported physical activity, eating habits and use of complementary medicine in breast cancer survivors. *BMC Cancer, 13*, 153. doi:10.1186/1471-2407-13-153

Thorpy, M.J., & Roth, T. (2013). Toward a classification of medications for sleep and circadian rhythm disorders. *Nature and Science of Sleep, 5*, 143–145. doi:10.2147/NSS.S55679

Tittle, M., McMillan, S., & Hagan, S. (2003). Validating the brief pain inventory for use with surgical patients with cancer. *Oncology Nursing Forum, 30*, 325–330. doi:10.1188/03.ONF.325-330

Tracy, B., & Morrison, R.S. (2013). Pain management in older adults. *Clinical Therapeutics, 35*, 1659–1668. doi:10.1016/j.clinthera.2013.09.026

U.S. Drug Enforcement Administration. (2002). A joint statement from 21 health organizations and the Drug Enforcement Administration. Promoting pain relief and preventing abuse of pain medications: A critical balancing act. *Journal of Pain and Symptom Management, 24*, 147. doi:10.1016/S0885-3924(02)00472-4

Vallance, K., Liu, W., Mandrell, B.N., Panetta, J.C., Gattuso, J., Hockenberry, M., … Hinds, P. (2010). Mechanisms of dexamethasone-induced disturbed sleep and fatigue in paediatric patients receiving treatment for ALL. *European Journal of Cancer, 46*, 1848–1855. doi:10.1016/j.ejca.2010.03.026

Vallejo, R., Barkin, R., & Wang, V. (2011). Pharmacology of opioids in the treatment of chronic pain syndromes. *Pain Physician, 14*, E343–E360.

Vallerand, A.H., Musto, S., & Polomano, R.C. (2011). Nursing's role in cancer pain management. *Current Pain and Headache Reports, 15*, 250–262. doi:10.1007/s11916-011-0203-5

Vallerand, A., Pieper, B., Crawley, J., Nordstrom, C., & Dinardo, E. (2013). The prevalence of pain and its association with psychosocial factors for indigent adults enrolled in a primary care clinic. *Clinical Journal of Pain, 29*, 917–923. doi:10.1097/AJP.0b013e31827c7b30

van den Beuken-van Everdingen, M.H.J., de Rijke, J.M., Kessels, A.G., Schouten, H.C., van Kleef, M., & Patijn, J. (2007). Prevalence of pain in patients with cancer: A systematic review of the past 40 years. *Annals of Oncology, 18*, 1437–1449. doi:10.1093/annonc/mdm056 van Dongen, M., van Rossum, E., Kessels, A., Sielhorst, H., & Knipschild, P. (2003). Ginkgo for elderly people with dementia and age-associated memory impairment: A randomized clinical trial. *Journal of Clinical Epidemiology, 56*, 367–376. doi:10.1016/S0895-4356(03)00003-9

Vearncombe, K.J., Rolfe, M., Wright, M., Pachana, N.A., Andrew, B., & Beadle, G. (2009). Predictors of cognitive decline after chemotherapy in breast cancer patients. *Journal of the International Neuropsychological Society, 15*, 951–962. doi:10.1017/S1355617709990567

Verstappen, C.C., Heimans, J.J., Hoekman, K., & Postma, T.J. (2003). Neurotoxic complications of chemotherapy in patients with cancer: Clinical signs and optimal management. *Drugs, 63*, 1549–1563. doi:10.2165/00003495 -200363150-00003

Von Ah, D., Jansen, C., Allen, D.H., Schiavone, R.M., & Wulff, J. (2011). Putting evidence into practice: Evidence-based interventions for cancer and cancer treatment-related cognitive impairment. *Clinical Journal of Oncology Nursing, 15*, 607–615. doi:10.1188/11.CJON.607-615

Walker, S. (2010). Pain. In J. Eggert (Ed.), *Cancer basics* (pp. 485–510). Pittsburgh, PA: Oncology Nursing Society.

Wefel, J.S., Kesler, S.R., Noll, K.R., & Schagen, S.B. (2015). Clinical characteristics, pathophysiology, and management of noncentral nervous system cancer-related cognitive impairment in adults. *CA: A Cancer Journal for Clinicians, 65*, 123–138. doi:10.3322/caac.21258

Wefel, J.S., Lenzi, R., Theriault, R., Buzdar, A.U., Cruickshank, S., & Meyers, C.A. (2004). 'Chemobrain' in breast carcinoma? A prologue. *Cancer, 101*, 466–475. doi:10.1002/cncr.20393

Wefel, J.S., & Schagen, S.B. (2012). Chemotherapy-related cognitive dysfunction. *Current Neurology and Neuroscience Reports, 12*, 267–275. doi:10.1007/s11910-012-0264-9

Wefel, J.S., Vardy, J., Ahles, T., & Schagen, S.B. (2011). International Cognition and Cancer Task Force recommendations to harmonise studies of cognitive function in patients with cancer. *Lancet Oncology, 12*, 703–708. doi:10.1016/ S1470-2045(10)70294-1

Weis, J. (2011). Cancer-related fatigue: Prevalence, assessment and treatment strategies. *Expert Review of Pharmacoeconomics and Outcomes Research, 11*, 441–446. doi:10.1586/erp.11.44

Wengström, Y., Rundström, C., Geerling, J., Pappa, T., Weisse, I., Williams, S.C., … Rustøen, T. (2014). The management of breakthrough cancer pain—educational needs a European nursing survey. *European Journal of Cancer Care, 23*, 121–128. doi:10.1111/ecc.12118

Wong, D.L., & Baker, C.M. (1988). Pain in children: Comparison of assessment scales. *Pediatric Nursing, 14*, 9–17.

World Health Organization. (1996). *Cancer pain relief with a guide to opioid availability* (2nd ed.). Albany, NY: Author.

Wu, L., Diefenbach, M., Gordon, W., Cantor, J., & Cherrier, M. (2012). Cognitive problems in patients on androgen deprivation therapy: A qualitative pilot study. *Urologic Oncology, 31*, 1533–1538. doi:10.1016/j.urolonc.2012.07.003

Yellen, S.B., Cella, D.F., Webster, K.A., Blendowski, C., & Kaplan, E. (1997). Measuring fatigue and other anemia-related symptoms with the Functional Assessment of Cancer Therapy (FACT) measurement system. *Journal of Pain and Symptom Management, 13*, 63–74. doi:10.1016/S0885-3924(96)00274-6

Yennurajalingam, S., Frisbee-Hume, S., Palmer, J.L., Delgado-Guay, M.O., Bull, J., Phan, A.T., … Bruera, E. (2013). Reduction of cancer-related fatigue with dexamethasone: A double-blind, randomized, placebo-controlled trial in patients with advanced cancer. *Journal of Clinical Oncology, 31*, 3076–3082. doi:10.1200/JCO.2012.44.4661

Yennurajalingam, S., Palmer, J.L., Zhang, T., Poulter, V., & Bruera, E. (2008). Association between fatigue and other cancer-related symptoms in patients with advanced cancer. *Supportive Care in Cancer, 16*, 1125–1130. doi:10.1007/ s00520-008-0466-5

CHAPTER 11

Myelosuppression and Second Malignancies

Brenda K. Shelton, DNP, RN, APRN-CNS, CCRN, AOCN®

Introduction

Bone marrow suppression is defined as a reduction in the production and maturation of all blood cell lines, resulting in leukopenia, thrombocytopenia, and anemia in peripheral blood (Camp-Sorrell, 2011). It is one of the most common and potentially life-threatening clinical complications experienced by patients with cancer (Irwin, Erb, Williams, Wilson, & Zitella, 2013; Watts, 2009). It often has been coined "the silent complication" because of the absence of clinical findings with initial cell depletion until the lack of hematopoietic cells results in clinical disorders, such as infection and bleeding. *Myelosuppression* is a term used interchangeably with *aplasia* (without cells), although it may loosely correlate to suppression of only the myelocytic cell line when used in direct care practice. The depth of aplasia (also termed *nadir*) is associated with its severity score (usually grades 0–4) and the length of time the blood counts remain suppressed (Shelton, 2011).

Oncology advanced practice nurses (APNs) possess expert knowledge of the risk factors, timing, clinical features, assessment scales, prevention strategies, and multidisciplinary management of myelosuppression. Within this text, general concepts of bone marrow suppression are addressed first, followed by specific findings and management associated with suppression of each cell line, and then general principles of patient management for all disorders as a group.

Bone Marrow Suppression

Etiology

More than 50% of patients with cancer will experience bone marrow suppression during the course of their disease (Bow, 2013; Erb & Vogel, 2013; National Comprehensive Cancer Network® [NCCN®], 2014a, 2014b). Bone marrow suppression often is the result of (a) systemic cancer, (b) cancer treatment, (c) comorbid health conditions, or (d) a combination of these factors. Nutraceuticals and herbal agents (e.g., winter cherry, kava kava, St. John's wort, evening primrose, ivy leaf) also may contribute to myelosuppression and even interfere with the therapeutic effects of antineoplastic chemotherapy or radiation therapy (Chiu, Yau, & Epstein, 2009; Memorial Sloan Kettering Cancer Center, n.d.; National Center for Complementary and Integrative Health, n.d.).

Specific health factors are documented to enhance the risk for significant bone marrow suppression when concomitant with cancer or its therapy. These risks include advanced age (older than 65 years); poor nutritional status; preexisting autoimmune disease, diabetes mellitus, gastrointestinal disorders, liver disease, or hematopoietic diseases; and substance abuse (NCCN, 2014c; Shelton, 2013). The contribution of myelosuppression to increased morbidity and reduced quality of life is well defined in the literature (Ahn & Lee, 2012; Shitara et al., 2011). Because of this, knowledge and skills regarding management of myelosuppression are essential for oncology APNs.

Cancer-Induced Bone Marrow Suppression

Cancer-induced bone marrow suppression occurs from three major mechanisms: (a) dysfunctional hematopoietic cells within the bone marrow, (b) bone marrow infiltration with tumor, and (c) general exhaustion of bone marrow reserves (Schrijvers, 2011; Whichard, Sarkar, Kimmel, & Corey, 2010). Hematologic malignancies, such as leukemias and multiple myeloma, involve a defect of a specific blood cell type. The cancer manifests as overproduction of immature or poorly functioning cells in a specific cell line, resulting in overcrowding of the marrow compartment with suppression of other cell production. Lymphomas often present as extramedullary disease but can infiltrate the bone marrow, leading to decreased function of the cell lines. Solid tumor malignancies with the highest propensity to infiltrate the bone marrow in the course of metastasis include melanoma and cancers of the breast, lung, kidney, and prostate (NCCN, 2014c; Whichard et al., 2010). Nonspecific cancer-induced myelosuppression can occur with prolonged chronic illness, malnutrition, chronic infection, liver metastases, or gastrointestinal involvement (NCCN, 2014b).

Chemotherapy-Induced Bone Marrow Suppression

As the most rapidly dividing cells of the body, the bone marrow is most frequently and consistently affected by cancer chemotherapy agents. Each antineoplastic agent has predictable specific cell-line–suppressing effects, timing of its effects, and severity of suppression. The degree of bone marrow suppression is a guide for selection of an agent or combination of agents to use in a treatment plan, the dosage to be delivered, and the frequency of administration. A few chemotherapy agents (most notably the nitrosoureas) affect the pluripotent stem cells, thereby affecting all cell lines. A summary of common antineoplastic agents and their typical myelosuppressive properties is presented in Table 11-1. Oncology APNs need to consider this information when prescribing chemotherapy regimens, performing patient monitoring, ascertaining the need for hematopoietic growth factors, and providing staff nurse consultation for management of myelosuppression.

Cell cycle–nonspecific agents, such as nitrosoureas, have the most potent and longest effect on myelosuppression. Agents such as anthracyclines and alkylating agents are cell cycle active, phase nonspecific, and result in moderate myelosuppression. Phase-specific agents, such as antimetabolites and vinca alkaloids, have the shortest degree of suppression. The only chemotherapy agents that are completely nontoxic to the bone marrow are steroidal hormones (Georgiou, Foster, & Xian, 2010; Polovich, Olsen, & LeFebvre, 2014).

Table 11-1. Common Myelosuppressive Chemotherapy Agents

Drug Class	Degree of Myelosuppression	Nadir (Days)	Duration of Myelosuppression (Days)
Alkylating agents (e.g., cyclophosphamide, melphalan)	Moderate	10–21	18–40
Anthracyclines (e.g., doxorubicin)	Severe	6–13	21–24
Antifolates (e.g., methotrexate)	Severe	7–14	14–21
Antipurines (e.g., fludarabine)	Moderate	7–14	14–21
Antipyrimidines (e.g., 5-fluoropyrimidine/ 5-fluorouracil)	Severe	7–14	21–24
Antitumor antibiotics (nonanthracycline) (e.g., bleomycin)	Moderate	10–21	17–28
Camptothecins (e.g., topotecan)	Moderate	4–7	6–12
Epipodophyllotoxins (e.g., etoposide)	Moderate	5–15	22–28
Nitrosoureas (e.g., carmustine)	Severe	26–60	35–85
Plant alkaloids (e.g., vincristine)	Mild–moderate	4–9	7–21
Proteasome inhibitors (e.g., bortezomib)	Mild–moderate	Unknown	Unknown
Taxanes (e.g., paclitaxel)	Moderate	8–12	15–21
Tyrosine kinase inhibitors (e.g., imatinib)	Neutropenia only	Unknown	Unknown
Agents with unique myelosuppressive features (timing, depth of aplasia)			
Alemtuzumab	Moderate–severe	Unknown	Unknown
Arsenic trioxide	Mild–moderate	Unknown	Unknown
Asparaginase	Moderate	10–20	10–20
Bendamustine	Severe	14–20	21–35
Brentuximab	Moderate	14	21
Busulfan	Severe	11–30	24–54
Carboplatin	Severe	16	21–25
Dacarbazine	Severe	21–28	28–35
Denileukin diftitox	Severe	4–15	Unknown
Hydroxyurea	Moderate	7	14–21
Mithramycin	Mild	5–10	10–18
Mitomycin	Moderate	28–42	42–56
Nitrogen mustard	Severe	7–14	28
Procarbazine	Moderate	25–36	35–50
Rituximab	Moderate	77–204	Length of therapy
Temozolomide	Moderate	21–28	28–50
Tositumomab + iodine	Moderate	8–15	Length of therapy
Yttrium-90 ibritumomab tiuxetan	Moderate	8–20	Length of therapy

Note. Based on information from Barber et al., 2011; Camp-Sorrell, 2011; Chan et al., 2012; Chang & Kahl, 2012; Dixit et al., 2012; Dunleavy et al., 2010; Georgiou et al., 2010; Gualberto, 2012; Hincks et al., 2011; Kalaycio, 2009; Kim et al., 2011; Koukourakis et al., 2009; National Comprehensive Cancer Network, 2014a, 2014b; Polovich et al., 2014; Shane & Shelton, 2004; Tesfa & Palmblad, 2011.

The normal proliferation rate of erythrocytes, platelets, and leukocytes determines the severity and timing of suppression following exposure to a toxin. Granulocytes typically live only 6–8 hours; platelets survive an average of 5–7 days; and erythrocytes live approximately 120 days. Depletion of the cell line is directly related to the normal turnover rate of the cell line after the antineoplastic agent destroys normal regrowth mechanisms. Leukopenia usually is the earliest indicator of bone marrow suppression, occurring about 7–15 days after treatment, but is the quickest to recover in most circumstances. When affected, platelets have the longest nadir, persisting for more than 20 days in many patients (Polovich et al., 2014; Shelton, 2013). Because of their long life span, red cells only present serious problems in patients receiving highly suppressing erythrocytic agents, such as anthracyclines or platinols, unless a bleeding problem also exists (Polovich et al., 2014). The onset of anemia often is delayed, occurring in the second or third cycle of therapy. Response to stimulating therapies may require four to eight weeks (Hinkel, Li, & Sherman, 2010; NCCN, 2014a).

Radiation-Induced Bone Marrow Suppression

Radiation therapy less frequently causes bone marrow suppression. However, myelosuppression occurs following radiation therapy when the treatment field involves marrow-producing tissue or with doses greater than 15 Gy (American Cancer Society, 2012; Kulkarni, Ghosh, Hauer-Jensen, & Kumar, 2010). Myelosuppression peaks in the third week of radiation therapy and often manifests as aplasia occurring simultaneously in all cell lines rather than sequentially as seen with chemotherapy. The recovery period is less predictable because radiation treatments may be required for several additional weeks after the onset of marrow suppression (Kulkarni et al., 2010). Marrow suppression usually is considered to be a dose-limiting toxicity of therapy and warrants a break from radiation until blood counts recover. Use of traditional preventive and supportive measures, such as hematopoietic growth factors, has not been well defined for use in radiation-induced myelosuppression.

Pathophysiology of Hematopoiesis

Hematopoiesis usually is confined to the proximal ends of long or flat bones of the body where the red bone marrow is found. These areas include the sternum, vertebrae, ribs, ileum, and skull. Extramedullary hematopoiesis is characterized by cell production that is re-expanded back into the long bones, spleen, or liver. This occurs with chronic hematopoietic disorders and hematologic malignancies. Adults have one to two liters of bone marrow, consisting primarily of reticular tissues and hemopoietic progenitor cells. The reticular tissue and hemocytoblasts form a framework of sinusoids, which feed into the marrow drainage system and venous system of the body. The reticular tissue provides support and nutrition for developing blood cells and secretes several colony-stimulating factors. The hemocytoblast, or colony-forming unit, is the pluripotent stem cell. Pluripotent stem cells express the CD34+ surface protein or antigen that has receptors for stem cell growth factors promoting proliferation (Whichard et al., 2010). Once "committed," the hemocytoblast becomes a progenitor cell for a specific hemopoietic cell line. These cell lines are erythroid (red cells), granulocytic (phagocytic white blood cells [WBCs]), monocytic (macrophage) cells, lymphoid (specific immunity white cells), and megakaryocytic (platelets). Commitment, or differentiation and maturation, occurs as a result of the acquisition or loss of specific growth factor receptors and the action of cytokines (Guberski, 2013; Haase, 2010; Whichard et al., 2010).

Hematopoietic growth factors are glycoprotein hormones that regulate the proliferation, differentiation, maturation, and activation of progenitor and mature blood cells to optimally meet the body's hematopoietic needs. Each growth factor has a specific receptor, and the receptor's presence on the cell surface varies with cell lineage and stage of differentiation. Existing identified hematopoietic growth factors include interleukins (ILs) 1, 3, 5, and 6, granulocyte macrophage–colony-stimulating factor, granulocyte–colony-stimulating factor, macrophage–colony-stimulating factor, stem cell factor, thrombopoietin, and erythropoietin (Held & Gundert-Remy, 2010). Normally, mature blood cells, except for platelets, enter the bloodstream by migrating through the epithelial lining of the sinusoids. Platelets are directly launched into the bloodstream via their maturation site in the sinusoid wall (Nayak, Rai, & Gupta, 2012).

Assessment

Patients with bone marrow suppression are likely to present with an array of symptoms related to the specific hematopoietic cell line or lines affected. These cell-specific findings are addressed under the headings of leukopenia, thrombocytopenia, and anemia. Patients with myelosuppression often reveal nonspecific symptoms that are present and noticeable even before low blood counts are noted. General constitutional symptoms reported by patients with myelosuppression include anorexia, fatigue, myalgias, and cognitive dysfunction (Camp-Sorrell, 2011; Erb & Vogel, 2013; Shelton, 2012). Because these symptoms are vague and nonspecific, they may not be immediately seen as indicative of myelosuppression unless astute clinicians recognize the timing associated with the predicted nadir.

Focused physical examination for evidence of infection and bleeding is performed routinely in patients at risk for myelosuppression. Anemia does not usually produce unique symptoms. Fever is the most common symptom of infection. Common inflammatory symptoms, such as swelling and purulent exudate, may not be present with neutropenia (Shelton, 2013; Watts, 2009). Localized pain, open and nonhealing wounds, and organ dysfunction, such as hypoxia, are more common manifestations of infections in myelosuppressed patients. Skin, mucous membrane, and soft tissue bleeding usually is present with significant thrombocytopenia (Bow, 2013; Shelton, 2012, 2013; Thienelt & Calverley, 2009). Petechiae and ecchymoses of soft tissues, mucosal bleeding, or occult blood in emesis, urine, or stool warrants assessment of the platelet count (Shelton, 2012). Anemia is most likely to present as fatigue or weakness, but cardiovascular compromise may occur (NCCN, 2014a).

Suspected myelosuppression is always first confirmed with a laboratory test, the complete blood count (CBC) (Shelton, 2012, 2013; Wahed & Dasgupta, 2015). Components of the CBC include the hematocrit, hemoglobin, total red blood cell (RBC) and WBC counts, RBC indices, WBC differential, platelet count, and blood cell morphologies. These components are addressed in the specific lineage disorders in the following sections. The National Cancer Institute (NCI) Common Terminology Criteria for Adverse Events (CTCAE) (NCI Cancer Therapy Evaluation Program [CTEP], 2010) can be used to grade toxicity for these hematologic parameters (see http://evs.nci.nih.gov/ftp1/CTCAE/About.html). An abnormal CBC may necessitate further diagnostic tests. When all cells are diminished, results are inconclusive for a specific disorder, thus necessitating a search for the etiology. If an error in cell production is suspected, a bone marrow aspiration and biopsy will be performed (Goroll & Mulley, 2009; Shelton, 2012). In many settings, oncology APNs perform this diagnostic test. If abnormal destruction is likely, cell survival studies (e.g., RBC survival studies performed with nuclear-tagged RBCs infused and followed by body scans) and hemolysis studies (e.g., direct bilirubin, schistocytes by smear) are indicated (Erb & Vogel, 2013).

Leukopenia

Definition and Etiology

Leukopenia is a reduced number of circulating leukocytes (WBCs) (Bow, 2013; Nayak et al., 2012). The two major types of WBCs are granulocytes and agranulocytes. Granulocytes include neutrophils, eosinophils, and basophils. Agranulocytes include lymphocytes and monocytes. The functions of these cells vary, and the specific cell deficiency may predict the nature of the immune defect and potential infectious complications (Wahed & Dasgupta, 2015). For example, neutrophils are the primary phagocytic responder and the only leukocyte that can be released in an immature form (band). As such, granulocytes (especially the neutrophil) are responsible for the body's response against bacterial invaders. Monocytes spend little time in the circulating serum before they differentiate into tissue macrophages, and hence, serum deficiencies are not well defined in clinical practice. Lymphocytes respond to specific immune threats and are important for recognition of foreign proteins, such as transplanted tissue or atypical antigens (e.g., viruses). APNs identify which cells are deficient or dysfunctional and translate this knowledge to predict and possibly prevent specific infectious complications. Table 11-2 demonstrates specific types of leukopenia and immune cell defects with expected infectious complications.

Neutropenia is a decrease in the number of circulating neutrophils. Disagreement exists as to what level of deficiency constitutes definitive neutropenia, but it may be best viewed as a continuum of severity based on the depth of the deficiency (Bow, 2013; Wahed & Dasgupta, 2015; White & Ybarra, 2014). The condition becomes definable when the absolute neutrophil count (ANC) is less than $1,500/mm^3$ (NCI CTEP, 2010). An ANC less than $1,000/mm^3$ is the threshold for moderate severity with increased risk for infection and commonly is used as a marker of the breakpoint for chemotherapy-induced neutropenia (Flowers et al., 2013; NCCN, 2014b). Neutropenia warranting infection prevention precautions or implementation of preventive bone marrow growth factors occurs when the ANC is less than $500/mm^3$ (NCI CTEP, 2010; NCCN, 2014b), or when the count is less than $1,000/mm^3$ and anticipated to reduce below $500/mm^3$ within the next 48 hours (Scialdone, 2012; White & Ybarra, 2014). Neutropenia occurs in diseases involving bone marrow production, as a result of excess destruction by autoimmune mechanisms, with certain marrow-toxic treatments, or with increased consumption during chronic illness. A diminished number of neutrophils alters the body's defenses against bacterial invaders. Disorders such as diabetes mellitus impair neutrophil function without necessarily reducing circulating numbers, causing similar clinical effects (Shelton, 2012).

Lymphocytopenia is a reduction in the number of lymphocytes in the blood. The suppression of T-lymphocyte function results in reduced ability to recognize foreign tissue, malignant cells, atypical microbes, and viruses (Wahed & Dasgupta, 2015). Lymphocytopenia is seen most commonly in AIDS and organ transplant immunosuppression. The CD4 molecular surface antigen is the target for HIV retroviral incorporation that leads to cell destruction of all cells with this marker. This marker is found on T4 lymphocytes and some macrophages. Cell destruction most often is detected by the absolute number of helper T4 lymphocytes (also called T4 count or absolute lymphocyte count). AIDS is classified by the CD4 count and the presence of other defining clinical syndromes, such as opportunistic infections, immunologic cancers, and neurologic disease (Relf, Shelton, & Jones, 2013). Other etiologies of lymphocytopenia include therapeutic suppression to reduce rejection of a transplanted organ, chronic use of corticosteroids, recent history

Table 11-2. Specific White Blood Cell Defects and Common Infectious Complications

Defect	High-Risk Patient Conditions	Common Infectious Complications
Granulocytopenia	Chronic infection/inflammation Diabetes mellitus Malnutrition Post chemotherapy Medications (allopurinol, chloramphenicol, flucytosine, trimethoprim-sulfamethoxazole, antiretrovirals, antineoplastic agents)	Bacterial infections for 3–7 days and throughout period of neutropenia Atypical bacterial infections after 7–10 days Fungal infections after 10–14 days Risk rises exponentially after 10 days; by day 21, almost all are infected.
Lymphopenia	Blood transfusions HIV disease IV drug use Medications (allopurinol, anesthetic agents, antipsychotic agents [clozapine], beta-lactam antibiotics, carbamazepine, chlorpromazine, corticosteroids, ganciclovir, immunosuppressive agents, propylthiouracil, ticlopidine, trimethoprim-sulfamethoxazole) Viral infection	Atypical and opportunistic infections Reactivation of dormant colonizations (e.g., *Pneumocystis jiroveci*, herpes simplex) Fungal infections
Immunoglobulin deficiency	Chronic illness Immunosuppressive therapy Severe malnutrition Recent transplant (solid organ or hematopoietic stem cell)	Sinus and pulmonary infections from a variety of sources
Asplena (from splenectomy)	Spleen removed	Infections with encapsulated organisms normally cleared by the spleen (e.g., pneumococcus, streptococcus)

Note. Based on information from Centers for Disease Control and Prevention, 2011; Dale & Welte, 2011; Friese, 2007; Irwin et al., 2013; National Comprehensive Cancer Network, 2014c; Nayak et al., 2012; Shelton, 2011, 2013; Wahed & Dasgupta, 2015.

of viral infection, or an unexplained phenomenon that occurs with IV drug use or malnutrition (Wahed & Dasgupta, 2015). Lymphocyte dysfunction has been associated with genetic abnormalities (e.g., congenital T-lymphocyte suppression, combined immunodeficiency syndrome) and Hodgkin lymphoma (Watts, 2009).

Assessment

Clinical assessment for neutropenia without concomitant infection may prove daunting because of the absence of specific symptoms. For this reason, researchers attempt to identify specific variables that predict the risk for neutropenia-related infection, better known as *neutropenic fever*. If clinicians can predict which patients are at high or low risk for severe infection with neutropenia, then they can implement proactive measures to minimize neutropenia and prevent infection. Alternatively, patients with low risk for serious infection during neutropenia may have febrile episodes managed by less resource-intensive care (Flowers et al., 2013; Teuffel, Ethier, Alibhai, Beyene, & Sung, 2011; Teuffel & Sung, 2012). Figure 11-1 outlines variables known to increase the risk of a neutropenic event leading to serious infection and sepsis. Specific disease-related variables for higher risk of infection also have been identified in therapy for breast cancer and lymphoma, where neutropenic infections causing decreased dose density (delays in therapy cycles or reductions in chemotherapy dose) can affect long-term remission rates and survival outcomes (Lyman, 2009; Yang, Savin, & Green, 2012). These are defined within Figure 11-1 (Blay et al., 1998; Blot et al., 2001; Hayes, 2001; Intragumtornchai, Sutheesophon, Sutcharitchan, & Swasdikul, 2000; Lyman, Lyman, & Agboola, 2005; NCCN, 2014c; Silber et al., 1998).

General—Patient Factors
- Age > 65 years
- Poor performance status
- Poor nutritional status
- History of severe neutropenia with similar treatment regimen
- Extensive previous chemotherapy
- Previous radiation therapy to marrow-containing bone
- Open wounds
- Active tissue infection
- Advanced or uncontrolled cancer
- Body surface area < 2/m²

General—Diagnostic Test Findings
- Preexisting neutropenia or lymphocytopenia
- Low albumin level
- Elevated lactate dehydrogenase (LDH) or serum albumin level < 3.5 mg/dl
- Elevated alkaline phosphatase
- Hyperglycemia
- Elevated bilirubin
- Low pretreatment neutrophil or lymphocyte count
- Bone marrow involvement with tumor

Early-Stage Breast Cancer
- Myelosuppression present after first cycle of therapy
- Doxorubicin and taxane combination
- Concurrent radiation therapy
- Preexisting bone marrow involvement

Non-Hodgkin Lymphoma
- Albumin < 3.5 mg/dl
- Bone marrow involvement
- Elevated LDH
- Advanced age (> 65 years)
OR
- International Prognostic Index > 2. Count one point for each variable present:
  - Advanced age (> 65 years)
  - Poor performance status (Karnofsky scale score < 50%)
  - LDH elevated > 300
  - Extranodal sites of disease (any = 1)
  - Stage of disease > II

Figure 11-1. Factors Influencing Risk of Serious Infection With Neutropenia

---

Note. Based on information from Blay et al., 1998; Blot et al., 2001; Intragumtornchai et al., 2000; Lyman, 2009; Lyman et al., 2005; Madsen et al., 2002; National Comprehensive Cancer Network, 2014c; Shelton, 2011; Silber et al., 1998; White & Ybarra, 2014.

Fever is the cardinal symptom of infection, although the degree of immunosuppression also may blunt the patient's ability to mount a fever response (White & Ybarra, 2014). NCCN defines fever as a single oral temperature (or equivalent) of 38.3°C (101°F) or 38°C (100.4°F) or higher over one hour (NCCN, 2014c). Subnormal body temperature also may be a significant indicator of leukopenia-related infection; however, the specific clinical implications are not well described (Shelton, 2011). It is proposed that subnormal body temperature is reflective of more severe sepsis or the presence of gram-negative organisms, but these speculations are not yet supported by research findings (NCCN, 2014c). Temperature assessment in neutropenic patients should take place at least four times per day and with any onset of symptoms of infection.

Inflammatory symptoms, such as erythema-enhanced capillary permeability, swelling, or pus formation, may not always be present in patients with leukopenia because of the absence of WBCs to produce inflammation. Fatigue is common even without infectious complications. Leukopenia beyond seven days is thought to significantly increase the risk of infection, and virtually all who are leukopenic beyond 21 days become infected (NCCN, 2014c). As a result of many antimicrobial and growth factor advances, mortality from neutropenia-induced infections has decreased from 21% to 7% in the past two decades (NCCN, 2014c).

When WBC responses are adequate, inflammatory symptoms can occur within the affected organ or body part. Organ-specific signs and symptoms of infection may be predicted by considering the clinical effects of introducing fluid extravasation and large numbers of WBCs into that organ or body space (Shane & Shelton, 2004). Possible organ-specific inflammatory symptoms include the presence of WBCs, causing increased intracranial pressure or nuchal rigidity, cloudy urine, purulent sputum or hypoxia, wound drainage or dehiscence, and development of effusions. Recognition of these symptoms, even with a single fever, may provide a targeted and focused intervention. Oncology APNs must ensure that patients, family, and staff understand the importance of assessing every open orifice, uncovering wounds to evaluate drainage, and looking for any abnormal organ function.

Diagnostic Testing

Serum tests are the primary diagnostic method used to detect leukopenia. The total WBC count and differential determines whether the number of WBCs is adequate to combat infection and mount inflammatory responses to injury. A low WBC count signals the probability of reduced neutrophil efficacy. Normally, the total WBC count is 5,000–10,000/mm^3, composed mostly of neutrophils, although the percentage of each cell line may assist in defining the specific immune deficit and predicting the type of infection the patient is most likely to develop. The ANC is indicative of the number of neutrophils available to combat infection. It is calculated by using the WBC differential with the formula in Figure 11-2. The frequency of ANC monitoring will vary depending on the individual patient. Oncology APNs have the expertise to consider the therapeutic regimen and patient-based variables to identify a plan for monitoring the complete WBC and differential based on expected values and planned interventions.

The CD4 count reflects the absolute number of CD4 molecule–containing cells, which primarily are helper T-lymphocyte cells but also include monocytes (Relf et al., 2013). CD4 counts lower than 500/mm^3 are considered a significant risk factor for opportunistic infection. CD4 counts are used for diagnosis, treatment planning, and evaluation of therapeutic response to treatment for AIDS. However, monitoring these numbers, despite abnormal values, has not proved to be helpful in the management of patients on corticosteroids or receiving organ transplant rejection inhibitors (NCCN, 2014c). Recent studies of lymphopenia with reduced CD4+ counts in patients with brain tumors and receiving concomitant temozolomide

---

Total number of white blood cells × % neutrophils = absolute neutrophil count

Example: 3,800 × 0.52 = 1,976 cells/mm^3

Calculation of the absolute neutrophil count provides the clinician with valuable information on the severity of leukopenia. The total number of white blood cells is multiplied by the percentage of neutrophils detected. This provides an absolute neutrophil count that can be applied to the toxicity scale.

Figure 11-2. Calculation of the Absolute Neutrophil Count

---

and radiation suggest that certain patients receiving combination chemotherapy and radiation may exhibit more pronounced lymphopenia and infection risk (Grossman et al., 2011).

In patients with leukopenia without a clear etiology, hematologic malignancies or marrow infiltration by other cancers is suspected. A bone marrow aspiration with or without bone marrow biopsy may reveal specific pathogenic disorders, such as myelofibrosis, myelodysplasia, leukemia, or aplastic anemia. The bone marrow aspirate is obtained from the posterior iliac crest or sternum. Most patients require pain medication or sedation to tolerate the discomfort of this procedure (Shelton, 2012). Normal bone marrow is easily aspirated without being extremely painful, but for most patients with hematologic disorders with a lack of bone marrow cells, the pain associated with attempts to aspirate from a dry marrow is difficult to tolerate. The pain associated with a dry aspirate is thought to be related to the degree of suction imposed in an attempt to obtain a specimen. Once 30–150 ml of red bone marrow is aspirated, it is smeared on pathology slides and sent to specialty hematology laboratories for genetic testing, flow cytometry, and cytopathology. Results usually are available in two to three days and may direct the plan of care. The bone marrow aspirate site is covered with a sterile dressing, and pain medication may be administered for a few days. If the patient has thrombocytopenia or bleeding, this site may require additional pressure, ice, or topical hemostatics.

Infection that is potentially severe, sepsis, and septic shock are possible complications of leukopenia and require assessment. Chapter 15 discusses sepsis and septic shock in greater detail.

Prevention and Management

Leukopenia is best treated by reversing the underlying cause. Most cancer-related leukopenia is an anticipated and unavoidable effect of cancer therapy and therefore not preventable. APNs review patients' medication profile and discuss any medications or alternative therapies that might enhance or prolong bone marrow suppression of WBCs. In some circumstances, other therapies with fewer marrow-suppressing effects may be available. Common offending prescriptive agents include allopurinol, antipsychotic agents (clozapine), beta-lactam antibiotics, carbamazepine, chlorpromazine, ganciclovir, phenytoin, propylthiouracil, ticlopidine, trimethoprim-sulfamethoxazole, and valproic acid (Schwartzberg, 2006; White & Ybarra, 2014). Vitamin E and echinacea are complementary and alternative therapies implicated in the development or worsening of leukopenia (de Lemos, John, Nakashima, O'Brien, & Taylor, 2004).

The best strategy for overall management of cancer- or treatment-induced leukopenia is prevention of infection. Patients who are at risk or who are predicted to develop any level of leukopenia are taught methods of preventing infection and how to recognize the early symptoms to ensure prompt, aggressive management of any infection that may occur. Common infection prevention practices are described in Table 11-3. Because many interventions are based on scientific principles of infectious disease but do not have a high level of scientific evi-

Table 11-3. Infection Prevention Strategies

Objective	Strategy	Evidence Base
Avoid exposure to infection risks.	Avoid exposures (e.g., avoiding crowds, limiting contact with small children or pets, screening visitors).	High
	Bathe and change linens daily; perform oral care 3–4 times daily and perineal care twice daily.	High
	Wear a high-particulate filter mask for exposure to construction.	High
	Avoid close contact with fresh flowers in standing water or soil. Avoid gardening unless wearing gloves and high-particulate filter mask.	High
	Cook or clean foods thoroughly before consumption. Store freshly made (preservative-free) foods no longer than 2–3 days under refrigeration. Avoid purchased foods with possible contamination (e.g., seafood, eggs, mayonnaise) unless circumstances of preparation are known.	High (except neutropenic diet)
	Change IV tubing daily if blood or parenteral nutrition is infused via that line. Avoid use of stopcocks in IV lines.	High
	Prescribe prophylactic and therapeutic antimicrobial agents. Assess variables influencing absorption or blood levels. Perform peak or trough levels as ordered.	High
	Use high-efficiency particulate air–filtered/negative-pressure rooms to reduce risk of acquiring airborne fungal pathogens.	High
	Keep windows closed.	Moderate
	If moderate to high risk of respiratory infection transmission is possible, wear masks, changing every 30 minutes during contacts.	Moderate
	Control blood glucose levels.	Moderate
	Follow a neutropenic diet (i.e., cooked foods only).	Low
	Consume bottled water or processed drinks only.	Low
Control environmental risks of microbial invasion.	Follow strict hand washing and hand hygiene between patient contacts or procedures. Provide hand hygiene products in the hospital setting for patients and families.	High
	Group together patients with leukopenia, or provide a private room.	High
	Clean all multipurpose equipment (e.g., oximeter probes, infusion pumps, electronic thermometers) between patient uses. Use single-use equipment and supplies whenever possible.	High

(Continued on next page)

Table 11-3. Infection Prevention Strategies *(Continued)*

Objective	Strategy	Evidence Base
Control environmental risks of microbial invasion. *(cont.)*	Consider immunizations required because of lymphocyte suppression. Do not use nasal inoculation for influenza immunization. Pneumococcal and meningitis vaccines may be indicated in some cases. Vaccinate healthcare professionals against influenza.	High
	Maintain clean living environment (e.g., no food waste on table and countertops).	Moderate
	Ensure sterile management of vascular access devices in the hospital. Follow institutional protocols for clean versus sterile home management of vascular access devices.	Moderate
	Perform incentive spirometry, and encourage deep breathing and coughing and ambulation as much as tolerated to prevent atelectasis.	Moderate
	Cover open lesions with sterile dressing. Change daily if drainage is present.	Moderate
	Apply prophylactic antimicrobial powders or ointments in areas at high risk for infection (e.g., skin folds, perineal area).	Low
	Change oxygen therapy equipment if it is visibly contaminated or if obvious breaks in integrity exist.	Low
Avoid invasive procedures.	Avoid rectal procedures (e.g., rectal temperature).	Moderate
	Use in-line endotracheal/tracheal tube suction systems with a flush port to clean the catheter after each use.	Moderate
	Consider enteral feeding rather than parenteral feeding. Even minimal use of gastrointestinal tract helps to maintain mucosal integrity, eliminating the need for high dextrose via IV line.	Moderate
	Use sterile procedure for an invasive procedure.	–
Implement measures to lessen severity or longevity of leukopenia.	Give hematopoietic growth factors between 24–72 hours postchemotherapy in individuals older than age 65 or those with chemotherapy regimens likely to produce neutropenia in > 20% of patients.	High
	Maintain good general health measures regarding nutrition, rest, and sleep.	Moderate
	Administer IV immunoglobulin as indicated (immunoglobulin G levels < 300 mcg/dl).	Low

Note. Based on information from Bartley, 2000; Bow, 2013; Boyce & Pettit, 2002; Centers for Disease Control and Prevention, 2011; Fox & Freifeld, 2012; Gardner et al., 2008; Irwin et al., 2013; Kroger et al., 2011; Lyman, 2009; Lyman & Kleiner, 2011; Lyman et al., 2005; Machado, 2005; National Comprehensive Cancer Network, 2014c; Sehulster & Chinn, 2003; Shelton 2012; Tomblyn et al., 2009; van Dalen et al., 2012; White & Ybarra, 2014.

dence, interventions are labeled with the level of research-based evidence to support implementation.

Prophylactic antimicrobial agents are administered in specific circumstances in which the risk of infection and benefit of therapy outweigh the risk of developing antimicrobial resistance. The clinical indications for prophylactic antimicrobial therapy are defined by national standards, although some additional high-risk patients also may benefit from this practice (Gafter-Gvili et al., 2012; Herbst et al., 2009; Pascoe & Steven, 2009; Wingard, Eldjerou, & Leather, 2012). Patients with prolonged neutropenia receive prophylaxis against gastrointestinal gram-negative organisms and *Candida*, and patients with prolonged lymphopenia may receive prophylaxis against *Pneumocystis jiroveci* and cytomegalovirus (Flowers et al., 2013; NCCN, 2014c). Oncology APNs often are responsible for implementing and assessing these specific interventions.

The clinical severity of leukopenia can be reduced by administration of growth factors (Aapro et al., 2011; Flowers et al., 2013; NCCN, 2014b) or immune globulin (NCCN, 2014c). Evidence suggests that at-risk patients should receive growth factor prophylaxis prior to the first cycle of therapy, as the highest risk of complications is associated with the first cycle of therapy (Crea, Giovannetti, Zinzani, & Danesi, 2009; Flowers et al., 2013; Herbst et al., 2009; Puhalla, Bhattacharya, & Davidson, 2012). Recent research using delayed administration of growth factors at the onset of fever during neutropenia has been inconclusive. This practice is uncommon but driven by individual prescriber preference (Bennett, Djulbegovic, Norris, & Armitage, 2013; Cooper, Madan, Whyte, Stevenson, & Akehurst, 2011; Page & Liles, 2011; Velasco, 2011). Specific dosages and administration procedures are available in current medication resources.

In patients who become infected while neutropenic, immediate administration of broad-spectrum antimicrobials remains the most essential therapy (Flowers et al., 2013; Freifeld et al., 2011; NCCN, 2014c; Saloustros, Tryfonidis, & Georgoulias, 2011). Outpatient antimicrobials may be used to treat febrile episodes in patients with a lower risk of sepsis, including children without respiratory symptoms, patients with suspected community-acquired infection, patients with nonhematologic malignancies or absence of active malignant disease, patients with expected neutropenia nadir of less than seven days or nadir not expected to drop below 500/mm³, and patients with no comorbid health conditions (NCCN, 2014b, 2014c). Severe infection with an expected delay in WBC recovery may be treated with granulocyte transfusions (Rimajova, Sopko, Martinka, Kubalova, & Mistrik, 2012; Stanworth et al., 2005).

Thrombocytopenia

Definition and Etiology

Thrombocytopenia is defined as inadequate numbers of circulating platelets available to participate in the initial phase of clotting. Clotting itself requires the integration of platelets, coagulation proteins made in the liver, calcium, and cytokines and inflammatory stimulators. The absence of platelets alone can result in life-threatening hemorrhage, as platelets are the first responders to a break in tissue integrity, and platelet aggregation is the triggering event for formation of a final fibrin clot (Wahed & Dasgupta, 2015). The degree of depletion reflects the severity of deficit (see Kuter, 2015; NCI CTEP, 2010). Many general medicine clinicians use the threshold of a platelet count less than 100,000/mm³, although this is considered to be too conservative for cancer therapy–related toxicity (Kuter, 2015). Thrombocytopenia is not usually considered to be clinically significant until platelet counts drop to less than 50,000/mm³, which is CTCAE toxicity grade 3 (Liebman, 2014; NCI CTEP, 2010; Shelton, 2012). Patients receiving therapeutic anticoagulation or undergoing surgical procedures are maintained with counts at or above 50,000/mm³, although most patients receiving oncologic/hematologic care require platelet transfusions when their level is less than 10,000/mm³ (Liebman, 2014; Vadhan-Raj, 2009) or at higher levels if they are symptomatic. Thrombocytopenia is the most common cause of bleeding in patients with cancer; however, this risk only increases significantly as the counts decrease below 25,000/mm³ (Liebman, 2014; Vadhan-Raj, 2009). Oncology APNs assess the risk for and presence of thrombocytopenia.

Thrombocytopenia may occur because of decreased production or function, consumption, or blood loss (see Table 11-4). The most common etiologies of abnormal production of platelets are chemotherapy and radiation therapy. The chemotherapy agents most likely to produce significant thrombocytopenia are the platinols (Kuter, 2015; Polovich et al., 2014). Medications such as histamine blockers or antiviral agents are well known for their effects on platelet production and are used cautiously in patients with cancer (Shelton, 2012). Some nutraceuticals and herbal agents are known to increase the risk of bleeding, although bleeding is more often related to interference with hepatic coagulation protein production or activity than to interference with platelets. Agents to avoid in patients with thrombocytopenia include vitamin E, garlic, ginkgo biloba, and ginger (de Lemos et al., 2004; Memorial Sloan Kettering Cancer Center, n.d.).

Blood loss–related or consumption thrombocytopenia occurs when platelets are lost with overt bleeding or are consumed in a microvascular bleeding process, such as disseminated intravascular coagulation. Blood losses less than 500 ml appear to be the threshold at which clotting factors also are depleted (Despotis, Zhang, & Lublin, 2007; Waters, 2014). In patients with large blood losses, significant thrombocytopenia occurs.

Assessment

Because platelets are the first responders to breaks in vascular integrity (usually occurring first in skin and soft tissues), symptoms such as petechiae (tiny purplish-red dots) and ecchymoses (bruises) occur. Petechiae and ecchymoses can occur with minor injury, dependent pressure (e.g., from lying on one area), or gravitational pressure (e.g., an arm hanging alongside the bed rail) in fragile vessels with inadequate coagulation factors (Shelton, 2012). Overt bleeding from wounds or body orifices or around existing tubes occurs immediately after injury to the vasculature if platelets are inadequate, as the platelet plug is the first step of the clotting cascade. Clinical bleeding events delayed 20 minutes to two hours indicate coagulation protein deficit, not necessarily thrombocytopenia (Waters, 2014). When large vessels are opened for any reason, spontaneous, severe, and continuous bleeding can occur. Organ-specific bleeding is most common in sites with a large mucosal or epithelial surface area, such as the gastrointestinal tract (oral, oropharynx, nasopharynx, gastric, rectal), urinary tract, or lungs (Shelton, 2012). Assessment for occult and overt blood in all excrement and exudates may reveal sources of bleeding. All sources of secretions and excrement (e.g., nasogastric secretions, urine, stool, sputum, nasal drainage, vaginal discharge) are examined for evidence of blood. Mucous membranes, such as in the oral cavity or gastrointestinal tract, particularly are prone to spontaneous bleeding with thrombocytopenia because vessels are so close to the membrane surface (Shelton, 2012). Additionally, bleeding may be evidenced by organ dysfunction, such as pulmonary crackles with hypoxemia or enlarged and tender liver with hepatic enzyme elevation.

Under some circumstances, circulating platelet levels are reduced because of abnormal sequestration rather than decreased production or loss (Liebman, 2014; Waters, 2014). The liver and spleen, which normally remove abnormal or senescent platelets, may inappropriately filter normal platelets from circulation. An enlarged and tender liver or spleen indicates that abnormal or fragmented cells are being captured by these organs. Excessive removal can be a normal compensatory mechanism when cell fragments are present, such as with massive

Table 11-4. Causes of Thrombocytopenia

Pathophysiologic Mechanism	Etiologic Factors
Abnormal production of platelets in the bone marrow	Alcohol Allopurinol Antineoplastic chemotherapy Aplastic anemia Burns Catecholamines Chloramphenicol Flucytosine Histamine-2 blockers Histoplasmosis Hormones Nutritional deficits Radiation (ionizing and nonionizing) exposure Thiazide diuretics
Interference with platelet function	Aminoglycosides Catecholamines Dextran Diabetes mellitus Hepatic cirrhosis Hyperthermia Hypothermia Loop diuretics Malignant lymphomas Nonsteroidal anti-inflammatory drugs Phenothiazines Salicylates Sarcoidosis Scleroderma Systemic lupus erythematosus Thyrotoxicosis Tricyclic antidepressants Uremia Vitamin E
Blood loss	Epistaxis Gastrointestinal bleed Hematuria Hemoptysis Retroperitoneal bleed (spontaneous or from blunt trauma) Vascular injury
Consumptive process	Disseminated intravascular coagulation Heart valves Heat stroke Large-bore IV catheters (e.g., balloon pump, dialysis catheters) Large tumor masses Sepsis-induced consumption Sulfonamides Transfusions Trimethoprim-sulfamethoxazole

(Continued on next page)

Table 11-4. Causes of Thrombocytopenia *(Continued)*

Pathophysiologic Mechanism	Etiologic Factors
Immunologic destruction of platelets	Heparin Immune thrombocytopenic purpura or thrombotic thrombocytopenic purpura Mononucleosis Vaccinations Viral illness

Note. Based on information from Andres et al., 2009; Fogarty & Dunbar, 2013; Kuter, 2015; Nayak et al., 2012; Polovich et al., 2014; Rodgers, 2009; Rome, 2007; Salacz et al., 2007; Shane & Shelton, 2004; Shelton, 2013; Wahed & Dasgupta, 2015.

---

thromboses. This usually is accompanied by jaundice as a manifestation of abnormal hemolysis (Shelton, 2013).

Although thrombocytopenia is a clear myelosuppressive toxicity, many medications and disease states alter platelet function, cause similar complications, or exacerbate symptoms associated with thrombocytopenia. In patients with mild to moderate thrombocytopenia who have excess bleeding, these factors are considered and treated. Common causes of platelet dysfunction include acetaminophen, alcohol, aminoglycosides, beta-blockers, dextran, diuretics (loop, thiazide), hypothermia, nonsteroidal anti-inflammatory drugs, penicillin, phenothiazines, rifampin, salicylates, tricyclic antidepressants, unfractionated heparin, uremia, and valproic acid (Shelton, 2013).

The defining feature of thrombocytopenia is a low platelet count, although other diagnostic tests may help to differentiate the specific etiology of platelet depletion or clarify an etiology for symptoms present with thrombocytopenia. If thrombocytopenia is related to blood loss, commensurate decreases in hemoglobin and hematocrit usually are present (Relf et al., 2013). Platelet production disorders usually are not independent of other hematopoietic cells; therefore, anemia and leukopenia usually accompany thrombocytopenia. When hepatosplenic sequestration occurs, serum bilirubin levels are increased, and blood cell smears show schistocytes (fragmented RBCs) (Shelton, 2013). Coagulation factor tests such as fibrinogen level, prothrombin time, partial thromboplastin time, fibrin degradation products, or antithrombin III levels will reveal coagulation abnormalities that may contribute to bleeding diatheses (Shelton, 2013).

Prevention and Management

When possible, serious thrombocytopenia is prevented with chemotherapy or radiation therapy dose adjustment. When this compromises possible response, platelet growth factor may be administered. The bone marrow growth factor currently approved by the U.S. Food and Drug Administration to stimulate bone marrow production of platelets is oprelvekin (IL-11). This agent is administered 6–24 hours after the last chemotherapy dose. The most common adverse effect is fluid retention, although thrombosis also is possible (Kim, Singh, & Arlen, 2014). It is important to evaluate the thrombotic risk prior to prescription of this agent.

Other factors are known to deplete platelet levels and can be avoided or minimized with proactive interventions. Avoidance of temperature extremes, rigors or seizures, and large-bore invasive lines can reduce platelet consumption (Kuter, 2015; Salacz, Lankiewicz, & Weissman, 2007). Preventing bleeding from other causes also is an important supportive intervention. Hepatic coagulation factors may be supported with administration of vitamin K (phytonadione) or plasma transfusions. Prevention of severe bleeding complications with general care measures is equally important, particularly when patients may be transfusion refractory as a result of antibody alloimmunization (Shelton, 2012). Patients with low platelet counts require elevation of the head of their bed (to reduce the risk of increased intracranial pressure–induced capillary hemorrhage), reduction of invasive procedures, and a safe, clutter-free environment. Patients are advised to protect their hands and feet from injury, to use only electric razors, and to avoid physical activities that increase risk of injury (Shelton, 2012).

Optimal management of thrombocytopenia involves determining the minimal tolerable and safe platelet count for each patient. Each patient has an individualized platelet threshold for transfusion based on his or her clinical needs and complications (Benjamin & Anderson, 2002; Kuter, 2015; Liebman, 2014). For example, patients with existing uremia that alters platelet quality may require a high platelet count, as would individuals who are receiving therapeutic heparin for a recent pulmonary embolism. Patients with open wounds or erosive malignant masses also might require higher platelet counts to prevent bleeding.

Thrombocytopenia-induced bleeding often involves the skin, mucous membranes, and soft tissues. Local procoagulant interventions or agents may be effective in preventing serious or persistent bleeding and often are initiated by APNs who are familiar with broader treatment options for bleeding (Shelton, 2013). The most common and inexpensive measure is application of ice or pressure to the site of bleeding. This causes vasoconstriction and reduces blood loss but does not prevent bleeding from recurring. Other supportive local measures to decrease bleeding from specific sites include topical agents, such as absorbable gelatin sponges, topical thrombin, oxidized cellulose, microfibrillar collagen hemostat, or hydrophilic polymer with ferrate powder (Shelton, 2012).

Systemic treatments for bleeding involve stimulation of the body's normal processes to produce factors or agents known to decrease the bleeding tendency. Their specific indications, dosing, administration procedures, and evaluation of responses are directed by the APN. Epsilon aminocaproic acid blocks plasminogen breakdown of plasmin (Shelton, 2013). Somatostatin (octreotide) enhances the activity of a normally occurring gastrointestinal enzyme with a procoagulant effect (Shelton, 2013). It may be used for management of gastrointestinal bleeding. High-dose estrogen also has been used to enhance normal clotting mechanisms, but its efficacy for use in bleeding patients is not established (Shelton, 2013). Because few effective therapies exist for platelet-induced bleeding, systemic therapies are targeted to enhance clotting via a mechanism other than the platelet arm.

Nursing management of bleeding risk or actual bleeding is supportive. No directed activities are used only with thrombocytopenia, other than platelet transfusions or platelet growth factor (IL-11/oprelvekin) (Modery-Pawlowski et al., 2013). Clinical studies with thrombopoietin were not as promising as anticipated (Kim et al., 2014), although the thrombopoietin receptor agonist romiplostim has been licensed for use in immune thrombocytopenia and shows promising long-term benefit in chronic immune thrombocytopenia (Kuter et al., 2013). Successful management of immune-mediated thrombocytopenia with splenectomy or rituximab has been well established (Ghanima, Godeau, Cines, & Bussel, 2012). Table 11-5 describes bleeding precautions and patient education strategies. Platelet transfusions often are administered to patients with cancer and thrombocytopenia. Whenever possible, single-donor platelet products are administered to reduce exposure to foreign antigens and development of platelet antibodies that cause transfusion refractoriness. Platelets produce more reactions than RBCs because of the potential presence of WBCs within the product (Rodriguez & Gobel, 2011). Febrile and allergic reactions are common; however, a specific antigen rarely can be identified (Rodriguez & Gobel, 2011). Patients with a history of

Table 11-5. Management of Thrombocytopenia

Objective	Strategy	Evidence Base
Prevent overt bleeding.	Limit invasive procedures.	High
	Avoid medications that affect coagulation factors and increase bleeding risks.	High
	Discourage strenuous activity, contact sports, or situations placing patient at high risk for injury (e.g., motorcycle riding).	Moderate
Prevent occult bleeding.	Use electric razors for shaving.	High
	Keep the head of the bed elevated at all times. Do not use Trendelenburg positioning for hypotension; weigh risks and benefits of its use for central line insertion.	Moderate
	Maintain oral hygiene, preventing gingivitis.	Moderate
	Avoid unnecessary venipunctures.	Moderate
	Use alternate site for automatic blood pressure cuff. Reset maximum inflation pressure when possible.	Moderate
	Monitor and aggressively treat hypertension.	Moderate
	Allow patient out of bed only with assistance until physical therapy evaluation. Pad bedrails if patient is in danger of injuring self on the bedrails.	Low
	Avoid rectal procedures.	Low
	Avoid intramuscular injections.	Low
	Maintain hydration of mucous membranes (nares, mouth, lips) with saline nose spray, fluid intake, humidified oxygen, and frequent oral care.	Low
	Use paper tape, or tape to barrier (e.g., DuoDerm®) to prevent skin tears.	Low
	Help to avoid constipation and straining for bowel movement.	Low
	Use red rubber catheters and lubricant with endotracheal, tracheal, or nasotracheal suctioning. Do not insert catheter beyond the end of the airway, and avoid insertion until resistance (indicates that catheter is potentially injuring the carina).	Low
Manage bleeding episodes.	Administer blood components as ordered; monitor for transfusion reactions. When possible, used matched platelets to reduce risk of alloimmunization.	High
	Use local hemostatic agents (e.g., Gelfoam®, Surgicel™, topical thrombin) to achieve skin and soft tissue hemostasis.	Moderate
	Apply ice or pressure to site of bleeding.	Moderate

(Continued on next page)

Table 11-5. Management of Thrombocytopenia *(Continued)*

Objective	Strategy	Evidence Base
Manage bleeding episodes. *(cont.)*	Assess fluid loss episodes by monitoring intake and output, central venous pressure, weight, and orthostatic vital signs. Weigh bloody dressings to estimate actual blood lost.	Moderate
	Hemorrhagic cystitis may require IV hydration, continuous bladder irrigations, and intrabladder hemostatic agents.	Moderate

Note. Based on information from Kuter, 2015; Nayak et al., 2012; Polovich et al., 2014; Rodriguez & Gobel, 2011; Rodgers, 2009; Salacz et al., 2007; Shane & Shelton, 2004; Shelton, 2012; Vadhan-Raj, 2009; Wahed & Dasgupta, 2015.

reactions are likely to receive premedications of acetaminophen and diphenhydramine prior to platelet transfusion. Single-donor platelet products usually have 6–10 units per transfusion. Each transfusion packet is estimated to provide a 20%–50% increase in platelet count (Benjamin & Anderson, 2002). Platelet transfusions do not require the same ABO/Rh compatibility as RBC products unless the patient weighs less than 40 kg or platelet transfusion volume exceeds 600 ml of unmatched platelets or plasma in a 24-hour period (Khan et al., 2007). The ABO antigen is found on RBCs, and antibodies to these antigens are found in plasma. Patients with an A or B antigen possess antibodies to other antigens and cannot receive RBCs with other antibodies. Patients with AB antigens have no antibodies and may receive any blood type. Patients with O blood type have no antibodies and may donate blood to any individual. ABO/Rh compatibility of platelets, plasma, and RBC products is core knowledge for oncology APNs (see Table 11-6).

Anemia

Definition and Etiology

Anemia is most often defined by the serum levels of circulating RBCs (hematocrit) or their oxygen-carrying capacity (hemoglobin). National standards define anemia as a reduction of hemoglobin or hematocrit by one-third or more of normal (initial screening in patients with hemoglobin levels less than 11 g/dl) (Koury & Lichtman, 2010; NCCN, 2014a). This definition is exclusively dependent on laboratory values and may not be a true reflection of this clinical syndrome without evidence of symptoms related to reduced oxygen-carrying capacity. Anemia is reported in 40%–75% of patients with cancer, but the wide variance of incidence is attributed to the variable definition (Erb & Vogel, 2013). Actual values and patient tolerance vary, and many patients with cancer slowly develop anemia and therefore tolerate much lower values without cardiopulmonary compromise. Because the life span of an RBC is up to 120 days, this hematopoietic element usually is depleted last when the source of dysfunction is within the bone marrow. Anemia in cancer or cancer therapy is common and is definitively linked to compromised quality of life and reduced survival (NCCN, 2014a). The optimal hemoglobin level and rate and method of correction continue to be debated (NCCN, 2014a).

Anemia in patients with cancer usually is categorized by the physiologic/etiologic mechanism, although it often is multifactorial. Common etiologic mechanisms include deficient or abnormal production, blood-loss anemia, hemolytic anemia, or cancer-associated anemia

Table 11-6. Blood Product Compatibility

Recipient's Blood Group	RBC Antigen	Serum Antibody	Compatible Donors: RBC Transfusions	Compatible Donors: Platelet or Plasma Transfusions
A	A	Anti-B	A and O	A and AB
B	B	Anti-A	B and O	B and AB
AB (universal recipient)	A and B	Neither anti-A nor anti-B	A, B, AB, O	AB
O	Neither	Anti-A and anti-B	O (universal donor)	A, B, AB, O

RBC—red blood cell

Note. Based on information from Carson et al., 2012.

(Shelton, 2012; Tefferi, Hanson, & Inwards, 2005). RBC production depends on a number of nutritional factors and precursor components. Nutritional anemias (iron deficiency, folate deficiency, vitamin B_{12} deficiency, inadequate transferrin) are common even among patients without cancer and should be considered when patients initially present with anemia (Shelton, 2012). Nutritional deficits occur in patients with cancer because of nausea and vomiting, fatigue and malaise, dysphagia, malabsorption syndromes, and gastric or bowel resection. Patients often receive gastric acid inhibitors (e.g., proton pump inhibitors), placing them at risk for vitamin B_{12} deficiency (Shelton, 2012). Inadequate production of RBCs may result from bone marrow infiltration with tumor, although leukopenia and thrombocytopenia are likely to precede anemia when this is the etiologic mechanism. More recent evidence also suggests that inflammation plays a major role in chronic anemia of malignancy and aging (Adamson, 2008; Ferrucci & Balducci, 2008).

RBCs normally are sensitized and removed by the spleen when they are senescent, deformed, or dysfunctional. The spleen can become oversensitized by the development of RBC autoantibodies that detect normal RBCs as foreign tissue and then signal splenic macrophages to remove and destroy them (Shelton, 2012). In addition, RBC autoantibodies may be circulating in the serum and initiate extrasplenic hemolysis. Abnormal sequestration in the spleen or intravascular hemolysis results in hemolytic anemia. Hemolytic anemia is commonly a secondary disorder, arising as a complication of liver and splenic disease, autoimmune disorders, viral infections, malignancy, bone marrow transplantation, or drug toxicity (Nayak et al., 2012). Additionally, transfusion reactions can cause hemolysis, although a persistent hemolytic anemia is unusual in these situations. One indication of recent blood loss or hemolysis is the presence of excessive reticulocytes (Tefferi et al., 2005). Reticulocytes are the immediate precursor cell for mature RBCs and are released early into circulation when the supply is inadequate. The reticulocyte count reflects the degree of bone marrow reserve and amount of replacement RBCs needed. The normal reticulocyte volume is less than 2% of the total RBC count, but in blood loss or hemolysis, it may be as high as 4%–8% of the total RBC count (Shelton, 2012).

Cancer-associated anemia is a syndrome of chronic anemia that persists beyond the time reasonable for cancer therapy–induced anemia and occurs in the absence of bone marrow disease. It is speculated to be partly attributable to an escalated metabolic rate and tumor-related hemolysis (Adamson, 2008; Ferrucci & Balducci, 2008). In one study, blunted responses to normal human erythropoietin were noted in patients with persistent anemia, suggesting that anemia is not always the result of erythropoietin deficiency and amenable to erythropoietin replacement therapy (NCCN, 2014a). Recent recognition of complications of erythropoietin replacement therapy has resulted in limitations in its use with cancer-related rather than therapy-related anemia (NCCN, 2014a).

Assessment

Patients with anemia are first assessed for a past medical-surgical history that suggests other correctable etiologic factors. A dietary history may reveal areas for nutritional interventions. The most important nutrients for the production of RBCs are iron, folate, vitamin B_{12}, and protein (Schrijvers, 2011; Wahed & Dasgupta, 2015). However, even with immediate nutritional replacement therapy, new RBC production may require two to four weeks (Goroll & Mulley, 2009). Assessing patients' surgical history identifies individuals with lower gastric or duodenal surgeries that resulted in hydrochloric acid and intrinsic factor depletion, leading to vitamin B_{12} deficiency (pernicious anemia). Because hemoglobin levels are partly dependent on muscle mass, anemia can develop when muscle atrophy and disuse syndrome occur (Wahed & Dasgupta, 2015). Hypermetabolism, such as with chronic infection, breaks down proteins for energy and may cause anemia (Goroll & Mulley, 2009). Hormones serve to regulate RBC production. When androgen or estrogen levels are manipulated in reproductive organ malignancies (e.g., ovarian, uterine, breast, testicular, prostate), RBC abnormalities can occur. Anemia is most often associated with increased estrogen or decreased androgen (Shelton, 2012).

A thorough medication history can reveal the potential etiology of marrow suppression, nutritional deficits, or hemolysis. Most antimetabolite, alkylating, and antibiotic antineoplastic agents given for more than one monthly cycle will induce anemia (Polovich et al., 2014). Other medications known to induce anemia that may be administered to patients with cancer include allopurinol, amphotericin B, antidysrhythmics (e.g., procainamide, quinidine), anticonvulsants (e.g., phenytoin, carbamazepine), antihypertensives (e.g., methyldopa), chloramphenicol, flucytosine, isoniazid, reverse transcriptase inhibitors, and trimethoprim-sulfamethoxazole (Nayak et al., 2012; Shelton, 2012). Independent risk factors for development of anemia in patients with cancer include female gender; older age; lower initial hemoglobin in females; breast, lung, and gynecologic malignancies; and treatment with platinol agents (NCCN, 2014a).

The physical signs of anemia are manifested as symptoms of inadequate oxygen delivery, compensatory symptoms to counteract hypoxia, and other symptoms of reduced RBC function (see Table 11-7). Diagnostic evaluation always begins with examination of the CBC, with particular attention to the hematocrit and hemoglobin, as these are the most direct measurements of RBC depletion. In addition to the hematocrit and hemoglobin, the RBC indices reported with the CBC may provide helpful diagnostic information. The mean corpuscular volume (MCV) detects the size or mass of the RBC. Young or immature cells are larger in size and cause increased MCV. Higher MCV is present with recent blood loss that increases release of reticulocytes, which are larger than mature RBCs. More macrocytic cells (folate and B_{12} deficiency) indicate more immature cells, also causing elevated MCV (Nayak et al., 2012; Uthman, n.d.). The mean corpuscular hemoglobin (MCH) and mean corpuscular hemoglobin concentration (MCHC) detect the relative amount of iron and oxygen saturation of the hemoglobin molecule. The MCH and MCHC are decreased in iron deficiency or hemoglobinopathies. Suspected iron deficiency from a low MCH is followed by assessment for decreased serum iron levels and high total iron-binding capacity in combination with low transferrin saturation or increased soluble transferrin receptor (Hinkel et al., 2010; Pieracci & Barie, 2006). When hemolysis is suspected, in addition to lower hemoglobin lev-

Table 11-7. Signs and Symptoms of Anemia

Pathophysiologic Mechanism	Signs/Symptoms
Inadequate oxygen delivery	Hypoxemia (decreased arterial oxygen level, decreased oxygen saturation) Dyspnea/air hunger Angina/ischemic changes on 12-lead electrocardiogram Neurologic symptoms—cognitive dysfunction, dizziness, blurred vision Oliguria Decreased bowel sounds, decreased motility, paralytic ileus, constipation Hypotension (systolic) Central cyanosis notable under eyelids, inside lips Capillary refill < 3 seconds
Compensatory mechanism for tissue hypoxia	Tachypnea, use of accessory muscles in increased ventilation Tachycardia Full bounding pulses Cool or diaphoretic extremities Cardiac murmurs
Inadequate blood viscosity/insulation	Orthostasis (heart rate increase > 20 bpm or blood pressure decrease > 40 mm Hg, or blood pressure systolic < 90 mm Hg) when moving from lying to sitting or sitting to standing Hypotension Hypothermia
Indicators of hemolysis	Enlarged and tender liver or spleen Jaundice

Note. Based on information from Cella, 1997; National Comprehensive Cancer Network, 2014a; Nayak et al., 2012; Shelton, 2012; Wahed & Dasgupta, 2015.

els and elevated bilirubin, an increased percentage of reticulocytes and decreased transferrin and haptoglobin are present (Coyne, 2006; Nayak et al., 2012; Pieracci & Barie, 2006). In patients with cancer, the assumption that anemia is related entirely to cancer or its treatment may lead to weeks of ineffective therapy. To ensure that precursor proteins are adequate for production of heme molecules and RBCs, baseline ferritin levels are assessed at the onset of therapy or the beginning of erythropoietin treatment. Erythropoietin levels have not been proved to be accurate for monitoring the efficacy of RBC stimulation therapies, although as many as 20%–30% of individuals with apparent erythropoietin deficiency do not respond to erythropoiesis-stimulating agents, suggesting a more complex etiology (Baribeault & Auerbach, 2011; NCCN, 2014a). On occasion, the mystery of anemia can be solved by administration of indium-tagged RBCs with a follow-up nuclear scan to determine whether those cells are lost via a damaged vessel or taken up by a spleen that is inappropriately hemolyzing (Shelton, 2012). This most commonly is used for patients presumed to have a vascular bleed without a diagnosable source. RBC morphologic abnormalities also may be helpful in providing diagnostic clues and triggering more extensive testing. For example, Howell-Jolly bodies are highly indicative of hepatic disease, and schistocytes may be present with disseminated intravascular coagulation (Shelton, 2012). Unique types of anemia (e.g., sickle-cell anemia, paroxysmal nocturnal hemoglobinuria, thalassemia) can be detected through other specialized serum and urine laboratory tests. Oncology APNs must be familiar with the medical-surgical and cancer-related causes and clinical signs of anemia and able to differentiate key diagnostic test results and treatments for each type of anemia. An overview of these findings is outlined in Table 11-8.

Prevention and Management

Anemia is a common and often unavoidable complication associated with cancer and cancer therapies. However, in the initial evaluation of a patient with cancer, a thorough assessment of nutritional status and comorbid disease conditions can reveal the presence of preexisting anemia or risk factors for its development. Early nutritional assessment can permit iron or folate replacement therapy at the onset, preventing lengthy unsuccessful treatment with erythropoiesis-stimulating factors. Patients who begin therapy with depleted iron precursors (transferrin, ferritin) or iron stores (iron-binding capacity/iron saturation) also may demonstrate inadequate responses to erythropoietin-stimulating agents (Hinkel et al., 2010). Oral iron replacement therapy is frequently ineffective because of iron's poor oral absorption; therefore, IV iron may be administered to high-risk patients (Baribeault & Auerbach, 2011; Schrijvers, 2011). Iron replacement is recommended if the ferritin level is less than 800 ng/ml and the transferrin saturation is lower than 20% (Hinkel et al., 2010). Nutritional supplementation with foods high in iron, such as organ meats, beans, nuts, and green vegetables, or those high in B vitamins, such as green vegetables and enriched cereals and grains, may enhance restoration of nutrition.

Table 11-8. Abnormal Clinical Findings of Specific Types of Anemia

Type of Anemia	Clinical Findings	Diagnostic Test Results
Suppressed bone marrow production of red blood cells (RBCs)	Infection, bleeding, and fatigue; degree/severity and marrow suppression will predict symptoms.	Bone marrow aspiration/biopsy shows low level of erythroblasts and other RBC precursors. Serum leukopenia, thrombocytopenia, and anemia
Folate-deficiency anemia	Fatigue, paresthesias, headache, difficulty concentrating/cognitive impairment	Decreased serum folate level (< 4 mg/dl) Decreased hemoglobin Increased mean corpuscular volume (MCV)
Iron-deficiency anemia	Fatigue, headache, smooth red tongue (painful), cracks in corners of the mouth, pica	Decreased hemoglobin Decreased MCV, decreased mean corpuscular hemoglobin/mean corpuscular hemoglobin concentration Decreased ferritin Decreased or normal serum iron Increased total iron-binding capacity Decreased transferrin saturation
Hemolytic anemia	Enlarged and tender liver and/or spleen, jaundice, pruritus	Decreased transferrin Deceased haptoglobin Increased urine urobilinogen levels Increased schistocytes RBC survival studies—indium-tagged RBCs administered and scanned for abnormal hepatic or splenic uptake

Note. Based on information from Erb & Vogel, 2013; George-Gay & Parker, 2003; National Comprehensive Cancer Network, 2014a; Nayak et al., 2012; Shelton, 2012; Uthman, n.d.; Wahed & Dasgupta, 2015.

Although chemotherapy and radiation therapy are known etiologies of anemia, the contribution of other medications to this complication often is overlooked. Anemia can potentially be prevented or reduced in severity by elimination of medications such as allopurinol or trimethoprim-sulfamethoxazole (NCCN, 2014a). Oxygen administration is used frequently to supplement other therapies for anemia and will optimize the delivery of oxygen to tissues that may be compromised because of anemia's effects; however, this is not useful if the patient is not concomitantly hypoxic (Haase, 2010).

When anemia cannot be avoided with passive measures, recombinant erythropoietin, a stimulating growth factor for RBCs, may be administered. Given as an IV infusion or subcutaneous injection, it supports RBC regrowth and hemoglobin maintenance in two to four weeks (NCCN, 2014a; Rizzo et al., 2010). The most up-to-date prescribing information is provided in medications resources. Baseline iron, ferritin, transferrin, and iron-binding protein values provide information regarding variables that may interfere with the efficacy of erythropoietin replacement therapy. Although erythropoietin is given to stimulate bone marrow production and commitment of RBCs, no clear benefit results from monitoring erythropoietin levels during treatment. Studies attempting to increase hemoglobin levels to 14–15 mg/dl for the purpose of increasing quality of life or tumor oxygenation to improve responses to therapy have shown no clear benefit and increased incidence of thrombotic cardiovascular events (Hinkel et al., 2010; NCCN, 2014a; Rizzo et al., 2010). Meta-analyses of use of these agents to support red cell growth have shown that use of erythropoiesis-stimulating agents within tightly defined clinical indications can reduce transfusions, but if the hemoglobin exceeds 12 mg/dl, they may increase the risk of venous thromboembolism, decrease overall survival, and possibly alter tumor progression (Bohlius, Tonia, & Schwarzer, 2011; Vansteenkiste, Wauters, Elliott, Glaspy, & Hedenus, 2013). Current recommendations are to first determine if the patient requires immediate correction of anemia by transfusion. The goals of cancer therapy must be weighed against potential risks when considering erythropoietic therapy (Bohlius et al., 2011; NCCN, 2014a).

Blood transfusion remains a common management strategy for anemia from all causes. The risk of transfusion-transmitted infection (e.g., hepatitis, cytomegalovirus, Epstein-Barr virus), immunosuppression (e.g., lymphocyte dysfunction), and complications of banked and preserved blood (e.g., hypothermia, hypocalcemia, hyperammonemia, hyperkalemia, acidosis) must be weighed against potential benefit (Carson et al., 2012; Galel, Nguyen, Fontaine, Goodnough, & Viele, 2009; Mercadante et al., 2009). Concentrated RBC products are used more often than whole blood because of the higher risk for reactions from blood products not filtered for WBCs and platelets. The bedside nurse ensures blood compatibility prior to hanging a blood product (see Table 11-6), and the patient is closely monitored for febrile, allergic, or hemolytic reactions. National recommendations suggest use of blood transfusions to attain a goal hemoglobin of 7–8 mg/dl in asymptomatic patients and approximately 8 mg/dl in symptomatic patients (Carson et al., 2012; NCCN, 2014a; Rizzo et al., 2010). Each unit of packed RBCs can be expected to increase the hemoglobin 1 mg/dl (Carson et al., 2012; Schrijvers, 2011). Blood alternatives, such as perfluochemicals suspended in albumin or stroma-free hemoglobin, may be administered in patients with contraindications for blood derivatives (Mercadante et al., 2009; Schrijvers, 2011).

Iron overload is an adverse effect of concern for patients with anemia who are treated with iron replacement, erythropoiesis-stimulating agents, or blood transfusions (Bacon, Adams, Kowdley, Powell, & Tavill, 2011; Erb & Vogel, 2013; Fleming & Ponka, 2012; Kwiatkowski, 2011). Clinical findings associated with this syndrome include fatigue, joint pain, impotence, or osteoporosis. Diagnosis is made with a serum ferritin greater than 1,000 ng/ml and hemochromatosis noted on liver biopsy (Erb & Vogel, 2013). Management includes use of iron-chelating agents such as tris-hydroxamate deferoxamine (DFO) (Greenberg et al., 2009).

Patients with concomitant neurologic, cardiovascular, or pulmonary compromise are likely to be provided oxygen therapy in an attempt to alleviate symptoms. Excess oxygen therapy can cause absorption atelectasis and hypoventilation. Mild to moderate aerobic exercise has shown promise as a supportive therapy for patients with anemia-related fatigue (NCCN, 2014a). The suggested regimen consists of 15–30 minutes of aerobic exercise three times a week.

Evaluation of Outcomes

Patients with myelosuppression related to cancer or its therapies present with variable complex symptoms. Although they adversely affect quality of life, these toxicities today account for less than 4% of cancer-related deaths (NCCN, 2014a). In some cases, the highest-risk patients are identified early in their treatment, and adjustment of the dose or schedule and initiation of supportive therapies allow for amelioration of myelotoxicity. For most patients, bone marrow suppression is temporary, and deficits return to normal upon completion of therapy. This knowledge is used to plan assessment, management, and follow-up care. As in all therapy toxicities, a few documented situations exist in which blood counts do not return to their pretreatment values. This is more common with high-dose therapies for hematologic malignancies where the targeted malignant cell line is within the bone marrow (Erb & Vogel, 2013). Acute leukemia induction therapy and hematopoietic stem cell transplantation have the highest risk for prolonged marrow suppression affecting one of the identified cell lines.

Implications for Oncology Advanced Practice Nurses

APNs are key resources for staff nurses and patients in developing an understanding of their clinical experiences with myelosuppression and the individual variables of management. The APN's broad knowledge base assists others in translating risk factors and the timing of myelosuppression to develop patient-specific plans of care. Implementation of preventive and treatment strategies is a key role of APNs in the management of myelosuppression. Finally, APNs play a pivotal role in developing facility-wide policies, procedures, staff education, and patient education that integrates evidence-based interventions for management of anemia in this vulnerable patient population.

Second Malignancies

Definition

A malignancy is considered a "second" malignancy when arising from mutations produced by prior exposure to a carcinogen. As an adverse effect of therapy, this eliminates inclusion of those cancers related to common risk factors or genetic changes alone (see Chapters 1 and 2) or second primary malignancies due to intrinsic risk factors. The rate of occurrence of second malignancies is higher in children (approximately 4%), solid organ transplant recipients (approximately 2%–3%), and patients who have received radiation therapy (approximately 1.5%–3%), although significant variation exists based on both treatment and host risk factors (Curtis et al., 2006; Maule et al., 2007; Oeffinger, Baxi, Friedman, & Moskowitz, 2013). People at greatest risk for development of second malignancies are young females and those who have received radiation therapy or high-dose cell cycle–nonspecific chemotherapy, although second malignancies have been reported in childhood cancer survivors of any type of cancer (Jazbec, Todorovski, & Jereb, 2007; Ottaviani, Robert, Huh, Palla, & Jaffe, 2013). The risk for second malignancies increases steadily with time after exposure, particularly for survivors of childhood cancer (Farioli, Violante, Mattioli, Curti, & Kriebel, 2013; Landier & Smith, 2011).

Most conventional antineoplastic therapies are successful because of their ability to destroy specific cells. The more nonspecific the action, the greater the number of normal cells that are damaged. In more targeted therapies, fewer normal cells are damaged, and latent carcinogenicity is less frequent. Second malignancies occur as a consequence of chemotherapy, radiation therapy, or T-cell suppression. Most second malignancies are myeloid, lymphoid, or soft tissue in origin, although a few highly aggressive forms of glioma, cervical cancer, rectal cancer, mesothelioma, and non-small cell lung cancer are associated with specific exposures (Chaturvedi et al., 2007; Farioli et al., 2013; Rugge, 2013). Children most often experience second cancers of the brain, bone, and thyroid (Wilson, Cohn, Johnston, & Ashton, 2010). Sarcomas are the most common malignancy related to radiation exposure (Landier & Smith, 2011; Schwartz et al., 2014). Second malignancies are associated with more rapid and uncontrolled growth, higher number of genetic mutations, resistance to treatment, and poor prognosis, although the latter is less clear (Chang et al., 2007; Larson, 2007; Oeffinger et al., 2013).

Etiology

The three main causes of second malignancies are chemotherapy, radiation therapy, and T-lymphocyte suppression (Inman, Frigola, Dong, & Kwon, 2007). The greater the therapy's nonspecific destruction, the higher the potential for second malignancy. This late effect also is related to dosage, length of exposure, and the level of growth and development of individual patients (Dantal & Pohanka, 2007). Children have the highest incidence of second malignancies, although it is unclear whether this is related to a higher mutation rate, longevity of survival, or iatrogenic growth hormones enhancing mutagenesis (Dantal & Pohanka, 2007; Woodmansee et al., 2013). Childhood cancers most often associated with second cancers are acute leukemia, brain tumors, Hodgkin lymphoma, retinoblastoma, and soft tissue sarcoma (Armstrong, 2010; Wilson et al., 2010). Treatment of acute leukemia in children is specifically associated with later brain tumors and thyroid cancer (Perkins, DeWees, Shinohara, Reddy, & Frangoul, 2013).

Radiation therapy has long been associated with risk of second malignancies. Cumulative radiation doses in excess of 30 Gy reportedly have a more significant risk than lesser doses (Schwartz et al., 2014), although even these data have been refuted (de Gonzalez et al., 2013). It has been suggested that photon therapy is more likely to induce second malignancies because of increased exposure to adjacent organs; however, recent trials were not able to validate this theory (Bekelman, Schultheiss, & De Gonzalez, 2013; Chung et al., 2013). Newer radiation therapies designed to preserve normal tissues, such as intensity-modulated radiation therapy and tomography, may reduce risk for second malignancies, but data are not mature enough to validate this theory (Kim, D.W., et al., 2013; Zaghloul, 2013).

Clearly, immunosuppressive drugs targeting T lymphocytes are more carcinogenic than those affecting cytokines such as tumor necrosis factor (Dantal & Pohanka, 2007). Additionally, a dose relationship exists that is seen more commonly in patients who received prolonged immunosuppressive therapy, as with those receiving a mismatched renal transplant, or those receiving multiple high-dose agents, as with heart-lung transplant (Bakker, van Imhoff, Verschuuren, & van Son, 2007; Chang et al., 2007). Another higher-risk group of patients are individuals who have received long-term corticosteroids, such as those with autoimmune disease. A summary of second malignancies according to their etiologic factors is listed in Table 11-9.

Table 11-9. Second Malignancies

Second Malignancy	Potential Etiologic Factors
Acute leukemia	Alkylating agents, especially with high doses or cumulative doses Antimetabolites Antitumor antibiotics Corticosteroids Epipodophyllotoxins
Bladder cancer	Radiation therapy for prostate cancer
Brain tumors	Therapeutic radiation for other cancers
Cervical cancer, invasive	HIV infection
Hepatoma	Androgen therapy
Kaposi sarcoma	HIV infection Transplant immunosuppression
Kidney cancer	Brain tumor therapies Cisplatin, especially in treatment for testicular cancer
Leukemia	Antitumor antibiotics Breast cancer treatment Lymphoma treatment Post-transplant immunosuppression Prostate cancer treatment
Lung cancer	HIV infection Therapeutic radiation for other cancers
Lymphoproliferative disorder (pre-malignant condition)	Corticosteroids Post-transplantation
Mesothelioma	Thoracic radiation for lung neoplasms (primary and secondary)
Neuroectodermal tumors	Growth hormone replacement after childhood cancers Therapeutic radiation for other cancers
Non-Hodgkin lymphoma	Alkylating agents Antimetabolites Antitumor antibiotics Cyclosporine Radiation therapy Tacrolimus
Rectal cancer	HIV infection
Salivary gland cancer	Head and neck radiation, especially in children
Sarcoma (soft tissue)	Therapeutic radiation for other cancers
Sebaceous tumors	Tacrolimus
Skin cancer (basal cell, squamous cell, melanoma)	Azathioprine Brachytherapy Sun/tanning bed exposure

(Continued on next page)

Table 11-9. Second Malignancies *(Continued)*	
Second Malignancy	**Potential Etiologic Factors**
Thyroid cancer	Brain tumor therapies Cisplatin-based regimens Therapeutic radiation

Note. Based on information from Abern et al., 2013; American Cancer Society, 2012; Bakker et al., 2007; Bhatia, 2013; Bhatia et al., 2007; Boukheris et al., 2013; Bowers et al., 2013; Fung et al., 2013; Kim, C.J., et al., 2013; Kim, D.W., et al., 2013; Lear et al., 2007; Perkins, Fei, et al., 2013; Rugge, 2013; Schwartz et al., 2014; Shinohara et al., 2014; Situm et al., 2007; Vajdic et al., 2006; Van den Broek et al., 2014; Wilson et al., 2013; Xu et al., 2013.

Pathophysiology

Second malignancies arise from damaged DNA that is unable to provide a normal RNA replication chain for normal cell division and maturation (Inman et al., 2007; Situm, Buljan, Bulic, & Simic, 2007). Despite clear chromosomal changes indicative of high risk for second malignancies, some individuals do not develop this complication. This suggests that DNA damage without impaired immune surveillance systems may not result in malignancy (Bakker et al., 2007; Situm et al., 2007). This is supported by the evidence that the highest-risk medications for development of second malignancies are those that are nonspecific in their action and likely to suppress lymphocyte activity. The chemotherapy agents that are used extensively in management of autoimmune disease (e.g., cyclophosphamide, methotrexate) are well-known carcinogens. Common chromosomal abnormalities associated with development of second malignancies include chromosome 5, 7, 22, and 23 deletions and translocations, trisomy 8, and complex karyotypes (Chang et al., 2007; Kim, C.J., et al., 2013; Larson, 2007). Sarcoma as a second malignancy occurs more frequently in a previous radiation portal (Schwartz et al., 2014). Out-of-field radiation exposure has also been documented in children and linked to later cancers of the breast, lung, and thyroid (Kourinou, Mazonakis, Lyraraki, Stratakis, & Damilakis, 2013; Strodtbeck et al., 2013). Mesothelioma occurs at a higher incidence in patients who have received radiation to the pleura (Farioli et al., 2013).

The average time from carcinogenic exposure to development of second malignancy varies dramatically from 13–36 months in patients receiving breast cancer treatment (Kaplan, Malmgren, & De Roos, 2013) to 10–15 years in survivors of childhood cancers (Wilson et al., 2010). Variables such as dose and exposure, as well as individual factors, cause variations of 2–20 years (Armstrong, 2010; Bowers et al., 2013; Oeffinger et al., 2013; Wilson et al., 2010).

Assessment

Because myeloproliferative, lymphoid, and soft tissue malignancies are most common, assessment of higher-risk patients includes periodic, thorough physical examinations and evaluation of any new, unexplained masses or enlarged lymph nodes. In many cases, the first symptoms of a second malignancy involve dysfunction of the hematopoietic cells with one of the cytopenias. Bone marrow or lymph node evaluation reveals malignant cells, and flow cytometry yields chromosomal abnormalities.

Prevention and Management

Reduced use of cell cycle–nonspecific chemotherapy agents, use of a more precise radiation delivery method, and decreased use of potent T-lymphocytic suppressive agents can reduce the likelihood of second malignancy after cancer treatment (Oeffinger et al., 2013; Rugge, 2013).

This strategy may be impractical in cases of life-threatening malignancy, but it is an option in solid organ transplant or autoimmune disease where other therapy options exist. Limiting radiation exposure through use of intensity modulation and radiation blocks to reduce exposure of normal structures has been effective at reducing radiation exposure and long-term risk for second malignancies (Hudson et al., 2009; Oeffinger et al., 2013).

Surveillance for potential malignancies is recommended in cancer survivors. Methods usually include periodic physical examinations with focus on masses or organ dysfunction and routine CBC and chemistry tests (Hudson et al., 2009).

When a patient presents with a second malignancy, the cytogenetics of the malignancy must be evaluated. This permits a choice of therapy based on knowledge of these resistant malignancies. The most potent available therapy often is implemented to ensure a rapid and comprehensive response.

Evaluation of Outcomes

An optimal outcome for patients with second malignancies is usually cancer control. Few of these resistant malignancies can be cured because of the extensiveness of cytogenetic abnormalities (Larson, 2007). After definitive therapy, follow-up computed tomography scans and bone marrow biopsies are completed to assess response. At times, follow-up tissue samples to validate eradication of a chromosome abnormality or viral antigen may be helpful, but these are difficult to obtain in every clinical situation.

Implications for Oncology Advanced Practice Nurses

APNs need to be aware of therapies that predispose patients to develop a second malignancy and may direct patients for more frequent follow-up. It may be impractical at the onset of cancer or autoimmune therapy to discuss the possibility of future malignancy, although this often is included in informed consent documents. It is ideal to discuss this risk and potential implications at a time when patients are stable and anxiety is less acute. Individuals experiencing second malignancies will require education and emotional support to assist them in making treatment decisions and understanding the prognostic implications of their decisions.

Conclusion

Myelosuppression and second malignancies after cancer treatment remain significant clinical concerns for oncology APNs. Myelosuppression is common and is the source of significant morbidity and mortality among all types and ages of patients with cancer. This complication encompasses risk for infection from neutropenia, bleeding from thrombocytopenia, and the myriad adverse effects related to anemia. Interventions to prevent or ameliorate the adverse effects of myelosuppression are nursing sensitive in nature and in the domain of independent or collaborative nursing practice. Oncology APNs can provide direct guidance for best practice in prevention and management of this complication while also providing staff education and addressing systems issues affecting care of these patients. Second malignancies are a rare but serious complication of cancer care. Oncology APNs must be knowledgeable of risk factors and screening and detection techniques that can enhance outcomes for these patients. Assisting in development of survivorship care plans for patients at highest risk for second malignancies can ensure that proper screening leads to early diagnosis and management when second malignancies occur. The role of the oncology APN involving the patient, nurse, and system spheres provides opportunities to enhance the care of all patients experiencing myelosuppression or second malignancies during and after cancer care.

Case Study

M.C. is a 67-year-old woman who presents with abdominal distension and palpable groin lymphadenopathy. She has a past medical history of smoking, hypertension, and a four-year history of immune thrombocytopenic purpura without known risk factors. Lymph node biopsy revealed follicular large cell lymphoma, stage IVB. The APN notes that despite an enlarged abdomen, the patient reports unintentional weight loss of 20 pounds over two months, profound fatigue, back pain, and night sweats. On physical examination, the APN notes a palpable liver and spleen. The APN realizes that M.H. has several risk factors for bone marrow suppression even before cancer treatment begins.

1. What are these risk factors?
   - In light of her advanced disease, she may have bone marrow involvement, and her age, malnourished state, and chronic diseases also may contribute to myelosuppression. Upon further assessment, the APN discovers that M.H. has a history of ongoing thrombocytopenia without hemorrhagic episodes. Physical assessment reveals pale oral mucosal membranes with two small aphthous ulcers inside the lower lip, cool extremities, slow capillary refill, weak and thready pedal pulses, and truncal petechiae. The microscopic urine shows RBCs and WBCs.
   - M.H.'s initial CBC results are as follows.

Blood Counts	Patient's Values	Normal
RBCs	2.9 cells/mm^3	$3.5–5 \times 10^6$/mm^3
MCV	100 mcg/mm^3	80–96 mcg/mm^3
MCH	27 pg/cell	26–34 pg/cell
MCHC	31 g/dl	31–37 g/dl
Hematocrit	29%	35%–45%
Hemoglobin	10.2 mg/dl	12–15 mg/dl
WBCs	3,800/mm^3	5,000–10,000/mm^3
Neutrophils	52%	33%–75%
Basophils	1%	2%–6%
Eosinophils	1%	1%–5%
Bands	3%	< 20%
Monocytes	6%	1%–10%
Lymphocytes	42%	12%–44%
Platelet count	34,000/mm^3	150,000–250,000/mm^3
Morphology/atypical cells	Hypochromia, megaloblasts	–

   - After examination of this blood work, the APN realizes that M.H. has a preexisting anemia.

2. What is the most likely type of anemia revealed in this CBC?
   - The type of anemia revealed by this CBC is megaloblastic (large immature cells) anemia as indicated by the MCV, and morphology indicates either folate or B_{12} deficiency. Her baseline anemia with increased MCV and hypochromic, macrocytic cells prompted a pretreatment assessment of ferritin and folate levels. Ferritin levels were low normal, and the folate level was 2 mg/dl, a value lower than normal. M.H. is prescribed a daily multivitamin with iron. M.H.'s current hemoglobin of 10.2 mg/dl does not require intervention at this time but warrants close observation of response to nutritional supplementation and expected chemotherapy suppression. Correction of nutritional anemias is essential prior to consideration for erythropoiesis-stimulating agents.
3. What is M.H.'s ANC based on this laboratory work?
   - To calculate, multiply the total number of WBCs by the percentage of neutrophils: ANC = 3,800 × 0.52 = 1,976/mm³. M.H.'s ANC is slightly abnormal. It is concerning that she is older, has chronic illnesses, and has a starting baseline leukopenia and neutropenia prior to initiating therapy, therefore placing her at considerable risk for protracted chemotherapy-induced neutropenia and its complications. M.H. is prescribed rituximab with CHOP (cyclophosphamide, doxorubicin, vincristine, and prednisone) chemotherapy.
4. Based on these WBC and neutrophil counts, what prophylactic measures will be implemented with the first cycle of chemotherapy to minimize the effects of myelosuppression?
   - Because of her baseline WBC suppression, pegfilgrastim was administered 24 hours after the first cycle of chemotherapy. She and her family received extensive education on prevention of infection at home. After her second cycle of chemotherapy, she reported profound fatigue, altered cognition, and an inability to perform normal self-care activities. At that time, her hemoglobin was 9.9 mg/dl, and an erythropoiesis-stimulating agent was prescribed. Given her symptomatology and clearly persistent anemia after nutritional supplementation, the risks and benefits of an erythropoiesis-stimulating agent were discussed and informed consent was obtained. The patient was aware that erythropoiesis-stimulating agents can increase blood viscosity and have been associated with hypertension, hypercoagulability, and increased mortality in some patients. After four weeks and a modest increase in hemoglobin, M.H. begins IV iron supplementation with her erythropoiesis-stimulating factor, with successful normalization of RBC counts.
5. Would the APN transfuse M.H. with RBCs while waiting for the erythropoietin to begin marrow stimulation?
   - This hemoglobin level of 9.9 mg/dl does not require RBC transfusions unless clinical evidence exists of tissue ischemia or cardiovascular compromise (e.g., abdominal pain with bowel ischemia and elevated lactate dehydrogenase, cardiac ischemia on electrocardiogram, chest pain, intractable tachycardia associated with hypotension).
   - Between the second and third cycle, M.H. develops a fever of 38.3°C (101°F) with accompanying epistaxis. Her platelet count is stable at 26,000/mm³, but occult blood in the stool and urine prompts the clinicians to consider platelet transfusion. She is admitted to the hospital for fluids and IV antibiotics. She receives platelet transfusions, but her platelet count does not rise. After resolution of her infectious episode, the bleeding resolves spontaneously, causing the clinicians to suspect that bleeding was related to altered platelet quality from fever and infection.

Key Points

Myelosuppression

- Oncology APNs must consider the following when prescribing chemotherapy regimens: patient monitoring, need for hematopoietic growth factors, and staff nurse consultation for management of myelosuppression.

- Patients at high risk for development of severe myelosuppression (and potential candidates for preventive measures) include those with advanced age (older than 65 years); poor nutritional status; preexisting autoimmune disease, diabetes mellitus, gastrointestinal disorders, liver disease, or hematopoietic diseases; and substance abuse.
- Independent risk factors for development of anemia in patients with cancer include female sex; older age; lower initial hemoglobin in females; breast, lung, and gynecologic malignancies; and treatment with platinol agents.
- The normal proliferation rate of erythrocytes, platelets, or leukocytes determines the severity and timing of suppression following exposure to a toxin such as chemotherapy. Depletion of the cell line is directly related to the normal turnover rate of the cell line after the antineoplastic agent destroys normal regrowth mechanisms.
- Granulocytes live about six to eight hours, with leukopenia occurring about 7–15 days after treatment.
- Platelets live about 5–7 days; they have the longest nadir and may persist for more than 20 days.
- Erythrocytes live about 120 days; the onset of anemia usually occurs following the second or third cycle of therapy.
- The ANC is indicative of the number of neutrophils available to combat infection. It is calculated by multiplying the total number of WBCs by the percentage of neutrophils detected.
- Radiation therapy may cause bone marrow suppression, but less frequently than chemotherapy. Myelosuppression can occur following radiation therapy when the treatment field involves marrow-producing tissue or with doses greater than 1,500 cGy. Myelosuppression peaks in the third week of radiation therapy and often manifests as aplasia occurring simultaneously in all cell lines rather than sequentially as seen with chemotherapy.

Second Malignancies

- Most second malignancies are myeloid, lymphoid, or soft tissue in origin; more rare are highly aggressive forms of glioma, cervical cancer, rectal cancer, mesothelioma, and non-small cell lung cancer. Sarcomas are the most common malignancy related to radiation exposure.
- The incidence of second malignancies is highest in children (approximately 4%), approximately 2%–3% in solid organ transplant recipients, and approximately 1.5%–3% in patients receiving radiation therapy. People at greatest risk are females treated for Hodgkin disease between ages 10 and 15 and males with acute lymphoblastic leukemia treated between ages 4.6 and 6.6 (Wilson et al., 2010). The risk for second malignancies increases steadily with time after exposure, particularly for survivors of childhood cancer.
- Evidence exists that medications with the highest risk for causing the development of second malignancies are nonspecific in their action and are likely to suppress lymphocyte activity, such as agents used in the management of autoimmune disease (e.g., cyclophosphamide, methotrexate).
- The average time from carcinogenic exposure to development of second malignancy varies from 13 months to 20 years, dependent on treatment modality, dose, and exposure, as well as individual factors.

Recommended Resources for Oncology Advanced Practice Nurses

- AABB (formerly the American Association of Blood Banks) Services and Standards: www .aabb.org

- Centers for Disease Control and Prevention: www.cdc.gov
- Leukemia and Lymphoma Society: www.leukemia-lymphoma.org
- Memorial Sloan Kettering Cancer Center: About Herbs, Botanicals and Other Products: www.mskcc.org/cancer-care/integrative-medicine/about-herbs-botanicals-other-products
- National Center for Complementary and Integrative Health: https://nccih.nih.gov
- NCI CTEP: http://ctep.cancer.gov

References

Aapro, M.S., Bohlius, J., Cameron, D.A., Dal Lago, L., Donnelly, J.P., Kearney, N., … Zielinski, C. (2011). 2010 update of EORTC guidelines for the use of granulocyte-colony stimulating factor to reduce the incidence of chemotherapy-induced febrile neutropenia in adult patients with lymphoproliferative disorders and solid tumours. *European Journal of Cancer, 47,* 8–32. doi:10.1016/j.ejca.2010.10.013

Abern, M.R., Dude, A.M., Tsivian, M., & Coogan, C.L. (2013). The characteristics of bladder cancer after radiotherapy for prostate cancer. *Urologic Oncology, 31,* 1628–1634. doi:10.1016/j.urolonc.2012.04.006

Adamson, J.W. (2008). The anemia of inflammation/malignancy: Mechanisms and management. *American Society of Hematology Education Program Book, 2008,* 159–165. doi:10.1182/asheducation-2008.1.159

Ahn, S., & Lee, Y.S. (2012). Predictive factors for poor prognosis febrile neutropenia. *Current Opinion in Oncology, 24,* 376–380. doi:10.1097/CCO.0b013e328352ead2

American Cancer Society. (2012). Second cancers caused by cancer treatment. Retrieved from http://www.cancer.org/cancer/cancercauses/othercarcinogens/medicaltreatments/secondcancerscausedbycancertreatment/second-cancers-caused-by-cancer-treatment-toc

Andres, E., Dali-Youcef, N., Serraj, K., & Zimmer, J. (2009). Recognition and management of drug-induced cytopenias: The example of idiosyncratic drug-induced thrombocytopenia. *Expert Opinion on Drug Safety, 8,* 183–190. doi:10.1517/14740330902784162

Armstrong, G.T. (2010). Long-term survivors of childhood central nervous system malignancies: The experience of the Childhood Cancer Survivor Study. *European Journal of Paediatric Neurology, 14,* 298–303. doi:10.1016/j.ejpn.2009.12.006

Bacon, B.R., Adams, P.C., Kowdley, K.V., Powell, L.W., & Tavill, A.S. (2011). Diagnosis and management of hemochromatosis: 2011 practice guideline by the American Association for the Study of Liver Diseases. *Hepatology, 54,* 328–354. doi:10.1002/hep.24330

Bakker, N.A., van Imhoff, G.W., Verschuuren, E.A.M., & van Son, W.J. (2007). Presentation and early detection of post-transplant lymphoproliferative disorder after solid organ transplantation. *Transplant International, 20,* 207–218. doi:10.1111/j.1432-2277.2006.00416.x

Barber, N.A., Afzal, W., & Akhtari, M. (2011). Hematologic toxicities of small molecule tyrosine kinase inhibitors. *Targeted Oncology, 6,* 203–215. doi:10.1007/s11523-011-0202-9

Baribeault, D., & Auerbach, M. (2011). Iron replacement therapy in cancer-related anemia. *American Journal of Health-System Pharmacy, 68*(10, Suppl. 1), S4–S14. doi:10.2146/ajhp110039

Bartley, J.M. (2000). APIC state-of-the-art report: The role of infection control during construction in health care facilities. *American Journal of Infection Control, 28,* 156–169. doi:10.1067/mic.2000.106055

Bekelman, J.E., Schultheiss, T., De Gonzalez, A.B. (2013). Subsequent malignancies after photon versus proton radiation therapy. *International Journal of Radiation Oncology, Biology, Physics, 87,* 10–12. doi:10.1016/j.ijrobp.2013.05.016

Benjamin, R.J., & Anderson, K.C. (2002). What is the proper threshold for platelet transfusion in patients with chemotherapy-induced thrombocytopenia? *Critical Reviews in Oncology/Hematology, 42,* 163–171. doi:10.1016/S1040-8428(01)00182-2

Bennett, C.L., Djulbegovic, B., Norris, L.B., & Armitage, J.O. (2013). Colony-stimulating factors for febrile neutropenia during cancer therapy. *New England Journal of Medicine, 368,* 1131–1139. doi:10.1016/j.ijrobp.2012.09.001

Bhatia, S. (2013). Therapy-related myelodysplasia and acute myeloid leukemia. *Seminars in Oncology, 40,* 666–675. doi:10.1053/j.seminoncol.2013.09.013

Bhatia, S., Krailo, M.D., Chen, Z., Burden, L., Askin, F.B., Dickman, P.S., … Miser, J.S. (2007). Therapy-related myelodysplasia and acute myeloid leukemia after Ewing sarcoma and primitive neuroectodermal tumor of bone: A report from the Children's Oncology Group. *Blood, 109,* 46–51. doi:10.1182/blood-2006-01-023101

Blay, J., Gomez, F., Sebban, C., Bachelot, T., Biron, P., Guglielmi, C., … Philip, T. (1998). The International Prognostic Index correlates to survival in patients with aggressive lymphoma in relapse: Analysis of the PARMA trial. *Blood, 92,* 3562–3568. Retrieved from http://www.bloodjournal.org/content/92/10/3562.long

Blot, F., Cordonnier, C., Buzin, A., Nitenberg, G., Schlemmer, B., & Bastuji-Garin, S. (2001). Severity of illness scores: Are they useful in febrile neutropenic adult patients in hematology wards? A prospective multicenter study. *Critical Care Medicine, 29,* 2125–2131. doi:10.1097/00003246-200111000-00013

Bohlius, J., Tonia, T., & Schwarzer, G. (2011). Twist and shout: One decade of meta-analyses of erythropoiesis-stimulating agents in cancer patients. *Acta Haematologica, 125,* 55–67. doi:10.1159/000318897

Boukheris, H., Stovall, M., Gilbert, E.S., Stratton, K.L., Smith, S.A., Weathers, R., ... Inskip, P.D. (2013). Risk of salivary gland cancer after childhood cancer: A report from the Childhood Cancer Survivor Study. *International Journal of Radiation Oncology, Biology, Physics, 85,* 776–783. doi:10.1016/j.ijrobp.2012.06.006

Bow, E.J. (2013). Infection in neutropenic patients with cancer. *Critical Care Clinics, 29,* 411–441. doi:10.1016/j.ccc.2013.03.002

Bowers, D.C., Nathan, P.C., Constine, L., Woodman, C., Bhatia, S., Keller, K., ... Bashore, L. (2013). Subsequent neoplasms of the CNS among survivors of childhood cancer: A systematic review. *Lancet Oncology, 14,* e321–e328. doi:10.1016/S1470-2045(13)70107-4

Boyce, J.M., & Pettit, D. (2002). Guideline for hand hygiene in health-care settings: Recommendations of the Healthcare Infection Control Practices Advisory Committee and the HICPAC/SHEA/APIC/IDSA Hand Hygiene Task Force. Society for Healthcare Epidemiology of America/Association for Professionals in Infection Control/Infectious Diseases Society of America. *Morbidity and Mortality Weekly Report: Recommendations and Reports, 51*(RR-16), 1–45.

Camp-Sorrell, D. (2011). Chemotherapy toxicities and management. In C.H. Yarbro, D. Wujcik, & B.H. Gobel (Eds.), *Cancer nursing: Principles and practice* (7th ed., pp. 458–503). Burlington, MA: Jones & Bartlett Learning.

Carson, J.L., Grossman, B.J., Kleinman, S., Tinmouth, A.T., Marques, M.B., Fung, M.K., ... Djulbegovic, B. (2012). Red blood cell transfusion: A clinical practice guideline from the AABB. *Annals of Internal Medicine, 157,* 49–58. doi:10.7326/0003-4819-157-1-201206190-00429

Cella, D. (1997). The Functional Assessment of Cancer Therapy-Anemia (FACT-An) Scale: A new tool for the assessment of outcomes in cancer anemia and fatigue. *Seminars in Hematology, 34*(3, Suppl. 2), 13–19.

Centers for Disease Control and Prevention. (2011). *Basic infection control and prevention plan for outpatient oncology settings.* Retrieved from http://www.cdc.gov/hai/pdfs/guidelines/basic-infection-control-prevention-plan-2011.pdf

Chan, A., Verma, S., Loibl, S., Crawford, J., Choi, M.R., Dreiling, L., & Vandenberg, T. (2012). Reporting of myelotoxicity associated with emerging regimens for the treatment of selected solid tumors. *Critical Reviews in Oncology/Hematology, 81,* 136–150. doi:10.1016/j.critrevonc.2011.03.003

Chang, C., Storer, B.E., Scott, B.L., Bryant, E.M., Shulman, H.M., Flowers, M.E., ... Deeg, H.J. (2007). Hematopoietic cell transplantation in patients with myelodysplastic syndrome or acute myeloid leukemia arising from myelodysplastic syndrome: Similar outcomes in patients with de novo disease and disease following prior therapy or antecedent hematologic disorders. *Blood, 110,* 1379–1387. doi:10.1182/blood-2007-02-076307

Chang, J.E., & Kahl, B.S. (2012). Bendamustine for treatment of chronic lymphocytic leukemia. *Expert Opinion on Pharmacotherapy, 13,* 1495–1505. doi:10.1517/14656566.2012.693163

Chaturvedi, A.K., Pfeiffer, R.M., Chang, L., Goedert, J.J., Biggar, R.J., & Engels, E.A. (2007). Elevated risk of lung cancer among people with AIDS. *AIDS, 21,* 207–213. doi:10.1097/QAD.0b013e3280118fca

Chiu, J., Yau, T., & Epstein, R.J. (2009). Complications of traditional Chinese/herbal medicines (TCM)—A guide for perplexed oncologists and other cancer caregivers. *Supportive Care in Cancer, 17,* 231–240. doi:10.1007/s00520-008-0526-x

Chung, C.S., Yock, T.I., Nelson, K., Xu, Y., Keating, N.L., & Tarbell, N.J. (2013). Incidence of second malignancies among patients treated with proton versus photon radiation. *International Journal of Radiation Oncology, Biology, Physics, 87,* 46–52. doi:10.1016/j.ijrobp.2013.04.030

Cooper, K.L., Madan, J., Whyte, S., Stevenson, M.D., & Akehurst, R.L. (2011). Granulocyte colony-stimulating factors for febrile neutropenia prophylaxis following chemotherapy: Systematic review and meta-analysis. *BMC Cancer, 11,* 404. doi:10.1186/1471-2407-11-404.

Coyne, D. (2006). Iron indices: What do they really mean? *Kidney International, 69*(Suppl. 101), S4–S8. doi:10.1038/sj.ki.5000404

Crea, F., Giovannetti, E., Zinzani, P.L., & Danesi, R. (2009). Pharmacologic rationale for early G-CSF prophylaxis in cancer patients and role of pharmacogenetics in treatment optimization. *Critical Reviews in Oncology/Hematology, 72,* 21–44. doi:10.1016/j.critrevonc.2008.10.014

Curtis, R.E., Freedman, D.M., Ron, E., Ries, L.A.G., Hacker, D.G., Edwards, B.K., ... Fraumeni, J.F., Jr. (Eds.). (2006). *New malignancies among cancer survivors: SEER cancer registries, 1973–2000* (NIH Pub No. 05-5302). Bethesda, MD: National Cancer Institute.

Dale, D.C., & Welte, K. (2011). Cyclic and chronic neutropenia. In G.H. Lyman & D.C. Dale (Eds.), *Cancer Treatment and Research: Vol. 157. Hematopoietic growth factors in oncology* (pp. 97–108). doi:10.1007/978-1-4419-7073-2_6

Dantal, J., & Pohanka, E. (2007). Malignancies in renal transplantation: An unmet medical need. *Nephrology Dialysis Transplantation, 22*(Suppl. 1), i4–i10. doi:10.1093/ndt/gfm085

de Gonzalez, A.B., Gilbert, E., Curtis, R., Inskip, P., Kleinerman, R., Morton, L., … Little, M.P. (2013). Second solid cancers after radiation therapy: A systematic review of the epidemiologic studies of the radiation dose-response relationship. *International Journal of Radiation Oncology, Biology, Physics, 86,* 224–233. doi:10.1016/j.ijrobp.2012.09.001

de Lemos, M.L., John, L., Nakashima, L., O'Brien, R.K., & Taylor, S.C. (2004). Advising cancer patients on natural health products—A structured approach. *Annals of Pharmacotherapy, 38,* 1406–1411. doi:10.1345/aph.1E062

Despotis, G.J., Zhang, L., & Lublin, D.M. (2007). Transfusion risks and transfusion-related pro-inflammatory response. *Hematology/Oncology Clinics of North America, 21,* 147–161. doi:10.1016/j.hoc.2006.11.002

Dixit, S., Baker, L., Walmsley, V., & Hingorani, M. (2012). Temozolomide-related idiosyncratic and other uncommon toxicities: A systematic review. *Anti-Cancer Drugs, 23,* 1099–1106. doi:10.1097/CAD.0b013e328356f5b0

Dunleavy, K., Tay, K., & Wilson, W.H. (2010). Rituximab-associated neutropenia. *Seminars in Hematology, 47,* 180–186. doi:10.1053/j.seminhematol.2010.01.009

Erb, C.H., & Vogel, W. (2013). Management of the complications of hematologic malignancies. In M. Olsen & L.J. Zitella (Eds.), *Hematologic malignancies in adults* (pp. 537–648). Pittsburgh, PA: Oncology Nursing Society.

Farioli, A., Violante, F.S., Mattioli, S., Curti, S., & Kriebel, D. (2013). Risk of mesothelioma following external beam radiotherapy for prostate cancer: A cohort analysis of SEER database. *Cancer Causes and Control, 24,* 1535–1545. doi:10.1007/s10552-013-0230-0

Ferrucci, L., & Balducci, L. (2008). Anemia of aging: The role of chronic inflammation and cancer. *Seminars in Hematology, 45,* 242–249. doi:10.1053/j.seminhematol.2008.06.001

Fleming, R.E., & Ponka, P. (2012). Iron overload in human disease. *New England Journal of Medicine, 366,* 348–359. doi:10.1056/NEJMra1004967

Flowers, C.R., Seidenfeld, J., Bow, E.J., Karten, C., Gleason, C., Hawley, D.K., … Ramsey, S.D. (2013). Antimicrobial prophylaxis and outpatient management of fever and neutropenia in adults treated for malignancy: American Society of Clinical Oncology clinical practice guideline. *Journal of Clinical Oncology, 31,* 794–810. doi:10.1200/JCO.2012.45.8661

Fogarty, P.F., & Dunbar, C.E. (2013). Thrombocytopenia. In G. Rodgers & N. Young (Eds.), *Bethesda handbook of hematology* (3rd ed., pp. 269–284). Philadelphia, PA: Wolters Kluwer Health/Lippincott Williams & Wilkins.

Fox, N., & Freifeld, A.G. (2012). The neutropenic diet reviewed: Moving toward a safe food handling approach. *Oncology, 26,* 572–575, 580, 582.

Freifeld, A.G., Bow, E.J., Sepkowitz, K.A., Boeckh, M.J., Ito, J.I., Mullen, C.A., … Wingard, J.R. (2011). Executive summary: Clinical practice guideline for the use of antimicrobial agents in neutropenic patients with cancer: 2010 update by the Infectious Diseases Society of America. *Clinical Infectious Diseases, 52,* 427–431. doi:10.1093/cid/ciq147

Friese, C. (2007). Prevention of infection in patients with cancer. *Seminars in Oncology Nursing, 23,* 174–183. doi:10.1016/j.soncn.2007.05.002

Fung, C., Fossa, S.D., Milano, M.T., Oldenburg, J., & Travis, L.B. (2013). Solid tumors after chemotherapy or surgery for testicular nonseminoma: A population-based study. *Journal of Clinical Oncology, 31,* 3807–3814. doi:10.1200/JCO.2013.50.3409

Gafter-Gvili, A., Fraser, A., Paul, M., Vidal, L., Lawrie, T.A., van de Wetering, M.D., … Leibovici, L. (2012). Antibiotic prophylaxis for bacterial infections in afebrile neutropenic patients following chemotherapy. *Cochrane Database of Systematic Reviews, 2012*(1). doi:10.1002/14651858.CD004386.pub3

Galel, S.A., Nguyen, D.D., Fontaine, M.J., Goodnough, L.T., & Viele, M.K. (2009). Transfusion medicine. In J.P. Greer, J. Foerster, G.M. Rodgers, F. Paraskevas, B. Glader, D.A. Arber, & R.T. Means Jr. (Eds.), *Wintrobe's clinical hematology* (12th ed., pp. 672–721). Philadelphia, PA: Wolters Kluwer Health/Lippincott Williams & Wilkins.

Gardner, A., Mattiuzzi, G., Faderl, S., Borthakur, G., Garcia-Manero, G., Pierce, S., … Estey, E. (2008). Randomized comparison of cooked and noncooked diets in patients undergoing remission induction therapy for acute myeloid leukemia. *Journal of Clinical Oncology, 26,* 5684–5688. doi:10.1200/JCO.2008.16.4681

George-Gay, B., & Parker, K. (2003). Understanding the complete blood count with differential. *Journal of PeriAnesthesia Nursing, 18,* 96–117. doi:10.1053/jpan.2003.50013

Georgiou, K.R., Foster, B.K., & Xian, C.J. (2010). Damage and recovery of the bone marrow microenvironment induced by cancer chemotherapy—Potential regulatory role of chemokine CXCL12/receptor CXCR4 signalling. *Current Molecular Medicine, 10,* 440–453. doi:10.2174/156652410791608243

Ghanima, W., Godeau, B., Cines, D.B., & Bussel, J.B. (2012). How I treat immune thrombocytopenia: The choice between splenectomy or a medical therapy as a second-line treatment. *Blood, 120,* 960–969. doi:10.1182/blood-2011-12-309153

Goroll, A.H., & Mulley, A.G., Jr. (2009). Evaluation of anemia. In A.H. Goroll & A.G. Mulley Jr. (Eds.), *Primary care medicine: Office evaluation and management of the adult patient* (6th ed., pp. 627–636). Philadelphia, PA: Wolters Kluwer Health/Lippincott Williams & Wilkins.

Greenberg, P.L., Rigsby, C.K., Stone, R.M., Deeg, H.J., Gore, S.D., Millenson, M.M., … Kumar, P. (2009). NCCN task force: Transfusion and iron overload in patients with myelodysplastic syndromes. *Journal of the National Comprehensive Cancer Network, 7*(Suppl. 9), S1–S16.

Grossman, S.A., Ye, X., Lesser, G., Sloan, A., Carraway, H., Desideri, S., & Piantadosi, S. (2011). Immunosuppression in patients with high-grade gliomas treated with radiation and temozolomide. *Clinical Cancer Research, 17,* 5473–5480. doi:10.1158/1078-0432.CCR-11-0774

Gualberto, A. (2012). Brentuximab vedotin (SGN-35), an antibody–drug conjugate for the treatment of CD30-positive malignancies. *Expert Opinion on Investigational Drugs, 21,* 205–216. doi:10.1517/13543784.2011.641532

Guberski, T.D. (2013). Anatomy and physiology of the hematological and immune systems. In P.G. Morton & D.K. Fontaine (Eds.), *Critical care nursing: A holistic approach* (10th ed., pp. 1021–1033). Philadelphia, PA: Wolters Kluwer Health/Lippincott Williams & Wilkins.

Haase, V.H. (2010). Hypoxic regulation of erythropoiesis and iron metabolism. *American Journal of Physiology—Renal Physiology, 299,* F1–F13. doi:10.1152/ajprenal.00174.2010

Hayes, N.A. (2001). Analyzing current practice patterns: Lessons from Amgen's Project ChemoInsight. *Oncology Nursing Forum, 28*(Suppl. 2), 11–16.

Held, T.K., & Gundert-Remy, U. (2010). Pharmacodynamic effects of haematopoietic cytokines: The view of a clinical oncologist. *Basic and Clinical Pharmacology and Toxicology, 106,* 210–214. doi:10.1111/j.1742–7843.2009.00514.x

Herbst, C., Naumann, F., Kruse, E.-B., Monsef, I., Bohlius, J., Schulz, H., & Engert, A. (2009). Prophylactic antibiotics or G-CSF for the prevention of infections and improvement of survival in cancer patients undergoing chemotherapy. *Cochrane Database of Systematic Reviews, 2009*(1). doi:10.1002/14651858.CD007107.pub2

Hincks, I., Woodcock, B.E., & Thachil, J. (2011). Is rituximab-induced late-onset neutropenia a good prognostic indicator in lymphoproliferative disorders? *British Journal of Haematology, 153,* 411–413. doi:10.1111/j.1365-2141.2010.08563.x

Hinkel, J.M., Li, E.C., & Sherman, S.L. (2010). Insights and perspectives in the clinical and operational management of cancer-related anemia. *Journal of the National Comprehensive Cancer Network, 8*(Suppl. 7), S38–S55.

Hudson, M.M., Mulrooney, D.A., Bowers, D.C., Sklar, C.A., Green, D.M., Donaldson, S.S., … Robison, L.L. (2009). High-risk populations identified in Childhood Cancer Survivor Study investigations: Implications for risk-based surveillance. *Journal of Clinical Oncology, 27,* 2405–2414. doi:10.1200/JCO.2008.21.1516

Inman, B.A., Frigola, X., Dong, H., & Kwon, E.D. (2007). Costimulation, coinhibition and cancer. *Current Cancer Drug Targets, 7,* 15–30. doi:10.2174/156800907780006878

Intragumtornchai, T., Sutheesophon, J., Sutcharitchan, P., & Swasdikul, D. (2000). A predictive model for life-threatening neutropenia and febrile neutropenia after the first course of CHOP chemotherapy in patients with aggressive non-Hodgkin's lymphoma. *Leukemia and Lymphoma, 37,* 351–360. Retrieved from http://informahealthcare.com/doi/abs/10.3109/10428190009089435

Irwin, M., Erb, C., Williams, C., Wilson, B.J., & Zitella, L.J. (2013). *Putting evidence into practice: Improving oncology patient outcomes; Prevention of infection.* Pittsburgh, PA: Oncology Nursing Society.

Jazbec, J., Todorovski, L., & Jereb, B. (2007). Classification tree analysis of second neoplasms in survivors of childhood cancer. *BMC Cancer, 7,* 27. doi:10.1186/1471-2407-7-27

Kalaycio, M. (2009). Bendamustine: A new look at an old drug. *Cancer, 115,* 473–479. doi:10.1002/cncr.24057

Kaplan, H., Malmgren, J., & De Roos, A.J. (2013). Risk of myelodysplastic syndrome and acute myeloid leukemia post radiation treatment for breast cancer: A population-based study. *Breast Cancer Research and Treatment, 137,* 863–867. doi:10.1007/s10549-012-2386-9

Khan, H., Belsher, J., Yilmaz, M., Afessa, B., Winters, J.L., Moore, S.B., … Gajic, O. (2007). Fresh-frozen plasma and platelet transfusions are associated with development of acute lung injury in critically ill medical patients. *Chest, 131,* 1308–1314. doi:10.1378/chest.06-3048

Kim, C.J., Freedman, D.M., Curtis, R.E., de Gonzalez, A.B., & Morton, L.M. (2013). Risk of non-Hodgkin lymphoma after radiotherapy for solid cancers. *Leukemia and Lymphoma, 54,* 1691–1697. doi:10.3109/10428194.2012.753543

Kim, D.W., Chung, W.K., Shin, D., Hong, S., Park, S.H., Park, S.-Y., … Yoon, M. (2013). Risk of second cancer from scattered radiation of intensity-modulated radiotherapies with lung cancer. *Radiation Oncology, 8,* 47. doi:10.1186/1748-717X-8-47

Kim, J.W., Singh, N.K., & Arlen, P.M. (2014). Hematopoietic growth factors. In J. Abraham, J.L. Gulley, & C.J. Allegra (Eds.), *Bethesda handbook of clinical oncology* (4th ed., pp. 439–447). Philadelphia, PA: Wolters Kluwer Health/Lippincott Williams & Wilkins.

Kim, W.-H., Yoon, S.H., Kim, C.-Y., Kim, K.-J., Lee, M.M., Choe, G., … Kim, H.-J. (2011). Temozolomide for malignant primary spinal cord glioma: An experience of six cases and a literature review. *Journal of Neuro-Oncology, 101,* 247–254. doi:10.1007/s11060-010-0249-y

Koukourakis, G.V., Kouloulias, V., Zacharias, G., Papadimitriou, C., Pantelakos, P., Maravelis, G., … Kouvaris, J. (2009). Temozolomide with radiation therapy in high grade brain gliomas: Pharmaceuticals considerations and efficacy; A review article. *Molecules, 14,* 1561–1577. doi:10.3390/molecules14041561

Kourinou, K.M., Mazonakis, M., Lyraraki, E., Stratakis, J., & Damilakis, J. (2013). Scattered dose to radiosensitive organs and associated risk for cancer development from head and neck radiotherapy in pediatric patients. *European Journal of Medical Physics, 29,* 650–655. doi:10.1016/j.ejmp.2012.08.001

Koury, M.J., & Lichtman, M.A. (2010). Structure of the marrow and the hematopoietic microenvironment. In K. Kaushansky, M.A. Lichtman, E. Beutler, T.J. Kipps, U. Seligsohn, & T.J. Prchal (Eds.), *Williams hematology* (8th ed., pp. 41–73). New York, NY: McGraw-Hill.

Kroger, A.T., Sumaya, C.V., Pickering, L.K., & Atkinson, W.L. (2011). General recommendations on immunization: Recommendations of the Advisory Committee on Immunization Practices (ACIP). *Morbidity and Mortality Weekly Report: Recommendations and Reports, 60*(RR02), 1–60. Retrieved from http://www.cdc.gov/mmwr/preview/mmwrhtml/rr6002a1.htm?s_cid=rr6002a1_e

Kulkarni, S., Ghosh, S.P., Hauer-Jensen, M., & Kumar, K.S. (2010). Hematological targets of radiation damage. *Current Drug Targets, 11,* 1375–1385. doi:10.2174/1389450111009011375

Kuter, D.J. (2015). Managing thrombocytopenia associated with cancer chemotherapy. *Oncology, 29,* 282–294. Retrieved from http://www.cancernetwork.com/oncology-journal/managing-thrombocytopenia-associated-cancer-chemotherapy

Kuter, D.J., Bussel, J.B., Newland, A., Baker, R.I., Lyons, R.M., Wasser, J., … Jun, S. (2013). Long-term treatment with romiplostim in patients with chronic immune thrombocytopenia: Safety and efficacy. *British Journal of Haematology, 161,* 411–423. doi:10.1111/bjh.12260

Kwiatkowski, J.L. (2011). Management of transfusional iron overload—Differential properties and efficacy of iron chelating agents. *Journal of Blood Medicine, 2,* 135–149. doi:10.2147/JBM.S13065

Landier, W., & Smith, S. (2011). Late effects of cancer treatment. In C.H. Yarbro, D. Wujcik, & B.H. Gobel (Eds.), *Cancer nursing: Principles and practice* (7th ed., pp. 1755–1779). Burlington, MA: Jones & Bartlett Learning.

Larson, R.A. (2007). Is secondary leukemia an independent poor prognostic factor in acute myeloid leukemia? *Best Practice and Research: Clinical Haematology, 20,* 29–37. doi:10.1016/j.beha.2006.10.006

Lear, W., Dahlke, E., & Murray, C.A. (2007). Basal cell carcinoma: Review of epidemiology, pathogenesis, and associated risk factors. *Journal of Cutaneous Medicine and Surgery, 11,* 19–30.

Liebman, H.A. (2014). Thrombocytopenia in cancer patients. *Thrombosis Research, 133*(Suppl. 2), S63–S69. doi:10.1016/S0049-3848(14)50011-4

Lyman, G.H. (2009). Impact of chemotherapy dose intensity on cancer patient outcomes. *Journal of the National Comprehensive Cancer Network, 7,* 99–108. Retrieved from http://www.jnccn.org/content/7/1/99.long

Lyman, G.H., & Kleiner, J.M. (2011). Summary and comparison of myeloid growth factor guidelines in patients receiving cancer chemotherapy. *Cancer Treatment and Research, 157,* 145–165. doi:10.1007/978-1-4419-7073-2_9

Lyman, G.H., Lyman, C.H., & Agboola, O. (2005). Risk models for predicting chemotherapy-induced neutropenia. *Oncologist, 10,* 427–437. doi:10.1634/theoncologist.10-6-427

Machado, C.M. (2005). Reimmunization after hematopoietic stem cell transplantation. *Expert Review of Vaccines, 4,* 219–228. doi:10.1586/14760584.4.2.219

Madsen, K., Rosenman, M., Hui, S., & Breitfeld, P. (2002). Value of electronic data for model validation and refinement: Bacteremia risk in children with fever and neutropenia. *Journal of Pediatric Hematology/Oncology, 24,* 256–262. doi:10.1097/00043426-200205000-00008

Maule, M., Scelo, G., Pastore, G., Brennen, P., Hemminki, K., Tracey, E., … Boffetta, P. (2007). Risk of second malignant neoplasms after childhood leukemia and lymphoma: An international study. *Journal of the National Cancer Institute, 99,* 790–800. doi:10.1093/jnci/djk180

Memorial Sloan Kettering Cancer Center. (n.d.). About herbs, botanicals and other products. Retrieved from http://www.mskcc.org/cancer-care/integrative-medicine/about-herbs-botanicals-other-products

Mercadante, S., Ferrera, P., Villari, P., David, F., Giarratano, A., & Riina, S. (2009). Effects of red blood cell transfusion on anemia-related symptoms in patients with cancer. *Journal of Palliative Medicine, 12,* 60–63. doi:10.1089/jpm.2008.0139

Modery-Pawlowski, C.L., Tian, L.L., Pan, V., McCrae, K.R., Mitragotri, S., & Gupta, A.S. (2013). Approaches to synthetic platelet analogs. *Biomaterials, 34,* 526–541. doi:10.1016/j.biomaterials.2012.09.074

National Cancer Institute Cancer Therapy Evaluation Program. (2010). *Common terminology criteria for adverse events* [v.4.03]. Retrieved from http://ctep.cancer.gov/protocolDevelopment/electronic_applications/ctc.htm

National Center for Complementary and Integrative Health. (n.d.). Health topics A–Z. Retrieved from http://nccam.nih.gov/health/atoz.htm

National Comprehensive Cancer Network. (2014a, July). *NCCN Clinical Practice Guidelines in Oncology (NCCN Guidelines®): Cancer- and chemotherapy-induced anemia* [v.2.2015]. Retrieved from http://www.nccn.org/professionals/physician_gls/pdf/anemia.pdf

National Comprehensive Cancer Network. (2014b). *NCCN Clinical Practice Guidelines in Oncology (NCCN Guidelines®): Myeloid growth factors* [v.2.2014]. Retrieved from http://www.nccn.org/professionals/physician_gls/pdf/myeloid_growth.pdf

National Comprehensive Cancer Network. (2014c). *NCCN Clinical Practice Guidelines in Oncology (NCCN Guidelines®): Prevention and treatment of cancer-related infections* [v.2.2014]. Retrieved from http://www.nccn.org/professionals/physician_gls/pdf/infections.pdf

Nayak, R., Rai, S., & Gupta, A. (2012). *Essentials in hematology and clinical pathology.* New Delhi, India: Jaypee Medical Publishers.

Oeffinger, K.C., Baxi, S.S., Friedman, D.N., & Moskowitz, C.S. (2013). Solid tumor second primary neoplasms: Who is at risk, what can we do? *Seminars in Oncology, 40,* 676–689. doi:10.1053/j.seminoncol.2013.09.012

Ottaviani, G., Robert, R.S., Huh, W.W., Palla, S., & Jaffe, N. (2013). Sociooccupational and physical outcomes more than 20 years after the diagnosis of osteosarcoma in children and adolescents: Limb salvage versus amputation. *Cancer, 119,* 3727–3736. doi:10.1002/cncr.28277

Page, A.V., & Liles, W.C. (2011). Colony-stimulating factors in the prevention and management of infectious diseases. *Infectious Disease Clinics of North America, 25,* 803–817. doi:10.1016/j.idc.2011.07.007

Pascoe, J., & Steven, N. (2009). Antibiotics for the prevention of febrile neutropenia. *Current Opinion in Hematology, 16,* 48–52. doi:10.1097/MOH.0b013e32831ac543

Perkins, S.M., DeWees, T., Shinohara, E.T., Reddy, M.M., & Frangoul, H. (2013). Risk of subsequent malignancies in survivors of childhood leukemia. *Journal of Cancer Survivorship, 7,* 544–550. doi:10.1007/s11764-013-0292-8

Perkins, S.M., Fei, W., Mitra, N., & Shinohara, E.T. (2013). Late causes of death in children treated for CNS malignancies. *Journal of Neuro-Oncology, 115,* 79–85. doi:10.1007/s11060-013-1197-0

Pieracci, F.M., & Barie, P.S. (2006). Diagnosis and management of iron-related anemias in critical illness. *Critical Care Medicine, 34,* 1898–1905. doi:10.1097/01.CCM.0000220495.10510.C1

Polovich, M., Olsen, M., & LeFebvre, K.B. (Eds.). (2014). *Chemotherapy and biotherapy guidelines and recommendations for practice* (4th ed.). Pittsburgh, PA: Oncology Nursing Society.

Puhalla, S., Bhattacharya, S., & Davidson, N.E. (2012). Hematopoietic growth factors: Personalization of risks and benefits. *Molecular Oncology, 6,* 237–241. doi:10.1016/j.molonc.2012.03.001

Relf, M.V., Shelton, B.K., & Jones, K.M. (2013). Common immunological disorders. In P.G. Morton & D.K. Fontaine (Eds.), *Critical care nursing: A holistic approach* (10th ed., pp. 1094–1132). Philadelphia, PA: Wolters Kluwer Health/Lippincott Williams & Wilkins.

Rimajova, V., Sopko, L., Martinka, J., Kubalova, S., & Mistrik, M. (2012). Granulocyte transfusions. *Bratislavské Lekárske Listy, 113,* 175–181. doi:10.4149/BLL_2012_041

Rizzo, J.D., Brouwers, M., Hurley, P., Seidenfeld, J., Arcasoy, M.O., Spivak, J.L., … Somerfield, M.R. (2010). American Society of Clinical Oncology/American Society of Hematology clinical practice guideline update on the use of epoetin and darbepoetin in adult patients with cancer. *Journal of Clinical Oncology, 28,* 4996–5010. doi:10.1200/JCO.2010.29.2201

Rodgers, G.M. (2009). Thrombocytopenia: Pathophysiology and classification. In J.P. Greer, J. Foerster, G.M. Rodgers, F. Paraskevas, B. Glader, D.A. Arber, & R.T. Means Jr. (Eds.), *Wintrobe's clinical hematology* (12th ed., pp. 1289–1291). Philadelphia, PA: Wolters Kluwer Health/Lippincott Williams & Wilkins.

Rodriguez, A.L., & Gobel, B.H. (2011). Bleeding. In C.H. Yarbro, D. Wujcik, & B.H. Gobel (Eds.), *Cancer nursing: Principles and practice* (7th ed., pp. 745–771). Burlington, MA: Jones & Bartlett Learning.

Rome, S.I. (2007). Nursing management: Hematologic problems. In S.L. Lewis, M.M. Heitkemper, S.R. Dirkson, P.G. O'Brien, & L. Bucher (Eds.), *Medical-surgical nursing: Assessment and management of clinical problems* (7th ed., pp. 684–737). Philadelphia, PA: Elsevier Mosby.

Rugge, M. (2013). Secondary cancer prevention: The clinico-pathological priority for the next decade. *Best Practice and Research: Clinical Gastroenterology, 27,* 157–158. doi:10.1016/j.bpg.2013.04.005

Salacz, M.E., Lankiewicz, M.W., & Weissman, D.E. (2007). Management of thrombocytopenia in bone marrow failure: A review. *Journal of Palliative Medicine, 10,* 236–244. doi:10.1089/jpm.2006.0126

Saloustros, E., Tryfonidis, K., & Georgoulias, V. (2011). Prophylactic and therapeutic strategies in chemotherapy-induced neutropenia. *Expert Opinion on Pharmacotherapy, 12,* 851–863. doi:10.1517/14656566.2011.541155

Schrijvers, D. (2011). Management of anemia in cancer patients: Transfusions. *Oncologist, 16*(Suppl. 3), 12–18. doi:10.1634/theoncologist.2011-S3-12

Schwartz, B., Benadjaoud, M.A., Cléro, E., Haddy, N., El-Fayech, C., Guibout, C., … de Vathaire, F. (2014). Risk of second bone sarcoma following childhood cancer: Role of radiation therapy treatment. *Radiation and Environmental Biophysics, 53,* 381–390. doi:10.1007/s00411-013-0510-9

Schwartzberg, L.S. (2006). Neutropenia: Etiology and pathogenesis. *Clinical Cornerstone, 8*(Suppl. 5), S5–S11. doi:10.1016/S1098-3597(06)80053-0

Scialdone, L. (2012). Overview of supportive care in patients receiving chemotherapy: Antiemetics, pain management, anemia, and neutropenia. *Journal of Pharmacy Practice, 25,* 209–221. doi:10.1177/0897190011431631

Sehulster, L.M., & Chinn, R.Y. (2003). Guidelines for environmental infection control in health-care facilities: Recommendations of CDC and the Healthcare Infection Control Practices Advisory Committee (HICPAC). *Morbidity and Mortality Weekly Report: Recommendations and Reports, 52*(RR10), 1–42. Retrieved from http://www.cdc.gov/mmwr/preview/mmwrhtml/rr5210a1.htm

Shane, K., & Shelton, B.K. (2004). Myelosuppression. In B.K. Shelton, C.R. Ziegfeld, & M.M. Olsen (Eds.), *Manual of cancer nursing* (pp. 309–352). Philadelphia, PA: Wolters Kluwer Health/Lippincott Williams & Wilkins.

Shelton, B.K. (2011). Infection. In C.H. Yarbro, D. Wujcik, & B.H. Gobel (Eds.), *Cancer nursing: Principles and practice* (7th ed., pp. 713–744). Burlington, MA: Jones & Bartlett Learning.

Shelton, B.K. (2012). Hematology and oncology problems. In J. Foster & S.S. Prevost (Eds.), *Advanced practice nursing of adults in acute care* (pp. 591–651). Philadelphia, PA: F.A. Davis.

Shelton, B.K. (2013). The hematologic and immunologic systems. In R.D. Dennison (Ed.), *Pass CCRN* (4th ed., pp. 636–684). Philadelphia, PA: Elsevier.

Shinohara, E.T., DeWees, T., & Perkins, S.M. (2014). Subsequent malignancies and their effect on survival in patients with retinoblastoma. *Pediatric Blood and Cancer, 61,* 116–119. doi:10.1002/pbc.24714

Shitara, K., Matsuo, K., Oze, I., Mizota, A., Kondo, C., Nomura, M., … Muro, K. (2011). Meta-analysis of neutropenia or leukopenia as a prognostic factor in patients with malignant disease undergoing chemotherapy. *Cancer Chemotherapy and Pharmacology, 68,* 301–307. doi:10.1007/s00280-010-1487-6

Silber, J.H., Fridman, M., DiPaolo, R.S., Erder, M.H., Pauly, M.V., & Fox, K.R. (1998). First-cycle blood counts and subsequent neutropenia, dose reduction, or delay in early-stage breast cancer therapy. *Journal of Clinical Oncology, 16,* 2392–2400.

Situm, M., Buljan, M., Bulic, S.O., & Simic, D. (2007). The mechanisms of UV radiation in the development of malignant melanoma. *Collegium Antropologicum, 31*(Suppl. 1), 13–16.

Stanworth, S.J., Massey, E., Hyde, C., Brunskill, S.J., Navarette, C., Lucas, G., … Paulus, U. (2005). Granulocyte transfusions for treating infections in patients with neutropenia or neutrophil dysfunction. *Cochrane Database of Systematic Reviews, 2005*(3). doi:10.1002/14651858.CD005339

Strodtbeck, K., Sloan, A., Rogers, L., Fisher, P.G., Stearns, D., Campbell, L., & Barnholtz-Sloan, J. (2013). Risk of subsequent cancer following a primary CNS tumor. *Journal of Neuro-Oncology, 112,* 285–295. doi:10.1007/s11060-013-1063-0

Tefferi, A., Hanson, C.A., & Inwards, D.J. (2005). How to interpret and pursue an abnormal complete blood count in adults. *Mayo Clinic Proceedings, 80,* 923–936. doi:10.4065/80.7.923

Tesfa, D., & Palmblad, J. (2011). Late-onset neutropenia following rituximab therapy: Incidence, clinical features and possible mechanisms. *Expert Review of Hematology, 4,* 619–625. doi:10.1586/EHM.11.62

Teuffel, O., Ethier, M.C., Alibhai, S.M., Beyene, J., & Sung, L. (2011). Outpatient management of cancer patients with febrile neutropenia: A systematic review and meta-analysis. *Annals of Oncology, 22,* 2358–2365. doi:10.1093/annonc/mdq745

Teuffel, O., & Sung, L. (2012). Advances in management of low-risk febrile neutropenia. *Current Opinion in Pediatrics, 24,* 40–45. doi:10.1097/MOP.0b013e32834c4b12

Thienelt, C.D., & Calverley, D.C. (2009). Thrombocytopenia caused by immunologic platelet destruction. In J.P. Greer, J. Foerster, G.M. Rodgers, F. Paraskevas, B. Glader, D.A. Arber, & R.T. Means Jr. (Eds.), *Wintrobe's clinical hematology* (12th ed., pp. 1292–1313). Philadelphia, PA: Wolters Kluwer Health/Lippincott Williams & Wilkins.

Tomblyn, M., Chiller, T., Einsele, H., Gress, R., Sepkowitz, K., Storek, J., … Boeckh, M.A. (2009). Guidelines for preventing infectious complications among hematopoietic cell transplantation recipients: A global perspective. *Biology of Blood and Marrow Transplantation, 15,* 1143–1238. doi:10.1016/j.bbmt.2009.06.019

Uthman, E. (n.d.). Blood cells and the CBC. Retrieved from http://web2.airmail.net/uthman/blood_cells.html

Vadhan-Raj, S. (2009). Management of chemotherapy-induced thrombocytopenia: Current status of thrombopoietic agents. *Seminars in Hematology, 46*(1, Suppl. 2), S26–S32. doi:10.1053/j.seminhematol.2008.12.007

Vajdic, C.M., McDonald, S.P., McCredie, M.R.E., van Leeuwen, M.T., Stewart, J.H., Law, M., … Grulich, A.E. (2006). Cancer incidence before and after kidney transplantation. *JAMA, 296,* 2823–2831. doi:10.1001/jama.296.23.2823

van Dalen, E.C., Mank, A., Leclercq, E., Mulder, R.L., Davies, M., Kersten, M.J., & van de Wetering, M.D. (2012). Low bacterial diet versus control diet to prevent infection in cancer patients treated with chemotherapy causing episodes of neutropenia. *Cochrane Database of Systematic Reviews, 2012*(9). doi:10.1002/14651858.CD006247.pub2

van den Broek, E.C., Liu, L., Posthuma, E.F.M., Janssen-Heijnen, M.L.G., Coebergh, J.W.W., & Soerjomataram, I. (2014). Increased risk of chronic lymphocytic leukaemia among cancer survivors in the Netherlands: Increased detection, causal factors or both? *Annals of Hematology, 93,* 157–162. doi:10.1007/s00277-013-1929-4

Vansteenkiste, J., Wauters, I., Elliott, S., Glaspy, J., & Hedenus, M. (2013). Chemotherapy-induced anemia: The story of darbepoetin alfa. *Current Medical Research and Opinion, 29,* 325–337. doi:10.1185/03007995.2013.766593

Velasco, R.P. (2011). Review of granulocyte colony-stimulating factors in the treatment of established febrile neutropenia. *Journal of Oncology Pharmacy Practice, 17,* 225–232. doi:10.1177/1078155210374129

Wahed, A., & Dasgupta, A. (2015). *Hematology and coagulation: A comprehensive review for board preparation, certification and clinical practice.* Philadelphia, PA: Elsevier.

Waters, J.H. (2014). Role of the massive transfusion protocol in the management of haemorrhagic shock. *British Journal of Anaesthesia, 113,* ii3–ii8. doi:10.1093/bja/aeu379

Watts, R.G. (2009). Neutropenia. In J.P. Greer, J. Foerster, G.M. Rodgers, F. Paraskevas, B. Glader, D.A. Arber, & R.T. Means Jr. (Eds.), *Wintrobe's clinical hematology* (12th ed., pp. 1527–1547). Philadelphia, PA: Wolters Kluwer Health/Lippincott Williams & Wilkins.

Whichard, Z.L., Sarkar, C.A., Kimmel, M., & Corey, S.J. (2010). Hematopoiesis and its disorders: A systems biology approach. *Blood, 115,* 2339–2347. doi:10.1182/blood-2009-08-215798

White, L., & Ybarra, M. (2014). Neutropenic fever. *Emergency Medicine Clinics of North America, 32,* 549–561. doi:10.1016/j.emc.2014.04.002

Wilson, C.L., Cohn, R.J., Johnston, K.A., & Ashton, L.J. (2010). Late mortality and second cancers in an Australian cohort of childhood cancer survivors. *Medical Journal of Australia, 193,* 258–261.

Wilson, C.L., Ness, K.K., Neglia, J.P., Hammond, S., Shnorhavorian, M., Leisenring, W.L., … Armstrong, G.T. (2013). Renal carcinoma after childhood cancer: A report from the Childhood Cancer Survivor Study. *Journal of the National Cancer Institute, 105,* 504–508. doi:10.1093/jnci/djt014

Wingard, J.R., Eldjerou, L., & Leather, H. (2012). Use of antibacterial prophylaxis in patients with chemotherapy-induced neutropenia. *Current Opinion in Hematology, 19,* 21–26. doi:10.1097/MOH.0b013e32834da9bf

Woodmansee, W.W., Zimmermann, A.G., Child, C.J., Rong, Q., Erfurth, E.M., Beck-Peccoz, P., … Robison, L.L. (2013). Incidence of second neoplasm in childhood cancer survivors treated with GH: An analysis of GeNeSIS and HypoCCS. *European Journal of Endocrinology, 168,* 565–573. doi:10.1530/EJE-12-0967

Xu, Y., Wang, H., Zhou, S., Yu, M., Wang, X., Fu, K., … Wang, P. (2013). Risk of second malignant neoplasms after cyclophosphamide-based chemotherapy with or without radiotherapy for non-Hodgkin lymphoma. *Leukemia and Lymphoma, 54,* 1396–1404. doi:10.3109/10428194.2012.743657

Yang, B.B., Savin, M.A., & Green, M. (2012). Prevention of chemotherapy-induced neutropenia with pegfilgrastim: Pharmacokinetics and patient outcomes. *Chemotherapy, 58,* 387–398. doi:10.1159/000345626

Zaghloul, M.S. (2013). Intensity modulated radiotherapy (IMRT) for pediatric cancer patients: The advantage and fear of second malignant neoplasm. *Journal of the Egyptian National Cancer Institute, 25,* 1–3. doi:10.1016/j.jnci.2012.11.002

CHAPTER 12

Cardiac and Pulmonary Toxicities

Marianne J. Davies, DNP, MSN, APRN, ACNP, AOCNP®

Introduction

Survival rates in patients with cancer have significantly increased over the past two decades with the advancement of therapeutic treatment options. The risk of developing cardiopulmonary toxicities has increased as a result of new therapeutic options and the aging of cancer survivors (Magnano, Cibrian, González, & Bosch, 2014). This chapter will review the potential toxicities that patients may develop following treatment with chemotherapy, biologic therapy, and radiation therapy. It will highlight the proposed etiology, risk factors, diagnosis, and treatment recommendations.

Cardiac Toxicities

Cardiotoxicities are a common side effect and toxicity of cancer therapy. Different patterns of cardiac dysfunction are seen, and some can be serious and life threatening. Several antineoplastic and targeted treatments can lead to cardiotoxicity. Radiation therapy to the heart or surrounding region may lead to cardiotoxicity. Schlitt, Jordan, Vordemark, Schwamborn, and Thomssen (2014) reported a 10-fold increase in cardiovascular disease in patients treated with chemotherapy or radiation therapy over the general population. Cancer also may metastasize into the heart and its surrounding structures or present as a primary cardiac tumor (angiosarcoma).

Historically, the most frequent cardiotoxicity was left ventricular dysfunction leading to congestive heart failure (CHF). However, several patterns of dysfunction have emerged as a result of new treatment regimens and drug classifications. Toxicities may present immediately or develop over a course of months (acute) to years (chronic) (Geiger, Lange, Suhl, Heinemann, & Stemmler, 2010). Acute changes include arrhythmias, electrocardiogram (ECG) changes, coronary artery spasms, angina, myocardial infarction, and blood pressure changes. Delayed toxicities include CHF and cardiomyopathy. Structural changes to the heart also can develop, such as pericardial effusion, cardiac tamponade, and pericardial fibrosis. Pericardial effusion and cardiac tamponade are covered in Chapter 16. Pericardial fibrosis will not be covered in this chapter. Cardiotoxicity may preclude patients from available treatment options if they develop a cancer recurrence (Cardinale, Bacchiani, Beggiato, Colombo, & Cipolla, 2013).

Etiology, Pathophysiology, and Risk Factors

Medications such as antineoplastics, biologic therapies, and supportive care used for cancer therapy are major risk factors for the development of acute and chronic cardiotoxicity, as is a personal or familial history of heart disease (Schlitt et al., 2014). See Table 12-1 for specific examples of agents associated with cardiotoxicity and related nursing implications.

Coronary ischemia and symptoms of angina pectoris can develop with the administration of pyrimidine antimetabolites 5-fluorouracil (5-FU) and capecitabine, as a result of vasospasm or endothelial injury. Patients may report nonspecific or angina symptoms of chest pain with radiation to the neck. Associated ECG changes may be present. The incidence is 1%–68% for 5-FU and 3%–9% for capecitabine (Yeh & Bickford, 2009). The onset

Table 12-1. Cardiac Toxicities Associated With Chemotherapy, Targeted Therapy, and Biotherapy

Drug	Toxicities	Nursing Implications
Aldesleukin (Proleukin®)	Death Myocardial ischemia Myocardial infarction Tachycardia Arrhythmias Hypotension Reduced vascular resistance	Side effects are probably a result of capillary leak syndrome. Patients with preexisting heart disease are at greater risk. Cardiac functioning can be determined by thallium stress testing.
Alemtuzumab (Campath®)	Decreased ejection fraction Heart failure Arrhythmias including tachycardia Myocardial infarction Acute cardiac insufficiency Cardiac arrest Cardiomyopathy	–
All-trans-retinoic acid, also known as tretinoin (Vesanoid®)	Pericardial effusions Myocardial ischemia/ infarction Arrhythmias Hypertension Cardiac failure Cardiac arrest Heart murmur Myocarditis Pericarditis Secondary cardiomyopathy	Impaired myocardial contractility and transient hypotension as part of retinoic acid-acute promyelocytic leukemia syndrome. Occurs within first month of treatment. Treat with steroids (10 mg every 12 hours for maximum of 3 days or until resolution of symptoms).

(Continued on next page)

Table 12-1. Cardiac Toxicities Associated With Chemotherapy, Targeted Therapy, and Biotherapy *(Continued)*

Drug	Toxicities	Nursing Implications
Androgen deprivation therapy	Increased fasting lipid and glucose levels Prolonged QTc interval Coronary heart disease Sudden cardiac death	Long-term therapy may not increase risk of cardiovascular side effects over short-term therapy. Monitor for development of comorbidities that can increase risk of cardiac disease (i.e., diabetes and obesity). Low-fat diet and exercise as preventive measures.
Anthracyclines • Daunorubicin • Doxorubicin • Doxorubicin liposomal • Epirubicin • Idarubicin • Mitoxantrone	Arrhythmias Pericarditis and myocarditis Cardiomyopathy with left ventricular dysfunction and/or heart failure that is cumulative and dose-dependent Doxorubicin liposomal has similar side effect profile as standard doxorubicin but at a lower incidence.	Baseline cardiac ejection fraction with MUGA scan or echocardiogram before therapy and periodically thereafter. Most manufacturers recommend dose reductions for hepatic impairment. See package inserts for specific recommendations. Each agent has different lifetime cumulative dose to prevent cardiotoxicity, especially CHF. Previous anthracyclines and heart disease are factored into lifetime cumulative dose. Assess for cardiac signs and symptoms at baseline, prior to each treatment, and throughout treatment. ECG changes (decrease of $\geq$ 30% in limb lead QRS voltage) and decrease in LVEF may precede CHF and other cardiomyopathy. Avoid exceeding lifetime doses. Endomyocardial biopsy is definitive diagnostic tool for diagnosis of myocardial injury. Cardiotoxicity defined as > 20% baseline decrease of LVEF if stayed in normal range or > 10% baseline decrease of LVEF if became abnormal. Doxorubicin liposomal: 500–550 mg/m^2; 450–500 mg/m^2 if receiving radiation therapy to the mediastinum or administration of other cardiotoxic agents such as cyclophosphamide. Daunorubicin: 550 mg/m^2, 400 mg/m^2 if prior radiation therapy including heart. Epirubicin: 900 mg/m^2. Contraindicated if severe myocardial insufficiency, recent myocardial infarction, or severe arrhythmias. Lower doses if concomitant radiation therapy or history of cardiovascular disease. Idarubicin: Cumulative dose not identified. Mitoxantrone: 140 mg/m^2. Higher risk for cardiotoxicity if radiation therapy to mediastinal/pericardial area. Special guidelines exist for patients with multiple sclerosis. Cardiotoxicity can occur any time after completion of therapy. Pediatric patients develop cardiotoxicity over a period of 15–20 years. Consider use of cardioprotectant agent, dexrazoxane, where benefits of doxorubicin therapy are present. Do NOT administer with trastuzumab.

(Continued on next page)

Table 12-1. Cardiac Toxicities Associated With Chemotherapy, Targeted Therapy, and Biotherapy *(Continued)*

Drug	Toxicities	Nursing Implications
Arsenic trioxide	QTc prolongation T-wave inversion Torsades de pointes Heart block Sudden death	Perform cardiac assessment at baseline and throughout treatment. Weekly ECGs are done to assess QTc interval. Twice-weekly electrolytes and coagulation studies (more if abnormality noted). Replete electrolytes. Keep potassium > 4 mmol/L and magnesium > 1.8 mg/ml but not above normal levels. Monitor renal function. Discontinue drugs that prolong QTc interval prior to starting therapy. Hold therapy if QTc interval exceeds 500 ms until interval falls below 450 ms.
Axitinib (Inlyta®)	Hypertension	Monitor BP at baseline and prior to each treatment. Monitor after therapy is complete, as hypertension can develop in delayed setting. Median time to onset of hypertension was within one month of start. Patients with hypertension: Monitor BP at home and report elevations. Initiate antihypertensives if BP elevation is grade 2 or higher. Follow dose reduction and discontinuation schedule per package insert.
Bevacizumab (Avastin®)	Hypertension Left ventricular dysfunction and/or heart failure Arterial thromboembolic events leading to cardiac ischemia Myocardial infarction	Monitor BP at baseline and prior to each treatment. Monitor after therapy is complete, as hypertension can develop in delayed setting. Patients with hypertension: Monitor BP at home and report elevations. Initiate antihypertensives if BP elevation is grade 2 or higher. Preexisting hypertension: More aggressive monitoring and escalation of antihypertensive medications, including dose increases and additional antihypertensive medications. Follow American Heart Association guidelines for management of hypertensive medications. It may be necessary to interrupt or stop bevacizumab therapy.
Bleomycin	Chest pain Pericarditis Myocardial ischemia Myocardial infarction Coronary artery disease	Cardiotoxicities are uncommon but occur more when drug is used in combination with other antineoplastic agents.
Busulfan	Pericardial and myocardial fibrosis Tachycardia Hypertension/hypotension	Fibrosis usually appears 4–9 years after the exposure to cumulative doses > 600 mg. IV busulfan can induce tachycardia and BP changes not usually seen with oral administration.

(Continued on next page)

Table 12-1. Cardiac Toxicities Associated With Chemotherapy, Targeted Therapy, and Biotherapy *(Continued)*

Drug	Toxicities	Nursing Implications
Cabozantinib (Cometriq®)	Hypertension	Monitor BP at baseline and prior to each treatment. Monitor after therapy is complete, as hypertension can develop in delayed setting. Patients with hypertension: Monitor BP at home and report elevations. Initiate antihypertensives if BP elevation is grade 2 or higher.
Capecitabine (Xeloda®)	Angina chest pain Substernal chest pain Arrhythmias are rare	Toxicities are more common in people with history of coronary artery disease. Interrupt treatment and administer anti-anginal treatment. Obtain cardiac enzyme, troponin, creatinine kinase, and electrolyte levels, ECG, chest x-ray, and pulse oximetry. Proceed with cardiology referral. May be possible to rechallenge at lower dose.
Cisplatin (Platinol®)	Arrhythmias (ST-T changes, left bundle branch block, acute ischemic events) Bradycardia Hypertension Cardiomyopathy Myocardial infarction	Replete electrolytes as needed.
Crizotinib (Xalkori®)	QTc prolongation; bradycardia	Hold treatment if QTc > 500 ms; permanently discontinue if seen with arrhythmia, heart failure, or torsades de pointes. Use with caution if patients are receiving other drugs that inhibit cytochrome P450 3A4 (CYP3A4) and known to cause bradycardia.
Cyclophosphamide (Cytoxan®)	Left ventricular dysfunction and/or heart failure Pericardial effusion Pericarditis	Risk factors include lymphoma diagnosis, older age, and possibly a history of higher doses of anthracyclines and abnormal ejection fraction. May potentiate doxorubicin-induced cardiotoxicity. May be fatal.
Cytarabine	Pericarditis with pericardial effusion and tamponade	Cardiotoxicities are rare and may be schedule dependent and occur if drug is used with other cardiotoxic agents. Corticosteroids might be beneficial.
Dasatinib (Sprycel®)	Chest pain Pericardial effusion CHF Left ventricular dysfunction QTc prolongation	Use with caution in patients with QTc prolongation and congenital long QT syndrome and in patients taking antiarrhythmic medication or medications that prolong QTc interval or anthracyclines. Correct hypokalemia and hypomagnesemia. Monitor for CHF and treat appropriately.

(Continued on next page)

**Table 12-1. Cardiac Toxicities Associated With Chemotherapy,
Targeted Therapy, and Biotherapy *(Continued)***

Drug	Toxicities	Nursing Implications
Eribulin (Halaven®)	QTc prolongation	Correct hypokalemia and hypomagnesemia before initiating eribulin. Obtain ECG monitoring if patients have CHF, bradyarrhythmias, or are taking drugs that prolong QTc interval. Avoid in patients with congenital long QT syndrome.
Erlotinib (Tarceva®)	Cardiac ischemia Myocardial infarction	Cardiotoxicities are rare.
Estramustine (Emcyt®)	Coronary ischemia Myocardial infarction	Estramustine contains estrogen-like compound that promotes clotting.
Etoposide (Toposar®)	Angina Hypotension and hypertension Myocardial infarction	Treat cardiotoxicities quickly.
Fludarabine	Hypotension Chest pain Pericardial effusion Heart failure Arrhythmia	When fludarabine is used in combination with melphalan, severe cardiotoxicity may develop. Heart failure and arrhythmias are rare.
5-Fluorouracil (Adrucil®)	Coronary artery thrombosis Coronary vasoconstriction Angina Myocardial infarction Arrhythmias Sudden death	Interrupt treatment and administer anti-anginal treatment. Obtain cardiac enzyme, troponin, creatinine kinase, and electrolyte levels, ECG, chest x-ray, and pulse oximetry. Proceed with cardiology referral. May be possible to rechallenge patients at a lower dose.
Ifosfamide (Ifex®)	Arrhythmias ECG changes Cardiogenic shock CHF	Cardiotoxicities are dose related, infrequent, and reversible with medical care.
Imatinib (Gleevec®)	Left ventricular dysfunction, heart failure	Determine LVEF at baseline and periodically during therapy. Reduced LVEF can occur as early as 1 month into therapy or delayed (more than a year into therapy). Close monitoring if history of or risk factors for cardiac disease. Risk is higher for cardiogenic shock/left ventricular dysfunction when starting imatinib if high eosinophils.
Interferon (Intron® A)	Cardiomyopathy Arrhythmias Hypotension Myocardial infarction Myocardial ischemia	Preexisting heart disease increases the risk of infarctions and ischemia. Arrhythmias are common; additional risk factors include prior cardiac history and dose of interferon.

(Continued on next page)

Table 12-1. Cardiac Toxicities Associated With Chemotherapy, Targeted Therapy, and Biotherapy *(Continued)*

Drug	Toxicities	Nursing Implications
Ixabepilone (Ixempra®)	Arrhythmias Left ventricular dysfunction	Cardiotoxicity is higher with concurrent capecitabine. Caution if history of cardiac disease. Discontinue cardiac ischemia or compromised cardiac function.
Lapatinib (Tykerb®)	Left ventricular dysfunction; Heart failure; QTc prolongation	Measure baseline LVEF and during treatment. Discontinue lapatinib if LVEF grade 2 or greater or if LVEF goes below normal. Reduced dose if given in combination with capecitabine or letrozole when restarting lapatinib. Administer cautiously if patients have or develop QTc prolongation.
Lenvatinib (Lenvima™)	Hypertension	Monitor BP at baseline and prior to each treatment. Monitor after therapy is complete, as hypertension can develop in delayed setting. Patients with hypertension: Monitor BP at home and report elevations. Initiate antihypertensives if BP elevation is grade 2 or higher.
Methotrexate	Syncope Chest pain Arrhythmias Myocardial infarction	Cardiotoxicities are rare.
Mitomycin C	Heart failure	Dose-dependent cardiotoxicity if doses greater than 30 mg/m^2 and may be exacerbated if coadminister doxorubicin 150 mg/m^2.
Nilotinib (Tasigna®)	QTc prolongation Ischemic heart disease	Correct hypokalemia and hypomagnesemia, and monitor regularly. Avoid administration with strong CYP3A4 inhibitors. Use with caution in patients with hepatic impairment. Obtain ECG at baseline, 7 days after starting nilotinib, and regularly thereafter.
Pazopanib (Votrient®)	Hypertension and hypertensive crisis QTc interval prolongation Torsades de pointes CHF and decreased LVEF	Monitor BP weekly initially, then every 2–4 weeks. Manage hypertension quickly. Perform baseline echocardiogram, ECG, and electrolytes and continue monitoring as clinically indicated.
Pertuzumab (Perjeta®)	CHF and decreased LVEF	Perform baseline echocardiogram, ECG, and electrolytes and continue monitoring as clinically indicated.
Ponatinib (Iclusig®)	Hypertension	Monitor BP weekly initially, then every 2–4 weeks. Manage hypertension quickly.
Ramucirumab (Cyramza®)	Hypertension	Monitor BP weekly initially, then every 2–4 weeks. Manage hypertension quickly.

(Continued on next page)

Table 12-1. Cardiac Toxicities Associated With Chemotherapy, Targeted Therapy, and Biotherapy *(Continued)*

Drug	Toxicities	Nursing Implications
Regorafenib (Stivarga®)	Myocardial ischemia and infarction Hypertension	Hold drug for cardiac ischemia/infarction. May resume after resolution. Monitor BP weekly initially, then every 2–4 weeks. Manage hypertension quickly.
Rituximab (Rituximab®)	Arrhythmias	Toxicities are uncommon. Discontinue if serious or life-threatening cardiac arrhythmias develop. Cardiac monitoring is recommended.
Sorafenib (Nexavar®)	Hypertension Arrhythmias Coronary syndrome Myocardial infarction	Monitor BP at baseline and at least weekly during first 6 weeks of therapy. Monitor BP throughout drug therapy. Hypertension may occur at any point during therapy. Teach patients to monitor BP at home and report BP elevations. Hold therapy for systolic BP > 200 mm Hg or diastolic BP > 100 mm Hg. Initiate antihypertensive medications immediately at onset of hypertension.
Sunitinib (Sutent®)	Hypertension QTc interval prolongation Torsades de pointes Left ventricular dysfunction Myocardial infarction Myocardial ischemia	Monitor BP at baseline and at least weekly during the first cycle of therapy. Continue to monitor BP during the 2 weeks off therapy and throughout treatment. Teach patients to monitor BP at home and report elevations. Hold therapy for systolic BP > 200 mm Hg or diastolic BP > 100 mm Hg. Initiate antihypertensive medications immediately at onset of hypertension. Perform cardiac assessment, including LVEF function, at baseline and throughout therapy.
Taxanes • Docetaxel (Taxotere®) • Paclitaxel (Taxol®) • Nanoparticle albumin-bound paclitaxel (Abraxane®)	Left ventricular dysfunction and/or heart failure, may occur within 48 hours of administration Hypotension Coronary vasoconstriction Chest pain—angina Arrhythmias Bradycardia Cardiovascular collapse Abnormal heart conduction	Toxicity increases when given with other cardiotoxic chemotherapy, such as doxorubicin.
Trastuzumab (Herceptin®)	Left ventricular dysfunction and heart failure Arrhythmias Cardiomyopathy	Hold treatment if > 16% decline in LVEF from pretreatment or > 10% decrease from pretreatment and now abnormal value until recovery. May rechallenge. Monitor LVEF every 3 months during treatment. If no recovery for more than 8 weeks, do not rechallenge. Provide medical management of cardiomyopathy and heart failure.

(Continued on next page)

Table 12-1. Cardiac Toxicities Associated With Chemotherapy, Targeted Therapy, and Biotherapy *(Continued)*

Drug	Toxicities	Nursing Implications
Vandetanib (Caprelsa®)	Hypertension; QTc interval prolongation; torsades de pointes	ECG at baseline and 2–4 weeks and 8–12 weeks and every 3 months after starting treatment; avoid drugs that prolong QTc interval; Black box warning to correct hypocalcemia, hypokalemia, and hypomagnesemia prior to drug administration. Do not start drug if QTc interval is > 450 ms, congenital long QT syndrome, bradyarrhythmias, history of torsades de pointes, or uncompensated heart failure. Dose reduce for renal impairment.
Vemurafenib (Zelboraf®)	QTc prolongation leading to ventricular arrhythmias, including torsades de pointes	Withhold drug if QTc > 500 ms or long QT syndrome or if patients are taking other medications known to prolong QTc. Reduce doses if withheld previously for QTc prolongation. Obtain ECG at day 15, monthly for 3 months, and then as needed. Use with caution in patients receiving other drugs that inhibit CYP3A4.
Vorinostat (Zolinza®)	QTc prolongation	Monitor by ECG and avoid other drugs that cause QTc prolongation.
Ziv-aflibercept (Zaltrap®)	Hypertension	Grade 3–4 hypertension risk. Unsure if safe with NYHA class III or IV CHF. May need adjustment of existing antihypertensive or multidrug therapy. Onset of hypertension with first 2 cycles. Monitor BP minimum every 2 weeks. Discontinue treatment or dose reduce until BP controlled.

BP—blood pressure; CHF—congestive heart failure; ECG—electrocardiogram; LVEF—left ventricular ejection fraction; ms—millisecond; MUGA—multigated acquisition; NYHA—New York Heart Association; QTc—corrected QT

Note. Based on information from Albini et al., 2010; ARIAD Pharmaceuticals, Inc., 2014; Astellas Pharma US, Inc., & Genentech, Inc., 2012; AstraZeneca Pharmaceuticals LP, 2014; Bair et al., 2013; Baxter, 2013; Bayer Healthcare Pharmaceuticals Inc., 2013; Bayer Healthcare Pharmaceuticals, Inc., & Onyx Pharmaceuticals, Inc., 2013; Bedford Laboratories, 2008, 2013a, 2013b; Bonita & Pradhan, 2013; Bristol-Myers Squibb Co., 2007, 2011a, 2011b, 2013, 2014; Cardinale, Colombo, Lamantia, et al., 2010; Cardinale, Colombo, Torrisi, et al., 2010; Celgene Corp., 2013; Cephalon, Inc., 2010; Eisai Inc., 2013, 2015; Exelixis, Inc., 2012; Geiger et al., 2010; Genentech, Inc., 2013a, 2013b, 2013c, 2014a, 2014b, 2015; Genzyme Corp., 2009; GlaxoSmithKline, 2013, 2014; Janssen Products, LP, 2013; Merck & Co., Inc., 2013, 2014; Monsuez et al., 2010; Nazer et al., 2011; Novartis Pharmaceuticals Corp., 2014a, 2014b; Pfizer Inc., 2011, 2013a, 2013b, 2014a, 2014b, 2014c; Prometheus Laboratories Inc., 2012; Regeneron Pharmaceuticals, Inc., & Sanofi-Aventis U.S. LLC, 2013; Ryberg, 2013; Sagent Pharmaceuticals, 2011; Sanofi-Aventis, 2013; Schlitt et al., 2014; Senkus & Jassem, 2011; Smith et al., 2010; Teva Pharmaceuticals, 2009, 2012a, 2012b, 2012c, 2012d, 2013; Yeh & Bickford, 2009.

may be from hours to five days. Mortality associated with 5-FU is 2.2%–13% (Yeh & Bickford, 2009). Risk is increased with doses greater than 800 mg/m², continuous infusion, preexisting coronary artery disease, concurrent use of radiation, or concurrent use of anthracyclines (Yeh & Bickford, 2009). Coronary vasoconstriction and myocardial ischemia also are noted with paclitaxel and docetaxel. Small molecule tyrosine kinase inhibitors (TKIs) may inhibit downstream kinases that are essential to myocardial repair. Myocardial ischemia has been noted with erlotinib, an epidermal growth factor receptor (EGFR) inhibitor. Acute coronary syndrome and coronary vasospasm have been documented with sorafenib (Yeh & Bickford, 2009).

Arterial thromboembolic events (ATEs) may occur with the use of monoclonal antibodies. Monoclonal antibodies that inhibit vascular endothelial growth factor (VEGF), such as bevacizumab, can cause ATEs with an incidence of 3%–19%. Several meta-analyses have documented the increase in ATEs and risk of myocardial ischemia with use of VEGF inhibitors (Bair, Choueiri, & Moslehi, 2013). Blocking VEGF may decrease the endothelial cells' ability to regenerate, leading to alterations in the vascular lining. The median time to onset is three months. Risk is increased with age greater than 65 and previous thrombotic events (Bair et al., 2013).

TKIs, specifically VEGF signaling pathway inhibitors, lead to decreased nitric oxide synthesis and increased vascular resistance. This, in turn, leads to vasoconstriction, which results in hypertension. VEGF promotes endothelial cell structure; thus, blocking VEGF leads to endothelial dysfunction (Bair et al., 2013). The incidence is 8%–25% with aflibercept, axitinib, bevacizumab, cabozantinib, pazopanib, ramucirumab, regorafenib, sorafenib, sunitinib, and vandetanib. Damage is increased with uncontrolled hypertension (Bonita & Pradhan, 2013). If hypertension is left untreated, hypertensive encephalopathy has developed with bevacizumab and vandetanib.

Arrhythmias, including QTc prolongation, have developed following the administration of antineoplastics, targeted agents, and supportive care agents. The pathophysiology of QTc prolongation is unknown. Caution should be used when antineoplastics and targeted agents are administered concurrently with other drugs that cause QTc prolongation. Antineoplastic agents associated with arrhythmias include arsenic trioxide, 5-FU, ixabepilone, paclitaxel, docetaxel, anthracyclines, and cyclophosphamide. Targeted agents include crizotinib, eribulin, lapatinib, pazopanib, sunitinib, vandetanib, and vorinostat (Bonita & Pradhan, 2013; Ewer & Ewer, 2013; Maitland et al., 2010; Steingart et al., 2012). Crizotinib and ceritinib, anaplastic lymphoma kinase (ALK) inhibitors used in the treatment of advanced or metastatic non-small cell lung cancer with the *EML4-ALK* oncogene, can lead to QTc prolongation. Treatment interruption is recommended if the QTc interval is more than 500 milliseconds during treatment, and permanent discontinuation is recommended if arrhythmias result from the prolonged QTc interval (Pfizer Inc., 2013b). Vandetanib, a multitargeted TKI used for treatment of thyroid cancer, can lead to prolonged QTc interval, torsades de pointes, and sudden death. Vandetanib is only available through a restricted access program because of its significant cardiotoxic profile. Serotonin antagonist antiemetics (ondansetron, granisetron, dolasetron, and palonosetron) may cause transient ECG changes including increased PR interval, QRS complex duration, and QTc interval. Methadone, used in the treatment of cancer-related pain, can cause prolongation of the QTc interval and place patients at risk for torsades de pointes (Chou et al., 2014).

Coronary artery disease can result from androgen deprivation therapy (ADT) used in men with locally advanced or metastatic prostate cancer. ADT reduces testosterone to castration levels and results in altered lipid profiles, such as increased cholesterol, thereby increasing the incidence of cardiac disease. With ADT, the incidence of myocardial infarction, coronary heart disease, and sudden cardiac death increases (Keating, O'Malley, Freedland, & Smith, 2010). Long-term survivors of testicular carcinoma treated with bleomycin, etoposide, and cisplatin (BEP regimen) are at increased risk for developing coronary artery disease (Haugnes et al., 2012).

Heart failure may occur with anthracycline administration as an acute, early, or late onset. Heart failure caused by acute toxicity is usually reversible. Early onset occurs within the first year following treatment. Late onset occurs more than one year after treatment and can occur as late as 10 years following completion of therapy (Bonita & Pradhan, 2013; Bowles et al., 2012; Yeh & Bickford, 2009). The mechanism of action has been hypothesized to be free radical oxygen formation, leading to myocardial fibrosis. However, several theories are being explored evaluating interference of topoisomerase II beta, an enzyme in DNA that is the target of several chemotherapy agents (Geiger et al., 2010; Yeh & Bickford, 2009). Anthracycline toxicity risk is associated with an age younger than 4 years and older than 65 years; cumulative doses of more than 550 mg/m^2; higher single dose; IV bolus versus infusion; concurrent chemotherapy with paclitaxel, cyclophosphamide, or trastuzumab; concurrent radiation therapy; and prior mediastinal radiation (Aapro et al., 2011; Bonita & Pradham, 2013; Cardinale & Sandri, 2010; Lipshultz et al., 2010). Heart failure may develop within 48 hours of taxane administration. Alkylating agents may cause direct endothelial injury and myocardial necrosis, leading to delayed heart failure and pericarditis (Al-Hashmi et al., 2012).

Trastuzumab is a monoclonal antibody that targets human epidermal growth factor receptor 2 (HER2). It is used in the treatment of HER2/neu-positive breast cancer. It can cause cardiomyopathy as a result of inhibition of cardiomyocyte repair. Trastuzumab alters myocyte survival pathways that rely on ErbB2 to ErbB4 receptors, leading to irreversible loss of myocytes (Geiger et al., 2010). Cardiac dysfunction is usually asymptomatic with decreased left ventricular ejection fraction (LVEF); however, heart failure can develop (Fiùza, 2009). The incidence of cardiotoxicity is 8%–27% with trastuzumab, depending on whether it is used with anthracyclines or paclitaxel (Ades et al., 2014). Patients with breast cancer who receive trastuzumab following anthracycline therapy are at increased risk for irreversible systolic dysfunction, with incidence as high as 28% (Seicean et al., 2013). The risk is increased with preexisting cardiac disease, age older than 50 years, previous or concurrent treatment with anthracycline, and higher body mass index (Bowles et al., 2012).

Small molecule TKIs can lead to heart failure resulting from inhibition of kinases essential to myocyte repair. Lapatinib is a small molecule TKI that targets HER2 and EGFR. It is used in combination with capecitabine in the treatment of HER2-positive breast cancer. The risk of cardiotoxicity is approximately 2%, lower than that of trastuzumab. Dasatinib, a multitargeted TKI, is used in the treatment of Philadelphia chromosome–positive chronic myeloid leukemia (CML) and acute lymphoblastic leukemia, with a 2%–4% incidence of heart failure (Yeh & Bickford, 2009). Imatinib is used to treat CML and gastrointestinal stromal tumors, with a risk of heart failure risk of 0.55–1.7% (Turrisi et al., 2010). Sunitinib, also a multitargeted TKI, is used in the treatment of metastatic renal cell cancer and gastrointestinal stromal tumors. It can lead to early cardiotoxicity in 4%–11% of patients, including potentially irreversible heart failure. The risk is increased in patients previously treated with an anthracycline and with a history of coronary artery disease (Monsuez, Charniot, Vignat, & Artigou, 2010). Bortezomib, a proteasome inhibitor used in treatment of multiple myeloma, leads to heart failure in 8% of patients (Yeh & Bickford, 2009).

Radiation therapy to the mediastinum and heart region may lead to pericarditis or myocardial infarction as acute toxicities. Late toxicities include cardiomyopathy and coronary artery disease. The pathophysiology is due to damage of the blood vessels causing inflammation with narrowing of the capillaries, leading to fibrosis. Damage to the endothelial cell membranes leads to myocyte death, ischemia, and fibrosis. Coronary artery disease results from injury to the coronary arteries (Darby et al., 2013). Fibrosis can occur in the pericardium, myocardium, or valves, leading to restrictive cardiomyopathy reduced diastolic cardiac function. Fibrosis of valves may progress 10–20 years after completion of therapy. Fibrosis of the conduction system may lead to arrhythmias (Wethal et al., 2009).

The risk of injury to the heart from radiation therapy increases with a larger volume of the heart exposed, high-dose fractions, concomitant cardiotoxic drugs (anthracyclines, trastuzumab), younger age at time of radiation, history of coronary artery disease, smoking, and hypertension (Darby et al., 2013). Patients with left-sided breast cancer who receive radiation therapy can develop cardiotoxicities that include coronary artery disease, cardiomyopathy, pericardial disease, valve dysfunction, and arrhythmias (Darby et al., 2013). In a case-controlled study of 2,168 patients receiving low-dose radiation for breast cancer, participants were found to be at increased risk, with onset from less than 5 to greater than 20 years. The risk is increased with higher overall doses of radiation. The presence of certain factors, including circulatory disease, diabetes, left-sided breast cancer, and smoking history, increased the risk (Copeland et al., 2013; Jaworski, Mariani, Wheeler, & Kaye, 2013; Perk et al., 2012). Patients with Hodgkin lymphoma who receive radiation therapy to portals above the diaphragm are at increased risk for development of valve dysfunction, angina pectoris, and myocardial infarction. The median time to development is 19 years after treatment. The risk is increased when radiation was delivered in childhood and with concurrent use of anthracyclines (Mulrooney et al., 2009).

Presenting Signs and Symptoms

Acute cardiotoxicities produce an abrupt onset of signs and symptoms, such as acute chest pain, pain radiating to the left arm or neck, shortness of breath, dyspnea on exertion, decreased or increased blood pressure, irregular or rapid heart rate, impaired cognition, and impaired oxygen exchange, or the toxicities can be asymptomatic (Berardi et al., 2013).

Chronic cardiotoxicity from CHF presents with signs of fluid overload, peripheral and pulmonary edema, jugular venous distension, shortness of breath, dyspnea on exertion, pulmonary rales, tachycardia, and inadequate tissue profusion. Patients may remain asymptomatic until severe damage has occurred (Berardi et al., 2013).

Prevention

Advanced practice nurses (APNs) should routinely screen patients for preexisting cardiac abnormalities. Patients should be encouraged to discontinue smoking and provided with resources to assist with smoking cessation. A baseline ECG and lipid panel should be obtained prior to initiation of cardiotoxic treatments. Pretreatment screening for blood pressure and LVEF should be completed in all patients prior to initiation of cardiotoxic agents. Cardiac abnormalities, such as hypertension and congestive heart failure, should be controlled prior to initiation of therapy. Pretreatment values may influence cumulative dosing of cardiotoxic therapies. VEGF inhibitors are contraindicated in patients with a history of uncontrolled angina, recent myocardial ischemia or infarction, uncontrolled arrhythmia, uncontrolled hypertension, or significant QTc interval prolongation (Le, Cao, & Yang, 2014). A risk assessment should be conducted prior to the initiation of these targeted therapies.

Multigated acquisition (MUGA) scan or echocardiogram can be used to assess LVEF. Normal LVEF is considered to be greater than 50%. In patients with borderline LVEF function (40%–50%), treatment should proceed with caution, weighing the risks and benefits as well as the patient's wishes. Patients receiving anthracyclines are monitored at baseline and periodically during treatment. Monitoring after suggested cumulative doses and then before each additional dose is recommended. Long-term monitoring is essential. Cardiotoxicity from anthracyclines may develop within the first year after completion of therapy; however, it may take up to 10–20 years to be evident (Suter & Ewer, 2013). Manufacturer guidelines for trastuzumab recommend monitoring at 3, 5, and 15 months after the initiation of trastuzumab (Genentech, Inc., 2014a). Protection from anthracycline cardiotoxicity involves limiting the lifetime cumulative dose of doxorubicin to 450–550 mg/m^2, epirubicin to 900 mg/m^2, and mitoxantrone to 140 mg/m^2 (Bonita & Pradhan, 2013). Substitution of doxorubicin with an analog, such as epirubicin or mitoxantrone, has a decreased rate of cardiotoxicity. Infusion of doxorubicin versus bolus treatment and use of liposomal pegylated formulation (Doxil®) have demonstrated decreased cardiotoxicity (Smith et al., 2010).

Use of a cardioprotective agent should be considered in patients who will benefit from ongoing treatment with an anthracycline such as doxorubicin. Dexrazoxane is an intravenously administered ethylenediaminetetraacetic acid–like chelator that binds to free iron and reduces the risk of doxorubicin-induced cardiotoxicity when administered prior to doxorubicin therapy. It is recommended only in patients with metastatic breast cancer receiving greater than 300 mg/m^2 of doxorubicin who will benefit from further treatment (Hensley et al., 2009). This limitation was prompted by fears of potential interference with doxorubicin's antitumor effect or potential development of secondary malignancies in the adjuvant setting. However, these have not been demonstrated in randomized clinical trials (Cardinale et al., 2013).

Medication reconciliation should be completed on all patients to assess for other drugs that have the potential to cause QTc prolongation. APNs should assess for potential drug-drug interactions, particularly drugs that are metabolized by the cytochrome P450 3A4 (CYP3A4) pathway, as they may inhibit or accelerate metabolism of either drug or potentiate side effects (Chen & Parameswaran, 2013).

Older adult patients are at particular risk because of comorbid medical conditions and risk of interactions from polypharmacy. Older adult patients should undergo rigorous cardiac pre-screening, with evaluation of preexisting cardiac diagnoses prior to cancer therapy. Consideration should be made to use less cardiotoxic agents or doses that do not reach upper cumulative levels, with more frequent monitoring for toxicity (Aapro et al., 2011).

Beta-blockers, such as carvedilol and nebivolol, have demonstrated reduced left ventricular dysfunction in patients receiving doxorubicin therapy (Cardinale et al., 2013). Biomarker assessment may help identify patients who are at risk for developing cardiotoxicity following anticancer therapy. In a clinical trial of 473 patients treated with high-dose doxorubicin and cyclophosphamide, 114 patients (24%) were found to have elevated levels of troponin I. These patients were randomized to receive enalapril or observation. Enalapril reduces left ventricular end-systolic wall dysfunction. The enalapril-treated group demonstrated no change in LVEF, while those not receiving the drug had a progressive reduction in LVEF (p < 0.001) and high incidence of heart failure (p < 0.001) and arrhythmias (p < 0.001) requiring treatment (Colombo, Sandri, Salvatici, Cipolla, & Cardinale, 2014). Enalapril also demonstrated improved left ventricular function in pediatric patients treated with doxorubicin, with a sustained effect of 6–10 years (Kalam & Marwick, 2013; Lipshultz et al., 2010).

Assessment and Diagnosis

Early detection of cardiotoxicity is essential for optimal treatment and recovery, as most patients will be asymptomatic for years (Bonita & Pradhan, 2013; Cardinale, Colombo, Lamantia, et al., 2010). A thorough cardiac evaluation includes assessment of heart rate, blood pressure, heart sounds (S3 gallop), jugular veins, weight gain (2 kg or more in a week), breath sounds, and edema (abdominal ascites, peripheral edema, and pulmonary edema). Patient complaints of excessive fatigue, shortness of breath, and new-onset dyspnea must be fully evaluated. Complaints of new-onset chest pain are evaluated by assessment of troponin level every eight hours to diagnose an acute myocardial infarction or other ischemic event. An ECG is performed to assess for dysrhythmias, and pulse oximetry is obtained to assess for hypoxia. Blood gases and cardiac neurohormones, such as atrial natriuretic peptide (ANP) and B-type natriuretic peptide (BNP) levels, may be helpful (Chowdhury, Kehl, Choudhary, & Maisel, 2013).

A MUGA scan or echocardiogram should be routinely scheduled beginning five years after treatment for patients who have received more than 35 Gy of radiation therapy exposure and for those who have received greater than 300 mg/m² of anthracyclines. Echocardiograms are noninvasive; however, they have operator variability. MUGA scans reduce variability but provide limited information about diastolic function and expose patients to radioactivity. However, these tests are insensitive, as changes in ejection fraction are demonstrated after significant damage to the myocardium has occurred and are poorly correlated to myocyte damage or repair (Bonita & Pradhan, 2013; Cardinale et al., 2013; Tan & Scherrer-Crosbie, 2014; Wethal et al., 2009). However, both modalities are acceptable and predictive of cardiotoxicity development (Sawaya et al., 2011). It is important to use the same modality at each evaluation to track a patient's progress over time (Hofstatter, Saadati, Russell, & Russell, 2011). Myocardial strain imaging, or deformation imaging, may detect early functional changes in myocardial function and predict future left ventricular dysfunction (Sawaya et al., 2011).

Troponin and BNP can be useful in monitoring for cardiotoxicity. Troponin is a protein found in the heart muscle. It is released into circulation when cardiomyocyte necrosis or damage is present, which also occurs with unstable angina, myocardial ischemia, and myocardial infarction (O'Brien, 2008). Monitoring of troponin levels is cost effective, more sensitive, and has less patient risk than echocardiogram/MUGA scan in identifying early cardiac damage (Cardinale et al., 2013). Elevated troponin levels indicate early myocyte damage in patients treated with high-dose chemotherapy regimens and are a predicator of future left ventricular damage (Cardinale et al., 2013; Sawaya et al., 2011). Troponin levels can be detected as soon as days after chemotherapy administration (Geiger et al., 2010). Troponin level elevations also have been seen in patients treated with standard anthracycline chemotherapy doses and with newer targeted agents such as trastuzumab (Cardinale, Colombo, Torrisi, et al., 2010). Lipshultz et al. (2010) reported increased troponin levels in pediatric patients with lymphoblastic leukemia treated with doxorubicin and cyclophosphamide, lasting several months. Those with elevations had an increase in late cardiotoxicities at five years (Lipshultz et al., 2010). Correlating troponin I and BNP with measures of LVEF may assist with early detection and prediction of patients who are at risk for cardiotoxicity (Sawaya et al., 2011).

ANP and BNP are released by the atrium and ventricles in the heart, respectively, when excessive stretch occurs, as it does with CHF (Geiger et al., 2010). These peptides help maintain blood volume and blood vessel diameter. BNP elevation of greater than 400 pg/ml is highly sensitive and correlated with echocardiogram confirmation of myocardial dysfunction. Elevation of BNP is associated with anthracycline toxicity (Cardinale & Sandri, 2010; Sawaya et al., 2011). Levels below 100 pg/ml are more indicative of fluid volume overload than CHF (Colombo et al., 2014).

Patients receiving VEGF inhibitors require active monitoring of their blood pressure. The National Cancer Institute (NCI) recommends monitoring be done weekly for one month, then every two to three weeks. The Common Terminology Criteria for Adverse Events (CTCAE) can be used to grade hypertensive toxicity (NCI Cancer Therapy Evaluation Program, 2010; see http://evs.nci.nih.gov/ftp1/CTCAE/About.html for grading scale). Antihypertensives should be initiated if grade 2–3 toxicity manifests. Grade 2 indicates moderate toxicity requiring medical intervention. Grade 3 hypertension is more severe and requires a more aggressive therapy to avoid progression to grade 4 toxicity or even death from stroke or other complications of untreated hypertension. Treatment is permanently discontinued if refractory hypertension or a hypertensive crisis occurs. Angiotensin-converting enzyme (ACE) inhibitors are recommended as first-line treatment. Calcium channel blockers should be avoided because they compete with metabolism via the CYP3A4 pathway with several VGEF inhibitors (Maitland et al., 2010; Nazer, Humphreys, & Moslehi, 2011).

A 12-lead ECG is performed for assessment of arrhythmias, complaints of chest pain, and other abnormalities. Patients who are at risk for arrhythmias should have close monitoring via ECG at regular intervals. Monitoring of QTc interval is important to identify early development of ischemic changes (Steingart et al., 2012).

If patients receiving 5-FU therapy develop angina pain during treatment, the infusion is stopped. Diagnostic studies such as ECG, chest x-ray, pulse oximetry, and troponin levels are recommended. A cardiology consult is recommended prior to resuming treatment. Nitroglycerine 0.8 mg sublingual may be useful in preventing cardiac arterial vasoconstriction in patients receiving bolus 5-FU therapy (Südhoff et al., 2004).

Early identification of heart failure prior to the demonstration of symptoms, using New York Heart Association criteria (Dolgin, 1994), is essential following completion of anthracycline therapy. Initiation of ACE inhibitors with or without beta-blockers is critical to reversal of left ventricular dysfunction within two months of treatment (Cardinale, Colombo, Lamantia, et al., 2010; Seicean et al., 2013). Heart failure caused by trastuzumab is reversible with standard heart failure therapy. Treatment can be resumed when cardiac abnormalities resolve (Cardinale, Colombo, Torrisi, et al., 2010).

Evidence-Based Treatment Strategies

Standard therapies used to treat acute and chronic CHF include ACE inhibitors, angiotensin receptor blockers, beta-blockers, vasodilators, and diuretics. ACE inhibitors are recommended as first-line therapy to improve cardiac function in patients who develop anthracycline-induced CHF (Haq et al., 1985; Jensen, Skovsgaard, & Nielsen, 2002; Ryberg et al., 1998). Patients with lymphoma had less heart failure when treated with metoprolol, although the effect was not statistically significant, leaving the authors to suggest that more research on the use of ACE inhibitors and beta-blockers is needed to determine preventive strategies (Georgakopoulos et al., 2010). However, there is a lack of data to support the long-term effects in slowing progressive dysfunction (Kalam & Marwick, 2013). No specific evidence-based guidelines currently exist for the management of anthracycline- and trastuzumab-induced heart failure in patients with cancer (Cardinale et al., 2013; Yeh & Bickford, 2009). Therefore, treatment of CHF should be based on standard American Heart Association recommendations (Yancy et al., 2013). Unless contraindicated, patients should be started on an ACE inhibitor and a beta-blocker (Fadol, 2013; Yeh & Bickford, 2009).

Treatment of hypertension should follow American Heart Association guidelines. Medications include ACE inhibitors, thiazide diuretics, beta-blockers, and calcium channel blockers (Woods, Lech, & Fadol, 2013). Several antihypertensive agents may inhibit metabolism of targeted therapies, thus increasing their potential toxicity. In addition, targeted therapies such as TKIs may inhibit metabolism of antihypertensives, requiring dose reductions (Chen & Parameswaran, 2013; Yeh & Bickford, 2009). Consultation with a cardiologist is warranted in all patients with chemotherapy-related cardiotoxicities.

Patients who develop valvular dysfunction may be at risk for endocarditis. Therefore, prophylactic treatment with antibiotics is recommended before invasive procedures (Habib et al., 2009).

Evaluation of Outcomes

Patients should receive education about the potential acute and chronic side effects of therapy prior to cancer treatment to ensure informed consent for treatment. Patients should have a cardiac history, physical examination, and LVEF evaluation at baseline, prior to each dose of cardiotoxic drug, and after therapy is completed. Part of the cardiac history includes assessing for preexisting cardiac disease and performing a full medication reconciliation to minimize the risk of drug interactions that may lead to cardiotoxicity. Oncology APNs also need to review initiation of any new medications (including supplements and over-the-counter medications).

APNs will review early signs and symptoms of toxicity with patients and instruct them to report these to the healthcare team promptly. Signs and symptoms to report include edema, shortness of breath, palpitations, exercise fatigue, and tachycardia. APNs assess and evaluate cardiac function with review of symptom history (onset, duration, and intensity), physical examination, and vital signs. Patients may need to undergo evaluation testing with ECG, MUGA scan, or echocardiogram, along with blood tests, including troponin, ANP, and BNP levels. At the first sign of cardiotoxicity, APNs should initiate appropriate interventions to prevent further cardiac decompensation. The benefits of ongoing therapy are weighed against the risk of worsening cardiac status or the development of life-threatening cardiotoxicity or death.

Implications for Oncology Advanced Practice Nurses

Oncology APNs must be knowledgeable about the risk of cardiotoxicity with anthracyclines, targeted therapies, other antineoplastic agents, and radiation therapy. Cardiotoxicities are cumulative for many agents. When cardiotoxic chemotherapy drugs are used in combination with other cardiotoxic agents or radiation therapy to the chest, the toxicity can be additive. Oncology APNs must perform a thorough baseline cardiac history and physical examination prior to the start of therapy. Assessment should continue throughout therapy and lifelong, as toxicity can develop at any time during or after treatment. Survivorship care plans can provide direction regarding the need for regular cardiovascular assessment. Recommendations for surveillance after treatment vary from yearly to every five years, depending on cumulative risk factors (Carver, Szalda, & Ky, 2013).

APNs must be prepared to educate patients on the side effect profile of each therapy, the potential risks, and the need for long-term follow-up. Counseling patients in maintaining a healthy lifestyle, including nutrition, exercise, smoking cessation, and reduction of lipid levels, can help reduce the risk of late effects such as coronary artery disease (Aapro et al., 2011; Haugnes et al., 2012; Knobf & Coviello, 2011). APNs should collaborate with cardiologists who are knowledgeable about cancer and its treatment to maximize patient care, particularly through the use of detailed risk-assessment evaluations (Albini et al., 2010; Hofstatter et al., 2011).

Pulmonary Toxicities

Pulmonary toxicities are common in cancer therapy. Different patterns of pulmonary dysfunction result following administration of several antineoplastic agents, targeted therapies, and radiation therapy. Some are serious and life threatening. Additional patterns of pulmonary dysfunction have emerged with the development of new treatment regimens and use of novel drugs. Although pulmonary toxicity is rare with most chemotherapy agents, drug-induced interstitial lung disease (ILD) is the most common toxicity overall, which involves the interstitium (between capillaries and alveolar space) of the lungs. Injury may also occur to the pleura, the airways, the pulmonary vasculature, the mediastinum, and the neuromusculature (Chapman, 2010; Ryu, 2010; Schwaiblmair et al., 2012).

Idiopathic interstitial pneumonia is a generic term that encompasses many diseases. This group of diseases is defined by involvement of the pulmonary interstitium more so than the alveolar spaces or airways. Recently, the classification of idiopathic interstitial pneumonia has been updated according to the groupings of major, rare, and unclassified. The *major* group includes diseases such as idiopathic pulmonary fibrosis, idiopathic nonspecific interstitial pneumonia, respiratory bronchiolitis-associated ILD, desquamative interstitial pneumonia, cryptogenic organizing pneumonia (formerly referred to as bronchiolitis obliterans organizing pneumonia, or BOOP), and acute interstitial pneumonia. The *rare* category includes idiopathic lymphoid interstitial pneumonia and idiopathic pleuroparenchymal fibroelastosis (Antoniou et al., 2014; Chapman, 2010; Travis et al., 2013).

The most common pulmonary toxicities are capillary leak syndrome; dyspnea; bronchospasm; ILD, specifically cryptogenic organizing pneumonia; acute respiratory distress syndrome (ARDS); interstitial pneumonitis; and pulmonary fibrosis. The pattern of presentation may be acute or delayed. The damage may be reversible if prompt medical attention is initiated. However, toxicity may be permanently disabling and lead to death if left undiagnosed and untreated. Each of the toxicities will be reviewed in this chapter.

Etiology, Pathophysiology, and Risk Factors

Capillary leak syndrome results from extravasation of plasma proteins and fluid into the extravascular space. It is characterized by edema, hypoproteinemia, and hemoconcentration. Capillary leak syndrome may be seen with bevacizumab, an inducer of vascular permeability; bortezomib; docetaxel; gemcitabine; granulocyte–colony-stimulating factor; interferon; interleukin-2; interleukin-11; and VEGF (Gardini et al., 2013; Hsiao, Wang, Chang, & Pei, 2010; Kai-Feng, Hong-Ming, Hai-Zhou, Li-Rong, & Xi-Yan, 2011; Lesterhuis et al., 2009; Samlowski et al., 2011; Shinohara, 2011; Xu, Zhao, & Tang, 2013; Yabe et al., 2010). It is also a complication of stem cell transplantation. Resolution of symptoms may or may not occur with discontinuation of the drug.

Dyspnea is associated with bortezomib, carfilzomib, lapatinib, sunitinib, and sorafenib (Barber & Ganti, 2011). The etiology is not understood, and it often is accompanied by other pulmonary symptoms. Infusion-related bronchospasm has occurred with cetuximab, etoposide, gemcitabine, mitomycin C, panitumumab, taxanes (paclitaxel, docetaxel), and vinca alkaloids (vincristine, vinblastine, vinorelbine) (Achermann et al., 2012; Barber & Ganti, 2011; Chua, Peters, Loneragan, & Clarke, 2009; Gardini et al., 2013).

Acute lung injury with diffuse alveolar damage can occur with mitomycin C and bleomycin. It is associated with high concentrations of inspired oxygen related to oxidative stress and the body's inability to protect against the toxic effects of oxygen damage (Schwaiblmair et al., 2012). Pleural effusions can occur in 20% of patients treated with dasatinib, especially when twice-daily dosing was used. Therefore, once-daily dosing is now used for dasatinib (Brixey & Light, 2010; Latagliata et al., 2013). Dasatinib also is associated with pulmonary hypertension (Orlandi, Rocca, Pazzano, & Ghio, 2012).

Cryptogenic organizing pneumonia can be a fatal pulmonary toxicity of methotrexate, gemcitabine, and rituximab (Hardak et al., 2012; Kawsar, Spiro, Cocco, & Daw, 2011; Lioté, Lioté, Séroussi, Mayaud, & Cadranel, 2010). The onset may occur after the first infusion or after several cycles (Hadjinicolaou, Nisar, Parfrey, Chilvers, & Östör, 2012). Rare cases of cryptogenic organizing pneumonia have been reported following thoracic irradiation (Fahim, Campbell, & Hart, 2012).

Several antineoplastic agents, molecular-targeted agents, and immunotherapies are associated with the development of ILD and interstitial pneumonitis. Noninfectious pneumonitis may develop as an autoimmune response to medication or T-cell-mediated hypersensitivity (Albiges et al., 2012; Grünwald et al., 2013). Antineoplastic agents associated with ILD and pneumonitis are listed in Figure 12-1. Pneumotox (http://pneumotox.com) is a regularly updated website that lists drugs implicated with specific pulmonary toxicity (Pneumotox, n.d.).

Rituximab can lead to the organizing pneumonia mentioned previously, as well as ILD fibrosis, and ARDS (Lioté et al., 2010). A systematic review of the literature identified 121 patients across several studies with ILD. ILD occurred more often in men and people between the ages of 50 and 60. Onset may occur after the first infusion or after several cycles and has been fatal (Hadjinicolaou et al., 2012).

Interstitial pneumonitis is a toxicity seen with molecular-targeted therapies. Targeted therapies are inhibitors or blockers of various targets, including EGFR inhibitors, TKIs, mammalian target of rapamycin inhibitors, VEGF inhibitors, proteasome inhibitors, and ALK inhibitors. The field of targeted therapies is growing rapidly with frequent introduction of new agents. Targeted therapies associated with pneumonitis are shown in Figure 12-2. Interstitial pneumonitis can be a treatment-limiting toxicity of immunotherapy agents (e.g., nivolumab pembrolizumab), agents targeting programmed death-1 receptor, and ipilimumab, an agent targeting the cytotoxic T-lymphocyte-associated antigen 4 (Brahmer et al., 2012; Hamid & Carvajal, 2013; Wolchok et al., 2013). Supportive medications, such as beta-blockers, ciprofloxacin, trimethoprim-sulfamethoxazole, and statins, can produce pneumonitis (Pneumotox, n.d.).

The risk and severity of interstitial pneumonitis are increased with the concurrent use of pulmonary toxic therapies, higher dosing, and dose-dense administration schedules of antineoplastic agents. The risk also is increased with cigarette smoking, age older than 70 years, very young age, preexisting pulmonary disease, prior history of radiation to the lungs, and high fraction of inspired oxygen (Dang et al., 2013; Hamid & Carvajal, 2012; Kharofa & Gore, 2013; Venkatramani et al., 2013). See Figure 12-3 for a more complete listing of risk factors for

• Anastrozole	• Cytarabine	• Methotrexate
• Bleomycin	• Docetaxel	• Mitomycin C
• Busulfan	• Fludarabine	• Paclitaxel
• Carmustine	• Gemcitabine	• Sorafenib
• Cyclophosphamide	• Interferon alpha	• Temozolomide

Figure 12-1. Antineoplastic Agents* Associated With Interstitial Lung Disease or Pneumonitis

* List is not all-inclusive.

Note. Based on information from Barber & Ganti, 2011; Chi et al., 2012; Disel et al., 2010; Gurram et al., 2013; Horiuchi-Yamamoto et al., 2012; Maldonado et al., 2007; Paulik et al., 2012; Tamura et al., 2013.

• Bortezomib	• Everolimus	• Rapamycin
• Cetuximab	• Gefitinib	• Rituximab
• Crizotinib	• Imatinib	• Temsirolimus
• Dasatinib	• Lenalidomide	• Thalidomide
• Erlotinib	• Panitumumab	• Trastuzumab

Figure 12-2. Targeted Therapies* Associated With Pneumonitis

* List is not all-inclusive.

Note. Based on information from Achermann et al., 2012; Albiges et al., 2012; Amraoui et al., 2013; Barber & Ganti, 2011; Bergeron et al., 2007; Dabydeen et al., 2012; Hoag et al., 2009; Iacovelli et al., 2012; Kang et al., 2011; Pepels et al., 2009; Tamura et al., 2013; Timm & Kolesar, 2013; Yamaguchi et al., 2012.

- Cigarette smoking
- Age
  - Older than 65 years
  - Very young age
- Ethnicity
- Preexisting pulmonary disease
- Radiation therapy
  - Prior radiation therapy
  - Concurrent with chemotherapy
  - Larger doses
  - Larger area of radiation
- High-dose oxygen therapy
- Gender (varies by drug)
- Drug-drug interactions
- Certain chemotherapy agents
  - Bleomycin
  - Carmustine
  - Cyclophosphamide
  - Lomustine

- Certain cardiovascular medications
  - Amiodarone
  - Statins
- Anti-inflammatories
  - Acetylsalicylic acid
  - Methotrexate
  - Nonsteroidal anti-inflammatory drugs
- Antimicrobials
  - Amphotericin B
  - Nitrofurantoin
  - Sulfasalazine
  - Sulfonamides
- Biologics
  - Anti-CD20 antibodies
  - Recombinant interferon alpha
  - T-cell antiproliferative agents such as cetuximab, bevacizumab, alemtuzumab, and trastuzumab
  - Tumor necrosis factor–alpha

Figure 12-3. Risk Factors for Pulmonary Toxicity Related to Cancer Treatment

Note. Based on information from Dang et al., 2013; Kharofa et al., 2012; Schwaiblmair et al., 2012; Venkatramani et al., 2013.

pulmonary toxicity, including the drugs most commonly implicated in drug-induced interstitial lung disease (DILD).

Radiation therapy causes cytotoxic damage to DNA, producing free radicals and cytokine release. These in turn cause damage to pneumocyte and endothelial cells, leading to a diffuse inflammatory process of pneumonitis (Dang et al., 2013). Pneumonitis typically develops within 4–12 weeks after treatment completion. Cella et al. (2014) reported that 9 out of 69 patients (13%) developed lung changes related to radiation therapy for Hodgkin lymphoma at a median of 10 months (range 9–18). The risk of pneumonitis increases when radiation is administered as concurrent therapy with radiosensitizing antineoplastic agents such as cyclophosphamide, irinotecan, gemcitabine, mitomycin C, taxanes (docetaxel, paclitaxel), and antifolates (pemetrexed) (Graves, Siddiqui, Anscher, & Movsas, 2010; Marks et al., 2010; Tsoutsou, 2014; Yazbeck, Villaruz, Haley, & Socinski, 2013). Pneumonitis also may develop in patients who receive sequential treatment with doxorubicin, etoposide, gemcitabine, paclitaxel, pemetrexed, and sunitinib following prior radiation therapy to a lung field (Barber & Ganti, 2011; Hochstrasser et al., 2012; Sadowska, Specenier, Germonpre, & Peeters, 2013; Seidel et al., 2010; Umemura et al., 2011; Yuasa et al., 2013). This phenomenon of radiation damage that is subclinical but develops later as a result of certain chemotherapy is referred to as *radiation recall*. It has produced latent dermatitis and pneumonitis (Forschner et al., 2014). Limited information exists in the literature describing the relationship of certain chemotherapy agents and radiation recall pneumonitis. Figure 12-4 lists agents that have been associated with radiation recall pneumonitis. The total volume of lung tissue irradiated and dose of radiation are the most significant risk factors for the development of pneumonitis (Dang et al., 2013; Marks et al., 2010; Venkatramani et al., 2013; Yazbeck et al., 2013).

Pulmonary fibrosis is a latent effect from radiation therapy. It may develop following resolution of acute pneumonitis or independently (Yazbeck et al., 2013). It also can result from treat-

• Docetaxel	• Gefitinib	• Sunitinib
• Doxorubicin	• Gemcitabine	• Trastuzumab
• Erlotinib	• Paclitaxel	• Vemurafenib
• Etoposide		

Figure 12-4. Chemotherapy Associated With Radiation Recall Pneumonitis

Note. Based on information from Arakawa et al., 2011; Castellano et al., 2003; Ding et al., 2011; Forschner et al., 2014; Kataoka et al., 1992; Lee et al., 2014; Ma et al., 1993; Malik et al., 2011; Merchant et al., 2012; Miya et al., 2003; Onal et al., 2012; Schwarte et al., 2007; Schweitzer et al., 1995; Seidel et al., 2010; Togashi et al., 2010; Yuasa et al., 2013.

ment with antineoplastics, including bleomycin, cetuximab, cyclophosphamide, methotrexate, mitomycin C, nitrosoureas, and panitumumab. Fibrosis may develop within 6–12 months or after a lengthy latent period. It is related to larger volume of lung irradiated, cumulative dosing (more than 20 Gy), very young and older age, high fraction of inspired oxygen, chronic obstructive pulmonary disease, and cigarette smoking (Barber & Ganti, 2011; Schwaiblmair et al., 2012).

ARDS has been linked to high-dose chemotherapy regimens, immunosuppression, and neutropenia, particularly in stem cell transplantation (Barber & Ganti, 2011). Lung damage sustained by these treatments leads to accumulation of fluid in the interstitial space and alveoli and predisposes patients to sepsis, which is the leading cause of ARDS. The syndrome leads to poor gas exchange and poor pulmonary compliance and may progress to pulmonary hypertension. Patients with hematologic malignancies, large thoracic tumor volume, and neutropenia are at increased risk for developing ARDS (Boeck et al., 2009; Mokart et al., 2012; Tükoğlu et al., 2013).

Presenting Signs and Symptoms

The symptoms associated with treatment-induced ILD, pneumonitis, fibrosis, and ARDS may begin with nonspecific reports of fever, chills, breathlessness, nonproductive cough, dyspnea, chest pain, and malaise (Achermann et al., 2012). These nonspecific signs and symptoms can make diagnosis of pulmonary toxicity very challenging. Patients may be asymptomatic, demonstrating ground-glass, linear and nodular opacities on radiographs. However, symptoms may progress rapidly if no intervention is initiated. On physical examination, tachypnea and use of accessory muscles may be noted. Occasional moist rales, pleural friction rub, or wheezing may be auscultated. In severe cases, hypoxia, respiratory insufficiency, cyanosis, pulmonary hypertension, acute cor pulmonale, and death may result (Dabydeen et al., 2012; Graves et al., 2010). Patients with capillary leak syndrome may have generalized edema and hypotension (Kai-Feng et al., 2011). DILD may present with digital clubbing and auscultation of respiratory crackles (Schwaiblmair et al., 2012). The onset of symptoms for each of the pulmonary toxicities is variable from days to weeks to months.

Prevention

Pulmonary function tests may be indicated before the administration of pulmonary toxic drugs. Pulmonary toxic treatments should be limited or used with extreme caution in patients with baseline chronic obstructive pulmonary disease or severe pulmonary fibrosis.

Various strategies have been used in the administration of radiation therapy to prevent or minimize pulmonary toxicity. Intensity-modulated radiation therapy and stereotactic body radiation therapy are approaches to minimize exposure of normal lung tissue to radiation while increasing delivery of dosing to cancer within the lung region (Graves et al., 2010; Oh, Ahn, Kim, & Pyo, 2013; Yazbeck et al., 2013). Alternative dosing schedules, such as hypofractionated (twice-daily dosing) radiation, have been employed as well (Cannon et al., 2013; Kobayashi et al., 2010; Oh et al., 2013). Amifostine, pentoxifylline, and ACE inhibitors have been used as cytoprotectants to minimize pneumonitis with mixed results and are not included in American Society of Clinical Oncology (ASCO) clinical practice guidelines (Graves et al., 2010; Kharofa, Cohen, Tomic, Xiang, & Gore, 2012; Yazbeck et al., 2013).

Assessment and Diagnosis

A thorough history and assessment of patients prior to treatment to obtain baseline pulmonary function is essential. The objective of the history and physical is to meticulously rule out other causes of pulmonary symptoms because ILD is a diagnosis of exclusion. A health history should include inquiry about prior pulmonary diagnoses, chest irradiation, exposures to pulmonary toxic agents, medication reconciliation, and smoking history. Because the time to onset ranges widely, this information may not prove very useful, but acute onset time is a characteristic of acute pneumonitis (Schwaiblmair et al., 2012). Pulmonary evaluation includes temperature, respiratory rate, heart rate, breath sounds, and oxygen saturation. Oxygen saturation should be measured at rest and with ambulation if possible to assess for exercise-induced hypoxia. Patient complaints of chest pressure, wheezing, shortness of breath, cough, and malaise should be fully evaluated. Early detection of pulmonary toxicity is essential for optimal treatment and recovery. Pulmonary evaluation should be completed prior to each treatment and then routinely following completion of therapy. Determination of baseline characteristics of increased risk will prove useful for both prevention and early detection of pulmonary toxicities.

The diagnosis of pneumonitis and other pulmonary toxicities is primarily a clinical diagnosis. Laboratory tests, diagnostic imaging, and interventional diagnostic procedures can help support and differentiate a pulmonary diagnosis but may not be particularly helpful in direct diagnosis of ILD. Laboratory tests include complete blood count, coagulation studies, BNP, blood cultures, sputum cultures, and virology. Microbiology and virology testing is obtained to rule out infectious pneumonia. A chest x-ray may be normal in the early stages of dysfunction. It may reveal diffuse haziness, ground-glass infiltrates, or opacities with progression of toxicity (Graves et al., 2010). DILD may present with drug-induced eosinophilia and presence of antinuclear antibody, anti-cytoplasmic antibody, and anti–glomerular basal membrane autoantibody elevated titers that support an autoimmune versus a nonautoimmune condition (Schwaiblmair et al., 2012). A computed tomography (CT) scan, preferably high-resolution CT, may show ground-glass consolidation or reticular opacities with pneumonitis (Achermann et al., 2012; Dabydeen et al., 2012; Tamura et al., 2013; Torrisi et al., 2011). Diffuse patchy nodules, volume loss with areas of consolidation, and discrete hazy areas are common in previously irradiated areas, indicating DILD (Schwaiblmair et al., 2012). Lobular dense consolidation may result with progression of inflammatory processes (Albiges et al., 2012). Pulmonary function tests are helpful for characterizing the pattern (obstructive, restrictive) and severity of respiratory impairment. Bronchoscopy with bronchoalveolar lavage (BAL) may be required to obtain cell cultures from the airways to help rule out infection and disease progression, as opposed to treatment toxicity. Lymphocytosis may be evident in the BAL with inflammatory processes (Grünwald et al., 2013). The ultimate diagnosis of ILD may be made after clinical improvement occurs with removal of the suspected offending agent or recurrence of ILD symptoms with rechallenge of the offending drug.

Evidence-Based Treatment Strategies

Once the offending agent is suspected or identified, treatment of pulmonary toxicity depends on severity of impairment. For asymptomatic pneumonitis, patients may continue with treatment if therapeutic effect is noted. If minor symptoms are present, interruption of therapy should be considered until symptoms resolve, which usually is expected. With severe symptoms, therapy should be discontinued, and patients should be treated with supportive care and steroids (Dabydeen et al., 2012; Seruga, Gan, & Knox, 2009). Other management strategies include limiting the cumulative dose of bleomycin to 400 units and minimizing the use of supplemental oxygen therapy in patients receiving drugs known to cause pulmonary toxicity (e.g., bleomycin, mitomycin C, nitrosoureas) (Froudarakis et al., 2013). Strategies for the prevention of pulmonary toxicities have shown mixed results and are not currently standard practice recommended by ASCO. Patients need to be risk stratified very carefully for their ability to receive potentially pulmonary toxic therapies.

Glucocorticoid therapy is initiated to treat moderate to severe symptoms of pneumonitis, with the goal of suppressing inflammation to prevent fibrosis. In general, treatment is empiric rather than evidence based. No randomized clinical trials have been conducted on the effectiveness of glucocorticoid therapy for the management of chemotherapy- or radiation-induced pulmonary toxicity, yet this is the standard treatment approach. Prednisone (0.75–1 mg/kg) is given orally daily or at doses of 60–100 mg orally daily for 2 weeks, with taper over 3–12 weeks until improvement. Patients with grade 3 pneumonitis (according to the CTCAE [NCI Cancer Therapy Evaluation Program, 2010]) should be admitted to the hospital for IV glucocorticoid therapy and supportive care. IV methylprednisolone (2–5 mg/kg/day in divided doses) may be required initially for severe symptoms (Achermann et al., 2012; Albiges et al., 2012; Graves et al., 2010; Grünwald et al., 2013; Gurram, Pulivarthi, & McGary, 2013; Yazbeck et al., 2013). Patients with grade 3 pneumonitis should be admitted to the hospital for monitoring of their respiratory status and disease progression. Patients may demonstrate clinical improvement within days of steroid initiation; however, radiographic improvement may not be seen for weeks to months (Hadjinicolaou et al., 2012). Steroids are expected to stop the inflammatory process and further lung damage, but it will not reverse lung tissue that has already died and fibrosed. Patients who are treated with steroids should be considered for a pneumococcal vaccine and annual influenza virus vaccine because of their risk for additional immunosuppression. Reactivation of tuberculosis also must be considered in this patient population (Schwaiblmair et al., 2012).

Supportive therapy may include oxygen support; however, extreme caution should be used with high concentrations of inspired oxygen in patients who have received bleomycin because of the risk of developing ARDS (Aakre, Efem, Wilson, Kor, & Eisenach, 2014). Empiric antibiotic therapy may be used with corticosteroid therapy. Bronchodilators are prescribed if evidence of bronchoconstriction is present.

The ACE inhibitors lisinopril and captopril may be effective in treating radiation pneumonitis (Kharofa & Gore, 2013). Pentoxifylline (400 mg TID) has been used as vascular therapy to help decrease fibrosis secondary to radiation therapy (Westbury & Yarnold, 2012).

Prognosis for recovery from ILD depends on early removal of the offending agent and initiation of supportive treatment. Prognostic variables include the specific drug; the physiologic, pathologic, and clinical severity of lung disease; and the amount of irreversible damage. For example, amiodarone is associated with a 40%–50% mortality rate even with early withdrawal of the drug and supportive treatment with steroids, as opposed to 15% in methotrexate-induced ILD (Schwaiblmair et al., 2012).

Evaluation of Outcomes

Patients should receive education about the potential for acute, delayed, and chronic side effects of cancer therapy prior to initiation of treatment to ensure informed consent. Patients should have a pulmonary history and physical examination performed at baseline, prior to each dose of pulmonary toxic drug, and at routine intervals following completion of therapy. The history should include preexisting pulmonary diagnoses and treatments. APNs should complete a full medication review to identify any medications with potential for pulmonary toxicity. They also should instruct patients to consult with the healthcare team prior to the initiation of new medications, including naturopathic and over-the-counter treatments.

APNs need to review early signs and symptoms of toxicity with patients and instruct them to report these to the healthcare team. Signs and symptoms include fever, chills, cough, breathlessness, chest pressure, wheeze, and tachypnea. APNs should assess and evaluate pulmonary function with review of symptom history (onset, duration, and intensity), physical examination, and vital signs. Patients may need to undergo pulmonary function tests and have a baseline chest radiograph or CT obtained. At the first sign of pulmonary toxicity, the healthcare team should undertake appropriate interventions to prevent further respiratory compromise. The benefits of ongoing therapy are weighed against the risk of worsening pulmonary status or the development of life-threatening toxicity or death.

Implications for Oncology Advanced Practice Nurses

Oncology APNs can play a pivotal role in the management of patients who are at risk for pulmonary toxicity. APNs must be knowledgeable about the risk of pulmonary toxicities with chemotherapy agents, targeted agents, immunotherapies, and radiation therapy. APNs should conduct a thorough history and physical examination before the start of treatment to help identify those patients who might be at increased risk. APNs should encourage smoking cessation and educate patients to maintain a healthy lifestyle to decrease the risk of long-term toxicities (Demark-Wahnefried, Rock, Patrick, & Byers, 2008). APNs should be actively involved in the screening of at-risk patients for pulmonary toxicities at each visit. Early diagnosis and treatment are critical to the successful management of pneumonitis and other pulmonary toxicities.

APNs should be prepared to educate patients about the potential for pulmonary toxicities while on therapy. Patients must be educated about the early signs of pulmonary toxicity and instructed to contact a healthcare provider if they develop cough, dyspnea, or fever. APNs can help communicate the potential for toxicities to other members of the patient's healthcare team.

If a patient is diagnosed with pneumonitis or other pulmonary toxicities, close clinical follow-up is essential. If a patient is clinically stable to be managed as an outpatient, the APN should conduct a physical examination every two weeks until symptoms resolve. Repeat CT scans should be obtained at two weeks, four weeks, and intermittently until complete resolution of radiographic pneumonitis.

Conclusion

Cardiac and pulmonary toxicities are potential complications in the acute and delayed setting for patients being treated for cancer. Toxicity may result from chemotherapy, biotherapy, or radiation therapy. Cardiotoxicities include heart failure, hypertension, arrhythmias, valve disease, ECG changes, coronary artery spasms, angina, myocardial infarction, and cardiomyopathy. Structural changes to the heart can also develop, such as pericardial effusion, cardiac tamponade, and pericardial fibrosis. Pulmonary toxicities include capillary leak syndrome, dyspnea, ILD, interstitial pneumonitis, fibrosis, organizing pneumonia, and ARDS. Oncology APNs play a crucial role in the evaluation of patients who are at risk for the development of toxicity. Early recognition is essential for successful management of cardiac and pulmonary toxicities. Patient education is critical to the safe management of patients receiving cardiotoxic and pulmonary toxic therapies.

Case Study

J.C. is a 72-year-old man diagnosed with multiple myeloma. His treatment regimen is bortezomib administered as subcutaneous injection of 1.3 mg/m^2 days 1, 4, 8, 11, 22, 25, 29, and 32 of a 42-day treatment cycle for four cycles, followed by 1.3 mg/m^2 days 1, 8, 22, and 29 of a 42-day treatment cycle for five cycles. This will be administered in conjunction with melphalan and prednisone.

1. What information should the APN obtain in a history and examination of J.C. prior to the start of therapy to screen for risk of pulmonary toxicity?
   • The APN should review the patient's past medical history, including prior pulmonary diagnoses (e.g., tuberculosis, chronic obstructive pulmonary disease, prior chest irradiation), medication review, and current review of symptoms. Physical examination should include assessment of vital signs, pulmonary sounds, and oxygen saturation.
2. J.C. has a history of hypercholesterolemia treated with a statin. He has a 60-pack-year history of smoking, having quit upon his recent myeloma diagnosis. He reports that he rarely has seen his primary care physician. What preliminary testing might be indicated for J.C. prior to the start of therapy?
   • The APN should consider obtaining baseline pulmonary function tests and chest radiograph.
3. Prior to cycle 5 of treatment, J.C. reports an increase in shortness of breath, dry nonproductive cough, and malaise. He has also noted ankle edema. What further evaluation should the APN conduct?
   • The APN should complete a full physical examination, including assessment of vital signs and oxygen saturation. The APN suspects capillary leak syndrome and potential pneumonitis. A chest radiograph is indicated; however, a high-resolution CT scan is preferred. Further dosing of bortezomib should be held until evaluation is completed.
4. J.C. has patchy ground-glass opacities on CT scan. Oxygen saturation has decreased to 88% on room air. J.C. reports an increase in effort of breathing. What treatment should the APN recommend?
   • J.C. has been on low-dose prednisone. He is immunosuppressed and at high risk for progression of symptoms and potential ARDS. He is admitted to the hospital for glucocorticoid administration and supportive care. Further treatment with bortezomib will be evaluated upon recovery of symptoms.

Key Points

Cardiac Toxicities

• Anthracyclines are therapeutically effective antineoplastic agents when the following criteria are met: baseline cardiotoxicity assessments, tracking of lifetime cumulative doses, ongoing patient assessment, and close monitoring.

- Cardiotoxicities include CHF, arrhythmias, hypertension, ECG changes, coronary artery spasms, angina, myocardial infarction, cardiomyopathy, and coronary artery disease, which may develop at any time during or immediately following treatment and for the remainder of the patient's life. Structural changes to the heart also can develop, such as valve disease, pericardial effusion, cardiac tamponade, and pericardial fibrosis.
- Monitoring of blood pressure, LVEF function with MUGA or echocardiogram, and ECG is crucial to the successful use of anthracyclines.

Pulmonary Toxicities

- Interstitial pneumonitis is a common pulmonary toxicity of several antineoplastic and targeted agents, as well as radiation therapy, used in the treatment of cancer.
- Symptoms of pulmonary toxicity are nonspecific, including nonproductive cough, mild to progressive dyspnea, and low-grade fever.
- The onset of pulmonary toxicity is variable; it can develop after one treatment to several months following therapy.
- Management of pulmonary toxicities includes interruption of therapy, glucocorticoid administration, and supportive care.

Recommended Resources for Oncology Advanced Practice Nurses

Cardiac Toxicities

- American Heart Association: www.heart.org (resources available at Healthcare/Research page)
- CardioOnc.org: www.cardioonc.org
- *Cardiotoxicity of Oncologic Treatments*, an open-access book edited by M. Fiuza, published in 2012: www.intechopen.com/books/cardiotoxicity-of-oncologic-treatments
- NCI CTCAE: http://ctep.cancer.gov/protocolDevelopment/electronic_applications/ctc.htm
- New York Heart Association Classification for Congestive Heart Failure: www.heart.org/HEARTORG/Conditions/HeartFailure/AboutHeartFailure/Classes-of-Heart-Failure_UCM_306328_Article.jsp

Pulmonary Toxicities

- ASCO: www.cancer.net/navigating-cancer-care/side-effects/shortness-breath-or-dyspnea
- Oncology Nursing Society Putting Evidence Into Practice resource on dyspnea: www.ons.org/practice-resources/pep/dyspnea
- Pneumotox: http://pneumotox.com

References

Aakre, B.M., Efem, R.I., Wilson, G.A., Kor, D.J., & Eisenach, J.H. (2014). Postoperative acute respiratory distress syndrome in patients with previous exposure to bleomycin. *Mayo Clinic Proceedings, 89*, 181–189. doi:10.1016/j.mayocp.2013.11.007

Aapro, M., Bernard-Marty, C., Brain, E.G.C., Batist, G., Erdkamp, F., Krzemieniecki, K., … Wedding, U. (2011). Anthracycline cardiotoxicity in the elderly cancer patient: A SIOG expert position paper. *Annals of Oncology, 22*, 257–267. doi:10.1093/annonc/mdq609

Achermann, Y., Frauenfelder, T., Obrist, S., Zaugg, K., Corti, N., & Günthard, H.F. (2012). A rare but severe pulmonary side effect of cetuximab in two patients. *BMJ Case Reports.* doi:10.1136/bcr-03-2012-5973

Ades, F., Zardavas, D., Pinto, A.C., Criscitiello, C., Aftimos, P., & de Azambuja, E. (2014). Cardiotoxicity of systemic agents used in breast cancer. *Breast, 23*, 317–328. doi:10.1016/j.breast.2014.04.002

Albiges, L., Chamming's, F., Duclos, B., Stern, M., Motzer, R.J., Ravaud, A., & Camus, P. (2012). Incidence and management of mTOR inhibitor-associated pneumonitis in patients with metastatic renal cell carcinoma. *Annals of Oncology, 23*, 1943–1953. doi:10.1093/annonc/mds115

Albini, A., Pennesi, G., Donatelli, F., Cammarota, R., De Flora, S., & Noonan, D.M. (2010). Cardiotoxicity of anticancer drugs: The need for cardio-oncology and cardio-oncological prevention. *Journal of the National Cancer Institute, 102*, 14–25. doi:10.1093/jnci/djp440

Al-Hashmi, S., Boels, P.J.M., Zadjali, F., Sadeghi, B., Sällström, J., Hultenby, K., … Hassan, M. (2012). Busulphan-cyclophosphamide cause endothelial injury, remodeling of resistance arteries and enhanced expression of endothelial nitric oxide synthase. *PLOS ONE, 7*, e30897. doi:10.1371/journal.pone.0030897

Amraoui, K., Belhadj, K., Maître, B., Jannière-Nartey, C., & Dupuis, J. (2013). Pulmonary toxicity after long-term treatment with lenalidomide in two myeloma patients. *European Respiratory Review, 22*(127), 93–95. doi:10.1183/09059180.00001912

Antoniou, K.M., Margaritopoulos, G.A., Tomassetti, S., Bonella, F., Costabel, U., & Poletti, V. (2014). Interstitial lung disease. *European Respiratory Review, 23*(131), 40–54. doi:10.1183/09059180.00009113

Arakawa, H., Johkoh, T., Sakai, F., Kusumoto, M., Hataji, O., & Taguchi, O. (2011). Exacerbation of radiation fibrosis with erlotinib: Another pattern of radiation recall phenomenon. *Japanese Journal of Radiology, 29*, 587–589. doi:10.1007/s11604-011-0590-x

ARIAD Pharmaceuticals, Inc. (2014). *Iclusig® (ponatinib)* [Package insert]. Cambridge, MA: Author.

Astellas Pharma US, Inc., & Genentech, Inc. (2012). *Tarceva® (erlotinib)* [Package insert]. South San Francisco, CA: Author.

AstraZeneca Pharmaceuticals LP. (2014). *Caprelsa® (vandetanib)* [Package insert]. Wilmington, DE: Author.

Bair, S.M., Choueiri, T.K., & Moslehi, J. (2013). Cardiovascular complications associated with novel angiogenesis inhibitors: Emerging evidence and evolving perspectives. *Trends in Cardiovascular Medicine, 23*, 104–113. doi:10.1053/j.seminoncol.2013.01.004

Barber, N.A., & Ganti, A.K. (2011). Pulmonary toxicities from targeted therapies: A review. *Targeted Oncology, 6*, 235–243. doi:10.1007/s11523-011-0199-0

Baxter. (2013). *Cyclophosphamide* [Package insert]. Deerfield, IL: Author.

Bayer HealthCare Pharmaceuticals Inc. (2013). *Stivarga® (regorafenib)* [Package insert]. Wayne, NJ: Author.

Bayer HealthCare Pharmaceuticals, Inc., & Onyx Pharmaceuticals, Inc. (2013). *Nexavar® (sorafenib)* [Package insert]. Whippany, NJ: Bayer HealthCare Pharmaceuticals, Inc.

Bedford Laboratories. (2008). *Cytarabine* [Package insert]. Bedford, OH: Author.

Bedford Laboratories. (2013a). *Daunorubicin hydrochloride injection* [Package insert]. Bedford, OH: Author.

Bedford Laboratories. (2013b). *Mitomycin* [Package insert]. Bedford, OH: Author.

Berardi, R., Caramanti, M., Savini, A., Chiorrini, S., Pierantoni, C., Onofri, A., … Cascinu, S. (2013). State of the art for cardiotoxicity due to chemotherapy and to targeted therapies: A literature review. *Critical Reviews in Oncology/Hematology, 88*, 75–86. doi:10.1016/j.critrevonc.2013.02.007

Bergeron, A., Réa, D., Levy, V., Picard, C., Meignin, V., Tamvurini, J., … Rousselot, P. (2007). Lung abnormalities after dasatinib treatment for chronic myeloid leukemia: A case series. *American Journal of Respiratory and Critical Care Medicine, 176*, 814–818. doi:10.1164/rccm.200705-715CR

Boeck, S., Metzeler, K.H., Hausmann, A., Baumann, A., Gallmeier, E., Parhofer, K.G., & Stemmler, H.-J. (2009). Cisplatin-based chemotherapy for pulmonary metastasized germ cell tumors of the testis—Be aware of acute respiratory distress syndrome. *Onkologie, 32*, 125–128. doi:10.1159/000197728

Bonita, R., & Pradhan, R. (2013). Cardiovascular toxicities of cancer chemotherapy. *Seminars in Oncology, 40*, 156–167. doi:10.1053/j.seminoncol.2013.01.004

Bowles, E.J.A., Wellman, R., Feigelson, H.S., Onitilo, A.A., Freedman, A.N., Delate, T., … Wagner, E.H. (2012). Risk of heart failure in breast cancer patients after anthracycline and trastuzumab treatment: A retrospective cohort study. *Journal of the National Cancer Institute, 104*, 1293–1305. doi:10.1093/jnci/djs317

Brahmer, J.R., Tykodi, S.S., Chow, L.Q., Hwu, W.J., Drake, C.J., Camacho, L.H., … Wigginton, J.M. (2012). Safety and activity of anti-PD-L1 antibody in patients with advanced cancer. *New England Journal of Medicine, 366*, 2455–2465. doi:10.1056/NEJMoa1200694

Bristol-Myers Squibb Co. (2007). *Ifex® (ifosfamide)* [Package insert]. Princeton, NJ: Author.

Bristol-Myers Squibb Co. (2011a). *Ixempra® (ixabepilone)* [Package insert]. Princeton, NJ: Author.

Bristol-Myers Squibb Co. (2011b). *Taxol® (paclitaxel)* [Package insert]. Princeton, NJ: Author.

Bristol-Myers Squibb Co. (2013). *Etopophos® (etoposide phosphate)* [Package insert]. Princeton, NJ: Author.

Bristol-Myers Squibb Co. (2014). *Sprycel® (dasatinib)* [Package insert]. Princeton, NJ: Author.

Brixey, A.G., & Light, R.W. (2010). Pleural effusions due to dasatinib. *Current Opinion in Pulmonary Medicine, 16,* 351–356. doi:10.1097/MCP.0b013e328338c486

Cannon, D.M., Mehta, M.P., Adkison, J.B., Khuntia, D., Traynor, A.M., Tomé, W.A., … Cannon, B.M. (2013). Dose-limiting toxicity after hypofractionated dose-escalated radiotherapy in non-small-cell lung cancer. *Journal of Clinical Oncology, 31,* 4343–4348. doi:10.1200/JCO.2013.51.5353

Cardinale, D., Bacchiani, G., Beggiato, M., Colombo, A., & Cipolla, C.M. (2013). Strategies to prevent and treat cardiovascular risk in cancer patients. *Seminars in Oncology, 40,* 186–198. doi:10.1053/j.seminoncol.2013.01.008

Cardinale, D., Colombo, A., Lamantia, G., Colombo, N., Civelli, M., DeGiacomi, G., … Cipolla, C.M. (2010). Anthracycline-induced cardiomyopathy: Clinical relevance and response to pharmacologic therapy. *Journal of the American College of Cardiology, 55,* 213–220. doi:10.1016/j.jacc.2009.03.095

Cardinale, D., Colombo, A., Torrisi, R., Sandri, M.T., Civelli, M., Salvatici, M., … Cipolla, C.M. (2010). Trastuzumab-induced cardiotoxicity: Clinical and prognostic implications of troponin I evaluation. *Journal of Clinical Oncology, 28,* 3910–3916. doi:10.1200/JCO.2009.27.3615

Cardinale, D., & Sandri, M.T. (2010). Role of biomarkers in chemotherapy-induced cardiotoxicity. *Progress in Cardiovascular Diseases, 53,* 121–129. doi:10.1016/j.pcad.2010.04.002

Carver, J.R., Szalda, D., & Ky, B. (2013). Asymptomatic cardiac toxicity in long-term cancer survivors: Defining the population and recommendations for surveillance. *Seminars in Oncology, 40,* 229–238. doi:10.1053/j.seminoncol.2013.01.005

Castellano, D., Hitt, R., Ciruelos, E., Cortés-Funes, H., & Colomer, R. (2003). Biweekly vinorelbine and gemcitabine: A phase I dose-finding study in patients with advanced solid tumors. *Annals of Oncology, 14,* 783–787. doi:10.1093/annonc/mdg196

Celgene Corp. (2013). *Abraxane® (paclitaxel protein-bound particles for injectable suspension)* [Package insert]. Summit, NJ: Author.

Cella, L., Liuzzi, R., D'Avino, V., Conson, M., Di Biase, A., Picardi, M., … Pacelli, R. (2014). Pulmonary damage in Hodgkin's lymphoma patients treated with sequential chemo-radiotherapy: Predictors of radiation-induced lung injury. *Acta Oncologica, 53,* 613–619. doi:10.3109/0284186X.2013.850739

Cephalon, Inc. (2010). *Trisenox® (arsenic trioxide)* [Package insert]. Frazer, PA: Author.

Chapman, J.T. (2010). Interstitial lung disease. Retrieved from http://www.clevelandclinicmeded.com/medicalpubs/diseasemanagement/pulmonary/interstitial-lung-disease/#f0010

Chen, C.L., & Parameswaran, R. (2013). Managing the risks of cardiac therapy in cancer patients. *Seminars in Oncology, 40,* 210–217. doi:10.1053/j.seminoncol.2013.01.006

Chi, D.C., Brogan, F., Turenne, I., Zelonis, S., Schwartz, L., & Saif, M.W. (2012). Gemcitabine-induced pulmonary toxicity. *Anticancer Research, 32,* 4147–4149. Retrieved from http://ar.iiarjournals.org/content/32/9/4147.long

Chou, R., Cruciani, R.A., Fiellin, D.A., Compton, P., Farrar, J.T., Haigney, M.C., … Zelter, L. (2014). Methadone safety: A clinical practice guideline from the American Pain Society and College on Problems of Drug Dependence, in collaboration with the Heart Rhythm Society. *Journal of Pain, 15,* 321–337. doi:10.1016/j.jpain.2014.01.494

Chowdhury, P., Kehl, D., Choudhary, R., & Maisel, A. (2013). The use of biomarkers in the patient with heart failure. *Current Cardiology Reports, 15,* 372. doi:10.1007/s11886-013-0372-4

Chua, W., Peters, M., Loneragan, R., & Clarke, S. (2009). Cetuximab-associated pulmonary toxicity. *Clinical Colorectal Cancer, 8,* 118–120. doi:10.3816/CCC.2009.n.019

Colombo, A., Sandri, A.T., Salvatici, M., Cipolla, C.M., & Cardinale, D. (2014). Cardiac complications of chemotherapy: Role of biomarkers. *Current Treatment Options in Cardiovascular Medicine, 16,* 313. doi:10.1007/s11936-014-0313-6

Copeland, K.A., Hosmane, V.R., Jurkovitz, C., Kolm, P., Bowen, J., DiSabatino, A., … Doorey, A.J. (2013). Frequency of severe valvular disease caused by mediastinal radiation among patients undergoing valve surgery in a community-based, regional academic medical center. *Clinical Cardiology, 36,* 217–221. doi:10.1002/clc.22106

Dabydeen, D.A., Jagannathan, J.P., Ramaiya, N., Krajewski, K., Schutz, F.A.B., Cho, D.C., … Choueiri, T.K. (2012). Pneumonitis associated with mTOR inhibitors therapy in patients with metastatic renal cell carcinoma: Incidence, radiographic findings and correlation with clinical outcome. *European Journal of Cancer, 48,* 1519–1524. Retrieved from http://www.ejcancer.com/article/S0959-8049(12)00275-4/abstract

Dang, J., Li, G., Ma, L., Diao, R., Zang, S., Han, C., … Yao, L. (2013). Predictors of grade ≥ 2 and ≥ 3 radiation pneumonitis in patients with locally advanced non-small cell lung cancer treated with three-dimensional conformal radiotherapy. *Acta Oncologica, 52,* 1175–1180. doi:10.3109/0284186X.2012.747696

Darby, S.C., Ewertz, M., McGale, P., Bennet, A.M., Blom-Goldman, U., Brønnum, D., … Hall, P. (2013). Risk of ischemic heart disease in women after radiotherapy for breast cancer. *New England Journal of Medicine, 368,* 987–998. doi:10.1056/NEJMoa1209825

Demark-Wahnefried, W., Rock, C.L., Patrick, K., & Byers, T. (2008). Lifestyle interventions to reduce cancer risk and improve outcomes. *American Family Physician, 77,* 1573–1578.

Ding, X., Ji, W., Li, J., Zhang, X., & Wang, L. (2011). Radiation recall pneumonitis induced by chemotherapy after thoracic radiotherapy for lung cancer. *Radiation Oncology, 6,* 24. doi:10.1186/1748-717X-6-24

Disel, U., Paydas, S., Yavuz, S., & Karakoc, E. (2010). Severe pulmonary toxicity associated with fludarabine and possible contribution of rituximab. *Chemotherapy, 56,* 89–93. doi:10.1159/000305255

Dolgin, M. (1994). *Nomenclature and criteria for diagnosis of diseases of the heart and great vessels* (9th ed.). Boston, MA: Little, Brown.

Eisai Inc. (2013). *Halaven® (eribulin mesylate)* [Package insert]. Woodcliff Lake, NJ: Author.

Eisai Inc. (2015). *Lenvima™ (lenvatinib)* [Package insert]. Woodcliff Lake, NJ: Author.

Eli Lilly and Co. (2015). *Cyramza® (ramucirumab)* [Package insert]. Indianapolis, IN: Author.

Ewer, M.S., & Ewer, S.M. (2013). Enigmas regarding the true extent and impact of tyrosine kinase inhibitor-related cardiotoxicity. *Expert Opinion on Drug Safety, 12,* 611–614. doi:10.1517/14740338.2013.828033

Exelixis, Inc. (2012). *Cometriq® (cabozantinib)* [Package insert]. South San Francisco, CA: Author.

Fadol, A.P. (2013). Heart failure in patients with cancer. In A.P. Fadol (Ed.), Cardiac complications of cancer therapy (pp. 159–194). Pittsburgh, PA: Oncology Nursing Society.

Fahim, A., Campbell, A.P., & Hart, S.P. (2012). Bronchiolitis obliterans organizing pneumonia: A consequence of breast radiotherapy. *BMJ Case Reports.* doi:10.1136/bcr.10.2011.4987

Fiùza, M. (2009). Cardiotoxicity associated with trastuzumab treatment of HER-2+ breast cancer. *Advances in Therapy, 26*(Suppl. 1), S9–S17. doi:10.1007/s12325-009-0048-z

Forschner, A., Zips, D., Schraml, C., Röcken, M., Iordanou, E., Leiter, U., … Meier, F. (2014). Radiation recall dermatitis and radiation pneumonitis during treatment with vemurafenib. *Melanoma Research, 24,* 512–516. doi:10.1097/CMR.0000000000000078

Froudarakis, M., Hatzimichael, E., Kyriazopoulou, L., Lagos, K., Pappas, P., Tzakos, A.G., … Briasoulis, E. (2013). Revisiting bleomycin from pathophysiology to safe clinical use. *Critical Reviews in Oncology/Hematology, 87,* 90–100. doi:10.1016/j.critrevonc.2012.12.003

Gardini, A.C., Aquilina, M., Oboldi, D., Lucchesi, A., Carloni, S., Tenti, E., … Frassineti, G.L. (2013). Separate episodes of capillary leak syndrome and pulmonary hypertension after adjuvant gemcitabine and three years later after nab-paclitaxel for metastatic disease. *BMC Cancer, 13,* 542. doi:10.1186/1471-2407-13-542

Geiger, S., Lange, V., Suhl, P., Heinemann, V., & Stemmler, H.-J. (2010). Anticancer therapy induced cardiotoxicity: Review of the literature. *Anti-Cancer Drugs, 21,* 578–590. doi:10.1097/CAD.0b013e3283394624

Genentech, Inc. (2013a). *Avastin® (bevacizumab)* [Package insert]. South San Francisco, CA: Author.

Genentech, Inc. (2013b). *Rituxan® (rituximab)* [Package insert]. South San Francisco, CA: Author.

Genentech, Inc. (2013c). *Xeloda® (capecitabine)* [Package insert]. South San Francisco, CA: Author.

Genentech, Inc. (2014a). *Herceptin® (trastuzumab)* [Package insert]. South San Francisco, CA: Author.

Genentech, Inc. (2014b). *Zelboraf® (vemurafenib)* [Package insert]. South San Francisco, CA: Author.

Genentech, Inc. (2015). *Perjeta® (pertuzumab)* [Package insert]. South San Francisco, CA: Author.

Genzyme Corp. (2009). *Campath® (alemtuzumab)* [Package insert]. Cambridge, MA: Author.

Georgakopoulos, P., Roussou, P., Matsakas, E., Karavidas, A., Anagnostopoulos, N., Marinakis, T., … Ahimastos, A. (2010). Cardioprotective effect of metoprolol and enalapril in doxorubicin-treated lymphoma patients: A prospective, parallel-group, randomized, controlled study with 36-month follow-up. *American Journal of Hematology, 85,* 894–896. doi:10.1002/ajh.21840

GlaxoSmithKline. (2013). *Tykerb® (lapatinib)* [Package insert]. Research Triangle Park, NC: Author.

GlaxoSmithKline. (2014). *Votrient® (pazopanib)* [Package insert]. Research Triangle Park, NC: Author.

Graves, P.R., Siddiqui, F., Anscher, M.S., & Movsas, B. (2010). Radiation pulmonary toxicity: From mechanisms to management. *Seminars in Radiation Oncology, 20,* 201–207. doi:10.1016/j.semradonc.2010.01.010

Grünwald, V., Weikert, S., Pavel, M.E., Hörsch, D., Lüftner, D., Janni, W., … Weber, M.M. (2013). Practical management of everolimus-related toxicities in patients with advanced solid tumors. *Onkologie, 36,* 295–302. doi:10.1159/000350625

Gurram, M.K., Pulivarthi, S., & McGary, C.T. (2013). Fatal hypersensitivity pneumonitis associated with docetaxel. *Tumori, 99,* e100–e103. doi:10.1700/1334.14814

Habib, G., Hoen, B., Tornos, P., Thuny, F., Prendergast, G., Vilacosta, I., … Zamorano, J.L. (2009). Guidelines on the prevention, diagnosis, and treatment of infective endocarditis (new version 2009): The Task Force on the Prevention, Diagnosis, and Treatment of Infective Endocarditis of the European Society of Cardiology (ESC). Endorsed by the European Society of Clinical Microbiology and Infectious Diseases (ESCMID) and by the International Society of Chemotherapy (ISC) for Infection and Cancer. *European Heart Journal, 30,* 2369–2413. doi:10.1093/eurheartj/ehp285

Hadjinicolaou, A.V., Nisar, M.K., Parfrey, H., Chilvers, E.R., & Östör, A.J.K. (2012). Non-infectious pulmonary toxicity of rituximab: A systematic review. *Rheumatology, 51,* 653–662. doi:10.1093/rheumatology/ker290

Hamid, O., & Carvajal, R.D. (2013). Anti-programmed death-1 and anti-programmed death-ligand 1 antibodies in cancer therapy. *Expert Opinion on Biological Therapy, 13,* 847–861. doi:10.1517/14712598.2013.770836

Haq, M.M., Legha, S.S., Choksi, J., Hortobagyi, G.N., Benjamin, R.S., Ewer, M., & Ali, M. (1985). Doxorubicin-induced congestive heart failure in adults. *Cancer, 56,* 1361–1365. doi:10.1002/1097-0142(19850915)56:6<1361::AID-CNCR2820560624>3.0.CO;2-S

Hardak, E., Oren, I., Dann, E.J., Yigla, M., Faibish, T., Rowe, J.M., & Avivi, I. (2012). The increased risk for pneumocystis pneumonia in patients receiving rituximab-CHOP-14 can be prevented by the administration of trimethoprim/sulfamethoxazole: A single-center experience. *Acta Haematologica, 127,* 110–114. doi:10.1159/000334113

Haugnes, H.S., Bosl, G.J., Boer, H., Gietema, J.A., Brydøy, M., Oldenburg, J., … Fosså, S.D. (2012). Long-term and late effects of germ cell testicular cancer treatment and implications for follow-up. *Journal of Clinical Oncology, 30,* 3752–3763. doi:10.1200/JCO.2012.43.4431

Hensley, M.L., Hagerty, K.L., Kewalramani, T., Green, D.M., Meropol, N.J., Wasserman, T.H., … Schuchter, L.M. (2009). American Society of Clinical Oncology 2008 clinical practice guideline update: Use of chemotherapy and radiation therapy protectants. *Journal of Clinical Oncology, 27,* 127–145. doi:10.1200/JCO.2008.17.2627

Hoag, J.B., Azizi, A., Doherty, T.J., Lu, J., Willis, R.E., & Rund, M.E. (2009). Association of cetuximab with adverse pulmonary events in cancer patients: A comprehensive review. *Journal of Experimental and Clinical Cancer Research, 28,* 113. doi:10.1186/1756-9966-28-113

Hochstrasser, A., Benz, G., Joerger, M., Templeton, A., Brutsche, M., & Früh, M. (2012). Interstitial pneumonitis after treatment with pemetrexed: A rare event? *Chemotherapy, 58,* 84–88. doi:10.1159/000336131

Hofstatter, E., Saadati, H., Russell, K., & Russell, R. (2011). Clinical vignettes: Integrated care of cancer patients by oncologists and cardiologists. *Current Cardiology Reviews, 7,* 258–261. doi:10.2174/157340311799960654

Horiuchi-Yamamoto, Y., Gemma, A., Taniguchi, H., Inoue, Y., Sakai, F., Johkoh, T., … Kudoh, S. (2012). Drug-induced lung injury associated with sorafenib: Analysis of all-patient post-marketing surveillance in Japan. *International Journal of Clinical Oncology, 18,* 743–749. doi:10.1007/s10147-012-0438-0

Hsiao, S.C., Wang, M.C., Chang, H., & Pei, S.N. (2010). Recurrent capillary leak syndrome following bortezomib therapy in a patient with relapsed myeloma. *Annals of Pharmacotherapy, 44,* 587–589. doi:10.1345/aph.1M585

Iacovelli, R., Palazzo, A., Mezi, S., Morano, F., Naso, G., & Cortesi, E. (2012). Incidence and risk of pulmonary toxicity in patients treated with mTOR inhibitors for malignancy: A meta-analysis of published trials. *Acta Oncologica, 51,* 873–879. doi:10.3109/0284186X.2012.705019

Janssen Products, LP. (2013). *Doxil® (doxorubicin hydrochloride liposome injection)* [Package insert]. Horsham, PA: Author.

Jaworski, C., Mariani, J.A., Wheeler, G., & Kaye, D.M. (2013). Cardiac complications of thoracic irradiation. *Journal of the American College of Cardiology, 61,* 2319–2328. doi:10.1016/j.jacc.2013.01.090

Jensen, B.V., Skovsgaard, T., & Nielsen, S.L. (2002). Functional monitoring of anthracycline cardiotoxicity: A prospective, blinded, long-term observational study of outcome in 120 patients. *Annals of Oncology, 13,* 699–709. doi:10.1093/annonc/mdf132

Kai-Feng, W., Hong-Ming, P., Hai-Zhou, L., Li-Rong, S., & Xi-Yan, Z. (2011). Interleukin-11-induced capillary leak syndrome in primary hepatic carcinoma patients with thrombocytopenia. *BMC Cancer, 11,* 204. doi:10.1186/1471-2407-11-204

Kalam, K., & Marwick, T.H. (2013). Role of cardioprotective therapy for prevention of cardiotoxicity with chemotherapy: A systematic review and meta-analysis. *European Journal of Cancer, 49,* 2900–2909. doi:10.1016/j.ejca.2013.04.030

Kang, J.J., Park, J.S., Kim, D.W., Lee, J., Jeong, Y.J., Choi, S.M., … Yim, J.J. (2011). Adverse pulmonary reactions associated with the use of monoclonal antibodies in cancer patients. *Respiratory Medicine, 106,* 443–450. doi:10.1016/j.rmed.2011.11.009

Kataoka, M., Kawamura, M., Nishiyama, Y., Higashino, H., Fujii, T., Mogami, H., … Hamamoto, K. (1992). A case with delayed-onset radiation pneumonitis suspected to be induced by oral etoposide. *Nihon Igaku Hōshasen Gakkai Zasshi, 52,* 641–645.

Kawsar, H.I., Spiro, T.P., Cocco, A., & Daw, H.A. (2011). BOOP as a rare complication of gemcitabine therapy. *BMJ Case Reports.* doi:10.1136/bcr.04.2011.4055

Keating, N.L., O'Malley, A.J., Freedland, S.J., & Smith, M.R. (2010). Diabetes and cardiovascular disease during androgen deprivation therapy: Observational study of veterans with prostate cancer. *Journal of the National Cancer Institute, 102,* 39–46. doi:10.1093/jnci/djp404

Kharofa, J., Cohen, E.P., Tomic, R., Xiang, Q., & Gore, E. (2012). Decreased risk of radiation pneumonitis with incidental concurrent use of angiotensin-converting enzyme inhibitors and thoracic radiation therapy. *International Journal of Radiation Oncology, Biology, Physics, 84,* 238–243. doi:10.1016/j.ijrobp.2011.11.013

Kharofa, J., & Gore, E. (2013). Symptomatic radiation pneumonitis in elderly patients receiving thoracic irradiation. *Clinical Lung Cancer, 14,* 283–287. doi:10.1016/j.cllc.2012.10.005

Knobf, M.T., & Coviello, J. (2011). Lifestyle interventions for cardiovascular risk reduction in women with breast cancer. *Current Cardiology Reviews, 7,* 250–257. doi:10.2174/157340311799960627

Kobayashi, H., Uno, T., Isobe, K., Ueno, N., Walanabe, M., Harada, R., … Ito, H. (2010). Radiation pneumonitis following twice daily radiotherapy with concurrent carboplatin and paclitaxel in patients with stage III non-small-cell lung cancer. *Japanese Journal of Clinical Oncology, 40,* 464–469. doi:10.1093/jjco/hyp190

Latagliata, R., Breccia, M., Fava, C., Stagno, F., Tiribelli, M., Luciano, L., … Alimena, G. (2013). Incidence, risk factors and management of pleural effusions during dasatinib treatment in unselected elderly patients with chronic myelogenous leukaemia. *Hematological Oncology, 31,* 103–109. doi:10.1002/hon.2020

Le, D.L., Cao, H., & Yang, L.X. (2014). Cardiotoxicity of molecular-targeted drug therapy. *Anticancer Research, 34,* 3243–3249.

Lee, H.E., Jeong, N.J., Lee, Y., Seo, Y.J., Kim, C.D., Lee, J.H., & Im, M. (2014). Radiation recall dermatitis and pneumonitis induced by trastuzumab (Herceptin®). *International Journal of Dermatology, 53,* e159–e160. doi:10.1111/j.1365-4632.2012.05788.x

Lesterhuis, W.J., Rennings, A.J., Leenders, W.P., Nooteboom, A., Punt, C.J., Sweep, F.C., … Van der Meer, J.W. (2009). Vascular endothelial growth factor in systemic capillary leak syndrome. *American Journal of Medicine, 122,* e5–e7. doi:10.1016/j.amjmed.2009.01.020

Lioté, H., Lioté, F., Séroussi, B., Mayaud, C., & Cadranel, J. (2010). Rituximab-induced lung disease: A systematic literature review. *European Respiratory Journal, 35,* 681–687. doi:10.1183/09031936.00080209

Lipshultz, S.E., Scully, R.E., Lipsitz, S.R., Sallan, S.E., Silverman, L.B., Miller, T.L., … Colan, S.D. (2010). Assessment of dexrazoxane as a cardioprotectant in doxorubicin-treated children with high-risk acute lymphoblastic leukemia: Long-term follow-up of a prospective, randomized, multicentre trial. *Lancet Oncology, 11,* 950–961. doi:10.1016/S1470-2045(10)70204-7

Ma, L.D., Taylor, G.A., Wharam, M.D., & Wiley, J.M. (1993). Recall pneumonitis: Adriamycin potentiation of radiation pneumonitis in two children. *Radiology, 187,* 465–467. doi:10.1148/radiology.187.2.8475291

Magnano, L.C., Cibrian, N.M., González, X.A., & Bosch, X. (2014). Cardiac complications of chemotherapy: Role of prevention. *Current Treatment Options in Cardiovascular Medicine, 16,* 312. doi:10.1007/s11936-014-0312-7

Maitland, M.L., Bakris, G.L., Black, H.R., Chen, H.X., Durand, J.-B., Elliott, W.J., … Cardiovascular Toxicities Panel, Convened by the Angiogenesis Task Force of the National Cancer Institute Investigational Drug Steering Committee. (2010). Initial assessment, surveillance, and management of blood pressure in patients receiving vascular endothelial growth factor signaling pathway inhibitors. *Journal of the National Cancer Institute, 102,* 596–604. doi:10.1093/jnci/djq091

Maldonado, F., Limper, A.H., Lim, K.G., & Aubrey, M.C. (2007). Temozolomide-associated organizing pneumonitis. *Mayo Clinic Proceedings, 82,* 771–773. doi:10.1016/S0025-6196(11)61197-X

Malik, S.M., Collins, B., Pishvaian, M., Ramzi, P., Marshall, J., & Hwang, J. (2011). A phase I trial of bexarotene in combination with docetaxel in patients with advanced solid tumors. *Clinical Lung Cancer, 12,* 231–236. doi:10.1016/j.cllc.2011.03.024

Marks, L.B., Bentzen, S.M., Deasy, J.O., Kong, F.M., Bradley, J.D., Vogelius, I.S., … Jackson, A. (2010). Radiation dose-volume effects in the lung. *International Journal of Radiation Oncology, Biology, Physics, 76,* S70–S76. doi:10.1016/j.ijrobp.2009.06.091

Merchant, M.S., Geller, J.I., Baird, K., Chou, A.J., Galli, S., Charles, A., … Mackall, C.L. (2012). Phase I trial and pharmacokinetic study of lexatumumab in pediatric patients with solid tumors. *Journal of Clinical Oncology, 30,* 4141–4147. doi:10.1200/JCO.2012.44.1055

Merck & Co., Inc. (2013). *Zolinza® (vorinostat)* [Package insert]. Whitehouse Station, NJ: Author.

Merck & Co., Inc. (2014). *Intron® A (interferon alfa-2b, recombinant)* [Package insert]. Whitehouse Station, NJ: Author.

Miya, T., Ono, Y., Tanaka, H., Koshiishi, Y., & Goya, T. (2003). [Radiation recall pneumonitis induced by gefitinib (Iressa): A case report]. *Nihon Kokyūki Gakkai Zasshi, 41,* 565–568.

Mokart, D., van Craenenbroeck, T., Lambert, J., Textoris, J., Brun, J.P., Sannini, A., … Blache, J.L. (2012). Prognosis of acute respiratory distress syndrome in neutropenic cancer patients. *European Respiratory Journal, 40,* 169–176. doi:10.1183/09031936.00150611

Monsuez, J.J., Charniot, J.C., Vignat, N., & Artigou, J.Y. (2010). Cardiac side-effects of cancer chemotherapy. *International Journal of Cardiology, 144,* 3–15. doi:10.1016/j.ijcard.2010.03.003

Mulrooney, D.A., Yeazel, M.W., Kawashima, T., Mertens, A.C., Mitby, P., Stovall, M., … Leisenring, W.M. (2009). Cardiac outcomes in a cohort of adult survivors of childhood and adolescent cancer: Retrospective analysis of the Childhood Cancer Survivor Study cohort. *BMJ, 339,* b4606. doi:10.1136/bmj.b4606

National Cancer Institute Cancer Therapy Evaluation Program. (2010). *Common terminology criteria for adverse events* [v.4.03]. Retrieved from http://ctep.cancer.gov/protocolDevelopment/electronic_applications/ctc.htm

Nazer, B., Humphreys, B.D., & Moslehi, J. (2011). Effects of novel angiogenesis inhibitors for the treatment of cancer on the cardiovascular system: Focus on hypertension. *Circulation, 124,* 1687–1691. doi:10.1161/CIRCULATIONAHA.110.992230

Novartis Pharmaceuticals Corp. (2014a). *Gleevec® (imatinib mesylate)* [Package insert]. East Hanover, NJ: Author.

Novartis Pharmaceuticals Corp. (2014b). *Tasigna® (nilotinib)* [Package insert]. East Hanover, NJ: Author.

O'Brien, P.J. (2008). Cardiac troponin is the most effective translational safety biomarker for myocardial injury in cardiotoxicity. *Toxicology, 245,* 206–218. doi:10.1016/j.tox.2007.12.006

Oh, D., Ahn, Y.C., Kim, B., & Pyo, H. (2013). Hypofractionated three-dimensional conformal radiation therapy alone for central located cT1-3N0 non-small-cell lung cancer. *Journal of Thoracic Oncology, 8,* 624–629. doi:10.1097/JTO.0b013e31828cb6db

Onal, C., Abali, H., Koc, Z., & Kara, S. (2012). Radiation recall pneumonitis caused by erlotinib after palliative definitive radiotherapy. *Onkologie, 35,* 191–194. doi:10.1159/000337616

Orlandi, E.M., Rocca, B., Pazzano, A.S., & Ghio, S. (2012). Reversible pulmonary arterial hypertension likely related to long-term, low-dose dasatinib treatment for chronic myeloid leukaemia. *Leukemia Research, 36,* e4–e6. doi:10.1016/j.leukres.2011.08.007

Paulik, A., Grim, J., & Filip, S. (2012). Predictors of irinotecan toxicity and efficacy in treatment of metastatic colorectal cancer. *Acta Medica, 55,* 153–159.

Pepels, M.J., Boomars, K.A., van Kimmenade, R., & Hupperets, P.S. (2009). Life-threatening interstitial lung disease associated with trastuzumab: Case report. *Breast Cancer Research and Treatment, 113,* 609–612. doi:10.1007/s10549-008-9966-8

Perk, J., De Backer, G., Gohlke, H., Graham, I., Reiner, Z., Verschuren, W.M., … Zannad, F. (2012). European guidelines on cardiovascular disease prevention in clinical practice (version 2012). The Fifth Joint Task Force of the European Society of Cardiology and Other Societies on Cardiovascular Disease Prevention in Clinical Practice (constituted by representatives of nice societies and by invited experts). *European Heart Journal, 33,* 1635–1701. doi:10.1714/1264.13964

Pfizer Inc. (2011). *Methotrexate* [Package insert]. New York, NY: Author.

Pfizer Inc. (2013a). *Inlyta® (axitinib)* [Package insert]. New York, NY: Author.

Pfizer Inc. (2013b). *Xalkori® (crizotinib)* [Package insert]. New York, NY: Author.

Pfizer Inc. (2014a). *Ellence® (epirubicin)* [Package insert]. New York, NY: Author.

Pfizer Inc. (2014b). *Emcyt® (estramustine)* [Package insert]. New York, NY: Author.

Pfizer Inc. (2014c). *Sutent® (sunitinib malate)* [Package insert]. New York, NY: Author.

Pneumotox. (n.d.). The drug-induced respiratory disease website. Retrieved from http://pneumotox.com

Prometheus Laboratories Inc. (2012). *Proleukin® (aldesleukin)* [Package insert]. San Diego, CA: Author.

Regeneron Pharmaceuticals, Inc., & Sanofi-Aventis U.S. LLC. (2013). *Zaltrap® (ziv-aflibercept)* [Package insert]. Bridgewater, NJ: Sanofi-Aventis U.S. LLC.

Ryberg, M. (2013). Cardiovascular toxicities of biological therapies. *Seminars in Oncology, 40,* 168–177. doi:10.1053/j.seminoncol.2013.01.002

Ryberg, M., Nielsen, D., Skovsgaard, T., Hansen, J., Jensen, B.V., & Dombernowsky, P. (1998). Epirubicin cardiotoxicity: An analysis of 469 patients with metastatic breast cancer. *Journal of Clinical Oncology, 16,* 3502–3508.

Ryu, J.H. (2010). Chemotherapy-induced pulmonary toxicity in lung cancer patients. *Journal of Thoracic Oncology, 5,* 1313–1314. doi:10.1097/JTO.0b013e3181e9dbb9

Sadowska, A.M., Specenier, P., Germonpre, P., & Peeters, M. (2013). Antineoplastic therapy-induced pulmonary toxicity. *Expert Review of Anticancer Therapy, 13,* 997–1006. doi:10.1586/14737140.2013.817684

Sagent Pharmaceuticals. (2011). *Fludarabine* [Package insert]. Schaumburg, IL: Author.

Samlowski, W.E., Kondapaneni, M., Tharkar, S., McGregor, J.R., Lauback, V.E., & Salvemini, D. (2011). Endothelial nitric oxide synthase is a key mediator of interleukin-2-induced hypotension and vascular leak syndrome. *Journal of Immunotherapy, 34,* 419–427. doi:10.1097/CJI.0b013e31821dcb50

Sanofi-Aventis U.S. LLC. (2013). *Taxotere® (docetaxel)* [Package insert]. Bridgewater, NJ: Author.

Sawaya, H., Sebag, I.A., Plana, J.C., Januzzi, J.L., Ky, B., Cohen, V., … Scherrer-Crosbie, M. (2011). Early detection and prediction of cardiotoxicity in chemotherapy-treated patients. *American Journal of Cardiology, 107,* 1375–1380. doi:10.1016/j.amjcard.2011.01.006

Schlitt, A., Jordan, K., Vordemark, D., Schwamborn, J., & Thomssen, C. (2014). Cardiotoxicity and oncological treatments. *Deutsches Arzteblatt International, 111,* 161–168. doi:10.3238/arztebl.2014.0161

Schwaiblmair, M., Behr, W., Haeckel, T., Märkl, B., Foerg, W., & Berghaus, T. (2012). Drug induced interstitial lung disease. *Open Respiratory Medicine Journal, 6,* 63–74. doi:10.2174/1874306401206010063

Schwarte, S., Wagner, K., Karstens, J.H., & Bremer, M. (2007). Radiation recall pneumonitis induced by gemcitabine. *Strahlentherapie und Onkologie, 183,* 215–217. doi:10.1007/s00066-007-1688-z

Schweitzer, V.G., Juillard, G.J.F., Bajada, C.L., & Parker, R.G. (1995). Radiation recall dermatitis and pneumonitis in a patient treated with paclitaxel. *Cancer, 76,* 1069–1072. doi:10.1002/1097-0142(19950915)76:6<1069::AID-CNCR2820760623>3.0.CO;2-7

Seicean, S., Seicean, A., Alan, N., Plana, J.C., Budd, G.T., & Marwick, T.H. (2013). Cardioprotective effect of β-adrenoceptor blockade in patients with breast cancer undergoing chemotherapy: Follow-up study of heart failure. *Circulation: Heart Failure, 6,* 420–426. doi:10.1161/CIRCHEARTFAILURE.112.000055

Seidel, C., Janssen, S., Karstens, J.H., Welte, T., Morgan, M., Ganser, A., & Grünwald, V. (2010). Recall pneumonitis during systemic treatment with sunitinib. *Annals of Oncology, 21,* 2119–2120. doi:10.1093/annonc/mdq444

Senkus, E., & Jassem, J. (2011). Cardiovascular effects of systemic cancer treatment. *Cancer Treatment Reviews, 37,* 300–311. doi:10.1016/j.ctrv.2010.11.001

Seruga, B., Gan, H.K., & Knox, J.J. (2009). Managing toxicities and optimal dosing of targeted drugs in advanced kidney cancer. *Current Oncology, 16*(Suppl. 1), S52–S59.

Shinohara, K. (2011). Systemic capillary leak syndrome caused by granulocyte colony-stimulating factor [Letter to the editor]. *Internal Medicine, 50,* 2259. doi:10.2169/internalmedicine.50.5647

Smith, L.A., Cornelius, V.R., Plummer, C.J., Levitt, G., Verrill, M., Canney, P., & Jones, A. (2010). Cardiotoxicity of anthracycline agents for the treatment of cancer: Systematic review and meta-analysis of randomized controlled trials. *BMC Cancer, 10,* 337. doi:10.1186/1471-2407-10-337

Steingart, R.M., Bakris, G.L., Chen, H.X., Chen, M.-H., Force, T., Ivy, S.P., … Tang, W.H.W. (2012). Management of cardiac toxicity in patients receiving vascular endothelial growth factor signaling pathway inhibitors. *American Heart Journal, 163,* 156–163. doi:10.1016/j.ahj.2011.10.018

Südhoff, T., Enderle, M.-D., Pahlke, M., Petz, C., Teschendorf, C., Graeven, U., & Schmiegel, W. (2004). 5-Fluorouracil induces arterial vasocontractions. *Annals of Oncology, 15,* 661–664. doi:10.1093/annonc/mdh150

Suter, T.M., & Ewer, M.S. (2013). Cancer drugs and the heart: Importance and management. *European Heart Journal, 34,* 1102–1111. doi:10.1093/eurheartj/ehs181

Tamura, M., Saraya, T., Fujiwara, M., Hiraoka, S., Yokoyama, T., Yano, K., … Goto, H. (2013). High-resolution computed tomography findings for patients with drug-induced pulmonary toxicity, with special reference to hypersensitivity pneumonitis-like patterns in gemcitabine-induced cases. *Oncologist, 18,* 454–459. doi:10.1634/theoncologist.2012-0248

Tan, T.C., & Scherrer-Crosbie, M. (2014). Cardiac complications of chemotherapy: Role of imaging. *Current Treatment Options in Cardiovascular Medicine, 16,* 296. doi:10.1007/s11936-014-0296-3

Teva Pharmaceuticals. (2009). *Idarubicin* [Package insert]. Irvine, CA: Author.

Teva Pharmaceuticals. (2012a). *Adrucil® (fluorouracil injection)* [Package insert]. Irvine, CA: Author.

Teva Pharmaceuticals. (2012b). *Mitoxantrone injection* [Package insert]. Irvine, CA: Author.

Teva Pharmaceuticals. (2012c). *Platinol® (cisplatin)* [Package insert]. Irvine, CA: Author.

Teva Pharmaceuticals. (2012d). *Vesanoid® (all-trans retinoic acid)* [Package insert]. Irvine, CA: Author.

Teva Pharmaceuticals. (2013). *Bleomycin* [Package insert]. Irvine, CA: Author.

Timm, A., & Kolesar, J.M. (2013). Crizotinib for the treatment of non-small-cell lung cancer. *American Journal of Health-System Pharmacy, 70,* 943–947. doi:10.2146/ajhp120261

Togashi, Y., Masago, K., Mishima, M., Fukudo, M., & Inui, K. (2010). A case of radiation recall pneumonitis induced by erlotinib, which can be related to high plasma concentration. *Journal of Thoracic Oncology, 5,* 924–925. doi:10.1097/JTO.0b013e3181dab0dd

Torrisi, J.M., Schwartz, L.H., Gollub, M.J., Ginsberg, M.S., Bosl, G.J., & Hricak, H. (2011). CT findings of chemotherapy-induced toxicity: What radiologists need to know about the clinical and radiologic manifestations of chemotherapy toxicity. *Radiology, 258,* 41–56. doi:10.1148/radiol.10092129

Travis, W.D., Costabel, U., Hansell, D.M., King, T.E., Jr., Lynch, D.A., Nicholson, A.G., … Valeyre, D. (2013). An official American Thoracic Society/European Respiratory Society Statement: Update of the international multidisciplinary classification of the idiopathic interstitial pneumonias. *American Journal of Respiratory and Critical Care Medicine, 188,* 733–748. doi:10.1164/rccm.201308-1483ST

Tsoutsou, P.G. (2014). The interplay between radiation and the immune system in the field of post-radical pneumonitis and fibrosis and why it is important to understand it. *Expert Opinion on Pharmacotherapy, 13,* 1781–1783. doi:10.1517/14656566.2014.938049

Tükoğlu, M., Erdem, G.U., Suyani, E., Sancar, M.E., Yalçin, M.M., Aygencel, G., … Sucak, G. (2013). Acute respiratory distress syndrome in patients with hematological malignancies. *Hematology, 18,* 123–130. doi:10.1179/1607845412Y.0000000038

Turrisi, G., Montagnani, F., Grotti, S., Marinozzi, C., Bolognese, L., & Fiorentini, G. (2010). Congestive heart failure during imatinib mesylate treatment. *International Journal of Cardiology, 145,* 148–150. doi:10.1016/j.ijcard.2009.07.006

Umemura, S., Yamane, H., Suwaki, T., Katoh, T., Yano, T., Shiote, Y., … Kamei, H. (2011). Interstitial lung disease associated with gemcitabine treatment in patients with non-small-cell lung cancer and pancreatic cancer. *Journal of Cancer Research and Clinical Oncology, 137,* 1469–1475. doi:10.1007/s00432-011-1013-1

Venkatramani, R., Kamath, S., Wong, K., Olch, A.J., Malvar, J., Sposto, R., … Mascarenhas, L. (2013). Correlation of clinical and dosimetric factors with adverse pulmonary outcomes in children after lung irradiation. *International Journal of Radiation Oncology, Biology, Physics, 86,* 942–948. doi:10.1016/j.ijrobp.2013.04.03

Westbury, C.B., & Yarnold, J.R. (2012). Radiation fibrosis-current clinical and therapeutic perspectives. *Clinical Oncology, 24,* 657–672. doi:10.1016/j.clon.2012.04.001

Wethal, T., Lund, M.B., Edvardsen, T., Fosså, S.D., Pripp, A.H., Holte, H., … Fosså, A. (2009). Valvular dysfunction and left ventricular changes in Hodgkin's lymphoma survivors. A longitudinal study. *British Journal of Cancer, 101,* 575–581. doi:10.1038/sj.bjc.6605191

Wolchok, J.D., Kluger, H., Callahan, M.K., Postow, M.A., Rizvi, N.A., Lesokhin, A.M., … Sznol, M. (2013). Nivolumab plus ipilimumab in advanced melanoma. *New England Journal of Medicine, 369,* 122–133. doi:10.1056/NEJMoa1302369

Woods, M.L., Lech, T., & Fadol, A.P. (2013). Hypertension in patients with cancer. In A.P. Fadol (Ed.), *Cardiac complications of cancer therapy* (pp. 95–107). Pittsburgh, PA: Oncology Nursing Society.

Xu, X.-J., Zhao, H.Z., & Tang, Y.M. (2013). Efficacy and safety of adoptive immunotherapy using anti-CD19 chimeric antigen receptor transduced T-cells: A systematic review of phase I clinical trials. *Leukemia and Lymphoma, 54,* 255–260. doi:10.3109/10428194.2012.715350

Yabe, H., Yabe, M., Koike, T., Shimizu, T., Morimoto, T., & Kato, S. (2010). Rapid improvement of life-threatening capillary leak syndrome after stem cell transplantation by bevacizumab. *Blood, 115,* 2723–2724. doi:10.1182/blood-2009-11-247056

Yamaguchi, T., Sasaki, M., & Itoh, K. (2012). Bortezomib-induced pneumonitis during bortezomib retreatment in multiple myeloma. *Japanese Journal of Clinical Oncology, 42,* 637–639. doi:10.1093/jjco/hys074

Yancy, C.W., Jessup, M., Bozkurt, B., Butler, J., Casey, D.E., Jr., Drazner, M.H., … Wilkoff, B.L. (2013). 2013 ACCF/AHA guideline for the management of heart failure: A report of the American College of Cardiology Foundation/American Heart Association Task Force on Practice Guidelines. *Circulation, 128,* e240–e327. doi:10.1161/CIR.0b013e31829e8776

Yazbeck, V.Y., Villaruz, L., Haley, M., & Socinski, M.A. (2013). Management of normal tissue toxicity associated with chemoradiation (primary skin, esophagus and lung). *Cancer Journal, 19,* 231–237. doi:10.1097/PPO.0b013e31829453fb

Yeh, E.T.H., & Bickford, C.L. (2009). Cardiovascular complications of cancer therapy: Incidence, pathogenesis, diagnosis, and management. *Journal of the American College of Cardiology, 53,* 2231–2247. doi:10.1016/j.jacc.2009.02.050

Yuasa, T., Kitsukawa, S., Sukegawa, G., Yamamoto, S., Kudo, K., Miyazawa, K., … Yonese, J. (2013). Early onset recall pneumonitis during targeted therapy with sunitinib. *BMC Cancer, 13,* 3. doi:10.1186/1471-2407-13-3

CHAPTER 13

Gastrointestinal, Genitourinary, and Hepatic Toxicities

Colleen M. O'Leary, MSN, RN, AOCNS®

Introduction

Every body system is vulnerable to cancer and cancer treatments. Dysfunction or toxicities occur by direct tumor effects or by treatment of the tumor. Direct tumor effects occur secondary to the mass effect created by the tumor, lymphatic invasion, or tumor invasion of adjacent body structures. Treatments for the tumor may cause local or systemic toxicities. It is beyond the scope of this chapter to encompass all of the possible tumor effects or treatment toxicities for each of these body systems; therefore, select toxicities from the gastrointestinal (GI), genitourinary (GU), and hepatic systems will be addressed.

Gastrointestinal Toxicities

GI side effects and toxicities are common in patients with cancer undergoing chemotherapy, radiation therapy, and molecular-targeted therapies. All parts of the GI tract can be affected. These include the esophagus, causing esophagitis; the upper GI tract, causing mucositis, nausea and vomiting, taste changes, and anorexia; and the colon, causing diarrhea, graft-versus-host disease (GVHD), colitis, and constipation. Toxicities can vary in severity for different people and with different therapies. Early recognition of these toxicities is important to provide optimal treatment. Table 13-1 provides a review of these toxicities.

Esophagitis

Definition and Incidence

Esophagitis, inflammation of the esophageal wall, occurs commonly in patients with lung and esophageal cancers. Because of the areas involved in the radiation field, as well as com-

Table 13-1. Gastrointestinal Toxicities in Patients With Cancer

Symptom	Incidence	Signs and Symptoms	Risk Factors	Pathophysiology	Prevention Strategies
Esophagitis	Most common with lung and esophageal cancer	Odynophagia Dysphagia Heartburn Epigastric pain Candidiasis	RT for lung or esophageal cancers Chemoradiotherapy with doxorubicin, bleomycin cyclophosphamide and/or cisplatin Immunocompromise	Cell destruction from chemoradiotherapy Candida albicans, herpes simplex virus, cytomegalovirus, varicella-zoster virus, oral bacterial flora	Few prevention strategies have been shown to be effective.
Anorexia/ cachexia	60%–80% of patients are affected	Loss of appetite Involuntary weight loss of 5% or more, loss of muscle mass, loss of adipose tissue, fatigue and weakness, early satiety	Advanced cancer Solid tumor (most often GI and lung) Chronic illness such as pulmonary diseases and congestive heart failure Very young Very old Multimodal therapy Medications	Multifactorial problem including obstruction of the GI tract, proinflammatory cytokines such as IL-6, IL-1, and TNF-α release resulting in metabolic dysfunction and early satiety. Neurohormonal abnormalities affecting the hypothalamic appetite center Psychosocial issues such as depression, anxiety, fear, grief, fatigue, pain, and reaction to body image	Dietary education and counseling by advanced practice nurses and registered dietitians at diagnosis and as needed throughout cancer trajectory Dietary caloric and nutritional supplements Small, frequent meals Avoid odors. Baseline nutritional assessments on all patients Encourage physical activity Control nausea and vomiting, mucositis, dry mouth, and taste changes.

(Continued on next page)

Table 13-1. Gastrointestinal Toxicities in Patients With Cancer *(Continued)*

Symptom	Incidence	Signs and Symptoms	Risk Factors	Pathophysiology	Prevention Strategies
Nausea and vomiting	Anticipatory: 10%–54% Chemotherapy-induced: 70%–80% (dependent on the emetogenicity of chemotherapy agent) RT-induced: 50%–80% (dependent on RT site and dose, fractionation, volume and technique)	Anticipatory, acute, delayed, and chronic nausea and vomiting	History of poorly controlled CINV Younger than 50 years Female gender High levels of anxiety prior to or during treatment Feeling warm, hot, dizzy or sweaty after chemotherapy Susceptibility to motion sickness History of pregnancy-induced nausea and vomiting Generalized weakness after chemotherapy Little to no alcohol consumption Advanced stage of disease Fatigue Pain Tumor burden Strong taste disturbances Poor performance status Concomitant medical conditions (obstruction, pancreatitis, hepatic metastasis, hypercalcemia, infection) RT to the abdomen Concomitant chemotherapy Radiation dose and frequency	Several neurotransmitters and their receptors are involved in the process of nausea and vomiting. Neurotransmitters include serotonin released from the GI tract and sending signals via the peripheral afferent pathway to the 5-HT receptor. The CTZ in the brain is stimulated. Stimulation of the CTZ results in signals being sent to the VC in the brain that precipitates vomiting. Other neurotransmitters include dopamine, histamine, and substance P, which play a role in delayed emesis.	Pharmacologic: Dependent on the emetogenic level of risk • Low risk: single agent • Moderate risk: combination of $5-HT_3$ and dexamethasone ± NK_1, ± anxiolytic • High risk: combination of $5-HT_3$, dexamethasone, and NK_1, ± anxiolytic

(Continued on next page)

Table 13-1. Gastrointestinal Toxicities in Patients With Cancer (Continued)

Symptom	Incidence	Signs and Symptoms	Risk Factors	Pathophysiology	Prevention Strategies
Mucositis	Adjuvant chemotherapy: 10% Primary chemotherapy: 40% Stem cell transplant: 80% Head and neck RT: 100%	May affect any area of the GI tract from the mouth to the anus and any other mucous membranes in the body Patients develop pain or discomfort in the affected areas.	Antimetabolite, antitumor antibiotic, alkylating agents, and plant alkaloid chemotherapy agents Biologic agents: IL-2 and interferon N Drugs or therapies that alter mucous membranes: oxygen therapy, anticholinergics, phenytoin, and steroids Neutropenia Total body irradiation or RT to the head and neck Dental disease or poor oral hygiene Ill-fitting dentures Advanced age and youth History of alcohol and/or tobacco use Poor nutrition Consumption of irritating foods Dehydration Head and neck cancer Leukemia, lymphoma, stem cell transplant Methotrexate for prophylaxis of GVHD Hepatic or renal impairment Multimodal therapies that damage the mucosa	A multistep process involving oxidative stress and the production of reactive oxygen species by RT or chemotherapy, production of signaling factors, damage to DNA, cell death at the basal layer followed by proinflammatory cytokines, ulceration, and then healing.	See the 2005 MASCC/ISOO mucositis guidelines (www. mascc.org/media/Resource_centers/Guidelines_table_12_Oct_05.pdf). Cryotherapy may be used with edatrexate bolus or 5-fluorouracil bolus Dental care, routine tooth cleansing and flossing, patient education, and bland rinses, such as saline and baking soda, are needed. All patients who will receive head and neck RT need pretreatment dental evaluation. Amifostine may be used with head and neck RT for reducing xerostomia. Midline radiation blocks and 3-D RT. Hematopoietic stem cell transplantation: low-level laser therapy at centers with trained staff, cryotherapy with high-dose melphalan, IV palifermin

(Continued on next page)

Table 13-1. Gastrointestinal Toxicities in Patients With Cancer (Continued)

Symptom	Incidence	Signs and Symptoms	Risk Factors	Pathophysiology	Prevention Strategies
Constipation	2%–27% of general population 40% of patients with cancer	Straining, small, round stools Feeling that rectum still has stool Feeling of rectal blockage Abdominal or rectal discomfort or pain Nausea and vomiting Impaction Hemorrhoids	Opioid therapy Other medications Vinca alkaloids, especially vincristine Thalidomide Low-fiber diet Low fluid intake Lack of activity Increased age	Multifactorial problem related to prolongation of GI transit time, absorption of water, reduced fiber consumption, medications, reduced mobility, and comorbidities Symptom of the cancer itself	Patient education related to use of laxatives and stool softeners administered on a regular basis Dietary manipulations to increase fiber and fluid intake Avoiding more than three days without having a stool Regular exercise Diaphragmatic breathing and abdominal muscle exercises GVHD Dietary changes including lactose intolerance, intake of caffeine, alcohol, or spicy, fatty foods Irritable bowel syndrome Ulcerative colitis Diverticulitis Malabsorption Partial bowel obstruction Anxiety and stress
Diarrhea	50%–80% of patients receiving chemotherapy and/or RT	Increase in frequency of stools Increase in liquid nature of stools Abdominal pain and cramping Fecal incontinence	RT to the pelvis, abdomen or lower thoracic and lumbar spine 5-FU in combination with high-dose leucovorin Weekly bolus 5-FU Paclitaxel Dactinomycin Dacarbazine Capecitabine	Chemotherapy and RT damage the mucosal lining of the GI tract, reducing its absorptive capacity and resulting in short GI transit times for food and fluids, reduced nutrient and fluid absorption, and increased bowel output.	Patient education on use of loperamide for all patients starting irinotecan therapy Patient education for all patients at risk for diarrhea needs to include dietary manipulation to reduce fiber, information on maintenance of fluid and electrolyte balance, and signs

(Continued on next page)

Table 13-1. Gastrointestinal Toxicities in Patients With Cancer (Continued)

Symptom	Incidence	Signs and Symptoms	Risk Factors	Pathophysiology	Prevention Strategies
Diarrhea (cont.)			Interleukin-2 Interferons Immunosuppression Intestinal resection or gastrectomy Manipulation of bowel during surgery Intestinal infection secondary to mucositis and neutropenia	Several types of diarrhea may develop, including malabsorptive, osmotic, secretory, and infectious. Can be acute or chronic.	and symptoms to report to healthcare provider.

CINV—chemotherapy-induced nausea and vomiting; CTZ—chemoreceptor trigger zone; 5-FU—5-fluorouracil; 5-HT—5-hydroxytryptamine; GI—gastrointestinal; GVHD—graft-versus-host disease; IL—interleukin; RT—radiation therapy; 3-D—three-dimensional; TNF-α—tumor necrosis factor-alpha; VC—vomiting center

Note. Based on information from Andrew et al., 2008; Avritscher et al., 2004; Barasch & Peterson, 2003; Benson et al., 2004; Bjordal et al., 2011; Camilleri, 2011; Caro et al., 2007; Conlon, 2010; Cunningham, 2014; Davila & Bresalier, 2008; Dianliang, 2009; Fearon, 2012; Giralt et al., 2008; Goebel, 2010; Granda-Cameron & Lynch, 2010; Johnson et al., 2007; Multinational Association of Supportive Care in Cancer/International Society for Oral Oncology, 2013; National Cancer Institute, 2013a, 2013b, 2013c, 2013d; National Comprehensive Cancer Network, 2015b; National Digestive Diseases Information Clearinghouse, n.d.; National Institute on Deafness and Other Communication Disorders, 2014; O'Rourke et al., 2010; Polovich et al., 2014; Roscoe et al., 2010; Shoemaker et al., 2011; Sonis, 2007; Strassels et al., 2010; Sykes, 2006; Thompson, 2012; Tipton, 2014; Tisdale, 2009, 2010; Underhill et al., 2015; Warr et al., 2011; Werner-Wasik et al., 2010; Worthington et al., 2011; Yavuzsen et al., 2009.

mon use of concurrent radiation and chemotherapy, radiation-induced esophagitis occurs most often in the treatment of lung and esophageal cancers. In patients receiving concurrent chemotherapy and radiation therapy to the thoracic area, 15%–25% will experience esophagitis within 90 days of treatment initiation (Werner-Wasik, Yorke, Deasy, Nam, & Marks, 2010). Acute esophagitis, occurring in less than 90 days of treatment, ranges from being asymptomatic, to mild dysphagia with ability to eat normally, to life-threatening symptoms requiring surgical intervention (National Cancer Institute [NCI] Cancer Therapy Evaluation Program [CTEP], 2010).

Presenting Signs and Symptoms

Common symptoms of esophagitis include difficulty swallowing or inability to swallow (dysphagia) that may be accompanied by pain with swallowing (odynophagia) (Davila & Bresalier, 2008; National Institute on Deafness and Other Communication Disorders, 2014; O'Rourke, Roqué, Bernadó, & Macbeth, 2010; Werner-Wasik et al., 2010). Patients also may complain of a cotton feel in the mouth, decreased ability to taste, and heartburn. Complaints of retrosternal chest pain are common with radiation-induced esophagitis (O'Rourke et al., 2010; Werner-Wasik et al., 2010). Candidiasis often accompanies esophagitis. The most familiar symptom of candidiasis is oral thrush manifested by white plaques or lesions on the tongue, cheeks, and roof of mouth. However, the absence of oral thrush does not necessarily exclude the diagnosis of esophagitis (Davila & Bresalier, 2008).

Risk Factors and Etiology

In patients with cancer who are immunocompromised, viral, fungal, or bacterial invasion is often the cause of esophagitis. Fungal infection by *Candida albicans* is the most common cause of esophageal candidiasis in immunocompromised patients (Davila & Bresalier, 2008). Common viral causes of esophagitis in patients with cancer include herpes simplex virus (HSV), cytomegalovirus (CMV), and, less common, varicella-zoster virus (VZV) (Davila & Bresalier, 2008).

Immunocompromised patients, including those with cancer, are at a higher risk for experiencing esophagitis. Radiation therapy for lung or esophageal cancer places patients at a higher risk for esophagitis. Chemotherapy including doxorubicin, bleomycin, cyclophosphamide, and cisplatin carries a higher risk of esophagitis (Davila & Bresalier, 2008). Induction chemotherapy increases the risk of esophagitis compared to standard radiation alone. The addition of chemotherapy to radiation increases the risk of esophagitis (O'Rourke et al., 2010).

Pathophysiology

The cells of healthy esophageal mucosa continually turn over and renew. When a patient receives chemotherapy or radiation therapy that includes the esophagus in the field, these rapidly growing esophageal cells are affected. The basal epithelial layer is affected most often, causing a thinning of the mucosa, which can lead to exposed tissue (Bradley & Movsas, 2004). Bacteria, viruses, and fungi, including *Candida albicans*, HSV, CMV, and VZV, invade the healthy esophageal mucosa, causing additional epithelial injury (Davila & Bresalier, 2008).

Prevention Strategies

Although few prevention strategies exist for esophagitis, several studies have attempted to define the most appropriate dose and volume of radiation to reduce the incidence of esophagitis (Werner-Wasik et al., 2010). These studies have been unable to identify the best threshold for dosing or volume. Doses as high as 74 Gy with concurrent chemotherapy are generally accepted as safe (Stinchcombe et al., 2008; Werner-Wasik et al., 2010).

Diagnosis and Assessment

Diagnosis should be done via endoscopy with biopsy, which shows small vesicle formations.

Evidence-Based Treatment Strategies

Although empiric antifungal therapy is appropriate with common symptoms, endoscopy should be performed if the symptoms do not improve. In immunocompromised patients with fungal infection, systemic therapy should be used as opposed to topical therapy (Davila & Bresalier, 2008). Treatment should include IV antivirals, including acyclovir or ganciclovir initially. After clinical improvement, patients are often switched to oral therapy. The bacterial forms of esophagitis are usually from a variety of bacteria found in the oral flora. Broad-spectrum antibiotics are effective in treating these infections.

Implications for Oncology Advanced Practice Nurses

Knowledge of the incidence of esophagitis is important for advanced practice nurses (APNs) to be able to anticipate and effectively treat it. Left unchecked, esophagitis can progress to life-threatening symptoms. Assessment of the severity of esophagitis is imperative. The Common Terminology Criteria for Adverse Events (CTCAE) grades esophagitis on a scale of 1–5 (NCI CTEP, 2010). APNs should be aware of not only the grading of the toxicity but also the recommendations regarding each grade. According to the CTCAE, grade 1, defined as asymptomatic, only requires observation. Grade 2 involves altered eating with recommendation of oral supplementation. Patients with grade 3 have severely impaired swallowing requiring a feeding tube. Total parenteral nutrition with or without hospitalization is indicated. Grade 4 requires urgent surgical interventions to address life-threatening consequences, and grade 5 is defined as death (NCI CTEP, 2010). Thorough assessment with prompt intervention is imperative. Educating patients and families about the symptoms of esophagitis and the interventions is within the scope of APN practice.

Anorexia and Cachexia

Definition and Incidence

Anorexia is defined as the abnormal loss of appetite for food (NCI, 2013c). It has been suggested that anorexia is not a single symptom but part of a more complex symptom that occurs in conjunction with other GI symptoms, including taste change, altered eating patterns, and food aversions (Yavuzsen et al., 2009). If left untreated, anorexia can lead to weight loss, muscle wasting, and malnutrition known as cachexia. It is estimated that 60%–80% of patients with cancer experience cancer anorexia-cachexia syndrome (CACS) (Goebel, 2010; Yavuzsen et al., 2009). In addition, about 20% of cancer deaths can be attributed to CACS rather than from the cancer itself (Hopkinson, Wright, & Foster, 2008).

Presenting Signs and Symptoms

Clinical manifestations of anorexia include an unintentional loss of more than 5% of usual weight, loss of appetite, loss of muscle mass, loss of adipose tissue, fatigue, and weakness. Body changes seen in anorexia are primarily a result of loss of adipose tissue. If left untreated, it can progress to CACS, where there is equal loss of adipose tissue and muscle (Tisdale, 2009, 2010). Patients with CACS have a poorer performance status, muscle wasting, fatigue, reduced mobility, and respiratory complications (Granda-Cameron & Lynch, 2010).

Risk Factors and Etiology

Risk factors for CACS include advanced cancer, tumor type, chronic illness, age, and multimodal treatment (Cunningham, 2014). Very young and very old patients, patients with pulmonary and cardiac comorbidities, and patients with solid tumors, especially GI and lung cancers, are at greater risk. In addition, evidence has shown that genetic factors play a role in the risk for CACS (Dianliang, 2009). Although lung and GI cancers pose a greater risk, not all patients develop CACS. Patients with these types of cancers who also have single mutations have increased production of interleukin (IL)-1, IL-6, and IL-10, which may increase susceptibility to cachexia (Fearon, 2012; Dianliang, 2009).

Patients receiving chemotherapy often experience taste alterations during treatment, which can be caused by direct injury of the taste buds by the chemotherapy. This inhibits mitosis in replicating receptor cells, causing an alteration in taste acuity (Henkin, 1994). Some agents disperse into the saliva, causing patients to complain of tasting the drug when it is injected. It is important to recognize that taste alterations may affect patients' desire to eat, and if left untreated, it may lead to more severe anorexia or cachexia.

A number of physiologic and psychological processes work together in the etiology of CACS. Psychological effects of depression, anxiety, fear grief, fatigue, and pain contribute to CACS (Polovich, Olsen, & LeFebvre, 2014). In addition, obstruction of the GI tract can lead to malabsorption, nausea, vomiting, and pain. Proinflammatory cytokines released by the tumor, including IL-6, IL-1, and tumor necrosis factor-alpha, can cause metabolic abnormalities and satiety. Neurohormonal abnormalities seen in cancer can directly affect the hypothalamic appetite center.

Pathophysiology

The process of CACS involves a variety of complex factors. When an increased expenditure of energy occurs along with decreased energy intake, several immunologic, neuroendocrine, and metabolic pathways lead to anorexia and eventual weight loss. Tumors release increased production of cytokines IL-1 and IL-6, which trigger the brain to experience early satiety and anorexia. These cytokines also have a direct catabolic effect on skeletal muscle wasting (Andrew, Kirkpatrick, Holden, & Hawkins, 2008; Caro, Laviano, & Pichard, 2007). In addition, patients' fear, grief, fatigue, pain, anxiety, and reaction to changes in body image can lead to anorexia (Polovich et al., 2014).

Prevention Strategies

Nutritional screening with a valid and reliable tool is essential to identify those at risk for anorexia early in their course of treatment (Cunningham, 2014). Dietary education and counseling throughout the cancer trajectory is important to assist patients in maintaining appropriate intake. Monitoring and recording weekly weights will help to identify issues early. Other strategies that may be effective in preventing appetite loss include encouraging small, frequent meals, providing an attractive setting for meals, encouraging physical activity, and using measures to control nausea and vomiting, mucositis, dry mouth, and taste changes (Polovich et al., 2014).

Diagnosis and Assessment

Patients determined to be at risk for anorexia should undergo a comprehensive nutritional assessment. This includes a thorough medical and dietary history, as well as anthropometric measurements, body composition analysis, evaluations of selected biometric markers, and assessment for any symptoms that may interfere with eating (Cunningham, 2014).

Medical and dietary history should include current medical conditions, weight and weight changes, medications, treatment schedule, and tolerance of treatment. Anthropometric measurements include body mass index, height, weight, skinfold thickness, tricep skinfold measures, and mid-arm muscle circumference. These measurements indicate dimensions, proportions, and ratios of the body. A body composition analysis measures lean body mass and fat mass. Laboratory values to monitor include serum albumin to measure protein stores, serum prealbumin to measure protein depletion, and serum transferrin to reflect the body's ability to make serum proteins (Polovich et al., 2014).

Evidence-Based Treatment Strategies

Pharmacologic interventions found to be effective include the use of corticosteroids such as dexamethasone, methylprednisolone, prednisolone, hydrocortisone, and fludrocortisone and the progestins medroxyprogesterone and megestrol acetate (Underhill, Caron, Ramsdell, Rogers, & Wolles, 2015). Nonpharmacologic interventions include enteral and parenteral nutritional supplementation and nutritional counseling. Interventions to encourage food intake include patient education regarding the use of herbs and spices, as well as cool foods (to avoid odors) and the avoidance of unpleasant odors.

Enteral nutrition administered via gastric or intestinal feeding tubes allows for correction of negative nutritional status while still maintaining gut function. Parenteral nutrition should be reserved for patients who have a dysfunctional GI tract. Patients receiving parenteral nutrition are at an increased risk for sepsis and catheter occlusion (Bosaeus, 2008; Dy et al., 2008).

The use of nutritional counseling from APNs in conjunction with a registered dietitian has been shown to be effective in sustaining nutritional intake (Underhill et al., 2015). The counseling includes good nutritional practices where food may be modified to meet individual preferences.

Implications for Oncology Advanced Practice Nurses

APNs can be vital in ensuring early assessment and interventions to prevent CACS. The effects of nutritional interventions should be closely monitored and adjusted as needed. Ensuring that patients and families are educated about potential nutritional problems, along with self-care measures, is important.

Nausea and Vomiting

Definition and Incidence

Nausea and vomiting remain common and potentially serious side effects of cancer therapy. Not only do nausea and vomiting negatively affect the patients' quality of life, but they also may hinder their ability to comply with treatment. Nausea and vomiting can lead to other debilitating issues, such as anorexia, decreased performance status, metabolic imbalance, wound dehiscence, esophageal tears, and nutritional deficiency (Fernández-Ortega et al., 2012).

It is important to know the different terms used when discussing nausea and vomiting. *Nausea* is the unpleasant subjective experience that is described as a "wavelike" feeling occurring in the stomach or the back of the throat that may be accompanied by vomiting (NCI, 2013b). *Retching* is described as a rhythmic contraction of the esophagus, diaphragm, and abdominal muscles in an attempt to eject stomach contents. Retching without vomiting is known as *dry heaves* (NCI, 2013b). *Vomiting* is the forceful expulsion of gastric, duodenal, or jejunal contents through the mouth (NCI, 2013b). Both chemotherapy and radiation therapy can cause nausea and vomiting. Chemotherapy-induced nausea and vomiting (CINV) occurs in 70%–80% of patients receiving chemotherapy (Kurtin, 2010) and can be classified as anticipatory, acute, or delayed. Anticipatory nausea and vomiting occurs in 10%–40% of patients, with nausea being more prevalent than vomiting (Kurtin, 2010). Incidence depends on the type of chemotherapy used as well as the dose and intensity.

Radiation-induced nausea and vomiting (RINV) occurs most often with radiation to the GI tract, liver, or brain. Incidence of RINV is approximately 90% when there is a large radiation field including the upper and mid-abdomen. This decreases to 15% when the radiation field includes lower body fields (Tipton, 2014).

Presenting Signs and Symptoms

Anticipatory nausea and vomiting usually occurs after three or four cycles of chemotherapy where CINV was inadequately controlled. Acute nausea and vomiting starts within minutes to hours after administration of chemotherapy and can last up to 24 hours depending on the agent (NCI, 2013b). Delayed nausea and vomiting occurs at least 24 hours after chemotherapy and may last up to six days.

Nausea and vomiting usually are not exhibited independently. Often they are found in conjunction with other symptoms. These include anorexia, fatigue, taste disturbances, and weight loss. It is important to identify all symptoms in the cluster and address each.

Risk Factors and Etiology

Nausea and vomiting can have a variety of etiologies. Chemotherapy, radiation therapy, use of other emetogenic medications, and the cancer itself may cause nausea and vomiting. Nausea and vomiting are more prevalent in advanced cancer and in terminally ill patients with cancer. This could be the result of other end-of-life conditions, including intestinal obstruction, liver impairment, kidney dysfunction, hypercalcemia, dehydration, and brain metastasis (Dy & Apostol, 2010).

Risk factors for CINV and RINV include patient- and treatment-related factors. Patient-related factors include female gender, age younger than 55, history of CINV or RINV, history of emesis with pregnancy, history of motion sickness, low alcohol intake, decreased performance status, anxiety, pretreatment expectation of nausea, fluid or electrolyte imbalance, constipation, infection, kidney disease, and use of opioids (National Comprehensive Cancer Network® [NCCN®], 2015b; Roscoe et al., 2010; Shoemaker, Estfan, Induru, & Walsh, 2011; Thompson, 2012; Warr, Street, & Carides, 2011). Treatment-related risk factors include the emetogenicity of the chemotherapy drug, the dose schedule, route and rate of administration of chemotherapy, concurrent chemotherapy and radiation therapy, radiation site, field size, and radiation dose and frequency (NCCN, 2015a; Roscoe et al., 2010; Shoemaker et al., 2011; Thompson, 2012; Warr et al., 2011).

Pathophysiology

Several neurotransmitters and their receptors are involved in the process of nausea and vomiting. These neurotransmitters, such as serotonin released from the GI tract, send signals via the afferent pathway to the 5-hydoxytryptamine (5-HT_3) receptor. The chemoreceptor trigger zone in the brain is then stimulated, resulting in signals being sent to the vomiting center to initiate vomiting. Other neurotransmitters with a role in nausea and vomiting include dopamine, histamine, and substance P, which play a role in delayed nausea and vomiting (Tipton, 2014).

Prevention Strategies

NCCN recommends starting antiemetic therapy prior to the start of cancer therapy. The type of antiemetic therapy used for prevention of acute and delayed nausea and vomiting is dependent on the emetogenicity of the chemotherapy or the field of radiation (NCCN, 2015a). For low-risk emetogenic agents, it is recommended to use a single agent, such as a steroid, metoclopramide, prochlorperazine, or a 5-HT_3 antagonist. Patients receiving moderately emetogenic chemotherapy should be premedicated with a combination of a 5-HT$_3$ antagonist, a steroid, plus or minus an NK$_1$ antagonist, and plus or minus an anxiolytic. Highly emetogenic chemotherapy should be prevented with a combination of a 5-HT$_3$ antagonist, a steroid, and an NK$_1$ antagonist, plus or minus an anxiolytic and proton pump inhibitor. Anticipatory nausea and vomiting should be prevented using an anxiolytic. Nonpharmacologic preventive techniques include relaxation, hypnosis, guided imagery, music therapy, and acupuncture or acupressure (NCCN, 2015a). For patients receiving radiation to the upper abdomen as well as total body irradiation, pretreatment should include a 5-HT$_3$ antagonist plus or minus a steroid.

Diagnosis and Assessment

Self-assessment and report is the cornerstone of assessment for nausea and vomiting. APNs should question patients regarding nausea and vomiting prior to and throughout each treatment. Several tools are available for self-assessment of nausea and vomiting. These include the Index of Nausea, Vomiting, and Retching (INVR) and the Multinational Association of Supportive Care in Cancer (MASCC) Antiemesis Tool (MAT) (Tipton, 2009). The INVR measures the frequency, severity, and distress of CINV, whereas the MAT measures frequency and severity both acutely and on days 2–4. A visual analog scale also may be used to measure nausea and vomiting.

A thorough history and physical can help to determine risk for nausea and vomiting. Physical assessment should include a focused abdominal assessment including auscultation of bowel sounds and palpation for tenderness, hepatomegaly, splenomegaly, ascites, and masses (Tipton, 2014). Diagnostic tests can help to determine dehydration, renal function, electrolyte imbalance, and hepatic function, all of which may lead to nausea and vomiting.

Evidence-Based Treatment Strategies

Treatment of nausea and vomiting is based on the same principles as prevention of nausea and vomiting. Depending on the emetogenicity of the chemotherapy or the field of radiation, NCCN guidelines are the same as for prevention. Nonpharmacologic interventions include complementary measures and structured education. Complementary interventions that have been shown to be helpful in treating nausea and vomiting include behavioral interventions, massage, music or art therapy, acupressure or acupuncture, and dietary modifications (Tipton, 2014). These measures can enhance the effectiveness of antiemetics. Ginger has been shown to be effective in managing nausea and vomiting because some components of ginger are 5-HT$_3$ antagonists (Ryan et al., 2012; Wickham, 2012; Zick et al., 2009).

Implications for Oncology Advanced Practice Nurses

Assessment of nausea and vomiting should begin with a thorough history and physical by the APN. Identification of risk factors is critical in determining the potential incidence of nausea and vomiting. Determining the emetogenicity of chemotherapy regimens is crucial in deciding what interventions to employ. Keeping updated on the recommendations of experts, including the NCCN guidelines, is imperative, as novel agents continue to be developed. Structured education regarding the use of antiemetics, as well as complementary interventions, can assist patients in tolerating nausea and vomiting.

Mucositis

Definition and Incidence

Mucosal damage affecting the GI tract is a common toxicity of both antineoplastic and radiation therapy. The terms *mucositis* and *stomatitis* have been used interchangeably; however, true mucositis begins at the lips and ends at the rectum. Oral mucositis is the most commonly studied mucositis and is associated with significant pain that not only decreases patients' ability to eat but also adversely affects their quality of life. Other areas in the GI tract affected by mucositis include the esophagus, stomach, and small and large intestines. Depending on what area is affected, symptoms may include pain, ulceration, nausea, vomiting, diarrhea, and rectal bleeding (Capp et al., 2009). Other systemic effects of both oral and GI mucositis include fatigue, malnutrition, sepsis, and occasionally death (Aprile, Ramoni, Keefe, & Sonis, 2008). For the purposes of this chapter, *mucositis* will refer to oral mucositis.

It is estimated that 10% of patients receiving adjuvant chemotherapy and 40% of those receiving primary chemotherapy experience mucositis (NCI, 2013d). Additionally, 80% of patients receiving stem cell transplant and 100% of patients with head and neck cancer experience mucositis (Bjordal et al., 2011).

Presenting Signs and Symptoms

The pattern of mucositis varies depending on the individual as well as the chemotherapy regimen being used. However, in general, patients receiving standard-dose chemotherapy begin to show visible signs of mucositis four to five days after initial treatment and peaks within two weeks (Raber-Durlacher, Elad, & Barasch, 2010). Stem cell transplant recipients experience mucositis three to five days after conditioning regimens, and patients with head and neck cancer who are receiving chemotherapy and radiation therapy show manifestations of mucositis during the second week of therapy (Raber-Durlacher et al., 2010). Clinical signs of mucositis begin with tender, reddened areas in the mouth that can progress to large painful lesions throughout the oral mucosa.

Risk Factors and Etiology

Mucositis can be the result of chemotherapy, targeted agents, or radiation therapy. Risks for oral mucositis can be divided into patient-, treatment-, and disease-related factors. Patient-related factors include advanced age and youth, history of alcohol or tobacco use, poor nutrition, poor oral health, reduced salivary flow, low body mass index (less than 20 for males and less than 19 for females), decreased renal function, high levels of oral microflora, and female gender (Wujcik, 2014). Treatment-related risk factors include the use of antimetabolites, antitumor antibiotics, alkylating agents, plant alkaloids, and the biologics IL-2 and interferon N (Avritscher, Cooksley, & Elting, 2004; Barasch & Peterson, 2003). Also included are drugs that alter mucous membranes, such as oxygen therapy, anticholinergics, phenytoin, and steroids. Additionally, high-dose chemotherapy regimens; allogeneic stem cell transplant; radiation to the head, neck, thorax, and abdomen; and use of chemotherapy along with radiation therapy are risk factors in the development of mucositis. Disease-related factors include neutropenia, dehydration, head and neck cancer, leukemia, lymphoma, and hepatic or renal dysfunction (Polovich et al., 2014).

Pathophysiology

Mucositis occurs via specific phases of development (Sonis, 2007). In the initiation phase, the mucosa appears normal, but DNA damage is occurring. This is followed by the primary damage response phase, in which proinflammatory cytokines amplify the injury. Patients are still unaware of damage. The third phase is the signaling or amplification phase, in which the cytokines continue to damage cells. Patients begin to experience pain in the ulceration phase, when ulcers penetrate through the epithelium. The final stage is healing, in which the epithelium begins to restore and normal cellular processes return. However, when patients continue treatment, the healing phase may never fully develop.

Prevention Strategies

Good oral care is the only strategy with strong evidence for prevention of oral mucositis. Oral care protocols should include routine brushing of the teeth with a soft toothbrush, regular flossing, and use of bland rinses to remove debris and bacteria (Eilers, Harris, Henry, & Johnson, 2014; MASCC/International Society for Oral Oncology [ISOO], 2013). No evidence supports that specific oral care protocols are any more effective than good routine oral care (Worthington et al., 2011). Oral cryotherapy has been shown to be effective with the use of bolus 5-fluorouracil, bolus edatrexate, and high-dose melphalan for the prevention of mucositis. Some evidence supports the benefit of cryotherapy with other agents and keratinocyte growth factor; however, all these trials were assessed as being at either high or unclear risk of bias (Worthington et al., 2011). Weak evidence exists for the use of low-energy laser treatments for the prevention of oral mucositis (Worthington et al., 2011). Midline radiation blocks and three-dimensional radiation treatments can be used with radiation therapy to the head and neck (MASCC/ISOO, 2013; Oncology Nursing Society, 2012).

Diagnosis and Assessment

The first point of assessment for oral mucositis is the patients themselves. It is important to teach patients to perform daily self-assessment for any erythema, edema, lesions, bleeding, tingling, or pain. They should be taught to report any new symptoms. Several assessment tools are available. One of the most widely used is the Oral Assessment Guide by Eilers and associates (Eilers, Berger, & Petersen, 1988). This guide assesses voice, swallowing, lips, tongue, saliva, mucous membranes, gingiva, and teeth or dentures on a scale of 1–3. The Oral Mucositis Assessment Scale assesses for erythema and ulcerations throughout the oral cavity (Sonis et al., 1999). Other assessment tools include the Oral Mucosa Rating Scale, the Oral Mucositis Index, and the Western Consortium for Cancer Nursing Research Oral Mucositis Assessment (Brown, 2011). The CTCAE includes a scale for oral mucositis that grades severity of oral mucositis from 1 (asymptomatic or mild) to 5 (death) (NCI CTEP, 2010). Regardless of which tool is being used, APNs need to know that the tool is not only reliable and valid, but also useful in their particular clinical setting.

Evidence-Based Treatment Strategies

Pain management is paramount when treating oral mucositis. The use of topical anesthetics and analgesics should be attempted prior to initiation of systemic medications. If the pain is not controlled, nonsteroidal anti-inflammatory drugs can be added followed by opioids until pain is controlled. The MASCC/ISOO guidelines recommend that patient-controlled analgesia with opioids be used for patients with severe mucositis (MASCC/ISOO, 2013). Topical hemostatic agents can be used for thrombocytopenic patients experiencing bleeding from mucositis, especially when the platelet count falls below 20,000/mm^3 (Wujcik, 2014). It is important to monitor nutritional intake because mucositis can deter patients from eating. Feeding tubes may be necessary if the mucositis becomes so severe that the patient can no longer eat. Recombinant keratinocyte growth factors have been shown to reduce the severity and duration of mucositis in patients receiving high-dose chemotherapy (Rodríguez-Caballero et al., 2012; Worthington et al., 2011).

Implications for Oncology Advanced Practice Nurses

APNs who are caring for patients with oral mucositis need to be prepared to help prevent, identify, and treat the problem. Ensuring that patients are informed of preventive measures is key. Consulting with dental experts in addition to the APN's thorough assessment is advised. Providing early treatment, including adequate pain control, can be vital in decreasing further decline. Use of valid and reliable assessment tools is vital in determining further interventions. APNs should be involved in further research regarding interventions to prevent and manage oral mucositis.

Constipation

Definition and Incidence

Constipation is a condition in which a person has fewer than three bowel movements a week or has bowel movements with stools that are hard, dry, and small, making them painful or difficult to pass (National Digestive Diseases Information Clearinghouse, n.d.). Constipation in patients with cancer can be the presenting problem of cancer, a side effect of their treatment, or a sign of disease progression (Polovich et al., 2014). Between 2% and 27% of the population suffers from constipation, which can significantly affect their quality of life (Sanchez & Bercik, 2011). The incidence of constipation in patients with cancer is equally as troublesome. However, not many recent studies have specifically focused on constipation in people with cancer. The Assessment, Information, Management (AIM) Higher Initiative was a study aimed at improving symptoms of anemia, neutropenia, nausea and vomiting, diarrhea, and constipation (Johnson, Moore, & Fortner, 2007). In this study, 40% of patients reported experiencing constipation during their most recent chemotherapy cycle.

Presenting Signs and Symptoms

Constipation can present with a variety of symptoms, some of which can be vague. Common symptoms include small, hard bowel movements, leakage of soft, liquid stool that looks like diarrhea, stomachache or cramps, frequent passing of gas or belching, and feeling bloated, full, or sluggish.

Risk Factors and Etiology

Constipation is caused by decreased motility of the large intestine, which can be a result of altered strength of contractions, poor muscle tone within the colon, or sensory changes in the anus and rectum. Several chemotherapy agents cause decreased motility, including vinca alkaloids. Vincristine, vinorelbine, and vinblastine can lead to decreased peristalsis by causing neurologic toxicities that affect the smooth muscles of the GI tract. Chemotherapy agents that cause increased nausea and vomiting can inadvertently cause constipation, with decreased food intake slowing peristalsis in the GI tract. The primary cause of medication-induced constipation is the use of opioids, which act directly on the mu receptors, again slowing peristalsis (Camilleri, 2011; Strassels, Maxwell, & Iyer, 2010). Other causes of constipation include alterations in diet, immobility, alterations in anatomy, and neuroendocrine disturbances. Patients receiving radiation therapy for gynecologic cancers will at times have constipation induced to prevent bowel movements while brachytherapy implants are in place. Normal bowel movements should return several days after therapy (Haylock, Curtiss, & Massey, 2014).

Risk factors for constipation are consistent with the etiologies listed. Patients are at a higher risk of constipation because of the cancer itself when the tumor causes mechanical pressure on the bowel. Damage to spinal cords from T8 to L3 can put people at great risk because this is where the nerves are that innervate the bowel. In addition, decreased mobility, dehydration, and a low intake of dietary fiber increase the risk for constipation (Polovich et al., 2014). Some metabolic and endocrine disorders put patients at greater risk, including hypercalcemia, Addison disease, hypo- or hyperthyroidism, Cushing syndrome, hypokalemia, and diabetes (NCI, 2013a). Use of certain medications puts patients at greater risk as well. These medications include neurotoxic chemotherapy such as vinca alkaloids, oxaliplatin, taxanes, thalidomide, anticholinergic medications, diuretics, opioids, aluminum- and calcium-based antacids, calcium and iron supplements, tricyclic antidepressants, antihypertensives, anxiolytics, 5-HT$_3$ antagonists, phenothiazines, and nonsteroidal anti-inflammatory drugs (NCI, 2013a).

Pathophysiology

To understand the pathophysiology of constipation, nurses need to understand normal bowel function. The intestines are divided into the small intestine, which includes the duodenum, jejunum, and the ileum; and the large intestine, which includes the ascending, transverse, and descending colon and the rectum. The small intestine absorbs nutrients from food, and the large intestine absorbs water from food and forms stool. Stomach contents stay in the small intestine for two to four hours, whereas they remain in the large intestine for 24–48 hours as they travel through the colon. The jejunum and the rest of the large intestine are responsible for absorbing fluid that passes through the bowels. Finally, the colon and abdominal muscles help to move the stool to the rectum and anus (Sykes, 2006). When factors such as decreased mobility, medications, or fluid and electrolyte imbalances in patients with cancer affect the normal function of the bowel, constipation can ensue depending on which of the functions is disrupted.

Prevention Strategies

A combination of pharmacologic and nonpharmacologic interventions are used to prevent constipation. Prophylactic bowel management protocols along with anticipation and assessment are critical. Instructing patients to increase consumption of dietary fiber and fluid intake to include eight 8 oz servings a day can be effective, unless the constipation is caused by opioids. Active and passive exercise can be helpful if patients can tolerate it. Providing privacy for patients while in the hospital and stressing the need for activity will help to prevent constipation.

Diagnosis and Assessment

A thorough history of patients' bowel pattern, dietary changes, and medications, along with a physical examination, can identify possible causes of constipation. Normal bowel pattern and any recent changes should be determined. Dietary intake should be assessed for amount and types of food eaten. Medications should be reviewed for any potential offending agents. Assessment of associated symptoms would include distension, flatus, cramping, or rectal fullness. Daily activity levels should be assessed, as well as anxiety and depression. Physical examination should include abdominal assessment with bowel sounds, tenderness, and distension. A digital rectal examination is done to rule out fecal impaction at the level of the rectum (NCI, 2013a).

Evidence-Based Treatment Strategies

The NCCN palliative care guidelines outline specific recommendations for the management of constipation (NCCN, 2015b). First and foremost is to attempt to determine the cause of constipation, such as electrolyte imbalances or comorbidities. Additionally, clinicians need to check for impaction and obstruction. If impaction and obstruction are ruled out, add titrate bisacodyl 10–15 mg TID to achieve one non-forced bowel movement every one to two days. If constipation persists, add another laxative such as bisacodyl suppository, polyethylene glycol, lactulose, sorbitol, magnesium hydroxide, or magnesium citrate. Consideration of prokinetic agents such as metoclopramide is recommended. For patients who are impacted, administer a glycerin suppository with or without a mineral oil enema. Manual disimpaction should be done following administration of an analgesic with or without an anxiolytic (NCCN, 2015b).

Implications for Oncology Advanced Practice Nurses

Constipation continues to be underaddressed in patients with cancer. APNs should thoroughly assess for signs of constipation throughout the treatment trajectory. Prevention is paramount to provide the best quality of life. Bowel patterns as well as potential risks for constipation should be monitored routinely. Educating patients in regard to preventive measures can help to forgo the need for additional interventions. If constipation develops, prompt management is required to ensure that it does not progress to further obstruction and potentially life-threatening outcomes.

Diarrhea

Definition and Incidence

Diarrhea is generally defined as an increase in the number of stools or the liquidity of stools, and can be life threatening in patients with cancer if left untreated. Ranging from grade 1, described as an increase of less than four stools per day over baseline or a mild increase in ostomy output over baseline, to grade 5, causing death, the CTCAE is most frequently used to describe the degree of diarrhea (NCI CTEP, 2010). The incidence of diarrhea varies and depends on factors such as the location of disease, treatment modality and course, use of other medications, and other patient-related considerations. Chemotherapy-induced diarrhea is estimated to affect 50%–80% of patients (Benson et al., 2004). The chemotherapy agent most commonly associated with diarrhea is 5-fluorouracil. Other agents with the highest risk of inducing diarrhea include irinotecan, alone or in combination with 5-fluorouracil; paclitaxel; dactinomycin; dacarbazine; and capecitabine (Polovich et al., 2014). Approximately 50% of patients receiving radiation to the pelvis or abdomen experience diarrhea, with the incidence increasing if they are receiving concurrent chemotherapy (Giralt et al., 2008). Diarrhea is common following hematopoietic stem cell transplantation, largely as a result of GVHD, GI surgical resection and surgical alteration of the GI tract also may result in diarrhea (Muehlbauer & Lopez, 2014). Diarrhea is described as osmotic, malabsorptive, secretory, exudative, or infectious and can be acute or chronic. Acute diarrhea occurs within 2–48 hours of the causative factor and lasts for 7–14 days or less. Chronic diarrhea is defined as lasting at least four weeks (Conlon, 2010).

Presenting Signs and Symptoms

Diarrhea can present as large volumes of stool that can vary in color and consistency depending on their origin. Small bowel diarrhea usually is lighter in color, watery, frothy, greasy appearing, and with large volumes with intermittent cramping (Conlon, 2010). Conversely, diarrhea that is smaller in volume, dark in color with little odor, soft, jelly-like, and mixed with mucus or blood originates in the large bowel (Conlon, 2010). Other symptoms that accompany diarrhea include abdominal pain, cramping and tenderness, urge to defecate, perineal discomfort, incontinence, dizziness, orthostatic symptoms, lethargy, nausea, vomiting, fever, and rectal bleeding (Conlon, 2010; NCI, 2013a). Symptoms are classified as complicated or uncomplicated depending on the grade of toxicity along with accompanying symptoms.

Risk Factors and Etiology

In patients with cancer, diarrhea is usually a result of treatment, including surgery, radiation therapy, and most often, chemotherapy. Surgery to the GI tract and radiation to the pelvis, abdomen, or lower thoracic and lumbar spines can result in diarrhea. Postsurgical complications that can lead to diarrhea include increased transit time, gastroparesis, fat malabsorption, lactose intolerance, fluid and electrolyte imbalance, and dumping syndrome (NCI, 2013a). The dose, fractionation, volume of bowel irradiated, and concomitant chemotherapy are factors that influence the risk of diarrhea with radiation therapy (NCI, 2013a).

Several chemotherapy agents pose a risk for diarrhea (Polovich et al., 2014). Those with the highest risk of diarrhea include capecitabine, dacarbazine, dactinomycin, 5-fluorouracil, irinotecan, and paclitaxel. Other chemotherapy agents that could cause diarrhea include cisplatin, cytarabine, docetaxel, floxuridine, fludarabine, hydroxyurea, idarubicin, mitoxantrone, oxaliplatin, pemetrexed, pentostatin, and topotecan. Biotherapy agents associated with diarrhea are IL-2 and interferons, whereas the targeted agents that can cause diarrhea are bortezomib, dasatinib, erlotinib, gefitinib, imatinib, lapatinib, lenalidomide, monoclonal antibodies, sunitinib, temsirolimus, thalidomide, and vorinostat (Muehlbauer & Lopez, 2014). Other risk factors for diarrhea include GVHD; inflammatory conditions such as diverticulitis, irritable bowel syndrome, and ulcerative colitis; malabsorption, partial bowel obstruction; and anxiety and stress (NCI, 2013a; Polovich et al., 2014).

Pathophysiology

Osmotic diarrhea is usually related to injury to the gut, dietary factors, or digestive problems. Water is pulled into the bowel from the osmotic pressure of unabsorbed particles, resulting in increased stool volume and weight (Conlon, 2010). Malabsorptive diarrhea occurs as a result of a combination of mechanical and biochemical mechanisms. When the mucosal integrity of the bowel is altered, malabsorption of fluid occurs. Surgical procedures such as gastrectomy reduce mucosal surface, causing enzyme deficiencies and leading to reduced absorption (Conlon, 2010). Secretory diarrhea happens when the intestines secrete more fluids and electrolytes than can be absorbed, leading to the production of a large volume of fluid and electrolytes in the small bowel and resulting in large stool volumes (Polovich et al., 2014). Diarrhea associated with GVHD and diarrhea with pelvic irradiation are examples of secretory diarrhea. When the intestinal epithelium is disturbed, allowing excess mucus, serum, protein, or blood into the GI tract, inflammation occurs, leading to exudative diarrhea (Conlon, 2010). Systemic fever, pus, blood, or mucus in the stool is seen with infectious diarrhea. As the infectious agent invades the intestinal mucosa, hydrostatic pressure in the blood vessels cause water and electrolytes, protein, mucus, and cells to accumulate in the bowel (Conlon, 2010). *Clostridium difficile* (*C. difficile*) is the most common infectious agent related to diarrhea in hospitalized patients (Davila & Bresalier, 2008).

Diagnosis and Assessment

The first step in assessment of diarrhea is a thorough review of patient risk factors and history. Focused assessment should include previous health history, bowel pattern, current antineoplastic regimen, medication history, anxiety and stress, and any alternative therapies (Conlon, 2010; Muehlbauer & Lopez, 2014; NCI, 2013a). An abdominal examination includes evaluation for rebound tenderness, guarding, hypoactive or hyperactive bowel sounds, and stool collection. Questioning patients regarding patterns of diarrhea will help to determine the grade and severity of diarrhea. The NCI CTCAE for diarrhea is a useful tool in determining severity. This scale rates severity based on the number of stools, whether with or without a colostomy. Grade 1 is an increase of less than four stools per day over baseline or mild increase in ostomy output. Grade 2 is an increase of four to six stools per day or moderate increase in ostomy output. Grade 3 includes an increase of seven or more stools per day, incontinence, or a severe increase in ostomy output, limiting self-care. Hospitalization is indicated for grade 3 diarrhea. Grade 4 diarrhea brings life-threatening consequences where urgent intervention is indicated, and grade 5 is death (NCI CTEP, 2010).

Several diagnostic tests can help in determining the etiology of diarrhea. Stool analysis can be performed to detect bacteria, fungus, ova and parasites, blood, and fecal leucocytes. *C. difficile* in patients with diarrhea can be confirmed with a series of three stool specimens, although it often is diagnosed with the first specimen (Conlon, 2010). A complete blood count should be used to determine the presence of infection, and blood chemistry can be useful in determining electrolyte imbalances. Abdominal radiographic imaging can be used to determine GI obstruction or fecal impaction. Endoscopy or colonoscopy with biopsy is useful in evaluating for GI abnormalities (American Society for Gastrointestinal Endoscopy Standards of Practice Committee et al., 2010).

Evidence-Based Treatment Strategies

Therapy-induced diarrhea should be treated with standard doses of over-the-counter loperamide per package instructions (4 mg after first loose stool and then 2 mg after each diarrhea episode, up to 16 mg/day) (Wilkes & Barton-Burke, 2012). Two types of diarrhea are associated with irinotecan. Acute diarrhea occurs within 24 hours of the infusion and is cholinergic in origin. It responds to atropine 0.25–1 mg IV or subcutaneous and may be prevented if atropine is given as a premedication in patients with prior early diarrhea (Wilkes & Barton-Burke, 2012). Late diarrhea (occurring 24 hours or more after irinotecan) is treated with aggressive loperamide therapy (4 mg after first evidence of diarrhea, followed by 2 mg every 2 hours until diarrhea-free for 12 hours; 4 mg can be used every 4 hours during the night) (Wilkes & Barton-Burke, 2012). Patients receiving a fluorouracil- or irinotecan-based regimen who develop diarrhea require oral loperamide therapy. Other antidiarrheal agents include octreotide (100–150 mcg subcutaneously every eight hours or 25–50 mcg/hour as an IV infusion, dose titrated to response). Loperamide is stopped when starting other agents, such as octreotide or paregoric. In addition to medication, dietary manipulations are necessary to manage diarrhea, although dietary manipulations alone are not effective for irinotecan-induced and other chemotherapy-induced diarrhea.

Many foods labeled as "sugar free" contain sugar alcohols that act like osmotic laxatives, worsen diarrhea, and should be avoided (Muehlbauer & Lopez, 2014). Modifying the diet to eliminate food items that worsen diarrhea, such as fiber, most dairy products (especially milk), caffeine, and fatty foods, which may increase intestinal motility, can help to control diarrhea (Muehlbauer & Lopez, 2014).

Discontinuing oral antibiotics is the first step in treating diarrhea associated with *C. difficile*; this will resolve diarrhea in about 25% of cases (Winkeljohn, 2011). If the diarrhea continues, metronidazole 250 mg orally four times a day or 500 mg orally three times a day should be initiated and continue for 10 days (Hall, 2010). Some research has indicated that vancomycin 125–500 mg orally four times a day for 10 days is more effective to use in patients with cancer (Schieszer, 2009). Investigation of a number of probiotic microorganisms has produced conflicting outcomes for their use in managing *C. difficile* infections. Certain probiotics have been recommended for the prophylaxis of radiation therapy–induced diarrhea. These include *Lactobacillus casei* 96 ml three times a day and VSL#3® (a patented probiotic mixture) one capsule three times a day (Visich & Yeo, 2010). For patients with diarrhea and vomiting and resultant dehydration, replacement of fluids and electrolytes should occur as needed. Education for all patients at risk for diarrhea needs to include dietary manipulations to reduce fiber, information on maintenance of fluid and electrolyte balance, and signs and symptoms to report to healthcare providers (Conlon, 2010).

Implications for Oncology Advanced Practice Nurses

APNs monitor patients to minimize and prevent GI side effects and toxicities and to minimize their effects if they occur. The prevention or treatment of side effect recurrence with additional and ongoing therapy needs to be considered. GI toxicities and side effects are common reactions to treatment. APNs need to manage GI side effects aggressively to achieve a positive outcome in patients' quality of life. Consultation with a gastroenterologist may be appropriate for patients who do not respond to treatment as expected.

Genitourinary Toxicities

The GU system includes the kidneys, bladder, ureters, urethra, renal pelvis, and the lymphatic system in both males and females; and the prostate, testes, and penis in males, and the cervix, vagina, vulva, uterus, fallopian tubes, and ovaries in females ("Urogenital System," 2015). Obstruction of a ureter by tumor is an example of direct tumor effect. An example of a direct treatment effect is the surgical removal of the ovaries. Cystitis, loss of libido, erectile dysfunction, dyspareunia, and ovarian failure are examples of toxicities caused by systemic treatments. Bladder cancer and its treatment may cause toxicities such as cystitis, bleeding, contracture, infection, inadequate bladder emptying, loss of fullness sensation, and urinary frequency and incontinence. Almost any bladder toxicity may be interrelated to sexual functioning and reproduction by effects caused by bladder resection, urinary diversions, or body image changes related to these. In addition, almost any cancer treatment and many other cancers, particularly those that affect the pelvis, can cause sexual and reproductive dysfunction. This section will focus on sexual dysfunction and infertility.

Sexual Dysfunction

Definition and Incidence

Sexuality is a global term that encompasses sexual functioning but also values, beliefs, attitudes, behaviors, intimacy, practices, body image, feelings and emotions, gender identity, societal roles, reproduction, and sexual orientation. Sexual functioning as a component of human sexuality refers to the sexual response as conceptualized by Masters and Johnson (1966) and Kaplan (1979). *Sexual dysfunction* is a broad term that includes dyspareunia, anorgasmia, loss of libido, penile atrophy, vaginal dryness, introital stenosis, vaginal stenosis, ovarian failure, erectile dysfunction, ejaculatory difficulties, menopausal symptoms, and recurrent vaginal infections. Generally, the most common type of sexual dysfunction in men is premature ejaculation. In men with cancer, erectile dysfunction is the most common form of sexual dysfunction (Flynn et al., 2011; NCI, 2013a). The most common types of sexual dysfunction reported in women are decreased libido, vaginal dryness, and dyspareunia (American Psychiatric Association, 2013; Falk & Dizon, 2013; Krychman & Millheiser, 2013). The most common type of sexual problem in both sexes is decreased libido (Krychman & Millheiser, 2013).

The Patient-Reported Outcomes Measurement Information System (PROMIS®), along with NCI, developed 16 focus groups with more than 100 participants to determine the relevance of cancer treatment on sexuality and sexual health. This study found that treatment-related symptoms affected sexual function both physically and psychologically in 100% of the participants (Flynn et al., 2011). The American Cancer Society (ACS) predicts that 468,040 new GU cancers will be diagnosed in the United States in 2015; approximately 70% of these cases will be of the genital system and about 30% of the urinary system (ACS, 2015). Numerous studies have documented sexual dysfunction following oncologic pelvic surgery, with the incidence of sexual dysfunction varying from 15% to almost 100% (Diaz & Close, 2010; Ginsberg, 2010; Lara, de Andrade, Consolo, & Romão, 2012). In patients with prostate cancer, penile deformities and erectile dysfunction are the most common adverse effects (Chung & Brock, 2013).

In patients with testicular cancer, ejaculatory dysfunction was the most commonly reported adverse event (Diaz & Close, 2010). Even in nonpelvic cancers, such as breast cancer, sexual dysfunction may occur (Anderson, 2013; Falk & Dizon, 2013; Flynn et al., 2011; Krychman & Millheiser, 2013; Pinto, 2013).

Presenting Signs and Symptoms

Signs of sexual dysfunction can result from the side effects of cancer therapy. Symptoms such as fatigue and body image changes can be precursors to sexual dysfunction. Symptoms of sexual dysfunction vary according to the patient, gender, type of cancer, and treatment. In women with cancer, complaints include decreased libido, hot flashes, difficulty becoming aroused, difficulty achieving orgasm, vaginal dryness, discharge, irritation, loss of sensation, dissatisfaction with body image, dyspareunia, less frequent intercourse, and inability to relax and enjoy sex (Flynn et al., 2011; Krychman & Millheiser, 2013). Vaginal dryness is the most commonly reported symptom in women, whereas erectile dysfunction is the most commonly reported in men (Flynn et al., 2011). Men may complain of erectile dysfunction, ejaculatory difficulty (anejaculation, premature ejaculation, dry ejaculation), decreased libido, hot flashes, difficulty with arousal, difficulty achieving orgasm, loss of sensation, poor body image, less frequent intercourse, and less pleasure in sex (Flynn et al., 2011; Krychman & Millheiser, 2013; NCI, 2013a). Psychosocial complaints might include feelings of decreased femininity or masculinity, anger, worry, embarrassment about the body, anxiety about relationships, fear of rejection, depression, fear of cancer recurrence, performance anxiety, and grief about the diagnosis and resultant life changes (Krebs, 2014).

Risk Factors and Etiology

Sexual dysfunction can occur in any patient with any cancer receiving any type of treatment, including surgery, radiation, chemotherapy, immunotherapy, and hormonal therapy. Surgical treatment for cancer (particularly of the GU systems) changes the anatomy, and permanent or temporary sexual dysfunction may occur as a result of the removal of sexual organs, altered functioning of GU systems, or damage to neurovascular structures (both sympathetic and parasympathetic fibers). Surgical resection can cause body image changes that affect sexuality. Oophorectomy causes hormonal disruption and reproductive failure. Women undergoing surgery for cervical, uterine, or vaginal cancer may experience vaginal stenosis, decreased sensation, decreased vaginal lubrication, fibrosis, or development of scar tissue (Krychman & Millheiser, 2013).

Surgery in men also may cause sexual dysfunction. Patients with testicular cancer who have undergone retroperitoneal lymph node dissection (RPLND) may have anejaculation (NCI, 2013a). Surgery for urologic cancer may leave men with penile deformities, fibrosis, or atrophy. The most common sexual dysfunction in men with cancer is erectile dysfunction as a result of neurogenic or vasculogenic damage. Patients also experience difficulties with ejaculation, ability to maintain an erection, and orgasm. Dysfunction may be temporary; research suggests that some men who have undergone radical prostatectomy may recover erectile function more than two years after the surgical intervention (Chung & Brock, 2013).

Radiation therapy may cause sexual dysfunction in both genders. In women, vaginal fibrosis, contractures, range-of-motion difficulties, skin changes, dyspareunia, lymphedema, shortened vaginal vault, and decreased lubrication and sensitivity may occur if the pelvic area is irradiated (Krychman & Millheiser, 2013). In men who receive radiation therapy to the pelvic region, blood vessels and nerves needed for erection may become fibrotic, causing erectile dysfunction that can be temporary or permanent. Other commonly reported complications of pelvic radiation in men include diarrhea, incontinence, decreased frequency of erection, and inability to lubricate or reach orgasm; concerns about infertility can lead to sexual dysfunction (Krebs, 2014; Sadovsky et al., 2010). Radiation toxicities vary according to radiation type, field, and dose. Up to 80% of both men and women who undergo radiation therapy report mild to severe fatigue regardless of the site of radiation (Flynn et al., 2011). This intense tiredness affects sexual function by decreasing desire and ability to sustain pleasurable sexual positions, as well as an inability to continue intercourse long enough to attain orgasm.

Pharmacologic treatments for cancer, including chemotherapy, hormonal manipulations, and immunotherapy, also may cause sexual dysfunction in patients with cancer. Chemotherapy can result in innumerable physical symptoms that affect sexual functioning and sexuality (Krychman & Millheiser, 2013). Uncontrolled nausea, vomiting, diarrhea, fatigue, mucositis, dysuria, hot flashes, sleep disorders, vaginal dryness or discharge, and constipation may influence libido, the desire for sexual intimacy, or the ability to have an orgasm. Effects of chemotherapy, such as alopecia, depression, emotional lability, body image changes, and weight changes, also negatively affect sexuality. Dysfunction varies according to the pharmacologic agent, dose, and length of treatment (Azim, Peccatori, de Azambuja, & Piccart, 2011). When chemotherapy is combined with another modality of treatment, sexual dysfunction may be exacerbated. A study of patients with breast cancer younger than age 40 found that not only did chemotherapy affect all phases of the sexual response cycle, but the effect was particularly devastating to young women who were also dealing with issues of infertility (Gilbert, Ussher, & Perz, 2010; Kedde, van de Wiel, Schultz, & Wijsen, 2013; Ochsenkuhn et al., 2011).

Other causes of sexual dysfunction in patients with cancer exist as well. Comorbid diseases, such as diabetes or depression, may cause or contribute to changes in sexual function. Numerous medications negatively affect sexual functioning (see Figure 13-1). Aging influences sexual dysfunction, particularly in regard to dyspareunia, with 17%–30% of menopausal women experiencing decreased vaginal lubrication (Nishimoto & Mark, 2010), but does not appear to be related to overall sexual health. Psychological distress, including depression, body image issues, anxiety, fear, and underlying psychiatric illnesses, may cause sexual dysfunction (Krychman & Millheiser, 2013).

Some identified risk factors for sexual dysfunction are aging, female gender, postmenopausal status in women, and poor performance status. The presence of sexual dysfunction prior to a cancer diagnosis is a risk factor for sexual dysfunction during and after a cancer diagnosis. Poor self-image and having a colostomy or stoma are associated with increased risk. Treatments such as GI or GU surgery and radiation to the pelvis, the anatomic nature of the cancer, and advanced disease are risk factors. Certain comorbidities, including depression, increase the risk for sexual dysfunction. Psychosocial issues, such as poor communication with partner, lack of social support, history of rape or sexual abuse, and a more recent diagnosis of cancer, also are risk factors (Krebs, 2014; Krychman & Millheiser, 2013; Nishimoto & Mark, 2010). See Table 13-2 for a list of causes of sexual dysfunction in patients with cancer.

• Anabolic steroids	• Aromatase inhibitors
• Androgen deprivation therapy	• Gabapentin
• Antiemetics (prochlorperazine, metoclopramide, scopolamine)	• Histamine (H_2) receptor antagonists
	• Opioids
• Antihistamines	• Selective serotonin reuptake inhibitors
• Antihypertensives	• Tricyclic antidepressants

Figure 13-1. Medications That May Cause or Contribute to Sexual Dysfunction

Note. Based on information from Manolis & Doumas, 2012; Wilkes & Barton-Burke, 2012.

Table 13-2. Causes of Sexual Dysfunction in Patients With Cancer

Cause	Examples
Psychological factors	Stress Depression Body image changes Fears (of death, cancer return)
Physical symptoms	Pain Fatigue Sleep disorders Urinary tract symptoms Gastrointestinal symptoms
Pharmacologic agents	Opioids Chemotherapy Psychotropic agents
Genitourinary structural changes	Penectomy Vulvectomy Urethrectomy Radical cystectomy Radical prostatectomy Radical hysterectomy Retroperitoneal lymph node dissection
Endocrine dysfunction	Bilateral orchiectomy Bilateral oophorectomy Androgen deprivation therapy
Neurologic damage	Damage to neural pathways (superior hypogastric plexus, inferior hypogastric plexus, pudendal, cavernosal and pelvic splanchnic nerves) from tumor encroachment or surgical resection Spinal cord lesion
Vascular damage	Damage to vasculature from pelvic radiation or surgical injury causing arterial insufficiency Venous leak allowing blood to leak from rigid penis

Note. Based on information from American Psychiatric Association, 2013; Chung & Brock, 2013; Falk & Dizon, 2013; Flynn et al., 2011; Krychman & Millheiser, 2013; Pinto, 2013.

Pathophysiology

Sexual dysfunction in patients with cancer can result from changes in gonadal function or in the sexual response cycle. Normally, the hypothalamus secretes gonadotropin-releasing hormone (GnRH), which triggers the anterior pituitary gland to produce follicle-stimulating hormone (FSH) and luteinizing hormone (LH). When FSH and LH are present, the ovaries are stimulated to produce estrogen and progesterone in women, while the testes produce testosterone in men. When blood levels of FSH and LH are adequate, production stops (Deneris & Huether, 2012; Dirksen, 2011; Latendresse & McCance, 2012). The sexual response cycle, first described by Masters and Johnson in 1966, includes four stages—excitement, plateau, orgasm, and resolution—which involve stages of muscle contraction and vasoconstriction (Masters & Johnson, 1966). Both gonadal function and the sexual arousal cycle can be altered by a variety of factors, including the cancer itself, individual patient factors, or treatment side effects as discussed previously.

Prevention Strategies

Treatment strategies exist that can decrease the risk of sexual dysfunction. For instance, in rectal cancer, sphincter-preserving surgery eliminates the need for a colostomy. In some GI or GU cancers, nerve-sparing procedures are possible, thus preserving patients' ability to have sexual intercourse and achieve orgasm. Nerve-sparing RPLND often preserves sexual functioning and fertility (Mezvrishvili & Managadze, 2006). In bladder cancer, the development of a "neobladder" allows maintenance of normal voiding patterns (Kanematsu, Yamamoto, & Ogawa, 2007). The choice of treatment modality may determine post-treatment sexual dysfunction. For example, radical prostatectomy in men with prostate cancer causes more erectile dysfunction than other therapies, such as brachytherapy (Snyder, Stock, Buckstein, & Stone, 2012).

Diagnosis and Assessment

Sexual dysfunction is difficult to quantify, and no uniform method of measurement exists. Multiple factors are considered, including anatomic, hormonal, physiologic, psychological, cognitive, behavioral, relational, and cultural factors. APNs can be more effective and comfortable with sexual health assessment when using a systematic and consistent set of open-ended questions with every patient, adapting these questions to each patient's unique situation. Clinicians need to be respectful of sexual orientation and cultural and religious values. Whenever possible, they should include the patient's partner's perspective.

The physical examination serves to further drive the diagnostic process. In men, this includes appraisal of hair patterns (assess for poor beard, slight underarm or pubic hair), testicular volume, prostate findings, height and body proportions, and breasts (for possible gynecomastia). The penis and testicles are examined for fibrosis, atrophy, or varicocele. In women, assessment of hair patterns (female pubic, facial, and underarm hair distribution) and examination of the breasts are performed. Pelvic and adnexal examination includes inspection for any signs of infection and attempts to elicit pain with cervical manipulation or during adnexal examination. A rectal examination is necessary for both men and women, assessing for rectocele, hemorrhoids, or other abnormalities. Figures 13-2 and 13-3 list diagnostic tests to consider in men and women, respectively. Hormonal tests, such as testosterone levels, and glucose and thyroid testing may indicate endocrinopathy, such as hypopituitarism, hyperthyroidism, or adrenal tumors. GnRH stimulation testing assesses pituitary reserve. A semen analysis includes semen volume; a lowered volume might indicate a partial obstruction of the ejaculatory ducts or retrograde ejaculation. The pH level of semen may indicate infection, blockage of seminal vesicles, or prostate abnormalities. Postejaculate urine analysis evaluates for retrograde ejaculation, which commonly is seen in patients with diabetes or after RPLND.

Figure 13-3 lists diagnostic tests to consider in women. Increased prolactin levels might indicate a pituitary or hypothalamus disorder. Higher levels of prolactin are associated with decreases in libido in both sexes (Krebs, 2014). FSH and LH levels assess pituitary function, gonadal function, and menopausal status. Excessive testosterone production in women might indicate adrenal or ovarian tumors, polycystic ovarian disease, and virilization. The Pap test, which rules out precancerous and cancerous conditions, also is used for hormonal assessment and to diagnose inflammatory diseases. Other diagnostic testing to rule out medical conditions causing sexual dysfunction may be indicated.

A sexual frequency baseline is established, and continuing assessment throughout the disease trajectory is required. Cancer or its treatments can exacerbate a preexisting problem; therefore, sexual function assessment must include evaluation of precancer sexual functioning (Krebs, 2014). The sexual function assessment includes inquiry regarding feelings of inadequacy, anxiety regarding sexual performance, depression, expectations, current relation-

- Semen analysis
- Testicular biopsy
- Luteinizing hormone*
- Testosterone assays
- Postejaculate urinalysis
- Follicle-stimulating hormone*

- Human chorionic gonadotropin
- Gonadotropin-releasing hormone stimulation testing
- Cultures for infection or sexually transmitted infections
- RigiScan® (TIMM Medical Technologies, Inc.) (determines the extent of erectile dysfunction)

Figure 13-2. Diagnostic Tests in the Workup of Sexual Dysfunction in Men

* These are ordered if serum testosterone is low; if both are appropriately elevated, then primary testicular failure is identified.

Note. Based on information from Krebs, 2014.

- Prolactin
- Prolactin level
- Serum estradiol
- Cervical Pap test
- Luteinizing hormone
- Testosterone assays

- Follicle-stimulating hormone
- Urinalysis and culture if indicated
- Human chorionic gonadotropin
- Photoplethysmography (quantifies sexual excitement)
- Cultures for infections and sexually transmitted diseases

Figure 13-3. Diagnostic Tests in the Workup of Sexual Dysfunction in Women

Note. Based on information from Krebs, 2014.

ships and levels of intimacy, previous sexual activity, religious and cultural beliefs, and partner expectations and anxieties (Krebs, 2014). Any history of sexual abuse or rape should be ascertained. Any report of pain in the genital regions requires careful assessment.

Assessment models can assist clinicians in obtaining more in-depth information. The ALARM and BETTER models are communication tools that may be used by oncology APNs to serve as reminders about information to request from patients. The ALARM model, which includes activity, libido, arousal, resolution, and medical data, tends to be of limited use to oncology nurses whose focus is on assessing patient concerns and providing support to them (Krebs, 2014). The BETTER model, reviewed in Figure 13-4, presents an acronym to guide clinicians through the assessment and patient education process, ending with documentation. Table 13-3 reviews tools that may be useful in clinical trials assessing sexual health in patients with cancer. Degrees of sexual dysfunction can be measured using the NCI CTCAE (see http://evs.nci .nih.gov/ftp1/CTCAE/CTCAE_4.03_2010-06-14_QuickReference_5x7.pdf), which not only categorizes the degree of toxicity but also makes recommendations for interventions (NCI CTEP, 2010).

B—Bring up the topic.
E—Explain your concern about sexuality as a key component of quality of life.
T—Tell patients about appropriate resources to assist them.
T—Assess timing, acknowledging that patients may ask for information as they are ready to receive it.
E—Educate patients about potential sexual toxicities that could occur as a result of cancer or its treatments and management options.
R—Record (document) your assessments and interventions in the medical record.

Figure 13-4. The BETTER Model for Sexual Health Assessment

Note. Based on information from Mick et al., 2004.

Table 13-3. Assessment Tools for Sexual Health and Function

Tool	Description
Derogatis Interview for Sexual Functioning (DISF) and DISF-SR (self-report) (Derogatis, 1987)	Measures quality of sexual functioning in five domains; 26-item interview
Sexual Adjustment Questionnaire (SAQ) (Waterhouse & Metcalfe, 1986)	Assesses impact of cancer or surgery on sexual function over a period of time; available in male and female versions
International Index of Erectile Function (IIEF) (Rosen et al., 1999)	Is a 15-item self-report that addresses five domains of function postoperatively; available in a 5-item short form
Changes in Sexual Functioning Questionnaire (Clayton et al., 1997)	Consists of 35 items that assess five domains of sexual functioning; 20-minute interview
Female Sexual Function Index (FSFI) (Rosen et al., 2000)	Evaluates arousal, orgasm, satisfaction, and pain using brief questionnaire
Sexual Health Inventory for Men (SHIM) (Day et al., 2001)	Addresses screening, diagnosis, and evaluation of severity of erectile dysfunction; widely used and easily administered

Evidence-Based Treatment Strategies

Interventions in men: Management for erectile dysfunction often includes oral medications. Sildenafil, vardenafil, and tadalafil all inhibit phosphodiesterase type 5, increasing guanosine monophosphate. This enhances the effects of nitric oxide in response to sexual stimulation and leads to smooth muscle relaxation and vasodilation in the corpus cavernosum, resulting in increased blood flow and erection. Common side effects include headache, dyspepsia, back pain, myalgia, nasal congestion, vision color changes, and flushing (Bayer Healthcare Pharmaceuticals Inc. & GlaxoSmithKline, 2014; Eli Lilly and Co., 2014; Pfizer Inc., 2010). However, if severe neurogenic damage has occurred, erectogenic agents are ineffective. They may be less effective in situations where libido is low, such as in patients treated with androgen-ablative therapy. A contraindication for sildenafil, vardenafil, and tadalafil is concomitant use with nitrates, such as nitroglycerin, sodium nitroprusside, and amyl nitrite (Bayer Healthcare Pharmaceuticals Inc. & GlaxoSmithKline, 2014; Eli Lilly and Co. 2014; Pfizer Inc., 2010).

Other interventions for erectile dysfunction include use of a penile vacuum erection device (VED), pharmacologic vasodilator injections or suppositories, and penile prostheses. However, patients often discontinue these interventions because of their inconvenience and difficulty in use. Dropout rates for VEDs are 20%–50%, whereas the dropout rate for vasodilator injections is closer to 40% (Pahlajani, Raina, Jones, Ali, & Zippe, 2012). Some of the concerns patients have described include discomfort, cumbersome use, and cold erection (Pahlajani et al., 2012).

Interventions in women: The treatment of menopausal symptoms (such as hot flashes, vaginal dryness, and negative emotional and cognitive states) often improves sexual functioning. Systemic or topical estrogen therapy is the most common management strategy; however, it may be contraindicated in patients with hormonally responsive cancers. Little, if any, systemic absorption of estrogen is reported with the estradiol-impregnated ring, and it may be helpful in minimizing menopausal symptoms. Vaginal lubricants or moisturizers may be used for vaginal dryness but often are not as effective as estrogen therapy. Hot flashes can be treated with a combination of medications such as belladonna, ergotamine, phenobarbital, vitamin E, or venlafaxine (Kaplan & Mahon, 2014; Morrow, Mattair, & Hortobagyi, 2011; North American Menopause Society, 2012). In women with decreased libido, androgen replacement therapy may be considered (Jordan, Hallam, Molinoff, & Spana, 2011). This type of therapy, as with estrogen therapy, may be contraindicated in some patients. Table 13-4 lists possible interventions for female sexual dysfunction and potential concerns related to each intervention. One concern is an increased risk of cardiovascular events and breast cancer with the use of hormones. Side effects of other pharmacologic treatments that can cause concern or discontinuation of treatment are dry mouth, dizziness, and difficulty concentrating. In addition, non-pharmacologic therapies can cause mucosal irritation, are often cumbersome, and require long-term patient commitment.

General interventions: Selective serotonin reuptake inhibitors often are used in the oncology population. Sexual dysfunction is a common side effect of these agents. Drug holidays, dose decreases, change of antidepressant, the use of erectile agents such as sildenafil, and the addition of bupropion or other pharmacologic agents prior to sexual activity are potential interventions (Krychman & Millheiser, 2013). Because sexual dysfunction in cancer survivors often has both biologic and psychogenic causes, an approach that involves several types of interventions may be more successful. Few evidence-based interventions are available for the management of sexual dysfunction in patients with cancer. The evidence source for many interventions may be case studies or opinions of expert authorities, agencies, or panels. In addition to specific interventions, psychosocial support is a vital part of sexual rehabilitation (Brotto, Yule, & Breckon, 2010). Information and support from clinicians decrease the negative impact of sexual dysfunction (Krebs, 2014). Patients often want and need practical evidence-based information in language they understand with sensitivity to culture, race, age, religion, and socioeconomic factors. At times, referral to a sexual health specialist is necessary. The role of oncology APNs in this case is to coordinate the referral and to follow up as necessary to ensure patients' needs are being met.

Implications for Oncology Advanced Practice Nurses

Sexual dysfunction is a common occurrence in patients with cancer, regardless of gender, and it negatively affects quality of life. It is likely to become more common as patients live longer and treatments become more complex. It may present at any time during the cancer trajectory. Oncology APNs possess skills that enable thorough evaluation, accurate diagnosis, and individualized, compassionate management. Although sexual function may not be the primary focus of oncologic care, acknowledgment of sexuality as an important component of quality of life and the treatment of sexual dysfunction are vital in the comprehensive and holistic care of patients with cancer. Myths held by both clinicians and patients can impede sexual health discussions (see Figure 13-5). Time limitations, feelings of discomfort or embarrassment, or absence of perceived need are not sufficient reasons for neglecting this aspect of health. Oncology APNs need to have knowledge regarding treatment techniques that minimize sexual toxicities and state-of-the-art interventions for the management of sexual dysfunction.

Early identification of patients at risk for sexual dysfunction can guide treatment decisions, and prophylactic measures may be possible. Many useful tools for assessment of sexual functioning exist. Interventions are individualized and range from simple to complex strategies. Few interventions have been validated in patients with cancer by clinical research. However, regardless of the intervention, patients require permission for discussion, reassurance, and support for optimal sexual health throughout their disease course.

Educational information includes the impact of cancer, treatment, and side effects of treatment on sexual health; fertility issues; management of sexual dysfunction; and available support services. APNs proactively begin with basic, factual information at the patient's level of understanding and then proceed to more sensitive or difficult topics. Just providing information validates patient concerns. Safer sex practices should be emphasized. Listening to

Table 13-4. Interventions in Female Sexual Dysfunction*

Dysfunction	Intervention	Concerns
Altered libido	Hormonal manipulation	May be contraindicated in some patients with cancer; may increase risk of breast cancer and cardiovascular events; estrogen must be given with progestin if uterus is intact
	Testosterone	Is under study; little is known about minimum levels of androgens required for female sexual functioning; may increase risk of breast cancer and heart disease
	Bupropion (for patients on antidepressants or opioids)	May cause concentration difficulties, sleep disturbance, and tremors
Hot flashes	Hormonal manipulation	As previously described
	Clonidine (transdermal or oral)	May cause dry mouth, dizziness, sedation, weakness, hypotension, and constipation
	Venlafaxine	May cause sexual dysfunction; may increase risk of suicide in patients with major depressive disorders
Vaginal dryness	Estrogen therapy	May be contraindicated in some patients with cancer; may increase risk of breast cancer and cardiovascular events; oral estrogen must be given with progestin if uterus is intact
	Lubricants/moisturizers	Can cause local irritation; may be messy or cumbersome; can stain clothing
Vaginal fibrosis, stenosis, scarring, or shortening	Vaginal dilators	Must be used daily for 10–15 minutes with lubricant; is cumbersome; has low adherence
Dyspareunia	Analgesia	Could contribute to sexual dysfunction; has sedative effects
	Topical anesthetic agents	Has potential for mucosal irritation
	Kegel exercises	Requires patient education and commitment to do exercises
	Alternate coital positions	—

* The level of evidence of these interventions varies significantly.

Note. Based on information from Herbenick et al., 2011; Jordan et al., 2011; Kaplan & Mahon, 2014; Morrow et al., 2011; North American Menopause Society, 2012; Roth et al., 2010.

- Older people are uninterested in sex.
- After cancer, one should just be "happy to be alive."
- Birth control is not necessary during cancer treatment.
- Abstinence from sexual activity will help to cure cancer.
- Sex is the last thing on the mind of a patient with cancer.
- Engaging in sexual contact will cause cancer to progress.
- Sexual contact should be avoided because cancer is contagious.
- Sexual health interventions are outside the clinical realm of oncology clinicians.

Figure 13-5. Myths Regarding Sexuality in Patients With Cancer

Note. Based on information from Brotto et al., 2010; Krebs, 2014.

the patient will give the APN clues about the significance of certain issues. Reassurance, support, and hope are needed throughout the cancer trajectory. Anticipatory guidance and education specific to the patient's treatment are necessary. Any effective education or intervention requires sensitivity to cultural issues, religious beliefs, and sexual orientation.

Reproductive Dysfunction: Infertility

Definition and Incidence

Cancer and its treatment may threaten fertility in both men and women. In 2015, there will be an estimated 810,170 new cases of cancer in women and 848,200 in men (ACS, 2015). Of these cases, 6% of men and 10% of women will be younger than age 45 (ACS, 2015). Infertility usually is defined as the inability to conceive after one year of intercourse without contraception. However, this definition does not fully meet the needs of many patients facing cancer treatment–related infertility. Many patients want to be parents following cancer treatment, and the fear of possible infertility causes distress for them (Peate, Meiser, Hickey, & Friedlander, 2009; Rosen, Rodriguez-Wallberg, & Rosenzweig, 2009; Tschudin & Bitzer, 2009). Rates of infertility following a cancer diagnosis vary depending on the cancer, its location, extent, and treatment, as well as individual patient characteristics. The effects on fertility may be transient, permanent, or late effects. An American Society of Clinical Oncology panel of experts found that available evidence suggests that fertility preservation is very important to many people with cancer (Loren et al., 2013). It is the responsibility of oncology health professionals to identify patients at risk for infertility, to adequately inform patients of the risk, and to understand the fertility preservation options available (Pentheroudakis, Orecchia, Hoekstra, & Pavlidis, 2010). Yet, many patients report that fertility issues were never discussed with them during their cancer diagnosis and treatment (Clayman, Harper, Quinn, Shah, & Reinecke, 2011; Forman, Anders, & Behera, 2010; Quinn et al., 2009).

The incidence of infertility following a cancer diagnosis is difficult to quantify. Research evaluating infertility rates generally reports incidence of azoospermia and amenorrhea, but these are not always adequate to quantify infertility. For example, in women, infertility may occur as a result of a decrease in ovulatory reserve, even though the woman maintains or resumes cyclic menses. Therefore, merely assessing amenorrhea following cancer treatment could give an inaccurate estimate of infertility. With the five-year expected survival rate of 68% for adult cancers and 83% for childhood cancers (NCI Surveillance, Epidemiology, and End Results Program, 2015), the aforementioned rates of cancer in people under 45 years of age, and the variability of infertility with cancer, it is clear that current infertility rates may be well underrated.

Presenting Signs and Symptoms

Amenorrhea is a presenting complaint of many women with infertility. Couples who are unable to become pregnant after a year are considered to be infertile. Women may report menopausal symptoms such as hot flashes and mood variations. Various symptoms of sexual dysfunction also may be present in both men and women.

Risk Factors and Etiology

The greatest risk for infertility in both men and women is associated with chemotherapy treatment, particularly the alkylating agents (Jensen, Morbeck, & Coddington, 2011; NCI, 2013e). Total body irradiation associated with hematopoietic stem cell transplantation is a major risk factor for infertility. Preexisting fertility problems, advancing age (particularly in women), and treatments affecting the reproductive organs increase the risk for infertility (NCI, 2013e).

Fertility may be compromised by the cancer itself or by treatment of the cancer. Chemotherapy and radiation therapy effects are dose dependent. The dose, frequency, route, and duration of chemotherapy influence the risk of infertility. The effects of radiation on fertility depend on the size and location of the radiation field and the total dose. The patient's age, sex, pretreatment fertility, and type of cancer also influence post–cancer diagnosis fertility (Jensen et al., 2011; NCI, 2013e). Cancer involving a reproductive organ often requires treatment that may result in infertility, such as surgical resection.

Pathophysiology

Hormonal regulation guides the process of fertility, beginning with the hypothalamus releasing GnRH. This hormone regulates LH and FSH, thereby regulating gonadal hormone secretion. An imbalance of any of these hormones could impair fertility. (See Pathophysiology section under sexual dysfunction earlier in chapter.)

Prevention Strategies

The prevention of cancer-related infertility begins with a discussion between clinicians and patients about the likelihood that the cancer or cancer treatment might cause infertility (Jensen et al., 2011; Krebs, 2014). Prevention of ovarian morbidity includes using less-toxic agents, lowering dosages, or abstaining from radiation therapy if deemed appropriate (Kelvin, Kroon, & Ogle, 2012). Another preventive measure is the application of external lead shields during radiation therapy to gonadal organs (NCI, 2013e).

Diagnosis and Assessment

Assessment of the risk for infertility must begin at the initial cancer diagnosis and be communicated with patients prior to treatment initiation. The male physical examination includes the same evaluation as for sexual dysfunction, with careful assessment for lesions, varicoceles, and absence of vas deferens. Laboratory assessment is similar as well, with the addition of semen analysis including semen volume, sperm concentration, motility, and morphology. FSH, LH, prolactin, and testosterone levels may be assessed. Women should be questioned about amenorrhea and menopausal symptoms. For premenopausal women, a sexual and menstrual history should be taken. The female physical examination is similar to that noted previously for sexual dysfunction. Laboratory assessment of fertility in women includes measurements of FSH and estradiol.

Evidence-Based Treatment Strategies

Some female interventions are menstrual cycle dependent and thus might delay cancer treatment by several weeks. Early referral to a fertility specialist may minimize delay. (See Tables 13-5 and 13-6 for a review of fertility preservation interventions.)

Table 13-5. Options for Male Fertility Preservation

Intervention	Description
Sperm cryopreservation	Freezing of sperm, ideally collected prior to start of treatment; most common intervention; most insurance companies do not cover
Gonadal shielding during radiation therapy	Use of shielding to prevent radiation to testes
Conservative surgical or radiation approaches	Surgical expertise required; limited selection of patients; for early-stage disease only; procedures experimental only
Testicular tissue cryopreservation and reimplantation	Freezing of testicular or germ cells and implanting following cancer treatment
Testis xenografting	Investigational
Spermatogonial isolation	Investigational

Note. Based on information from Center for Reproductive Medicine and Infertility, 2007; Donnez et al., 2010; Ginsberg et al., 2010; Jensen et al., 2011; Silber et al., 2010.

Embryo cryopreservation is the most common and successful form of fertility preservation in women. A sperm donor is required. This procedure generally takes several weeks to complete, as women must undergo hormonal stimulation and then egg harvesting. In vitro fertilization (IVF) is performed with donor sperm, and the embryos are frozen, with implantation occurring at a later time (Donnez et al., 2010; Ginsberg et al., 2010; Jensen et al., 2011; Silber et al., 2010). Human embryos can survive the freezing and thawing process up to 95% of the time, with pregnancy rates of greater than 60% when multiple embryos are available (Jensen et al., 2011). In women with hormonally responsive cancers, hormonal stimulation with agents such as letrozole or tamoxifen may be used (Jensen et al., 2011). Unfertilized oocyte cryopreservation is another fertility preservation option. One advantage of this procedure is that no sperm donor is required. Ovarian stimulation and the oocyte harvesting procedures are similar to that of embryo cryopreservation, but no IVF occurs prior to freezing (Donnez et al., 2010; Ginsberg et al., 2010; Jensen et al., 2011; Silber et al., 2010). With more recent advances in technology, oocytes can survive the freezing process 50%–60% of the time, with fertilization rates of 60%–70% using intracytoplasmic sperm injection (Jensen et al., 2011). However, live birth rates are lower than with frozen embryos (Jensen et al., 2011).

Ovarian tissue cryopreservation may be an option for women with a hormonally responsive cancer (Donnez et al., 2010; Ginsberg et al., 2010; Jensen et al., 2011; Silber et al., 2010). However, it is still considered investigational. The advantages of this procedure are that tissue can be obtained with minimal delay of cancer therapy, no partner is required at the time of harvesting, and the transplanted tissue maintains its ability to produce endogenous hormones, which eliminates the need for hormone replacement therapy (Donnez et al., 2010; Ginsberg et al., 2010; Jensen et al., 2011; Silber et al., 2010). An ovary or part of an ovary is removed. The outer surface is divided into smaller strips, which are cryopreserved and stored. Following the patient's recovery from cancer treatment, the strips are transplanted back to the remaining ovary or to a more superficial area in the abdomen, thus restoring estrogen production.

Ovarian suppression with GnRH analogs during chemotherapy is a controversial, investigational method of fertility preservation. This involves the coadministration of GnRH analogs

Table 13-6. Options for Female Fertility Preservation

Intervention	Description
Embryo cryopreservation	Most common and successful intervention; requires two weeks of ovarian stimulation with follicle-stimulating hormone from onset of menses; oocytes are collected by ultrasound-guided transvaginal needle aspiration under sedation, then oocytes are fertilized in vitro and cryopreserved; most insurance companies do not cover; requires sperm donor
Oophoropexy (transposition of ovaries)	Surgical repositioning of ovaries out of pelvic radiation field
Gonadal shielding	Use of shielding to prevent radiation to reproductive organs
Conservative surgical or radiation approaches such as sparing resections and trachelectomy	Surgical expertise required; limited selection of patients; for early-stage disease only; removal of cervix, but preservation of the uterus; increased risk for midtrimester losses and preterm birth
Intensity-modulated radiation therapy	Radiation therapy technique used for pelvic radiation to precisely shape the field of treatment to minimize dose to the ovaries; ovaries are still at risk from scatter radiation; does not protect from gonadotoxic chemotherapy
Oocyte cryopreservation	Investigational; freezing of unfertilized eggs; requires two weeks of ovarian stimulation with follicle-stimulating hormone from onset of menses; thawed later and fertilized in vitro; useful if patient has no partner or has religious or ethical objections to embryo freezing
Ovarian tissue cryopreservation	Investigational; advantage of no ovarian stimulation or donor required; ovarian tissue is removed, frozen, and, at later date, reimplanted; potential for reintroduction of cancer cells
Ovarian suppression by gonadotropin-releasing hormone agonist or antagonist	Investigational and controversial; given during chemotherapy; potential for cancer cell stimulation

Note. Based on information from Donnez et al., 2010; Ginsberg et al., 2010; Jensen et al., 2011; Silber et al., 2010.

during chemotherapy and suppression of ovarian function, thus protecting the ovary from cytotoxic effects (Jensen et al., 2011).

In men, sperm cryopreservation is the most commonly used method of fertility preservation. This ideally is done before beginning chemotherapy. The most common barrier found for this procedure is the lack of information about this as an option (Williams, 2010).

Referrals for counseling are indicated for some patients, as cancer-related infertility may be associated with psychosocial distress (Kelvin, Kroon, & Ogle, 2012). Ethical considerations also should be addressed. Directions for future disposition of the stored embryos, oocytes, ovarian tissue, and sperm should be clear in case of the patient's death. Other ethical concerns include harm to future offspring (such as physical health effects or psychological health effects) and balancing cancer risks with the desire for fertility.

Implications for Oncology Advanced Practice Nurses

Infertility is a risk of cancer and its therapy. Patients must be informed of this risk. Many patients undergoing cancer treatment may desire fertility preservation. It is a responsibility of oncology APNs to be knowledgeable about these options and to provide patients with this information. APNs can provide resources to patients, and referral to an infertility specialist early in the cancer trajectory is desirable. Referral for psychological counseling may be in order. Patients require information about risks of cancer recurrence if fertility preservation is undertaken. APNs must be aware of and willing to address the potential ethical issues that could arise related to treatments for infertility.

Hepatic Toxicities

Definition and Incidence

Hepatotoxicity is generally defined as a state of toxic damage to the liver or a tendency or ability to cause hepatotoxicity. Björnsson, Bergmann, Björnsson, Kvaran, and Olafsson (2013) further defined hepatotoxicity or liver injury as elevation of at least three times the upper limit of alanine aminotransferase (ALT) and twice the upper limit of alkaline phosphatase, whether or not clinical hepatitis is present. Hepatitis is an acute or chronic inflammatory injury to the liver caused by a toxin or a virus. Cirrhosis may be defined as fibrotic and nodular tissue formation that distorts the normal anatomic structure of the liver and may be caused by toxins, bacteria, or viruses. Cholestasis is a compromised flow or complete blockage of bile flow into the duodenum. Sinusoidal obstructive syndrome (SOS), previously referred to as veno-occlusive disease, is associated with hepatic venous obstruction from perisinusoidal damage, with dilation and congestion leading to hepatic fibrosis.

Polovich et al. (2014) summarized the incidence of hepatotoxicity related to chemotherapy and biotherapy and reported ranges of less than 1% to 84% depending on the specific agent. Acetaminophen is the leading cause of acute liver failure. Even therapeutic doses of acetaminophen may cause significant increases in liver enzymes, which commonly manifests as jaundice. Hepatotoxicity following an overdose of acetaminophen is the leading cause for drug-induced liver injury (DILI) in both the United States and the United Kingdom (Russmann, Kullak-Ublick, & Grattagliano, 2009). Most other drugs have an idiosyncratic aspect to hepatotoxicity, with risk of acute liver injury being less than 1 per 10,000 exposed patients (Russmann et al., 2009). More than 900 toxins, including drugs and herbals, have been identified and account for approximately 20%–40% of DILI (Mehta, 2012).

Presenting Signs and Symptoms

Edema, pruritus, jaundice, malaise, headache, anorexia, ecchymosis, low-grade fever, muscle and joint aches, and urine and stool color changes (such as clay-colored stools in liver injury) are the most common presenting signs and symptoms of DILI. Jaundice is a presenting sign when late-stage disease is present in metabolic liver diseases such as hemochromatosis (Mehta, 2012).

Risk Factors and Etiology

Hepatotoxicity is influenced by the chemical property of the drug, individual genetics, and environmental factors. Examples of these influences include age, gender, family history of hereditary liver diseases, prior tumor involvement of the liver, prior radiation therapy to the liver or right side of abdomen, the use of other drugs (including illicit drugs) or alcohol, cirrhosis, and comorbidities such as HIV, diabetes, and prior or current hepatitis (Fregonese &

Stolk, 2008; Polovich et al., 2014). Resembling alcoholic liver disease, nonalcoholic steatohepatitis (NASH) happens in those who either do not drink or drink very little alcohol. NASH can progress to cirrhosis and is associated with obesity, diabetes, and insulin resistance. It is the second most common cause of hepatic injury after viruses and alcohol use and is the most common cause of cryptogenic cirrhosis or cirrhosis caused by unknown etiology. NASH can be induced by chemotherapy agents such as tamoxifen (National Digestive Diseases Information Clearinghouse, 2012).

Hepatocellular dysfunction most likely occurs from viral hepatitis, hepatic metastasis, antidepressants, hormonal agents, and chemotherapy agents such as asparaginase, cytarabine, high-dose interferons and regular-dose interferon beta, streptozocin, thalidomide, flutamide, 6-thioguanine, and imatinib mesylate (Fregonese & Stolk, 2008; Polovich et al., 2014) (see Table 13-7). Other chemotherapy agents also may contribute to hepatotoxicity when administered in high doses, such as busulfan, carmustine, cyclophosphamide, cytarabine, dactinomycin (especially in frequent cycles), methotrexate, and mitomycin. Asparaginase has one of the highest risks for hepatotoxicity (Fregonese & Stolk, 2008; Polovich et al., 2014).

Chronic low-dose methotrexate has been reported to cause portal fibrosis that can progress to full-blown cirrhosis, potentially through the disruption of the homeostasis of folate (a B vitamin that contributes to cellular purine and thymidine synthesis) (Fregonese & Stolk, 2008; Polovich et al., 2014). Although methotrexate used for cancer treatment can cause acute and reversible liver damage, long-term and consistent use, especially for nonmalignant diseases such as rheumatoid arthritis, can lead to irreversible hepatic fibrosis. In a systematic review of studies published before May 2006 (Zorzi et al., 2007), fluorouracil was associated with hepatic steatosis (a benign mild case of nonalcoholic fatty liver disease), which often progresses to a potentially fatal outcome. NASH has been linked to the administration of irinotecan, particularly in overweight and obese patients (those with a body mass index exceeding 25 kg/m^2) and patients with metabolic syndrome. NASH also may increase postoperative morbidity. NASH can progress to fibrosis or cirrhosis and, ultimately, liver failure (Zorzi et al., 2007). SOS is associated with the administration of chemotherapy agents such as cytarabine, cyclophosphamide, dacarbazine, mitomycin, 6-mercaptopurine, oxaliplatin, and 6-thioguanine, as well as high doses of busulfan, carmustine, cyclophosphamide, and mitomycin for stem cell transplantation (Davila & Bresalier, 2008; Fregonese & Stolk, 2008; Polovich et al., 2014).

Many supportive medications used in cancer care can be risk factors in the development of hepatotoxicity. Amoxicillin-clavulanic acid is one of the most frequent drugs associated with liver toxicity, but antiretrovirals also are problematic (Chang & Schiano, 2007). Acetaminophen can lead to acute hepatitis. Chlorpromazine may cause acute cholestasis. Tamoxifen, a medication commonly used in breast cancer, is linked to the development of NASH. Fibrosis and cirrhosis have been reported with the use of methotrexate. Busulfan and cyclophosphamide are occasionally associated with SOS (Fregonese & Stolk, 2008; Polovich et al., 2014). Seeff (2007) listed nitrofurantoin, minocycline, clometacin, methyldopa, and oxyphenisatine as drugs associated with liver injury. Drugs for which autoimmune hepatitis associations have been less compelling include atomoxetine, diclofenac, fenofibrate, 3-hydroxy-3-methyl-glutaryl coenzyme A reductase inhibitors (e.g., atorvastatin, rosuvastatin, simvastatin). Herbal drugs associated with hepatotoxicity include Dai-saiko-to, germander, 3,4-methylenedioxymethamphetamine (Ecstasy), *Morinda citrifolia* or noni juice, dihydralazine, and tienilic acid.

Herbal drugs can damage hepatocytes directly through parent herbal preparation or indirectly by its metabolites that may be toxic, mutagenic, or carcinogenic. Examples include quercetin, safrole, methyl eugenol, estragole, pulegone in the mint group, teucrin A in *Teucrium chamaedrys* found in dietary supplements, echimidine, and jacobine (Zhou, Xue, Yu, & Wang, 2007).

Table 13-7. Chemotherapy Drugs Associated With Hepatotoxicity

Drug	Associated Hepatotoxicities
Asparaginase	Increased AST/ALT Increased bilirubin Increased alkaline phosphatase Reversible Hepatocellular damage High potential for hepatotoxicity
Bevacizumab	Increased bilirubin
Bortezomib	Increased AST/ALT Increased bilirubin Reversible Veno-occlusive disease
Busulfan	Cholestatic disease Hepatocellular damage Veno-occlusive disease High potential at high dose
Capecitabine	Increased AST/ALT Increased bilirubin Increased alkaline phosphatase
Carboplatin	Increased AST/ALT Increased bilirubin Increased alkaline phosphatase Reversible
Carmustine	Increased AST/ALT Increased bilirubin Increased alkaline phosphatase Reversible Veno-occlusive disease
Cisplatin	Increased AST/ALT Increased bilirubin Reversible Cholestatic disease Hepatocellular damage
Cyclophosphamide	Increased AST/ALT Increased bilirubin Reversible Veno-occlusive disease
Cytarabine	Increased AST/ALT Increased bilirubin Cholestatic disease High potential for hepatotoxicity
Dacarbazine	Increased AST/ALT
Dactinomycin	Increased AST/ALT Hepatocellular damage Veno-occlusive disease

(Continued on next page)

Table 13-7. Chemotherapy Drugs Associated With Hepatotoxicity *(Continued)*

Drug	Associated Hepatotoxicities
Daunorubicin	Increased bilirubin
Denileukin diftitox	Increased AST/ALT Reversible
Docetaxel	Increased AST/ALT Increased alkaline phosphatase
Doxorubicin	Increased AST/ALT Increased bilirubin
Etoposide	Increased AST/ALT Increased bilirubin Hepatocellular damage High potential for hepatotoxicity
Floxuridine	Increased AST/ALT Increased bilirubin Increased alkaline phosphatase High potential for hepatotoxicity
Fluorouracil	Increased AST/ALT Increased bilirubin Increased alkaline phosphatase Reversible Hepatocellular damage High potential for hepatotoxicity
Flutamide	Increased AST/ALT Increased bilirubin Reversible Hepatocellular damage Cholestatic disease
Gefitinib	Increased AST/ALT Increased bilirubin Increased alkaline phosphatase
Gemcitabine	Increased AST/ALT Increased bilirubin Increased alkaline phosphatase
Gemtuzumab ozo-gamicin	Increased AST/ALT Increased bilirubin Increased alkaline phosphatase Veno-occlusive disease
Ifosfamide	Increased AST/ALT Increased bilirubin Increased alkaline phosphatase
Imatinib	Increased AST/ALT Increased bilirubin Increased alkaline phosphatase

(Continued on next page)

Table 13-7. Chemotherapy Drugs Associated With Hepatotoxicity *(Continued)*

Drug	Associated Hepatotoxicities
Interferon alpha	Increased AST/ALT Increased alkaline phosphatase High potential at high dose
Interleukin-2	Increased AST/ALT Increased bilirubin Increased alkaline phosphatase Reversible Cholestatic disease
Irinotecan	Increased AST/ALT Increased bilirubin Increased alkaline phosphatase
Lomustine	Increased AST/ALT Increased bilirubin Increased alkaline phosphatase Reversible Hepatocellular damage High potential at high dose
Megestrol	Cholestatic disease
Melphalan	Increased AST/ALT Increased bilirubin Veno-occlusive disease
Mercaptopurine	Increased AST/ALT Increased bilirubin Increased alkaline phosphatase Reversible Hepatocellular damage Cholestatic disease High potential at high dose
Methotrexate	Increased AST/ALT Increased bilirubin Reversible High potential for hepatotoxicity
Mithramycin	Hepatocellular damage High potential for hepatotoxicity
Mitoxantrone	Increased AST/ALT Increased bilirubin Reversible
Oxaliplatin	Increased AST/ALT Increased bilirubin Veno-occlusive disease
Paclitaxel	Increased AST/ALT Increased bilirubin Increased alkaline phosphatase

(Continued on next page)

Table 13-7. Chemotherapy Drugs Associated With Hepatotoxicity *(Continued)*

Drug	Associated Hepatotoxicities
Procarbazine	Increased AST/ALT Increased bilirubin
Streptozocin	Increased AST/ALT High potential for hepatotoxicity
Tamoxifen	Increased AST/ALT Increased bilirubin Hepatocellular damage
Thioguanine	Increased AST/ALT Increased bilirubin Veno-occlusive disease
Topotecan	Increased AST/ALT Increased bilirubin
Vinblastine	Increased AST/ALT Increased bilirubin
Vincristine	Increased AST/ALT Increased bilirubin Increased alkaline phosphatase High potential for hepatotoxicity
Vinorelbine	Increased AST/ALT Increased bilirubin

ALT—alanine aminotransferase; AST—aspartate aminotransferase

Note. Based on information from Fregonese & Stolk, 2008; Polovich et al., 2014.

Herbal drugs may be indirectly responsible for liver injury by competing for liver metabolism of concurrently used medications. Herbal drugs often are metabolized by the same cytochrome P450s (CYPs) that standard medications use, and some herbal drugs conjugate enzymes to reactive agents that are associated with drug toxicity. Many complementary and alternative substances that cause indirect hepatotoxicity, including flavonoids (e.g., quercetin) and alkenylbenzenes (e.g., safrole, methyl eugenol, estragole) are metabolized to a genotoxic substance. Some herbals, such as capsaicin, glabridin (from licorice root), oleuropein (in olive oil), daily sulfone (in garlic), and resveratrol (in red wine), can inhibit CYPs and thus can contribute to herb-drug interactions. This interaction also may be responsible for inhibiting CYPs so that a desired response of less-toxic metabolites from standard medications is formed (Zhou et al., 2007).

Case reports exist of hepatotoxicity related to the administration of epidermal growth factor receptor inhibitors, including cases of severe hepatitis from gefitinib and erlotinib. Generally, serum transaminases returned to baseline normal after the drug was discontinued (Ramanarayanan & Scarpace, 2007).

Pathophysiology

The liver is responsible for the metabolism of fats, proteins, and carbohydrates. It also converts drugs into active metabolites or nontoxic substances for excretion. Pathophysiologic changes related to hepatotoxicity are of a neoplastic, inflammatory, or fibrotic nature. Kupffer cells, macrophages of the liver, respond to toxins by releasing inflammatory substances, growth factors, reactive oxygen ions, free radicals, and peroxides. This release of substances regulates acute hepatocyte injury and other chronic responses of the liver, which includes hepatocellular carcinoma, through a multistep process of DNA damage that alters cell growth so that mutations are allowed to continue (Roberts et al., 2007). Damaged hepatocytes cannot metabolize or eliminate bilirubin, synthesize many of the coagulation factors, synthesize glucose, uptake lactate acid, or moderate intracellular lactate generation from anaerobic glycolysis (Roberts et al., 2007).

Disruption in bilirubin consists of either overproduction, reduction in uptake or conjugation, or decreased flow by cell mechanisms, such as intrahepatic cholestasis, or by duct obstruction, such as extrahepatic cholestasis (Roesser, 2014). Portal inflammation and biliary injury occurs from a hypersensitivity-induced autoimmune reaction, probably within the canaliculi of the bile ducts (Watanabe et al., 2007). Certain drugs, such as chlorpromazine, are more likely to produce hepatotoxicity in the form of cholestasis including portal inflammation and biliary damage (Watanabe et al., 2007). Signs and symptoms of cholestasis may occur three to four weeks after the drug is discontinued. This latent onset may be a result of the slow repair and regeneration potential of cholangiocytes (Watanabe et al., 2007). SOS, commonly found in patients who have had a stem cell transplant, occurs from blockage of venous circulation in the centrilobular and sublobular hepatic blood vessels from certain chemicals, such as busulfan and cyclophosphamide. A great deal of individual variation exists in the metabolism of IV cyclophosphamide, which modifies the risk of SOS for each person. If SOS develops, it is presumed to occur from the formation of acrolein, a toxic metabolite to the sinusoidal endothelial cells in the liver (Polovich et al., 2014).

Prevention Strategies

Routine monitoring of aminotransferases, specifically ALT, can be used to identify potential hepatotoxicity in high-risk individuals. If an immune-mediated hepatotoxicity manifests shortly after therapy is initiated with a rapid onset of symptoms, the offending agent may need to be discontinued. Assessment for and discontinuation of any other hepatotoxic drugs also is indicated. It may be necessary to adjust the dose of chemotherapy if hepatic function is affected. Similar reactions in the patient's history and subsequent successful treatment are verified, including discontinuation of the offending drug. Other potential causes of hepatotoxicity, such as alcohol use, must be ruled out. The patient should be instructed to follow a low-fat, high-glucose diet containing vitamin B and C (Polovich et al., 2014). The Invader® (Hologic, Inc., 2011) is a molecular assay on the uridine-5'-diphosphate-glucuronosyltransferase 1A1 (UGT1A1) enzyme that is used to determine whether genetic variations exist that will affect how drugs that use this enzyme are metabolized and excreted. To date, this test is used with patients receiving irinotecan. It is the beginning of a new age of drug personalization that may provide information about individualized, accurate therapeutic dosing for individuals while potentially avoiding harmful effects such as hepatotoxicity (Hologic, Inc., 2011).

Diagnosis and Assessment

Once the diagnosis of liver injury has been made through a history, physical examination, and abnormal laboratory parameters, the cause of the injury must be considered. Testing occurs using viral serology or liver imaging and by evaluating for the presence of potentially offending drugs. A cardiovascular evaluation also is in order.

Physical assessment of the skin should include assessing for the presence of jaundice, ecchymosis, and petechiae. Neurologic examination should include level of orientation and mental status. An abdominal assessment should include bowel sounds, liver and spleen, ascites, and venous distension.

Medical history should include the dose, route, and duration of the potentially offending drug, as well as previous administration. Because the idiosyncrasy of drugs varies, history should include all medications for the past three months. In general, the onset of hepatic dysfunction occurs anywhere from 5 to 90 days (Mehta, 2012). Excluding other potential diagnoses such as acute viral hepatitis, autoimmune hepatitis, cholecystitis, cholangitis, and alcoholic liver disease is essential (Mehta, 2012). Medical history also should include history of organ transplant, hepatitis, exposure to infected individuals, and any hereditary liver diseases (Polovich et al., 2014).

Serum aminotransferases aspartate aminotransferase (AST) and ALT are used most frequently and typically are elevated with liver damage that includes injury and necrosis. Hepatocyte or bile duct damage usually is detected using the serum aminotransferases and cholestasis if alkaline phosphatase (ALP) is elevated. The highest values of serum ALP are associated with cholestatic liver diseases. Elevations in serum bilirubin, urine bilirubin, and urobilinogen may contribute to the diagnosis of abnormal liver transport of substances from circulation. Serum albumin and coagulation factors detect abnormalities of liver metabolism and synthesis. A decrease in serum albumin occurs in patients with cirrhosis and ascites. Serum albumin levels typically are normal in viral hepatitis, DILI, and obstructive jaundice. Immunoglobulins and serologic tests for viral hepatitis may help with the diagnosis of liver injury but do not contribute information about liver function (Mehta, 2012). ALT is more specific for liver damage than AST because this substance is more localized in the liver than any other area of the body. AST is a more general test for liver damage; however, it is more sensitive in alcohol-related liver damage and muscle damage.

The gamma-glutamyl transpeptidase (GGT) level is used as a diagnostic value in hepatobiliary disease but also can indicate renal failure, myocardial infarction, pancreatic disease, and diabetes mellitus. The result of the GGT test is influenced if the patient is taking phenytoin or is drinking alcohol (Mehta, 2012). In summary, elevations in AST, ALT, and bilirubin are detectable in hepatocellular dysfunction. Prolonged prothrombin and thrombin times also may be indicators of compromised renal function resulting from injury and especially have been noted after asparaginase administration. Many of the abnormal laboratory tests return to normal after the drug is discontinued. A positive dechallenge is a 50% fall in serum transaminase levels within eight days of stopping the drug (Mehta, 2012). See Table 13-8 for laboratory values seen in hepatotoxicity.

Abdominal ultrasounds are relatively inexpensive and useful to detect dimensions of the hepatobiliary tree and view the gallbladder, bile ducts, and hepatic tumors. A computed tomography (CT) scan will delineate focal hepatic lesions 1 cm or larger and some diffuse conditions. It also can be used to visualize adjacent structures in the abdomen. Magnetic resonance imaging is more sensitive than a CT scan for determining metastasis, hemangioma, hepatoma, or other liver lesions. The portal vein, hepatic veins, and biliary tract can be visualized without contrast injections (Mehta, 2012).

Liver biopsy can determine the etiology of the hepatotoxicity and the pathology of masses or lesions identified after imaging (Mehta, 2012). Liver biopsy can prove to be definitive, especially if clinical signs of hepatotoxicity are present but serologic, autoimmune, metabolic, and other measures fail to yield diagnostic information. Biopsy also is used to verify DILI and rule out hepatocellular carcinoma, infiltrative disorders, cirrhosis, and viral hepatitis. Cultures may be obtained on liver biopsy tissue to determine the success of therapy for metabolic or viral liver disease. A liver biopsy is not essential in every case, but can serve to provide supportive evidence.

Table 13-8. Laboratory Values Seen in Hepatotoxicity

Hepatocellular Damage	Seen In	Comments
Liver Injury		
ALT (previously known as SGPT)	Mild elevations in fatty liver, NASH, chronic viral hepatitis, DILI, chronic hepatitis C Moderate elevations with DILI, hepatitis C, acute and chronic hepatitis, autoimmune disease Highest elevations in viral-, drug-, or toxin-induced damage	Highest concentrations in liver; most cost-effective AST:ALT < 1 = viral hepatitis AST:ALT > 1 = liver metastases or liver congestion from chemotherapy Elevated ALT, normal ALP and GGT = hepatitis Elevated ALP and GGT and normal ALP = biliary cirrhosis
AST (previously known as SGOT)	More specific for alcohol abuse, MI	AST:ALT > 2 = alcoholic liver disease
Obstruction	–	AST/ALT > 300 u/L acute biliary obstruction, rapid peak and decline in lab values over 24–72 hours
ALP	Highest levels seen in cholestatic disease	More diagnostic when used with other findings
Bili	Biliary cirrhosis, hepatic failure, prolonged fasting, hemorrhage, hemolytic diseases, pernicious anemia	–
GGT	Cholelithiasis and other biliary tract disease, chronic alcoholism, renal disease, obesity, diabetes mellitus, COPD, MI, pancreatic disease Persistent and significant increase in nonalcoholic liver disease, alcoholic liver disease, chronic hepatitis, and cirrhosis	Correlates with ALP levels If elevated with AST:ALT > 2 more diagnostic of alcoholic liver disease
Liver Transport Capacity		
Serum bilirubin	Conjugated—elevated with hepatobiliary disease even if total bilirubin is normal Unconjugated—elevated hemolysis and Gilbert syndrome	–
Ability of Liver to Metabolize Drug		
Plasma clearance of substances metabolized by liver	–	Plasma clearance is the most important pharmacokinetic parameter because it is the only one that controls the overall drug exposure. It is the parameter used to determine the dosage required to maintain an average steady-state plasma concentration.

(Continued on next page)

Table 13-8. Laboratory Values Seen in Hepatotoxicity *(Continued)*

Hepatocellular Damage	Seen In	Comments
Liver Synthesis Function—extent of injury or function of liver		
Albumin	Ascites, cirrhosis, nephritic syndrome, protein-losing enteropathy, burns	Most important plasma protein made by the liver Tells more about the severity of liver disease but is affected by protein loss in urine or gastrointestinal tract
PT	Liver failure Indicates deficiency of ≥ 1 liver synthe-sized factor	Frequent fluctuations in levels, so ideal monitoring tool INR and increased bili = poor prognosis in nonacetaminophen acute liver failure and poor prognosis in severe alcoholic hepatitis; jaundice also adds to confirmation of prognosis
INR	More specific for vitamin K deficiency; also seen in DIC and with warfarin therapy	–
Coagulation factors	Full liver failure indicated by < 20% of normal factor V; indicates very poor prognosis	–
Assists With Accurate Diagnosis—does not assess liver function		
Ig level	Increased serum globulin level indicates nonspecific chronic liver disease Increased IgG = autoimmune hepatitis Increased IgM = primary biliary cirrhosis	–
Autoantibody levels	Primary biliary cirrhosis, autoimmune hepatitis	–
Serologic tests for viral hepatitis	–	–

ALP—alkaline phosphatase; ALT—alanine aminotransferase; AST—aspartate aminotransferase; bili—bilirubin; COPD—chronic obstructive pulmonary disease; DIC—disseminated intravascular coagulation; DILI—drug-induced liver injury; GGT—gamma-glutamyl transpeptidase; Ig—immunoglobulin; IgG—immunoglobulin G; IgM—immunoglobulin M; INR—international normalized ratio; MI—myocardial infarction; NASH—nonalcoholic steatohepatitis; PT—prothrombin time; SGOT—serum glutamic oxaloacetic transaminase; SGPT—serum glutamic pyruvic transaminase

Note. Based on information from Mehta, 2012; Toutain & Bousquet-Mélou, 2004.

Evidence-Based Treatment Strategies

Treatment of hepatotoxicity includes removal of the offending agent, if known, or otherwise treating the cause to stop the liver injury from progressing and to prevent irreversible damage. Frequent monitoring of laboratory values is an important intervention to monitor treatment effectiveness. APNs need to consider referral to a gastroenterologist for a more complex and inexplicable course of hepatotoxicity.

Silymarin (extract of milk thistle) is a commonly used herb in cancer care because of its anti-inflammatory and antifibrotic effects (Verma & Thuluvath, 2007). It also is known as a liver tonic. It is thought to prevent or reverse hepatotoxicity of damaging drug metabolites or other toxins. Several experimental and clinical trials have shown that the membrane-stabilizing and antioxidant activity of silymarin promotes hepatocyte regeneration, reduces inflammatory reactions, and inhibits fibrogenesis (Féher & Lengyel, 2012). However, unclear or conflicting support exists for the use of milk thistle in acute viral hepatitis, cancer prevention, or drug- or toxin-induced hepatotoxicity.

Implications for Oncology Advanced Practice Nurses

Oncology APNs have resources available to objectively evaluate the outcome of treating hepatotoxicity. The inadequacy of many of the methods to measure hepatotoxicity and the latency of symptom onset in many types of liver injury, especially if the injury is drug induced, make it necessary for APNs to monitor serial liver function testing following baseline testing at the first visit and correlate it with the history and physical examination findings.

Liver injury may remain subclinical in nature or produce only subtle signs and symptoms. More than 900 toxins, including drugs and herbs, have been implicated in DILI, many of which include medications used in the treatment and support of patients with cancer (Pandit, Sachdeva, & Bafna, 2012). Oncology APNs have frequent contact with patients with cancer who are at high risk for hepatotoxicity because of their history, cancer diagnosis, or treatment. APNs must screen high-risk individuals for liver disease and monitor their status closely for early signs of liver injury. APNs can order appropriate diagnostic and monitoring studies and make gastroenterology consults in a timely fashion to aid in prevention and early diagnosis. Patients and families will require assistance to understand the results of their tests.

Conclusion

Cancer or cancer treatment may cause GI, GU, and hepatic toxicities. Furthermore, people with cancer often have comorbidities that increase the risk of toxicity. Some toxicities can be prevented or lessened by astute observation with the goal to discover and treat any adverse reaction early enough to prevent irreversible damage. Oncology APNs must be knowledgeable in the presenting signs and symptoms, prevention, diagnosis and assessment, and evidence-based treatment strategies for these toxicities to deliver high-quality patient care and preserve patients' quality of life.

Case Study

J.C. is a 39-year-old woman diagnosed with stage IIB breast cancer that was estrogen receptor positive, progesterone receptor negative, and HER2 overexpressed. She has completed a lumpectomy and is undergoing chemotherapy treatment with doxorubicin and cyclophosphamide followed by a taxane. Beginning at the start of the taxane, she will also receive 52 weeks of treatment with trastuzumab. Following chemotherapy, she will receive radiation to the breast with a boost to the tumor bed.

During one of her clinic visits, J.C. relates that she is worried about her sexual relationship with her husband. She has noticed that her libido has declined since her diagnosis and that sexual intercourse has become painful.

1. The APN understands the importance of an assessment of sexual function, including such things as hormonal, physiologic, psychological, cognitive, behavioral, relational, and cultural factors as well as physical assessment in order to obtain a correct diagnosis. What information should the oncology APN obtain in the sexual history?
   - It is important to establish a baseline of sexual functioning prior to J.C.'s diagnosis when conducting a sexual history, as cancer and its treatment could exacerbate any previous problem. The APN would inquire about feelings of inadequacy, anxiety in regard to sexual performance, depression, and expectations, as well as her partner's expectations and anxieties. Specific questions about dyspareunia and libido should be posed to J.C. The ALARM and the BETTER models are useful to assist in performance of a thorough sexual history.
   - Upon further exploration, J.C. relates that she is experiencing vaginal dryness that contributes to dyspareunia. She also states that she no longer feels attractive because of her surgery and believes that her husband no longer finds her appealing. She is experiencing fatigue from her chemotherapy treatments as well.

2. What are some specific interventions that the APN could recommend?
   - The oncology APN realizes that J.C. is experiencing sexual dysfunction caused by treatment side effects as well as an alteration in self-image. The nurse schedules a meeting with the patient and her husband to discuss their feelings together. For vaginal dryness, the oncology APN might recommend a water-based lubricant. The nurse suggests that scheduling intimate times when J.C.'s fatigue level is low might be beneficial. Because J.C. has had some difficulties with mucositis after chemotherapy, the APN asks about vaginal irritation or lesions, which J.C. denies.

3. J.C. tells the APN that her friend experienced vaginal dryness following her hysterectomy and that taking estrogen relieved this. She asks the APN to prescribe this for her. What should the APN do?
   - The oncology APN discusses the benefits and risks of systemic or topical estrogen therapy for menopausal symptoms such as vaginal dryness. The nurse admits that this is the most common management strategy but that it may be contraindicated in patients with hormonally responsive cancer, noting that J.C.'s cancer is estrogen receptor positive. Following this discussion, J.C. decides to try vaginal lubricants for a month and that if they do not prove helpful, a vaginal estrogen agent may be considered.
   - During the follow-up visit with J.C. and her husband, the APN facilitates a discussion of sexual expectations and any anxieties that either J.C. or her husband are experiencing since her diagnosis. In an effort to counteract the fatigue that J.C. experiences during treatment, she and her husband determine when she has more energy during the chemotherapy cycle. They decide to plan a special romantic evening during this time.

Key Points

Gastrointestinal Toxicities

- GI toxicities can result from chemotherapy, radiation therapy, and molecular-targeted therapies.
- GI toxicities affect all areas of the GI tract.
- Many of the GI toxicities affect the patients' quality of life and also may lower their ability to comply with treatment.

- Consultation with a gastroenterologist may be appropriate for patients who do not respond to treatment as expected.

Genitourinary Toxicities

- Sexual dysfunction and infertility are common side effects of cancer and cancer therapy.
- Sperm and embryo cryopreservation often are viable options for fertility preservation.
- The ALARM and BETTER models are communication tools that may be used to elicit in-depth information. The PLISSIT model guides the clinician's dialogue and intervention.
- Despite potentially effective preventive measures and treatments for sexual dysfunction and infertility, patients with cancer continue to report limited communications about sexual health with their clinicians.

Hepatic Toxicities

- The major types of liver disease pathology include hepatocellular, cholestatic, and a mixture of both.
- The major causes of liver injury include several commonly used drugs, such as acetaminophen, methotrexate, asparaginase, and tamoxifen.
- The most common presenting signs and symptoms of DILI include edema, pruritus, jaundice, malaise, headache, anorexia, ecchymosis, low-grade fever, muscle and joint aches, and urine and stool color changes.
- The most frequent laboratory studies used to assist in diagnosis and monitoring of liver injury are the serum aminotransferases AST and ALT.

Recommended Resources for Oncology Advanced Practice Nurses

Gastrointestinal Toxicities

- NCCN guidelines for managing nausea and vomiting in patients with cancer: www.nccn.org/professionals/physician_gls/pdf/antiemesis.pdf
- NCI CTCAE grading scale for toxicities: http://evs.nci.nih.gov/ftp1/CTCAE/CTCAE_4.03_2010-06-14_QuickReference_5x7.pdf
- NCI PDQ® information summary for health professionals on oral complications of chemotherapy and head and neck radiation: www.cancer.gov/cancertopics/pdq/supportivecare/oralcomplications/HealthProfessional
- Oncology Nursing Society Putting Evidence Into Practice resources, which evaluate the evidence on interventions for common toxicities, including anorexia, CINV, constipation, diarrhea, and mucositis: www.ons.org/practice-resources/pep

Genitourinary Toxicities

- American Cancer Society. (2013). Sexuality for the man with cancer. Available at www.cancer.org/acs/groups/cid/documents/webcontent/002910-pdf.pdf
- American Cancer Society. (2013). Sexuality for the woman with cancer. Available at www.cancer.org/acs/groups/cid/documents/webcontent/002912-pdf.pdf

- Katz, A. (2007). *Breaking the silence on cancer and sexuality: A handbook for healthcare providers.* Pittsburgh, PA: Oncology Nursing Society.
- Livestrong Fertility, part of the Livestrong Foundation, assists patients with cancer with infertility and provides information, resources, and financial assistance: www.livestrong.org/we-can-help/fertility-services
- Turnbull, G. (2009). *Intimacy after ostomy surgery guide.* Available at www.ostomy.org/uploaded/files/ostomy_info/uoaa_sexuality_en.pdf

Hepatic Toxicities

- National Academy of Clinical Biochemistry *Laboratory Medicine Practice Guidelines*: www.aacc.org/science-and-research/practice-guidelines/hepatic-injury
- NCCN Guidelines® for Hepatobiliary Cancers: www.nccn.org/professionals/physician_gls/pdf/hepatobiliary.pdf

References

American Cancer Society. (2015). *Cancer facts and figures 2015.* Retrieved from http://www.cancer.org/research/cancerfactsstatistics/cancerfactsfigures2015/index

American Psychiatric Association. (2013). *Diagnostic and statistical manual of mental disorders* (5th ed.). Washington, DC: Author.

American Society for Gastrointestinal Endoscopy Standards of Practice Committee, Shen, B., Khan, K., Ikenberry, S.O., Anderson, M.A., Banerjee, S., … Dominitz, J.A. (2010). The role of endoscopy in the management of patients with diarrhea. *Gastrointestinal Endoscopy, 71,* 887–892. doi:10.1016/j.gie.2009.11.025

Anderson, J.L. (2013). Acknowledging female sexual dysfunction in women with cancer. *Clinical Journal of Oncology Nursing, 17,* 233–235. doi:10.1188/13.CJON.233-235

Andrew, I., Kirkpatrick, G., Holden, K., & Hawkins, C. (2008). Audit of symptoms and prescribing in patients with the anorexia-cachexia syndrome. *Pharmacy World and Science, 30,* 489–496. doi:10.1007/s11096-008-9192-9

Aprile, G., Ramoni, A., Keefe, D., & Sonis, S. (2008). Application of distance matrices to define associations between acute toxicities in colorectal cancer patients receiving chemotherapy. *Cancer, 112,* 284–292. doi:10.1002/cncr.23182

Avritscher, E.B.C., Cooksley, C.D., & Elting, L.S. (2004). Scope and epidemiology of cancer therapy-induced oral and gastrointestinal mucositis. *Seminars in Oncology Nursing, 20,* 3–10. doi:10.1053/j.soncn.2003.10.002

Azim, H.A., Peccatori, F.A., de Azambuja, E., & Piccart, M.J. (2011). Motherhood after breast cancer: Searching for la dolce vita. *Expert Review of Anticancer Therapy, 11,* 287–298. doi:10.1586/era.10.208

Barasch, A., & Peterson, D.E. (2003). Risk factors for ulcerative oral mucositis in cancer patients: Unanswered questions. *Oral Oncology, 39,* 91–100. doi:10.1016/S1368-8375(02)00033-7

Bayer Healthcare Pharmaceuticals Inc. & GlaxoSmithKline. (2014). *Levitra® (vardenafil)* [Package insert]. Retrieved from https://www.gsksource.com/pharma/content/dam/GlaxoSmithKline/US/en/Brands/LEVITRA/pdf/Levitra_PI.PDF

Benson, A.B., III, Ajani, J., Catalano, R.B., Engelking, C., Kornblau, S.M., Martenson, J.A., Jr., … Wadler, S. (2004). Recommended guidelines for the treatment of cancer treatment-induced diarrhea. *Journal of Clinical Oncology, 22,* 2918–2926. doi:10.1200/JCO.2004.04.132

Bjordal, J.M., Bensadoun, R.J., Tunèr, J., Frigo, L., Gjerde, K., & Lopes-Martins, R.A. (2011). A systematic review with meta-analysis of the effect of low-level laser therapy (LLLT) in cancer therapy-induced oral mucositis. *Supportive Care in Cancer, 19,* 1069–1077. doi:10.1007/s00520-011-1202-0

Björnsson, E.S., Bergmann, O.M., Björnsson, H.K., Kvaran, R.B., & Olafsson, S. (2013). Incidence, presentation, and outcomes in patients with drug-induced liver injury in the general population of Iceland. *Gastroenterology, 144,* 1419–1425. doi:10.1053/j.gastro.2013.02.006

Bosaeus, I. (2008). Nutritional support in multimodal therapy for caner cachexia. *Supportive Care in Cancer, 16,* 447–451. doi:10.1007/s00520-007-0388-7

Bradley, J., & Movsas, B. (2004). Radiation esophagitis: Predictive factors and preventive strategies. *Seminars in Radiation Oncology, 14,* 280–286. doi:10.1016/j.semradonc.2004.06.003

Brotto, L.A., Yule, M., & Breckon, E. (2010). Psychological interventions for the sexual sequelae of cancer: A review of the literature. *Journal of Cancer Survivorship, 4,* 346–360. doi:10.1007/s11764-010-0132-z

Brown, C. (2011). Oral mucositis. In C.H. Yarbro, D. Wujcik, & B.H. Gobel (Eds.), *Cancer nursing: Principles and practice* (7th ed., pp. 807–817). Burlington, MA: Jones & Bartlett Learning.

Camilleri, M. (2011). Opioid-induced constipation: Challenges and therapeutic opportunities. *American Journal of Gastroenterology, 106,* 835–842. doi:10.1038/ajg.2011.30

Capp, A., Inostroza-Ponta, M., Bill, D., Moscato, P., Lai, C., Christie, D., … Denham, J.W. (2009). Is there more than one proctitis syndrome? A revisitation using data from the TROG 96.01 trial. *Radiotherapy and Oncology, 90,* 400–407. doi:10.1016/j.radonc.2008.09.019

Caro, M.M.M., Laviano, A., & Pichard, C. (2007). Nutritional intervention and quality of life in adult oncology patients. *Clinical Nutrition, 16,* 289–301. doi:10.1016/j.clnu.2007.01.005

Center for Reproductive Medicine and Infertility. (Ed.). (2007). *Cancer and fertility resource guide 2007–2008.* New York, NY: Author.

Chang, C.Y., & Schiano, T.D. (2007). Review article: Drug hepatotoxicity. *Alimentary Pharmacology and Therapeutics, 25,* 1135–1151. doi:10.1111/j.1365-2036.2007.03307.x

Chung, E., & Brock, G. (2013). Sexual rehabilitation and cancer survivorship: A state of art review of current literature and management strategies in male sexual dysfunction among prostate cancer survivors. *Journal of Sexual Medicine, 10*(Suppl. 1), 102–111. doi:10.1111/j.1743-6109.2012.03005.x

Clayman, M.L., Harper, M., Quinn, G.P., Shah, S., & Reinecke, J. (2011). The status of oncofertility resources at NCI-designated comprehensive cancer centers. *Journal of Clinical Oncology, 29*(Suppl. 580), Abstract 9123. Retrieved from http://meetinglibrary.asco.org/content/77605-102

Clayton, A., McGarvey, E., & Clavet, G. (1997). The Changes in Sexual Functioning Questionnaire (CSFQ): Development, reliability, and validity. *Psychopharmacology Bulletin, 33,* 731–745.

Conlon, B. (2010). Malnutrition and malabsorptive diarrhea in pancreatic cancer. *Oncology Nutrition Connection, 18*(4), 10–21.

Cunningham, R.S. (2014). The cancer cachexia syndrome. In C.H. Yarbro, D. Wujcik, & B.H. Gobel (Eds.), *Cancer symptom management* (4th ed., pp. 351–384). Burlington, MA: Jones & Bartlett Learning.

Davila, M., & Bresalier, R.S. (2008). Gastrointestinal complications of oncologic therapy. *Nature Clinical Practice: Gastroenterology and Hepatology, 5,* 682–696. doi:10.1038/ncpgasthep1277

Day, D., Ambegaonker, A., Harriot, K., & McDaniel, A. (2001). A new tool for predicting erectile dysfunction. *Advances in Therapy, 18,* 131–139. doi:10.1007/BF02850301

Deneris, A., & Huether, S.E. (2012). Structure and function of the reproductive system. In S.E. Huether & K.L. McCance (Eds.), *Understanding pathophysiology* (5th ed., pp. 774–798). St. Louis, MO: Elsevier Mosby.

Derogatis, L. (1987). The Derogatis Stress Profile (DSP): Quantification of psychological stress. *Advances in Psychosomatic Medicine, 17,* 30–54.

Dianliang, Z. (2009). Probing cancer cachexia-anorexia: Recent results with knockout, transgene and polymorphisms. *Current Opinion in Clinical Nutrition and Metabolic Care, 12,* 227–231. doi:10.1097/MCO.0b013e328329d14b

Diaz, V.A., Jr., & Close, J.D. (2010). Male sexual dysfunction. *Primary Care: Clinics in Office Practice, 37,* 473–489, vii–viii. doi:10.1016/j.pop.2010.04.002

Dirksen, S.R. (2011). Nursing assessment: Reproductive system. In S.L. Lewis, S.R. Dirksen, M.M. Heitkemper, L. Buscher, & I.M. Camera (Eds.), *Medical-surgical nursing: Assessment and management of clinical problems* (8th ed., pp. 1287–1305). St. Louis, MO: Elsevier Mosby.

Donnez, J., Jadoul, P., Squifflet, J., Van Langendonckt, A., Donnez, O., Van Eyck, A.S., … Dolmans, M.M. (2010). Ovarian tissue cryopreservation and transplantation in cancer patients. *Best Practice and Research. Clinical Obstetrics and Gynaecology, 24,* 87–100. doi:10.1016/j.bpobgyn.2009.09.003

Dy, S.M., & Apostol, C.C. (2010). Evidence-based approaches to other symptoms in advanced cancer. *Cancer Journal, 16,* 507–513. doi:10.1097/PPO.0b013e3181f45877

Dy, S.M., Lorenz, K.A., Naeim, A., Sanati, H., Walling, A., & Asch, S.M. (2008). Evidence-based recommendations for cancer fatigue, anorexia, depression and dyspnea. *Journal of Clinical Oncology, 26,* 3886–3895. doi:10.1200/JCO.2007.15.9525

Eilers, J., Berger, A.M., & Petersen, M.C. (1988). Development, testing and application of the oral assessment guide. *Oncology Nursing Forum, 15,* 325–330.

Eilers, J., Harris, D., Henry, K., & Johnson, L.A. (2014). Evidence-based interventions for cancer treatment–related mucositis: Putting evidence into practice. *Clinical Journal of Oncology Nursing, 18*(Suppl. 6), 80–96. doi:10.1188/14 .CJON.S3.80-96

Eli Lilly and Co. (2014). *Cialis® (tadalafil)* [Package insert]. Retrieved from http://pi.lilly.com/us/cialis-pi.pdf

Falk, S.J., & Dizon, D.S. (2013). Sexual dysfunction in women with cancer. *Fertility and Sterility, 100,* 916–921. doi:10.1016/j.fertnstert.2013.08.018

Fearon, K.C. (2012). The 2011 ESPEN Arvid Wretlind lecture: Cancer cachexia: The potential impact of translational research on patient-focused outcomes. *Clinical Nutrition, 31,* 577–582. doi:10.1016/j.clnu.2012.06.012

Féher, J., & Lengyel, G. (2012). Silymarin in the prevention and treatment of liver diseases and primary liver cancer. *Current Pharmaceutical Biotechnology, 13,* 210–217. doi:10.2174/138920112798868818

Fernández-Ortega, P., Caloto, M.T., Chirveches, E., Marquilles, R., San Francisco, J., Quesada, A., … Llombart-Cussac, A. (2012). Chemotherapy-induced nausea and vomiting in clinical practice: Impact on patients' quality of life. *Supportive Care in Cancer, 20,* 3131–3148. doi:10.1007/s00520-012-1448-1

Flynn, K.E., Jeffery, D.D., Keefe, F.J., Porter, L.S., Shelby, R.A., Fawzy, M.R., … Weinfurt, K.P. (2011). Sexual functioning along the caner continuum: Focus group results from the Patient-Reported Outcomes Measurement Information System (PROMIS®). *Psycho-Oncology, 20,* 378–386. doi:10.1002/pon.1738

Forman, E.J., Anders, C.K., & Behera, M.A. (2010). A nationwide survey of oncologists regarding treatment-related infertility and fertility preservation in female cancer patients. *Fertility and Sterility, 94,* 1652–1656. doi:10.1016/j.fertnstert.2009.10.008

Fregonese, L., & Stolk, J. (2008). Hereditary alpha-1-antitrypsin deficiency and its clinical consequences. *Orphanet Journal of Rare Diseases, 3,* 16. Retrieved from http://www.ojrd.com/content/3/1/16

Gilbert, E., Ussher, J.M., & Perz, J. (2010). Sexuality after breast cancer: A review. *Maturitas, 66,* 397–407. doi:10.1016/j.maturitas.2010.03.027

Ginsberg, J.P., Carlson, C.A., Lin, K., Hobbie, W.L., Wigo, E., Wu, X., … Kolon, T.F. (2010). An experimental protocol for fertility preservation in prepubertal boys recently diagnosed with cancer: A report of acceptability and safety. *Human Reproduction, 25,* 37–41. doi:10.1093/humrep/dep371

Ginsberg, T.B. (2010). Male sexuality. *Clinics in Geriatric Medicine, 26,* 185–195. doi:10.1016/j.cger.2010.02.007

Giralt, J., Regadera, J.P., Verges, R., Romero, J., de la Fuente, I., Biete, A., … Dieleman, L.A. (2008). Effects of probiotic lactobacillus casei DN-114 001 in prevention of radiation-induced diarrhea: Results from multicenter, randomized, placebo-controlled nutritional trial. *International Journal of Radiation Oncology, Biology, Physics, 71,* 1213–1219. doi:10.1016/j.ijrobp.2007.11.009

Goebel, M. (2010). Anorexia-cachexia syndrome in advanced cancer. *Journal of Palliative Medicine, 13,* 627–628. doi:10.1089/jpm.2010.9828

Granda-Cameron, C., & Lynch, M.P. (2010). Cancer cachexia. In C.G. Brown (Ed.), *A guide to oncology symptom management* (pp. 65–89). Pittsburgh, PA: Oncology Nursing Society.

Hall, D. (2010). Catching on to *C. difficile*: What you need to know about the causes, treatment and prevention of this dangerous infection. *American Nurse Today, 5*(7), 12–14.

Haylock, P.J., Curtiss, C., & Massey, R.L. (2014). Constipation. In C.H. Yarbro, D. Wujcik, & B.H. Gobel (Eds.), *Cancer symptom management* (4th ed., pp. 161–183). Burlington, MA: Jones & Bartlett Learning.

Henkin, R.I. (1994). Drug-induced taste and smell disorders: Incidence, mechanisms and management related primarily to treatment of sensory receptor dysfunction. *Drug Safety, 11,* 318–377.

Herbenick, D., Reece, M., Hensel, D., Sanders, S., Jozkowski, K., & Fortenberry, J.D. (2011). Association of lubricant use with women's sexual pleasure, sexual satisfaction, and genital symptoms: A prospective daily diary study. *Journal of Sexual Medicine, 8,* 202–212. doi:10.1111/j.1743-6109.2010.02067.x

Hologic, Inc. (2011). Invader® chemistry. Retrieved from http://www.invaderchemistry.com/invader_applications/invader-ugt1a1.html

Hopkinson, J.B., Wright, D.N., & Foster, C. (2008). Management of weight loss and anorexia. *Annals of Oncology, 19*(Suppl. 7), vii289–vii293. doi:10.1093/annonc/mdn452

Jensen, J.R., Morbeck, D.E., & Coddington, C.C., III. (2011). Fertility preservation. *Mayo Clinic Proceedings, 86,* 45–49. doi:10.4065/mcp.2010.0564

Johnson, G.D., Moore, K., & Fortner, B. (2007). Baseline evaluation of the AIM higher initiative: Establishing the mark from which to measure. *Oncology Nursing Forum, 34,* 729–734. doi:10.1188/07.ONF.729-734

Jordan, R., Hallam, T.J., Molinoff, P., & Spana, C. (2011). Developing treatments for female sexual dysfunction. *Clinical Pharmacology and Therapeutics, 89,* 137–141. doi:10.1038/clpt.2010.262

Kanematsu, A., Yamamoto, S., & Ogawa, O. (2007). Changing concepts of bladder regeneration. *International Journal of Urology, 14,* 673–678. doi:10.1111/j.1442-2042.2007.01768.x

Kaplan, H. (1979). *Disorders of sexual desire and other new concepts and techniques in sex therapy.* New York, NY: Brunner/Mazel Publications.

Kaplan, M., & Mahon, S. (2014). Hot flash management: Update of the evidence for patients with cancer. *Clinical Journal of Oncology Nursing, 18*(Suppl. 6), 59–67. doi:10.1188/14.CJON.S3.59-67

Kedde, H., van de Wiel, H.B.M., Schultz, W.C.M.W., & Wijsen, C. (2013). Sexual dysfunction in young women with breast cancer. *Supportive Care in Cancer, 21,* 271–280. doi:10.1007/s00520-012-1521-9

Kelvin, J.F., Kroon, L., & Ogle, S.K. (2012). Fertility preservation for patients with cancer. *Clinical Journal of Oncology Nursing, 16,* 205–210. doi:10.1188/12.CJON.205-210

Krebs, L. (2014). Altered body image and sexual health. In C.H. Yarbro, D. Wujcik, & B.H. Gobel (Eds.), *Cancer symptom management* (4th ed., pp. 507–540). Burlington, MA: Jones & Bartlett Learning.

Krychman, M., & Millheiser, L.S. (2013). Sexual health issues in women with cancer. *Journal of Sexual Medicine, 10*(Suppl. 1), 5–15. doi:10.1111/jsm.12034

Kurtin, S.E. (2010). Chemotherapy-induced nausea and vomiting: Clinical updates. *Oncology Pharmacist, 3,* 44–45.

Lara, L.A.S., de Andrade, J.M., Consolo, F.D., & Romão, A.P.M.S. (2012). Women's poorer satisfaction with their sex lives following gynecologic cancer treatment. *Clinical Journal of Oncology Nursing, 16,* 273–277. doi:10.1188/12.CJON .273-277

Latendresse, G., & McCance, K.L. (2012). Alterations of the reproductive systems, including sexually transmitted infections. In S.E. Huether & K.L. McCance (Eds.), *Understanding pathophysiology* (5th ed., pp. 799–870). St. Louis, MO: Elsevier Mosby.

Loren, A.W., Mangu, P.B., Beck, L.N., Brennan, L., Magdalinski, A.J., Partridge, A.H., … Oktay, K. (2013). Fertility preservation for patients with cancer: American Society of Clinical Oncology clinical practice guideline update. *Journal of Clinical Oncology, 31,* 2500–2510. doi:10.1200/JCO.2013.49.2678

Manolis, A., & Doumas, M. (2012). Antihypertensive treatment and sexual dysfunction. *Current Hypertension Reports, 14,* 285–292. doi:10.1007/s11906-012-0276-5

Masters, W., & Johnson, V. (1966). *Human sexual response.* St. Louis, MO: Little, Brown.

Mehta, N. (2012). Drug-induced hepatotoxicity. Retrieved from http://emedicine.medscape.com/article/169814 -overview

Mezvrishvili, Z., & Managadze, L. (2006). Complications of nerve sparing retroperitoneal lymph node dissection. *Georgian Medical News, 132,* 20–23.

Mick, J., Hughes, M., & Cohen, M. (2004). Using the BETTER model to assess sexuality. *Clinical Journal of Oncology Nursing, 8,* 84–86. doi:10.1188/04.CJON.84-86

Morrow, P.K.H., Mattair, D.N., & Hortobagyi, G.N. (2011). Hot flashes: A review of pathology and treatment modalities. *Oncologist, 16,* 1658–1664. doi:10.1634/theoncologist.2011-0174

Muehlbauer, P.M., & Lopez, R.C. (2014). Diarrhea. In C.H. Yarbro, D. Wujcik, & B.H. Gobel (Eds.), *Cancer symptom management* (4th ed., pp. 185–205). Burlington, MA: Jones & Bartlett Learning.

Multinational Association of Supportive Care in Cancer/International Society for Oral Oncology. (2013). Updated clinical guidelines for the prevention and treatment of oral mucositis. Retrieved from http://www.mascc.org/ mucositis-guidelines

National Cancer Institute. (2013a). Gastrointestinal complications (PDQ®). Retrieved from http://www.cancer.gov/ cancertopics/pdq/supportivecare/gastrointestinalcomplications/HealthProfessional/page2

National Cancer Institute. (2013b). Nausea and vomiting (PDQ®). Retrieved from http://www.cancer.gov/cancertopics/ pdq/supportivecare/nausea/Patient

National Cancer Institute. (2013c). Nutrition in cancer care (PDQ®). Retrieved from http://www.cancer.gov/ cancertopics/pdq/supportivecare/nutrition/HealthProfessional

National Cancer Institute. (2013d). Oral complications of chemotherapy and head and neck radiation. Retrieved from http://www.cancer.gov/cancertopics/pdq/supportivecare/oralcomplications/HealthProfessional/page5

National Cancer Institute. (2013e). Sexuality and reproductive issues (PDQ®). Retrieved from http://www.cancer.gov/ about-cancer/treatment/side-effects/sexuality-fertility-women/sexuality-pdq#section/_13

National Cancer Institute Cancer Therapy Evaluation Program. (2010). *Common terminology criteria for adverse events* [v.4.03]. Retrieved from http://evs.nci.nih.gov/ftp1/CTCAE/CTCAE_4.03_2010-06-14_QuickReference _5x7.pdf

National Cancer Institute Surveillance, Epidemiology, and End Results. (2015). Table 2.8: 5-Year relative and period survival by race, sex, diagnosis year and age. Retrieved from http://seer.cancer.gov/csr/1975_2012/browse_csr.php ?sectionSEL=2&pageSEL=sect_02_table.08.html

National Comprehensive Cancer Network. (2015a). *NCCN Clinical Practice Guidelines in Oncology (NCCN Guidelines®): Antiemesis* [v.1.2015]. Retrieved from http://www.nccn.org/professionals/physician_gls/pdf/antiemesis.pdf

National Comprehensive Cancer Network. (2015b). *NCCN Clinical Practice Guidelines in Oncology (NCCN Guidelines®): Palliative care* [v.1.2015]. Retrieved from http://www.nccn.org/professionals/physician_gls/pdf/palliative.pdf

National Digestive Diseases Information Clearinghouse. (n.d.). Constipation: Definition and facts for constipation. Retrieved from http://www.niddk.nih.gov/health-information/health-topics/digestive-diseases/constipation/Pages/ definition-facts.aspx

National Digestive Diseases Information Clearinghouse. (2012). Nonalcoholic steatohepatitis. Retrieved from http:// digestive.niddk.nih.gov/ddiseases/pubs/nash

National Institute on Deafness and Other Communication Disorders. (2014). Dysphagia. Retrieved from http://www .nidcd.nih.gov/health/voice/pages/dysph.aspx

Nishimoto, P.W., & Mark, D.D. (2010). Altered sexuality patterns. In C.G. Brown (Ed.), *A guide to oncology symptom management* (pp. 423–455). Pittsburgh, PA: Oncology Nursing Society.

North American Menopause Society. (2012). The 2012 hormone therapy position statement of the North American Menopause Society. *Menopause, 19,* 257–271. Retrieved from http://www.ncbi.nlm.nih.gov/pmc/articles/PMC3443956

Ochsenkuhn, R., Hermelink, K., Clayton, A.H., von Schonfeldt, V., Gallwas, J., Ditsch, N., … Kahlert, S. (2011). Menopausal status in breast cancer patients with past chemotherapy determines long-term hypoactive sexual desire disorder. *Journal of Sexual Medicine, 18,* 1486–1494. doi:10.1111/j.1743-6109.2011.02220.x

O'Rourke, N., Roqué, M.R.I., Bernadó, N.F., & Macbeth, F. (2010). Concurrent chemoradiotherapy in non-small cell lung cancer. *Cochrane Database of Systematic Reviews, 2010*(6). doi:10.1002/14651858.CD002140.pub3

Pahlajani, G., Raina, R., Jones, S., Ali, M., & Zippe, C. (2012). Vacuum erection devices revisited: Its emerging role in the treatment of erectile dysfunction and early penile rehabilitation following prostate cancer therapy. *Journal of Sexual Medicine, 9,* 1182–1189. doi:10.1111/j.1743-6109.2010.01881.x

Pandit, A., Sachdeva, T., & Bafna, P. (2012). Drug-induced hepatotoxicity: A review. *Journal of Applied Pharmaceutical Science, 2*(5), 233–243. doi:10.7324/JAPS.2012.2541

Peate, M., Meiser, B., Hickey, M., & Friedlander, M. (2009). The fertility-related concerns, needs and preferences of younger women with breast cancer: A systematic review. *Breast Cancer Research and Treatment, 116,* 215–223. doi:10.1007/s10549-009-0401-6

Pentheroudakis, G., Orecchia, R., Hoekstra, H.J., & Pavlidis, N. (2010). Cancer, fertility and pregnancy: ESMO clinical practice guidelines for diagnosis, treatment and follow-up. *Annals of Oncology, 21*(Suppl. 5), v266–v273. doi:10.1093/annonc/mdq198

Pfizer Inc. (2010). *Viagra® (sildenafil)* [Package insert]. New York, NY: Author.

Pinto, A.C. (2013). Sexuality and breast cancer: Prime time for young patients. *Journal of Thoracic Disease, 5*(Suppl. 1), S81–S86. doi:10.3978/j.issn.2072-1439.2013.05.23

Polovich, M., Olsen, M., & LeFebvre, K.B. (Eds.). (2014). *Chemotherapy and biotherapy guidelines and recommendations for practice* (4th ed.). Pittsburgh, PA: Oncology Nursing Society.

Quinn, G.P., Vadaparampil, S.T., Lee, J.-H., Jacobsen, P.B., Bepler, G., Lancaster, J., … Albrecht, T.L. (2009). Physician referral for fertility preservation in oncology patients: A national study of practice behaviors. *Journal of Clinical Oncology, 27,* 5952–5957. doi:10.1200/JCO.2009.23.0250

Raber-Durlacher, J.E., Elad, S., & Barasch, A. (2010). Oral mucositis. *Oral Oncology, 46,* 452–456. doi:10.1016/j.oraloncology.2010.03.012

Ramanarayanan, J., & Scarpace, S.L. (2007). Acute drug induced hepatitis due to erlotinib. *Journal of the Pancreas, 8,* 39–43. Retrieved from http://www.joplink.net/prev/200701/06.html

Roberts, R.A., Ganey, P.E., Ju, C., Kamendulis, L.M., Rusyn, I., & Klaunig, J.E. (2007). Role of the Kupffer cell in mediating hepatic toxicity and carcinogenesis. *Toxicological Sciences, 96,* 2–15. doi:10.1093/toxsci/kfl173

Rodríguez-Caballero, A., Torres-Lagares, D., Robles-García, M., Pachón-Ibáñez, J., González-Padilla, D., & Gutiérrez-Pérez, J.L. (2012). Cancer treatment-induced oral mucositis: A critical review. *International Journal of Oral and Maxillofacial Surgery, 41,* 225–238. doi:10.1016/j.ijom.2011.10.011

Roesser, K.A. (2014). Hepatotoxicity. In D. Camp-Sorrell & R.A. Hawkins (Eds.), *Clinical manual for the oncology advanced practice nurse* (3rd ed., pp. 663–671). Pittsburgh, PA: Oncology Nursing Society.

Roscoe, J.A., Morrow, G.R., Colagiuri, B., Heckler, C.E., Pudlo, B.D., Colman, L., … Jacobs, A. (2010). Insight in the prediction of chemotherapy-induced nausea. *Supportive Care in Cancer, 18,* 869–876. doi:10.1007/s00520-009-0723-2

Rosen, A., Rodriguez-Wallberg, K.A., & Rosenzweig, L. (2009). Psychosocial distress in young cancer survivors. *Seminars in Oncology Nursing, 25,* 268–277. doi:10.1016/j.soncn.2009.08.004

Rosen, R.C., Brown, C., Heiman, J., Leiblum, S., Meston, C., Shabsigh, R., … D'Agostino, R., Jr. (2000). The Female Sexual Function Index (FSFI): A multidimensional self-report instrument for the assessment of female sexual function. *Journal of Sex and Marital Therapy, 26,* 191–208. doi:10.1080/009262300278597

Rosen, R.C., Cappelleri, J.C., Smith, M.D., Lipsky, J., & Peña, B.M. (1999). Development and evaluation of an abridged, 5-item version of the International Index of Erectile Function (IIEF-5) as a diagnostic tool for erectile dysfunction. *International Journal of Impotence Research, 11,* 319–326.

Roth, A.J., Carter, J., & Nelson, C.J. (2010). Sexuality after cancer. In J.C. Holland, W.S. Breitbart, & P.B. Jacobsen (Eds.), *Psycho-oncology* (2nd ed., pp. 245–250). New York, NY: Oxford University Press.

Russmann, S., Kullak-Ublick, G.A., & Grattagliano, I. (2009). Current concepts of mechanisms in drug-induced hepatotoxicity. *Current Medicinal Chemistry, 16,* 3041–3053. doi:10.2174/092986709788803097

Ryan, J.L., Heckler, C.E., Roscoe, J.A, Dakhil, S.R., Kirshner, J., Flynn, P.J., … Morrow, G.R. (2012). Ginger (*Zingiber officinale*) reduces acute chemotherapy-induced nausea: A URCC CCOP study of 576 patients. *Supportive Care in Cancer, 20,* 1479–1489. doi:10.1007/s00520-011-1236-3

Sadovsky, R., Basson, R., Krychman, M., Morales, A.M., Schover, L., Wang, R., & Incrocci, L. (2010). Cancer and sexual problems. *Journal of Sexual Medicine, 7,* 349–373. doi:10.1111/j.1743-6109.2009.01620.x

Sanchez, M.I.P., & Bercik, P. (2011). Epidemiology and burden of chronic constipation. *Canadian Journal of Gastroenterology, 25*(Suppl. B), 11B–15B. Retrieved from http://www.ncbi.nlm.nih.gov/pmc/articles/PMC3206560

Schieszer, J. (2009). *C. difficile* infection on the rise in cancer patients. *Clinical Oncology News: Current Practice.* Retrieved from http://www.clinicaloncology.com

Seeff, L.B. (2007). *AASLD-FDA-NIH-PhRMA-Hepatotoxicity special interest group meeting. 2007 presentations.* Retrieved from http://archive.is/j5IKF

Shoemaker, L.K., Estfan, B., Induru, R., & Walsh, T.D. (2011). Symptom management: An important part of cancer care. *Cleveland Clinic Journal of Medicine, 78*, 25–34. doi:10.3949/ccjm.78a.10053

Silber, S., Kagawa, N., Kuwayama, M., & Gosden, R. (2010). Duration of fertility after fresh and frozen ovary transplantation. *Fertility and Sterility, 94*, 2191–2196. doi:10.1016/j.fertnstert.2009.12.073

Snyder, K.M., Stock, R.G., Buckstein, M., & Stone, N.N. (2012). Long-term potency preservation following brachytherapy for prostate cancer. *BJU International, 110*, 221–225. doi:10.1111/j.1464-410X.2011.10800.x

Sonis, S.T. (2007). Pathobiology of oral mucositis: Novel insights and opportunities. *Journal of Supportive Oncology, 5*(9, Suppl. 4), 3–11.

Sonis, S.T., Eilers, J.P., Epstein, J.B., LeVeque, F.G., Liggett, W.H., Jr., Mulagha, M.T., … Wittes, J.P. (1999). Validation of a new scoring system for the assessment of clinical trial research of oral mucositis induced by radiation or chemotherapy: Mucositis Study Group. *Cancer, 85*, 2103–2113. doi:10.1002/(SICI)1097-0142(19990515)85:10<2103::AID-CNCR2>3.0.CO;2-0

Stinchcombe, T.E., Lee, C.B., Moore, D.T., Rivera, M.P., Halle, J., Limentani, S., … Socinski, M.A. (2008). Long-term follow-up of a phase I/II trial of dose escalating three-dimensional conformal thoracic radiation therapy with induction and concurrent carboplatin and paclitaxel in unresectable stage IIIA/B non-small cell lung cancer. *Journal of Thoracic Oncology, 3*, 1279–1285. doi:10.1097/JTO.0b013e31818b1971

Strassels, S.A., Maxwell, T.L., & Iyer, S. (2010). Constipation in persons receiving hospice care. *Journal of Pain and Symptom Management, 40*, 810–820. doi:10.1016/j.jpainsymman.2010.03.018

Sykes, N.P. (2006). The pathogenesis of constipation. *Journal of Supportive Oncology, 4*, 213–218.

Thompson, N. (2012). Optimizing treatment outcomes in patients at risk for chemotherapy-induced nausea and vomiting. *Clinical Journal of Oncology Nursing, 16*, 309–313. doi:10.1188/12.CJON.309-313

Tipton, J.M. (2009). Chemotherapy-induced nausea and vomiting. In L.H. Eaton & J.M. Tipton (Eds.), *Putting evidence into practice: Improving oncology patient outcomes* (pp. 63–69). Pittsburgh, PA: Oncology Nursing Society.

Tipton, J. (2014). Nausea and vomiting. In C.H. Yarbro, D. Wujcik, & B.H. Gobel (Eds.), *Cancer symptom management* (4th ed., pp. 213–233). Burlington, MA: Jones & Bartlett Learning.

Tisdale, M.J. (2009). Mechanisms of cancer cachexia. *Physiological Reviews, 89*, 381–410. doi:10.1152/physrev.00016.2008

Tisdale, M.J. (2010). Cancer cachexia. *Current Opinion in Gastroenterology, 26*, 146–151. doi:10.1097/MOG.0b013e3283347e77

Toutain, P.L., & Bousquet-Mélou, A. (2004). Plasma clearance. *Journal of Veterinary Pharmacology and Therapeutics, 27*, 415–425. doi:10.1111/j.1365-2885.2004.00613.x

Tschudin, S., & Bitzer, J. (2009). Psychological aspects of fertility preservation in men and women affected by cancer and other life-threatening diseases. *Human Reproduction Update, 15*, 587–597. doi:10.1093/humupd/dmp015

Underhill, M.L., Caron, P., Ramsdell, M.J., Rogers, B., & Wolles, B. (2015). Putting Evidence Into Practice: Anorexia. Retrieved from https://www.ons.org/practice-resources/pep/anorexia

Urogenital system. (2015). In *Encyclopedia Britannica*. Urogenital system anatomy. Retrieved from http://www.britannica.com/science/urogenital-system

Verma, S., & Thuluvath, P.J. (2007). Complementary and alternative medicine in hepatology: Review of the evidence of efficacy. *Clinical Gastroenterology and Hepatology, 5*, 408–416. doi:10.1016/j.cgh.2006.10.014

Visich, K.L., & Yeo, T.P. (2010). The prophylactic use of probiotics in the prevention of radiation therapy-induced diarrhea. *Clinical Journal of Oncology Nursing, 14*, 467–473. doi:10.1188/10.CJON.467-473

Warr, D.G., Street, J.C., & Carides, A.D. (2011). Evaluation of risk factors predictive of nausea and vomiting with current standard-of-care antiemetic treatment: Analysis of phase 3 trial of aprepitant in patients receiving Adriamycin-cyclophosphamide-based chemotherapy. *Supportive Care in Cancer, 19*, 807–813. doi:10.1007/s00520-010-0899-5

Watanabe, N., Takashimizu, S., Kojima, S., Kagawa, T., Nishizaki, Y., Mine, T., & Matsuzaki, S. (2007). Clinical and pathological features of a prolonged type of acute intrahepatic cholestasis. *Hepatology Research, 37*, 598–607. doi:10.1111/j.1872-034X.2007.00115.x

Waterhouse, J., & Metcalfe, M.C. (1986). Development of the sexual adjustment questionnaire. *Oncology Nursing Forum, 13*(3), 53–59.

Werner-Wasik, M., Yorke, E., Deasy, J., Nam, J., & Marks, L.B. (2010). Radiation dose-volume effects in the esophagus. *International Journal of Radiation Oncology, Biology, Physics, 76*, S86–S93. doi:10.1016/j.ijrobp.2009.05.070

Wickham, R. (2012). Evolving treatment paradigms for chemotherapy-induced nausea and vomiting. *Cancer Control, 19*(Suppl. 2), 2–9.

Wilkes, G.M., & Barton-Burke, M. (Eds.). (2012). *Oncology nursing drug handbook* (12th ed.). Burlington, MA: Jones & Bartlett Learning.

Williams, D.H., IV. (2010). Sperm banking and the cancer patient. *Therapeutic Advances in Urology, 2*, 19–34. doi:10.1177/1756287210368279

Winkeljohn, D. (2011). *Clostridium difficile* infection in patients with cancer. *Clinical Journal of Oncology Nursing, 15*, 215–217. doi:10.1188/11.CJON.215-217

Worthington, H.V., Clarkson, J.E., Bryan, G., Furness, S., Glenny, A.-M., Littlewood, A., … Khalid, T. (2011). Interventions for preventing oral mucositis for patients with cancer receiving treatment. *Cochrane Database of Systematic Reviews, 2011*(4). doi:10.1002/14651858.CD000978.pub5

Wujcik, D. (2014). Mucositis. In C.H. Yarbro, D. Wujcik, & B.H. Gobel (Eds.), *Cancer symptom management* (4th ed., pp. 403–415). Burlington, MA: Jones & Bartlett Learning.

Yavuzsen, T., Walsh, D., Davis, M.P., Kirkova, J., Jin, T., LeGrand, S., … Haddad, A. (2009). Components of the anorexia-cachexia syndrome: Gastrointestinal symptom correlates of cancer anorexia. *Supportive Care in Cancer, 17*, 1531–1541. doi:10.1007/s00520-009-0623-5

Zhou, S.-F., Xue, C.C., Yu, X.Q., & Wang, G. (2007). Metabolic activation of herbal and dietary constituents and its clinical and toxicological implications: An update. *Current Drug Metabolism, 8*, 526–553. doi:10.2174/138920007781368863

Zick, S.M., Ruffin, M.T., Lee, J., Normolle, D.P., Siden, R., Alrawi, S., & Brenner, D.E. (2009). Phase II trial of encapsulated ginger as a treatment for chemotherapy-induced nausea and vomiting. *Supportive Care in Cancer, 17*, 563–572. doi:10.1007/s00520-008-0528-8

Zorzi, D., Laurent, A., Pawlik, T.M., Lauwer, G.Y., Vauthey, J.N., & Abdalla, E.K. (2007). Chemotherapy-associated hepatotoxicity and surgery for colorectal liver metastasis. *British Journal of Surgery, 94*, 274–286. doi:10.1002/bjs.5719

CHAPTER 14

Neurologic, Ocular, and Dermatologic Toxicities

Vanna M. Dest, MSN, APRN-BC, AOCN®

Introduction

Patients with cancer experience neurologic, ocular, and dermatologic toxicities throughout the course of their disease and treatment. Neurologic toxicities are common and range from mild, reversible conditions, such as peripheral neuropathy, to life-threatening conditions, such as leukoencephalopathy. They may result from the disease itself, its treatment, or comorbidities. Ocular toxicities are less common and also may stem from the cancer itself, cancer-related treatment, or other medications. Although ocular toxicities are rare, they present a serious risk for vision loss and reduced quality of life. Dermatologic symptoms are common in patients with cancer and have received increased attention in recent years with the introduction of targeted therapies and immunotherapy in the treatment of cancer. Skin effects result from other cancer treatment modalities as well, such as chemotherapy, radiation, and stem cell transplantation.

Oncology advanced practice nurses (APNs) must be well informed in the etiology, signs and symptoms, incidence, prevention, diagnosis and assessment, and management of these toxicities. Patient education is essential in enabling prompt identification and management of neurologic, ocular, and dermatologic toxicities.

Neurologic Toxicities

Definition and Incidence

Neurologic symptoms are common in patients with cancer and usually represent the cancer itself, coagulopathy, infection, metabolic/nutritional imbalances, or the toxic effects of cancer-related therapies such as chemotherapy and radiation therapy. Nearly 50% of people with cancer will present to the emergency department with neurologic symptoms (Baldwin, Živković, & Lieberman, 2012). For patients receiving neurotoxic chemotherapy, 20%–40% will experience peripheral neurotoxicities (Travis et al., 2014). Neurotoxicity related to cancer itself includes the diagnosis of primary brain and spinal tumors, metastatic disease to the brain and spine, and paraneoplastic syndrome, which is related to the underlying cancer and immunologic mechanisms. Cancer treatment modalities such as radiation therapy, chemotherapy, and hematopoietic stem cell transplantation (HSCT) can cause a variety of neurotoxic effects, including encephalopathy, myelopathy, and neuropathies. Neuropathies are common, dose-limiting side effects of several commonly used chemotherapy agents. Many neurotoxicities, such as peripheral neuropathy, may be annoying and interfere with daily living but can be reversible. However, other conditions, such as leukoencephalopathy and paraneoplastic syndromes, can be potentially life threatening.

Neurotoxicity describes the adverse effects caused in the central nervous system (CNS), peripheral nervous system, autonomic nervous system, or sensory organs. The severity of the neurotoxicity will depend on variables related to the offending agent, the duration of exposure, and the individual experiencing the neurotoxicity (Arlien-Søborg & Simonsen, 2011). Primary and metastatic tumors of the nervous system, including the brain and spine, are fairly common in the cancer population. Primary brain tumors in adults are rare and make up about 2% of all malignancies. In contrast, brain tumors are the second most common tumor in children (Huttner, 2012). It is estimated that about 22,850 cases that include the brain and spine will be diagnosed in 2015 (Siegel, Miller, & Jemal, 2015). Brain metastases are very common and usually originate from lung, breast, melanoma, renal, and colon cancers. It is estimated that up to 40% of patients with cancer will develop one or more brain metastases throughout the cancer trajectory (Butowski, 2011). Primary spinal cord tumors are rare but can cause significant neurologic damage (Mechtler & Nandigam, 2013). About 5%–10% of patients with cancer will develop spinal metastases (Yoshihara & Yoneoka, 2014).

Paraneoplastic neurologic syndromes are relatively rare and poorly understood. *Paraneoplastic neurologic syndrome* is defined as a dysfunction of the nervous system that develops acutely or subacutely and originates distant from the original site of cancer or cancer metastasis. The central, peripheral, and autonomic nervous systems can be affected (Didelot & Honnorat, 2014; Kannoth, 2012). It is estimated that less than 1% of patients with cancer will develop a paraneoplastic neurologic syndrome, but this is dependent on the type of cancer and the definition used to describe paraneoplastic neurologic syndromes. In more than 50% of people diagnosed with paraneoplastic neurologic syndrome, a diagnosis of cancer followed (Braik, Evans, Telfer, & McDunn, 2010; Pelosof & Gerber, 2010). Other cancers (a) produce neuroendocrine proteins, such as in small cell lung cancer (SCLC) and neuroblastoma; (b) contain neuronal components, such as in teratomas; (c) involve immunoregulatory organs, such as in thymomas; or (d) affect immunoglobulin production, such as in lymphomas and myeloma (Damek, 2010; Pelosof & Gerber, 2010).

Cancer treatment–related neurotoxicity is caused by the acute and chronic effects of radiation therapy, chemotherapy, and/or HSCT. The majority of patients diagnosed with cancer will receive some form of chemotherapy, and approximately 66% of patients with cancer will receive radiation therapy throughout the cancer trajectory (American Society for Radiation Oncology, 2012). The incidence of chemotherapy-induced peripheral neuropathy is about 38% in patients receiving multiple agents. This number is variable and depends on chemotherapy agents and regimen, duration of therapy, and assessment methods (Cavaletti et al., 2010, 2013; Cavaletti & Zanna, 2002; Hershman et al., 2014). In the United States, more than 18,000 HSCTs are performed every year (Živković & Abdel-Hamid, 2010). About 10%–40% of transplant recipients will develop a significant neurologic complication (Živković & Abdel-Hamid, 2010).

Etiology and Presenting Signs and Symptoms

Neurotoxicities may be correlated with primary cancers, metastasis, or treatment. Primary cancers and metastases related to the central, peripheral, and autonomic nervous system are more likely to cause neurotoxicity. Brain metastases are commonly caused by cancers of the lung, breast, melanoma, kidney, and colon. Common presenting symptoms of primary or metastatic brain tumors include seizure activity, headaches, and nausea/vomiting. Symptoms are also dependent on the location of the brain that is affected. The frontal lobe controls personality, intellect, judgment, abstract thinking, mood, and affect. The parietal lobe controls sensory perception and spatial relations. The temporal lobe controls hearing, memory, and speech, and the occipital lobe controls sight. The cerebellum controls coordination and balance (Keogh & Henson, 2012).

Primary spinal tumors are uncommon but are classified by where they arise. The two main classifications are *extradural*, or originating from outside the spine, and *intradural*, or originating from inside the dura mater. The most common primary spinal tumors include ependymoma, astrocytoma, meningioma, and lymphoma. Spinal metastases are commonly caused by cancers of the breast, lung, prostate, and multiple myeloma. Common presenting symptoms of primary or metastatic spinal tumors include pain that is localized or radicular in nature, sensory impairment with numbness and tingling, motor impairment, and bladder or bowel dysfunction. Pain usually is the first symptom, whereas motor impairment and bladder or bowel dysfunction are late signs. The key is to diagnosis and treat toxicities quickly to maintain neurologic function (Mechtler & Nandigam, 2013).

The most common paraneoplastic neurologic syndromes are caused by the cancer and are related to immunologic mechanisms within the body. Immune cross-reactivity exists between tumor cells and components of the nervous system, resulting in production of tumor-directed antibodies, also referred to as *onconeural antibodies*. Onconeural antibodies may affect any part of the central or peripheral nervous system and may mimic any neurologic complication of cancer. The symptoms can be severe in nature, but prompt diagnosis and treatment may result in stabilization or improvement of symptoms. Treatment of the underlying malignancy will minimize neurologic compromise (Kannoth, 2012; Pelosof & Gerber, 2010; Rosenfeld & Dalmau, 2010).

The majority of paraneoplastic syndromes develop within days to weeks and either stabilize or progress. CNS syndromes often have prodromic gastrointestinal (GI) and respiratory viral symptoms, which then progress to neurologic symptoms. The etiology of the prodrome is unclear but may be related to release of antibodies. Paraneoplastic neurologic syndromes can affect the CNS, the neuromuscular junction, or the peripheral nervous system. Depending on the affected nervous system, paraneoplastic neurologic syndromes symptoms may include cognitive changes, personality changes, ataxia, cranial nerve deficits, weakness, or numbness. See Table 14-1 for the common paraneoplastic neurologic syndromes in cancer.

Despite the technological and treatment planning advances, radiation therapy to the brain and spinal cord can cause acute and chronic neurologic effects and neurotoxicity. The effects of radiation therapy depend on the volume of irradiated tissue, total dose delivered, dose per fraction, and duration of treatment. For example, larger volume of tissue treated, larger fraction size (greater than 200 cGy), and longer length of radiation therapy contribute to increased neurotoxicity. Other factors that may increase the risk of neurotoxicity include older age or younger age; concomitant medical conditions such as diabetes or vascular disease; chemotherapy; and genetic predisposition of the tumor. Genetic predisposition can include rare familial syndromes such as neurofibromatosis, Li-Fraumeni syndrome, and Cowden syndrome (Ricard et al., 2012). Smoking, excess alcohol consumption, and poor diet have been associated with risk of head and neck cancer and also for development of neurocognitive dysfunction (Lawrence et al., 2010; Welsh et al., 2014). The effects are generally categorized by time of appearance after radiation therapy is delivered, such as acute, early delayed, and late delayed. The pathophysiology of radiation therapy–induced neurotoxicity includes the development of

Table 14-1. Common Paraneoplastic Neurologic Syndromes in Cancer

Paraneoplastic Syndrome	Cancer Diagnosis	Signs and Symptoms
Central Nervous System		
Cerebellar degeneration	Breast cancer Hodgkin lymphoma Ovarian cancer Small cell lung cancer (SCLC)	Prodrome of dizziness Nausea/vomiting Visual disturbances (blurred vision, diplopia, oscillopsia [objects in visual field oscillate]) Gait difficulties (truncal and limb ataxia) Dysarthria Dysphagia
Limbic encephalitis	Breast cancer Germ cell tumors of the testis Hodgkin lymphoma SCLC Teratomas of the ovary Thymoma	Mood changes Hallucinations Memory loss Seizures Hypothalamic symptoms (i.e., hyperthermia, somnolence, endocrine dysfunction)
Neuromuscular Junction		
Lambert-Eaton myasthenic syndrome: Disorder of neuromuscular junction characterized by impaired acetylcholine release from the presynaptic motor terminal	Adenocarcinomas Cervical cancer Lymphomas Prostate cancer SCLC (3%–5%)	Fatigue Bilateral leg weakness Muscle aches Vague paresthesias Dry mouth (xerostomia)
Myasthenia gravis	Thymoma	Weakness of voluntary muscles Diaphragmatic weakness
Peripheral Nervous System		
Autonomic neuropathy	SCLC Thymoma	Panautonomic neuropathy Gastrointestinal dysfunction Dry eyes/mouth Bowel/bladder dysfunction Altered pupillary light reflexes Constipation Nausea/vomiting Dysphagia Weight loss Abdominal distension
Subacute peripheral sensory neuropathy	Breast cancer Hodgkin lymphoma Lung cancer (usually SCLC; 70%–80%) Ovarian cancer Sarcomas	Paresthesias Pain that begins in upper extremities first Ataxia Decreased sensory sensation Deep tendon reflexes decreased or absent

Note. Based on information from Braik et al., 2010; Damek, 2010; Pelosof & Gerber, 2010; Rosenfeld & Dalmau, 2010.

necrosis occurring one to two years later, which is caused by ischemia secondary to blood vessel damage, as well as demyelination and oligodendrocyte dysfunction (Lawrence et al., 2010; Pradat & Delanian, 2013). See Table 14-2 for common neurologic complications of radiation therapy based on the time period after therapy completion.

Radiation therapy can affect the brain, spinal cord, cranial nerves, and nerve plexuses. The most common radiation therapy–induced neurotoxicities are also categorized by time of presentation after completion of radiation therapy. The most common neurotoxicities are listed in Table 14-3 with clinical manifestations.

Chemotherapy-induced neurotoxicities are common complications of many chemotherapy agents and dose-limiting effects. They may be acute or chronic in nature and may affect both the central and peripheral nervous systems. These effects can be mild or life threatening. Neurotoxicity may result from direct toxic effects on the nervous system cells, as well as indirectly from the metabolic or cerebrovascular effects caused by antineoplastic drugs. The blood-brain barrier may prevent many agents from affecting the nervous system. Other risk factors include advancing age, administration of multiple agents, route of administration, dose, and impaired clearance, as well as radiation therapy, which may cause decreased integrity of the blood-brain barrier. Hence, the blood-brain barrier may be more vulnerable (Rinne, Lee, & Wen, 2012;

Table 14-2. Common Neurologic Complications Categorized by Time of Onset After Completion of Radiation Therapy (RT)

Site	Acute (< 4 Weeks After RT)	Early Delayed (1–6 Months After RT)	Late Delayed (> 6 Months After RT)
Brain	Acute encephalopathy	Somnolence syndrome Worsening of preexisting symptoms Transitory cognitive impairment Subacute rhombencephalitis (occurs 1–3 months after RT, leading to symptoms such as ataxia, dysarthria, diplopia, and nystagmus)	Focal brain radionecrosis Cognitive impairment and leukoencephalopathy Secondary brain tumors
Spinal cord	–	Lhermitte phenomenon (electric shock–like waves shooting down spine when head is flexed forward)	Focal spinal radionecrosis Progressive myelopathy Spinal hemorrhage
Cranial nerves	–	Hearing loss Anosmia Ageusia (loss of taste)	Hearing loss Visual loss Lower cranial nerve paralysis
Peripheral nerves	Paresthesias	Brachial or lumbosacral transitory plexopathy	Brachial or lumbosacral irreversible plexopathy Malignant nerve sheath tumors Lower motor neuron syndrome

Note. Based on information from Dropcho, 2010; Soussain et al., 2009.

Table 14-3. Overview of Radiation Therapy–Induced Neurotoxic Conditions

Neurotoxic Conditions	Signs and Symptoms
Acute encephalopathy • Occurs within 2 weeks after beginning cranial radiation therapy (RT) • Often occurs just a few hours after first fraction • Seen with fraction doses > 3 Gy • Occurs in 5% of patients within a few days after stereotactic radiosurgery	Drowsiness Dysarthria Fever Headache Nausea/vomiting Worsening of preexisting neurologic deficits
Somnolence syndrome • Occurs mainly in children, approximately 50% of cases • More severe in children younger than 3 years old • Presents 3–8 weeks after cranial RT • Symptom resolution within 3–6 weeks	Drowsiness Excessive sleep Fever Headache Irritability Nausea Transient papilledema
Tumor pseudoprogression syndrome • Occurs within 6–12 weeks after cranial RT • Occurs within weeks of completing RT and receiving temozolomide • Difficult to determine tumor progression • Imaging may be normal or show edema and contrast enhancement within tumor bed	Worsening of presenting neurologic focal symptoms such as headache, nausea, visual disturbances, motor weakness, or speech disturbances, or may be asymptomatic
Cerebral injury • Most common neurotoxicity • Occurs at any age; may be more problematic in pediatric population • Diffuse cortical atrophy, ventricular dilation, and abnormalities in white matter shown on imaging • Imaging abnormalities progress over time • Correlated to higher doses of RT, large volume, and increasing age of patient	Cognitive impairment/dysfunction such as memory loss and decrease in functional ability
Focal brain necrosis • Severe reaction to RT affecting the white matter of the brain or spinal cord, producing necrosis and vascular injury • Occurs within 1–2 years after completing RT • Incidence of 3%–24% • Can mimic tumor recurrence • Dependent on total dose, fraction size, and volume treated • Possibly increased risk with history of diabetes, advancing age, and history of chemotherapy • Imaging is challenging; MRI spectroscopy preferred	Focal neurologic deficits Intracranial hypertension Seizures May be asymptomatic

(Continued on next page)

Table 14-3. Overview of Radiation Therapy–Induced Neurotoxic Conditions *(Continued)*

Neurotoxic Conditions	Signs and Symptoms
Cognitive dysfunction and leukoencephalopathy • Most common late effect • Occurs several years after RT • Occurs with RT but exacerbated by the presence of brain tumors, brain tumor progression, chemotherapy, encephalomyelitis, and endocrine dysfunction • Possibly increased risk with advancing age, large fraction doses (greater than 2 Gy/day), large volume of irradiated tissue, combined treatment with chemotherapy, and vascular conditions such as diabetes and hypertension • Thought to be caused by an inflammatory response, impairment of neuron function, and decreased neurogenesis	Attention deficits Executive function deficits Judgment deficits Short-term memory loss Visual motor deficits
Cerebrovascular disease • Usually occurs 5–10 years after RT • Stenosis/occlusion of cerebral arteries resulting from RT to tumors within the brain and head/neck region	Difficulty speaking Dizziness Headache Mental fogginess Motor weakness Visual problems
Radiation-induced central nervous system tumors • Most common in childhood survivors of brain tumors or leukemia • 10-fold increase in risk of developing a meningioma; usually occurred 15 years after RT • 7-fold increase in risk of developing a glioma; usually occurred 5 years after RT	Headache Nausea Other symptoms dependent on location of tumor
Cranial nerve injury • Optic and hypoglossal nerves commonly affected by RT • Optic neuropathy usually presenting within 12–18 months after RT; occurs with RT to orbit, sinus, nasopharynx, pituitary adenoma, and craniopharyngioma • Hypoglossal palsy usually developing 2–10 years after head/neck RT	Optic neuropathy • Decreased/loss of visual acuity • Decreased/loss of visual field Hypoglossal palsy • Atrophy of tongue
Myelopathy • Most common form is transient; occurs 4–6 months after RT • Also referred to as Lhermitte phenomenon • Can also be delayed, occurring 1–2 years after RT	Lhermitte phenomenon • Paresthesias radiating down spine and lower extremities • Can be exacerbated by neck flexion or physical exertion Delayed myelopathy • Numbness or dysesthesias of lower extremities • Motor weakness • Sphincter dysfunction • Pain not an issue • Paraplegia/quadriplegia in 50% of patients

(Continued on next page)

Table 14-3. Overview of Radiation Therapy–Induced Neurotoxic Conditions *(Continued)*

Neurotoxic Conditions	Signs and Symptoms
Plexopathies • Can occur in any plexus included in RT field • Most common include brachial and lumbosacral • Can be reversible or progressive but more commonly seen as delayed • Brachial plexopathy most common in breast cancer (40%–75% of cases), lung cancer, and lymphoma; peak onset of 2–4 years after RT • Lumbosacral plexopathy possible after RT to the pelvis or para-aortic lymph nodes • Potential for delayed lumbosacral plexopathy occurring 5 years after RT	Brachial plexopathy • Numbness/paresthesias of hands and fingers • Motor weakness Lumbosacral plexopathy • Motor weakness from L2–S1 or L5–S1 • Atrophy • Loss of muscle stretch reflexes

Note. Based on information from Ballesteros-Zebadua et al., 2012; Brejt et al., 2013; Dropcho, 2010; Gibbs et al., 2009; Parvez et al., 2014; Pouleau et al., 2012; Prasanna et al., 2012; Rinne et al., 2012; Soussain et al., 2009.

Soussain et al., 2009). Neuropathy can occur in several forms, which include cerebellar, central, autonomic, and peripheral (see Table 14-4).

CNS neurotoxicities are serious but occur less frequently than peripheral neurotoxicities. Metabolic encephalopathy, meningitis, leukoencephalopathy, headaches, seizures, and other CNS toxicities have been reported. These effects can occur as a result of excitatory mechanisms and apoptosis in CNS progenitor cells. Drugs associated with central neurotoxicities include capecitabine, cisplatin, cyclophosphamide, cytarabine, 5-fluorouracil, ifosfamide, interferon, and methotrexate. The drug or its metabolite crosses the blood-brain barrier, leading to central neurotoxicities. Capecitabine is a prodrug for 5-fluorouracil and has been found to cause a multifocal leukoencephalopathy. Cisplatin may cause ototoxicity, which results in high-frequency sensorineural hearing loss and tinnitus (Miltenburg & Boogerd, 2014). Cytarabine at high doses ($1-3 \text{ g/m}^2$ every 12–24 hours) can cause an acute cerebellar syndrome. Symptoms include ataxia, dysarthria, nystagmus, lethargy, confusion, and possibly seizures (Miltenburg & Boogerd, 2014). 5-Fluorouracil can cause an acute cerebellar syndrome in about 5% of patients, which is manifested by acute onset of ataxia, dysmetria, dysarthria, and nystagmus. Ifosfamide is activated in the liver, forming ifosfamide mustard and acrolein. It can cause encephalopathy in 20%–30% of patients and may present as lethargy, confusion, hallucinations, cerebellar dysfunction, seizures, cranial nerve palsies, and extrapyramidal effects (Argyriou, Kyritsis, Makatsoris, & Kalofonos, 2014; Miltenburg & Boogerd, 2014). Interferon is a biologic agent that can cause peripheral neuropathy and other neurotoxicity at doses above 20 million units/m² (Fischer, Knobf, Durivage, & Beaulieu, 2003; Merck and Co., 2011). Common side effects include headaches, confusion, lethargy, and seizures. Methotrexate can cause aseptic meningitis with intrathecal administration. The presenting symptoms include headache, fever, nuchal rigidity, and seizures. High-dose methotrexate has been found to cause neurotoxicity, especially in patients being treated for CNS lymphoma or children with acute lymphoblastic leukemia. Common neurotoxic effects include somnolence, confusion, and seizures. A delayed effect may be leukoencephalopathy, which may be exacerbated with the use of radiation therapy (Hospira, 2011). Taxanes (e.g., paclitaxel, docetaxel) can cause visual disturbances, which include scintillating scotomas (partial alteration in the field of vision) during infusion and vision loss. Vincristine may cause oculomotor neuropathy, leading to ptosis and ophthalmoplegia (weakness or paralysis of one of the extraocular muscles) (Argyriou et al., 2014; Livshits, Rao, & Smith, 2014; Miltenburg & Boogerd, 2014).

Chemotherapy can affect the peripheral nervous system. The most common presentation is peripheral neuropathy, which is a general term for peripheral nerve damage. It can result in dose reduction or early drug discontinuation, as well as diminished quality of life and func-

Table 14-4. Types of Neurotoxicities Associated With Chemotherapy, Biotherapy, and Targeted Therapies

Type of Neurotoxicity	Area Affected	Signs and Symptoms
Cerebellar	Cerebellum	Ataxia Changes in reflexes Confusion, change in mental status, memory loss Diplopia Dysarthria Paresthesias
Central	Meningitis	Change in level of consciousness Fever Headache Nausea/vomiting
	Metabolic encephalopathy	Agitation Altered cranial nerve function Altered motor function Altered speech Altered thought processes Blurred vision Coma, seizures, lethargy/sleepiness Confusion, nightmares, restlessness Headache Paranoia, delusions/hallucinations Proteinuria Stupor, nausea/vomiting, aphasia Urinary incontinence
	Leukoencephalopathy	Altered mental status Neurologic deficits Sudden increase in blood pressure Vision loss/blindness
	Seizures	Aura Drooling Eye movements Involuntary movements Loss of bladder/bowel control Loss of consciousness Teeth clinching
Autonomic	Autonomic nervous system	Altered cardiac, vascular, gastrointestinal, respiratory, and endocrine function Constipation, ileus, urinary retention Erectile dysfunction Postural hypotension

(Continued on next page)

Table 14-4. Types of Neurotoxicities Associated With Chemotherapy, Biotherapy, and Targeted Therapies *(Continued)*

Type of Neurotoxicity	Area Affected	Signs and Symptoms
Peripheral	Peripheral, cranial, and spinal nerves	Altered motor function Altered sensory function (i.e., loss of heat and cold sensation, vibration and pain) Feeling of "pins and needles" in the glove-and-stocking distribution of the hands and feet, weakness, loss of muscle function, or loss of sensation or vibration; often starts distally and ascends up extremity. Loss of reflexes such as deep tendon reflexes Myalgias Neuropathies may be progressive with drug interruption or discontinuation Pain and altered temperature sensation resulting from small fiber neurotoxicity Proprioception and altered sense of vibration resulting from large fiber toxicity

Note. Based on information from Argyriou et al., 2014; Miltenburg & Boogerd, 2014; Schlegel, 2011; Soussain et al., 2009.

tional status (Hershman et al., 2014). The exact etiology of peripheral neuropathy is not fully understood. Multiple theories are summarized by Miltenburg and Boogerd (2014), including the hypothesis that because the nerve cell bodies of the peripheral motor axons are within the blood-brain barrier, they are protected from antineoplastic agent injury, unlike the efferent portions of the peripheral motor axons, which lie outside the blood-brain barrier. The motor nerves are less affected because they have more myelin protection than the smaller-diameter sensory nerves. Chemotherapy agents affect the nervous system in different ways and can occur from the level of sensory cell bodies in the dorsal root ganglion to the distal axon. Another mechanism is disruption of the microtubules, which are key to the axonal transport processes and critical for energy and material delivery. Preexisting diseases, such as diabetes, and combination therapy with known neurotoxic side effects may precipitate and exacerbate peripheral neuropathy.

Peripheral neuropathy can be sensory or motor in nature, although sensory is more common. Sensory neuropathy is caused by the effect on large sensory nerves leading to paresthesias, dysesthesias, and numbness in the hands and feet. Paresthesias usually are described as "pins and needles," and dysesthesias are described as painful, burning sensations. The neuropathy is usually bilateral, and the sensory loss is usually in a "glove and stocking" distribution with an ascending pattern (Miltenburg & Boogerd, 2014; Vilholm, Christensen, Zedan, & Itani, 2014). Vibration sense, touch, and proprioception may be altered, and pain may be present. The reduction or loss of deep tendon reflexes indicates greater toxicity (Hausheer, Schilsky, Bain, Berghorn, & Lieberman, 2006). Motor neuropathy is less common and is caused by damage to the smaller sensory fibers. It can cause motor weakness, autonomic symptoms, and incidental cranial nerve involvement (Miltenburg & Boogerd, 2014; Park et al., 2013).

Neuropathy also can be classified as acute or chronic. Acute neuropathy is a transient syndrome with an abrupt onset and can appear during or shortly after the first few infusions. It often presents with paresthesias, dysesthesias, or both. This is primarily seen with oxaliplatin and observed at higher doses of 130–180 mg/m^2 (Zedan, Hansen, Svenningsen, & Vilholm,

2014). Chronic and cumulative toxicity has a more gradual onset and takes longer to resolve. The incidence of peripheral neuropathies varies widely depending on the drugs administered. Common chemotherapy agents that can cause peripheral neuropathy include cisplatin, oxaliplatin, taxanes (e.g., paclitaxel, docetaxel), vincristine, thalidomide, and bortezomib. It is thought that cisplatin causes peripheral neuropathy by affecting the large myelinated sensory fibers, and symptoms will develop from injury to the dorsal root ganglion. With oxaliplatin, peripheral neuropathy can occur in two distinct neuropathy clusters: one occurs during or shortly after the first few infusions, whereas more cumulative sensory neuropathy may develop over time (Tofthagen, McAllister, & McMillan, 2011; Zedan et al., 2014). The taxanes can cause sensory neuropathy and affect the peripheral nerves by stabilizing the microtubule system, which is responsible for mitosis and intracellular transport of proteins from the axon and cell body (Carlson & Ocean, 2011; Smith, 2013). Vincristine-induced peripheral neuropathy is thought to develop from disruption of tubulin, causing axonal degeneration (Argyriou et al., 2014; Carlson & Ocean, 2011; Miltenburg & Boogerd, 2014). Bortezomib primarily affects small nerve fibers of the lower extremities and is more sensory in nature. All grades of peripheral neuropathy occur in about 38% of patients receiving bortezomib (Argyriou et al., 2014; Berkowitz & Walker, 2012; Millennium Pharmaceuticals, 2012; Miltenburg & Boogerd, 2014). Thalidomide has been associated with sensory neuropathy, which occurs in 3%–32% of patients (Argyriou et al., 2014; Cavaletti, 2014; Miltenburg & Boogerd, 2014). See Table 14-5 for more details regarding individual chemotherapy agents and their potential neurotoxicities.

Peripheral neuropathy develops in patients when cumulative doses of neurotoxic agents are reached. Cumulative doses leading to neurotoxicities vary with each agent, but in some patients, peripheral neuropathy may develop prior to reaching the cumulative dose. The APN must then consider dose reduction or discontinuation of the neurotoxic agent based on symptoms, function, and quality of life. See Table 14-6 for cumulative doses of neurotoxic antineoplastic agents.

Risk factors of peripheral neuropathy include advancing age, presence of paraneoplastic syndrome, alcohol abuse, thiamine or B complex deficiency, history of other comorbid diseases such as HIV, Lyme disease, diabetes, multiple sclerosis, Guillain-Barré syndrome, pernicious anemia, herpes zoster, or peripheral vascular disease, or traumatic injury causing neuropathy (Miltenburg & Boogerd, 2014).

HSCT causes many neurologic toxicities, which are thought to be related to the effects of chemotherapy or radiation therapy, metabolic abnormalities, organ failure, graft-versus-host disease (GVHD), infection, and myelosuppression. The most common neurotoxic effects include encephalopathy, headaches, seizures, cerebrovascular events, infections, and neuromuscular conditions. GVHD is a consequence of allogeneic transplantation that occurs from donor T cells attacking mismatched recipient antigens. It usually affects the skin, liver, eyes, and mouth. It also can cause neurologic conditions such as polymyositis, myasthenia gravis, and chronic inflammatory demyelinating polyneuropathy (Koeppen, Thirugnanasambanthan, & Koldehoff, 2014; Živković & Abdel-Hamid, 2010).

Other medications and substances, such as lithium, phenytoin, amiodarone, colchicine, lead, alcohol, and toluene, also can cause neurologic side effects (Chung, Prasad, & Lloyd, 2014; Walker, 2013).

Prevention Strategies

The development of neurologic symptoms is based on the cancer itself and the type of cancer treatment modalities used, as well as supportive care therapies. It is important that APNs have a good understanding and knowledge of the potential neurologic effects from cancer

Table 14-5. Neurotoxicities Associated With Chemotherapy, Biotherapy, and Targeted Therapies

Drug	Side Effect/Toxicity	Clinical Considerations
Asparaginase	Cerebellar dysfunction Encephalopathy	Uncommon; does not cross blood-brain barrier Encephalopathy associated with hepatotoxicity
Bevacizumab	Leukoencephalopathy	Discontinue drug. Monitor for symptom resolution and treat hypertension. No evidence to restart therapy if symptom resolution
Bortezomib	Peripheral neuropathy, more sensory-related side effects Symmetrical pain, burning, numbness, hyperesthesia	Dose dependent Threshold dose: > 16 mg/m^2 Peaks around the fifth cycle Improvement with dose reduction, interruption, discontinuation, or subcutaneous administration
Busulfan	Seizures	With high-dose therapy
Capecitabine	Leukoencephalopathy	Discontinue drug. Improvement in several days, but presentation differs from 5-fluorouracil
Carboplatin	Sensory neuropathy	Less frequent side effect compared to cisplatin Stroke-like syndromes with intra-arterial administration
Carmustine	Headache	With high doses
Cisplatin	Affect large peripheral nerve fibers with loss of proprioception and ataxia High-frequency hearing loss Lhermitte symptoms Vestibule patchy Encephalopathy (with intracarotid administration)	Cumulative doses of 300–500 mg/m^2 Risk factors: Dose, duration, and administration schedule Usually gradual presentation May worsen after therapy is complete or discontinued and usually improves with time
Cytarabine, high-dose	Altered mental status Cerebellar toxicity Peripheral neuropathy Seizures	Assess cerebellar toxicity at baseline and prior to each dose. Hold for changes in cerebellar function until symptoms resolve. Toxicity usually resolves with stopping therapy. Reduce dose in older adults or those with hepatic or renal dysfunction.
Cytarabine, liposomal (IT use)	Encephalopathy Sustained-release formulation causes aseptic meningitis and/or chemical arachnoiditis	Self-limiting Administer with dexamethasone 4 mg BID (IV or oral) on first day of chemotherapy and continue for total of 5 days.
Etoposide	Confusion Peripheral neuropathy Seizures	Uncommon; usually mild Assess for altered sensory and motor function prior to each cycle.

(Continued on next page)

Table 14-5. Neurotoxicities Associated With Chemotherapy, Biotherapy, and Targeted Therapies *(Continued)*

Drug	Side Effect/Toxicity	Clinical Considerations
5-Fluorouracil	Cerebellar toxicity Encephalopathy Seizures	Discontinue therapy. Steroids may be helpful. If toxicity is caused by dihydropyrimidine dehydrogenase deficiency, it may respond to high doses of thymidine (IV).
Fludarabine	Confusion Peripheral neuropathy Somnolence	Usually transient symptoms
Ifosfamide	Change in mental status (from mild confusion to profound obtundation); variable onset from hours to weeks after initiation of drug; usually reversible 2–3 days after drug stopped Encephalopathy (high doses) Peripheral neuropathy Toxicity because of drug metabolites crossing blood-brain barrier	Incidence < 20%; more common with earlier cycles Hold drug for changes in mental status. Adequate hydration and normal renal function are necessary to enhance excretion of drug's metabolite, chloroacetaldehyde. Other risk factors include length of administration, bolus infusion, oral administration, presence of acidosis, impaired liver function, prior isolation therapy, bulky abdominal disease, medications, poor performance status, and low serum albumin levels. Hold drug with neurotoxicity. Hydrate, provide supportive care, and monitor neurologic status. Methylene blue minimizes neurotoxic effects, usually 50 mg of 1%–2% solution.
Imatinib	Headache	Occurs in 10%–53% of patients
Interferon	Dementia Depression Headache Lethargy Neuropsychiatric effects Seizures	Assess for and provide patient education regarding neuropsychiatric side effects. Neuropsychiatric toxicity requires discontinuation of therapy. Risk is greater with prior neurologic or psychiatric diagnosis.
Interleukin	Neuropsychiatric side effects: Cognitive changes, delusions, hallucinations, and depression	With higher doses Reversible side effects
Methotrexate	Aseptic or arachnoiditis meningitis (intrathecal) Encephalopathy (high-dose IV) Leukoencephalopathy Lumbosacral radiculopathy Myelopathy Nerve palsy Seizures	Consider premedication with steroids. Neurotoxic effects may be acute, subacute, or delayed.

(Continued on next page)

Table 14-5. Neurotoxicities Associated With Chemotherapy, Biotherapy, and Targeted Therapies *(Continued)*

Drug	Side Effect/Toxicity	Clinical Considerations
Oxaliplatin	Acute pseudolaryngopharyngeal spasms Myotonia Peripheral neuropathy, especially sensory (acute or chronic)	Common; expected side effect Acute and sudden onset after treatment by exposure to cold Develops during infusion or up to 2 weeks later May minimize between cycles Affects hands, feet, digits, lips, mouth, and throat Mild to moderate in severity Cumulative chronic and persistent sensory neuropathy increases as cumulative dose increases. Other risk factors include time of infusion and baseline peripheral neuropathy. Fine motor movement may be affected. Reversible 6–8 months after therapy completed Provide patient education for self-care, avoidance of precipitating factors, and management. Advise patients to avoid cold air and cold foods/liquids, and to keep hands and feet warm. Acute laryngopharyngeal dysesthesias with exposure to cold Myotonia precipitated by cold
Procarbazine	Confusion Hallucinations Mild encephalopathy Peripheral neuropathy	Encephalopathy increases as dose increases. Procarbazine may potentiate sedative effects of narcotic analgesics and phenothiazines.
Retinoic acid	Headache Pseudotumor cerebri with visual field deficits and compromised color vision	Readily crosses blood-brain barrier Teratogenic effects in developing CNS
Rituximab	Dizziness Headache Leukoencephalopathy Myalgia Paresthesias	Not common Leukoencephalopathy may be associated with viral infections during therapy.
Steroids	Depression Encephalopathy Mania Myopathy Psychoses	Watch for steroid psychosis. Medication must be tapered.
Tamoxifen	Headache Ischemic stroke Keratopathy (noninflammatory disease of cornea) Retinopathy	Can exacerbate migraine headaches

(Continued on next page)

Table 14-5. Neurotoxicities Associated With Chemotherapy, Biotherapy, and Targeted Therapies *(Continued)*

Drug	Side Effect/Toxicity	Clinical Considerations
Taxanes (docetaxel/ paclitaxel)	Autonomic neurotoxicity (high doses) Large-fiber sensory neuropathy Peripheral sensory neuropathy Seizures Transient encephalopathy	Affects lower extremities more than upper extremities Paclitaxel causes more peripheral neuropathy than docetaxel. Greater risk with high cumulative doses of paclitaxel, higher doses over short infusion times, weekly dosing, preexisting neuropathies, or prior or concurrent administration of cisplatin Usually resolves with time
Thalidomide	Lethargy Peripheral neuropathy Sensory neuropathy Sleepiness	May not be reversible Dose-limiting toxicity Often begins after 1 year of starting drug or more acutely May also develop after therapy stopped May need to discontinue drug if peripheral neuropathy develops to prevent additional damage Neuropathy may present early. Dose at bedtime.
Vinblastine	Peripheral neuropathy	Affects lower extremities more than upper extremities
Vincristine	Ataxia Autonomic neuropathy Cranial nerve involvement (rare) Encephalopathy Peripheral neuropathy (common)	Affects lower extremities more than upper extremities Loss of deep tendon reflexes Progresses if therapy not discontinued Maximum dose per week of 2 mg Usually reversible but may worsen once therapy is stopped Peripheral neuropathy usually seen after 3–4 doses Worsens with cumulative doses of 15–20 mg Can produce paralysis at cumulative doses > 30 mg Autonomic neuropathy can cause constipation, abdominal pain, syncope, and orthostatic hypotension Must initiate bowel regimen
Vinorelbine	Peripheral neuropathy	Affects lower extremities more than upper extremities

Note. Based on information from Argyriou et al., 2014; Berkowitz & Walker, 2012; Livshits et al., 2014; Miltenburg & Boogerd, 2014; Rinne et al., 2012; Schlegel, 2011; Sioka et al., 2014.

treatments. No known preventive measures exist for neurotoxicities, but various interventions may minimize the severity. The severity of neurotoxicity is based on the type of chemotherapy agent, the use of multiple agents, the cumulative dose, the location of radiation therapy, the total dose and fraction size of radiation, the presence of other comorbid conditions, and advancing age. Peripheral neuropathy is the most common treatment-related neurotoxic effect and can negatively affect patients' quality of life. The American Society of Clinical Oncology (ASCO) recently published clinical guidelines for chemotherapy-induced peripheral neuropathy (Hershman et al., 2014). Despite the many trials that have studied agents to prevent chemotherapy-induced peripheral neuropathy, no evidence-based intervention has been found. Based on ASCO's recommendations, the following interventions should not be offered to patients: acetyl-L-carnitine, amifostine, amitriptyline, calcium and magnesium for patients

Table 14-6. Neurotoxic Antineoplastic Agents and Cumulative Doses

Neurotoxic Antineoplastic Agents	Cumulative Doses for Neurotoxicity
Bortezomib	Cumulative dose depends on grade/signs and symptoms. See package insert for recommendations on dose modifications based on grade of neuropathy.
Cisplatin	Peripheral sensory neuropathy is common with cumulative doses above 300 mg/m^2. With mild neuropathy, full-dose therapy is appropriate. With severe neuropathy and functional changes, dose reduction or discontinuation of drug is recommended.
Oxaliplatin	Neurotoxicity correlates to cumulative dose of 750–850 mg/m^2. Regimen schedule (every 3 weeks reported less neurotoxicity than every 2 weeks)
Taxanes (docetaxel/paclitaxel)	Dose dependent Paclitaxel: Neurotoxicity correlates with cumulative doses > 250 mg/m^2. Docetaxel: Neurotoxicity correlates with cumulative doses > 600 mg/m^2.
Vincristine	Neurotoxicity correlates with cumulative doses of 6–8 mg. Symptoms worsen with doses of 15–20 mg. Paralysis occurs at cumulative doses > 30 mg.

Note. Based on information from Berkowitz & Walker, 2012; Millennium Pharmaceuticals, 2012; Miltenburg & Boogerd, 2014; National Cancer Institute Cancer Therapy Evaluation Program, 2010; Park et al., 2013.

receiving oxaliplatin, diethyldithiocarbamate, glutathione for patients receiving paclitaxel or carboplatin, nimodipine, Org 2766, all-trans-retinoic acid, recombinant human leukemia inhibitory factor, vitamin E, and omega-3 fatty acids. In addition, the use of complementary and alternative medicine has not been established in the treatment of peripheral neuropathy (Hershman et al., 2014). Dose reduction and dose delay are also strategies to minimize or prevent neurotoxicity.

Therefore, assessment and management by the APN are crucial, especially to determine baseline neurologic function. Prompt interruption or discontinuation of therapy, dose reductions, or dose delays may be necessary to manage certain toxicities.

Diagnosis and Assessment

One of the most important roles of the APN is to assess and appropriately diagnose patients with cancer for disease- and treatment-related effects. With the common occurrence of neurologic complications and toxicities in this population, a complete and thorough neurologic history and physical examination are needed for safe patient care when treatment plans include neurotoxic agents. Both should be performed at initial consultation (baseline), throughout therapy, minimally before each dose of chemotherapy to assess for central and peripheral neuropathy, and when new symptoms arise. The use of standardized tools to document neuropathy is important for accuracy and appropriate determination of progression. Components of history taking should include presenting symptoms, past and current oncology treatment regimens (i.e., radiation therapy site, total dose and fraction size, chemotherapy agents, duration of treatment, and cumulative dose), medication profile, cognitive changes, history of neurologic symptoms (e.g., seizures, headaches, mental status changes, confusion), and history of other comorbid conditions, such as diabetes, movement disorders, and dementia (Kennedy & Zakaria, 2012).

No standardized approaches to the assessment of chemotherapy-induced neurotoxicity exist. However, a thorough neurologic examination should include assessment of mental status, cranial nerves, motor reflexes, sensation, coordination, and gait. APNs assess the severity and impact of the neurotoxicity on patients' quality of life and ability to function in daily life. See Table 14-7 for more details on a thorough neurologic examination for the evaluation of neurologic symptoms.

Paraneoplastic syndromes may produce central or peripheral neurotoxicities (Dropcho, 2010). SCLC is associated with a number of paraneoplastic syndromes that may have signs and symptoms similar to chemotherapy-induced neurotoxicities. Examples include hyponatremia-induced altered mental status changes and Lambert-Eaton myasthenic syndrome (Braik et al., 2010; Didelot & Honnorat, 2014). Lambert-Eaton myasthenic syndrome produces signs and symptoms such as fatigue, leg weakness, myalgias, and reduced deep tendon reflexes (Didelot & Honnorat, 2014).

Lymphomas may affect cranial nerves or nerve roots either through direct growth or paraneoplastic syndromes (McCoyd, Gruner, & Foy, 2014). Postural hypotension can occur from

Table 14-7. Components of Neurologic Examination

Assessment	Examination Details
Mental status	Perform Mini-Mental State Examination. Assess for • Level of awareness: Awake, alert • Attentiveness • Orientation: Person, place, and time • Speech and language: Fluency, comprehension, repetition, naming, reading, and writing • Memory: Registration, immediate recall, recent memory, and remote history • Higher intellectual function: General knowledge, abstraction, judgment, insight, and reasoning • Mood and affect.
Cranial nerves	Examine all cranial nerves (1–12). Perform visual acuity and funduscopic examination.
Motor	Assess muscle strength, effort, coordination, and extrapyramidal function. Tests of dexterity and coordination are most sensitive in determining upper motor neuron and cerebellar dysfunction. Assess for muscle atrophy, muscle tone, and movement disturbances.
Reflexes	Reflex tests are the most objective part of neurologic exam. Assess both motor and sensory function.
Sensation	Assess for vibration, joint position sense, temperature, light touch, double simultaneous stimulation, graphesthesia (the ability to recognize writing on the skin purely by the sensation of touch), stereognosis (the ability to perceive and recognize the form of an object in the absence of visual and auditory information by using tactile information), and Romberg test.
Coordination and gait	Assess truncal stability, fine finger movements, toe tapping, finger-nose-finger, heel-knee-shin, and rapid alternating movements. Observe gait and station.

Note. Based on information from Wills, 2012.

autonomic nervous system dysfunction. Spinal cord compression causes localized back pain, nerve root pain, and altered sensory and motor function below the area of the compression. If undiagnosed and untreated, spinal cord compression can progress to paralysis with significant morbidity, including incontinence, skin breakdown, and other hazards of immobility. Reversibility of the complications of spinal cord compression depends on time to treatment. Alcohol abuse and resultant malnutrition can cause peripheral neuropathies. Altered electrolyte levels, such as hypocalcemia, may produce signs and symptoms that mimic peripheral neuropathy. Hypercalcemia may cause altered mental status, seizures, and altered reflexes. Diagnostic workup may include serum chemistries, diagnosis of underlying malignancy, and imaging studies such as computed tomography (CT) or magnetic resonance imaging (MRI).

Common assessment findings with peripheral neuropathy may include absent or diminished Achilles reflex, absent or diminished vibration sensation at the great toe, and an abnormal Romberg test (Argyriou et al., 2014; Braik et al., 2010; Smith, 2013). In addition, the gold standard for neurophysiologic assessment includes the use of nerve conduction studies, which measure the amplitude and conduction velocity of sensory and motor fibers. A common finding in peripheral neuropathy is the reduction of compound sensory action potential.

In assessing cancer- or treatment-related symptoms, it is important to combine the findings of the history and physical examination and formulate the differential diagnosis. With the presentation of these neurologic symptoms, other diagnostic methods may be required. APNs must formulate a differential diagnosis for the presenting symptoms. They should consider differential diagnoses in patients with neurotoxicity, which may include paraneoplastic neurologic syndromes, metabolic disturbances, or diabetes-induced peripheral neuropathy.

Diabetes-induced peripheral neuropathy produces similar symptoms (Miltenburg & Boogerd, 2014; Vilholm et al., 2014). Diabetic neuropathy commonly affects the fingers, hands, arms, and feet and often is described as a "glove and stocking" neuropathy. In addition, sensory neuropathy is most common and typically starts in the distal feet and progresses proximally. Patients often experience numbness, tingling, aching, electric shock–like pain, allodynia (pain caused by stimuli that does not normally cause pain), or hyperesthesia. The pain may be constant, intermittent, or worse at night. Often, symptoms will improve with adequate glucose control (Berkowitz & Walker, 2012).

To diagnose most paraneoplastic neurologic syndromes, APNs need to address four clinical features: the presentation of neurologic symptoms before the diagnosis of cancer, the occurrence of similar syndromes without a cancer correlation, the absence of paraneoplastic antibodies, and the small size of associated tumors (Braik et al., 2010). See Table 14-8 for more details on diagnosis and management.

Treatment-related neurologic side effects are common with the peripheral nervous system being affected more than the CNS. The severity of the impairment is weighed against the benefits and risks of continued therapy, dose reductions, or treatment breaks. APNs need to be able to adequately and consistently assess the degree of neurotoxicity prior to each treatment and more frequently if warranted. Commonly used toxicity grading scales for neurologic disorders and symptoms include the World Health Organization scale, Eastern Cooperative Oncology Group (ECOG) scale, and National Cancer Institute (NCI) Cancer Therapy Evaluation Program's Common Terminology Criteria for Adverse Events (CTCAE). See NCI Cancer Therapy Evaluation Program (2010) for details on CTCAE grading of nervous system disorders commonly seen in the oncology population, including cognitive disturbance, leukoencephalopathy, peripheral motor neuropathy, and peripheral sensory neuropathy.

It is also important to assess functional status and quality of life when neurologic effects are present. Scales to assess function include the Functional Assessment of Cancer Therapy/Gynecologic Oncology Group–Neurotoxicity, the Functional Assessment of Cancer Therapy–

Taxane, the Peripheral Neuropathy Scale, oxaliplatin-associated neuropathy questionnaires, the Scale for Chemotherapy-Induced Long-Term Neurotoxicity, and the Patient Neurotoxicity Questionnaire (FACIT.org, n.d.). In addition, the APN may ask the patient to perform common activities such as writing his or her name, picking up small objects, buttoning buttons, and walking.

Quality-of-life assessment is also crucial in patients experiencing neurologic symptoms, whether they are disease or treatment related. Scales used to assess quality of life include the

Table 14-8. Paraneoplastic Neurologic Syndromes in Cancer: Diagnosis and Management

Paraneoplastic Syndrome	Diagnostic Testing	Medical Management
Central Nervous System		
Cerebellar degeneration	CSF analysis: May show pleocytosis, increased proteins, intrathecal synthesis of IgG, and oligoclonal bands MRI brain: May be normal initially and after months may show global cerebellar atrophy FDG-PET: May show increased metabolism in cerebellum during early stages and then decreased metabolism in late stages	IVIG Steroids Plasma exchange Cyclophosphamide Rituximab
Limbic encephalitis	EEG: Rules out status epilepticus FDG-PET: Detects hypermetabolism in temporal lobe MRI brain: May show temporal lobe dysfunction, either unilateral or bilateral CSF analysis: May show mild pleocytosis, increased proteins, intrathecal synthesis of IgG and oligoclonal bands	IVIG Steroids Plasma exchange Cyclophosphamide Rituximab
Neuromuscular Junction		
Lambert-Eaton myasthenic syndrome	EMG: May show low compound muscle action potentials	3,4-Diaminopyridine Guanidine Pyridostigmine Steroids Azathioprine IVIG Plasma exchange
Myasthenia gravis	EMG: May show decreased response to repetitive nerve stimulation	Thymectomy Pyridostigmine Steroids Azathioprine Cyclosporine A Tacrolimus Mycophenolate mofetil Rituximab Cyclophosphamide Plasma exchange IVIG

(Continued on next page)

**Table 14-8. Paraneoplastic Neurologic Syndromes in Cancer:
Diagnosis and Management (Continued)**

Paraneoplastic Syndrome	Diagnostic Testing	Medical Management
Peripheral Nervous System		
Autonomic neuropathy	Abdominal x-ray Barium studies: May show gastrointestinal dilation but no obstruction Esophageal manometry: May show achalasia or spasms	Supportive care • Hydration fluids • Salt intake • Fludrocortisone/midodrine • Caffeine
Subacute peripheral sensory neuropathy	Nerve conduction study: May reveal reduced or absent sensory nerve action potentials CSF analysis: May show mild pleocytosis, increased proteins, intrathecal synthesis of IgG, and oligoclonal bands	Steroids Cyclophosphamide IVIG Plasma exchange

CSF—cerebrospinal fluid; EEG—electroencephalogram; EMG—electromyogram; FDG-PET—fluorodeoxyglucose positron-emission tomography; IgG—immunoglobulin G; IVIG—intravenous immunoglobulin; MRI—magnetic resonance imaging

Note. Based on information from Pelosof & Gerber, 2010; Rosenfeld & Dalmau, 2010; Sioka et al., 2014; Soffietti et al., 2014.

European Organisation for Research and Treatment of Cancer QLQ-CIPN20, Spitzer Quality of Life Index, and Memorial Symptom Assessment Scale (Heutte, Plisson, Lange, Prevost, & Babin, 2014).

Evidence-Based Treatment Strategies

The treatment of paraneoplastic neurologic syndromes is dependent on whether there is a known diagnosis of cancer. If a patient presents with a classic paraneoplastic syndrome or has developed a subacute neurologic disability that is not explained by physical examination or laboratory evaluation, a paraneoplastic syndrome should be suspected. Further diagnostic testing must be performed including MRI, lumbar puncture with cerebrospinal fluid analysis, electrodiagnostic tests, and measurement of paraneoplastic antibodies in the serum. With the presence of paraneoplastic antibodies, as listed in Table 14-1, determination of the underlying cancer is crucial so that an appropriate treatment plan can be formulated. Treatment of the underlying cancer that is causing the paraneoplastic syndrome will resolve or minimize symptoms. In patients with a known diagnosis of cancer who present with neurologic symptoms, other causes need to be considered, such as brain or spinal metastases, before they are diagnosed with a paraneoplastic syndrome (Braik et al., 2010; Pelosof & Gerber, 2010). See Table 14-9 for details on the diagnosis and management of paraneoplastic neurologic syndromes.

Cancer treatment-related toxicities are many, and each has different assessment and management strategies. See Table 14-9 for details on the diagnosis and management of radiation therapy– and antineoplastic therapy–related neurotoxicities.

The management of peripheral neuropathy has gathered much attention and research over the past several years, mainly because of its very distressing effects, which can negatively affect individuals' quality of life. Symptom management and treatment of painful sensory peripheral neuropathies are important for patients' quality of life.

Table 14-9. Diagnosis and Management of Cancer Treatment–Related Neurotoxicities

Neurotoxicity	Diagnostic Testing	Medical Management
Radiation-Related Neurotoxicities		
Acute encepha-lopathy	MRI brain: Can be used to evaluate for herniation	Steroids
Somnolence syndrome	EEG: May show nonspecific diffuse slow waves	Steroids
Tumor pseudo-progression syndrome	MRI brain with spectroscopy: MRI may show increased edema, and contrast may enhance within tumor bed, which makes it difficult to distinguish between tumor progression Close follow-up with CT or MRI in 4–8 weeks	Steroids
Cerebral injury	MRI brain: Shows diffuse cortical atrophy, ventricular dilata-tion, and signal abnormalities in hemispheric white matter	Methylphenidate Modafinil Donepezil
Focal brain necrosis	MRI brain with spectroscopy: To determine perfusion Elevated choline:creatine ratios and choline:N-acetylaspartate are indicative of tumor rather than radiation necrosis.	Steroids Bevacizumab Surgical debulking
Cognitive dys-function and leu-koencephalopathy	MRI brain: Shows diffuse bilateral hyperintensity of the hemi-spheric white matter	Neuropsychologi-cal assessment
Myelopathy	MRI spine: Shows widening of the affected cord and abnor-mal signal intensity on T2-weighted images Abnormalities often extend beyond RT ports.	Steroids Pain management Hyperbaric oxygen therapy
Plexopathy	CT/MRI: Often can distinguish between RT brachial plexopa-thy and plexus metastases FDG-PET: Can be used to identify metastatic breast cancer to the brachial plexus if not clearly identified by CT or MRI Needle EMG testing: May be useful in diagnosing RT brachial plexopathy. Myokymia, the involuntary movement of mus-cles, is present in 50%–70% of patients with plexopathy.	Steroids Pain management
Chemotherapy-Related Neurotoxicities		
Seizures	CT/MRI brain: Can be used to evaluate for primary brain tumor or brain metastases EEG: Can be used to evaluate for electrical impulses	Steroids Anticonvulsants
Encephalopathy	MRI brain: May show reversible abnormalities in white matter of the occipital, parietal, and frontal lobes	Steroids
Leukoencepha-lopathy	MRI brain: May show diffuse bilateral hyperintensity of the hemispheric white matter	Antihypertensives Removal of caus-ative agent

CT—computed tomography; EEG—electroencephalogram; EMG—electromyogram; FDG-PET—fluorodeoxyglucose positron-emission tomography; MRI—magnetic resonance imaging; RT—radiation therapy

Note. Based on information from Braik et al., 2010; Didelot & Honnorat, 2014; Dropcho, 2010; Horska & Barker, 2010; Kannoth, 2012; Pelosof & Gerber, 2010; Soussain et al., 2009.

Over the years, many different agents have been studied in the treatment of peripheral neuropathy and include the use of anticonvulsants, selective serotonin reuptake inhibitors, serotonin-norepinephrine reuptake inhibitors, tricyclic antidepressants, opioids and topical lidocaine, menthol, capsaicin, and ketamine. Some of these have been supported by research but not supported as evidence-based (Trivedi, Silvestri, & Wolfe, 2013). ASCO recently published prevention and management guidelines for chemotherapy-induced peripheral neuropathy (Hershman et al., 2014). The Oncology Nursing Society's (ONS's) Putting Evidence Into Practice resource (Visovsky et al., 2014) details interventions to prevent or reduce the effects of peripheral neuropathy based on the level of evidence. See Figure 14-1 for details.

American Society of Clinical Oncology
Recommended for Practice
- Duloxetine: Start on 30 mg daily and titrate to 60 mg BID. Common side effects: nausea, dry mouth, headache, and somnolence.
- Tricyclic antidepressants: Reasonable options include nortriptyline and desipramine.
- Gabapentin: Start at 100 mg PO TID or 300 mg at bedtime and titrate to 1,800 mg/day in divided doses. Common side effects: ataxia, dizziness, fatigue, and somnolence.
- Topical gels containing baclofen (10 mg), amitriptyline HCl (40 mg), and ketamine (20 mg) (known as BAK)

No Recommendations Can Be Made
- Acetyl-L-carnitine had a positive phase III abstract but has not been published in peer-reviewed journals; a prevention trial suggested this agent was associated with worse outcomes.

Oncology Nursing Society
Putting Evidence Into Practice
Recommended for Practice
- Duloxetine, a serotonin-norepinephrine reuptake inhibitor, has been shown to be effective treatment for chemotherapy-induced peripheral neuropathy, especially with taxanes and oxaliplatin. The mechanism of action is inhibition of serotonin and norepinephrine reuptake in the central nervous system where antidepressant and pain inhibition are mediated.

Effectiveness Not Established
- Acupuncture
- Amifostine
- Amitriptyline
- BAK
- Bee venom
- Calcium and magnesium infusion
- Calcium channel blockers
- Cannabis/cannabinoids
- Carbamazepine
- Cutaneous stimulation
- Gabapentin and opioid combination
- Glutamine
- Glutathione
- Goshajinkigan
- KRN5500
- Nortriptyline
- Omega-3
- Palmitoylethanolamide
- Pregabalin
- Venlafaxine
- Vitamin E

Effectiveness Unlikely
- Lamotrigine

Not Recommended for Practice
- Carnitine/L-carnitine
- Human leukemia inhibitory factor

Figure 14-1. Evidence-Based Management Recommendations for Treatment of Chemotherapy-Induced Peripheral Neuropathy

---

Note. Based on information from Argyriou et al., 2014; Hershman et al., 2014; Miltenburg & Boogerd, 2014; Pfizer Inc., 2012; Smith et al., 2013; Visovsky et al., 2014.

Nonpharmacologic interventions may be used to complement the treatment of peripheral neuropathy. These may include cognitive and behavioral modifications, such as relaxation and guided imagery, distraction, cognitive reframing, and support groups, and physical measures, such as heat, cold, and massage therapy. However, none of these interventions are supported by evidence (Paice, 2009).

It is important for APNs to assess the functional status and ensure patient safety at home. This may include referral to a podiatrist for foot care, physical therapy, or occupational therapy to enhance strength and balance. For patients with a history of diabetes, it is essential that their diabetes be under control. Strength and coordination of the lower extremities are necessary for gait, but these can be affected with peripheral neuropathy. Progressive resistance training is the most effective intervention for increasing muscle strength and improving gait (Tofthagen, Visovsky, & Berry, 2012). The prevention of falls is also important in patients with peripheral neuropathy. Muscle-building exercises, ambulation, and strength and balance training have proved to be helpful in improving balance and ambulation and reducing fall risk. Patient and family education is extremely important and should include safety measures within and outside the home (see Table 14-10).

Evaluation of Outcomes

Neurotoxicity may occur with cancer itself or cancer-related treatments. APNs must continuously monitor patients' neurologic status at baseline and throughout the cancer trajectory. These symptoms and side effects can significantly reduce quality of life and functional status. The neurotoxicities can be central or peripheral in nature, with periph-

Table 14-10. Safety Measures for Patients Experiencing Chemotherapy-Induced Peripheral Neuropathy

Type of Measure	Recommendations
General self-care measures	Use zipper pulls and buttoners. Wear shoes with elastic shoe laces or Velcro straps. Wear closed-toed shoes. Wear gloves and socks in cold weather. Avoid jewelry with clasps.
Safety measures inside the home	Keep rooms well lighted. Illuminate stairs and hallways. Use a night-light in rooms. Avoid throw rugs. Be careful with extension cords. Remove furniture with sharp edges. Use rubber gloves when washing dishes. Use pot holders and oven mitts to handle hot kitchen dishes and pans.
Safety measures outside the home	Store garden tools appropriately. Place nails and screws in containers. Keep walkways free of clutter. Absorb all oil spills with sand or cat litter. Wear rubber shoes or work boots when working outside or in the garden.

Note. Based on information from Tofthagen et al., 2013.

eral neuropathy being more common. Antineoplastic therapy is tailored to patients' specific needs and problems caused by the cancer and resultant peripheral neuropathy side effects. Options include dose reductions, therapy interruptions or breaks, and discontinuation of therapy, in addition to measures to decrease severity of symptoms as well as self-care measures. Patient and family education is extremely important in minimizing risk and enhancing safety.

Implications for Oncology Advanced Practice Nurses

As neurotoxicity is a common and often expected side effect of cancer therapy, APNs must build routine evaluation of peripheral, cranial, and spinal nerves and CNS function into standard assessment and patient screening for toxicity and side effects.

Patient education is crucial to self-care management and coping. As such, it must be instituted with therapy and continued throughout therapy and after completion. Moreover, APNs need to be familiar with the medications used for symptom management to enhance quality of life.

Although less common than other side effects, ocular and neurologic toxicities have a profound effect on patients' quality of life, and some neurotoxicities are progressive and potentially life threatening if patients are not assessed and drug therapy interrupted. Oncology APNs need to follow the research and evidence-based practice findings to provide the highest quality in safe patient care. Baseline neurologic assessments and ongoing patient monitoring for the early onset of signs and symptoms of neurotoxicity should be performed prior to each dose of potentially neurotoxic therapy and follow-up visits to provide for safe patient care. Education for patients and families promotes self-care, which allows patients to take control of the side effects by avoiding precipitating events whenever possible. In addition, education allows patients to manage and report uncommon but potentially life-threatening toxicities.

Ocular Toxicities

Definition and Incidence

Ocular symptoms are relatively uncommon in patients with cancer but may be related to the cancer itself or cancer-related treatment modalities such as chemotherapy, radiation therapy, and HSCT, as well as other medications commonly used in the cancer population (Kheir, Sniegowski, El-Sawy, Li, & Esmaeli, 2014; Mesquida et al., 2010). Primary cancers of the eye are relatively uncommon but are considered a serious diagnosis given the potential for loss of vision. In addition, ocular toxicities are viewed in the same manner and have gained more attention as a serious side effect of cancer-related treatments.

Metastatic disease to the eye is rare. Most metastases arise in the uvea or within the orbit. Orbital metastasis occurs within the space adjacent to the eye and bony walls. It has been estimated that this occurs in 2%–3% of patients (Eagle, 2013; Perez, Saeed, Tan, & Cruz-Guillory, 2013; Voleti & Hubschman, 2013).

Another cause of ocular symptoms in patients with cancer is paraneoplastic syndromes. Visual paraneoplastic syndromes are less common, are difficult to diagnose, and generally affect the retina and optic nerve. Cancer treatment–related ocular toxicity is rare but is considered a significant event because of the potential for vision loss and diminished quality of life. Ocular side effects and toxicities produced by cancer therapy can occur with radiation therapy, chemotherapy agents, targeted agents, immunotherapy, HSCT, and supportive medications used in the cancer population.

Etiology and Presenting Signs and Symptoms

Common presenting symptoms of uveal melanoma may include blurred vision, presence of flashing lights (called *photopsia*), and visual field defects (Yonekawa & Kim, 2012). Presenting symptoms of orbital metastases may include proptosis, ptosis, diplopia, blurred vision, pain, and more prominent nodular eyelid and usually occur unilaterally. Proptosis is the forward displacement and entrapment of the eye from behind the eyelid. The majority of metastatic tumors to the eye are caused by cancers of lung, breast, GI tract, and prostate (Ng & Ilsen, 2010).

As with other paraneoplastic syndromes, visual paraneoplastic syndromes are related to immunologic mechanisms within the body as a result of tumor-directed antibodies. Cancer-associated retinopathy is the most common of the intraocular neoplastic syndromes and is most commonly associated with SCLC followed by gynecologic and breast cancers. Presenting symptoms are caused by cone photoreceptor dysfunction and are manifested by photosensitivity, photopsia, glare, reduced central vision, and impaired color perception. Paraneoplastic optic neuropathies are less common but also associated with SCLC. Often, paraneoplastic syndromes are associated with myelopathy and cerebellar degeneration. Patients may present with painless vision loss over days to weeks (Rahimy & Sarraf, 2013).

Radiation therapy can affect the retina, lens, conjunctiva, lacrimal apparatus, optic nerve, and eyelid. Common ocular effects include cataract development, retinopathy, keratoconjunctivitis, optic neuropathy, and visual impairment. The lens is the most radiosensitive structure of the eye and is a common late effect as a result of cataract development. The severity and interval of the development of radiation-induced cataracts are inversely related to dose. A smaller fraction size reduces the overall risk and delays onset. Therefore, a smaller fraction size is recommended to minimize risk. The time of development ranges from six months to many years, with a mean of two to three years. Single fractions of 2,000 cGy or a total dose of 8,000 cGy in divided doses can increase the incidence of cataracts. At higher doses, the development of cataracts can increase to 100% (Sanfilippo & Formenti, 2013). The risk also is correlated to age at time of treatment, total dose, and fractionation. In children, an increased risk of cataract development is seen with 1,000 cGy, whereas in adults, the risk increases with doses greater than 2,500 cGy. Cataract development also is very common in patients receiving total body irradiation in the HSCT population (Abdelkawi, 2012; Roberts, Chen, & Seropian, 2013; Sanfilippo & Formenti, 2013). Radiation retinopathy is a late effect of radiation therapy, which slowly progresses to occlusive retinal microangiopathy. Microangiopathy is a disease of the capillaries or very small blood vessels, which become thick and weak and may eventually bleed. The median time to presentation is approximately 2.6 years. Microangiopathy is thought to be caused by radiation injury to the vascular endothelial cells. The predictors of retinopathy are the total dose and fraction size delivered. Patients receiving more than 6,000 cGy are at greater risk. Hyperfractionation, or two fractions per day, has been found to reduce the risk of retinopathy by 50%. Other factors that may increase risk include diabetes and history of antineoplastic agents (Ainsbury et al., 2009; Hager & Seitz, 2014; Sanfilippo & Formenti, 2013).

Optic neuropathy is another late effect of radiation, which is also dose dependent. It may present months to years after radiation therapy, with a peak incidence in 18 months. Optic neuropathy is thought to be caused by radiation injury to the nerve fibers and usually presents as visual field deficits. The risk appears to increase with age, especially age older than 50

(Sanfilippo & Formenti, 2013). Other radiation-induced effects include lid epithelioma, lacrimal duct atrophy, dry eye, ptosis, orbital hypoplasia (decreased development of the orbit), and keratoconjunctivitis (ocular surface infection) (Pihos, 2013). These are all associated with total dose of radiation therapy greater than 5,000 cGy. Lid epithelioma is an eyelid mass, which is usually benign.

Chemotherapy or antineoplastic agents also can cause ocular toxicities. The ocular organs have a high degree of sensitivity to chemotherapy agents. The ocular toxicities are dependent on antineoplastic agent, dose, cumulative dose, and route of administration. Intra-arterial and intrathecal administration carry the greatest risk. Additional risk factors include concurrent use of other high-risk ocular toxic drugs and renal and hepatic insufficiency (Hager & Seitz, 2014; Livshits et al., 2014). The exact mechanism is not well understood, but the toxicities are thought to be caused by direct damage to the ocular structures. Possible effects of chemotherapy include cataract development, retinal opacities, lid and lacrimal disorders, optic neuritis, and inflammatory conditions such as blepharitis, conjunctivitis, uveitis, keratitis, and iritis (Agustoni et al., 2014). Targeted agents also cause ocular symptoms, including blepharitis, trichomegaly, conjunctivitis, dry eye, and epiphora. In addition, novel immunotherapy agents can cause ocular toxicity, although they are rare and reported in less than 1% of patients. These toxicities include uveitis, episcleritis, photophobia, pain, dryness of the eyes, and blurred vision (Howell, Lee, Bowyer, Fusi, & Lorigan, 2015). See Table 14-11 for details on common ocular toxicities caused by various chemotherapy agents, including targeted agents and immunotherapy.

Patients who have undergone HSCT also are at risk for ocular toxicities. In addition to the increased risk for cataracts, patients who undergo an allogeneic transplant are at risk for ocular GVHD. This occurs when the GVHD attacks the ocular tissue. The exact mechanism is not completely understood but is thought to be related to fibrous formation and atrophy of conjunctiva and cornea. Presenting symptoms include dry, painful, burning, irritated eyes; photophobia; blurred vision; and difficulty opening eyes in the morning secondary to secretions (Johnson, 2013; Shikari, Antin, & Dana, 2013).

Medications such as anticholinergics and antiepileptics also may affect ocular function by causing dryness of the eyes (Blomquist, 2011; Livshits et al., 2014). In addition, the use of steroids is very common in the oncology population and is linked to the development of increased ocular pressure, leading to glaucoma, cataracts, infection, and blurred vision. Bisphosphonate therapy is shown to cause ocular inflammation leading to conjunctivitis, uveitis, and keratitis (Kheir et al., 2014).

Prevention Strategies

The development of ocular symptoms is based on the cancer itself, the type of cancer-related treatment modalities used, and the supportive care therapies employed. It is important that APNs have a good understanding and knowledge of the potential ocular effects from cancer-related treatments. No known preventive measures exist for ocular toxicities, but various interventions may minimize the severity. The severity of ocular toxicity is based on various factors, which include the type of chemotherapy agent, the cumulative dose, the location of radiation therapy, the total dose and fraction size of radiation therapy, the presence of other comorbid medical conditions, and the patient's age. In the radiation arena, cataract development is best minimized by fractionation of radiation dose. Smaller fraction size is recommended. Customized lens shielding is not recommended during total body irradiation because of the risk of retro-ocular relapse in leukemia (Roberts et al., 2013). In addition, patients must be diligent about ongoing ophthalmology follow-up.

Table 14-11. Ocular Toxicities Associated With Chemotherapy, Targeted Therapy, and Immunotherapy Agents

Agent	Ocular Side Effects/Toxicities	Nursing Considerations
Antiandrogens	Eye pain Dry eyes Blurred vision Photosensitivity	Nilutamide can cause night blindness.
BCNU/carmustine	Blurred vision Conjunctival hyperemia Vision loss and microvascular changes with concurrent cisplatin and cyclophosphamide	Ocular symptoms occur in 70% of patients receiving intracarotid therapy.
BRAF inhibitors (e.g., sorafenib, vemurafenib, dabrafenib)	Development of solitary or multiple squamous cell carcinomas including near eyes	Squamous cell carcinomas develop in 6%–11% of patients on dabrafenib and 26% of patients on vemurafenib. Examine skin and eyelids on regular basis.
Busulfan	Cataracts Blurred vision Keratoconjunctivitis	Incidence and severity of cataracts increase with duration and total dose of therapy. Most common type is posterior subcapsular cataract. Mean duration to development is 113.5 months.
Capecitabine	Eye irritation	Ocular irritation occurs in 10% of patients.
Carboplatin	Blurred vision and blindness with intracarotid administration	Ocular effects are rare with carboplatin.
Cetuximab	Blepharitis Dry eye Trichomegaly (increased eyelash growth) Conjunctivitis Squamous blepharitis	
Chlorambucil	Keratitis	
Cisplatin	Toxicities related to neurotoxicity including neuritis, papilledema, blurred vision, and blindness High-dose therapy: Irreversible vision changes including changes in color vision and ocular pigment changes	Toxicities are associated with all routes of administration.

(Continued on next page)

Table 14-11. Ocular Toxicities Associated With Chemotherapy, Targeted Therapy, and Immunotherapy Agents *(Continued)*

Agent	Ocular Side Effects/Toxicities	Nursing Considerations
Cyclophosphamide	Blurred vision Keratoconjunctivitis Blepharoconjunctivitis (inflammation of eyelid and conjunctiva) Epiphora (excessive watering of eyes) Cataracts	–
Cytarabine	Excreted in tears, causing keratitis in high doses (corneal inflammation)	–
Docetaxel	Excreted in tears, causing eye irritation Canalicular inflammation and blockage of tear ducts with epiphora (excessive tearing) Erosive conjunctivitis Punctal stenosis	Weekly docetaxel is associated with epiphora and canalicular stenosis.
Doxorubicin	Increased tearing and conjunctivitis (rare)	–
Epidermal growth factor receptor inhibitors (e.g., cetuximab, gefitinib, panitumumab)	Trichomegaly	Trichomegaly develops 8–12 weeks after initiation of therapy.
Fludarabine	Associated with high doses	–
5-Fluorouracil	Drug excreted in tears Blurred vision Ocular pain Photophobia Itching Burning Excessive lacrimation Irreversible epiphora from canalicular obstruction Neuro-ophthalmologic toxicities such as nystagmus, neuropathy, and diplopia	Ocular toxicity occurs in 25%–38% of patients receiving single-agent or combined 5-fluorouracil.
Ifosfamide	Blurred vision Conjunctivitis	–
Imatinib	Periorbital edema Epiphora Subconjunctival hemorrhage	–

(Continued on next page)

Table 14-11. Ocular Toxicities Associated With Chemotherapy, Targeted Therapy, and Immunotherapy Agents *(Continued)*

Agent	Ocular Side Effects/Toxicities	Nursing Considerations
Immunotherapy agents (immune checkpoint inhibitors) • CTLA-4 inhibitors (e.g., ipilimumab, tremelimumab) • Anti–PD-1 antibodies (e.g., nivolumab, pembrolizumab, pidilizumab [CT-011]) • Anti–PD-L1 antibodies (e.g., MPDL3280A, BMS-936559, MEDI4736)	Photophobia Eye pain Dryness of eyes Blurred vision Uveitis Episcleritis (inflammatory condition affecting the episcleral tissue that lies between the sclera and conjunctiva)	Toxicity is reported in less than 1% of patients and usually occurs after two months of therapy.
Interferon	Neuropathy Retinopathy Retinal hemorrhage	—
Methotrexate	Excreted in tears Edema, pain, blurred vision, light sensitivity, conjunctivitis, and reduced tears Epiphora, reversible or irreversible	High-dose ocular toxicity occurs in 25% of patients within 2–7 days after IV administration. Intrathecal administration is associated with optic neuropathy.
Mitomycin C	Blurred vision	—
Oxaliplatin	May be related to neurotoxicity Pain, changes in vision and ptosis	—
Paclitaxel	Sensation of flashing lights during administration May be associated with vascular toxicity	—
Retinoids	Blepharoconjunctivitis Opacity of cornea Night blindness	—
Steroids	Infection Cataracts Glaucoma Blurred vision Retinal hemorrhage	Ocular toxicities are very common.
Tamoxifen	Corneal deposits Cataracts Retinopathy Keratopathy Decreased vision Neuritis Retinal hemorrhage	Corneal deposits develop in up to 72% of patients being treated with 20 mg/day for at least 6 months.

(Continued on next page)

Table 14-11. Ocular Toxicities Associated With Chemotherapy, Targeted Therapy, and Immunotherapy Agents *(Continued)*

Agent	Ocular Side Effects/Toxicities	Nursing Considerations
Trastuzumab	Dry eyes Increased tearing Blurred vision Conjunctivitis	–
Vinca alkaloids	Can cause cranial nerve neuro-toxicity, leading to symptoms of optic neuropathy, palsies, ptosis, vision loss, and night blindness	–

CTLA-4—cytotoxic T-lymphocyte associated antigen 4; PD-L1—programmed death-ligand 1; PD-1—programmed cell death protein 1

Note. Based on information from Agustoni et al., 2014; Bristol-Myers Squibb Co., 2011; Foroozan, 2010; Hager & Seitz, 2014; Howell et al., 2015; Kheir et al., 2014; Livshits et al., 2014; Naidoo et al., 2014; Pruitt, 2010; van der Noll et al., 2013.

Diagnosis and Assessment

APNs should consider referring patients, especially those with a history of eye disorders, diseases, or comorbidities such as hypertension or diabetes, for a baseline ocular examination. APNs should assess patients at baseline and prior to each treatment for ocular toxicities. Patients must be taught the signs and symptoms of ocular toxicities and instructed on the need to report them immediately. Patients who report a history of eye disease should be referred to an ophthalmologist. The diagnosis, assessment, and treatment of ocular disorders require immediate consultation with an ophthalmologist to perform an examination that includes pupil reflex, retinal examination, and an assessment of eye muscle function.

The diagnosis of ocular cancers is detected on routine eye examinations or when patients present with ocular symptoms. A dilated fundus is the most important factor in accurately diagnosing uveal melanoma. Melanomas often appear as pigmented, dome- or collar-button–shaped masses. Ultrasonography is important in diagnosing and monitoring uveal melanomas. The diagnosis of orbital metastases is made through case history, thorough eye examination, and imaging studies such as MRI or CT of the orbits. The diagnosis of ocular paraneoplastic syndromes mirrors the diagnosis of other ocular conditions and includes case history and thorough eye examination.

APNs should examine the conjunctiva for discoloration and moisture. The eyelids are examined for ptosis and the eyelashes for excess growth. An eye chart is used to assess for loss of vision, and color vision cards are helpful in assessing for loss of color vision. In addition, APNs should be suspicious of any new vision or eye complaints by patients because for many of the antineoplastics, ocular side effects and toxicities are uncommon or rarely reported. See Figure 14-2 for more details on history taking and physical examination in assessing ocular toxicities.

For patients at risk for or with ocular side effects and toxicities, patient education is important. When prescribing or caring for patients receiving drugs known to cause ocular toxicity, APNs need to provide drug-appropriate patient education on self-care management strategies for side effects. Dependent on the type and severity of the ocular toxicity, APNs should discuss safety issues such as not driving and being careful while using hazardous objects or while walking to reduce the risk of falling. Loose or hazardous objects such as throw rugs and items that obstruct pathways in the home should be removed or relocated so as to not become hazards.

History Taking Components
- Do you have eye discomfort or pain?
- Do you have dry eyes?
- Do you have any problems with your vision? Decreased visual acuity? Blurred vision? Double vision?
- Do you have sensitivity to light?
- Are your eyes irritated? Itchy? Burning?
- Do you have any drainage from your eyes?
- Do you have excessive tearing?
- Do you see flashing lights?

Physical Examination Highlights
- Inspect eyebrows for quantity, distribution, and dryness.
- Inspect eyelids for edema, color, lesions, condition, and direction of eyelashes, and adequacy and symmetry with which the eyelids close.
- Inspect lacrimal gland and lacrimal sac for swelling. Look for excessive tearing or dryness.
- Inspect conjunctiva and sclera for color, vascular pattern, nodules, and swelling.
- Inspect cornea and lenses for opacity.
- Inspect pupils for size, shape, and symmetry. Test for pupillary reaction to light.
- Assess extraocular eye movements.
- Perform an ophthalmoscopic examination to evaluate the retina, optic disc, arterioles, and veins.
- Perform a visual acuity test using Snellen chart.

Figure 14-2. History Taking and Physical Examination Components

Patients who wear contact lenses should avoid wearing them during therapy with high-dose cytarabine, methotrexate, 5-fluorouracil, and other drugs that are excreted in the tears. Other patients should be informed to immediately stop wearing contact lenses should any ocular effects develop, such as dry eyes or changes in vision. Table 14-12 summarizes the most common ocular toxicities and their presenting symptoms, assessment, and management.

Evidence-Based Treatment Strategies

The treatment of ocular tumors includes surgery and radiation therapy. Uveal melanomas are treated with enucleation for large tumors, but radiation therapy is the mainstay of treatment. The form of radiation therapy used is brachytherapy, also referred to as internal radiation. The commonly used isotope is iodine-125. Another form of radiation commonly used is proton beam radiation therapy (Augsburger, Corrêa, & Shaikh, 2009; Yonekawa & Kim, 2012).

Treatment of orbital metastases is generally performed for palliation and can include surgery, chemotherapy, hormonal therapy, and radiation therapy. Radiation therapy to the orbits is the mainstay of treatment for most patients. The total dose generally ranges from 2,000 to 4,000 cGy over two to four weeks (Ng & Ilsen, 2010). The management of ocular paraneoplastic syndromes includes treating the underlying disease, which is consistent with how other paraneoplastic syndromes are treated.

High-dose cytarabine ocular toxicities such as corneal irritation, eye pain, tearing, photophobia, blurred vision, conjunctival hyperemia, and foreign body sensation are common. Management includes glucocorticoid eyedrops to be initiated before high-dose therapy. This has been shown to decrease and even prevent the development of conjunctivitis or photophobia. Also, the combined use of saline eye washing with instillation of 0.1% sodium betamethasone phosphate eyedrops has been effective (Foroozan, 2010; Mori et al., 2011).

Docetaxel has also been associated with ocular toxicities secondary to secretion of drug in tears leading to epiphora, which causes inflammation of the lacrimal outflow system, fibrosis, and then canalicular stenosis. Epiphora is manifested by eye irritation, conjunctivitis, and tearing. Patients undergoing weekly docetaxel therapy have a 64% chance of developing epiphora, whereas those receiving docetaxel every three weeks have a 31% chance of developing epiphora (Esmaeli & Valero, 2013; Kheir et al., 2014; Zaveri & Cohen, 2014). Management of epiphora

Table 14-12. Diagnosis and Management of Common Ocular Toxicities

Ocular Condition	Presenting Symptoms	Diagnosis	Management
Blepharoconjunctivitis (conjunctivitis and inflammation of eyelid)	Red eyes Swelling of conjunctiva Epiphora	Physical exam	Topical or ophthalmologic drops or ointments
Cataracts	Decreased vision Glare	Visual acuity test	Surgical removal
Dry eyes	Itching Burning Tired eyes	Physical exam Schirmer test to determine if tear glands produce enough tears. (Calibrated strips of nontoxic filter paper are placed within lower eyelid. Both eyes are tested at same time. Patients are asked to keep eyes closed for 5 minutes. Wetting of less than 5 mm indicates deficient tear production.)	Artificial tears Topical steroids Topical cyclosporine
Excessive lacrimation (epiphora)/canalicular stenosis	Excessive tears Conjunctivitis Erythema and irritation of eyelid	Ophthalmic exam Schirmer test	Topical steroids Surgical procedures: Bicanalicular intubation (stent placed within lacrimal duct) or dacryocystorhinostomy (procedure that eliminates fluid and mucus from the lacrimal duct)
Graft-versus-host disease	Keratoconjunctivitis Dry, irritated eyes Photophobia Blurred vision	Physical exam Schirmer test Cytology	Preservative-free eyedrops Selective muscarinic agonists (pilocarpine, cevimeline orally) Cyclosporine eyedrops Topical steroids
Keratoconjunctivitis (combination of conjunctivitis and corneal inflammation)	Itching Ropy discharge Burning Photophobia Decreased vision	Physical exam	Topical/ophthalmologic drops or ointment Cyclosporine/tacrolimus ointment
Optic neuropathy	Vision loss Visual field deficits	Magnetic resonance imaging of the brain, including optic apparatus	No effective treatment
Retinopathy	Blurred vision Visual field changes	Ophthalmic exam Fluorescein angiography	Periodic follow-up if asymptomatic Laser therapy
Trichomegaly	Curling, lengthening, and rigidity of eyelashes	Physical assessment	No effective treatment

(Continued on next page)

Table 14-12. Diagnosis and Management of Common Ocular Toxicities (Continued)

Ocular Condition	Presenting Symptoms	Diagnosis	Management
Uveitis/episcle-ritis	Ocular pain Redness Photophobia Excessive tearing Decreased vision	Physical exam Ophthalmic exam	Topical steroids, usually prednisolone 1% for grade 1–2 toxicity; systemic corticosteroids and discontinuation of immunotherapy for grade 3–4 toxicity

Note. Based on information from Agustoni et al., 2014; Bielory & Bielory, 2010; Chen et al., 2014; Foroozan, 2010; Hager & Seitz, 2014; Howell et al., 2015; Johnson, 2013; Kheir et al., 2014; Pruitt, 2010.

includes a baseline ophthalmologic examination with probing and irrigation of the canalicular or nasolacrimal ducts by an ophthalmologist prior to the start of docetaxel. Epiphora resulting from docetaxel may respond to tobramycin 0.3% and dexamethasone 0.1% (TobraDex®, Alcon Laboratories, 2011) eyedrops administered in a combination solution, one drop four times a day for seven days followed by a tapering regimen over four weeks (Esmaeli & Valero, 2013). If the drops are effective, ongoing reevaluations by the ophthalmologist are needed every four to six weeks. If these medications are not effective, surgical intervention, such as probing and irrigation, may reveal narrowed canaliculi. Silicone tubes may be placed in the canaliculi to promote reabsorption of tears. Additional surgery and glass tube placement may be needed in severe cases (Esmaeli & Valero, 2013; Zaveri & Cohen, 2014). Artificial tears may be useful for dry eyes associated with docetaxel administration (Kheir et al., 2014; Zaveri & Cohen, 2014).

Evaluation of Outcomes

Patients should be monitored for ocular symptoms at diagnosis and for ocular toxicities prior to each treatment and at each follow-up appointment. Patients require follow-up with an ophthalmologist as recommended.

Implications for Oncology Advanced Practice Nurses

APNs need to maintain a high degree of suspicion for the development of ocular toxicities in patients with a new eye complaint and for patients receiving drugs associated with eye toxicities. Some ocular toxicities, their prevention, and treatment strategies are known, but for many agents, ocular side effects are rare or were previously reported as single case studies. Patients should have pretreatment ophthalmologic examinations when receiving drugs with known ocular toxicities.

Dermatologic Toxicities

Definition and Incidence

Dermatologic symptoms are common in the oncology population and can be related to the cancer itself; cancer-related treatment modalities such as chemotherapy, radiation therapy, and HSCT; and other medications commonly used in the cancer population. Dermatologic toxicities have gained more attention over the past several years with the advent of targeted therapies in the treatment of various cancers. Dermatologic toxicities can be disfiguring and cause interruption in treatment, especially when caused by combination radiation and chemotherapy. Toxicities may affect the hair, nails, and skin. When the skin barrier is compromised, patients are more susceptible to infection, more sensitive to allergens, and more vulnerable to radiation skin side effects (Bensadoun et al., 2013).

Cancer treatment–related dermatologic toxicities are caused by the acute and chronic effects of radiation therapy, chemotherapy, and HSCT. The majority of patients diagnosed with cancer will receive some form of chemotherapy, and approximately 66% of patients will receive radiation therapy throughout the cancer trajectory (American Society for Radiation Oncology, 2012). More than 90% of patients receiving radiation therapy will develop some type of skin reaction (McQuestion, 2010). The incidence of chemotherapy-induced dermatologic toxicities has increased and is dependent on the chemotherapy agents or regimen and the duration of therapy. Since the advent of targeted therapies and immunotherapy, the incidence of dermatologic side effects has increased (Robert, Sibaud, Mateus, & Cherpelis, 2012). Among recipients of HSCT, the most common dermatologic toxicity is GVHD. It is estimated that of the patients undergoing allogeneic HSCT, 20%–70% will develop acute GVHD and 60%–70% will develop chronic GVHD (Hymes, Alousi, & Cowen, 2012; Latchford, 2010). In addition, many medications cause cutaneous reactions, and it is estimated that 75%–95% of skin reactions are related to medications (Witt & Young, 2010).

Etiology and Presenting Signs and Symptoms

Paraneoplastic syndromes of the skin are considered dermatoses that are associated with malignancy (Silva & Danson, 2013). Some examples of dermatoses include acanthosis nigricans, dermatomyositis, paraneoplastic pemphigus, and Sweet syndrome. Acanthosis nigricans has been associated with adenocarcinomas but particularly GI malignancies. Dermatomyositis appears to be a precursor in the development of cancer and may be seen in breast, lung, gastric, genitourinary, and ovarian cancers. Paraneoplastic pemphigus has been identified in a variety of lymphoproliferative disorders such as non-Hodgkin lymphoma and chronic lymphocytic leukemia. Sweet syndrome is a prototype of the neutrophilic dermatoses. It is most commonly associated with acute myeloid leukemia but also can be drug induced by granulocyte–colony-stimulating factor and all-trans-retinoic acid (Shah, Jack, Liu, & Hopkins, 2011; Silva & Danson, 2013).

Dermatologic effects and toxicities produced by cancer therapy can occur with radiation therapy, chemotherapy agents, targeted agents, immunotherapy, and HSCT. Radiation-related skin reactions are common and are caused by the effect of radiation on rapidly dividing cells, which includes the integument. The epidermis is a radiosensitive organ and includes the outer cornified layer and the deeper basal layer, which are continually dividing. The basal layer of the epidermis contains stem cells that divide and differentiate into mature skin cells. The dermis, which is underlying the epidermis, contains blood vessels, nerves, glands, and hair follicles. With radiation, a fixed number of basal cells are damaged. The remaining cells become cornified and shed, leading to an imbalance of cells being damaged and those being produced. In addition, an inflammatory response occurs with the release of histamine and serotonin. Simultaneously, a vascular response with extracapillary cell injury and capillary dilation occurs. Radiation therapy also affects other constituents of the skin, such as the hair follicles and sweat and sebaceous glands. The hair follicles enter the resting phase of the cycle cell, and hair growth ceases. Sweat and sebaceous glands can be permanently damaged after radiation doses of 30 Gy (McQuestion, 2011). Treatment- and patient-related risk factors also contribute to the development of skin reactions with radiation therapy (see Figure 14-3).

Treatment-Related Risk Factors	Patient-Related Risk Factors
• Large volume of tissue being treated • Type of energy used resulting in higher skin dose (i.e., lower energy photons and electrons) • Use of tangential fields (i.e., breast) • Use of tissue equivalent or bolus material • Total dose of radiation delivered as defined by a larger fraction size (> 200 cGy) • Accelerated fractionation schedule • Longer treatment duration	• Areas of thin or smooth epidermis • Areas of skin-to-skin contact (i.e., skin folds, axillae, face, perineum) • Previous lymphocele aspiration • Areas of compromised skin integrity within the treatment fields • Presence of other medical comorbidities such as diabetes or renal failure • Poor nutritional status • Older age • Ethnicity • Concurrent chemotherapy, immunotherapy, or targeted therapy with radiation therapy • Other factors: Chronic sun and environmental exposure, smoking history

Figure 14-3. Treatment- and Patient-Related Risk Factors in the Development of Radiation Therapy–Associated Skin Reactions

Note. Based on information from McQuestion, 2010, 2011.

Radiation skin reactions are classified as acute or late/chronic effects. Acute effects are those that occur within the first three months of radiation therapy, whereas late effects may take months to years to develop after radiation therapy is completed. Late effects of radiation therapy have been associated with larger total dose and volume of irradiated tissue, fraction size greater than 200 cGy, history of prior or concurrent chemotherapy, older age, poor performance status, medical comorbidities such as diabetes and connective tissue disease, presence of radiation fibrosis, and presence of vascular and neural changes, as well as endocrine and growth-related factors (McQuestion, 2011). See Tables 14-13 and 14-14 for more details on acute and late skin reactions resulting from radiation therapy.

Dermatologic cells, including the skin, hair follicles, and nail matrix, are rapidly dividing cells and are vulnerable to chemotherapy, targeted agents, and immunotherapy. The most common dermatologic side effects with epidermal growth factor receptor (EGFR) inhibitors include papulopustular reactions, dry skin, nail alterations, alopecia, and anagen effluvium, the loss of growth-phase hairs. Hormonal therapy causes dry skin, hair alterations, and nail alterations. Novel immunotherapy agents, including ipilimumab and nivolumab, most commonly cause maculopapular rash, pruritus, hair depigmentation, and vitiligo (Choi, 2014; Howell et al., 2015). Traditional chemotherapy most often yields dry skin, hair changes, and nail alterations (Fabbrocini et al., 2012; Livshits et al., 2014). Alopecia is a common skin manifestation of systemic chemotherapy. Antineoplastic agents affect rapidly growing hair cells, also referred to as cells within the anagen phase. Chemotherapy causes the hair shaft to become more fragile, thus resulting in breakage. Some chemotherapy or higher doses of other chemotherapy can cause complete mitotic arrest, which results in atrophy of the hair root and loss of hair root bulbs. Other drugs cause bulb deformity and narrowing of hair shafts. The mechanism of hair loss is usually spontaneous, or hair is lost during combing or shampooing. The degree of hair loss varies from thinning hair to complete hair loss. The most common area for hair loss is the scalp; other hair follicles are usually less active and not as readily affected, such as the eyebrows, axillae, and pubic region. Alopecia depends on the type of chemotherapy, the use of combination of drugs, dosage, and the frequency and route of administration (Chon, Champion, Geddes, & Rashid, 2012). The use of bolus IV chemotherapy agents has immediate peak

Table 14-13. Acute Skin Reactions of Radiation Therapy

Skin Effect	Pathophysiology	Presenting Signs and Symptoms
Erythema	Result of capillary dilation in the dermis accompanied by edema	Generally occurs within the 2–3 weeks of radiation therapy Transient erythema can occur within 24 hours of starting radiation therapy Varying degrees of redness of skin in irradiated area
Hyperpigmentation	Melanin migration to the epidermal surface	Generally occurs after 2–4 weeks of beginning radiation therapy Varying degrees of tanning of irradiated skin
Dry desquamation	Decreased ability of basal layer to replace surface layers, causing epidermis to shed	Flaking of skin and dryness with potential for peeling
Moist desquamation	Extracapillary cell damage caused by increased capillary blood flow, hyperemia, and edema. This can result in dermal exposure with moistness, tenderness, redness, oozing, and leakage of serous fluid from radiation field. Risk factors include skin fold areas (i.e., axillae, inframammary area, groin).	Sloughing of skin with exudate and associated pain

Note. Based on information from Baney, 2011; Baney et al., 2011; McQuestion, 2010, 2011.

serum levels, which results in hair loss. IV infusions over several hours to days are associated with greater risk for alopecia. Low-dose IV infusions have a lesser risk for alopecia (Chon et al., 2012; Komen, Smorenburg, van den Hurk, & Nortier, 2013).

Hand-foot syndrome is also referred to as *palmar-plantar erythrodysesthesia* or *acral erythema.* The pathophysiology is not completely understood, but it is theorized to be caused by a direct toxic effect on the vasculature of the epidermis and dermis or by the accumulation of the chemotherapy agent in eccrine structures, leading to erythema of the palms and soles. The mechanism for hyperpigmentation is thought to be related to the toxic effects of chemotherapy on the melanocytes (Degen et al., 2010).

The pathophysiology of chemotherapy extravasation is caused by direct cellular toxicity when the toxic agent inadvertently leaks into surrounding tissue, but the exact sequence of injury is unknown and may be different for various agents. Risk factors for extravasation include administration device, type of treatment, patient-related characteristics, and clinician-related characteristics. Chemotherapy classified as an irritant will not cause tissue necrosis, but if chemotherapy is classified as a vesicant, some amount of tissue necrosis will occur (Fidalgo et al., 2012). A current listing of chemotherapy irritants and vesicants can be found in the ONS's *Chemotherapy and Biotherapy Guidelines and Recommendations for Practice* (Polovich, Olsen, & LeFebvre, 2014). Table 14-15 provides more details on the most common dermatologic toxicities and their causative chemotherapy agents.

Targeted therapies are relatively new agents being used in the treatment of various cancers. These therapies have emerged because of a better understanding of cellular processes, in particular tumor growth and development. These agents assist in preventing tumors from growing, metastasizing, and interfering with the patient's immune system. These targeted agents can be used as monotherapy or in combination with conventional chemotherapy. Their mechanism of action is targeted toward the cell membrane receptors, signaling pathways and proteins, enzymatic activity, and regulatory cell growth. It is proposed that these factors are aberrant or more prevalent in cancer cells than normal cells (Boucher, Olson, & Piperdi, 2011; Chanprapaph, Vachiramon, & Rattanakaemakorn, 2014; Fabbrocini et al., 2012; Robert et al., 2012).

The human epidermal growth factor receptor (HER1), also referred to as EGFR, plays a role in normal differentiation and development of epidermal keratinocytes, stimulating epidermal growth, inhibiting differentiation and inflammation, protecting against ultraviolet damage, and assisting in quicker wound healing. EGFR is expressed on normal epidermal and follicular keratinocytes, the basal layer of the epidermis, the outer root of the hair follicle, the sebaceous epithelium, the eccrine epithelium, and some connective tissues. The most common cancers that overexpress EGFR include head and neck, colorectal, breast, cervical, renal, esophageal, and lung. Overexpression of EGFR is found in up to 80% of non-small cell lung cancers (Silva & Danson, 2013). Skin manifestations are common in therapies that target epidermal growth factor signaling and pathways. The exact mechanism of rash development with agents is unknown, but it is suggested to be related to the inhibition of human keratinocytes. The cutaneous reactions are thought to be related to the inhibition of EGFR, which alters kera-

Table 14-14. Late Skin Effects of Radiation Therapy

Skin Effect	Pathophysiology	Presenting Signs and Symptoms
Photosensitivity	Destruction of melanocytes in the irradiated dermis, which reduces the skin's ability to protect itself from ultraviolet rays	Enhanced erythema of skin exposed to ultraviolet rays from direct sunlight and/or tanning beds
Xerosis	Caused by cutaneous injury to skin	Chronic dryness of irradiated area
Hypopigmentation Hyperpigmentation	Results from damage to melanocytes	Pigmentation changes may be hypopigmented (loss of pigment) or hyperpigmented (tanning effect).
Telangiectasia	Caused by damage and stretching of small blood vessels, which may occur if moist desquamation occurred during RT. Dose and fraction dependent.	Telangiectasia is characterized by reddened spider-like veins that are superficial.
Atrophy	Newly formed epidermis is thinner	Thin and fragile epidermis
Fibrosis	Fibroblasts, which are responsible for producing collagen, proliferate as a result of a cytokine cascade that causes increased extracellular matrix leading to development of fibrosis	Dense, hard, and uneven skin texture May appear as induration, thickened dermis, and edema.
Ulceration and necrosis	Same pathophysiology as fibrosis and impaired wound healing	Painful ulcers with red, raised edges and necrotic base. Usually shows little to no epithelialization or contractility.

Note. Based on information from Baney, 2011; Baney et al., 2011; McQuestion, 2010, 2011.

tinocyte proliferation, differentiation, and migration. Both monoclonal antibodies and small molecule tyrosine kinase inhibitors interfere with EGFR (Boucher et al., 2011; Eaby-Sandy & Lynch, 2014).

Dermatologic side effects of targeted therapies include papulopustular reaction, xerosis/pruritus, hand-foot syndrome, subungual splinter hemorrhages, fissures, telangiectasia, hyperpigmentation, hair changes, and paronychia with pyrogenic granuloma. Papulopustular reac-

Table 14-15. Common Dermatologic Effects of Chemotherapy and Their Causative Agents

Skin Manifestation	Pathophysiology and Presenting Symptoms	Causative Agents
Alopecia	Begins within 2–3 weeks of chemotherapy initiation Hair loss is temporary and reversible. Regrowth of hair generally takes 3–5 months but complete hair regrowth may take up to 1–2 years after chemotherapy is discontinued. Changes in hair color (lighter/darker), hair texture (thinner/coarser), and hair type (curly/straight) may be apparent with hair regrowth. Varying degrees of alopecia are described as minimal, moderate, or severe. Hair loss may be asymptomatic with the exception of psychological pain. Some patients may experience scalp itching and discomfort within 1–2 days prior to alopecia and during period of hair loss.	Bleomycin Cyclophosphamide Cytarabine Dactinomycin Daunorubicin Docetaxel Doxorubicin Etoposide 5-Fluorouracil Idarubicin Ifosfamide Interferon Irinotecan Mechlorethamine Methotrexate Mitoxantrone Paclitaxel Vincristine
Hand-foot syndrome	Dose and duration related Characterized by demarcated, tender erythematous plaques on palms of hands and soles of feet. Associated with pain and tingling of hands and feet which progresses to edema, erythema, tenderness to touch, and desquamation.	Capecitabine Docetaxel 5-Fluorouracil Liposomal doxorubicin
Hyperpigmentation	Discoloration of the skin, nails, and mucous membranes A common site is the nail surface, either transversely or longitudinally. Discoloration of the teeth The degree of hyperpigmentation can occur locally around the site of administration or generalized. Hyperpigmentation is common in darker skin. Hyperpigmented streaking of veins that are used for 5-fluorouracil infusion without evidence of extravasation or chemical phlebitis	Bleomycin Busulfan Carmustine Cyclophosphamide Dactinomycin Daunorubicin Doxorubicin Fluorouracil Hydroxyurea Methotrexate Thiotepa
Macular-papular rash	Characterized by ill-defined erythematous, macular-papular rash with associated pruritus	Bortezomib Docetaxel Gemcitabine Paclitaxel

(Continued on next page)

Table 14-15. Common Dermatologic Effects of Chemotherapy and Their Causative Agents *(Continued)*

Skin Manifestation	Pathophysiology and Presenting Symptoms	Causative Agents
Nail dystrophies	Dystrophies are transient and resolve slowly when treatment is discontinued. Complete resolution may take up to six months. Hyperpigmentation is common and occurs most often in African American individuals. The pattern of pigmentation is generally at the base of the nail and causes transverse ridges. Hyperpigmentation may be accompanied by nail raising and paronychia. Paronychia is an inflammation of the nail fold and is frequently caused by bacteria or fungus. Onycholysis, or partial separation of the nail plate, may also occur.	Bleomycin Capecitabine Cyclophosphamide Docetaxel Doxorubicin Paclitaxel Pemetrexed
Radiation recall	Acute inflammatory reaction confined to previously irradiated areas that can be triggered when certain chemotherapy agents are administered after RT Causes erythema, maculopapular eruptions, vesicular development, and desquamation within the previously irradiated site Can range from a mild rash to severe skin necrosis	Actinomycin D Bleomycin Capecitabine Carboplatin Cisplatin Dacarbazine Docetaxel Doxorubicin Etoposide Fluorouracil Gemcitabine Hydroxyurea Ifosfamide Interferon Melphalan Methotrexate Mitomycin Oxaliplatin Paclitaxel Tamoxifen Vinblastine Vinorelbine Other drugs: Antimicrobials, immunotherapy drugs, hormonal agents
Hypersensitivity	Type I hypersensitivity reactions can cause urticaria, angioedema, or anaphylaxis. Asparaginase reactions most commonly cause acute urticarial. Hypersensitivity reactions with paclitaxel are manifested with rash, hypotension, dyspnea, and bronchospasms.	Asparaginase Carboplatin Cisplatin Docetaxel Etoposide Mechlorethamine Oxaliplatin Paclitaxel

(Continued on next page)

Table 14-15. Common Dermatologic Effects of Chemotherapy and Their Causative Agents (Continued)

Skin Manifestation	Pathophysiology and Presenting Symptoms	Causative Agents
Chemotherapy extravasation	Infrequent side effect of chemotherapy administration Occurs in about 0.01%–7% of patients receiving peripheral IV chemotherapy and 0.3%–4.7% of patients with central venous access devices Inadvertent leakage of a drug or solution from a vein or unintentional injection into surrounding healthy, normal tissues, leading to skin and tissue damage Ranges from mild to severe tissue destruction, including erythema and ulceration Full-thickness skin necrosis with damage to underlying tendons, muscles, and neurovascular structures also can occur.	Vesicant agents: Cisplatin Dactinomycin Daunorubicin Doxorubicin Epirubicin Idarubicin Mechlorethamine Melphalan Mitomycin Paclitaxel Vinblastine Vincristine Vindesine Vinorelbine

Note. Based on information from Balagula et al., 2011; Burris & Hurtig, 2010; Chon et al., 2012; Dest, 2010; Fidalgo et al., 2012; Livshits et al., 2014; Vultaggio & Castells, 2014.

tion is the most common side effect of targeted therapies. The rash appears to be dose dependent and occurs in 45%–100% of patients (Chanprapaph et al., 2013; Fabbrocini et al., 2012; Qiao & Fang, 2012; Robert et al., 2012; Urban & Anadkat, 2013). The etiology and pathology of these rashes is unclear, so clinicians need to describe rashes in terms of appearance and location. Recommended terminology includes *pustular/papular rash*, *pustular eruption*, or *follicular and intrafollicular eruption* (Belum, Cercek, Sanz-Motilva, & Lacouture, 2013). Some clinicians may refer to this rash as *acneform*, which is considered incorrect by many experts. The mechanism of the rash is related to the role of EGFR in epidermal and pilosebaceous follicle homeostasis. A positive correlation exists between the occurrence and intensity of the rash and tumor response and overall survival (Robert et al., 2012). See Table 14-16 for more details on the dermatologic toxicities caused by targeted agents and Table 14-17 for details on specific targeted drugs, their indications, and the most common dermatologic effects.

The newest agents in cancer are the inhibitors of PD-1 or PD-L1, which allow cancers to be destroyed by the immune system by inhibiting cell surface proteins that tumor cells and tumor-infiltrating myeloid cells can express to inactivate T lymphocytes. Dermatologic effects of novel immunotherapy agents include maculopapular rash, pruritus, vitiligo, and hair depigmentation (Howell et al., 2015; Naidoo, Page, & Wolchok, 2014). See Table 14-18 for details on specific immunotherapy agents, common dermatologic effects, and management.

HSCT has made incredible progress since its implementation in clinical practice in the late 1960s with improved survival and decreased morbidity and mortality. Despite increased survival, patients can experience serious side effects and complications, specifically dermatologic effects, which occur in the allogeneic population. *Allogeneic* means the graft comes from a donor. Common dermatologic complications in this population include acute GVHD, chronic GVHD, and hand-foot syndrome. See Chapter 7 for a summary of pathophysiology, risk factors, and clinical manifestations of GVHD (Hymes et al., 2012; Latchford, 2010). Hand-foot syndrome also occurs in this population but is not as well documented as it is with some chemotherapy agents. The pathophysiology in HSCT is not well understood but is thought to be

Table 14-16. Common Dermatologic Effects of Targeted Agents

Skin Manifestation	Presenting Symptoms
Papulopustular reaction	Reaction occurs in more seborrheic areas and generally appears on the face, neck, shoulders, upper trunk, and scalp. Reaction is characterized by the presence of papulopustular lesions but very different from comedones or lesions associated with acne vulgaris. Rash may also be maculopapular in appearance. Rash is associated with pruritus. Rash typically appears within 1–3 weeks of the initiation of therapy and reaches its peak by 3–5 weeks. The severity of the rash is dependent on the agent and dosage. It has been suggested that presence and severity of rash are correlated with therapeutic outcome.
Xerosis/pruritus	Effects present as dry skin with flaking. Patients can experience increased skin fragility, bruising, and swelling over joints with associated fissures leading to increased tenderness. Xerosis/pruritus occurs within 1–3 months of therapy.
Hand-foot syndrome	Syndrome is also called *acral erythema* or *palmar-plantar erythrodysesthesia*. Effects occur on the palms of the hands and soles of the feet. Syndrome is characterized by erythema with associated edema and pain. Development of hand-foot syndrome may also be associated with the formation of hyperkeratosis and desquamation.
Subungual splinter hemorrhages	Single or multiple linear black or brown streaks Painless distal hemorrhages under the fingernails
Fissures	Altered skin integrity of lateral nail folds and/or distal finger tufts Occurs with paronychia
Telangiectasias	Appears behind the ears and on the face, chest, and extremities. Usually fades with time but may result with some hyperpigmentation
Hyperpigmentation	Hyperpigmentation occurs after resolution of papulopustular rash, or eczema can develop. Incidence may be higher in people with darker skin. Hyperpigmentation can occur in oral mucosa, nails, hair, and even on the back.
Hair changes	Changes are reported within 4–8 weeks of therapy and are transient. Manifestations include changes in scalp hair texture, which usually consists of curlier, more brittle hair and dry, pruritic scalp. Alopecia occurs but is less common. Growth of facial hair and eyelashes may increase. Increased eyelash growth is referred to as trichomegaly. Patients may exhibit curling, lengthening, and rigidity of eyelashes, as well as thickening and rigidity of eyebrows
Paronychia with pyrogenic granuloma	Nail changes are less frequent than rash but occur in 10%–15% of patients and are the second most common adverse reaction in patients receiving epidermal growth factor receptor inhibitors. Usually evident within 4–8 weeks from the initiation of therapy The nail fold of the thumb and great toe usually become inflamed and may develop into a pyogenic granuloma, also referred to as *paronychia*. Another nail manifestation is the formation of subungual splinter hemorrhage, which is a mass of blood that develops under the nail bed. Can lead to loss of nail(s)

Note. Based on information from Chanprapaph et al., 2014; Eaby-Sandy & Lynch, 2014; Fabbrocini et al., 2012; Koll-mannsberger & Mitchell, 2013; Reyes-Habito & Roh, 2014b; Robert et al., 2012; Urban & Anadkat, 2013; Wood, 2009.

Table 14-17. Targeted Therapies and Dermatologic Manifestations

Targeted Agent	Classification of Targeted Agent/ Target Molecule	Cancer Indications	Dermatologic Effect
Axitinib	Multikinase inhibitors	Renal cell	Alopecia Exanthematous eruptions Facial erythema Hand-foot syndrome Rash/desquamation Splinter subungual hemorrhages Xerosis
Bevacizumab	Vascular endothelial growth factor (VEGF) inhibitors	Advanced lung Breast Colorectal Renal cell	Altered wound healing Mucosal bleeding
Cetuximab	Epidermal growth factor receptor (EGFR) inhibitors	Advanced squamous cell carcinoma of head/neck Metastatic colorectal	Paronychia Rash
Dabrafenib	*BRAF* inhibitor	Brain tumors Colorectal Hairy cell leukemia Lung Melanoma Papillary thyroid	Alopecia Development of squamous cell proliferation Hand-foot syndrome Hyperkeratosis Photosensitivity Skin rash
Gefitinib	EGFR inhibitors	Advanced non-small cell lung cancer	Rash Paronychia
Imatinib	*BCR-ABL* inhibitors	Chronic myeloid leukemia	Acute generalized exanthematous pustulosis Photosensitivity Rash Sweet syndrome
Panitumumab	EGFR inhibitors	Metastatic colorectal	Paronychia Rash
Sorafenib	VEGF receptor multikinase inhibitor	Renal cell Hepatocellular	Alopecia Exanthematous eruptions (measles-like lesion) Facial erythema Hand-foot syndrome Rash/desquamation Splinter subungual hemorrhages Xerosis
Sunitinib	VEGF receptor tyrosine kinase inhibitor	Renal cell Gastrointestinal stromal tumor	Hair changes Hand-foot syndrome Maculopapular exanthems Phototoxicity Subungual hemorrhages

(Continued on next page)

Table 14-17. Targeted Therapies and Dermatologic Manifestations *(Continued)*

Targeted Agent	Classification of Targeted Agent/ Target Molecule	Cancer Indications	Dermatologic Effect
Vemurafenib	*BRAF* inhibitor	Brain Colorectal Hairy cell leukemia Lung Melanoma Papillary thyroid	Alopecia Development of squamous cell proliferation Hand-foot syndrome Hyperkeratosis Photosensitivity Skin rash

Note. Based on information from Belum, Patel, et al., 2013; Chanprapaph et al., 2014; Ishak et al., 2013; Robert et al., 2012.

Table 14-18. Immunotherapy Agents, Dermatologic Manifestations, and Management

Immunotherapy Agent	Dermatologic Manifestation	Management
Ipilimumab	Maculopapular rash Pruritus Vitiligo (melanoma-associated hypopigmentation)	Management of rash includes use of topical steroids, with or without antihistamines. Systemic corticosteroids can be used for higher-grade eruptions.
Nivolumab	Rash Pruritus Vitiligo Lichenoid dermatitis Blisters (when combined with ipilimumab)	Management of pruritus includes alcohol-free emollient creams, cool compresses, oatmeal baths, topical corticosteroids, and systemic antihistamines.
Pembrolizumab	Rash Pruritus Vitiligo Lichenoid dermatitis	No known prevention or treatment exists for vitiligo, but sun exposure should be limited to minimize photosensitivity.

Note. Based on information from Choi, 2014; Lacouture et al., 2014.

related to the direct effect of chemotherapy on the dermal structures (Latchford, 2010). See Chapter 7 for more details on dermatologic toxicities seen in the HSCT population.

Many dermatologic side effects can occur with commonly prescribed and administered medications in the oncology population. These range from asymptomatic rash to life-threatening effects, such as with Stevens-Johnson syndrome and toxic epidermal necrolysis. The incidence of drug reactions is higher in patients who are immunosuppressed, which includes patients with HIV, systemic lupus erythematosus, and lymphoma. Older adults also are at increased risk for developing drug eruptions. Different types of drug eruptions exist, but the most common are morbilliform and urticarial reactions. They account for 94% of all drug eruptions (Ahmed, Pritchard, & Reichenberg, 2013). Drug eruptions are classified by clinical and histologic characteristics. See Table 14-19 for details on the different types of cutaneous reactions that can occur with supportive medications used in oncology.

Table 14-19. Types of Cutaneous Reactions Seen With Supportive Medications Used in Oncology

Type of Cutaneous Eruption	Presenting Symptoms	Causative Agents	Management
Morbilliform eruptions	Rash with erythematous macules and/or papules, which can extend into larger plaques. Usually begins on trunk and occurs 1–2 weeks after initiation of causative agent.	Allopurinol Antibiotics: • Aminopenicillins • Cephalosporins • Sulfonamides Anticonvulsants Antihypertensives Anxiolytics Diuretics Nonsteroidal anti-inflammatory drugs (NSAIDs)	Stop causative agent. Administer topical steroids and systemic antihistamines.
Urticarial eruptions	Can be further defined into simple urticarial eruptions, those with angioedema/anaphylaxis, or serum sickness–like reactions. Angioedema consists of edematous, non-urticarial lesions that involve the epidermis, dermis, and subcutaneous tissue. Serum sickness–like reaction includes fever, arthralgia, and urticarial rash and usually presents 1–3 weeks after administration.	Antibiotics are common drugs responsible for urticarial eruptions: • Cephalosporins • Penicillins • Sulfonamides • Tetracyclines Drugs associated with angioedema: • Angiotensin-converting enzyme (ACE) inhibitors • Monoclonal antibodies • NSAIDs • Penicillins • Radiographic contrast media Drugs associated with serum sickness: • Amoxicillin • Ampicillin • Beta-blockers • Bupropion • Cefaclor • Cefprozil • Cephalexin • Ciprofloxacin • Doxycycline • Minocycline • Penicillin • Sulfonamide	Management of urticarial eruptions includes • Discontinue causative agent. • Administer systemic antihistamines. • Administer systemic corticosteroids for severe or refractory cases. Treatment of angioedema includes supportive care, maintaining airway, and epinephrine. Treatment of serum sickness includes discontinuation of causative agent and administration of systemic corticosteroids and antihistamines.

(Continued on next page)

Table 14-19. Types of Cutaneous Reactions Seen With Supportive Medications Used in Oncology *(Continued)*

Type of Cutaneous Eruption	Presenting Symptoms	Causative Agents	Management
Vasculitic eruptions	Caused by inflammation and necrosis of the vessel wall within the dermis and subcutaneous tissues. Presence of eosinophilia assists in confirming drug-induced etiology. Occurs 7–21 days after drug is administered.	Allopurinol Cephalosporins Cimetidine Fluoroquinolones NSAIDs Penicillin Sulfonamides	Discontinue causative agent. Institute leg elevation and compression. Administer colchicine, dapsone, corticosteroids, or immunosuppressants.
Fixed drug eruptions	Circumscribed, pruritic, erythematous, and dusky patches, single or multiple. The hallmark of a fixed drug eruption is geographic memory. Eruptions are most common in the perineal area, genital area, lips, palms of hands, and soles of feet. The reaction usually occurs within 2 days after initiation of causative agent.	Allopurinol Barbiturates Laxatives NSAIDs Sulfonamides Tetracyclines	Discontinue causative agent. Administer topical steroids and supportive care.
Acneform eruptions	Cutaneous reactions to a drug that produce lesions resembling acne vulgaris. Lesions appear as erythematous papules or erythematous pustules. They are not associated with comedones. They are typically seen on the face, trunk, and proximal extremities.	Androgens Corticosteroids Lithium Oral contraceptives	Discontinue causative agent. Apply benzoyl peroxide, topical retinoids, and topical antibiotics.
Acute generalized exanthematous pustulosis	Systemic pustular eruption associated with leukocytosis and fever. The onset is rapid but most commonly occurs in 2–7 days.	Acetylsalicylic acid Allopurinol Aminopenicillins Enalapril Griseofulvin Itraconazole Macrolides Vancomycin	Discontinue causative agent.

(Continued on next page)

Table 14-19. Types of Cutaneous Reactions Seen With Supportive Medications Used in Oncology (Continued)

Type of Cutaneous Eruption	Presenting Symptoms	Causative Agents	Management
Blistering eruptions	Include pemphigus, which consists of flaccid bullae that create crusted erosions; drug-induced bullous pemphigoid, which consists of bullae; and drug-induced linear immunoglobulin A (IgA) bullous dermatosis, which also consists of bullae. They are autoimmune disorders that can be induced by medications.	Drugs associated with pemphigus: • Captopril • Gold sodium thiomalate • Levodopa • Penicillamine • Penicillin • Phenobarbital • Piroxicam • Propranolol • Rifampin Drugs associated with bullous pemphigoid: • ACE inhibitors • Ampicillin • Chloroquine • Furosemide • Penicillin • Psoralen plus ultraviolet A light • Sulfasalazine Drugs associated with linear IgA bullous dermatosis: • Amiodarone • Atorvastatin • Captopril • Ceftriaxone • Diclofenac • Furosemide • Lithium • Metronidazole • Penicillin • Phenytoin • Piroxicam • Rifampin • Trimethoprim-sulfamethoxazole • Vancomycin	Discontinue causative agent. Administer systemic corticosteroids and/or other immunosuppressive agents.
Lichenoid eruptions	Uncommon eruptions that resemble lichen planus with shiny violaceous polygonal papules and plaques. They often occur in sun-exposed areas.	Antimalarials Beta-blockers Gold Lithium Methyldopa NSAIDs Penicillamines Phenylenediamine derivatives Sulfonylureas Thiazide diuretics	Management is symptomatic with topical corticosteroids.

(Continued on next page)

Table 14-19. Types of Cutaneous Reactions Seen With Supportive Medications Used in Oncology (Continued)

Type of Cutaneous Eruption	Presenting Symptoms	Causative Agents	Management
Stevens-Johnson syndrome and toxic epidermal necrolysis	Both are rare but have significantly high mortality rate. They present with erythematous macules, papules, vesicles, or plaques that develop duskiness and progressive bullous changes progressing to epithelial desquamation. The onset occurs 1–3 weeks after initiation of causative medication. Diagnosis is made by skin biopsy.	Allopurinol Aminopenicillins Anticonvulsants Barbiturates Carbamazepine Corticosteroids Lamotrigine NSAIDs Phenobarbital Phenytoin Trimethoprim-sulfamethoxazole Valproic acid	Discontinue causative agent. Hospitalize patients for wound care and symptomatic care. Use emollients and nonstick dressings to denude areas. Broad-spectrum antibiotics are not recommended. Use of steroids and immunomodulatory therapies is controversial.
Hypersensitivity syndrome (also referred to as drug reaction with eosinophilia and systemic symptoms, or DRESS), and drug-induced hypersensitivity syndrome	Presents as polymorphic cutaneous eruptions, which can be morbilliform or erythrodermic. Internal organs may be involved, including the liver, kidneys, heart, and lungs. Eruptions usually occur within 2–6 weeks after initiation of causative agent.	Allopurinol Carbamazepine Dapsone Gold salts Minocycline Phenytoin Sulfonamides Valproic acid	Discontinue causative agent. Institute systemic steroid therapy. Provide referral to various specialties based on organ involvement.

Note. Based on information from Ahmed et al., 2013; Roujeau et al., 2014.

Prevention Strategies

The development of dermatologic symptoms is based on the cancer itself and the type of cancer-related treatment modalities used, as well as supportive care therapies. It is important that APNs have a good understanding and knowledge of the potential dermatologic effects from cancer and cancer-related treatment. Photoprotective measures, such as avoiding the sun during peak midday hours (11 am–2 pm), using sunscreen (sun protection factor [SPF] 30 or greater), wearing protective clothing, and avoiding tanning beds, are recommended to decrease the incidence of nonmelanoma skin cancers and effects of photosensitivity (Council, 2013).

The severity of dermatologic toxicity depends on the type of chemotherapy agent, the use of multiple agents, cumulative dose, the location of radiation therapy, total dose and fraction size of radiation, the presence of other comorbid conditions, and advancing age. With radiation therapy, the use of intensity-modulated radiation therapy (IMRT) helps to minimize severity of skin reactions compared to conventional radiation therapy (see Chapter 6 for more information on this radiation therapy technique). Although no preventive measures are available for dermatologic toxicities with the use of chemotherapy or targeted agents, various interventions may minimize the severity (Gosselin et al., 2014; Williams, Carlson, Fuhrman, Robison,

& Shelton, 2014). Therefore, early assessment and management by APNs are crucial to allow for continuation of treatment. Prompt interruption or discontinuation of therapy, dose reductions, or dose delays may be necessary to manage certain toxicities.

Diagnosis and Assessment

Paraneoplastic syndromes associated with skin manifestations can occur with some cancers but are relatively rare. Acanthosis nigricans is characterized by pigmented, velvety plaques seen on both sides of the neck and intertriginous areas. Acanthosis palmaris or acquired pachydermatoglyphia involves palmar skin changes, including hyperkeratosis. Erythema gyratum repens is rare and presents with diffuse erythema bordered by desquamation. Acrokeratosis paraneoplastica also presents with erythema that includes scaly patches on the bridge of nose, helixes, and extremities. Acquired hypertrichosis lanuginosa is the presence of soft, long, thin, nonpigmented hair on the face and ears. Necrolytic migratory erythema is characterized by a pink, maculopapular rash. Leser-Trélat sign is manifested by an acute increase in the size and number of seborrheic keratoses. Dermatomyositis is characterized by periorbital erythema with poikilodermatous eruptions occurring on extensor surfaces. Poikiloderma is described as areas of hypopigmentation, hyperpigmentation, telangiectasia, and atrophy. Paraneoplastic pemphigus presents as painful stomatitis along with polymorphic cutaneous eruptions ranging from lichen planus–like or erythema multiforme–like lesions. Sweet syndrome is characterized by pyrexia, neutrophilia, and tender erythematous cutaneous lesions (Shah et al., 2011; Silva & Danson, 2013).

Radiation therapy and its related skin effects can cause significant acute and long-term consequences for patients, such as pain, pruritus, difficulty with movement or ambulation, sleep disturbances, and difficulty wearing certain clothing articles. This can add to their physical discomfort and decreased quality of life. In addition, body image changes may occur (Oddie et al., 2014). Chemotherapy, targeted therapies, and immunotherapy also can cause significant dermatologic side effects, leading to decreased quality of life, discomfort, and altered body image. The combination of chemotherapy and radiation therapy may have a synergistic effect on the incidence and severity of dermatologic effects (Bensadoun et al., 2013). See Chapter 6 for more detailed information on radiation therapy–related dermatologic side effects and recommendations for treatment.

One of the most important APN roles is to assess and appropriately diagnose patients with cancer for disease-related and treatment-related effects. With the common occurrence of dermatologic complications and toxicities in this population, a complete and thorough dermatologic history and physical examination are needed for safe patient care when treatment plans include treatments or agents that cause dermatologic toxicities. Both should be performed at initial consultation (baseline), throughout therapy, and minimally before each dose of chemotherapy or weekly during radiation therapy to assess for skin changes and toxicities. Components of history taking should include presenting symptoms, past and current oncology treatment regimens (i.e., radiation therapy site, total dose, and fraction size; duration of treatment and cumulative dose of chemotherapy, targeted agents, and immunotherapy), medication profile, allergies, occupational and recreational history, recent travel, contact history, and history of other comorbid conditions, such as diabetes, sarcoidosis, hyperthyroidism, and other endocrine abnormalities. A thorough dermatologic examination should be performed in a room that is warm and lighted with diffuse bright daylight. Artificial lighting with fluorescent lights can change the appearance of the skin and any lesions. The entire body must be inspected with attention to the hair, scalp, and nails. The skin must be assessed for any lesions, rashes, and altered skin integrity. If any lesions or rashes are noted, they must be described with appropriate terminology. See Table 14-20 for more details on a thorough dermatologic examination for the evaluation of any dermatologic symptoms.

Systemic chemotherapy agents can cause a wide array of dermatologic effects and toxicities. The skin and its constituents are rapidly dividing cells with epithelial, connective tissue, vascular, and neural components, which in turn can lead to skin manifestations present at diagnosis, during treatment, or as chronic effects of cancer and its treatment (Belum, Patel, Lacouture, & Rodeck, 2013; Reyes-Habito & Roh, 2014a, 2014b). Accurate assessment and differentiation of the etiology are challenging because of combined-modality and multidrug approaches. Management strategies of skin-related toxicities vary and are dependent on the causative agent. Early detection and treatment of these symptoms will assist with control, decrease morbidity, and permit continuation of therapy (Bensadoun et al., 2013).

APNs need to be able to adequately and consistently assess the degree of dermatologic toxicity prior to each treatment and more frequently if warranted. Commonly used toxicity grading scales for radiation-induced skin reactions include the Radiation Therapy Oncology Group Acute Radiation Morbidity Criteria, the Radiation-Induced Skin Reaction Assessment Scale, and the CTCAE. See NCI Cancer Therapy Evaluation Program (2010) for details on the CTCAE radiation dermatitis scale.

Commonly used toxicity grading scales for other dermatologic toxicities include the World Health Organization scale and the CTCAE. See NCI Cancer Therapy Evaluation Program

---

Table 14-20. Components of Dermatologic Examination

Assessment	Examination Details
Skin	Perform inspection of entire body, including flexor areas, extensor areas, and sun-exposed areas.
	Check for altered skin integrity.
	Describe characteristics of skin or skin lesions by the following.
	• Color
	• Configuration
	• Distribution
	• Lesion pattern
	• Type of lesion
	– Annular: Ring-shaped
	– Bulla: Vesicle > 0.5 cm
	– Cyst: Firm, raised encapsulated lesion; usually filled with liquid or semisolid material
	– Lichen: Thickening of skin with exaggerated skin markings
	– Macule: Circumscribed, flat lesion with change in color; < 1 cm
	– Nodule: Raised, firm lesion; > 0.5 cm
	– Papule: Raised, solid lesion; < 0.5 cm
	– Patch: Circumscribed, flat lesion; > 1 cm
	– Plaque: Circumscribed, raised superficial lesion with flat surface; > 0.5 cm
	– Pustule: Circumscribed, raised lesion filled with purulent exudate; size varies
	– Vesicle: Circumscribed, raised lesion filled with liquid or semisolid material
	– Wheal: Firm, raised, pink or red swelling of the skin; size and shape vary; associated pruritus; lasts less than 24 hours
Hair	Inspect for localized or generalized alopecia.
	Inspect for excessive hair growth on scalp, eyebrows, and eyelashes.
Nails	Inspect for color, ridges, dryness, fissures, and altered skin integrity.

Note. Based on information from Witt & Young, 2010.

(2010) for details on some of the CTCAE dermatologic disorders commonly seen in the oncology population, including alopecia, dry skin, hyperpigmentation, hand-foot syndrome, nail discoloration, nail infection, nail loss, nail ridging, pruritus, rash acneform, and rash maculopapular.

Evidence-Based Treatment Strategies

The treatment for dermatologic paraneoplastic syndromes is to treat the underlying disease after diagnosis is confirmed. Although dermatologic paraneoplastic syndromes are rare, they often are associated with GI tract, breast, lung, genitourinary, and ovarian cancers; lymphoproliferative disorders such as non-Hodgkin lymphoma and chronic lymphocytic leukemia; and acute myeloid leukemia (Shah et al., 2011).

The management of radiation-induced skin reactions has been a challenge in radiation therapy for years despite the advances in technology and radiation delivery. Many clinical trials have evaluated various agents in the prevention of radiation-related skin reactions. To date, no evidence-based information supports their use in practice. ONS's Putting Evidence Into Practice (Barney et al., 2011) described and categorized interventions to prevent or reduce the effects of radiation dermatitis based on the level of evidence. The only interventions recognized as recommended for practice were radiation therapy treatment planning, delivery that minimizes radiation skin reactions (i.e., IMRT), and skin hygiene and usual care practices, including gentle skin and hair washing with a mild pH-neutral soap (e.g., Dove®), moisturizing, and use of aluminum-free deodorant (Gosselin et al., 2014).

Success in treating chemotherapy extravasation includes early detection and diagnosis and individualized approaches based on the offending agent. Vidall, Roe, Dougherty, and Harrold (2013) have recommended the use of cooling followed by dexrazoxane for anthracycline extravasations in comparison to cooling followed by dimethyl sulfoxide. See Table 14-21 for details on evidence-based strategies for radiation dermatitis.

Despite the lack of evidence, oncology nurses and APNs recognize the need to manage the distressing effects of radiation-related skin toxicity. The objectives are to provide patient comfort, reduce discomfort and pain, maintain good hygiene, protect from trauma, and maintain body image. Moist desquamation can occur with radiation therapy and generally occurs in an area of a skin fold such as the neck, axillae, inframammary area, abdomen, and groin. The area should be cleansed with soap and water to naturally debride skin cells. APNs should consider use of specialized dressings. The choice of dressing should be based on principles of wound healing, assessment, comfort, need for dressing changes, product evaluation, and cost (McQuestion, 2010).

Patient and caregiver education is important to promote self-care behaviors and should include the following (Dreno et al., 2013; McQuestion, 2010).
- Wash skin using soap and lukewarm water in a bath or shower.
- Use mild soap such as Dove with thorough rinsing, and then pat dry with soft towel.
- Use unscented, lanolin-free, hydrophilic (water-based) lubricant or moisturizer on irradiated skin as long as skin is intact.
- Avoid use of cosmetic or perfumed products in irradiated area.
- Use aluminum-free deodorant.
- Do not use cornstarch or baby powder in area of skin folds.
- Wear loose-fitting clothing made of cotton or soft fabric.
- Protect skin from the sun or cold wind.
- Avoid the use of tapes, adhesives, or adhesive bandages on irradiated skin.
- Avoid the use of heating pads or ice packs on irradiated skin.

• Use an electric razor, if needed, and avoid straight-edge razors.
• Avoid swimming in lakes and chlorinated pools and using hot tubs or saunas.
• Avoid sun exposure and trauma to irradiated area, and use sunscreen with SPF 30 or greater.

Further research is needed in evaluating interventions for the prevention and management of radiation-related skin reactions.

Treatment-related dermatologic side effects are common and can occur with traditional chemotherapy, but particularly with the newer targeted agents. The severity of the impairment is weighed against the benefits and risks of continued therapy, dose reductions, or treatment

Table 14-21. Oncology Nursing Society Evidence-Based Management Recommendations for Radiation Dermatitis

Level of Evidence	Intervention
Recommended for practice	Use of intensity-modulated radiation therapy Gentle skin and hair washing with mild pH-neutral soap Use of aluminum-free deodorants
Likely to be effective	Calendula and silver sulfadiazine
Effectiveness not established	Anionic polar phospholipid cream Aquaphor® ATP cream Bepanthen—topical Cavilon™ No Sting Barrier Film Chamomile cream and almond ointment Dietary supplements such as zinc and vitamin C Epithelial growth factor Glutathione and anthocyanin (Ray-Gel®) Granulocyte macrophage–colony-stimulating factor–impregnated gauze Henna ointment Herbal medicine Honey-impregnated gauze Hyaluronic acid/sodium hyaluronate Hydrocolloid dressings LED light Lipiderm™ MASO65D (Xclair®) Oil in water emulsion Platelet gel Silver leaf dressing Sodium sucrose octasulfate Steroids—topical Sucralfate Theta cream Urea and hyaluronic acid—topical Urea-based topical Vitamin C Wheatgrass WOBE-MUGOS® Zinc/zinc supplements
Effectiveness unlikely	Aloe vera Trolamine (Biafine®)

Note. Based on information from Baney et al., 2011; Bensadoun et al., 2013; Dreno et al., 2013; Gosselin et al., 2014.

breaks. The management of chemotherapy-related dermatologic side effects has been well recognized and established (see Table 14-22).

Since the advent of targeted therapies, much attention has been placed on their potential to cause dermatologic toxicities. The management of skin-related manifestations continues to evolve, but few evidence-based interventions are available, as further research is needed. The ONS's Putting Evidence Into Practice project team (Williams et al., 2014) detailed interventions to prevent or reduce the effects of cutaneous reactions based on the level of evidence. They analyzed rash, xerosis, hand-foot syndrome (palmar-plantar erythrodysesthesia), and photosensitivity. They concluded that dose interruption or modification was likely to be effective. Other management strategies, including the use of antibiotics, benzoyl peroxide, corticosteroids, emollients/moisturizers, and sunscreen, were categorized as Effectiveness Not Established (Williams et al., 2014). More research is needed in evaluating interventions for the prevention and management of skin reactions resulting from targeted therapies.

Despite the preceding recommendations, management of these symptoms is empirical and based on expert advice and consensus. It is important to keep in mind that a positive correlation exists between the occurrence and intensity of the rash eruption and tumor response and overall survival. Therefore, the management of these skin reactions is geared toward patient comfort and enhanced quality and quantity of life. Table 14-23 outlines the proposed management of dermatologic manifestations caused by targeted therapies, which has been developed based on expert advice and consensus. A proactive approach is crucial in the management of these skin manifestations.

The management of dermatologic toxicities continues to evolve as experience and knowledge about this exciting new treatment grow. Present management guidelines have been developed on expert advice. See Table 14-18 for details.

The management of dermatologic toxicities in the HSCT population is serious and needs to be addressed without delay. Treatment of GVHD requires close collaboration with the transplant team. Prompt treatment may decrease the risk of skin breakdown, contracture formation, and permanent disability. See Table 14-24 for details regarding the management of dermatologic toxicities in HSCT.

The management of dermatologic manifestations secondary to medications is relatively straightforward. The management includes (a) removing and discontinuing the causative agent, (b) providing supportive care measures for the associated symptoms, such as pruritus, and (c) providing hydration, infection control, and pain management with life-threatening reactions, such as Stevens-Johnson syndrome or toxic epidermal necrolysis (Witt & Young, 2010).

Evaluation of Outcomes

Many dermatologic manifestations may be exhibited by the cancer itself or as a result of treatment, such as radiation therapy or systemic treatment. Oncology APNs must be able to recognize and, even more importantly, differentiate among the various skin manifestations. Another challenge lies in the management of these dermatologic manifestations. More evidence-based practice guidelines are needed for appropriate management and continuity of care, as well as improved quality of life, both physically and psychologically.

Implications for Oncology Advanced Practice Nurses

Dermatologic effects and toxicities are common but often less expected than other toxicities. APNs must continually assess patients for a wide array of dermatologic presentations. Patient education is essential to self-care, prevention, and early detection. Ongoing assessment and management are crucial in efforts to maintain or improve patients' quality of life.

Dermatologic toxicities are common and primarily caused by cancer-related treatments including radiation therapy, chemotherapy, targeted therapies, immunotherapy, and HSCT.

Table 14-22. Management of Chemotherapy-Related Dermatologic Side Effects

Side Effect	Management Recommendations
Alopecia	No preventive measures exist for alopecia. Nurses need to perform appropriate psychosocial assessments and provide interventions for distress in men and women, with attention to social and psychological ramifications and altered body image. Patients require education tailored to their chemotherapy regimen and degree of alopecia expected. Management strategies include the following. • Avoid use of dryers, straightening irons, hot rollers, or curling irons. • Protect scalp from the sun by wearing sunscreen and/or protective covering. • If total alopecia is present, cleanse and condition the scalp regularly. • Support the use of wigs, scarves, and hats. Insurance may reimburse for wigs (cranial prosthesis). • Support attendance to American Cancer Society's Look Good Feel Better program, which is designed to provide support and education for body image changes.
Hyperpigmentation	Instruct patients to avoid sunlight and to use sunscreen (sun protection factor ≥ 30). Topical retinoids, topical hydroquinone, and corticosteroids may be used, but effectiveness is not established, and this is not necessary if solitary sign or symptom. If no treatment is initiated, hyperpigmentation will resolve over time once chemotherapy is discontinued.
Hand-foot syndrome (also known as palmar-plantar erythrodysesthesia)	Topical ointments aid in skin hydration and maintenance of skin integrity. Over-the-counter interventions include Bag Balm®, Biafine®, and Aquaphor®. Syndrome may improve with dose reductions or treatment interruptions. Use of topical corticosteroids or anesthetics is not recommended because they may exacerbate symptoms.
Hypersensitivity	Patients should receive premedication with an antihistamine (i.e., diphenhydramine), corticosteroid (i.e., hydrocortisone, dexamethasone), and H_2 receptor antagonist (i.e., ranitidine). Docetaxel also is associated with hypersensitivity reactions. Measures used to minimize a hypersensitivity reaction include premedication with dexamethasone, which is continued for 3 days post-treatment.
Macular-papular rash	Topical corticosteroids (i.e., hydrocortisone 1% or higher ointment) and/or systemic corticosteroids and antihistamines are used for management. Systemic isotretinoin can be given if no response to antibiotics.
Radiation recall	Management strategies for radiation recall include • Topical ointments (Aquaphor®, Eucerin®) and steroid-based ointments • Removal of precipitating agent.

(Continued on next page)

Table 14-22. Management of Chemotherapy-Related Dermatologic Side Effects
(Continued)

Side Effect	Management Recommendations
Chemotherapy extravasation	Management of suspected or actual extravasation should include the following. • Ensure extravasation kit is readily available. • Stop infusion of chemotherapy. • Disconnect IV tubing and aspirate any residual chemotherapy. • Apply ice for all chemotherapy agents except vinca alkaloids. Apply ice for 15–20 minutes at least 4 times daily and elevate affected extremity. Apply heat if causative agent is vinca alkaloid. • Consider an antidote, if applicable. • Document event, including photographs. • Continue patient follow-up for at least two weeks with referral to plastic surgeon and physical therapy.
Nails	Nurses should instruct patients on the following. • Keep nails short. • Maintain good daily hygiene. • Avoid exposure to harmful chemicals and detergents. • Keep nails and hands moisturized and protect hands from irritants by wearing gloves and avoiding trauma or injury. • Avoid artificial or acrylic nails because of increased risk of injury or infection. Nail polish may be used, but nail polish remover may be harmful to nail surface. Biotin, a water-soluble B-complex vitamin, may improve overall nail condition. Recommended dose is 5 mg/day.

Note. Based on information from Bidoli et al., 2010; Cashman & Sloan, 2010; Chon et al., 2012; Dest, 2010; Reye-Habito & Roh, 2014a.

These toxicities adversely affect quality of life, especially in younger people and when a visible rash is present (Joshi et al., 2010). Oncology APNs need to follow the research and evidence-based practice findings to provide the highest quality, safe patient care. Baseline dermatologic assessments and ongoing monitoring for the early onset of signs and symptoms of skin toxicity should be performed prior to each dose of potentially dermatologic toxic therapy and follow-up visits to provide for safe patient care. Education for patients and their caregivers promotes self-care, which allows patients to take control of the side effects by avoiding precipitating events whenever possible. In addition, education allows patients to manage and report these toxicities.

Conclusion

Cancer and its various treatment modalities, as well as comorbidities and other medications, have the potential to cause neurologic, ocular, and dermatologic toxicities. Oncology APNs need to be vigilant in prevention and early identification and intervention to limit the negative effect on patients' quality of life and the potential for severe and life-threatening conditions. This includes baseline and routine assessment; symptom management, including dose reduction, treatment break, or drug discontinuation as indicated; referral as needed; and patient and caregiver education.

Table 14-23. Management of Targeted Therapy/Biotherapy–Related Dermatologic Side Effects

Side Effect	Management Recommendations
Papulopustular reaction	Skin should be moisturized and hydrated with emollient creams and ointments, such as Eucerin®, Cetaphil®, Aquaphor®, Bag Balm®, and Neutrogena Norwegian Formula®.
	Moisturizing products that contain alcohol, perfumes, or dyes should be avoided because of increased dryness and irritation.
	Skin must be protected from injury.
	Topical steroids, such as hydrocortisone 1% or clobetasol propionate ointment, may be used.
	If emollient creams are not effective, antihistamine therapy with diphenhydramine (Benadryl®) or hydroxyzine (Atarax®) can be tried.
	No evidence-based information is available about prophylactic use of topical or systemic antibiotics.
	Incidence of infection increases when lesions develop honey-crusted scabs or purulent drainage. Most common cause of infection is *Staphylococcus aureus*. Treatment of suspected infection includes topical antibiotics such as 1% clindamycin, erythromycin, metronidazole, or systemic antibiotics. Most appropriate antibiotics include minocycline, doxycycline, and tetracycline. Doxycycline is first-line therapy with dose of 100–200 mg/day for 4–8 weeks.
	Systemic corticosteroids may be used for severe skin reactions.
	Dose reduction may be needed for severe reaction or poor tolerability.
	Psychological status of patients needs to be addressed.
Xerosis/pruritus	Emollient creams, such as Aquaphor, Bag Balm, Eucerin, Kerasal®, and Neutrogena Norwegian Formula, can be used for dryness.
	Vitamin A or urea-based ointments may be used.
Hand-foot syndrome	Syndrome may improve with dose reductions or treatment interruptions.
	No evidence-based interventions are available.
	Emollients may help with dryness and cracking.
Subungual splinter hemorrhages	Manifestation is self-limiting and does not require intervention.
Fissures	Emollient creams, such as Aquaphor, Bag Balm, Eucerin, Kerasal, and Neutrogena Norwegian Formula, may be used.
Telangiectasias	No medical management has been shown to be effective.
Hyperpigmentation	No medical management has been established. Resolution occurs when therapy is completed.
Hair changes	No medical management has been established. Resolution occurs when therapy is completed.
Paronychia with pyrogenic granuloma	The mainstay of treatment is to decrease extent of granulation tissue. Management strategies include • Soaking of affected digit with soap and water followed by application of moisturizer • Use of topical corticosteroids • Use of systemic antibiotics, such as minocycline.

Note. Based on information from Boucher et al., 2011; Eaby-Sandy & Lynch, 2014; Kiyohara et al., 2013; Reyes-Habito & Roh, 2014b; Robert et al., 2012; Wood, 2009.

Table 14-24. Management of Dermatologic Toxicities in the Hematopoietic Stem Cell Transplantation Population

Side Effect	Management Recommendations
Acute graft-versus-host disease	The mainstay of prevention and treatment is the use of immunosuppressive drugs, such as • Cyclosporine: Total daily dose = 1.5 mg/kg IV every 12 hours • Corticosteroids: Dose varies from 0.5–2 mg/kg/day every 12 hours • Tacrolimus: Total daily dose = 1–2 mg PO every 12 hours • Mycophenolate mofetil: Dose ranges from 1–1.5 mg IV or PO every 12 hours • Methotrexate: 5–15 mg/m² IV on days 1, 3, 6, and 11 after transplant.
Chronic graft-versus-host disease	Immunosuppressive medications are the mainstay of prophylaxis and treatment. Ultraviolet light phototherapy may be used. The duration of therapy differs and can range from months to years.
Palmar-plantar erythrodysesthesia	No prevention strategies or evidence-based interventions are recommended.

Note. Based on information from Hymes et al., 2012; Latchford, 2010.

Case Study

   A.B. is 60-year-old man who presented with a several-month history of throat pain and a recently developed left-sided neck mass. His workup included an MRI of the neck, which revealed a 3.2 cm left tongue mass with an associated 2.3 cm left level II node, a 1 cm right level III node, and a 1.2 cm right periparotid enhancing nodule. A subsequent positron-emission tomography scan revealed a left base of tongue mass with extension to the floor of the oral cavity to the hyoid bone (maximum standardized uptake value [SUVm] 13.4), an adjacent right oropharynx mass with mild hypermetabolism, bilateral neck adenopathy including left level II (SUVm 6.2), left supraclavicular region with moderate to severe uptake, right level II and III with milder uptake, and right supraclavicular lymph node measuring less than 1 cm. There were no distant metastases. A fine needle aspiration was performed and confirmed squamous cell carcinoma. A direct laryngoscopy, esophagoscopy, and biopsy were performed, and final pathology revealed moderately differentiated squamous cell carcinoma, strongly human papillomavirus positive (p16), with skeletal muscle involvement and lymphovascular invasion present. He was staged as a cT2N2cM0 (stage IVA). Current ECOG status is 0. His past medical history includes hypertension, diverticulitis, and gastroesophageal reflux disease. His past surgical history includes colon resection for diverticulitis and basal cell carcinoma excised from his right upper arm and nose. He is married and has two children. He smoked 1–2 cigarettes per day for 10 years and drinks alcohol socially.

   He started concurrent chemoradiation with curative intent. He was scheduled to receive daily IMRT to the head and neck region for a total dose of 7,000 cGy over 35 fractions at 200 cGy per fraction with weekly cetuximab. During the first week, he received a loading dose of 400 mg/m² and then reduced to 250 mg/m² weekly.

   After cycle 1, he developed chills and fever and was advised to take diphenhydramine and acetaminophen. He also was placed on corticosteroids for five days. Week 2: A.B. received cetuximab and radiation therapy. He developed erythema of oropharyngeal region; skin was benign. Week 3: A.B. received cetuximab and radiation therapy; he began experiencing taste alterations and xerostomia. Skin examination revealed mild erythema of the neck and maculopapular rash on the nose, chin, and base of skull. Oral cavity examination revealed moderate erythema and patchy mucositis of left buccal mucosa. Week 4: A.B. was admitted for seven days secondary to confluent mucositis and dehydration. A percutaneous endoscopic gastrostomy tube was placed. Concurrent cetuximab and radiation therapy were put on hold. Week 5: The patient resumed radiation therapy and cetuximab. Week 6: The patient received concurrent cetuximab and radiation therapy; rash persists. Week 7: The patient received concurrent cetuximab and radiation therapy; his rash persists, but today is his last cycle of cetuximab.

1. How would the APN differentiate between radiation dermatitis and an EGFR inhibitor–induced dermatologic manifestation?
   • Radiation skin reaction is present within the radiation portal (bilateral neck region), whereas EGFR inhibitor–induced rash appears on face, neck, shoulders, upper trunk, and scalp.
2. How would the APN treat his maculopapular rash based on evidence-based management?
   • The APN would institute a treatment break or delay.
3. How would the APN treat his maculopapular rash based on expert advice and consensus?
   • Choices may include
     – Cleanse skin twice daily with gentle facial cleansing lotion (Cetaphil); allow to dry.
     – Apply clindamycin phosphate 1% lotion to affected area twice daily; allow to dry.
     – Apply clobetasol propionate 0.05% cream to affected area twice daily; allow to dry.
     – Apply emollient lotion as needed.
     – Add an oral antibiotic, such as minocycline 100 mg PO BID.
4. What evidence-based recommendations would the APN provide to minimize his radiation dermatitis?
   • The APN would recommend use of IMRT and gentle washing of the skin with mild pH soap.
5. When should the APN expect radiation dermatitis to begin? When would the APN expect EGFR inhibitor–induced rash to begin?
   • Radiation dermatitis begins within two to three weeks of starting radiation therapy; EGFR inhibitor–induced rash appears one to three weeks after initiation of treatment.

Key Points

Neurotoxicities

• Baseline and routine neurologic assessments are performed on all patients receiving neurotoxic agents.
• Assessment needs to include the central, peripheral, and autonomic nervous systems.
• Baseline peripheral neuropathy is documented to allow for monitoring of neurotoxicity throughout therapy.
• Therapy can be held, doses reduced, or the treatment plan altered for neurotoxicity.
• Many peripheral neuropathies and neurotoxicities are reversible.
• Holding the dose or giving a dose break may reduce the severity during therapy.
• Symptom management of peripheral neuropathy improves patients' quality of life.

Ocular Toxicities

• APNs need to maintain a high degree of suspicion for ocular toxicities, as they are more common than previously thought.

- APNs should perform baseline eye examinations on all patients who are to initiate chemotherapy.
- Patients who are anticipated to have ocular toxicities from therapy should see an ophthalmologist for assessment and evaluation prior to starting therapy.
- APNs should provide supportive medications and symptom management to palliate ocular symptoms.
- Patients with ocular complaints require prompt referral to an ophthalmologist.

Dermatologic Toxicities

- Baseline and routine dermatologic assessments are performed on all patients receiving radiation therapy and chemotherapy and biotherapy/targeted agents.
- APNs should provide supportive medications and symptom management to palliate dermatologic symptoms.
- Patients require referral to a dermatologist if they are experiencing severe dermatologic symptoms.
- A dose reduction or treatment break may reduce the severity of dermatologic symptoms.

Recommended Resources for Oncology Advanced Practice Nurses

Neurotoxicities

- Hershman, D.L., Lacchetti, C., Dworkin, R.H., Smith, E.M.L., Bleeker, J., Cavaletti, G., ... Loprinzi, C.L. (2014). Prevention and management of chemotherapy-induced peripheral neuropathy in survivors of adult cancers: American Society of Clinical Oncology clinical practice guideline. *Journal of Clinical Oncology, 32,* 1941–1967. doi:10.1200/JCO.2013.54.0914
- Neuropathy Association: www.neuropathy.org
- Tofthagen, C., & Irwin, M. (2014). Peripheral neuropathy. In M. Irwin & L.A. Johnson (Eds.), *Putting evidence into practice: A pocket guide to cancer symptom management* (pp. 201–210). Pittsburgh, PA: Oncology Nursing Society.
- Visovsky, C., Camp-Sorrell, D., Collins, M.L., Olson, E.K., Tofthagen, C.S., & Wood, S.K. (2014). Putting evidence into practice: Peripheral neuropathy. Retrieved from https://www.ons.org/practice-resources/pep/peripheral-neuropathy

Ocular Toxicities

- American Association of Ophthalmic Oncologists and Pathologists: www.aaoop.org
- International Society of Ocular Oncology: www.isoo.org

Dermatologic Toxicities

- Gosselin, T., McQuestion, M., Beamer, L., Feight, D., Merritt, C., Omabegho, M., & Shaftic, A. (2014). Putting evidence into practice: Radiodermatitis. Retrieved from https://www.ons.org/practice-resources/pep/radiodermatitis
- Gosselin, T.K., Omabegho, M., & Irwin, M. (2014). Radiodermatitis. In M. Irwin & L.A. Johnson (Eds.), *Putting evidence into practice: A pocket guide to cancer symptom management* (pp. 233–242). Pittsburgh, PA: Oncology Nursing Society.

- Johnson, L.A. (2014). Skin effects. In M. Irwin & L.A. Johnson (Eds.), *Putting evidence into practice: A pocket guide to cancer symptom management* (pp. 243–253). Pittsburgh, PA: Oncology Nursing Society.
- Williams, L., Carlson, J., Fuhrman, A., Robison, J., & Shelton, G. (2014). Putting evidence into practice: Skin reactions. Retrieved from https://www.ons.org/practice-resources/pep/skin-reactions

References

Abdelkawi, S. (2012). Lens crystallin response to whole body irradiation with single and fractionated doses of gamma radiation. *International Journal of Radiation Biology, 88,* 600–606. doi:10.3109/09553002.2012.695097

Agustoni, F., Platania, M., Vitali, M., Zilembo, N., Haspinger, E., Sinno, V., … Garassino, M.C. (2014). Emerging toxicities in the treatment of non-small cell lung cancer: Ocular disorders. *Cancer Treatment Reviews, 40,* 197–203. doi:10.1016/j.ctrv.2013.05.005

Ahmed, A.M., Pritchard, S., & Reichenberg, J. (2013). A review of cutaneous drug eruptions. *Clinics in Geriatric Medicine, 29,* 527–545. doi:10.1016/j.cger.2013.01.008

Ainsbury, E.A., Bouffler, S.D., Dörr, W., Graw, J., Muirhead, C.R., Edwards, A.A., & Cooper, J. (2009). Radiation cataractogenesis: A review of recent studies. *Radiation Research, 172,* 1–9. doi:10.1667/RR1688.1

Alcon Laboratories. (2011). *TobraDex® (tobramycin and dexamethasone)* [Package insert]. Fort Worth, TX: Author.

American Society for Radiation Oncology. (2012). Fast facts about radiation therapy. Retrieved from https://www.astro.org/News-and-Media/Media-Resources/FAQs/Fast-Facts-About-Radiation-Therapy/Index.aspx

Argyriou, A.A., Kyritsis, A.P., Makatsoris, T., & Kalofonos, H.P. (2014). Chemotherapy-induced peripheral neuropathy in adults: A comprehensive update of the literature. *Cancer Management and Research, 6,* 135–147. doi:10.2147/CMAR.S44261

Arlien-Søborg, P., & Simonsen, L. (2011). Chemical neurotoxic agents. In J.M. Stellman (Ed.), *Encyclopaedia of occupational health and safety* (4th ed.). Retrieved from http://www.ilo.org/iloenc/part-i/nervous-system/item/289-chemical-neurotoxic-agents

Augsburger, J.J., Corrêa, Z.M., & Shaikh, A.H. (2009). Effectiveness of treatments for metastatic uveal melanoma. *American Journal of Ophthalmology, 48,* 119–127. doi:10.1016/j.ajo.2009.01.023

Balagula, Y., Garbe, C., Myskowski, P.L., Hauschild, A., Rapoport, B.L., Boers-Doets, C.B., & Lacouture, M.E. (2011). Clinical presentation and management of dermatological toxicities of epidermal growth factor receptor inhibitors. *International Journal of Dermatology, 50,* 129–146. doi:10.1111/j.1365-4632.2010.04791.x

Baldwin, K.J., Živković, S.A., & Lieberman, F.S. (2012). Neurologic emergencies in patients who have cancer: Diagnosis and management. *Neurologic Clinics, 30,* 101–128. doi:10.1016/j.ncl.2011.09.004

Ballesteros-Zebadua, P., Chavarria, A., Celis, M.A., Paz, C., & Franco-Perez, J. (2012). Radiation-induced neuroinflammation and radiation somnolence syndrome. *CNS and Neurological Disorders—Drug Targets, 11,* 937–949. doi:10.2174/1871527311201070937

Baney, T. (Ed.). (2011). Radiodermatitis. In L.H. Eaton, J.M. Tipton, & M. Irwin (Eds.), *Putting evidence into practice: Improving oncology patient outcomes* (Vol. 2, pp. 49–56). Pittsburgh, PA: Oncology Nursing Society.

Baney, T., McQuestion, M., Bell, K., Bruce, S., Feight, D., Weis-Smith, L., & Haas, M. (2011). ONS PEP resource: Radiodermatitis. In L.H. Eaton, J.M. Tipton, & M. Irwin (Eds.), Putting evidence into practice: Improving oncology patient outcomes (Vol. 2, pp. 57–75). Pittsburgh, PA: Oncology Nursing Society.

Belum, V.R., Cercek, A., Sanz-Motilva, V., & Lacouture, M.E. (2013). Dermatologic adverse events to targeted therapies in lower GI cancers: Clinical presentation and management. *Current Treatment Options in Oncology, 14,* 389–404. doi:10.1007/s11864-013-0254-4

Belum, V.R., Patel, H.F., Lacouture, M.E., & Rodeck, U. (2013). Skin toxicity of targeted cancer agents: Mechanisms and intervention. *Future Oncology, 9,* 1161–1170. doi:10.2217/fon.13.62

Bensadoun, R.J., Humbert, P., Krutman, J., Luger, T., Triller, R., Rougier, A., … Dreno, B. (2013). Daily baseline skin care in the prevention, treatment, and supportive care of skin toxicity in oncology patients: Recommendations from a multinational expert panel. *Cancer Management and Research, 5,* 401–408. doi:10.2147/CMAR.S52256

Berkowitz, A., & Walker, S. (2012). Bortezomib-induced peripheral neuropathy in patients with multiple myeloma. *Clinical Journal of Oncology Nursing, 16,* 86–89. doi:10.1188/12.CJON.86-89

Bidoli, P., Cortnovis, D.L., Colombo, I., Crippa, A., Cicchiello, F., Villa, F., & Attomare, G. (2010). Isotretinoin plus clindamycin seem highly effective against severe erlotinib-induced skin rash in advanced non-small cell lung cancer. *Journal of Thoracic Oncology, 5,* 1662–1663. doi:10.1097/JTO.0b013e3181ec1729

Bielory, B., & Bielory, L. (2010). Atopic dermatitis and keratoconjunctivitis. *Immunology and Allergy Clinics of North America, 30,* 323–336. doi:10.1016/j.iac.2010.06.004

Blomquist, P.H. (2011). Ocular complications of systemic medications. *American Journal of the Medical Sciences, 342,* 62–69. doi:10.1097/MAJ.0b013e3181f06b21

Boucher, J., Olson, L., & Piperdi, B. (2011). Preemptive management of dermatologic toxicities associated with epidermal growth factor receptor inhibitors. *Clinical Journal of Oncology Nursing, 15,* 501–508. doi:10.1188/11.CJON.501-508

Braik, T., Evans, A.T., Telfer, M., & McDunn, S. (2010). Paraneoplastic neurological syndromes: Unusual presentations of cancer. A practical review. *American Journal of the Medical Sciences, 340,* 301–308. doi:10.1097/MAJ.0b013e3181d9bb3b

Brejt, N., Berry, J., Nisbet, A., Bloomfield, D., & Burkill, G. (2013). Pelvic radiculopathies, lumbosacral plexopathies, and neuropathies in oncologic disease: A multidisciplinary approach to a diagnostic challenge. *Cancer Imaging, 13,* 591–601. Retrieved from http://www.ncbi.nlm.nih.gov/pmc/articles/PMC3893894/pdf/ci130052.pdf

Bristol-Myers Squibb Co. (2011). *BiCNU® (carmustine for injection)* [Package insert]. Princeton, NJ: Author.

Burris, H.A., III, & Hurtig, J. (2010). Radiation recall with anticancer agents. *Oncologist, 15,* 1227–1237. doi:10.1634/theoncologist.2009-0090

Butowski, N. (2011). Medical management of brain metastases. *Neurosurgery Clinics of North America, 22,* 27–36. doi:10.1016/j.nec.2010.08.004

Carlson, K., & Ocean, A.J. (2011). Peripheral neuropathy with microtubule-targeting agents: Occurrence and management approach. *Clinical Breast Cancer, 11,* 73–81. doi:10.1016/j.clbc.2011.03.006

Cashman, M.W., & Sloan, S.B. (2010). Nutrition and nail disease. *Clinics in Dermatology, 28,* 420–425. doi:10.1016/j.clindermatol.2010.03.037

Cavaletti, G. (2014). Chemotherapy-induced peripheral neurotoxicity (CIPN): What we need and what we know. *Journal of the Peripheral Nervous System, 19,* 66–76. doi:10.1111/jns5.12073

Cavaletti, G., & Zanna, C. (2002). Current status and future prospects for the treatment of chemotherapy-induced peripheral neurotoxicity. *European Journal of Cancer, 38,* 1832–1837.

Cavaletti, G., Frigeni, B., Lanzani, F., Mattavelli, L., Susani, E., Alberti, P., … Bidoli, P. (2010). Chemotherapy-induced peripheral neurotoxicity assessment: A critical revision of the currently available tools. *European Journal of Cancer, 46,* 479–494.

Cavaletti, G., Cornblath, D.R., Merkies, I.S., Postma, T.J., Rossi, E., Frigeni, B., … Valsecchi, M.G. (2013). The Chemotherapy-Induced Peripheral Neuropathy Outcome Measures Standardization study: From consensus to the first validity and reliability findings. *Annals of Oncology, 24,* 454–462. doi:10.1093/annonc/mds329

Chanprapaph, K., Vachiramon, V., & Rattanakaemakorn, P. (2014). Epidermal growth factor receptor inhibitors: A review of cutaneous adverse events and management. *Dermatology Research and Practice, 2014,* Article ID 734249. doi:10.1155/2014/734249

Chen, J.J., Applebaum, D.S., Sun, G.S., & Pflugfelder, S.C. (2014). Atopic keratoconjunctivitis: A review. *Journal of the American Academy of Dermatology, 70,* 569–575. doi:10.1016/j.jaad.2013.10.036

Choi, J.N. (2014). Dermatologic adverse events to chemotherapeutic agents, Part 2: BRAF inhibitors, MEK inhibitors, and ipilimumab. *Seminars in Cutaneous Medicine and Surgery, 35,* 40–48.

Chon, S.Y., Champion, R.W., Geddes, E.R., & Rashid, R.M. (2012). Chemotherapy-induced alopecia. *Journal of the American Academy of Dermatology, 67,* e37–e47. doi:10.1016/j.jaad.2011.02.026

Chung, T., Prasad, K., & Lloyd, T.E. (2014). Peripheral neuropathy: Clinical and electrophysiological considerations. *Neuroimaging Clinics of North America, 24,* 49–65. doi:10.1016/j.nic.2013.03.023

Council, M.L. (2013). Common skin cancers in older adults: Approach to diagnosis and management. *Clinics in Geriatric Medicine, 29,* 361–372. doi:10.1016/j.cger.2013.01.011

Damek, D.M. (2010). Cerebral edema, altered mental status, seizures, acute stroke, leptomeningeal metastases, and paraneoplastic syndrome. *Hematology/Oncology Clinics of North America, 24,* 515–535. doi:10.1016/j.hoc.2010.03.010

Degen, A., Alter, M., Schenck, F., Satzger, I., Völker, B., Kapp, A., & Gutzmer, R. (2010). The hand-foot-syndrome associated with medical tumor therapy—Classification and management. *Journal der Deutschen Dermatologischen Gesellschaft, 8,* 652–661. doi:10.1111/j.1610-0387.2010.07449.x

Dest, V. (2010). Systemic therapy–induced skin reactions. In M.L. Haas & G.J. Moore-Higgs (Eds.), *Principles of skin care and the oncology patient* (pp. 141–166). Pittsburgh, PA: Oncology Nursing Society.

Didelot, A., & Honnorat, J. (2014). Chapter 78—Paraneoplastic disorders of the central and peripheral nervous systems. In J. Biller & J.M. Ferro (Eds.), *Handbook of clinical neurology* (Vol. 121, pp. 1159–1179). doi:10.1016/B978-0-7020-4088-7.00078-X

Dreno, B., Bensadoun, R.J., Humbert, P., Krutmann, J., Luger, T., Triller, R., … Seité, S. (2013). Algorithm for dermocosmetic use in the management of cutaneous side-effects associated with targeted therapy in oncology. *Journal of the European Academy of Dermatology and Venereology, 27,* 1071–1080. doi:10.1111/jdv.12082

Dropcho, E.J. (2010). Neurotoxicity of radiation therapy. *Neurologic Clinics, 28,* 217–234. doi:10.1016/j.ncl.2009.09.008

Eaby-Sandy, B., & Lynch, K. (2014). Side effects of targeted therapies: Rash. *Seminars in Oncology Nursing, 30,* 147–154. doi:10.1016/j.soncn.2014.06.001

Eagle, R.C., Jr. (2013). Ocular tumors: Triumphs, challenges and controversies. *Saudi Journal of Ophthalmology, 27,* 129–132. doi:10.1016/j.sjopt.2013.06.002

Esmaeli, B., & Valero, V. (2013). Epiphora and canalicular stenosis associated with adjuvant docetaxel in early breast cancer: Is excessive tearing clinically important? *Journal of Clinical Oncology, 31,* 2076–2077. doi:10.1200/JCO.2012.47.5897

Fabbrocini, G., Cameli, N., Romano, M.C., Mariano, M., Panariello, L., Bianca, D., & Monfrecola, G. (2012). Chemotherapy and skin reactions. *Journal of Experimental and Clinical Cancer Research, 31,* 50. doi:10.1186/1756-9966-31-50

FACIT.org. (n.d.). Questionnaires. Retrieved from http://www.facit.org/FACITOrg/Questionnaires

Fidalgo, J.A.P., Fabregat, L.G., Cervantes, A., Margulies, A., Vidall, C., & Roila, F. (2012). Management of chemotherapy extravasation: ESMO–EONS clinical practice guidelines *Annals of Oncology, 23*(Suppl. 7), vii167–vii173. doi:10.1093/annonc/mds294

Fischer, D.S., Knobf, M.T., Durivage, H.J., & Beaulieu, N.J. (2003). *The cancer chemotherapy handbook* (6th ed.). Philadelphia, PA: Elsevier Mosby.

Foroozan, R. (2010). Neuro-ophthalmic complications of chemotherapy. In *North American Neuro-Ophthalmology Society 2010 annual meeting syllabus* (pp. 299–316). Retrieved from http://www.nanosweb.org/files/Neuro-Ophthalmology.of.Cancer.pdf

Gibbs, I.C., Patil, C., Gerszten, P.C., Adler, J.R., & Burton, S.A. (2009). Delayed radiation-induced myelopathy after spinal radiosurgery. *Neurosurgery, 64*(Suppl.), A67–A72. doi:10.1227/01.NEU.0000341628.98141.B6

Gosselin, T., McQuestion, M., Beamer, L., Feight, D., Merritt, C., Omabegho, M., & Shaftic, A. (2014). Putting evidence into practice: Radiodermatitis. Retrieved from https://www.ons.org/practice-resources/pep/radiodermatitis

Hager, T., & Seitz, B. (2014). Ocular side effects of biological agents in oncology: What should the clinician be aware of? *OncoTargets and Therapy, 7,* 69–77. doi:10.2147/OTT.S54606

Hausheer, F.H., Schilsky, R.L., Bain, S., Berghorn, E.J., & Lieberman, F. (2006). Diagnosis, management, and evaluation of chemotherapy-induced peripheral neuropathy. *Seminars in Oncology, 33,* 15–49. doi:10.1053/j.seminoncol.2005.12.010

Hershman, D.L., Lacchetti, C., Dworkin, R.H., Smith, E.M.L., Bleeker, J., Cavaletti, G., … Loprinzi, C.L. (2014). Prevention and management of chemotherapy-induced peripheral neuropathy in survivors of adult cancers: American Society of Clinical Oncology clinical practice guideline. *Journal of Clinical Oncology, 32,* 1941–1967. doi:10.1200/JCO.2013.54.0914

Heutte, N., Plisson, L., Lange, M., Prevost, V., & Babin, E. (2014). Quality of life tools in head and neck oncology. *European Annals of Otorhinolaryngology, Head and Neck Diseases, 131,* 33–47. doi:10.1016/j.anorl.2013.05.002

Horska, A., & Barker, P. (2010). Imaging of brain tumors: MR spectroscopy and metabolic imaging. *Neuroimaging Clinics of North America, 20,* 293–310. doi:10.1016/j.nic.2010.04.003

Hospira. (2011). *Methotrexate* [Package insert]. Lake Forest, IL: Author.

Howell, M., Lee, R., Bowyer, S., Fusi, A., & Lorigan, P. (2015). Optimal management of immune-related toxicities associated with checkpoint inhibitors in lung cancer. *Lung Cancer, 88,* 117–123. doi:10.1016/j.lungcan.2015.02.007

Huttner, A. (2012). Overview of primary brain tumors: Pathologic classification, epidemiology, molecular biology, and prognostic markers. *Hematology/Oncology Clinics of North America, 26,* 715–732. doi:10.1016/j.hoc.2012.05.004

Hymes, S.R., Alousi, A.M., & Cowen, E.W. (2012). Graft-versus-host disease: Part I. Pathogenesis and clinical manifestations of graft-versus-host disease. *Journal of the American Academy of Dermatology, 66,* 515.e1–515.e18. doi:10.1016/j.jaad.2011.11.960

Ishak, R.S., Aad, S.A., Kyei, A., & Farhat, F.S. (2013). Cutaneous manifestations of anti-angiogenic therapy in oncology: Review with focus on VEGF inhibitors. *Critical Reviews in Oncology/Hematology, 90,* 152–164. doi:10.1016/j.critrevonc.2013.11.007

Johnson, N.I. (2013). Ocular graft-versus-host disease after allogeneic transplantation. *Clinical Journal of Oncology Nursing, 17,* 621–626. doi:10.1188/13.CJON.621-626

Joshi, S.S., Ortiz, S., Witherspoon, J.N., Rademaker, A., West, D.P., Anderson, R., … Lacouture, M.E. (2010). Effects of epidermal growth factor receptor inhibitor-induced dermatologic toxicities on quality of life. *Cancer, 116,* 3916–3923. doi:10.1002/cncr.25090

Kannoth, S. (2012). Paraneoplastic neurologic syndrome: A practical approach. *Annals of Indian Academy of Neurology, 15,* 6–12. doi:10.4103/0972-2327.93267

Kennedy, A., & Zakaria, R. (2012). Taking a neurological history. *Medicine, 40,* 403–408. doi:10.1016/j.mpmed.2012.05.006

Keogh, B.P., & Henson, J.W. (2012). Clinical manifestations and diagnostic imaging of brain tumors. *Hematology/Oncology Clinics of North America, 26,* 733–755. doi:10.1016/j.hoc.2012.05.002

Kheir, W.J., Sniegowski, M.C., El-Sawy, T., Li, A., & Esmaeli, B. (2014). Ophthalmic complications of targeted cancer therapy and recently recognized ophthalmic complications of traditional chemotherapy. *Survey of Ophthalmology, 59,* 493–502. doi:10.1016/j.survophthal.2014.02.004

Kiyohara, Y., Yamazaki, N., & Kishi, A. (2013). Erlotinib-related skin toxicities: Treatment strategies in patients with metastatic non-small cell lung cancer. *Journal of the American Academy of Dermatology, 69,* 463–472. doi:10.1016/j.jaad.2013.02.025

Koeppen, S., Thirugnanasambanthan, A., & Koldehoff, M. (2014). Neuromuscular complications after hematopoietic stem cell transplantation. Supportive Care in Cancer, 22, 2337–2341. doi:10.1007/s00520-014-2225-0

Kollmannsberger, C., & Mitchell, T. (2013). Selected toxicities of targeted therapies: Presentation and management. *Seminars in Oncology Nursing, 40,* 499–510. doi:10.1053/j.seminoncol.2013.05.011

Komen, M.M., Smorenburg, C.H., van den Hurk, C.J., & Nortier, J.W. (2013). Factors influencing the effectiveness of scalp cooling in the prevention of chemotherapy-induced alopecia. *Oncologist, 18,* 885–891. doi:10.1634/theoncologist.2012-0332

Lacouture, M.E., Wolchok, J.D., Yosipovitch, G., Kähler, K.C., Busam, K.J., & Hauschild, A. (2014). Ipilimumab in patients with cancer and the management of dermatologic adverse events. *Journal of the American Academy of Dermatology, 71,* 161–169. doi:10.1016/j.jaad.2014.02.035

Latchford, T.M. (2010). Cutaneous effects of blood and marrow transplantation. In M.L. Haas & G.J. Moore-Higgs (Eds.), Principles of skin care and the oncology patient (pp. 167–194). Pittsburgh, PA: Oncology Nursing Society.

Lawrence, Y.R., Li, X.A., el Naqa, I., Hahn, C.A., Marks, L.B., Merchant, T.E., & Dicker, A.P. (2010). Radiation dose–volume effects in the brain. *International Journal of Radiation Oncology, Biology, Physics, 76*(Suppl. 3), S20–S27. doi:10.1016/j.ijrobp.2009.02.091

Livshits, Z., Rao, R.B., & Smith, S.W. (2014). An approach to chemotherapy-associated toxicity. *Emergency Medicine Clinics of North America, 32,* 167–203. doi:10.1016/j.emc.2013.09.002

McCoyd, M., Gruner, G., & Foy, P. (2014). Chapter 69—Neurologic aspects of lymphoma and leukemias. In J. Biller & J.M. Ferro *(Eds.), Handbook of clinical neurology* (Vol. 120, pp. 1027–1043). doi:10.1016/B978-0-7020-4087-0.00069-3

McQuestion, M. (2010). Radiation-induced skin reactions. In M.L. Haas & G.J. Moore-Higgs (Eds.), *Principles of skin care and the oncology patient* (pp. 115–139). Pittsburgh, PA: Oncology Nursing Society.

McQuestion, M. (2011). Evidence-based skin care management in radiation therapy: Clinical update. *Seminars in Oncology Nursing, 22,* 163–173. doi:10.1016/j.soncn.2006.04.004

Mechtler, L.L., & Nandigam, K. (2013). Spinal cord tumors: New views and future directions. *Neurologic Clinics, 31,* 241–268. doi:10.1016/j.ncl.2012.09.011

Merck and Co. (2011). *Intron® A (interferon alfa-2b, recombinant for injection)* [Package insert]. Whitehouse Station, NJ: Author.

Mesquida, M., Sanchez-Dalmau, B., Ortiz-Perez, S., Pelegrín, L., Molina-Fernandez, J.J., Figueras-Roca, M., … Adán, A. (2010). Oxaliplatin-related ocular toxicity. *Case Reports in Oncology, 3,* 423–427. doi:10.1159/000322675

Millennium Pharmaceuticals. (2012). *Velcade® (bortezomib)* [Package insert]. Cambridge, MA: Author.

Miltenburg, N.C., & Boogerd, W. (2014). Chemotherapy-induced neuropathy: A comprehensive survey. *Cancer Treatment Reviews, 40,* 872–882. doi:10.1016/j.ctrv.2014.04.004

Mori, T., Kato, J., Yamane, A., Aisa, Y., Kawata, Y., Ichimura, M., … Okamoto, S. (2011). Prevention of cytarabine-induced kerato-conjunctivitis by eye rinse in patients receiving high-dose cytarabine and total body irradiation as a conditioning for hematopoietic stem cell transplantation. *International Journal of Hematology, 94,* 261–265. doi:10.1007/s12185-011-0912-x

Naidoo, J., Page, D.B., & Wolchok, J.D. (2014). Immune checkpoint blockade. *Hematology/Oncology Clinics of North America, 28,* 585–600. doi:10.1016/j.hoc.2014.02.002

National Cancer Institute Cancer Therapy Evaluation Program. (2010). *Common terminology criteria for adverse events* [v.4.03]. Retrieved from http://ctep.cancer.gov/protocolDevelopment/electronic_applications/ctc.htm

Ng, E., & Ilsen, P.F. (2010). Orbital metastases. *Optometry, 81,* 647–657. doi:10.1016/j.optm.2010.07.026

Oddie, K., Pinto, M., Jollie, S., Blasiak, E., Ercolano, E., & McCorkle, R. (2014). Identification of need for an evidence-based nurse-led assessment and management protocol for radiation dermatitis. *Cancer Nursing, 37,* E37–E42. doi:10.1097/NCC.0b013e3182879ceb

Paice, J.A. (2009). Clinical challenges: Chemotherapy-induced peripheral neuropathy. *Seminars in Oncology Nursing, 25*(2, Suppl. 1), S8–S19. doi:10.1016/j.soncn.2009.03.013

Park, S.B., Goldstein, D., Krishnan, A.V., Lin, C.S.-Y., Friedlander, M.L., Cassidy, J., … Kiernan, M.C. (2013). Chemotherapy-induced peripheral neurotoxicity: A critical analysis. *CA: A Cancer Journal for Clinicians, 63,* 419–437. doi:10.3322/caac.21204

Parvez, K., Parvez, A., & Zadeh, G. (2014). The diagnosis and treatment of pseudoprogression, radiation necrosis and brain tumor recurrence. *International Journal of Molecular Sciences, 15,* 11832–11846. doi:10.3390/ijms150711832

Pelosof, L.C., & Gerber, D.E. (2010). Paraneoplastic syndromes: An approach to diagnosis and treatment. *Mayo Clinic Proceedings, 85,* 838–854. doi:10.4065/mcp.2010.0099

Perez, V.L., Saeed, A.M., Tan, M., & Cruz-Guillory, F. (2013). The eye: A window to the soul of the immune system. *Journal of Autoimmunity, 45,* 7–14. doi:10.1016/j.jaut.2013.06.011

Pfizer Inc. (2012). *Neurontin® (gabapentin)* [Package insert]. New York, NY: Author.

Pihos, A.M. (2013). Epidemic keratoconjunctivitis: A review of current concepts in management. *Journal of Optometry, 6,* 69–74. Retrieved from http://www.ncbi.nlm.nih.gov/pmc/articles/PMC3880539/pdf/main.pdf

Polovich, M., Olsen, M., & LeFebvre, K.B. (Eds.). (2014). *Chemotherapy and biotherapy guidelines and recommendations for practice* (4th ed.). Pittsburgh, PA: Oncology Nursing Society.

Pouleau, H.-B. Sadeghi, N., Balériaux, D., Mélot, C., De Witte, O., & Lefranc, F. (2012). High levels of cellular proliferation predict pseudoprogression in glioblastoma patients. *International Journal of Oncology, 40,* 923–928. doi:10.3892/ijo.2011.1260

Pradat, P.-F., & Delanian, S. (2013). Chapter 43—Late radiation injury to peripheral nerves. In G. Said & C. Krarup (Eds.), *Handbook of clinical neurology* (Vol. 115, pp. 743–758). doi:10.1016/B978-0-444-52902-2.00043-6

Prasanna, P.G.S., Stone, H.B., Wong, R.S., Capala, J., Bernhard, E.J., Vikram, B., & Coleman, C.N. (2012). Normal tissue protection for improving radiotherapy: Where are the gaps? *Translational Cancer Research, 1,* 35–48. Retrieved from http://www.ncbi.nlm.nih.gov/pmc/articles/PMC3411185

Pruitt, A.A. (2010). Update on treatment of primary and secondary central nervous system tumors. In *North American Neuro-Ophthalmology Society 2010 annual meeting syllabus* (pp. 259–267). Retrieved from http://www.nanosweb.org/files/Neuro-Ophthalmology.of.Cancer.pdf#page=43

Qiao, J., & Fang, H. (2012). Hand-foot syndrome related to chemotherapy. *Canadian Medical Association Journal, 184,* E818. doi:10.1503/cmaj.111309

Rahimy, E., & Sarraf, D. (2013). Paraneoplastic and non-paraneoplastic retinopathy and optic neuropathy: Evaluation and management. *Survey of Ophthalmology, 58,* 430–458. doi:10.1016/j.survophthal.2012.09.001

Reyes-Habito, C.M., & Roh, E.K. (2014a). Cutaneous reactions to chemotherapeutic drugs and targeted therapy for cancer: Part I. Conventional chemotherapeutic drugs. *Journal of the American Academy of Dermatology, 71,* 203.e1–203.e12. doi:10.1016/j.jaad.2014.04.014

Reyes-Habito, C.M., & Roh, E.K. (2014b). Cutaneous reactions to chemotherapeutic drugs and targeted therapy for cancer: Part II. Targeted therapy. *Journal of the American Academy of Dermatology, 71,* 217.e1–217.e11. doi:10.1016/j.jaad.2014.04.013

Ricard, D., Idbaih, A., Ducray, F., Lahutte, M., Hoang-Xuan, K., & Delattre, J.-Y. (2012). Primary brain tumours in adults. *Lancet, 379,* 1984–1996. doi:10.1016/S0140-6736(11)61346-9

Rinne, M.L., Lee, E.Q., & Wen, P.Y. (2012). Central nervous system complications of cancer therapy. *Journal of Supportive Oncology, 10,* 133–141.

Robert, C., Sibaud, V., Mateus, C., & Cherpelis, B.S. (2012). Advances in the management of cutaneous toxicities of targeted therapies. *Seminars in Oncology, 39,* 227–240. doi:10.1053/j.seminoncol.2012.01.009

Roberts, K.B., Chen, Z., & Seropian, S. (2013). Total-body and hemibody irradiation. In E.C. Halperin, D.E. Wazer, C.A. Perez, & L.W. Brady (Eds.), *Perez and Brady's principles and practice of radiation oncology* (6th ed., pp. 339–350). Philadelphia, PA: Lippincott Williams & Wilkins.

Rosenfeld, M.R., & Dalmau, J. (2010). Update on paraneoplastic and autoimmune disorders of the central nervous system. *Seminars in Neurology, 30,* 320–331. doi:10.1055/s-0030-1255223

Roujeau, J.-C., Haddad, C., Paulmann, M., & Mockenhaupt, M. (2014). Management of nonimmediate hypersensitivity reactions to drugs. *Immunology and Allergy Clinics of North America, 34,* 473–487. doi:10.1016/j.iac.2014.04.012

Sanfilippo, N.J., & Formenti, S.C. (2013). Eye and orbit. In E.C. Halperin, D.E. Wazer, C.A. Perez, & L.W. Brady (Eds.), *Perez and Brady's principles and practice of radiation oncology* (6th ed., pp. 696–710). Philadelphia, PA: Wolters Kluwer Health/Lippincott Williams & Wilkins.

Schlegel, U. (2011). Central nervous system toxicity of chemotherapy. *European Association of NeuroOncology Magazine, 1*(1), 25–29.

Shah, A., Jack, A., Liu, H., & Hopkins, R.S. (2011). Neoplastic/paraneoplastic dermatitis, fasciitis, and panniculitis. *Rheumatic Disease Clinics of North America, 37,* 573–592.

Shikari, H., Antin, J.H., & Dana, R. (2013). Ocular graft-versus-host disease: A review. *Survey of Ophthalmology, 58,* 233–251. doi:10.1016/j.survophthal.2012.08.004

Siegel, R.L., Miller, K.D., & Jemal, A. (2015). *Cancer statistics, 2015. CA: A Cancer Journal for Clinicians, 65,* 5–29. doi:10.3322/caac.21254

Silva, S., & Danson, S. (2013). Targeted therapy and new anticancer drugs in advanced disease. *Thoracic Surgery Clinics, 23,* 411–419. doi:10.1016/j.thorsurg.2013.05.008

Sioka, C., Fotopoulos, A., & Kyritsis, A.P. (2014). Paraneoplastic immune-mediated neurological effects of systemic cancers. *Expert Review of Clinical Immunology, 10,* 621–630. doi:10.1586/1744666X.2014.901151

Smith, E.M.L. (2013). Current methods for the assessment and management of taxane-related neuropathy. *Clinical Journal of Oncology Nursing, 17*(Suppl. 1), 22–34. doi:10.1188/13.CJON.S1.22-34

Smith, E.M.L., Pang, H., Cimincione, C., Fleishman, S., Paskett, E.D., Ahles, T., … Shapiro, C.L. (2013). Effect of duloxetine on pain, function, and quality of life among patients with chemotherapy-induced painful peripheral neuropathy: A randomized clinical trial. *JAMA, 309,* 1359–1367. doi:10.1001/jama.2013.2813

Soffietti, R., Trevisan, E., & Rudà, R. (2014). Chapter 80—Neurologic complications of chemotherapy and other newer and experimental approaches. In J. Biller & J.M. Ferro (Eds.), *Handbook of clinical neurology* (Vol. 121, pp. 1199–1218). doi:10.1016/B978-0-7020-4088-7.00080-8

Soussain, C., Ricard, D., Fike, J.R., Mazeron, J.-J., Psimaras, D., & Delattre, J.-Y. (2009). CNS complications of radiotherapy and chemotherapy. *Lancet, 374,* 1639–1651. doi:10.1016/S0140-6736(09)61299-X

Tofthagen, C., McAllister, D., & McMillan, S. (2011). Peripheral neuropathy in patients with colorectal cancer receiving oxaliplatin. *Clinical Journal of Oncology Nursing, 15,* 182–188. doi:10.1188/11.CJON.182-188

Tofthagen, C., Visovsky, C., & Berry, D.L. (2012). Strength and balance training for adults with peripheral neuropathy and high risk of fall: Current evidence and implications for future research [Online exclusive]. *Oncology Nursing Forum, 39,* E416–E424. doi:10.1188/12.ONF.E416-E424

Tofthagen, C., Visovsky, C.M., & Hopgood, R. (2013). Chemotherapy-induced peripheral neuropathy: An algorithm to guide nursing management. *Clinical Journal of Oncology Nursing, 17,* 138–144. doi:10.1188/13.CJON.138-144

Travis, L.B., Fossa, S.D., Sesso, H.D., Frisina, R.D., Hermann, D.N., & Beard, C.J., … Dolan, M.E. (2014). Chemotherapy-induced peripheral neurotoxicity and ototoxicity: New paradigms for translational genomics. *Journal of the National Cancer Institute, 106*(5), dju044. doi:10.1093/jnci/dju044

Trivedi, J.R., Silvestri, N.J., & Wolfe, G.I. (2013). Treatment of painful peripheral neuropathy. *Neurologic Clinics, 31,* 377–403. doi:10.1016/j.ncl.2013.01.003

Urban, C., & Anadkat, M.J. (2013). A review of cutaneous toxicities from targeted therapies in the treatment of colorectal cancers. *Journal of Gastrointestinal Oncology, 4,* 319–327. doi:10.3978/j.issn.2078-6891.2013.033

van der Noll, R., Leijen, S., Neuteboom, G.H.G., Beijnen, J.H., & Schellens, J.H.M. (2013). Effect of inhibition of the FGFR-MAPK signaling pathway on the development of ocular toxicities. *Cancer Treatment Reviews, 39,* 664–672. doi:10.1016/j.ctrv.2013.01.003

Vidall, C., Roe, H., Dougherty, L., & Harrold, K. (2013). Dexrazoxane: A management option for anthracycline extravasations. *British Journal of Nursing, 22*(Suppl. 17), S6–S12. doi:10.12968/bjon.2013.22.Sup17.S6

Vilholm, O.J., Christensen, A.A., Zedan, A.H., & Itani, M. (2014). Drug-induced peripheral neuropathy. *Basic and Clinical Pharmacology and Toxicology, 115,* 185–192. doi:10.1111/bcpt.12261

Visovsky, C., Camp-Sorrell, D., Collins, M.L., Olson, E.K., Tofthagen, C.S., & Wood, S.K. (2014). Putting evidence into practice: Peripheral neuropathy. Retrieved from https://www.ons.org/practice-resources/pep/peripheral-neuropathy

Voleti, V.B., & Hubschman, J.-P. (2013). Age-related eye disease. *Maturitas, 75,* 29–33. doi:10.1016/j.maturitas.2013.01.018

Vultaggio, A., & Castells, M.C. (2014). Hypersensitivity reactions to biologic agents. *Immunology and Allergy Clinics of North America, 34,* 615–632. doi:10.1016/j.iac.2014.04.008

Walker, J. (2013). Cancer-related neurological toxicity: Peripheral neuropathy. In R. Hawkins & D. Camp-Sorrell (Eds.), *InPractice oncology nursing.* Retrieved from http://www.inpractice.com/textbooks/oncology-nursing/symptom-management/neurologic-toxicity/chapter-pages/page-3.aspx

Welsh, L.C., Dunlop, A.W., McGovern, T., McQuaid, D., Dean, J.A., Gulliford, S.L., … Newbold, K.L. (2014). Neurocognitive function after (chemo)-radiotherapy for head and neck cancer. *Clinical Oncology, 26,* 765–775. doi:10.1016/j.clon.2014.06.014

Williams, L., Carlson, J., Fuhrman, A., Robison, J., & Shelton, G. (2014). Putting evidence into practice: Skin reactions. Retrieved from https://www.ons.org/practice-resources/pep/skin-reactions

Wills, A. (2012). How to perform a neurological examination. *Medicine, 40,* 409–414. doi:10.1016/j.mpmed.2012.05.013

Witt, M.E., & Young, M. (2010). Common drug reactions with cutaneous manifestations. In M.L. Haas & G.J. Moore-Higgs (Eds.), *Principles of skin care and the oncology patient* (pp. 33–56). Pittsburgh, PA: Oncology Nursing Society.

Wood, L.S. (2009). Management of vascular endothelial growth factor and multikinase inhibitor side effects. *Clinical Journal of Oncology Nursing, 13*(Suppl. 6), 13–18. doi:10.1188/09.CJON.S2.13-18

Yonekawa, Y., & Kim, I.K. (2012). Epidemiology and management of uveal melanoma. *Hematology/Oncology Clinics of North America, 26,* 1169–1184. doi:10.1016/j.hoc.2012.08.004

Yoshihara, H., & Yoneoka, D. (2014). Trends in the surgical treatment for spinal metastasis and the in-hospital patient outcomes in the United States from 2000 to 2009. *Spine Journal, 14,* 1844–1849. doi:10.1016/j.spinee.2013.11.029

Zaveri, J., & Cohen, A.J. (2014). Lacrimal canaliculitis. *Saudi Journal of Ophthalmology, 28,* 3–5. doi:10.1016/j.sjopt.2013.11.003

Zedan, A.H., Hansen, T.F., Svenningsen, A.F., & Vilholm, O.J. (2014). Oxaliplatin-induced neuropathy in colorectal cancer: Many questions with few answers. *Clinical Colorectal Cancer, 13,* 73–80. doi:10.1016/j.clcc.2013.11.004

Živković, S.A., & Abdel-Hamid, H. (2010). Neurologic manifestations of transplant complications. *Neurologic Clinics, 28,* 235–251. doi:10.1016/j.ncl.2009.09.011

CHAPTER 15

Metabolic Emergencies

Diane G. Cope, PhD, ARNP-BC, AOCNP®

Introduction

Metabolic emergencies have a lower incidence rate in patients with cancer when compared to the more common side effects of pain, nausea, vomiting, and fatigue. However, when metabolic emergencies occur, they can be associated with significant morbidity and mortality. Advanced practice nurses (APNs) must be knowledgeable in recognizing risk factors for metabolic oncologic emergencies and the signs and symptoms of impending crisis in order to initiate immediate treatment to ameliorate devastating consequences and prevent mortality. This chapter will review the incidence, pathophysiology, assessment, and treatment strategies for disseminated intravascular coagulation, sepsis, tumor lysis syndrome, hypercalcemia of malignancy, syndrome of inappropriate antidiuretic hormone secretion, and anaphylaxis.

Disseminated Intravascular Coagulation

Disseminated intravascular coagulation (DIC) is an oncologic emergency characterized by overstimulation of normal coagulation that causes a paradoxical disorder of diffuse clotting and profuse hemorrhage. Although DIC is associated with a wide variety of clinical conditions, including myeloproliferative disorders and certain solid tumors, the most common clinical condition associated with DIC is sepsis and frequently is present in patients with cancer who present with neutropenic fever (Levi, 2009; Levi & Schmaier, 2014). APNs should be knowledgeable about the pathophysiology, diagnostic assessment, and treatment strategies for DIC to help prevent life-threatening consequences.

Definition and Incidence

DIC is a condition involving widespread activation of the normal coagulation system that causes intravascular formation of fibrin and thrombotic occlusion, resulting in diffuse clotting. Simultaneously, the depletion of platelets and coagulation proteins induces profuse hemorrhaging (Levi, 2009). DIC may be acute or chronic in nature. Acute DIC is associated with more bleeding, whereas chronic DIC is associated with thrombus formation (Levi & Schmaier, 2014). The exact incidence of DIC in patients with cancer is difficult to determine because of its numerous etiologies. However, approximately 10% of all patients with cancer are estimated to develop DIC (Gobel, 2011).

Presenting Signs and Symptoms

The most obvious sign of DIC is bleeding. Clinically, patients may have continuous oozing from body orifices, surgical wounds, and venipuncture sites. In addition, patients may have sclera and conjunctival bleeding, gingival bleeding, epistaxis, hemoptysis, ecchymosis, blood in the urine and stool, heavy prolonged vaginal bleeding, and petechiae. In more severe cases, intracranial, gastrointestinal (GI), genitourinary, pleural, and pericardial bleeding will occur (Arruda & High, 2012).

Other signs of DIC result from the simultaneous thrombosis that is occurring; however, signs of thrombosis are less clinically evident. The formation of fibrin and small clots obstruct the microvascular system and large vessels, thereby decreasing organ function, especially the central nervous system (CNS) and the cardiac, pulmonary, renal, hepatic, and dermatologic systems (Kaplan, 2013a). Skin involvement is the most obvious manifestation of thrombosis, including deep tissue bleeding and large subcutaneous hematomas that can develop into gangrene and tissue ischemia. Lung involvement may be manifested as shortness of breath, tachypnea, and diminished oxygen saturation. Renal involvement may be exhibited by hematuria and, later, anuria and oliguria. Other organ involvement may be seen, with signs such as hypotension; tachycardia; weak, thready pulse; and altered mental status and confusion (Gobel, 2011).

Risk Factors

DIC occurs as a result of an underlying condition; therefore, risk factors are related to the underlying condition. Numerous clinical conditions are associated with the development of DIC (see Table 15-1). Tissue damage and activation of the coagulation system can result from hematologic and hepatic abnormalities, trauma, vascular disorders, obstetric complications, metabolic acidosis, immune reactions, and prosthetic devices. In patients with cancer, specific malignancies and treatment-related consequences can place individuals at a higher risk for the development of DIC. The most common cause of DIC is septicemia, which occurs in approximately 30%–50% of patients with gram-negative sepsis (Kaplan, 2013a; Levi & Schmaier, 2014). Other microorganisms, such as fungi, viruses, and parasites, also may cause DIC. In patients with cancer, a higher risk of DIC is related to the underlying malignancy and sepsis. Leukemias, especially acute promyelocytic leukemia, and solid tumor malignancies (e.g., mucin-producing adenocarcinomas) are associated with DIC (Franchini, Di Minno, & Coppola, 2010). With sepsis, release of cytokines and activation of the coagulation pathway lead to release of bacterial endotoxins and cell membrane material that stimulates the inflammatory response, subsequently resulting in hypercoagulation and DIC (Levi, 2009). Hematologic malignancies and solid tumors are hypercoagulable states that release two tumor-derived mediators of DIC, a protease and tumor necrosis factor, which activate the clotting cascade (Kaplan, 2013a).

Pathophysiology

Normally, the body maintains a balanced state between clot formation, or thrombosis, and clot breakdown, or fibrinolysis (see Figure 15-1). When vascular or tissue injury occurs, the endothelium is damaged, and the procoagulant subendothelial tissue is uncovered. Vasocon-

Table 15-1. Conditions Underlying Disseminated Intravascular Coagulation

Clinical Condition	Specific Associated Dysfunction	Pathophysiologic Process
Bacterial infections	Gram-negative bacteria: Meningococcus, salmonella, *Pseudomonas* species, *Enterobacteriaceae*, *Haemophilus* Gram-positive bacteria: Pneumococcus, staphylococci, hemolytic streptococci	Initiation of coagulation by endotoxin-bacterial coated lipopolysaccharide. Endotoxin activates factor XII to factor XIIa and induces a platelet release reaction, causing endothelial sloughing, damage, and permeability and release of granulocyte procoagulant materials.
Viral infections	Varicella, hepatitis, cytomegalovirus, HIV	–
Parasitic infections	–	–
Malignancy	Hematologic • Acute promyelocytic leukemia • Acute myeloid leukemia • Acute lymphocytic leukemia • Chronic myeloid leukemia • Myeloproliferative diseases Solid tumors • Adenocarcinomas of the lung, breast, prostate, stomach, ovary, and gastrointestinal tract	Activation of coagulation with hemolysis, endothelial damage, and release of cytokines
Hematologic	Polycythemia rubra vera Heparin-induced thrombocytopenia with thrombosis	Hemolysis, hyperfibrinolysis, activation of coagulation, bleeding, and increased tendency for thrombosis and thromboembolism
Trauma	Burns Brain injury Fat embolism Massive tissue destruction	Microhemolysis with release of red cell membrane phospholipids or red cell adenosine diphosphate (ADP) with release of tissue and cellular enzymes into systemic circulation
Vascular disorders	Brain infarction, cerebrovascular accident, cerebral hemorrhage, large hemangioma, aortic aneurysm	Endothelial sloughing and activation of coagulation
Obstetric complications	Abruptio placentae, abortions, amniotic fluid embolism, hemorrhagic shock, dead fetus syndrome, preeclampsia	Release of placental enzymes, uterine tissue, and thromboplastin-like materials, which enter maternal systemic circulation and activate coagulation system
Intravascular hemolysis	Transfusion reactions, multiple transfusions of whole blood	Triggers intravascular coagulation with release of red cell ADP or red cell phospholipoprotein that activates the procoagulant system

(Continued on next page)

Table 15-1. Conditions Underlying Disseminated Intravascular Coagulation *(Continued)*

Clinical Condition	Specific Associated Dysfunction	Pathophysiologic Process
Hepatic failure	Obstructive jaundice, acute hepatic failure	Coagulation abnormalities seen with hepatic dysfunction and intrahepatic or extrahepatic cholestasis
Metabolic acidosis	–	Endothelial sloughing with activation of XII to XIIa, activation of XI to XIa, and platelet release reaction. Release of tumor necrosis factor, interleukins, and interferon activates the coagulation pathway. Decreased thrombomodulin and inhibition of thrombin-mediated activities. Antithrombosis from activation of protein C and S system with thrombus formation and end-organ damage.
Toxic and immunologic reactions	Snake or spider bites, recreational drugs, transplant rejections	Tissue and endothelial damage with circulating antigen-antibody complexes, endotoxemia, platelet damage and release, and hemolysis
Prosthetic devices	Aortic balloon-assist devices, LeVeen or Denver shunts	Thrombosis or thromboembolism with activation of the coagulation system

Note. Based on information from Gobel, 2011; Kaplan, 2013a; Levi & Schmaier, 2014.

striction and platelet attraction occur at the site, and a platelet plug is formed. The release of procoagulant substances and tissue factor activates the coagulation cascade. The coagulation cascade is a sequential activation of clotting factors that ends with the formation of a stable fibrin clot. When the coagulation cascade is initiated, the fibrinolytic pathway is activated. The fibrinolytic pathway controls for excessive clot formation and eventually dissolves the clot and repairs tissue (Kaplan, 2013a).

In DIC, the vascular endothelial injury causes overstimulation of the coagulation system and an imbalance between coagulation and fibrinolysis (see Figure 15-2). As a result of the overstimulation, excessive thrombin formation, consumption and depletion of clotting factors and platelets, and activation of the fibrinolytic pathway occur (Kaplan, 2013a; Levi & Schmaier, 2014). The excess thrombin formation enhances the conversion of plasminogen to plasmin, and fibrinolysis occurs. Fibrin degradation products that possess procoagulant activity increase and result in hemorrhage into the subcutaneous tissues, skin, and mucous membranes. Simultaneously, enhanced fibrin formation exists, with hypercoagulation and microvascular thrombosis resulting in end-organ damage (Franchini et al., 2010).

Prevention Strategies

For DIC, no interventional or treatment strategies are available that can prevent the process from occurring, except for strategies to treat the underlying disorder. Once DIC is suspected, APNs should facilitate the initiation of treatment immediately to prevent or reduce significant morbidity and mortality.

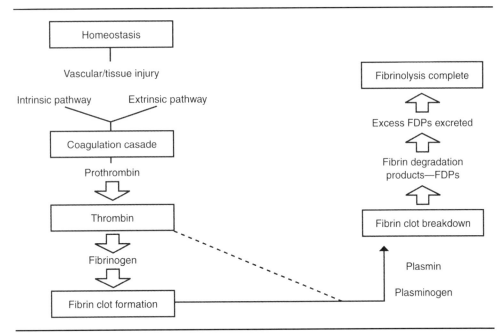

Figure 15-1. Normal Hemostasis

Note. From "Metabolic Emergencies" (p. 384), by B.H. Gobel in J.K. Itano and K.N. Taoka (Eds.), *Core Curriculum for Oncology Nursing* (4th ed.), 2005, St. Louis, MO: Elsevier. Copyright 2005 by Elsevier. Reprinted with permission.

Diagnosis and Assessment

DIC may have an abrupt or insidious onset, may be acute or chronic, and may be compensated or decompensated depending on the degree of consumption and utilization of the various procoagulant substances and platelets (Leung, 2015; Levi, Toh, Thachil, & Watson, 2009). Therefore, a thorough history and physical examination and review of laboratory studies are critical in diagnosing DIC.

The history should include a review of any risk factors associated with an increased risk of DIC as outlined in Table 15-1. Patient evaluation also should cover any prior history of bleeding tendencies, bleeding episodes, or history of blood clots, such as deep vein thrombosis (DVT) or pulmonary embolism.

The physical examination should evaluate for any signs and symptoms that may be seen with bleeding or thrombosis. This necessitates a thorough assessment of each organ system (see Table 15-2). Bleeding from at least three unrelated sites is highly suspicious for DIC (Levi & Schmaier, 2014).

No single laboratory test has significant sensitivity or specificity to diagnose DIC (Levi et al., 2009). The laboratory test results should be evaluated in correlation to the patient's clinical presentation and risk factors associated with DIC (see Table 15-3). The classic laboratory findings seen with DIC include prolonged clotting times (prothrombin time [PT], activated partial thromboplastin time [PTT], and thrombin time), increased levels of fibrin degradation products and D-dimers, low platelet count and fibrinogen levels, and low plasma levels of coagulation factors and coagulation inhibitors (such as antithrombin and protein C) (Kaplan, 2013a; Levi et al., 2009). The Scientific Subcommittee on DIC of the International Society on Thrombosis and Haemostasis has proposed a scoring system for the diagnosis of DIC (Toh & Hoots,

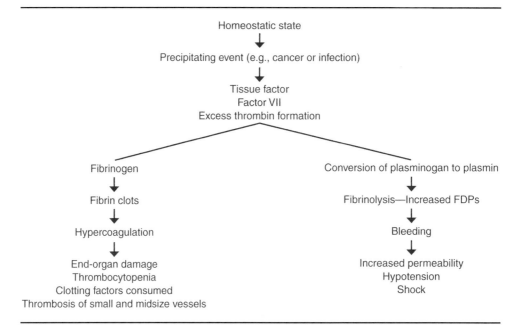

Figure 15-2. The Process of Disseminated Intravascular Coagulation

FDPs—fibrin degradation products

Note. From "Disseminated Intravascular Coagulation" (p. 931), by B.H. Gobel in C.H. Yarbro, D. Wujcik, & B.H. Gobel (Eds.), *Cancer Nursing: Principles and Practice* (7th ed.), 2011, Burlington, MA: Jones & Bartlett Learning. Copyright 2011 by Jones & Bartlett Learning. Reprinted with permission.

2007). The system consists of a five-step algorithm that designates a score based on the severity of abnormality of the platelet count, fibrin-related markers, PT, and fibrinogen level (see Figure 15-3). A score of 5 or greater is compatible with overt (or acute) DIC. This scoring system has recently been found to have a greater than 90% sensitivity and specificity in diagnosing DIC; however, the use of this algorithm is based on the presence of a known underlying disorder associated with DIC (Bakhtiari, Meijers, de Jonge, & Levi, 2004). Differential diagnoses may include hemolytic uremic syndrome or idiopathic thrombocytopenic purpura in addition to the numerous underlying disorders discussed previously.

Evidence-Based Treatment Strategies

Because of the wide variety of underlying disorders and clinical manifestations seen with DIC, treatment should be individualized to the specific patient presentation. The first priority in managing DIC is to treat the underlying disorder. Other goals of management include administration of replacement therapies aimed at reducing or ameliorating the hemorrhagic episodes, control of coagulation processes, and supportive care.

Replacement therapies are administered to replace deficiencies resulting from coagulation factors, inhibitors, and platelet consumption in an effort to reverse the hemorrhagic events associated with DIC (Levi et al., 2009). Fresh frozen plasma (FFP) and platelet transfusions are the standard blood components used in patients with significant bleeding. FFP is preferred over specific coagulation factor concentrates because it contains all of the deficient coagulation factors and inhibitors seen in DIC. The usual dose of FFP is 15 ml/kg IV

Table 15-2. Physical Assessment for Patients at Risk for Bleeding or Thrombosis

Organ	Assessment
CNS: Symptoms dependent on site and size of bleeding or clot	Headache, nausea/vomiting, retching, mental status changes (restlessness, confusion, lethargy, obtundation, coma), vertigo, seizures, changes in pupil size and reactivity; eye deviations, sensory or motor strength alterations, speech alterations, paralysis
Eyes	Visual disturbances—blurring, diplopia, absent or altered fields of vision, nystagmus, increased injections in sclera, conjunctival hemorrhage, periorbital edema; note if sclera are icteric
Nose	Petechiae, blood-tinged drainage, epistaxis
Mouth	Petechiae of oral mucosa, pain, dysphagia, hematemesis, bleeding gums/mucosa, blood-tinged secretions, ulcerations with frank bleeding
Upper gastrointestinal: esophagus/stomach	Dysphagia, hematemesis, blood-tinged secretions, substernal burning and pain, epigastric discomfort (burning, tenderness, or cramping), coffee ground emesis, nausea, vomiting, fever, weakness, anorexia, melena, hyperactive bowel sounds
Lower gastrointestinal: duodenum/anus	Pain (location, occurrence, duration, quality), nausea, vomiting, tarry stools, diarrhea, bowel sounds (hyper- or hypoactive), cramping, occult blood in stools, frank blood in stools (rectum or lower), blood around anus, frequency and quantity of stools, pain with bowel movements (hemorrhoids)
Lungs	Tachypnea, dyspnea, air hunger, respiration rate, depth, and exertion Crackles, rubs, wheezing, diminished breath sounds, hemoptysis (frothy BRB sputum—major airway bleeding), stridor, tickling in throat or chest with desire to cough
Cardiovascular	Tachycardia and hypotension (characteristic of anemia and acute blood loss) Changes in VS, color and temperature of extremities, peripheral pulses (present, quality), and changes in peripheral perfusion Pericardial effusions: dyspnea, cough, pain, orthopnea, venous distension, tamponade (muted heart sounds, hypotension, pulsus paradoxus, tachycardia, angina, palpitations)
Abdomen	Hepatomegaly (liver disease—possible coagulation disorder), RUQ pain, abdominal distension Splenomegaly (increased risk for bleeding): Assess for any trauma; if spleen ruptures, rapid hypovolemic shock ensues; left flank or left shoulder pain Retroperitoneal bleeding: vague abdominal complaints, ecchymoses over flank, occasional bulging flanks and tenderness; associated with hypovolemia
Genitourinary	Decreased urinary output caused by massive bleeding is associated with hypovolemia and shock Hematuria: dysuria, burning, frequency, pain on urination, suprapubic pain and cramping, gross blood in urine, clots Menorrhagia: suprapubic pain and cramping, gross blood in urine, clots (may need to straight catheterize female patients to distinguish between urinary or vaginal bleeding) Frequency and size of clots, number of sanitary napkins used and color of urine are important in measuring bleeding

(Continued on next page)

Table 15-2. Physical Assessment for Patients at Risk for Bleeding or Thrombosis
(Continued)

Organ	Assessment
Musculoskeletal	Bleeding into the joints is usually associated with alterations in coagulation; swollen, warm, sore joint with decreased mobility (active and passive ROM); usually unilateral; tapping the joint's synovial fluid is frequently required to distinguish infection from bleeding. Unilateral swelling of affected extremity, with or without positive Homan's sign
Skin	Petechiae, ecchymosis, purpura, hematoma; oozing from venipuncture sites, central lines, catheters, injection sites, incisional wounds, nasogastric tubes Gangrene, alterations in skin color (e.g., pallor, cyanosis), alterations in skin temperature

BRB—bright red blood; CNS—central nervous system; ROM—range of motion; RUQ—right upper quadrant; VS—vital signs

Note. Based on information from Friend & Pruett, 2004.

From "Bleeding and Thrombotic Complications" (p. 295), by A.L. Rodriguez in C.H. Yarbro, D. Wujcik, and B.H. Gobel (Eds.), *Cancer Symptom Management* (4th ed.), 2014, Burlington, MA: Jones & Bartlett Learning. Copyright 2014 by Jones & Bartlett Learning. Reprinted with permission.

and is indicated in patients with significant DIC-associated bleeding and a fibrinogen level below 100 mg/dl (Levi et al., 2009). However, evidence suggests that FFP at a dose of 30 ml/kg IV may be more effective in promoting complete correction of coagulation factor levels (Levi et al., 2009). Platelet transfusions should be given if the patient's platelet count is less than 20,000/mm³ or if the platelet count is less than 50,000/mm³ and the patient is actively bleeding. Washed packed red blood cells should be given if the patient's hemoglobin is less than 8 mg/dl. Washed packed blood cells are preferred over whole blood because they limit volume and immune complications (Gobel, 2011). Patients with severe hyperfibrinolysis and low fibrinogen levels may be treated with cryoprecipitate at a dosage of 1 U/10 kg (Levi et al., 2009).

Anticoagulant therapy is used when patients have persistent DIC four to six hours after receiving treatment for the underlying disorder and is aimed at reversing ongoing thrombosis, which can ultimately result in end-organ damage. Heparin acts to inhibit further thrombogenesis and prevent reaccumulation of a clot after spontaneous fibrinolysis (Arruda & High, 2012). The usual heparin dose is 80–100 U/kg subcutaneously every four to six hours or 20,000–30,000 U/day continuous IV infusion. Because of the high risk of excessive bleeding, heparin therapy requires close monitoring and is contraindicated in patients who have CNS disorders or open wounds or who have had recent surgery (Gobel, 2011). Antithrombin III also may be administered to increase the anticoagulation effects of heparin. Antithrombin III is indicated when significantly low levels of antithrombin III are present or in patients with severe DIC. The usual dose of antithrombin III consists of a loading dose of 100 U/kg IV over three hours followed by continuous infusion of 100 U/kg/day (Kaplan, 2013a). Patients receiving antithrombin III should be monitored closely for localized bleeding or hematoma, hypotension, and shock. As a result of the suppression of the fibrinolytic system in DIC, antifibrinolytic agents, such as epsilon-aminocaproic acid (EACA) or tranexamic acid, may be considered for patients who have severe hemorrhage after blood component replacement therapy. These agents are very effective fibrinolytic inhibitors and should only be given with concomitant heparin (Kitchens, 2009). EACA is given at a loading dose of 5–10 g IV, followed by a slow push of 2–4 g/hr for 24 hours, or until bleeding is controlled. EACA can cause ventricular arrhythmias,

Table 15-3. Laboratory Data in Disseminated Intravascular Coagulation (DIC)

Laboratory Test	Result	Comments
Prothrombin time	Prolonged	Prolonged, shortened, or normal Nonspecific in DIC; may be prolonged because of liver disease, vitamin K deficiency, obstructive biliary disease, or warfarin therapy
Activated partial thromboplastin time	Prolonged	Prolonged, shortened, or normal Decreased quantity of any coagulation factors Nonspecific in DIC; may be caused by heparin therapy, increased fibrin degradation products, and consumption of clotting factors
International normalized ratio	Prolonged	Prolonged, shortened, or normal Nonspecific in DIC Evaluates overall coagulation
Platelet count	Decreased	Frequent finding, but nonspecific in DIC Decreasing trend in serial platelet counts; may show steep drop Absolute platelet count less than 100,000/mm^3
Fibrin degradation products	Elevated	Indicates breakdown of fibrin and fibrinogen Elevated level may occur with surgery, obstetric complication, inflammation, and venous thromboembolism
D-dimer	Elevated	Elevated levels indicate hyperfibrinolysis. Common in DIC, trauma, recent surgery, inflammation, and venous thromboembolism
Antithrombin III level	Decreased	Anticoagulant activity inhibited Accelerated coagulation
Protein C	Decreased	Anticoagulant activity inhibited Accelerated coagulation
Thrombin time	Elevated	Estimate of plasma fibrinogen Prolonged with heparin, streptokinase, or urokinase therapy Prolonged in DIC, liver disease, or fibrinogen deficiency
Fibrinogen	Decreased	Plasma concentration of fibrinogen decreases very slowly; seen only in severe cases of DIC Nonspecific in DIC; may be low because of congenital or acquired hypofibrinogenemia, fibrinolysis, severe liver disease, malignant processes, or obstetrical trauma
Peripheral smear	Schistocytes (red cell fragments) present	Nonspecific finding in DIC
Plasminogen levels	Decreased	Hyperfibrinolysis
Alpha-2 antiplasmin levels	Decreased	Hyperfibrinolysis

(Continued on next page)

Table 15-3. Laboratory Data in Disseminated Intravascular Coagulation (DIC)
(Continued)

Laboratory Test	Result	Comments
Fibrinopeptide A level	Elevated	Indicates accelerated rate of fibrin formation and coagulation
Thrombin-antithrombin complex	Elevated	Indicates accelerated rate of fibrin formation and coagulation

Note. Based on information from Arruda & High, 2012; Franchini et al., 2006; Gobel, 2011; Saba & Morelli, 2006.

From "Disseminated Intravascular Coagulation" (p. 89), by M. Kaplan in M. Kaplan (Ed.), *Understanding and Managing Oncologic Emergencies: A Resource for Nurses* (2nd ed.), 2013, Pittsburgh, PA: Oncology Nursing Society. Copyright 2013 by Oncology Nursing Society. Reprinted with permission.

severe hypotension, and severe hypokalemia (Gobel, 2011). Tranexamic acid is given at a dose of 1–2 g IV every 8–12 hours (Gobel, 2011). Additional medical treatment strategies include IV hydration to treat hypotension and intracellular volume depletion and specific therapies for possible complications, such as acute renal failure, cardiac tamponade, hemothorax, intracerebral hematoma, and gangrene.

Implications for Oncology Advanced Practice Nurses

The care of patients with DIC is very complex and necessitates prompt treatment and close monitoring. It is critical that APNs recognize early signs and symptoms of DIC and either initiate or support the nursing staff in the pharmacologic management and supportive care of patients immediately. Nurses should assess vital signs, noting any hypotension, tachycardia, tachypnea, or temperature change, all of which may indicate bleeding. The physical examination enables APNs to identify any signs and symptoms of bleeding or thrombosis and to begin appropriate clinical interventions (Gobel, 2011; Kaplan, 2013a). Hemorrhaging or oozing from gums, suture lines, and IV sites, as well as epistaxis, hematuria, and hemoptysis, are all highly suggestive of DIC. Other less overt signs and symptoms of bleeding that may suggest DIC and should be continually monitored for are guaiac-positive stools, headache, joint and abdominal pain, skin petechiae, ecchymosis, purpura, or acral cyanosis (cyanosis of peripheral structures such as extremities, digits, metatarsals, and ears). Patients should have direct pressure placed on any areas of bleeding, and skin protective measures should be initiated to prevent further injury. Venipuncture and blood draw sticks should be kept to a minimum. For gingival oozing, patients should only use soft oral swabs (such as Toothettes®) and normal saline mouth rinses. Patients with epistaxis should have pressure placed on the bridge of the nose and be placed in an upright position. GI bleeding should be assessed carefully, and patients should be given stool softeners, along with a stool diary to record melenic stools and estimated blood loss.

Patients' fluid status is followed closely with intake and output monitoring to assess for early signs of acute renal failure. With any bleeding, patients should be well hydrated with IV fluids to maintain vascular pressure. Patients should increase fluid intake unless contraindicated.

Close assessment of signs or symptoms of thrombosis is necessary. Microvascular emboli of the skin or extremities may be evidenced by small necrotic lesions or skin mottling. DVT may present as unilateral extremity swelling with localized erythema. To help to prevent DVT, patients should have elevation of the extremity, passive or active range of motion performed

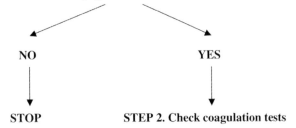

Step 1. Risk assessment

Does the patient have un underlying disorder known to be associated with DIC?

NO   YES

STOP   **STEP 2. Check coagulation tests**

Platelet count, PT, fibrinogen, soluble fibrin monomers, FDPs

STEP 3. Score global coagulation test results

- Platelet count (x10^9/L): >100 = 0; <100 = 1; <50 = 2

- PT (sec.): <3 = 0; >3 but >6 = 1; >6 = 2

- Fibrinogen (g/L): >1 = 0; <1 = 1

- Fibrin-related markers: no increase = 0; moderate increase = 2; strong increase = 3

STEP 4. Calculate score

STEP.5 If ≥ 5   STEP 5. If < 5

Compatible with overt DIC   Suggestive of non-overt DIC

Repeat scoring daily   Repeat after 1-2 days

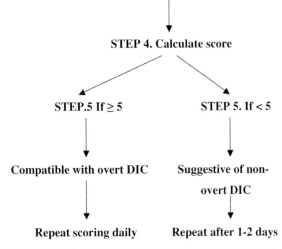

Figure 15-3. Diagnostic Algorithm and Scoring System for Disseminated Intravascular Coagulation (DIC)

FDPs—fibrin degradation products; PT—prothrombin time

Note. From "Recent Acquisitions in the Pathophysiology, Diagnosis and Treatment of Disseminated Intravascular Coagulation," by M. Franchini, G. Lippi, and F. Manzato, 2006, *Thrombosis Journal, 4,* p. 6. Retrieved from http://www.ncbi.nlm.nih.gov/pmc/articles/PMC1402263/pdf/1477-9560-4-4.pdf. Copyright 2006 by Franchini et al.; licensee BioMed Central Ltd. Reprinted from an open access article distributed under the terms of the Creative Commons Attribution License (http://creativecommons.org/licenses/by/2.0), which permits unrestricted use, distribution, and reproduction in any medium, provided the original work is properly cited.

on all extremities to prevent stasis, and avoidance of any restrictive clothing or compression of the posterior popliteal knee (Gobel, 2011).

Pharmacologic agents, as discussed in the treatment section, should be administered promptly to make every attempt to eradicate the process of DIC. APNs should evaluate the laboratory studies every eight hours to monitor treatment effectiveness and the need for additional therapy (Kaplan, 2013a).

Patients with acute DIC are critically ill and require intensive care monitoring. The overall disorder can be very frightening for both patients and their family members; therefore, significant social, spiritual, and psychological services may be required. Patients and family members should be kept informed and educated about the current clinical status, and the healthcare team should answer questions in a timely manner to reduce anxiety.

Sepsis

Sepsis is a complex interaction between an infecting microorganism and an individual's immune, inflammatory, and coagulation responses. Sepsis in patients with cancer is a life-threatening event, especially when patients are receiving chemotherapy and may be neutropenic. APNs can play a key role in prevention and also in directing immediate treatment to reverse the devastating clinical decline related to sepsis that can rapidly progress to death. Therefore, it is critical that APNs are knowledgeable about the pathophysiology and management of sepsis.

Definition and Incidence

Sepsis and *septic shock* are terms previously used to define a wide variety of inflammatory responses. In 1992, the term *systemic inflammatory response syndrome* (SIRS) was introduced (Bone et al., 1992). Infection/bacteremia is the presence of viable bacteria or fungi in the blood with positive blood cultures (Neviere, 2015). SIRS is the systemic response to infection and is described as two or more of the following: temperature higher than 38°C (100.4°F) or less than 36°C (96.8°F); heart rate greater than 90 beats/minute; respiratory rate greater than 20 breaths/minute; or a white blood cell count greater than 12,000/mm^3, less than 4,000/mm^3, or greater than 10% bands (Shelton, 2011). Sepsis is the systemic inflammatory response to a variety of clinical insults to the body and is manifested by two or more of the SIRS criteria. Sepsis occurs in response to an overwhelming bacterial infection that enters the bloodstream. Severe sepsis is associated with organ dysfunction, hypotension, and organ hypoperfusion. Septic shock is sepsis with hypotension/hypoperfusion that is unresponsive to aggressive fluid resuscitation with organ dysfunction (Dellinger et al., 2013; Neviere, 2015). Multiple organ dysfunction syndrome is the presence of dysfunction in more than one organ requiring aggressive treatment to maintain homeostasis (Dellinger et al., 2013; Neviere, 2015).

The incidence of sepsis among hospitalized patients in the United States is estimated at more than one million cases each year (Martin, 2012). The mortality rate associated with sepsis ranges from 12% to 50% in hospitalized patients (Neviere, 2015). Approximately 25% of patients with cancer will develop sepsis, with associated mortality estimated at 28% (Shelton, 2011).

Presenting Signs and Symptoms

The classic signs and symptoms of sepsis are fever, shaking chills and rigors, hypotension, tachycardia, tachypnea, and mental status changes. Patients who are neutropenic may present with no significant signs or symptoms of sepsis, with the exception of fever because of immunosuppression and depression of the normal phagocytic and inflammatory responses (National Comprehensive Cancer Network® [NCCN®], 2015). Additional manifestations depend on the stage of sepsis. Signs and symptoms of severe sepsis reflect the extensive vasodilation that is occurring in various organ systems, whereas the signs and symptoms of septic shock reflect the hypoperfusion and widespread alterations in circulation, tissue oxygenation, and organ dysfunction (see Figure 15-4).

Risk Factors

Risk factors associated with sepsis include infections of the pulmonary, cutaneous, renal, and GI organ systems; exposure to bacteria, fungi, and viruses; medical therapies; trauma; invasive devices; and miscellaneous risk factors, such as age, comorbidities, and frequent hospitalizations (see Figure 15-5). In patients with cancer, numerous factors may enhance individuals' susceptibility for infection. In healthy individuals, three immune defense mechanisms are present in the setting of infection (Shelton, 2011). The first line of defense is granulocytes, which phagocytize and kill bacteria. The second line of defense is cell-mediated immunity, which activates monocytes, macrophages, and T lymphocytes to eliminate pathogens, viruses, and malignant cells. The third line of defense is humoral immunity, which activates the B lymphocytes to produce antibodies specific to foreign bodies or antigens. All three of these mechanisms are affected in most patients with cancer because of either the cancer process or treatment. Patients with cancer undergoing treatment characteristically have granulocytopenia. Patients with hematologic cancers and patients undergoing stem cell transplantation have diminished function of T lymphocytes. Patients with multiple myeloma, Waldenström macro-

Severe Sepsis (Vasodilation)	Septic Shock (Hypoperfusion)
• Tachypnea	• Anemia
• Tachycardia	• Tachypnea
• Lactic acidosis	• Tachycardia
• Hyperglycemia	• Hypotension
• Bounding pulse	• Lactic acidosis
• Thrombocytopenia	• Hyperglycemia
• Decreased fibrinogen	• Elevated PT/PTT
• Decreased urine output	• Thrombocytopenia
• Dry, warm, flushed skin	• Lethargy or coma
• Leukopenia/leukocytosis	• Weak, thready pulse
• Anxiety, confusion, agitation	• Decreased fibrinogen
• Normal or elevated temperature	• Cold, clammy, pale skin
• Normal or low blood pressure	• Subnormal temperature
• Diminished breath sounds, rales	• Leukopenia/leukocytosis
• Increased fibrin degradation products	• Increased fibrin degradation products
• Decreased gastrointestinal (GI) motility, nausea	• Hyponatremia, hypokalemia, hypocalcemia
• Elevated prothrombin time (PT)/partial thromboplastin time (PTT)	• Decreased albumin, magnesium, phosphate
	• Diminished breath sounds, rales with pulmonary edema
	• Decreased GI motility, jaundice, elevated liver function tests
	• Anuria, elevated blood urea nitrogen/creatinine, acute renal failure

Figure 15-4. Signs and Symptoms of Severe Sepsis and Septic Shock

Note. Based on information from Dellinger et al., 2013; National Comprehensive Cancer Network, 2015; O'Leary, 2011.

System	Major Pathogens	Therapies	Invasive Devices	Other

Cutaneous
• Trauma
• Burns
• Skin or wound infections
• Abscesses
• Cysts
• Tumor involvement
Pulmonary
• Upper respiratory infections
• Sinus infections
• Pneumonia
Renal
• Lower urinary tract infections
• Upper urinary tract infections
Gastrointestinal
• Upper
  – Mucositis
  – Esophagitis
• Lower
  – Peritonitis
  – Diverticulitis
  – Cholelithiasis
  – Bowel infections
	Gram-positive bacteria
	• *Staphylococcus epidermidis*
	• *Staphylococcus aureus*
	• *Staphylococcus viridans*
	Gram-negative bacteria
	• *Escherichia coli*
	• *Klebsiella*
	• *Pseudomonas*
	• *Enterobacter*
	Fungi
	• *Candida*
	• *Aspergillus*
	Viruses
	• Herpes simplex
		Chemotherapy
		Radiation therapy
		Immunosuppressive agents
		Antibiotics
		Blood transfusions
		Splenectomy
		Surgical procedures
			Venous access devices
			Urinary catheters
			Gastrostomy tubes
			Nasogastric tubes
			Arterial catheters
			Ommaya reservoirs
			Chest tubes
			Surgical drainage tubes
				Age
				• < 1 year
				• > 65 years
				Comorbidities
				• Autoimmune disease
				• Diabetes mellitus
				• Renal disease
				• Alcoholism
				• HIV disease
				• Hepatic disease
				Frequent hospitalizations
				Malnutrition
				Neutropenia
				Trauma
				Exposure to gram-positive or gram-negative bacteria

Figure 15-5. Risk Factors Associated With Sepsis

Note. Based on information from Freifeld et al., 2011.

globulinemia, and chronic lymphocytic leukemia and patients who are asplenic or are receiving chemotherapy can have impaired B-lymphocyte function (Shelton, 2011).

Before the 1980s, the major documented pathogen in infected neutropenic patients was gram-negative organisms originating from bowel colonization (NCCN, 2015). Since that time, gram-positive bacteria (associated with the increasing use of venous access devices) and fungi have become more common causative agents for infection in neutropenic patients with fever (Bow, 2013).

Pathophysiology

The body's normal defense system works to recognize and destroy foreign bacteria and antigens. At the site of an injury, the endothelium secretes adherence molecules that attract leukocytes. Activation of polymorphonuclear leukocytes produces additional adhesion molecules that promote aggregation and margination to the vascular endothelium and is responsible for the cardinal signs of local inflammation, which include local vasodilation, hyperemia, and increased microvascular permeability. Lymphocytes also release cytokines, including tumor necrosis factor and interleukins, which are responsible for local vasodilation and increased vascular permeability to facilitate neutrophil saturation in the tissue and phagocytosis of bacteria (Gobel, Peterson, & Hoffner, 2013; Shelton, 2011).

Without this normal inflammatory response, microbes can enter the body's circulatory system and tissue and cause an uncontrolled inflammatory response. Endotoxins, associated with gram-negative bacteria, and exotoxins, associated with gram-positive bacteria, stimulate release of inflammatory substances. The inflammatory substances—macrophages, monocytes, neutrophils, and plasma cells—activate tumor necrosis factor and cytokines that promote tissue inflammation, extensive widespread vasodilation, decreased arterial and venous tone, and activation of the clotting mechanisms. As a result, capillary leak syndrome occurs with third-spacing of fluids, hypoperfusion and decreased oxygenation of tissue and organs, ischemia, cell death, and coagulopathies seen in sepsis (Gobel et al., 2013; Shelton, 2011).

Prevention Strategies

APNs can facilitate prevention strategies through ongoing, thorough assessment of patients receiving chemotherapy and immediate initiation of prophylactic treatment if any patient is identified as being at high risk for infection. Patients who are at high risk for infection, including patients with hematologic malignancies, stem cell transplant recipients, or patients expected to have prolonged neutropenia, should receive treatment with quinolone therapy for seven days (NCCN, 2015; Shelton, 2011). Standard therapy for any patient receiving antineoplastic treatment that poses more than a 20% risk of febrile neutropenia should include colony-stimulating factors (NCCN, 2015; Shelton, 2011). Patient and caregiver education should include instructions to prevent infection, such as practicing good hand-washing techniques, avoiding exposure to others with known infections, and knowing the signs and symptoms to report to healthcare providers (e.g., fever, cough, purulent sputum production, urinary complaints, nausea, vomiting, diarrhea, any skin erythema or open wounds).

Diagnosis and Assessment

Diagnosis of sepsis and septic shock is based on the patient's history, physical examination, and diagnostic studies. The history should include a complete review of the patient's cancer, treatment, any recent immunosuppressive or antibiotic agents, recent blood product administration, comorbidities, and insertion of invasive devices. Presenting symptoms may facilitate identification of the source of infection, and therefore the patient should be evaluated for any history of fever, cough with productive sputum, shortness of breath, weakness, mental status changes, syncope, burning on urination, urinary incontinence, oliguria, nausea, vomiting, or diarrhea (Gobel et al., 2013; Shelton, 2011). The physical examination should include complete vital signs with temperature, blood pressure, pulse rate, respiratory rate, and oxygen saturation. Sites of possible infection, such as the oral cavity, perianal region, skin wounds, or catheter exit sites, should be carefully evaluated. Although all systems require examination, the respiratory, cardiovascular, GI, and neurologic systems should receive special consideration, as review of these systems may provide specific data that contribute to the diagnosis and possible source of infection. On examination, patients with sepsis may present with adventitious or absent breath sounds, tachypnea, tachycardia, bounding pulse, abdominal tenderness with hypoactive or hyperactive bowel sounds, and generalized weakness with mental status changes.

Diagnostic studies include blood, urine, sputum, stool, and drainage cultures, complete blood count, complete metabolic panel, coagulation studies, pulse oximetry, chest x-ray, and electrocardiogram (ECG). The complete blood count in patients with sepsis may reflect an elevated or decreased white blood cell count (greater than $12,000/mm^3$ or less than $4,000/mm^3$); greater than 10% blasts; low hemoglobin level secondary to hemorrhage, hemodilution, or hemolysis;

and a low platelet count secondary to platelet destruction or decreased production of platelets (Dellinger et al., 2013; O'Leary, 2011). With both sepsis and septic shock, hyperglycemia will occur as a result of the compensatory anti-inflammatory response with gluconeogenesis and the reduction of insulin secretion (Dellinger et al., 2013). Hypoglycemia may be seen in prolonged septic shock. In addition, elevated blood urea nitrogen (BUN) and creatinine levels will occur as a result of dehydration or renal failure in both sepsis and septic shock. In septic shock, electrolyte alterations that may occur include decreased sodium, potassium, calcium, albumin, magnesium, and phosphate (O'Leary, 2011). Prolonged PT and PTT frequently are seen as a result of possible liver dysfunction and alterations in the coagulation pathway. Assessment of the pulmonary system will include pulse oximetry and chest x-ray. Pulse oximetry values will reflect hypoxia and poor oxygenation, and the chest x-ray may note the presence of pneumonia, effusions, or pulmonary edema. However, in patients with neutropenia, radiographic abnormalities may not be present (Lewis, Hendrickson, & Moynihan, 2011). Arterial blood gases can provide additional information regarding a patient's oxygenation and presence of respiratory alkalosis and metabolic acidosis. An ECG should be performed to rule out possible cardiac causes of hypotension and to evaluate for possible arrhythmias (O'Leary, 2011).

Differential diagnoses may include DIC, acute myocardial infarction, acute pulmonary embolus, acute pancreatitis, acute GI hemorrhage, tumor fever, and adverse drug reactions. Other differential diagnoses may involve metabolic or volemic alterations, such as diabetic ketoacidosis, diuretic-induced hypovolemia, and adrenal insufficiency.

Evidence-Based Treatment Strategies

Treatment for sepsis involves respiratory support, fluid resuscitation, inotropic and vasopressor agents, DVT prophylaxis, insulin therapy, antibiotic and antifungal agents, activated protein C, blood transfusion support, and nutritional and electrolyte replacement (O'Leary, 2011; Penack et al., 2011) (see Table 15-4). Once the diagnosis of severe sepsis has been made, intensive therapy should begin, and the patient should be admitted to the critical care unit for aggressive fluid resuscitation and continuous monitoring of blood pressure, mean arterial pressure (MAP), central venous pressure (CVP), venous oxygen saturation (ScvO$_2$), arterial saturation, and arterial blood gases. Initial resuscitation (within the first six hours after the diagnosis of severe sepsis) should maintain a CVP of 8–12 mm Hg, MAP of 65 mm Hg or greater, urine output greater than 0.5 ml/kg/hour, and ScvO$_2$ greater than 70% (Dellinger et al., 2013).

Patients should be assessed for an adequate airway, and initiation of oxygen therapy should occur immediately with continuous pulse oximetry monitoring to decrease the risk for acute lung injury and to decrease associated mortality (O'Leary, 2011). In patients with severe sepsis, intubation and mechanical ventilation may be required, as a majority of patients develop significant pulmonary complications secondary to pulmonary edema, poor gas exchange, encephalopathy, and altered level of consciousness. More than 50% of patients will develop acute respiratory distress syndrome, the most severe form of acute lung injury. Without correction, patients will progress and develop pulmonary fibrosis (Penack et al., 2011).

Because of the decreased vascular tone and third-spacing of fluid that occurs in sepsis, patients develop hypotension and decreased intracellular fluid. Rapidly administered fluid resuscitation is critical to replace intracellular fluid deficits and replenish organ perfusion. Fluid replacement may include colloids or crystalloids, such as normal saline or lactated Ringer's, and may necessitate large quantities—as much as 10 L within the first 24 hours. Although specific evidence-based guidelines do not exist pertaining to the type of fluid, crystalloids rapidly replace the extracellular volume; therefore, patients require larger volumes for intracellular resuscitation (Schmidt & Mandel, 2015). In patients with preexisting cardiac disease, fluid

Table 15-4. Treatment Strategies for Severe Sepsis

Treatment	Goals of Therapy
Respiratory Support	
Oxygen therapy	Venous oxygen saturation > 70%
Continuous pulse oximetry monitoring	
Intubation and ventilation as required	
Fluid Resuscitation	
May require up to 10 L in 24 hours	Central venous pressure of 8–12 mm Hg
Normal saline	Mean arterial pressure (MAP) > 65 mm Hg
Lactated Ringer's	Urine output > 0.5 ml/kg/hr
Albumin	Increase in blood pressure
	Decrease in pulse rate
	Improvement in organ function
Drug Therapy—Vasopressors	
Dopamine 2–25 mcg/kg/min IV	At lower doses: Vasodilation with increased urinary output and sodium excretion
	At higher doses: Vasoconstriction with increased cardiac contractility, blood pressure, and pulse
Norepinephrine 1–30 mcg/min IV	Vasoconstriction, increased MAP
Drug Therapy—Inotropics	
Phenylephrine 40–180 mcg/min IV	Vasoconstriction, increased blood pressure
Epinephrine 1–20 mcg/min IV	Vasoconstriction, increased MAP
Vasopressin 0.01–0.04 units/min IV	Vasoconstriction with decreased urine output and water retention
Dobutamine 5–15 mcg/kg/min IV	Vasoconstriction, increased cardiac contractility and heart rate
Low-Molecular-Weight Heparin	Deep vein thrombosis prophylaxis
Insulin	Maintain serum blood glucose levels at 80–110 mg/dl
Antibiotic Agents—Monotherapy	
Cefepime 2 g IV every 12 hours	Broad-spectrum antibacterial activity
Ceftazidime 2 g IV every 12 hours	
Imipenem/cilastatin 500 mg IV every 6 hours	
Meropenem 500–1,000 mg IV every 8 hours	
Piperacillin/tazobactam 3–4 g IV every 4–6 hours	
Antibiotic Agents—Double-Coverage Therapy	
Gentamicin 1 mg/kg IV every 8 hours plus antipseudomonal penicillin	Broad-spectrum antibacterial activity
Piperacillin/tazobactam plus cefepime or ceftazidime	
Ciprofloxacin 50 mg/kg IV every 4 hours plus piperacillin/tazobactam	
Vancomycin 500 mg IV every 6 hours if appropriate	

(Continued on next page)

Table 15-4. Treatment Strategies for Severe Sepsis *(Continued)*

Treatment	Goals of Therapy
Antifungal Agents	
Fluconazole 400 mg initial dose then 200 mg IV daily	Empiric antifungal for *Candida* organisms
Amphotericin B (test dose 1 mg) 1–1.5 mg/kg/day IV	Empiric antifungal for aspergillosis
Caspofungin 70 mg loading dose on first day followed by 50 mg/day IV	Empiric antifungal for aspergillosis
Metabolic and Electrolyte Replacement	
Enteral or parenteral nutrition 25–30 kcal/kg/usual body weight/day 1.3–2 g protein per kg/day 30%–70% of daily glucose caloric intake 15%–30% of daily lipid caloric intake Sodium, potassium, magnesium, calcium, phosphate, zinc: Maintain normal serum levels.	Nutritional and electrolyte support

Note. Based on information from Freifeld et al., 2011; Gobel et al., 2013.

replacement must be administered with caution, and close monitoring of patients' CVP is necessary to guide fluid resuscitation. Overall, an increase in blood pressure, decrease in pulse rate, and improvement in organ function demonstrates response to fluid replacement.

If fluid replacement does not achieve improvement in the patient's clinical status, the patient may have inadequate myocardial contractility or persistent vasodilation. If the patient appears to have persistent vasodilation, a vasopressor is appropriate to increase the blood pressure. If the patient has clinical signs of poor organ perfusion with cool extremities, an inotropic agent should be considered. Vasopressor agents, which include norepinephrine and dopamine, are adrenergic agonists and cause increased cardiac contractility and vasoconstriction in high doses. Inotropic agents (usually used as second-line drugs) include phenylephrine, epinephrine, vasopressin, or dobutamine (Dellinger et al., 2013; Schmidt & Mandel, 2015).

Transfusion support is necessary to control active bleeding and correct severe anemia. Platelets should be administered for acute bleeding or if the platelet count is less than 5,000/mm^3. Packed red blood cells should be administered for hemoglobin levels below 7 g/dl. Maintaining hemoglobin levels above 10 g/dl has not been shown to improve patients' outcome related to sepsis (Penack et al., 2011).

Empiric antibiotic therapy should be administered immediately after cultures have been obtained and patients have a high suspicion for sepsis. Patients with neutropenia who present with fever or any potential signs of infection should be immediately treated (within one hour) with a broad-spectrum antibiotic. A delay in treatment has been associated with significant mortality (Penack et al., 2011). According to the NCCN guidelines on the prevention and treatment of cancer-related infections, initial therapy should be based on the most common potentially infecting organism, the potential sites of infection, the antimicrobial susceptibilities of locally isolated pathogens, and the broad-spectrum antibacterial activity of the agent, as well as the patient's infection risk assessment, clinical instability such as hypotension or organ dysfunction, medication allergies, and previous antibiotic therapy history (NCCN, 2015). The NCCN guidelines present an assessment classification system, the Multinational Association of Supportive Care in Cancer, for identifying risk in neutropenic patients with cancer. Detailed discussion regarding this risk assessment classification system is beyond the scope of this chapter, and readers are referred to the NCCN guidelines for further information. Both monotherapy and double-coverage therapy have been found to be appropriate initial treatment for the management of febrile neutropenia (NCCN, 2015). Monotherapy may consist of cefepime, ceftazidime, imipenem and cilastatin, meropenem, or piperacillin and tazobactam. Double-coverage therapy may consist of an aminoglycoside plus antipseudomonal penicillin or an extended-spectrum antipseudomonal cephalosporin, or ciprofloxacin plus antipseudomonal penicillin (NCCN, 2015). The addition of empiric vancomycin to either monotherapy or to double-coverage therapy remains controversial. The use of vancomycin is indicated in some infections caused by gram-positive pathogens that can lead to rapid death; however, vancomycin is associated with an increased incidence of nephrotoxicity and hepatotoxicity. In addition, the increased use of vancomycin has led to a recent rise in vancomycin-resistant organisms (NCCN, 2015). Vancomycin may be considered for serious catheter-related infections, for known colonization with beta-lactam–resistant pneumococci or methicillin-resistant *Staphylococcus aureus*, for patients whose blood cultures are positive for gram-positive bacteria (prior to final identification and susceptibility testing), for patients who have been previously treated prophylactically with ciprofloxacin or trimethoprim-sulfamethoxazole, or for those patients with hypotension or septic shock without an identified pathogen (NCCN, 2015).

Empiric antifungal agents also should be considered in the treatment of sepsis in patients with cancer with proven or probable fungal infections that are unresponsive to broad-spectrum antibacterial agents. The most common fungal infections in patients with neutropenia are *Candida* and *Aspergillus* (NCCN, 2015). Fluconazole is indicated for patients with uncomplicated candidemia, and amphotericin B is indicated for treatment of aspergillosis. Amphotericin B is a common empiric antifungal and also is administered in patients who have been treated with broad-spectrum antibiotics and have persistent fevers (NCCN, 2015).

Severe sepsis and septic shock are manifested as a significant inflammatory response with the possibility of adrenal insufficiency that occurs with major illness. Corticosteroids are commonly used for adrenal insufficiency and for inflammatory diseases. However, corticosteroids, regardless of dose and duration of treatment, have shown no significant impact on mortality associated with sepsis and are not recommended as standard treatment but have shown at least mild effectiveness in treating the inflammatory response of sepsis (Kaufman & Mancebo, 2015). Use of corticosteroids may increase the risk of secondary infections.

Human activated protein C (APC), an anticoagulant and anti-inflammatory agent, has been has been used to reduce the high mortality rate associated with severe sepsis or septic shock. However, a recent updated Cochrane review found no evidence suggesting that APC should be used for treating patients with severe sepsis or septic shock. Additionally, APC was associated with a higher risk of bleeding and is not recommended in the treatment of septic shock (Martí-Carvajal, Solà, Gluud, Lathyris, & Cardona, 2012).

During this critical, prolonged clinical illness, patients will require nutritional support to meet metabolic requirements and electrolyte replacement. Enteral tube feedings are preferred over IV nutrition, which often is associated with significant complications such as infection. In addition to standard electrolyte replacement, patients will require insulin to treat hyperglycemia that occurs as a result of the decreased insulin secretion seen with severe illness (Dellinger et al., 2013).

Implications for Oncology Advanced Practice Nurses

APNs act as facilitators and coordinators of care for patients diagnosed with sepsis. APNs should be able to identify patients who are at high risk for infection and employ prevention strategies. All patient procedures should be performed using aseptic technique, especially those involving care of invasive devices. Recognition of the signs and symptoms of impending sepsis is critical so that appropriate treatment can be started immediately. In addition to the treatment strategies outlined in Table 15-4, APNs should promote patient safety and institute preventive measures that decrease further complications. Daily skin assessment is critical to evaluate for the presence of wounds, and patients should have skin protective devices in place as needed, such as mechanical floatation beds, sequential compression devices, and heel protectors. Patients experiencing altered mental status or agitation may require sedation to prevent injuries.

APNs also can facilitate the promotion of long-term care during the acute phase of illness. The long-term goal is resolution of infection and return to normal organ function; therefore, communication and environmental orientation should be maintained. Daily physical therapy can help prevent muscle atrophy and loss of physical function.

Family and caregiver support is critical during the patient's acute illness. Family members require ongoing information regarding the patient's status and should be educated about the rationale for procedures and treatments. Emotional support is of utmost priority, as the diagnosis of sepsis and its associated clinical manifestations can be frightening for family members. Family members also should be offered other supportive resources, such as social work and chaplain services. APNs should be prepared to discuss advance directives and appropriate palliative and hospice services, if necessary.

Tumor Lysis Syndrome

Tumor lysis syndrome (TLS) is characterized by electrolyte and metabolic disturbances caused by cell lysis as a result of chemotherapy, radiation therapy, biotherapy, or surgery. The release of intracellular products from the cell lysis overloads the body's normal homeostatic mechanisms. Without treatment, these metabolic disturbances can lead to acute renal failure, multiple organ failure, cardiac arrhythmias, and death. APNs should be knowledgeable about the pathophysiology, diagnosis, assessment, and treatment of TLS; however, of utmost importance is knowledge of preventive strategies.

Definition and Incidence

TLS is a metabolic oncologic emergency characterized by rapid cell lysis caused by surgery, radiation therapy, or the administration of chemotherapy or biotherapy. Following cell lysis, intracellular contents including potassium, phosphorus, and uric acid are released into the vascular system. The characteristic metabolic disturbances associated with TLS include hyperkalemia, hyperuricemia, hyperphosphatemia, and hypocalcemia.

The exact incidence of TLS is not known, but the incidence in high-grade non-Hodgkin lymphoma is approximately 40% (Howard, 2014). Although the incidence of TLS does not vary by age or gender, older patients are more at risk for TLS and have more significant complications when diagnosed with TLS because of preexisting renal dysfunction (Cairo & Bishop, 2004).

Presenting Signs and Symptoms

Patients with TLS present with signs and symptoms that are dependent on the degree of metabolic abnormalities. Hyperkalemia, defined as serum potassium levels above 6.5 mEq/L, is often the first metabolic abnormality, occurring 6–72 hours after the initiation of therapy and can produce symptoms that include nausea, vomiting, paresthesia, muscle weakness, paralysis, syncope, lethargy, muscle cramps, increased bowel sounds, and diarrhea. ECG changes can include bradycardia and/or tachycardia, P-wave and T-wave changes, and life-threatening arrhythmias, such as ventricular fibrillation (Coiffier, Altman, Pui, Younes, & Cairo, 2008; Howard, Jones, & Pui, 2011; Lydon, 2011).

Hyperuricemia is defined as serum uric acid levels above 10 mg/dl and can occur 24–48 hours after the initiation of therapy (McCurdy & Shanholtz, 2012). Symptoms of hyperuricemia are malaise, nausea, vomiting, diarrhea, anorexia, edema, flank pain, fatigue, weakness, oliguria, and anuria. Severe hyperuricemia, defined as uric acid levels above 20 mg/dl, can cause acute and chronic renal failure with extreme lethargy, extreme somnolence, seizures, paresthesias, endocarditis, azotemia, anuria, and hypertension (McCurdy & Shanholtz, 2012).

Hyperphosphatemia is defined as serum phosphorus levels above 5 mg/dl and usually occurs 24–48 hours after the initiation of therapy (Gobel, 2013). Symptoms of hyperphosphatemia generally are the result of compromised renal function and include azotemia, oliguria, anuria, and acute renal failure (Coiffier et al., 2008). With increasing phosphorus levels, symptoms of nausea, vomiting, diarrhea, seizures, numbness, tingling, muscle cramps, and muscle twitching can occur (Gobel, 2013).

Hypocalcemia occurs as a result of calcium-phosphorus binding that decreases ionized calcium in the systemic circulation and is defined as serum calcium levels less than 8.7 mg/dl, which usually occur 24–48 hours after initiation of therapy (Lydon, 2011). Symptoms of hypocalcemia include diarrhea, muscle cramps, muscle spasms, tetany, positive Chvostek sign (exhibited as facial muscle spasms following a tap on one side of the face), positive Trousseau sign (exhibited as upper-arm muscular spasms following pressure to the principal vessel and nerve of the limb), seizures, syncope, laryngospasm with stridor, and anorexia. Cardiac signs of hypocalcemia include hypotension, cardiac arrhythmias such as ventricular arrhythmias and prolonged QT wave, heart block and sudden death, and cardiac arrest. Mental status changes associated with TLS may include irritability, anxiety, confusion, depression, and hallucinations (Fojo, 2011).

Risk Factors

TLS occurs most frequently in patients with chemotherapy-sensitive lymphoproliferative malignancies, presenting with large bulky adenopathy or with elevated white blood cell counts, such as high-grade lymphomas or acute leukemias (Fojo, 2011). Patients with various types of solid tumors can experience TLS, but these are more rare and associated to a greater degree with large bulky tumors that are chemotherapy sensitive (see Figure 15-6). Other risk factors include an elevated serum uric acid level, an elevated lactate dehydrogenase (LDH) level, pre-existing renal dysfunction, and volume depletion (Coiffier et al., 2008; Lydon, 2011).

Several therapies may enhance metabolic abnormalities that contribute to the development of TLS (see Figure 15-7). Potassium and phosphorus oral supplements and enteral and parenteral nutrition can alter the normal electrolyte balance. Potassium-sparing diuretics have the potential for elevating serum potassium and enhancing dehydration. Concurrent nephrotoxic drugs, such as aminoglycosides, amphotericin B, nonsteroidal anti-inflammatory drugs (NSAIDs), and angiotensin-converting enzyme inhibitors, also can elevate serum potassium. Clindamycin contains potassium and phosphate and should be avoided (Gobel, 2013; Maloney, 2016).

Certain chemotherapy agents and radiation therapy have been associated with TLS. However, these clinical presentations have only been described as case reports. Patients with non-

Common or High-Risk Cancers	Less Common Cancers	Rare Cancers

• Acute leukemias
• Hodgkin lymphoma
• High-grade non-Hodgkin lymphoma (NHL)
	• Chronic leukemias
	• Other NHL
		• Solid tumors
		  – Breast
		  – Ovarian
		  – Lung
		• Soft tissue sarcomas
		• Thymoma
		• Metastatic melanoma
		• Seminoma
		• Neuroblastoma

Figure 15-6. Malignancies Associated With Tumor Lysis Syndrome

Note. Based on information from Fojo, 2011; Lydon, 2011.

small cell lung cancer have been diagnosed with TLS when treated with docetaxel (Ajzensz-tejn, Hegde, & Lee, 2006), with irinotecan and cisplatin (Persons, Garst, Vollmer, & Crawford, 1998), and with zoledronic acid (Kurt et al., 2005). TLS was documented in one patient with small cell lung cancer after receiving topotecan (Beriwal, Singh, & Garcia-Young, 2002) and in two patients with metastatic melanoma after receiving IV hydrocortisone (Beriwal et al., 2002; Habib & Saliba, 2002). In patients with multiple myeloma, TLS has been associated with tha-lidomide (Cany, Fitoussi, Boiron, & Marit, 2002; Fuente et al., 2004) and bortezomib (Jaskie-wicz, Herrington, & Wong, 2005). Patients receiving total body irradiation (Linck et al., 2003; Yamazaki et al., 2004) and palliative radiation (Fleming, Henslee-Downey, & Coffey, 1991) have experienced TLS.

Pathophysiology

TLS is characterized by electrolyte and metabolic disturbances as a result of cellular changes. Following chemotherapy administration, predominantly malignant cells undergo rapid cell lysis/death. Cell lysis releases intracellular components into the vascular circulation. These include potassium, phosphorus, and nucleic acid, all of which are believed to be in higher concentra-tions in cancerous cells compared to normal cells. Without prompt removal from the circula-tory system, a variety of untoward effects can develop, such as fatal cardiac arrhythmias. Nucleic acids, also released into the circulation, are further broken down into uric acid in the kidneys. Decreased renal function can cause an inability to adequately excrete uric acid, resulting in hyperuricemia, precipitation of urate crystals, and acute renal failure (Fojo, 2011; Lydon, 2011).

Diagnosis and Assessment

The diagnosis of TLS is based on clinical symptoms and laboratory findings. The exact tim-ing of the onset of TLS has not been defined but can range from hours to 14 days after che-

• Clindamycin • Enteral and parenteral nutrition • Potassium-sparing diuretics	• Concurrent nephrotoxic medications • Angiotensin-converting enzyme inhibitors • Potassium and phosphorus oral supplements

Figure 15-7. Therapies Enhancing Tumor Lysis Syndrome

Note. Based on information from Gobel, 2013.

motherapy administration (Gobel, 2013). A complete metabolic profile can identify the key laboratory values associated with TLS, which include potassium, phosphorus, calcium, and creatinine. The other key laboratory study that should be performed is uric acid. Typically, hyperkalemia is the initial sign of TLS.

Cairo and Bishop (2004) developed definitions of laboratory values and clinical TLS symptoms that aid in rapid assessment (see Figure 15-8). These definitions have been incorporated into the Cairo-Bishop risk grading classification, which assists in determining the need for aggressive prevention and treatment of TLS (see Table 15-5) (Cairo & Bishop, 2004). The first part of the grading classification is based on laboratory values. If two or more of these values are abnormal three days before or seven days after chemotherapy administration, more caution and earlier intervention and treatment may be necessary. The second part of the grading classification is based on clinical status. Clinical TLS is defined as laboratory TLS plus one or more of the clinical TLS categories.

The history and physical examination should include a thorough assessment for all presenting symptoms suggestive of TLS, which may include neurologic changes, GI complaints, urinary symptoms, and neuromuscular alterations (Lydon, 2011). The most significant physical examination abnormality may involve the neurologic and neuromuscular assessment. TLS can result in lethargy and generalized weakness associated with metabolic toxicities and hyperuricemia in addition to muscle weakness, muscle spasms, paresthesias, and positive Trousseau and Chvostek signs related to hypocalcemia and hyperkalemia that can progress to paralysis (Lydon, 2011). Other neurologic changes may consist of restlessness, irritability, confusion, lethargy, weakness, and possible seizures. GI complaints may include diarrhea, nausea, vomiting, anorexia, and abdominal cramping and pain associated with hyperuricemia and hyperkalemia. Reported symptoms associated with urinary effects may include flank pain, hematuria, oliguria, and anuria related to acute renal failure. Complete vital signs should be obtained, especially noting blood pressure and pulse changes. Hyperkalemia associated with TLS may result in hypotension and bradycardia; however, decreased renal function and fluid retention may result in hypertension. In the physical examination, lung assessment may reveal rales or rhonchi when auscultating breath sounds secondary to acute renal failure and fluid overload. Cardiac examination may reveal bradycardia in early TLS and tachycardia, arrhythmias, and ECG changes in more advanced TLS. Hyperactive bowel sounds may be noted on abdominal examination, with generalized abdominal tenderness on palpation secondary to hyperkalemia.

Evidence-Based Treatment Strategies

The most important factors in TLS are prevention and thorough assessment for stage of disease, concomitant therapies, comorbidities, renal function, and a complete review of laboratory values prior to initiating any type of treatment. For patients thought to be at high risk for TLS, prevention strategies include prophylactic hydration to maintain a urine output greater

Laboratory Tumor Lysis Syndrome	Clinical Tumor Lysis Syndrome
• Potassium: > 6 mEq/L or 25% increase from baseline • Phosphorus: > 6.5 mg/dl or 25% increase from baseline • Calcium: < 7 mg/dl or 25% decrease from baseline • Uric acid: > 8 mg/dl or 25% increase from baseline • Creatinine: 1.5 times the upper limit of normal	• Cardiac arrhythmias or sudden death • Seizures

Figure 15-8. Cairo-Bishop Definition of Laboratory and Clinical Tumor Lysis Syndrome

Note. Based on information from Cairo & Bishop, 2004.

Table 15-5. Cairo-Bishop Grading Classification of Tumor Lysis Syndrome

	Grade 0[a]	Grade I	Grade II	Grade III	Grade IV	Grade V
LTLS	–	+	+	+	+	+
Creatinine[b,c]	1.5 × ULN	1.5 × ULN	> 1.5–3.0 × ULN	> 3.0–6.0 × ULN	> 6.0 ULN	Death[d]
Cardiac arrhythmia[c]	None	Intervention not indicated	Non-urgent medical intervention indicated	Symptomatic and incompletely controlled medically or controlled with device (e.g., defibrillator)	Life-threatening (e.g., arrhythmia associated with CHF, hypotension, syncope, shock)	Death[d]
Seizure[c]	None	–	One brief generalized seizure; seizure(s) well controlled by anticonvulsants or infrequent focal motor seizures not interfering with activities of daily living	Seizure in which consciousness is altered; poorly controlled seizure disorder; with breakthrough generalized seizures despite medical intervention	Seizure of any kind which are prolonged, repetitive, or difficult to control (e.g., status epilepticus, intractable epilepsy)	Death[d]

Clinical tumour lysis syndrome (CTLS) requires one or more clinical manifestations along with criteria for laboratory tumour lysis syndrome (LTLS). Maximal CTLS manifestation (renal, cardiac, neuro) defines the grade.

[a] No laboratory tumour lysis syndrome (LTLS).

[b] Creatinine levels: patients will be considered to have elevated creatinine if their serum creatinine is 1.5 times greater than the institutional upper limit of normal (ULN) below age/gender defined ULN. If not specified by an institution, age/sex ULN creatinine may be defined as: > 1 < 12 years, both male and female, 61.6 μmol/L; ≥ 12 < 16 years, both male and female, 88 μmol/L; ≥ 16 years, female, 105.6 μmol/L; ≥ 16 years, male, 114.4 μmol/L.

[c] Not directly or probably attributable to a therapeutic agent (e.g., rise in creatinine after amphotericin administration).

[d] Attributive probably or definitely to CTLS.

Note. From "Tumour Lysis Syndrome: New Therapeutic Strategies and Classification," by M.S. Cairo and M. Bishop, 2004, *British Journal of Haematology, 127,* p. 6. doi:10.1111/j.1365-2141.2004.05094.x. Copyright 2004 by Blackwell Publishing Ltd. Reprinted with permission.

than 150–200 ml/hour and prophylactic rasburicase (Coiffier et al., 2008; Gobel, 2013). For those patients thought to be at intermediate risk for TLS, hydration plus allopurinol or rasburicase is recommended (Coiffier et al., 2008).

Once TLS has been diagnosed, each laboratory and clinical abnormality must be addressed (see Table 15-6). Patients may need to be admitted to the intensive care unit for cardiac monitoring based on laboratory value alterations and symptoms. Aggressive fluid hydration should be employed, if cardiac status permits, to maintain a urine output greater than 150–200 ml/hour. Loop and osmotic diuretics also should be considered if patients are not hypovolemic (Coiffier et al., 2008). Hyperphosphatemia can be normalized by restricting phosphate intake and administering phosphate-binding, aluminum hydroxide antacids. Calcium gluconate can

Table 15-6. Standard Treatment for Tumor Lysis Syndrome

Metabolic Abnormality	Treatment
Renal insufficiency	IV fluids: Normal saline 3 L/m²/day or enough to keep urine output > 100 ml/hr Diuresis with loop or osmotic diuretics Dialysis if renal failure
Hyperphosphatemia	Phosphate binders: Aluminum hydroxide 50–150 mg/kg/day Dialysis if renal failure
Hyperkalemia	Regular insulin 10 units IV Hypertonic glucose 50–100 ml IV Calcium gluconate or calcium chloride 100–200 mg IV Sodium bicarbonate 45 mEq IV Sodium polystyrene sulfonate 15–30 g every 6 hours PO or rectal Dialysis if renal failure
Hypocalcemia	Calcium gluconate 50–200 mg IV
Hyperuricemia	IV fluids: Normal saline 3 L/m²/day or enough to keep urine output > 100 ml/hr Rasburicase 0.05–2 mg/kg IV daily for 7 days Dialysis if renal failure

Note. Based on information from Cope, 2013; Lydon, 2011.

be administered for low calcium levels, although hypocalcemia usually is corrected following correction of phosphate levels. Calcium gluconate is usually reserved for patients who are symptomatic related to their hypocalcemia, and it should be used with caution in patients with severe hyperphosphatemia (Gobel, 2013). Furthermore, aggressive treatment for hyperkalemia should be instituted, as severe hyperkalemia can lead to fatal cardiac arrhythmias. Specific treatment includes the administration of calcium gluconate, sodium bicarbonate, sodium polystyrene sulfonate, insulin, loop diuretics, and dextrose.

The two pharmacologic agents used in practice for hyperuricemia are allopurinol, either oral or IV, and IV rasburicase. Allopurinol is used specifically to prevent TLS and should be initiated at least 24–48 hours prior to chemotherapy. Allopurinol acts to inhibit the conversion of the enzyme hypoxanthine, in the presence of xanthine oxidase, to xanthine to uric acid. Blocking the formation of uric acid and crystals may prevent renal insufficiency and failure. Allopurinol acts to reduce serum uric acid levels in two to three days. Side effects of allopurinol include rash, nausea, vomiting, hypersensitivity, and renal insufficiency and failure.

Rasburicase also may be used to lower serum uric acid levels and acts to oxidize uric acid to allantoin, a metabolite of uric acid that has a greater solubility than uric acid and therefore is easier to excrete. Rasburicase reduces serum uric acid levels within 24 hours and is used for both prevention and management of hyperuricemia. Side effects include hypersensitivity reaction, fever, nausea, vomiting, and headaches. Rasburicase is contraindicated in patients with glucose-6-phosphate dehydrogenase deficiency, as rasburicase can cause hemolytic anemia or methemoglobinemia in these patients (Sanofi-Aventis U.S. LLC, 2011).

Implications for Oncology Advanced Practice Nurses

APNs can play a key role in the prevention and management of TLS. Through initial assessment and identification of risk factors, APNs can recognize patients who are in need of prophylactic treatment and vigilant monitoring once chemotherapy has been initiated. Prior to treatment, laboratory values and urine pH should be reviewed to assess pretreatment kidney function, calcium, uric acid, potassium, and LDH levels to identify high-risk patients. Patients should be started on prophylactic hydration and diuresis, and medications such as allopurinol should be started at least 24–48 hours prior to therapy. After initiation of treatment, patient monitoring should include vital signs every four hours, electrolyte values every eight hours during the first 48–72 hours after chemotherapy administration, urinalysis to monitor urine pH every six to eight hours, strict intake and output measurement, daily weight and ECG, and seizure precautions if hypocalcemia occurs. Dialysis should be considered if treatment strategies do not improve metabolic abnormalities and renal failure. Early initiation of dialysis can avoid irreversible renal failure. Patients with persistent hypocalcemia, hyperuricemia, hyperkalemia, hyperphosphatemia, volume overload, and uremia should be evaluated for dialysis (Coiffier et al., 2008; Gobel, 2013). Phosphate and uric acid clearance rates are greater with hemodialysis in comparison to peritoneal dialysis and therefore are the preferred treatment approach. Patient and caregiver education should include risk factors for the development of TLS, signs and symptoms, goals of treatment, and dietary restrictions, including potassium and phosphorus. Patients should receive written instructions about prophylactic strategies, including allopurinol medication administration and the importance of this medication in their treatment, the importance of good hydration, and when to notify healthcare providers.

Hypercalcemia of Malignancy

Hypercalcemia can be induced by a variety of disorders, with the major causes being cancer and hyperparathyroidism. Hypercalcemia of malignancy may occur in patients with both solid tumors and hematologic malignancies and usually is associated with advanced disease. APNs should be knowledgeable of the risk factors, signs and symptoms, and treatment strategies for hypercalcemia in an effort to correct calcium levels, manage and treat symptoms, and provide quality-of-life care to patients.

Definition and Incidence

Hypercalcemia can be classified as mild, moderate, or severe, based on laboratory values. Mild hypercalcemia is defined as a serum calcium level of 12 mg/dl; moderate hypercalcemia is defined as a serum calcium level of 12–14 mg/dl; and severe hypercalcemia is defined as a serum calcium level greater than 14 mg/dl. Hypercalcemia occurs in an estimated 10%–40% of adults with cancer and to a lesser extent in children with cancer (estimated to occur in approximately 0.5%–1% of pediatric cancers) (Kaplan, 2011). Solid tumors such as squamous cell cancers of the lung and breast tumors and certain hematologic malignancies (e.g., multiple myeloma) are most frequently associated with hypercalcemia (see Table 15-7).

Presenting Signs and Symptoms

Patients with hypercalcemia present with a variety of symptoms that generally are nonspecific. Many symptoms may correlate to advanced disease and can be confounded by factors such as cancer treatment side effects, medications, and comorbidities. The most common symptoms are associated with calcium's action in the neuromuscular, GI, renal, and cardiovascular systems (Agraharkar, Dellinger, & Gangakhedkar, 2015). Patients may present with fatigue, weakness, anorexia, depression, vague abdominal pain, constipation, thirst, and polyuria. CNS impairment can be exhibited as delirium, disorientation, and hallucinations, which

Table 15-7. Incidence of Hypercalcemia by Tumor Type

Tumor Type	Incidence (%)
Breast cancer with bone metastases	30–40
Multiple myeloma	20–40
Squamous cell carcinoma of the lung	12.5–35
Unknown primary	7
Lymphoma/leukemia	Up to 50
Renal cancer	3–17
Squamous cell carcinoma of the head and neck	2.9–25

Note. Based on information from Kaplan, 2013b.

can progress to obtundation and stupor or coma as serum calcium levels increase. Cardiovascular changes associated with hypercalcemia are seen with ECG changes, including prolonged PR interval, widened QRS complex, shortened QT interval, shortened or absent ST segments, bundle branch block, and bradycardia. As calcium levels increase, widened T waves and ventricular arrhythmias may develop and progress to complete heart block, asystole, and cardiac arrest (Kaplan, 2013b).

Risk Factors

In addition to the diagnosis of cancer, specifically squamous cell cancer of the lung, breast cancer, and multiple myeloma, several other factors place patients at increased risk for hypercalcemia. Cancer-induced hypercalcemia most often occurs as a result of increased bone breakdown or resorption and destruction with the mobilization of calcium into the extracellular fluid and concurrent renal calcium clearance dysfunction. Patients with metastatic bone disease or renal insufficiency are at high risk for hypercalcemia (Kaplan, 2013b). Immobility, often associated with metastatic bone disease, can increase calcium resorption from bone (Agraharkar et al., 2015). Dehydration, anorexia, nausea and vomiting, fever, and renal failure can reduce renal blood flow and renal calcium excretion. Furthermore, certain medications, such as hormonal therapy and thiazide diuretics, may increase renal calcium reabsorption and precipitate or exacerbate hypercalcemia (Kaplan, 2013b).

Pathophysiology

Calcium in the body is responsible for numerous metabolic, physiologic, and structural mechanisms. Calcium regulates cardiac, smooth, and skeletal muscle contractility, transmission of nerve impulses, cell permeability, maintenance of normal clotting mechanisms, and bone remodeling and structure. Serum calcium levels indicate both ionized and bound forms, with bound forms composing the majority (99%) of the body's calcium in the bones and teeth. Ionized calcium is the active form (1%) in the serum and is bound to albumin, bicarbonate, and phosphate. Regulation of calcium levels is maintained by parathyroid hormone (PTH), 1,25-dihydroxyvitamin D, and calcitonin. Serum ionized calcium is regulated by PTH that is secreted by the parathyroid glands when serum ionized calcium is decreased. PTH acts on target cell receptors to increase renal tubular calcium reabsorption, enhance calcium resorption from mineralized bone and inhibit osteoblasts, and promote synthesis of 1,25-dihydroxyvitamin D, which increases intestinal absorption of calcium and phosphorus, resulting in an increase in serum calcium levels (Kaplan, 2011).

The primary causes of hypercalcemia of malignancy are humoral hypercalcemia of malignancy (HHM) or local osteolytic hypercalcemia (LOH). Patients with HHM may or may not have bone metastasis but can have tumors that secrete humoral factors consisting of hormones and cytokines that act systemically or locally to stimulate excessive calcium bone resorption and subsequent hypercalcemia (Kaplan, 2013b). The tumors most likely to be associated with HHM are squamous cell carcinomas of the head and neck, esophagus, cervix, or lung; renal carcinoma; ovarian carcinoma; endometrial carcinoma; and breast carcinoma (Makras & Papapoulos, 2009). A hormone that plays a key role in hypercalcemia in patients with solid tumors is parathyroid hormone–related protein (PTH-rP), which closely resembles PTH (McMahan & Linneman, 2009). Similar to PTH, PTH-rP increases osteoclast bone resorption, reduces bone formation, and stimulates the renal tubules to increase calcium resorption, with subsequent hypercalcemia and hypercalciuria resulting in impaired sodium and water resorption with polyuria and dehydration. The decreased fluid volume causes proximal tubular calcium and sodium resorption that further increases serum calcium concentrations. Increased calcium concentrations in the glomerular filtrate can result in nephrocalcinosis, or calcium precipitation in the renal tubules. PTH-rP secreted by tumors does not have normal negative feedback mechanisms; therefore, serum calcium levels increase without regulatory control. Other tumor-induced mediators of HHM, including interleukins 1 and 6, transforming growth factor (alpha and beta), epidermal growth factor, and tumor necrosis factor, stimulate osteoclastic bone resorption and can potentiate the effects of PTH-rP on osteoclast activity and calcium homeostasis (Makras & Papapoulos, 2009).

Local osteolytic hypercalcemia is caused by increased bone resorption from direct bone destruction by primary or metastatic tumors that release calcium into the systemic circulation. LOH usually is seen in advanced disease with extensive osteolytic bone metastases (Makras & Papapoulos, 2009; McMahan & Linneman, 2009). Tumor cells produce local cytokines, osteoclast-regulating factors, and PTH-rP that induce local bone resorption, osteoclast migration to the tumor site, osteolysis, and hypercalcemia (Kaplan, 2011; Makras & Papapoulos, 2009).

Diagnosis and Assessment

Patients presenting with vague symptoms of weakness, fatigue, malaise, and nausea and vomiting who also have known bone metastasis should be considered to be at high risk for hypercalcemia. Laboratory studies should be performed, including complete blood count, complete metabolic panel, phosphorus, magnesium, and PTH-rP, if available. Laboratory results that have a direct impact on hypercalcemia and treatment are calcium and phosphorus, which have an inverse relationship; BUN and creatinine, which are used to assess renal function; magnesium, which can exacerbate neuromuscular effects of hypercalcemia with decreased levels; and albumin, which is directly related to calcium levels. Serum calcium levels reflect ionized calcium levels, except in the presence of hypoalbuminemia. Patients with cancer often have hypoalbuminemia, and therefore the total serum calcium should be corrected for the albumin level by calculating as follows: measured serum calcium + (0.8 × 4 – measured serum albumin concentration).

The patient assessment should include a thorough history and physical examination. Several areas of the history may provide specific information that is directly related to hypercalcemia, such as symptoms, disease status and treatment, and medication record. Symptoms that have a rapid onset are more indicative of hypercalcemia of malignancy in comparison to a history of slower symptom onset, which is associated with hyperparathyroidism or other diseases. Disease status is important to assess, as more advanced disease and the presence of metastatic bone disease are risk factors for hypercalcemia. Medication records should be reviewed to note the use of any medications known to enhance hypercalcemia, such as hormonal therapy, thiazide diuretics, calcium, or vitamin D (Kaplan, 2013b).

The physical examination also may highlight specific abnormalities suggestive of hypercalcemia (see Table 15-8). Neurologic manifestations of hypercalcemia may be most prominent in patients presenting with lethargy and confusion that can progress to obtundation and coma as the calcium level continues to increase. Increased calcium levels cause slowing of gastric motility, which may be exhibited on physical examination as abdominal distension, and hypoactive bowel sounds, which correlate with complaints of nausea, vomiting, constipation, and indigestion. Renal system dysfunction is characterized by a reduction in urine concentration and polyuria. As a result, patients can be dehydrated with dry mucous membranes, poor skin turgor, increased thirst, and orthostatic hypotension. Hypercalcemia also causes cardiovascular abnormalities that can include bradycardia, hypertension, and ECG changes, such as a prolonged PR interval, a prolonged or widened QRS, a shortened QT interval, or widened T waves. Differential diagnosis can include TLS, hyperparathyroidism, adrenal insufficiency, hypophosphatemia, immobility, endocrine disorders, medication, dehydration, hyponatremia, and progressive disease.

Evidence-Based Treatment Strategies

Hypercalcemia usually occurs late in the disease trajectory. Therefore, before any treatment is initiated, the patient and family members or caregivers should receive information regarding the patient's overall prognosis and expected risks and benefits of treatment. Treatment for hypercalcemia may temporarily improve symptoms, although no ultimate effect on survival occurs (Kaplan, 2011). For any possible prolonged normalization of the serum calcium levels, antitumor therapy should be initiated. The decision to consider not initiating treatment is an option; however, proceeding with treatment also can improve quality of life.

Treatment for hypercalcemia initially focuses on fluid replacement and diuretics to improve renal calcium excretion followed by specific hypercalcemic treatment that inhibits bone resorption of calcium. The severity of hypercalcemia influences specific treatment

Table 15-8. Physical Examination Abnormalities Associated With Hypercalcemia

System	Abnormality
Neuromuscular	Decreased muscle strength and tone, decreased deep tendon reflexes
Neurologic	Fatigue, lethargy, confusion
Cardiovascular	Orthostatic hypotension, bradycardia, electrocardiogram changes such as prolonged PR interval and widened QRS intervals, shortened QT and ST intervals, broadened T wave, sinus bradycardia, and arrhythmias
Gastrointestinal	Anorexia, nausea, vomiting, abdominal tenderness and distension, hypoactive bowel sounds, constipation
Renal	Polyuria, polydipsia, nocturia, dehydration, decreased glomerular filtration rate

Note. Based on information from Agraharkar et al., 2015; Kaplan, 2011, 2013b.

strategies (see Table 15-9). Thiazide diuretics are not administered, as this class of diuretics increases renal tubular calcium absorption and may exacerbate hypercalcemia. Loop diuretics inhibit calcium resorption in the ascending loop of Henle and facilitate hypercalciuria. Agents that inhibit bone resorption include bisphosphonates, calcitonin, and gallium nitrate (see Table 15-10). Bisphosphonate therapy is the most frequently prescribed treatment because of its effectiveness in lowering serum calcium levels in comparison to calcitonin, plicamycin, and gallium nitrate. In addition, the action of calcitonin is limited, and plicamycin and gallium are no longer marketed in the United States (Wilkes & Barton-Burke, 2013).

Other antihypercalcemic therapies include corticosteroids and dialysis. Corticosteroids inhibit vitamin D metabolism, inhibit calcitriol-induced GI calcium absorption, and increase urinary calcium excretion. Steroid therapy is used most frequently with hematologic malignancies, although no evidence exists to support their effectiveness. The antihypercalcemic effect of corticosteroids may not be seen for days to weeks (Kaplan, 2013b), and long-term use may cause side effects such as immunosuppression, hyperglycemia, GI bleeding, and bone demineralization.

Dialysis is indicated for patients who require rapid lowering of the serum calcium level to prevent life-threatening side effects and have tumors that are chemotherapy sensitive. The effect of dialysis on lowering serum calcium is brief but can remove 200–2,000 mg of calcium in a 24–48-hour period (Siddiqui & Weissman, 2010).

Implications for Oncology Advanced Practice Nurses

APNs can play a key role in the management of hypercalcemia (see Figure 15-9). Prevention strategies are of utmost importance and include the identification of patients who are at risk for hypercalcemia, promotion of adequate hydration at all times, especially during chemotherapy, and education of patients and family members regarding signs and symptoms

Table 15-9. Hypercalcemia Treatment According to Severity

Serum Calcium Level	Treatment Strategies
Mild < 12 mg/dl	Administer IV hydration followed by observation. Treat with antiemetic agents. Limit sedative medications.
Moderate 12–13.5 mg/dl	Administer IV hydration: Normal saline (NS) 3,000–6,000 ml first 24 hours. After rehydration: Administer loop diuretics—furosemide 20–40 mg every 12 hours. Treat with antiemetic agents. Limit sedative medications. Implement bisphosphonate therapy (see Table 15-10).
Severe > 14 mg/dl	Administer IV hydration: NS 3,000–6,000 ml first 24 hours. After rehydration: Administer loop diuretics—furosemide 20–40 mg every 12 hours. Treat with antiemetic agents. Limit sedative medications. Implement bisphosphonate therapy (see Table 15-10).

Note. Based on information from Kaplan, 2011, 2013b.

Table 15-10. Pharmacologic Agents That Inhibit Bone Resorption

Agent	Dose	Mechanism of Action	Side Effects	Comments
Pamidronate	60–90 mg IV over 2 hours	Binds to hydroxyapatite in calcified bone to block dissolution of minerals and prevent release of calcium from bone Reduces number of osteoclasts	Transient low-grade temperature elevations Local reactions at infusion site	Onset of action within 24 hours with maximum effect in 7–10 days
Zoledronic acid	4 mg IV over at least 15 minutes	Inhibits bone resorption and inhibits tumor-related osteoclast activity	Nausea, vomiting, fever, chills, bone pain, and/ or arthralgias and myalgias, elevated creatinine	Onset of action within 24 hours, but can be up to 4–7 days
Calcitonin	4 IU/kg subcutaneous or intramuscular every 12 hours, with dose escalations after 1–2 days to 8 IU/kg every 12 hours to 8 IU/kg every 6 hours	Inhibits calcium and phosphorus resorption from bone Decreases renal calcium resorption	Mild nausea, transient cramping, abdominal pain, cutaneous flushing	Onset of action within 24–36 hours with brief effect
Plicamycin (no longer marketed in the United States)	25–30 mcg/kg IV over 30 minutes	Inhibits osteoclast RNA synthesis	Nausea, vomiting, thrombocytopenia, nephrotoxicity, flulike syndrome, dermatologic reactions, and stomatitis	Onset of action within 12 hours, with maximum response occurring 48 hours after administration and persisting for 3–7 days
Gallium nitrate	200 mg/m²/day IV over 24 hours for 5 days	Inhibits bone resorption and calcium release from bone	Nephrotoxicity	Given after adequate rehydration Onset of action within 24 hours and lasting for 7–8 days

Note. Based on information from Areva Pharmaceuticals Corp., 2012; Novartis Pharmaceuticals Corp., 2015; Wilkes & Barton-Burke, 2013.

that should be reported to healthcare providers. Patient instructions should reinforce the importance of maintaining an oral fluid intake of 3 L per day, the importance of performing weight-bearing activities, and the importance of standing at least four to six times per day. Patients who are bedridden should perform passive range-of-motion activities at least

Prevention Strategies
- Adequate hydration
- Identification of high-risk patients
- Patient safety to prevent injury and potential fractures

Patient and Family/Caregiver Education
- Symptoms to report to healthcare providers
  - Fatigue
  - Lethargy
  - Weakness
  - Confusion
  - Constipation
  - Nausea and vomiting

Symptom Management
- Confusion
- Constipation
- Nausea and vomiting

Hypocalcemic Agents
- Pamidronate 60–90 mg IV over 2 hours
- Zoledronic acid 4 mg IV over no less than 15 minutes
- Calcitonin 4 IU/kg subcutaneous or intramuscular every 12 hours
- Gallium nitrate 200 mg/m^2/day IV over 24 hours for 5 days

Figure 15-9. Hypercalcemia Management and the Advanced Practice Nurse Role

Note. Based on information from Kaplan, 2013b.

twice a day. Patients also should receive instruction about the importance of using assistive devices, such as canes, walkers, or handrails, to prevent falls and injuries. If a patient has any signs or symptoms of neurologic changes, even minor, living arrangements should be evaluated for the need of additional support. With each encounter, patients should be assessed for any signs and symptoms of hypercalcemia, and they should have laboratory studies performed at least every two to three weeks. Prompt diagnosis and treatment is critical to alleviate symptoms and enhance patients' quality of life. Once the diagnosis has been made, APNs should begin fluid hydration, diuretics, and bisphosphonate agents as previously discussed. Patients and family members will require psychological and social support, as patients may require other needs, such as hospice and palliative care (Kaplan, 2013b).

Syndrome of Inappropriate Antidiuretic Hormone Secretion

Syndrome of inappropriate antidiuretic hormone secretion (SIADH) is a fluid and electrolyte imbalance that is one of the most common underlying causes of hyponatremia in adults with cancer. Early recognition of this syndrome is critical because if it goes untreated, patients may experience life-threatening seizures, coma, and death. APNs should be able to identify patients who are at risk for SIADH in order to initiate prompt therapy and prevent an oncologic emergency.

Definition and Incidence

SIADH is defined as an endocrine paraneoplastic syndrome that causes an increased production and secretion of antidiuretic hormone (ADH), also known as vasopressin, and results in increased reabsorption of water in the renal tubules, fluid overload, water intoxication, dilutional hyponatremia, and inappropriately concentrated urine (Sterns, 2013a). An endocrine paraneoplastic syndrome is the abnormal ectopic production of hormones by malignant tumors. Although hyponatremia frequently is seen in the oncology setting, the incidence of SIADH is approximately 10% in patients with small cell lung cancer (Keenan, 2011) and 1%–2% in adults with cancer (Ellison & Berl, 2007; Pelosof & Gerber, 2010).

Presenting Signs and Symptoms

The presenting signs and symptoms of SIADH are directly related to the onset and degree of hyponatremia and subsequent water intoxication of intracellular fluids. The greatest effect is on the neurologic system because of swelling of brain cells. When SIADH has a rapid onset or if the serum sodium level is less than 110 mEq/L, acute neurologic symptoms related to cerebral edema, such as delirium, hypoactive reflexes, ataxia, gait disturbances, seizures, coma, and death, can occur (Keenan, 2011; Lough, 2010). With slower onset or if the serum sodium level is 125–134 mEq/L, patients may be asymptomatic (Ellison & Berl, 2007). Other abnormalities are exhibited in the cardiovascular, GI, renal, and musculoskeletal systems (see Table 15-11).

Risk Factors

Several factors are associated with an increased risk of SIADH, including malignancy, comorbidities, and medications (see Figure 15-10). The most common malignancy, accounting for approximately 80% of all cases of SIADH, is small cell lung cancer (Keenan, 2011). Other malignancies include non-small cell lung, head and neck, pancreatic, prostate, or colon cancer, lymphomas, thymoma, and primary brain tumors. Drug-induced SIADH is relatively common and can be caused by chemotherapy, narcotics, sedatives, antidepressants, general anesthetics, thiazide diuretics, and hypoglycemic agents.

Pathophysiology

Normally, ADH that is released from the posterior pituitary gland and is secreted in response to increased serum osmolality and decreased plasma volume regulates sodium and water in the body. Fluid and electrolytes maintain a homeostasis between the intracellular and extracellular compartments. When the extracellular fluid has a high osmolality, or concentration of solutes in the solution, water moves freely out of the intracellular compartment. With low osmolality, as seen with hyponatremia, water moves from the intracellular into the extracellular compartments. Arginine vasopressin, the biologic active form of ADH, is released in response to an increased serum osmolality. ADH acts on the V_2 receptors in the renal collecting ducts to increase water reabsorption and decrease urine output. When excess production of ADH occurs, increased water retention by the kidneys and increased body water cause expansion of the plasma volume or water intoxication (Lough, 2010; Sterns, 2015a).

SIADH develops because of tumors that produce and secrete ADH or by abnormal secretion of ADH from the pituitary gland as a result of inflammation, neoplasm, vascular lesions, or drugs (Keenan, 2011; Pelosof & Gerber, 2010). The uncontrolled secretion of ADH causes increased water reabsorption, decreased urine output, hyposmolality, and hyponatremia. The normal feedback mechanism for thirst is stimulated by increased plasma concentration and decreased renal perfusion that activates the renin-angiotensin-aldosterone system, causing additional water intake. The majority of the water is in the intracellular fluid; therefore, edema is not present.

Prevention Strategies

Any patient with cancer who presents with any of the risk factors listed in Figure 15-10 should be considered to be at risk for SIADH and requires frequent evaluation for signs, symp-

Table 15-11. Signs and Symptoms of Syndrome of Inappropriate Antidiuretic Hormone Secretion

Signs and Symptoms	Mild	Moderate	Severe
Sodium level (mEq/L)	125–134	115–124	< 115
General	May be nonspecific or none; weakness, fatigue, malaise	–	–
Neurologic	Headache	Confusion Disorientation Personality changes Hypoactive reflexes Altered mental status	Coma Ataxia Tremors Seizures Delirium Psychosis Papilledema Focal neurologic signs
Cardiovascular	–	–	No edema Normal skin turgor Usually normal pulse Usually normal blood pressure
Gastrointestinal	Thirst Nausea Diarrhea Anorexia Vomiting Abdominal cramping Moist mucous membranes	–	–
Renal	–	Oliguria (< 400 ml/24 hours) Weight gain Incontinence	–
Musculoskeletal	Muscle cramps	Myoclonus	–

Note. Based on information from Cope, 2013; Keenan, 2011.

toms, and laboratory abnormalities suggestive of SIADH. Patients receiving cancer treatment should have frequent evaluation of sodium, BUN, creatinine, uric acid, and phosphate levels (Keenan, 2011). Patients should report any nausea, vomiting, headaches, neurologic changes, decreased urine output, and weight gain of more than five pounds in one day. Family members also must note any signs and symptoms of neurologic changes in the patient and report these immediately to healthcare professionals.

Diagnosis and Assessment

Key factors in the history, physical examination, and laboratory results can assist APNs in diagnosing SIADH. A thorough history should be completed that assesses the onset of symptoms, disease status, comorbidities, and medications. Of significant concern are the neurologic symptoms that patients may exhibit, because of the potential for cerebral edema. Depending on the level of hyponatremia, patients may present with confusion, lethargy, irritability, and hyporeflexia. Abdominal examination may reveal generalized tenderness and hyperactive bowel sounds. Diagnostic studies should include a complete metabolic panel, serum osmolality, urine osmolality, thyroid function tests, and computed tomography (CT) scan of the head to rule out other etiologies for neurologic changes, such as brain tumors, hemorrhage, and edema (Ellison & Berl, 2007). With SIADH, serum osmolality will be decreased or less than 275 mOsm/kg, and urine osmolality will be increased or greater than 100 mOsm/kg water

Diagnosis		Medications		Other
Malignancy	**Nonmalignancy**	**Chemotherapy**	**Other**	Current nicotine
Bladder carcinoma	Acute intermittent	Cisplatin	Acetaminophen	use
Carcinoid tumor	porphyria	Cyclophospha-	Angiotensin-	History of smoking
Central nervous	AIDS	mide	converting	Idiopathic syn-
system tumors	Central nervous	Ifosfamide	enzyme inhib-	drome of inap-
• Primary	system disor-	Interferon—alpha	itors	propriate antid-
• Metastatic	ders	or gamma	Barbiturates	iuretic hormone
• Ewing sarcoma	• Cerebral	Melphalan (high	Chlorpropamide	secretion in older
Gastrointestinal	abscess	dose)	Dopaminergic	adults
cancer	• Cerebral hemor-	Vinca alkaloids	drugs	Pain
• Colon	rhage		General anes-	Positive pressure
• Duodenum	• Cerebral vascu-		thetic	respirators
• Esophagus	lar accident		Isoproterenol	Postoperative time
• Pancreas	• Encephalitis		Morphine	period
Gynecologic cancer	Guillain-Barré syn-		Nonsteroidal anti-	Stress
• Ovary	drome		inflammatory	Trauma
• Cervix	Lupus erythema-		drugs	
Head and neck	tosus		Opioids	
cancer	Pulmonary disor-		Oxytocin	
Hematologic can-	ders		Selective sero-	
cer	• Chronic obstruc-		tonin reuptake	
• Acute myeloid	tive pulmonary		inhibitors	
leukemia	disease		Somatostatin	
• Chronic lympho-	• Infections		Thiazide diuretics	
cytic leukemia	• Status asthmat-		Tricyclic antide-	
• Lymphoma	icus		pressants	
Lung cancer				
• Small cell				
• Non-small cell				
Mesothelioma				
Prostate cancer				
Thymic neuroblas-				
toma				
Thymoma				

Figure 15-10. Risk Factors Associated With Syndrome of Inappropriate Antidiuretic Hormone Secretion

Note. Based on information from Akalin et al., 2001; Chan, 1997; Finley, 1998; Garrett & Simpson, 1998; Haapoja, 2000; Hirshberg & Ben-Yehuda, 1997; Keenan, 1999; Kirch et al., 1997; Langer-Nitsche et al., 2000; Miaskowski, 1997; Miller, 2001; Otto, 1997; Poe & Taylor, 1989; Robertson, 2001.

From "Syndrome of Inappropriate Antidiuretic Hormone Secretion in Malignancy: Review and Implications for Nursing Management," by L.A. Langfeldt and M.E. Cooley, 2003, *Clinical Journal of Oncology Nursing, 7,* p. 427. Copyright 2003 by Oncology Nursing Society. Reprinted with permission.

(Sherlock & Thompson, 2010). Hyponatremia can have other etiologies in addition to SIADH. The differential diagnosis may include dehydration, fluid retention and overload, cardiac disease, drug-induced hypervolemia, Addison disease, adrenal insufficiency, hepatic and renal disorders, and thyroid disease (Keenan, 2011).

Evidence-Based Treatment Strategies

Treatment of SIADH is based on the onset and severity of hyponatremia, underlying pathology, and presenting symptoms. Treatment initially is focused on correction of the underlying cause because this usually will result in significant improvement in hyponatremia (Cope, 2013; Keenan, 2011; Verbalis, Goldsmith, Greenberg, Schrier, & Sterns, 2007). For mild SIADH with sodium levels above 120 mEq/L, fluid intake should be restricted to 800–1,000 ml/day, and limited IV hydration with isotonic saline should be administered. For moderate SIADH with sodium levels of 110–120 mEq/L, fluid intake should be restricted, and IV hydration, electrolytes, and diuretics should be administered. If hyponatremia does not resolve with fluid restriction and IV hydration, demeclocycline, lithium, or urea can be administered for mild or moderate hyponatremia (Zietse, van der Lubbe, & Hoorn, 2009). Demeclocycline interferes with the action of ADH on the renal tubules and promotes excretion of water. The usual dosage of demeclocycline is 600–1,200 mg/day orally (Zietse et al., 2009). Fluid restrictions are not required with the use of demeclocycline. Possible side effects of demeclocycline include nausea, photosensitivity, and renal dysfunction. Demeclocycline should be used with caution in patients with hepatic or renal insufficiency. Lithium also interferes with the action of ADH on the renal tubules. The usual dosage of lithium is 900–1,200 mg/day orally (Sherlock & Thompson, 2010). Side effects include nausea, vomiting, anorexia, weakness, and tremors. Urea acts by causing osmotic diuresis. The usual dosage of urea is 1–1.5 g/kg IV with the maximum dose of 120 g/day (Keenan, 2011). Side effects include nausea, vomiting, and anorexia.

For severe SIADH with sodium levels below 100 mEq/L, hypertonic (3%) saline solution should be administered to correct the sodium level by 0.5–1 mEq/L per hour with a target level of 125 mEq/L (Sherlock & Thompson, 2010). Rapid correction of hyponatremia is contraindicated and can result in brain damage and a permanent neurologic condition called central pontine myelinolysis or demyelination. Targeted treatment is another option with recent approval of vaptans—vasopressin-receptor antagonists that inhibit the effects of vasopressin water reabsorption (Sterns, 2015b). Tolvaptan, an oral agent, and conivaptan, an IV agent, are useful in patients with severe hyponatremia because of their ability to cause rapid elevation of serum sodium over one to two hours (Sterns, 2015b). Patients presenting with severe SIADH should be cared for in an intensive care setting because of the need for close monitoring while correcting sodium levels.

Implications for Oncology Advanced Practice Nurses

The priority for APN practice is prevention. APNs should evaluate patients who are at high risk for developing hyponatremia and SIADH and be able to recognize early clinical signs and symptoms. Immediate treatment is critical to prevent life-threatening side effects. Because SIADH may present with subtle changes that often are similar to other abnormalities, such as dehydration, chemotherapy side effects, and neurologic disorders, APNs need to focus on thorough assessment, history, physical examination, and close monitoring of laboratory studies that can indicate SIADH.

Patient and caregiver education also is a key component of the APN role. APNs should instruct patients to maintain adequate hydration throughout chemotherapy to prevent dehydration. They also need to instruct patients and caregivers to report abnormalities to health-care providers, including weight gain, anorexia, nausea, vomiting, weakness, headaches, mental status changes, increased thirst, and decreased urine output.

APNs should initiate therapy as soon as SIADH has been diagnosed. Patients will require detailed information, both verbal and written, regarding fluid restriction. APNs can assist patients in understanding the need for fluid restrictions and in scheduling fluid intake throughout the day. Patients also should receive a list of fluids and foods that are high in sodium and protein, such as beef and chicken broth and processed meats. For patients on fluid restrictions, patient education should include information regarding frequent mouth rinses and use of sugar-free gum or candy for dry mucous membranes. For patients requiring pharmacologic therapy, written instructions should be given about drug administration. Patients taking demeclocycline should be instructed to take the medication two times per day, avoid taking medications with meals, avoid sun exposure, apply sunscreen and protective clothing, and monitor for nausea, vomiting, signs of infection, and urinary output alterations. Patients taking lithium should be monitored for nausea, vomiting, anorexia, and any changes in neurologic status, such as tremors or weakness. Urea administration requires monitoring for nausea, vomiting, and anorexia. For patients who are symptomatic and require IV hydration, APNs should monitor sodium levels at least every eight hours to ensure gradual sodium level normalization. Patient safety is a major concern because of mental status changes and the possibility for seizures. Institution of seizure precautions and close patient monitoring are necessary to prevent patient injury.

Anaphylaxis

Anaphylaxis is an adverse immunologic response to exposure to an offending agent that can result in a life-threatening reaction. Anaphylactic reactions usually have a rapid onset with respiratory, cardiovascular, cutaneous, or GI manifestations. APNs should be cognizant of potential causative agents, clinical manifestations, and treatment protocols to prevent fatal allergic reactions that can occur in patients with cancer.

Definition and Incidence

Anaphylaxis and anaphylactoid reactions are allergic reactions from exposure to a causative agent (Eisenberg, 2013). Anaphylaxis is an allergic immunoglobulin E (IgE)-mediated, immediate hypersensitivity reaction, whereas anaphylactoid reactions are not IgE mediated. Both conditions are referred to as anaphylaxis because they have similar pathophysiologic processes and clinical manifestations (Lieberman et al., 2010).

The exact incidence of anaphylaxis is unknown because of variations in definition by practitioners, underdiagnosing, and underreporting of this clinical condition (Eisenberg, 2013; Lieberman et al., 2010). In the United States, approximately 1% of all emergency department visits involve anaphylaxis, with an estimated 500–1,000 fatal anaphylactic reactions per year (Neugut, Ghatak, & Miller, 2001).

Presenting Signs and Symptoms

Presenting signs and symptoms of anaphylaxis vary significantly among patients. The most common are urticaria, angioedema, flushing, and pruritus (Eisenberg, 2013). Anaphylactic manifestations can occur with the pulmonary, cardiovascular, GI, cutaneous, and neurologic systems (see Table 15-12).

Risk Factors

Several risk factors have been identified that can increase the likelihood of an anaphylactic reaction. These include a history of prior exposure to a particular agent, a history of prior anaphylactic episodes, gender, route of exposure, certain foods, certain medications and blood products, insect stings and bites, exposure to latex, and physical factors (Eisenberg, 2013; Mustafa, 2014).

The prior exposure history and prior anaphylactic episodes can increase the risk of anaphylaxis in an individual. The frequency and intensity of exposure and the time interval between exposures can affect anaphylactic risk. Interrupted exposure to an antigen and greater exposure to an antigen are associated with a higher risk of anaphylaxis. Individuals with a previous history of anaphylaxis to foods, antibiotics, insect bites, and radiographic contrast media are at increased risk for future reactions. Short time intervals between exposure and high doses of antigen given by a rapid absorption route also are factors that can increase an individual's risk for an anaphylactic reaction. When an antigen is administered intravenously, anaphylactic reactions are more common and more severe than with intramuscular, subcutaneous, or oral administration (Pagani, 2010).

Women in general have a higher rate of anaphylaxis than men and have a higher risk for anaphylactic reaction when exposed to aspirin, NSAIDs, latex, and neuromuscular blockers. Men have a higher risk of experiencing anaphylactic reactions to fire ants and insect stings because of occupational and recreational exposure (Mustafa, 2014).

Several foods are common causes of anaphylaxis, with food allergies affecting approximately 8% of children younger than three years of age and approximately 2% of adults (Cianferoni & Muraro, 2012). Common foods that cause anaphylaxis are cow's milk, eggs, fish, shellfish, peanuts, soy, and tree nuts. Other foods include bananas, beets, buckwheat, chamomile tea, citrus fruits, kiwis, mustard, pinto beans, potatoes, and rice (Tupper & Visser, 2010). Some food allergies, such as peanut, tree nut, and seafood, can be lifelong, although other food allergens can be resolved if the food is eliminated from the diet for one to two years (Cianferoni & Muraro, 2012).

Table 15-12. Signs and Symptoms of Anaphylaxis

System	Signs and Symptoms
Cutaneous	Flushing Urticaria Angioedema Lacrimation Diaphoresis Pruritus with or without rash
Pulmonary	Stridor Dyspnea Wheezing Rhinitis/rhinorrhea Nasal congestion Laryngeal edema Pulmonary arrest
Gastrointestinal	Diarrhea Abdominal pain Nausea and vomiting
Cardiovascular	Vertigo Syncope Hypotension Cardiac arrest Substernal pain Bradycardia/tachycardia
Neurologic	Seizures
Renal	Flank pain
Miscellaneous	Feelings of impending doom

Note. Based on information from Gobel & O'Leary, 2011; Van Gerpen, 2009.

The most common medications related to anaphylactic reactions are aspirin, NSAIDs, and beta-lactam antibiotics, such as penicillins, cephalosporins, and sulfonamides (Simons, 2010). Other medications include ciprofloxacin, insulin, iron dextran, mannitol, nitrofurantoin, opiates, streptokinase, thiopental, and vaccines (Ruppert, 2013). Certain chemotherapy agents also are more commonly associated with anaphylactic reactions. These include the asparaginases, cytarabine, etoposide, imatinib, levamisole, melphalan, mesylate, methotrexate, oxaliplatin, pemetrexed, platinum compounds, procarbazine, rituximab, taxanes, teniposide, topotecan, and trimetrexate (Camp-Sorrell, 2011). Blood products can include cryoprecipitate, immunoglobulin, plasma, and whole blood. Finally, radiographic contrast media, often used with diagnostic tests, can produce a wide variety of anaphylactic reactions.

Insect stings and bites are common causes of anaphylaxis and account for approximately 90–100 deaths per year in the United States (Centers for Disease Control and Prevention, 2012). Causative agents are fire ants and Hymenoptera insects, which include bees, wasps, hornets, yellow jackets, and sawflies (Ruppert, 2013).

Latex has become a significant occupational allergen because of universal precautions and the increased use of gloves. Individuals who have a latex allergy also are at higher risk for the development of allergies to bananas, kiwis, pears, pineapples, grapes, and papayas (Yunginger, 2009).

Physical factors may precipitate an anaphylactic reaction. These include cold temperatures and exercise. More vigorous exertion, such as running, tennis, dancing, skiing, and bicycling, are more likely to produce anaphylaxis than less vigorous exercise, such as walking and horseback riding (Ruppert, 2013).

Pathophysiology

Anaphylactic reactions result from activation and release of mediators from mast cells and basophils. Initially, the antigen-specific IgE (the agent causing the reaction) binds and sensitizes the mast cell to the antigen. In patients with cancer, examples of antigen-specific IgE are the chemotherapy agent, the chemotherapy agent's metabolite, or the vehicle that is used to dissolve the chemotherapy agent (Gobel & O'Leary, 2011). With subsequent exposure to the antigen, degranulation of the mast cells and basophils releases histamine, tryptase, prostaglandins, and platelet-activating factor. These mediators target receptors that stimulate anaphylactic responses such as pruritus, vascular permeability, mucosal edema, mucus production, and smooth muscle constriction (Kemp, 2012).

Prevention Strategies

Once an antigen has been identified as causing an anaphylactic reaction, the best preventive strategy is avoidance of the antigen. If appropriate, skin testing also can be performed for diagnostic purposes. Patient education is the most important preventive strategy. Patients should receive education about the risks of future anaphylaxis and avoidance strategies. For patients receiving chemotherapy known to cause hypersensitivity reactions that could result in anaphylaxis, APNs should ensure administration of medications used for prophylaxis for anaphylaxis, which include corticosteroids, H_1 and H_2 blockers, and an antipyretic (Gobel & O'Leary, 2011).

Diagnosis and Assessment

Diagnosis is primarily based on clinical manifestations. Classic signs and symptoms that have an acute onset and support the diagnosis of anaphylaxis include cutaneous reactions, laryngeal edema, bronchospasm, and hypotension (Tupper & Visser, 2010). Once the patient has received emergency treatment and is stabilized, a complete history and physical examination can be obtained. Any prior anaphylactic reactions should be documented in addition to any known allergies and list of foods, medications, activities, or exposure to any insects just prior to the anaphylactic event. The physical examination should assess vital signs and focus on the cutaneous, pulmonary, cardiovascular, GI, and neurologic systems (see Table 15-12). The differential diagnosis includes septic shock, vasovagal reaction, cardiogenic shock, hypovolemic shock, carcinoid syndrome, panic attack, hyperglycemia, hypoglycemia, foreign body aspiration, status asthmaticus, and pulmonary embolism.

Evidence-Based Treatment Strategies

The initial treatment for anaphylaxis is to stabilize the patient by maintaining the airway, providing oxygen administration at 8–10 L per minute unless contraindicated in patients with chronic obstructive pulmonary disease, placing the patient in a supine or Trendelenburg position, maintaining IV access and rapidly administering normal saline, and, in patients with cancer, stopping the infusion of the offending agent or chemotherapy drug. Pharmacologic therapy may include the administration of epinephrine, antihistamines, bronchodilators, or corticosteroids, depending on the severity of the anaphylactic reaction (see Table 15-13) (Joint Task Force on Practice Parameters, 2010).

Implications for Oncology Advanced Practice Nurses

APNs can play a critical role in the prevention, assessment, diagnosis, and treatment of anaphylactic reactions. In the oncology setting, the potential for anaphylaxis is great with the introduction of new medications. Furthermore, numerous chemotherapy agents and the solvents used for administration possess the potential for adverse reactions such as anaphylaxis.

APNs can identify patients at high risk for anaphylaxis by performing a complete assessment that includes identification of any known allergies or prior history of allergic reactions. Although some antineoplastic agents possess greater potential for allergic reactions, all patients receiving chemotherapy or biotherapy agents should be considered to be at risk for an anaphylactic reaction. Patients who are at risk should be educated about the potential for allergic reactions both in the supervised treatment setting and also at home. Patients and caregivers should receive written instructions about the signs and symptoms to report to healthcare providers.

Of paramount importance is the availability of proper equipment, including an emergency kit and medications to adequately treat patients who experience an anaphylactic reaction as a consequence of chemotherapy administration. Patient safety and stabilization once a reaction has occurred is critical, and APNs should be knowledgeable about the appropriate procedures for the treatment of anaphylaxis. APNs should reassure patients to reduce anxiety and fear throughout the anaphylactic reaction.

Evaluation of Outcomes

High-quality patient care is a result of evidence-based interventions and evaluation of outcomes. APNs can play a critical role in evaluating nursing-sensitive patient outcomes for patients experiencing or at risk for metabolic emergencies because of their direct involvement in facilitating patient care.

Table 15-13. Pharmacologic Treatment for Anaphylaxis

Agent	Dosage	Indication
Epinephrine intramuscular or sub-cutaneous	0.3–0.5 ml in anterior or lateral thigh If no response, may repeat every 5–15 minutes	Angioedema Hypotension Laryngeal edema
Diphenhydramine	25–50 mg IV over 10–15 minutes	Mucosal edema Mucus production
Ranitidine	1 mg/kg over 10–15 minutes	Mucosal edema
Famotidine	20 mg IV	Mucus production
Albuterol	2.5–5 mg in 3 ml saline via nebulizer	Bronchospasm
Methylprednisolone Dexamethasone	125 mg IV 20 mg IV	Bronchospasm
Crystalloid solution for IV infusion (maintain blood pressure)	–	–
If inadequate response to epi-nephrine and saline:		
Dopamine	5–20 mcg/kg/min	–
Norepinephrine	0.5–30 mcg/min	–

Note. Based on information from Joint Task Force on Practice Parameters, 2010; Mustafa, 2014; Ruppert, 2013.

Ultimately, the overall goal in the treatment of DIC is to prevent mortality and significantly reduce morbidity. Research on the most effective treatment for DIC is limited because of the numerous underlying disorders and the variance in clinical presentations. Currently, some treatments remain controversial, as discussed previously; however, the standard of treatment remains directed at the individual clinical presentation and severity of the DIC process.

The overall goal of treatment for sepsis and septic shock is to eradicate the infectious organism and prevent organ failure. Results of clinical trials involving antibiotic therapy have now provided evidence to facilitate specific antibiotic guidelines for the treatment of sepsis (NCCN, 2015). Other treatment strategies are based on individual clinical presentation to provide supportive care throughout the illness trajectory.

The priority in TLS is prevention; therefore, APNs' primary goal is to ensure that patients receive adequate oncologic therapy without complications. When TLS occurs, prompt treatment is imperative to correct metabolic abnormalities and ultimately prevent major irreversible complications, such as renal failure and cardiac arrest.

With hypercalcemia of malignancy, the main treatment goal is rapid reduction of serum calcium levels to resolve associated signs and symptoms. Outcome evaluation should include assessment of symptom resolution and decreasing serum and urinary calcium levels. In addition to aggressive hydration and symptom management, bisphosphonate therapy has been found to be very effective in hypercalcemia prevention and treatment (Kaplan, 2013b; Keenan, 2011).

The goal of treatment for SIADH is correction of hyponatremia and associated clinical manifestations. No randomized clinical trials exist to guide this therapy; however, the literature supports fluid restriction, IV hydration with hypertonic saline for severe hyponatremia, and pharmacologic agents such as demeclocycline, lithium, and urea.

The goal of treatment for anaphylaxis is to eradicate the allergic reaction and clinical manifestations and stabilize the patient. No randomized clinical trials exist, but the literature supports the clinical practice of using pharmacologic agents, including epinephrine, antihistamines, vasopressors, crystalloid IV solution, bronchodilators, and antiarrhythmic medications.

Conclusion

Metabolic oncologic emergencies, including DIC, sepsis, TLS, SIADH, hypercalcemia of malignancy, and anaphylaxis, can evolve rapidly. APNs have a unique role in providing direct continuous care for patients and family members throughout the disease and treatment trajectory. With advanced knowledge and understanding of the metabolic emergencies that can occur in patients with cancer, APNs can facilitate prevention strategies for patients at high risk for developing complications. APNs should employ treatment strategies immediately to prevent morbidity and mortality.

Case Study

L.M. is a 52-year-old woman who was diagnosed four years ago with stage IV small cell lung carcinoma with metastasis to the brain and bone. She originally received radiation therapy to the brain and received six cycles of cisplatin and irinotecan. Follow-up CT scans, bone scan, and positron-emission tomography scan showed that L.M. was in complete remission. She did well for two years, when follow-up CT scan showed a right hilar mass. L.M. was enrolled in a clinical trial with vinflunine. L.M. had significant side effects with this drug and experienced constipation and overwhelming fatigue. After two cycles, L.M. described herself as "completely worn out."

Two weeks after the second cycle of vinflunine, L.M.'s husband took her to the emergency department. Her husband reported that she was incoherent and her sentences and conversation were inappropriate. He also noticed that she had twitching and tremors of her hands, but he did not witness any seizure-like activity. L.M. denied experiencing any headaches, nausea, vomiting, or paresthesias. Neurologic examination demonstrated that L.M. was disoriented to person, place, and time and was unable to answer simple questions.

A complete metabolic panel revealed a serum sodium level of 117 mEq/L and a calcium level of 11.4 mg/dl. L.M. was admitted to the intensive care unit after her stay in the emergency department.

1. Based on L.M.'s history and clinical presentation, what should the APN include in the differential diagnosis?
   - The differential diagnosis would include
     - Metabolic abnormalities
     - Cerebrovascular accident
     - Recurrent brain metastasis
     - Chemotherapy side effects
     - Anemia related to chemotherapy
     - Hypoxia secondary to disease progression.
2. What diagnostic tests should be performed?

- Diagnostic tests should include both radiographic and laboratory studies. A magnetic resonance imaging study of the brain should be performed to rule out any neurologic abnormalities and possible recurrent metastasis. Laboratory tests should include a complete blood count to evaluate for anemia, as well as a complete metabolic profile to evaluate for any metabolic abnormalities that may be contributing to her neurologic changes.

3. Based on this assessment data, what abnormality is most likely the cause of L.M.'s signs and symptoms?
   - L.M. presents with moderate hyponatremia with a sodium level of 117 mEq/L. Sodium levels in this range can cause symptoms of altered mental status, confusion, and myoclonus. L.M. also presents with hypercalcemia and a calcium level of 11.4 mg/dl. Hypercalcemia can cause confusion and constipation.

4. What therapies should the APN expect to be initiated for SIADH and hypercalcemia?
   - The treatment for SIADH should include fluid restriction, isotonic saline IV hydration, and diuretic therapy. If the hyponatremia does not resolve with these treatments, demeclocycline, lithium, or urea may be administered, or the saline can be changed to a hypertonic solution. The treatment for hypercalcemia should include IV hydration and bisphosphonate therapy.
   - At the time of discharge, L.M.'s sodium level was 130 mEq/L and her calcium level was 9.7 mg/dl. L.M. was discharged on demeclocycline and started on bisphosphonate therapy as an outpatient. Prior to discharge, L.M. had CT scans that showed an enlarging right hilar mass and recurrent bone metastasis. L.M.'s husband was very anxious about taking his wife home and providing her care.

5. What should the APN include in the discharge plan?
   - The APN should first address the concerns of L.M.'s husband because he is the primary caregiver and will be responsible for understanding and executing the discharge instructions. L.M.'s husband should be given education about SIADH and hypercalcemia with explanations regarding why these are frequently seen in patients with cancer. The instructions should include signs and symptoms and what to report to the healthcare providers. Discharge instructions also should include to maintain a well-balanced diet and adequate fluid intake. Medication instructions should include dosage and frequency schedule for oral demeclocycline and the importance of continuing IV bisphosphonate therapy as an outpatient. The APN also should identify community resources for supportive care for L.M.'s husband, such as home health or hospice as needed.

Once discharged, L.M. continued to improve and saw her oncologist to discuss other treatment options. Her chemotherapy regimen was changed to etoposide and carboplatin. After two cycles, L.M.'s sodium level continued to improve to her current level of 132 mEq/L. A follow-up CT scan showed a decrease in the size of the hilar mass, showing a positive response to therapy. With the improvement in her disease and sodium level, her demeclocycline was discontinued. She continues on bisphosphonate therapy and has not had any further episodes of hypercalcemia.

Key Points

Disseminated Intravascular Coagulation

- Although a wide variety of clinical conditions are associated with DIC, the most common is sepsis.
- DIC is characterized by diffuse clotting and profuse hemorrhage.

- The classic laboratory findings are prolonged clotting times, increased levels of fibrin degradation product and D-dimers, low platelet count and fibrinogen levels, and low plasma levels of coagulation factors.
- Treatment strategies focus on treatment of the underlying disorder, administration of replacement therapies, and supportive care.

Sepsis

- Sepsis is a complex interaction between an infecting microorganism and the immune, inflammatory, and coagulation responses of an individual.
- Gram-positive bacteria and fungi are common causative agents for infection in neutropenic patients with fever.
- Treatment strategies involve respiratory support, fluid resuscitation, inotropic and vasopressor agents, DVT prophylaxis, insulin therapy, antibiotic and antifungal agents, activated protein C, blood transfusion support, and nutritional and electrolyte replacement.

Tumor Lysis Syndrome

- TLS is characterized by electrolyte and metabolic disturbances caused by cell lysis as a result of chemotherapy, radiation therapy, biotherapy, or surgery.
- The characteristic metabolic disturbances associated with TLS include hyperkalemia, hyperuricemia, hyperphosphatemia, and hypocalcemia.
- Prevention strategies for patients thought to be at high risk for TLS include allopurinol, fluid loading, and urinary alkalinization.
- Treatment strategies are aimed at correction of laboratory and metabolic abnormalities.

Hypercalcemia of Malignancy

- Hypercalcemia of malignancy occurs in patients with solid tumors and hematologic malignancies and usually is associated with advanced disease.
- Patients with hypercalcemia can present with a wide variety of signs and symptoms.
- Standard treatment strategies include fluid replacement, diuretics, and bisphosphonate therapy.

Syndrome of Inappropriate Antidiuretic Hormone Secretion

- SIADH is an endocrine paraneoplastic syndrome that causes increased ADH with fluid overload and dilutional hyponatremia.
- Signs and symptoms are related to the onset and degree of hyponatremia.
- Treatment strategies include correction of the underlying cause, oral fluid restriction, IV hydration, diuretics, and demeclocycline, lithium, or urea therapy.

Anaphylaxis

- Anaphylaxis is an adverse immunologic response to exposure to an offending agent.
- Offending agents may include certain foods, insect bites, latex, physical exertion, and certain medications and blood products.
- Classic signs and symptoms of anaphylaxis include cutaneous reactions, laryngeal edema, bronchospasm, and hypotension.

• Treatment strategies include stabilization of the patient, supportive care, rapid administration of normal saline, and pharmacologic therapy with epinephrine, antihistamines, bronchodilators, or corticosteroids.

Recommended Resources for Oncology Advanced Practice Nurses

Disseminated Intravascular Coagulation

• Medscape article with information regarding etiologies, diagnosis, workup, and treatment for DIC: http://emedicine.medscape.com/article/199627-overview
• UpToDate® professional-level topic review: "Clinical Features, Diagnosis, and Treatment of Disseminated Intravascular Coagulation in Adults": www.uptodate.com/contents/clinical -features-diagnosis-and-treatment-of-disseminated-intravascular-coagulation-in-adults (subscription required)

Sepsis

• International Sepsis Forum: http://internationalsepsisforum.com
• Society of Critical Care Medicine resources for patients and family members regarding sepsis: www.myicucare.org
• Surviving Sepsis Campaign, a website for patients, healthcare professionals, and the general public regarding sepsis information: www.survivingsepsis.org
• UpToDate professional-level topic review: "Evaluation and Management of Severe Sepsis and Septic Shock in Adults": www.uptodate.com/contents/evaluation-and-management-of -severe-sepsis-and-septic-shock-in-adults (full article viewable without subscription)

Tumor Lysis Syndrome

• Patients Against Lymphoma patient information regarding TLS, with additional website links: www.lymphomation.org/side-effect-tumor-lysis.htm
• UpToDate professional-level topic review: "Tumor Lysis Syndrome: Prevention and Treatment": www.uptodate.com/contents/tumor-lysis-syndrome-prevention-and-treatment (full article viewable without subscription)

Hypercalcemia of Malignancy

• Clinical Key: Professional-level topic review of the causes, diagnosis, and treatment of hypercalcemia: www.clinicalkey.com/topics/endocrinology/hypercalcemia.html
• UpToDate professional-level topic review: "Hypercalcemia of Malignancy": www.uptodate .com/contents/hypercalcemia-of-malignancy (subscription required)
• Novartis Pharmaceuticals patient website with information about hypercalcemia: www .novartis.ca/en/disease_conditions/C-D/index.shtml

Syndrome of Inappropriate Antidiuretic Hormone Secretion

• Medscape article providing a professional-level topic review of SIADH: http://emedicine .medscape.com/article/246650-overview

Anaphylaxis

- Patient information regarding anaphylactic reactions: http://foodallergies.about.com/od/foodallergysymptoms/a/Anaphylaxis-Overview.htm

References

Agraharkar, M., Dellinger, O.D., III, & Gangakhedkar, A.K. (2015, January 15). Hypercalcemia. Retrieved from http://emedicine.medscape.com/article/240681-overview

Ajzensztejn, D., Hegde, V.S., & Lee, S.M. (2006). Tumor lysis syndrome after treatment with docetaxel for non–small-cell lung cancer. *Journal of Clinical Oncology, 24,* 2389–2391. doi:10.1200/JCO.2005.02.8753

Akalin, E., Chandrakantan, A., Keane, J., & Hamburger, R.J. (2001). Normouricemia in the syndrome of inappropriate antidiuretic hormone secretion. *American Journal of Kidney Diseases, 37,* 1–3. doi:10.1016/S0272-6386(01)90005-8

Areva Pharmaceuticals Corp. (2012). Pamidronate disodium for injection [Package insert]. Elizabethtown, KY: Author.

Arruda, V.R., & High, K.A. (2012). Disseminated intravascular coagulation. In D.L. Longo, A.S. Fauci, D.L. Kasper, S.L. Hauser, J.L. Jameson, & J. Loscalzo (Eds.), *Harrison's principles of internal medicine* (18th ed., pp. 973–980). New York, NY: McGraw-Hill Medical.

Bakhtiari, K., Meijers, J.C., de Jonge, E., & Levi, M. (2004). Prospective validation of the International Society of Thrombosis and Haemostasis scoring system for disseminated intravascular coagulation. *Critical Care Medicine, 32,* 2416–2421. doi:10.1097/01.CCM.0000147769.07699.E3

Beriwal, S., Singh, S., & Garcia-Young, J.A. (2002). Tumor lysis syndrome in extensive-stage small-cell lung cancer. *American Journal of Clinical Oncology, 25,* 474–475. doi:10.1097/00000421-200210000-00010

Bone, R.C., Balk, R.A., Cerra, F.B., Dellinger, R.P., Fein, A.M., Knaus, W.A., … Sibbald, W.J. (1992). Definitions for sepsis and organ failure and guidelines for the use of innovative therapies in sepsis. The ACCP/SCCM Consensus Conference Committee. American College of Chest Physicians/Society of Critical Care Medicine. *Chest, 101,* 1644–1655. doi:10.1378/chest.101.6.1644

Bow, E.J. (2013). Infection in neutropenic patients with cancer. *Critical Care Clinics, 29,* 411–441. doi:10.1016/j.ccc.2013.03.002

Cairo, M.S., & Bishop, M. (2004). Tumour lysis syndrome: New therapeutic strategies and classification. *British Journal of Haematology, 127,* 3–11. doi:10.1111/j.1365-2141.2004.05094.x

Camp-Sorrell, D. (2011). Chemotherapy toxicities and management. In C.H. Yarbro, D. Wujcik, & B.H. Gobel (Eds.), *Cancer nursing: Principles and practice* (7th ed., pp. 458–503). Burlington, MA: Jones & Bartlett Learning.

Cany, L., Fitoussi, O., Boiron, J.M., & Marit, G. (2002). Tumor lysis syndrome at the beginning of thalidomide therapy for multiple myeloma. *Journal of Clinical Oncology, 20,* 2212. Retrieved from http://jco.ascopubs.org/content/20/8/2212.1.long

Centers for Disease Control and Prevention. (2012, February). Insects and scorpions. Retrieved from http://www.cdc.gov/niosh/topics/insects

Chan, T.Y. (1997). Drug-induced syndrome of inappropriate antidiuretic hormone secretion: Causes, diagnosis and management. *Drugs and Aging, 11,* 27–44. doi:10.2165/00002512-199711010-00004

Cianferoni, A., & Muraro, A. (2012). Food-induced anaphylaxis. *Immunology and Allergy Clinics of North America, 32,* 165–195. doi:10.1016/j.iac.2011.10.002

Coiffier, B., Altman, A., Pui, C.-H., Younes, A., & Cairo, M.S. (2008). Guidelines for the management of pediatric and adult tumor lysis syndrome: An evidence-based review. *Journal of Clinical Oncology, 26,* 2767–2778. doi:10.1200/JCO.2007.15.0177

Cope, D.G. (2013). Syndrome of inappropriate antidiuretic hormone secretion. In M. Kaplan (Ed.), *Understanding and managing oncologic emergencies: A resource for nurses* (2nd ed., pp. 411–431). Pittsburgh, PA: Oncology Nursing Society.

Dellinger, R.P., Levy, M.M., Rhodes, A., Annane, D., Gerlach, H., Opal, S.M., … Moreno, R. (2013). Surviving Sepsis Campaign: International guidelines for management of severe sepsis and septic shock: 2012. *Critical Care Medicine, 41,* 580–637. doi:10.1097/CCM.0b013e31827e83af

Eisenberg, S. (2013). Infusion reactions. In M. Kaplan (Ed.), *Understanding and managing oncologic emergencies: A resource for nurses* (2nd ed., pp. 199–255). Pittsburgh, PA: Oncology Nursing Society.

Ellison, D.H., & Berl, T. (2007). The syndrome of inappropriate antidiuresis. *New England Journal of Medicine, 356,* 2064–2072. doi:10.1056/NEJMcp066837

Finley, J.P. (1998). Syndrome of inappropriate ADH (SIADH). In C.R. Ziegfeld, B.G. Lubejko, & B.S. Shelton (Eds.), *Manual of cancer nursing* (pp. 431–435). Philadelphia, PA: Lippincott Williams & Wilkins.

Fleming, D.R., Henslee-Downey, P.J., & Coffey, C.W. (1991). Radiation induced acute tumor lysis syndrome in the bone marrow transplant setting. *Bone Marrow Transplantation, 8,* 235–236.

Fojo, A.T. (2011). Metabolic emergencies. In V.T. DeVita Jr., T.S. Lawrence, & S.A. Rosenberg (Eds.), *Cancer: Principles and practice of oncology* (9th ed., pp. 2142–2152). Philadelphia, PA: Wolters Kluwer Health/Lippincott Williams & Wilkins.

Franchini, M., Di Minno, M.N., & Coppola, A. (2010). Disseminated intravascular coagulation in hematologic malignancies. *Seminars in Thrombosis and Hemostasis, 36,* 388–403. doi:10.1055/s-0030-1254048

Franchini, M., Lippi, G., & Manzato, F. (2006). Recent acquisitions in the pathophysiology, diagnosis and treatment of disseminated intravascular coagulation. *Thrombosis Journal, 4,* 4. doi:10.1186/1477-9560-4-4

Freifeld, A.G., Bow, E.J., Sepkowitz, K.A., Boeckh, M.J., Ito, J.I., Mullen, C.A., … Wingard, J.R. (2011). Clinical practice guideline for the use of antimicrobial agents in neutropenic patients with cancer: 2010 update by the Infectious Diseases Society of America. *Clinical Infectious Diseases, 52*(4), e56–e93. doi:10.1093/cid/cir073

Friend, P.H., & Pruett, J. (2004). Bleeding and thrombotic complications. In C.H. Yarbro, M.H. Frogge, & M. Goodman (Eds.), *Cancer symptom management* (3rd ed., pp. 233–251). Burlington, MA: Jones & Bartlett Learning.

Fuente, N., Mañe, J.M., Barcelo, R., Muñoz, A., Perez-Hoyos, T., & Lopez-Vivanco, G. (2004). Tumor lysis syndrome in a multiple myeloma treated with thalidomide. *Annals of Oncology, 15,* 537. doi:10.1093/annonc/mdh116

Garrett, C.A., & Simpson, T.A., Jr. (1998). Syndrome of inappropriate antidiuretic hormone associated with vinorelbine therapy. *Annals of Pharmacotherapy, 32,* 1306–1309. doi:10.1345/aph.17278

Gobel, B.H. (2011). Disseminated intravascular coagulation. In C.H. Yarbro, D. Wujcik, & B.H. Gobel (Eds.), *Cancer nursing: Principles and practice* (7th ed., pp. 928–938). Burlington, MA: Jones & Bartlett Learning.

Gobel, B.H. (2013). Tumor lysis syndrome. In M. Kaplan (Ed.), *Understanding and managing oncologic emergencies: A resource for nurses* (2nd ed., pp. 433–459). Pittsburgh, PA: Oncology Nursing Society.

Gobel, B.H., & O'Leary, C. (2011). Hypersensitivity reactions to antineoplastic drugs. In C.H. Yarbro, D. Wujcik, & B.H. Gobel (Eds.), *Cancer nursing: Principles and practice* (7th ed., pp. 792–806). Burlington, MA: Jones & Bartlett Learning.

Gobel, B.H., Peterson, G.J., & Hoffner, B. (2013). Sepsis and septic shock. In M. Kaplan (Ed.), *Understanding and managing oncologic emergencies: A resource for nurses* (2nd ed., pp. 287–335). Pittsburgh, PA: Oncology Nursing Society.

Haapoja, I.S. (2000). Syndrome of inappropriate antidiuretic hormone. In C.H. Yarbro, M.H. Frogge, M. Goodman, & S.L. Groenwald (Eds.), *Cancer nursing: Principles and practice* (5th ed., pp. 913–919). Burlington, MA: Jones & Bartlett Learning.

Habib, G.S., & Saliba, W.R. (2002). Tumor lysis syndrome after hydrocortisone treatment in metastatic melanoma: A case report and review of the literature. *American Journal of the Medical Sciences, 323,* 155–157. doi:10.1097/00000441-200203000-00007

Hirshberg, B., & Ben-Yehuda, A. (1997). The syndrome of inappropriate antidiuretic hormone secretion in the elderly. *American Journal of Medicine, 103,* 207–273. doi:10.1016/S0002-9343(97)00250-7

Howard, S.C. (2014). Tumor lysis syndrome. In J.E. Niederhuber, J.O. Armitage, J.H. Doroshow, M.B. Kastan, & J.E. Tepper (Eds.), *Abeloff's clinical oncology* (5th ed., pp. 591–596). Philadelphia, PA: Elsevier.

Howard, S.C., Jones, D.P., & Pui, C.-H. (2011). The tumor lysis syndrome. *New England Journal of Medicine, 364,* 1844–1854. doi:10.1056/NEJMra0904569

Jaskiewicz, A.D., Herrington, J.D., & Wong, L. (2005). Tumor lysis syndrome after bortezomib therapy for plasma cell leukemia. *Pharmacotherapy, 25,* 1820–1825. doi:10.1592/phco.2005.25.12.1820

Joint Task Force on Practice Parameters. (2010). The diagnosis and management of anaphylaxis parameter: 2010 update. *Journal of Allergy and Clinical Immunology, 126,* 477–480. doi:10.1016/j.jaci.2010.06.022

Kaplan, M. (2011). Hypercalcemia of malignancy. In C.H. Yarbro, D. Wujcik, & B.H. Gobel (Eds.), *Cancer nursing: Principles and practice* (7th ed., pp. 939–963). Burlington, MA: Jones & Bartlett Learning.

Kaplan, M. (2013a). Disseminated intravascular coagulation. In M. Kaplan (Ed.), *Understanding and managing oncologic emergencies: A resource for nurses* (2nd ed., pp. 69–102). Pittsburgh, PA: Oncology Nursing Society.

Kaplan, M. (2013b). Hypercalcemia of malignancy. In M. Kaplan (Ed.), *Understanding and managing oncologic emergencies: A resource for nurses* (2nd ed., pp. 103–155). Pittsburgh, PA: Oncology Nursing Society.

Kaufman, D.A., & Mancebo, J. (2015). Corticosteroid therapy in septic shock [Literature review current through May 2015; topic last updated January 10, 2014]. Retrieved from http://www.uptodate.com/contents/corticosteroid-therapy-in-septic-shock

Keenan, A.M. (1999). Syndrome of inappropriate secretion of antidiuretic hormone in malignancy. *Seminars in Oncology Nursing, 15,* 160–167. doi:10.1016/S0749-2081(99)80003-5

Keenan, A.K.M. (2011). Syndrome of inappropriate antidiuretic hormone. In C.H. Yarbro, D. Wujcik, & B.H. Gobel (Eds.), *Cancer nursing: Principles and practice* (7th ed., pp. 1005–1013). Burlington, MA: Jones & Bartlett Learning.

Kemp, S.F. (2012). Anaphylaxis and serum sickness. In E.T. Bope & R.D. Kellerman (Eds.), *Conn's current therapy 2013* (pp. 64–68). Philadelphia, PA: Elsevier Saunders.

Kirch, C., Gachot, B., Germann, N., Blot, F., & Nitenberg, G. (1997). Recurrent ifosfamide-induced hyponatraemia. *European Journal of Cancer, 33,* 2438–2439. doi:10.1016/S0959-8049(97)00329-8

Kitchens, C.S. (2009). Thrombocytopenia and thrombosis in disseminated intravascular coagulation (DIC). *Hematology, 1,* 240–246. doi:10.1182/asheducation-2009.1.240

Kurt, M., Onal, I.K., Elkiran, T., Altun, B., Altundag, K., & Gullu, I. (2005). Acute tumor lysis syndrome triggered by zoledronic acid in a patient with metastatic lung adenocarcinoma. *Medical Oncology, 22,* 203–206. doi:10.1385/MO:22:2:203

Langer-Nitsche, C., Luck, H.J., & Heilmann, M. (2000). Severe syndrome of inappropriate antidiuretic hormone secretion with docetaxel treatment in metastatic breast cancer. *Acta Oncologica, 39,* 1001. doi:10.1080/028418600 50216007

Leung, L.L.K. (2015). Clinical features, diagnosis, and treatment of disseminated intravascular coagulation [Literature review current through May 2015; topic last updated November 17, 2014]. Retrieved from http://www.uptodate .com/contents/clinical-features-diagnosis-and-treatment-of-disseminated-intravascular-coagulation-in-adults

Levi, M.M. (2009). Disseminated intravascular coagulation in cancer patients. *Best Practice and Research Clinical Haematology, 22,* 129–136. doi:10.1016/j.beha.2008.12.005

Levi, M.M., & Schmaier, A.H. (2014). Disseminated intravascular coagulation. Retrieved from http://emedicine. medscape.com/article/199627-overview

Levi, M.M., Toh, C.H., Thachil, J., & Watson, H.G. (2009). Guidelines for the diagnosis and management of disseminated intravascular coagulation. British Committee for Standards in Haematology. *British Journal of Haematology, 145,* 24–33. doi:10.1111/j.1365-2141.2009.07600.x

Lewis, M.A., Hendrickson, A.W., & Moynihan, T.J. (2011). Oncologic emergencies: Pathophysiology, presentation, diagnosis, and treatment. *CA: A Cancer Journal for Clinicians, 61,* 287–314. doi:10.3322/caac.20124

Lieberman, P., Nicklas, R.A., Oppenheimer, J., Kemp, S.F., Lang, D.M., Bernstein, D.I., … Wallace, D. (2010). The diagnosis and management of anaphylaxis practice parameter: 2010 update. *Journal of Allergy and Clinical Immunology, 126,* 477–480. doi:10.1016/j.jaci.2010.06.022

Linck, D., Basara, N., Tran, V., Vucinic, V., Hermann, S., Hoelzer, D., & Fauser, A.A. (2003). Peracute onset of severe tumor lysis syndrome immediately after 4 Gy fractionated TBI as part of reduced intensity preparative regimen in a patient with T-ALL with high tumor burden. *Bone Marrow Transplantation, 31,* 935–937. doi:10.1038/sj.bmt.1704025

Lough, M.E. (2010). Endocrine disorders and therapeutic management. In L.D. Urden, K.M. Stacy, & M.E. Lough (Eds.), *Critical care nursing: Diagnosis and management* (6th ed., pp. 892–937). St. Louis, MO: Elsevier Mosby.

Lydon, J. (2011). Tumor lysis syndrome. In C.H. Yarbro, D. Wujcik, & B.H. Gobel (Eds.), *Cancer nursing: Principles and practice* (7th ed., pp. 1014–1028). Burlington, MA: Jones & Bartlett Learning.

Makras, P., & Papapoulos, S.E. (2009). Medical treatment of hypercalcaemia. *Hormones, 8,* 83–95. doi:10.14310/horm.2002.1225

Maloney, K.W. (2016). Metabolic emergencies. In J.K. Itano (Vol. ed.), *Core curriculum for oncology nursing* (5th ed., pp. 478–494). Philadelphia, PA: Elsevier.

Martí-Carvajal, A.J., Solà, I., Gluud, C., Lathyris, D., & Cardona, A.F. (2012). Human recombinant protein C for severe sepsis and septic shock in adult and paediatric patients. *Cochrane Database of Systematic Reviews, 2012*(12). doi:10.1002/14651858.CD004388.pub6

Martin, G.S. (2012). Sepsis, severe sepsis and septic shock: Changes in incidence, pathogens and outcomes. *Expert Review of Anti-Infective Therapy, 10,* 701–706. doi:10.1586/eri.12.50

McCurdy, M.T., & Shanholtz, C.B. (2012). Oncologic emergencies. *Critical Care Medicine, 20,* 1–11. doi:10.1097/CCM.0b013e31824e1865

McMahan, J., & Linneman, T. (2009). A case of resistant hypercalcemia of malignancy with a proposed treatment algorithm. *Annals of Pharmacotherapy, 43,* 1532–1538. doi:10.1345/aph.1L313

Miaskowski, C. (1997). Oncologic emergencies. In *Oncology nursing: An essential guide for patient care* (pp. 225–243). Philadelphia, PA: W.B. Saunders.

Miller, M. (2001). Syndrome of excess antidiuretic hormone release. *Critical Care Clinics, 17,* 11–23. doi:10.1016/S0749-0704(05)70149-4

Mustafa, S.S. (2014). Anaphylaxis. Retrieved from http://emedicine.medscape.com/article/135065-overview

National Comprehensive Cancer Network. (2015). *NCCN Clinical Practice Guidelines in Oncology (NCCN Guidelines®): Prevention and treatment of cancer-related infections* [v.2.2015]. Retrieved from http://www.nccn.org/professionals/physician_gls/pdf/infections.pdf

Neugut, A.I., Ghatak, A.T., & Miller, R.L. (2001). Anaphylaxis in the United States: An investigation into its epidemiology. *Archives of Internal Medicine, 161,* 15–21. doi:10.1001/archinte.161.1.15

Neviere, R. (2015). Sepsis and the systemic inflammatory response syndrome: Definitions, epidemiology, and prognosis [Literature review current through May 2015; topic last updated April 24, 2015]. Retrieved from http://www

.uptodate.com/contents/sepsis-and-the-systemic-inflammatory-response-syndrome-definitions-epidemiology-and-prognosis

Novartis Pharmaceuticals Corp. (2015). *Zometa® (zoledronic acid for injection)* [Package insert]. East Hanover, NJ: Author.

O'Leary, C. (2011). Septic shock. In C.H. Yarbro, D. Wujcik, & B.H. Gobel (Eds.), *Cancer nursing: Principles and practice* (7th ed., pp. 964–978). Burlington, MA: Jones & Bartlett Learning.

Otto, S. (1997). Syndrome of inappropriate antidiuretic hormone secretion. In *Oncology nursing* (3rd ed., pp. 463–474). St. Louis, MO: Mosby.

Pagani, M. (2010). The complex clinical picture of presumably allergic side effects to cytostatic drugs: Symptoms, pathomechanism, reexposure, and desensitization. *Medical Clinics of North America, 94,* 835–852. doi:10.1016/j.mcna.2010.03.002

Pelosof, L.C., & Gerber, D.E. (2010). Paraneoplastic syndromes: An approach to diagnosis and treatment. *Mayo Clinic Proceedings, 85,* 838–854. doi:10.4065/mcp.2010.0099

Penack, O., Buchheidt, D., Christopeit, M., von Lilienfeld-Toal, M., Massenkeil, G., Hentrich, M., ... Ostermann, H. (2011). Management of sepsis in neutropenic patients: Guidelines from the infectious diseases working party of the German Society of Hematology and Oncology. *Annals of Oncology, 22,* 1019–1029. doi:10.1093/annonc/mdq442

Persons, D.A., Garst, J., Vollmer, R., & Crawford, J. (1998). Tumor lysis syndrome and acute renal failure after treatment of non-small-cell lung carcinoma with combination irinotecan and cisplatin. *American Journal of Clinical Oncology, 21,* 426–429. doi:10.1097/00000421-199808000-00024

Poe, C.M., & Taylor, L.M. (1989). Syndrome of inappropriate antidiuretic hormone: Assessment and nursing implications. *Oncology Nursing Forum, 16,* 373–381.

Robertson, G.L. (2001). Antidiuretic hormone: Normal and disordered function. *Endocrinology and Metabolism Clinics of North America, 30,* 671–695. doi:10.1016/S0889-8529(05)70207-3

Ruppert, S.D. (2013). Recognizing and managing acute anaphylaxis. *Nurse Practitioner, 38,* 10–13. doi:10.1097/01.NPR.0000433082.01313.c2

Saba, H.I., & Morelli, G.A. (2006). The pathogenesis and management of disseminated intravascular coagulation. *Clinical Advances in Hematology and Oncology, 4,* 919–926.

Sanofi-Aventis U.S. LLC. (2011). *Elitek® (rasburicase)* [Package insert]. Bridgewater, NJ: Author.

Schmidt, G.A., & Mandel, J. (2015). Evaluation and management of severe sepsis and septic shock in adults [Literature review current through May 2015; topic last updated April 10, 2015]. Retrieved from http://www.uptodate.com/contents/evaluation-and-management-of-severe-sepsis-and-septic-shock-in-adults

Shelton, B.K. (2011). Infection. In C.H. Yarbro, D. Wujcik, & B.H. Gobel (Eds.), *Cancer nursing: Principles and practice* (7th ed., pp. 713–744). Burlington, MA: Jones & Bartlett Learning.

Sherlock, M., & Thompson, C.J. (2010). The syndrome of inappropriate antidiuretic hormone: Current and future management options. *European Journal of Endocrinology, 162,* S13–S18. doi:10.1530/EJE-09-1057

Siddiqui, F., & Weissman, D.E. (2010). Hypercalcemia of malignancy. *Journal of Palliative Medicine, 13,* 77–78. doi:10.1089/jpm.2010.9894

Simons, F.E.R. (2010). Anaphylaxis. *Journal of Allergy and Clinical Immunology, 125,* S161–S181. doi:10.1016/j.jaci.2009.12.981

Sterns, R.H. (2015a). Pathophysiology and etiology of the syndrome of inappropriate antidiuretic hormone secretion (SIADH) [Literature review current through May 2015; topic last updated July 15, 2014]. Retrieved from http://www.uptodate.com/contents/pathophysiology-and-etiology-of-the-syndrome-of-inappropriate-antidiuretic-hormone-secretion-siadh

Sterns, R.H. (2015b). Treatment of hyponatremia: Syndrome of inappropriate antidiuretic hormone secretion (SIADH) and reset osmostat [Literature review current through May 2015; topic last updated Jul 22, 2014]. Retrieved from http://www.uptodate.com/contents/treatment-of-hyponatremia-syndrome-of-inappropriate-antidiuretic-hormone-secretion-siadh-and-reset-osmostat

Toh, C.H., & Hoots, W.K. (2007). The scoring system of the Scientific and Standardisation Committee on Disseminated Intravascular Coagulation of the International Society on Thrombosis and Haemostasis: A 5-year overview. *Journal of Thrombosis and Haemostasis, 5,* 604–606. doi:10.1111/j.1538-7836.2007.02313.x

Tupper, J., & Visser, S. (2010). Anaphylaxis: A review and update. *Canadian Family Physician, 56,* 1009–1011.

Van Gerpen, R. (2009). Chemotherapy and biotherapy-induced hypersensitivity reactions. *Journal of Infusion Nursing, 32,* 157–165. doi:10.1097/NAN.0b013e3181a1a8ae

Verbalis, J.G., Goldsmith, S.R., Greenberg, A., Schrier, R.W., & Sterns, R.H. (2007). Hyponatremia treatment guidelines 2007: Expert panel recommendations. *American Journal of Medicine, 120*(11, Suppl. 1), S1–S21. doi:10.1016/j.amjmed.2007.09.001

Wilkes, G., & Barton-Burke, M. (2013). *2013 oncology nursing drug handbook.* Burlington, MA: Jones & Bartlett Learning.

Yamazaki, H., Hanada, M., Horiki, M., Kuyama, J., Sato, T., Nishikubo, M., … Inoue, T. (2004). Acute tumor lysis syndrome caused by palliative radiotherapy in patients with diffuse large B-cell lymphoma. *Radiation Medicine, 22,* 52–55.

Yunginger, J.W. (2009). Natural rubber latex allergy. In N.F. Adkinson, B.S. Bochner, W.W. Busse, S.T. Holgate, R.F. Lemanske, & F.E.R. Simons (Eds.), *Middleton's allergy: Principles and practice* (7th ed., Vol. 2, pp. 1019–1026). St. Louis, MO: Elsevier Mosby.

Zietse, R., van der Lubbe, N., & Hoorn, E.J. (2009). Current and future treatment options in SIADH. *NDT Plus, 2*(Suppl. 3), iii12–iii19. doi:10.1093/ndtplus/sfp154

CHAPTER 16

Structural Oncologic Emergencies

Marcelle Kaplan, MS, RN, AOCN®, CBCN®

Introduction

Oncologic emergencies are complications that can occur in patients with cancer as a result of the malignant process or secondary to antineoplastic therapies. Their appearance frequently signals advanced or recurrent disease but also may be the presenting sign of unsuspected malignancy (Kaplan, 2013). Prompt recognition and intervention are essential in helping patients maintain a reasonable quality of life and prevent progression to a life-threatening emergency. This chapter will describe four structural emergencies: superior vena cava syndrome, cardiac tamponade, spinal cord compression, and increased intracranial pressure.

Superior Vena Cava Syndrome

The superior vena cava (SVC) is the major vein that carries deoxygenated blood from the head, neck, upper chest, and arms to the right side of the heart. Obstruction or compression of the SVC leads to a spectrum of clinical findings called the superior vena cava syndrome (SVCS). Compression or blockage of the SVC impairs venous return to the right atrium from the head, thorax, and upper extremities and causes venous congestion and edema in these areas. Cardiac output decreases because of diminished blood return to the heart (Shelton, 2013). Causes of SVC obstruction can be divided into intrinsic or extrinsic factors. Intrinsic causes of SVCS include the presence of thrombosis or intraluminal tumor within the SVC. Extrinsic obstruction more commonly results from a locally advanced bronchogenic tumor or enlarged mediastinal lymph nodes (McKenzie, McTyre, Kunaprayoon, & Redmond, 2013; National Cancer Institute [NCI], 2014). SVCS can develop gradually or rapidly depending on the proliferation rate of the underlying malignancy. It becomes an emergency when symptoms are severe and result in decreased cardiac filling, cerebral edema, and respiratory distress (Feng & Pennell, 2012; Shelton, 2013). Advanced practice nurses (APNs) need to be alert to patients who are potentially at risk for SVCS, as well as be able to recognize it early so that interventions can be initiated before it becomes life threatening.

Incidence

SVCS was first described in 1757 in a patient who had a syphilitic aneurysm of the ascending aorta (Hunter, 1757). Until the advent of antibiotics, the most frequent causes of SVCS were syphilitic aortic aneurysms, tuberculous mediastinitis, and untreated infection (Drews & Rabkin, 2014). Annually, approximately 15,000 people in the United States develop SVCS, mostly due to the presence of cancer in the mediastinum (Yahalom, 2011). Malignant disease, especially right-sided lung cancer, is responsible for 70%–95% of cases (Drews & Rabkin, 2014; NCI, 2014; Nickloes et al., 2014). Small cell lung cancer (SCLC) is associated with the highest frequency of SVCS, primarily due to its usual occurrence in the central part of the lung and involvement with mediastinal lymph nodes (Nickloes et al., 2014). Squamous cell carcinoma of the lung has the next highest frequency, followed by adenocarcinoma of the lung, non-Hodgkin lymphoma (NHL), and large cell lung cancer (NCI, 2014). Although lung cancer confers the highest risk for SVCS, only 3%–10% of patients with lung cancer will develop SVCS (Theodore & Jablons, 2010). The male to female ratio is approximately 5:1 (Theodore & Jablons, 2010). Men have an increased incidence of SVCS because of higher lung cancer rates (Nickloes et al., 2014). SVCS is most common in adults between the ages of 50 and 70 (Nunnelee, 2007), who also have higher lung cancer rates. Patients with lymphoma and SVCS tend to be younger, as do those with SVCS due to nonmalignant causes (Beeson, 2014; Laskin, Cmelak, Meranze, Yee, & Johnson, 2014). Currently, nonmalignant causes of SVCS account for 20%–40% of cases, most often due to thrombosis formation related to the increasingly common use of intravascular devices, such as pacemakers and central venous catheters (Drews & Rabkin, 2014; Nickloes et al., 2014).

Signs and Symptoms

The clinical signs and symptoms of SVCS vary depending on the rapidity and extent of SVC obstruction (Shelton, 2013) (see Figure 16-1). Partial or complete SVC obstruction reduces venous blood return to the heart from the upper body, increases venous congestion, and decreases cardiac output. Partial obstruction may be asymptomatic or produce vague signs and symptoms that are often unrecognized, such as nasal congestion, which is often an early presenting symptom (Nickloes et al., 2014; Theodore & Jablons, 2010). SVCS is more likely to be life threatening when the obstruction is sudden, as collateral veins have not had time to develop. Rapid onset of symptoms is more likely to occur when intravascular thrombosis occludes the SVC (Nickloes et al., 2014).

SVCS that develops gradually produces signs and symptoms that reflect edema and venous engorgement. The most common signs and symptoms of SVCS are facial or neck swelling (82%), upper extremity swelling (68%), dyspnea (66%), cough (50%), and dilated chest vein collaterals (38%) (Brumbaugh, 2011). Symptoms of SVCS often are worse in the morning after the patient has been sleeping supine during the night. Patients also may notice that symptoms are exacerbated with positional changes, such as bending forward to put on shoes, coughing, or stooping (Laskin et al., 2014; Shelton, 2013). On arising, patients often report a sense of "fullness" in the head. Swelling in the face, neck, and arms may be present, causing shirt collars to be tight (Stoke sign). Women may develop breast swelling and have trouble removing their rings because of finger swelling. The symptoms usually improve after the patient has been upright for several hours, as gravity reduces the edema in the upper body (Shelton, 2013). Sleeping in

Early Signs and Symptoms	Late Signs and Symptoms
• Dyspnea • Chest pain • "Fullness" in head • Ruddy complexion • Facial swelling upon arising • Nonproductive cough, hoarseness • Redness and edema in conjunctivae • Venous distension in neck and upper chest • Swelling of neck, arms, and hands (Stoke sign)	• Stridor • Dysphasia • Hemoptysis • Tachycardia • Horner syndrome • Severe headache • Dizziness, syncope • Congestive heart failure • Changes in mental status • Decreased blood pressure • Severe respiratory distress • Visual disturbances, blurred vision

Figure 16-1. Signs and Symptoms of Superior Vena Cava Syndrome

Note. Based on information from Brumbaugh, 2011; Feng & Pennell, 2012; Nickloes et al., 2014; Nunnelee, 2007; Shelton, 2013.

an upright position may increase comfort. Patients with lung cancer or lymphoma most often experience dyspnea. Chest pain or discomfort and dysphagia also can occur (Brumbaugh, 2011; Laskin et al., 2014). Edema of the face, upper thorax, and extremities, periorbital and conjunctival edema, and cyanosis result in a purple frog–like appearance (Shelton, 2013). Increased venous pressures can cause chronic pleural and pericardial effusion as a result of impaired lymphatic drainage (Theodore & Jablons, 2010). Pleural effusions are common in SVCS due to both malignant and nonmalignant causes (Yahalom, 2011).

Late signs and symptoms of SVCS can be severe and life threatening. Respiratory symptoms can include stridor and respiratory distress. Involvement of the recurrent laryngeal nerve (cranial nerve X) by lymph nodes can result in a paralyzed true vocal cord, leading to dysphagia and hoarseness and placing the patient at risk for aspiration (Shelton, 2013). Late signs and symptoms related to the cardiovascular system can include tachycardia, decreased blood pressure, congestive heart failure, and cyanosis. Late symptoms of SVCS in the central nervous system (CNS) are related to cerebral edema and include severe headache, irritability, visual disturbances (blurred vision), dizziness, and syncope (Feng & Pennell, 2012). Mental status changes occur as SVCS progresses, including confusion, decreased consciousness, seizures, and coma, which can indicate increased intracranial pressure (Drews & Rabkin, 2014). Hemoptysis also may be present in patients with SVCS. Horner syndrome (unilateral ptosis, constricted pupil, and ipsilateral loss of sweating from pressure on the cervical sympathetic nerves) can occur rarely in SVCS (Brumbaugh, 2011).

Yu, Wilson, and Detterbeck (2008) have proposed a symptom grading system for SVCS based on the Common Terminology Criteria for Adverse Events of the NCI Cancer Therapy Evaluation Program (see Table 16-1). Symptoms included are directly related to the presence of SVCS rather than other factors and are divided into categories according to severity.

Risk Factors and Etiology

Both extrinsic and intrinsic factors can contribute to the development of SVCS. The presence of a tumor mass or enlarged lymph nodes in the mediastinum can exert extrinsic pressure against the SVC. SVC compression can be acute and complete or incomplete and gradual, depending on whether a thrombus is present in the lumen of the SVC in addition to an impinging extrinsic tumor (Nickloes et al., 2014). Risk factors for thrombosis formation include inti-

Table 16-1. Proposed Symptom Grading System for Superior Vena Cava Obstruction

Grade	Symptom Severity	Characteristics
0	Asymptomatic	Superior vena cava obstruction seen radiographically
1	Mild	Mild head or neck edema; cyanosis; plethora
2	Moderate	Moderate head or neck edema; signs of mild or moderate functional impairment, such as dysphagia, cough, and impaired movements of head, jaw, or eyelids; visual disturbances due to ocular edema
3	Severe	Cerebral edema causing headache or dizziness; mild to moderate laryngeal edema; syncope upon bending, reflecting reduced cardiac reserve
4	Life threatening	Significant cerebral edema causing confusion and obtundation; laryngeal edema leading to stridor and possible airway compression; symptoms reflecting significantly impaired cardiac function, such as unprovoked syncope, hypotension, or impaired renal function
5	Fatal	Death

Note. Based on information from Yu et al., 2008.

mal damage to the vein from central venous catheters, venous stasis from extrinsic compression, and a hypercoagulable state in patients with malignancy. Ahmann (1984) reviewed reports from several cancer centers of postmortem examinations performed on patients who received treatment for SVCS, typically with radiation therapy. These studies revealed that the presence of intravascular thrombus plus an extrinsic tumor was often associated with complete SVC obstruction. Extrinsic tumor without thrombus formation was more often associated with partial SVC obstruction, because of the development of collateral venous drainage pathways (Ahmann, 1984).

The most common etiology for the development of SVCS is mediastinal malignancy, typically right-sided lung cancers that compress the SVC in the right mediastinum, or enlarged mediastinal lymph nodes (commonly right paratracheal nodes) that obstruct upper venous return to the heart (McKenzie et al., 2013; Nickloes et al., 2014). SCLC is the most frequent cause of SVCS, followed by squamous cell carcinoma of the lung, and then adenocarcinoma of the lung (NCI, 2014; Yahalom, 2011). The appearance of SVCS is the presenting symptom in 10% of patients diagnosed with SCLC and 1.7% of patients diagnosed with non-small cell lung cancer (NSCLC) (McKenzie et al., 2013). NHL involving the mediastinum can cause SVCS in rare cases; diffuse large cell lymphoma and lymphoblastic lymphoma are the most common histologies (Yahalom, 2011).

Metastatic disease in the mediastinum accounts for approximately 5%–10% of cases of SVCS (Laskin et al., 2014). Breast cancer is the most common metastatic cause of SVCS. Metastatic thyroid tumors and melanoma are infrequent causes of SVCS (Theodore & Jablons, 2010). Other cancers that can cause SVCS include Kaposi sarcoma, thymoma, germ cell tumors, colon cancer, esophageal cancer, and mesothelioma (NCI, 2014).

The most common etiology of nonmalignant SVCS is thrombosis caused by the presence of an intravascular device, such as a central venous catheter or pacemaker (Drews & Rabkin, 2014). Mediastinal fibrosis is the second most common nonmalignant cause because of either previous radiation therapy to the mediastinum or infection from tuberculosis or histoplasmosis (Brumbaugh, 2011). Other rare benign causes of SVCS are thoracic aortic aneurysm, substernal goiter, large benign mediastinal masses, and congestive heart failure (Theodore & Jablons, 2010).

Pathophysiology

The SVC is the major vessel that carries venous drainage from the head, neck, upper extremities, and upper thorax to the right atrium of the heart (see Figure 16-2). It possesses several features that make it vulnerable to compression by a space-occupying lesion: thin walls, low-pressure blood flow, enclosure within a rigid compartment, and being surrounded by multiple lymph node chains. The SVC is located in the middle mediastinum surrounded by several relatively rigid structures, including the sternum, trachea, right bronchus, aorta, pulmonary artery, and vertebrae. In addition, it is completely encircled by chains of lymph nodes, including the perihilar and paratracheal lymph nodes, that drain the structures of the right thoracic cavity and the lower part of the left thorax (NCI, 2014; Shelton, 2013).

The junction of the right and left brachiocephalic (or innominate) veins forms the beginning of the SVC. The SVC extends for 6–8 cm, courses anteriorly to the right main bronchus, enters the pericardial sac, and terminates at the right atrium. The azygos vein empties into the SVC at the level of the mainstem bronchus. The azygos venous system is an important alternative pathway if the blockage is above its entrance to the SVC. Impaired venous drainage above the azygos vein causes less venous pressure, and the SVCS is less pronounced because of the distension and accommodation of the azygos system for the venous return from the upper body (Laskin et al., 2014; NCI, 2014). Blood flow in a patent azygos vein, which normally handles about 11% of the total venous return from the head, neck, and upper extremities, can compensate for SVC blockage by increasing capacity to 35% of the upper venous return (Theodore & Jablons, 2010) (see Figure 16-2). If the SVC obstruction occurs below the azygos vein, the manifestations of SVCS are more severe because the venous return must be shunted by way of the upper abdominal veins and the inferior vena cava (Laskin et al., 2014; NCI, 2014).

Prevention Strategies

Thrombus formation associated with intravascular devices can lead to SVCS of iatrogenic origin (Schifferdecker, Shaw, Piemonte, & Eisenhauer, 2005). Thrombolytic therapy followed by anticoagulation may provide benefit when the thrombus is detected early and extrinsic SVC compression is absent. Thrombolytic therapy is contraindicated in patients with a history of bleeding disorders, hemorrhagic stroke, and increased intracranial pressure or cerebral metastases (National Comprehensive Cancer Network® [NCCN®], 2014). Anticoagulation using unfractionated or low-dose heparin is initiated following thrombolysis to prevent recurrence. Bleeding precautions during both thrombolysis and anticoagulation are important for nurses to institute.

Diagnosis and Assessment

It is important for APNs to obtain patients' clinical history to determine the underlying cause of SVCS. The majority of SVCS cases are the result of malignancy; however, a small percentage of patients do not have cancer (Beeson, 2014; NCI, 2014). Identification of risk factors can help to develop the differential diagnosis. Smoking history, exposure to environmental or occupational carcinogens, previous cancer history, presence of central venous catheters or pacemakers, previous radiation to the thorax, and history of allergies and infections should be determined (Shelton, 2013).

Many of the physical examination findings of SVCS are specific to the syndrome, making clinical identification straightforward (Feng & Pennell, 2012; Yahalom, 2011) (see Figure 16-1). Physical examination reveals edema of the face, neck (causing shirt collars to be tight), upper thorax, breast, and upper extremities. Veins in the neck and upper extremities may be visibly dilated, and prominent collateral venous channels over the anterior chest and abdomen may be present (Feng & Pennell, 2012; Theodore & Jablons, 2010). Facial plethora (ruddy complexion of the face and cheeks) and periorbital and conjunctival edema often are present. Blood pressure may be high in the upper extremities, particularly on the right side, in contrast to the legs, where it is low. Compensatory tachycardia often is noted.

Late signs occur more commonly in rapidly progressive, severe SVCS, which accounts for less than 2% of cases (Drews & Rabkin, 2014). Cyanosis of the face or upper torso and engorged conjunctiva can occur. Stridor, tachypnea, tachycardia, and orthopnea are manifestations of respiratory distress. Mental status changes, visual changes, syncope, coma, seizures, and death can occur as a result of cerebral and laryngeal edema (Shelton, 2013).

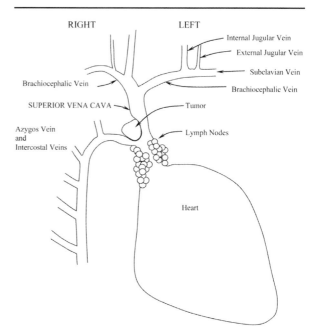

The superior vena cava (SVC) is formed by the merger of the left and right brachiocephalic (or innominate) veins in the upper mediastinum. They are the major veins returning blood to the SVC and are formed by the convergence of the corresponding internal jugular and subclavian veins.

Figure 16-2. Superior Vena Cava Obstruction With Azygos Venous System

Note. From "Superior Vena Cava Syndrome" (p. 389), by B. Shelton in M. Kaplan (Ed.), *Understanding and Managing Oncologic Emergencies: A Resource for Nurses* (2nd ed.), 2013. Copyright 2013 by Oncology Nursing Society. Reprinted with permission.

The diagnostic evaluation has two components: imaging and tissue diagnosis, as most causes of SVCS are attributable to malignancy. Standard chest radiographs, contrast-enhanced computed tomography (CT), and magnetic resonance imaging (MRI) are imaging modalities used for SVCS. Contrast venography, which previously was the mainstay of SVCS diagnosis, has largely been supplanted by the accuracy of contrast CT (Shelton, 2013) but is performed when interventions such as SVC stenting or surgical bypass are planned (Ganeshan, Hon, Warakaulle, Morgan, & Uberoi, 2009).

Chest x-ray often is the initial imaging method and is positive in more than 80% of SVCS cases. The most common findings on chest x-ray are a widened mediastinum, usually on the right, a right-sided chest mass, or SVC dilation and the presence of collateral vessels (Drews & Rabkin, 2014). Associated radiographic findings may include pleural effusion, lung lobe collapse, and cardiomegaly (NCI, 2014). However, chest x-ray cannot image a thrombus obstructing the SVC (Nickloes et al., 2014).

Contrast-enhanced spiral or multislice CT scan is a more effective imaging method to determine whether an extrinsic mass or an intraluminal thrombus is present (Feng & Pennell, 2012; Nickloes et al., 2014). A CT of the chest with contrast provides clear details about the SVC and its branches and the location of the obstruction and nearby critical structures, such as the bronchi and spinal cord. CT also is used to guide biopsy procedures via mediastinoscopy, bronchoscopy, or percutaneous fine needle aspiration (Nickloes et al., 2014). MRI can provide greater detail of the mediastinal structures and allows direct visualization of blood flow. MRI is generally used in patients who have contrast allergies or renal failure and is important when SVC stenting is anticipated (Nickloes et al., 2014; Nunnelee, 2007). Disadvantages of MRI include increased cost and scan time, as well as patient factors, such as an inability to lie flat for prolonged periods and claustrophobia. Urgent intervention is required to relieve the SVC obstruction in patients with severe or life-threatening airway or cardiac compromise, cerebral edema and/or hypotension, or spontaneous syncope.

Patients with SVCS attributable to tumor require a tissue diagnosis to determine tumor histology and develop an optimal treatment plan. The least invasive techniques possible are employed (Feng & Pennell, 2012). Sputum cytology is diagnostic in about 50% of patients with lung cancer. Cytology is as accurate as tissue diagnosis in SCLC; cytologic specimens are typically retrieved by bronchoscopy with brushings. If a pleural effusion is present, thoracentesis can be diagnostic in 70% of patients (Laskin et al., 2014; Yahalom, 2011). Palpable cervical or supraclavicular lymph nodes or a superficial mass may be biopsied for tissue diagnosis. A bone marrow biopsy may provide diagnosis in patients with NHL or SCLC, as these diseases often involve the bone marrow, and may assist in staging as well (Nunnelee, 2007). Mediastinoscopy, which was previously contraindicated because of concerns of bleeding risk in patients with SVCS, has been performed safely with a high success rate when less invasive measures do not result in a definitive diagnosis (Feng & Pennell, 2012; Yahalom, 2011).

Differential Diagnosis

Aortic aneurysm, tuberculosis, pneumonia, syphilis, acute respiratory distress syndrome, chronic obstructive pulmonary disease and emphysema, mediastinitis, pericarditis, and cardiac tamponade are other processes to consider in the differential diagnosis (Beeson, 2014; Nickloes et al., 2014). These processes can cause mediastinal changes resulting in symptoms associated with SVCS. A thorough history to evaluate for possible exposures and imaging studies can help to distinguish differences.

Evidence-Based Treatment Strategies

SVCS that develops acutely is a true emergency that requires prompt intervention for relief of symptoms. Treatment goals are alleviation of symptoms and treatment of the underlying disease. The etiology of the SVCS, the severity of symptoms, the patient's prognosis and treatment preference, the underlying malignancy, and the presence of thrombosis guide the treatment plan. Treatment is based on the cancer histology and disease stage and may include the use chemotherapy, radiation therapy, steroids, diuretics, thrombolytic therapy, or surgical intervention. Randomized clinical trials regarding the management of SVCS are scarce; most data come from retrospective case series (Feng & Pennell, 2012).

Chemotherapy is used for highly chemosensitive malignancies, such as SCLC, NHL, and germ cell tumors (Yahalom, 2011). The appearance of SVCS in patients with SCLC does not change their overall prognosis, and more than 80% will achieve a complete or partial response to treatment (Laskin et al., 2014). Improvement in symptoms usually occurs within

7–14 days (Laskin et al., 2014). Patients with NSCLC who develop SVCS have a poorer prognosis and a poorer response to chemotherapy unless they have cytogenetic markers indicating chemosensitivity (Shelton, 2013). Radiation therapy to palliate symptoms is usually more appropriate for patients with NSCLC (Drews & Rabkin, 2014). Chemotherapy, tailored to histologic subtypes, is the primary treatment for NHL complicated by SVCS because chemotherapy has both local and systemic effects. Radiation may be added as local consolidation therapy in patients with bulky early-stage diffuse large cell lymphoma (Yahalom, 2011). Chemotherapy may be used in combination with thoracic radiation in treating SCLC; the combination provides rapid relief of symptoms and appears to reduce the risk of SVCS recurrence compared to chemotherapy alone (Yahalom, 2011). The combination treatment will result in increased side effects, and patients need close monitoring (Shelton, 2013). An important issue when using chemotherapy in patients with SVCS is the route of delivery. Because of the venous stasis in the upper thorax, chemotherapy can become concentrated if it is delivered via the upper extremities. A central line through the femoral vein may be necessary for safe drug delivery.

Radiation therapy usually is delivered to palliate the signs and symptoms of SVCS (McKenzie et al., 2013) but is considered the treatment of choice for patients with SVCS caused by NSCLC (Yahalom, 2011). Radiation is initiated emergently if the patient's clinical status deteriorates rapidly (Shelton, 2013).

No specific evidence-based radiation dose schema exists for treating malignancy-associated SVCS. The radiation dose is determined by the tumor type, extent of disease, history of previous radiation in the area, and the patient's performance status (Laskin et al., 2014). Radiation therapy for SVCS is usually delivered with an initial two to four fractions of 300–400 cGy each to obtain rapid symptomatic relief. This is followed by standard daily dose fractions of 180–200 cGy to a total dose of 3,000–5,000 cGy, depending on tumor histology and disease extent (Yahalom, 2011). Various case study reports of radiation schedules using hypofractionated regimens, which deliver high doses in shorter periods, have indicated rapid and lasting responses with minimal toxicities (McKenzie et al., 2013; Yahalom, 2011). Recently, a published case study described the excellent outcome of the use of stereotactic body radiation therapy (SBRT), which delivers focused high-dose radiation therapy, in treating a patient with an uncommon presentation of early-stage NSCLC complicated by SVCS. SBRT was initiated to simultaneously palliate the SVCS and definitively treat the NSCLC. Resolution of the SVCS was rapid and effective and maintained at three-month follow-up (McKenzie et al., 2013). High rates of local control have been reported for early-stage lung cancer using SBRT, although determination of the optimal dose rates to prevent excessive toxicities in patients with centrally located lung tumors requires further investigation (McKenzie et al., 2013). Randomized clinical trials for optimal management of lung cancer–related SVCS are lacking.

Lymphomas are typically radiosensitive and may respond better to lower radiation doses than other tumor types. Radiation is delivered with curative intent to a total dose of 3,500–4,500 cGy, with daily fractions of 180–200 cGy over a four- to five-week period (Drews & Rabkin, 2014). Overall, patients may notice improvement in venous congestion within three to four days of treatment as a result of improved venous blood flow. Radiation therapy provides maximum symptom relief within three to four weeks in 70% of patients with lung cancer and 95% of patients with lymphoma (Drews & Rabkin, 2014; Nickloes et al., 2014). Better outcomes are seen in patients with lymphoma than in those with lung cancer (Shelton, 2013). The side effects of radiation depend on the total dose, the fraction dose, the amount of normal tissue in the radiation field, and whether concomitant chemotherapy is given. Short-term side effects of radiation include fatigue, skin erythema, cough, nausea, dysphagia, and heartburn (Brumbaugh, 2011). Rarely, bleeding or perforation of the SVC may occur (Shelton, 2013). Possible delayed side effects of radiation include pneumonitis, pulmonary fibrosis, brachial plexus damage, esophageal stenosis, cardiac changes, and spinal cord injury (Brumbaugh, 2011).

Supportive medical therapies may be employed to manage symptoms. Oxygen can be used to relieve dyspnea, and analgesics may be of benefit in patients with chest pain. Diuretics and steroids are commonly used to relieve laryngeal or cerebral edema, although no evidence exists to support their use (NCI, 2014; Nickloes et al., 2014). Patients receiving diuretic therapy need to be monitored for dehydration, which can lead to hypovolemia and further reduce venous return to the heart. Steroids generally are not recommended in patients with SVCS caused by lung cancer and should not be started in patients without a prior tissue diagnosis. Lymphomas respond so well to steroid therapy that diagnosis might be impossible after steroid initiation (Feng & Pennell, 2012).

Thrombolytic therapy is used to treat SVCS caused by catheter-induced thrombosis. The therapy should be initiated within five days of onset for maximum effectiveness. The thrombolytic agent is infused through the catheter or through a peripheral site to try to lyse the clot and is followed by heparin anticoagulation to prevent re-embolization (Vedantham, 2012). Thrombolysis should be avoided in patients with absolute risk factors for bleeding, such as history of hemorrhagic stroke or major trauma, surgery, or head injury in the previous three weeks, history of ischemic stroke in previous three months, intracranial tumor, or severe thrombocytopenia (NCCN, 2014). Streptokinase, urokinase, and recombinant tissue plasminogen activator (rtPA) are of value if used early in the thrombotic process (Yahalom, 2011). Treatment should follow recommendations for pulmonary embolism (Feng & Pennell, 2012). The most commonly used drug for fibrinolysis currently is rtPA (Vedantham, 2012). Febrile reactions are more common with rtPA, as are serious adverse events such as anaphylaxis and angioedema. Patients receiving rtPA require close monitoring during and immediately after the infusion, and emergency equipment should be readily available. If the cause of SVCS is catheter-induced thrombosis, removal of the catheter accompanied by heparin administration is indicated (Feng & Pennell, 2012). Patients should be monitored for bleeding, and blood products should be available in the event of hemorrhage. Randomized controlled clinical trials evaluating the outcomes of various therapeutic strategies for catheter-induced thrombosis are needed (NCCN, 2014).

Endovascular stent placement can rapidly relieve SVCS obstruction caused by malignancy; cyanosis is resolved immediately, and head and neck edema in a few days (Feng & Pennell, 2012). Because of the ease and safety of stent placement, the procedure has been recommended as a first choice for immediate relief of severe symptoms of malignancy-related SVC obstruction until the etiology can be determined and appropriate therapies instituted (Fagedet et al., 2013; Lanciego et al., 2009). In general, stenting is not appropriate for patients whose cancers can be anticipated to be cured or controlled, such as SCLC, which is very responsive to chemotherapy and radiation, or for those with SVCS associated with benign causes who have long life expectancies (Feng & Pennell, 2012).

Metal self-expanding stents are placed percutaneously by an interventional radiologist with the patient under conscious sedation and local anesthesia (Shelton, 2013). If thrombosis is extensive, thrombolytic therapy and balloon angioplasty may be performed prior to stent placement to allow for complete expansion of the vessel (Laskin et al., 2014; Yahalom, 2011). Rupture of the SVC is a rare but catastrophic complication of balloon angioplasty and may lead to cardiac tamponade. Equipment for emergency pericardiocentesis should be at hand during SVC angioplasty. A follow-up venogram confirms correct stent position, free blood flow, and absence of venous rupture. Consensus is lacking about the use of anticoagulant or antiplatelet therapy after stent placement (Laskin et al., 2014; NCI, 2014). The advantages of stenting is immediate response and symptom relief within a few days, in contrast to chemotherapy or radiation therapy, in which response may not be seen before three to four weeks. Stenting also does not interfere with initiation of subsequent antineoplastic therapies (Lanciego et al., 2009) and can be repeated if thrombosis recurs (Fagedet et al., 2013). Complication rates during and following stent placement procedures range from 0% to 19% and include bleeding (SVC rupture, hemorrhage, hemoptysis, epistaxis, hematoma at the insertion site), cardiac tamponade and cardiac failure, recurrent laryngeal palsy, infection, stent occlusion, pulmonary embolus, and stent migration into the right atrium causing cardiac arrhythmias (Ganeshan et al., 2009).

Surgical intervention is rare for malignant causes of SVCS and usually is reserved for patients with severe SVCS who have failed angioplasty and intravascular stenting (Laskin et al., 2014). A surgical bypass creates a circulation route around the SVC obstruction between the innominate or jugular vein on the left side to the right atrium. Autologous saphenous veins, synthetic materials, or tissue from the patient's pericardium may be used. This is an extensive surgical procedure and may not be feasible for patients with malignancy-associated SVCS. Thus, surgical intervention is most often reserved for SVCS caused by benign conditions, such as granulomatous disease, substernal goiter, or aortic aneurysm (Laskin et al., 2014). Postoperative complications include atrial fibrillation, stroke, respiratory failure, myocardial infarction, and Horner syndrome (Feng & Pennell, 2012).

Implications for Oncology Advanced Practice Nurses

SVCS is an obstructive complication seen in malignant and benign conditions. The most common malignancies associated with SVCS are SCLC and lymphoma. The onset typically is gradual, but it can develop rapidly. Early recognition and intervention is important to prevent progression to an emergency. Establishment of etiology is needed to determine the treatment plan. APNs can help to facilitate the recognition of early SVCS, establish a diagnosis, and implement intervention before it becomes a true emergency. APNs also should be aware that the use of vascular access devices increases the risk of SVCS.

Randomized controlled trials are lacking for optimal management of SVCS. NCCN (2014) provides guidelines for treating venous thromboembolic disease that address the indications and contraindications for thrombolytic and anticoagulant therapies and suggested strategies, drug regimens, and duration. Nursing management of patients with SVCS includes assessing cardiac, respiratory, and neurologic status, instituting measures to relieve symptoms, monitoring efficacy and side effects of treatment, providing comfort measures and emotional support, and allaying anxiety. Measures to promote oxygenation and perfusion include oxygen therapy, elevation of the head of the bed, activity restrictions, and anxiety management. Maintaining fluid balance is important to prevent dehydration, which could contribute to thrombus formation or fluid overload and increase the symptoms of SVCS. Evidence of airway obstruction, cardiac compromise, or changes in the patient's mental and neurologic status signals the need for emergent care (Shelton, 2013). IV access in the arms and arm blood pressure measurement should be avoided because of the presence of edema and elevated venous pressure (Nunnelee, 2007). Bowel management is needed to ensure patients avoid performing the Valsalva maneuver, which increases venous pressure. Patients require reassurance that the facial and periorbital edema and cyanosis will dissipate following treatment. Patient and caregiver education should be provided about the signs and symptoms of SVCS because of the possibility of relapse. Patients receiving anticoagulants require instruction regarding medication administration and signs of bleeding. Emotional support and counseling are important for patients and caregivers when SVCS occurs, as it may be the presenting sign of cancer or an indication of disease recurrence.

Cardiac Tamponade

Cardiac tamponade is a clinical syndrome resulting from compression of the heart caused by excessive accumulation of fluid, pus, gas, or blood in the pericardial sac, the space between the myocardium (the muscle of the heart) and the pericardium (the outer covering sac of the heart). Cardiac tamponade is most often caused by malignant disease and is a life-threatening oncologic emergency (Freter & Haddadin, 2014). The buildup of pericardial fluid causes extrinsic pressure on the heart chambers, resulting in decreased ventricular filling, decreased cardiac output, and compromised cardiac function (Story, 2013). Fluid collection around the heart is known as pericardial effusion and usually precedes cardiac tamponade. They are distinct entities. Pericardial effusion is the presence of abnormal fluid that often has no hemodynamic consequences, whereas cardiac tamponade causes increased intrapericardial pressure with potentially life-threatening hemodynamic consequences. Untreated, cardiac tamponade rapidly leads to cardiovascular collapse, shock, and death (Kwong & Nguyen, 2011; Story, 2013; Yarlagadda, 2015).

Incidence

The incidence of cardiac tamponade in the United States is 2 cases per 10,000 people (Yarlagadda, 2015). Malignancy is the most common cause, accounting for 30%–60% of all cases (Yarlagadda, 2015). About 13%–23% of patients with cancer will develop cardiac tamponade (Kaplow, 2011). Based on results of autopsy studies of patients with malignancies, lung cancer had the highest incidence of malignant pericardial effusions (33%), followed by breast cancer (25%), and then hematologic malignancies (15%), especially leukemia, Hodgkin lymphoma, and NHL (NCI, 2014). Occasionally, pericardial tamponade may be the presenting sign of cancer (Freter & Haddadin, 2014; Maisch, Ristic, & Pankuweit, 2010).

Nonmalignant conditions contribute to the incidence of cardiac tamponade and include uremia (10%–15% of cases), idiopathic pericarditis (5%–15%), infectious diseases (5%–10%), anticoagulation (5%–10%), and connective tissue diseases (2%–6%) (Yarlagadda, 2015). Prognosis for survival following malignancy-related cardiac tamponade is poor. Results of a study indicated a median survival of 150 days following diagnosis; 76% of patients died within one year (Kwong & Nguyen, 2011; Yarlagadda, 2015).

Signs and Symptoms

Cardiac tamponade may be missed in patients with pericardial effusion. These patients often are asymptomatic or have nonspecific symptoms that are attributed to disease progression or to other cardiac conditions (Freter & Haddadin, 2014; Kwong & Nguyen, 2014). The signs and symptoms of cardiac tamponade (see Figure 16-3) are variable and depend on the volume of fluid, how quickly it accumulates, and the patient's underlying cardiac status. Initially, patients with evolving cardiac tamponade are asymptomatic or have vague symptoms. Symptoms increase as the pericardial effusion becomes larger (Kaplow, 2013; Story, 2013). Dyspnea is the most common presenting symptom of cardiac tamponade (Freter & Haddadin, 2014; Grannis, Kim, & Lai, 2014). Dyspnea, tachycardia, and elevated jugular venous pressure were the most common clinical findings in a retrospective study of patients with cardiac tam-

Early Signs and Symptoms	Late Signs and Symptoms
• Dyspnea • Tachycardia • Anxiety/agitation • Muffled heart sounds • Pericardial friction rub • Venous jugular pressure elevation • Chest pain, relieved by leaning forward and intensified by lying supine	• Oliguria • Cyanosis • Tachypnea • Tachycardia • Peripheral edema • Pulsus paradoxus • Hepatojugular reflux • Altered level of consciousness • Beck triad—Classic signs of cardiac tamponade (elevated jugular venous pressure, hypotension, and distant heart sounds; may not all occur together)

Figure 16-3. Signs and Symptoms of Cardiac Tamponade

Note. Based on information from Freter & Haddadin, 2014; Grannis et al., 2014; Kaplow, 2013; Kwong & Nguyen, 2011; Story, 2013; Yarlagadda, 2015.

ponade (Roy, Minor, Brookhart, & Choudhry, 2007). Other common symptoms include chest pain, fatigue, apprehension/anxiety, restlessness, and orthopnea (Story, 2013). Chest pain is often described as "heaviness" and may be relieved by leaning forward and worsened by lying supine because of increased heart compression. Eventually, as fluid continues to accumulate over time or if it accumulates acutely and rapidly, the ability of the pericardium to compensate by stretching is overwhelmed, and the effects of cardiac tamponade increase in severity (Story, 2013). Heart sounds are distant or muffled, and a pericardial friction rub develops as a result of fluid accumulation and cardiac compression (Kaplow, 2013). Impairment of right atrial filling during diastole leads to increased venous pressure, systemic venous congestion, and right heart failure manifested by jugular vein distension, edema, and hepatomegaly (Brashers, 2013). Tachypnea, tachycardia, and peripheral edema develop. Anorexia, nausea, and vomiting may occur because of visceral venous congestion and venous stasis (Kaplow, 2013; Story, 2013).

Late signs and symptoms of cardiac tamponade include worsening cough, dyspnea, hoarseness, and dysphasia or hiccups resulting from mechanical compression of the esophagus, trachea, diaphragm, and adjacent nerves. Cardiac function becomes increasingly compromised as indicated by the appearance of pulsus paradoxus, a decrease in systolic blood pressure of greater than 10 mm Hg during inspiration. Pulsus paradoxus reflects reduced filling of the left ventricle during diastole and decreased cardiac output (Brashers, 2013). In general, pulsus paradoxus is seen mostly in nonmalignant conditions such as constrictive pericarditis (Story, 2013). The classic signs of cardiac tamponade, the Beck triad, occur as cardiac tamponade progresses. The Beck triad, which includes hypotension, muffled heart sounds, and elevated jugular venous pressure, reflects the rapid accumulation of pericardial fluid (Yarlagadda, 2015). Prolonged hypotension leads to decreased perfusion of the kidneys, resulting in oliguria, and decreased peripheral perfusion, leading to weakness, cyanosis, and cool and clammy extremities. Mental status changes can occur, including anxiety, confusion, restlessness, and decreased level of consciousness.

Risk Factors and Etiology

The major cause of pericardial effusion is malignancy or its treatment, but nonmalignant causes exist as well. Malignancy is the most common cause of cardiac tamponade, usually caused by bleeding into the pericardial sac (Spangler & Gentlesk, 2014). Malignant pericardial effusions can develop through direct extension into the pericardial sac of tumors growing close to the heart, especially lung cancer, breast cancer, and mediastinal lymphoma (Lewis et al., 2011). Metastatic spread to the pericardial sac occurs with cancers of the lung and breast, melanoma, lymphoma, and leukemia (Lewis, Hendrickson, & Moynihan, 2011; NCI, 2014). Overall, lung cancer has the highest risk of causing pericardial effusion (Lestuzzi, 2010). Other tumors that can metastasize to the heart include liver, gastric, esophageal, pancreatic, ovarian, and cervical malignancies. One-third of patients with metastases to the pericardium will die from cardiac tamponade (NCI, 2014). Patients with cancer who have preexisting disease in the mediastinum or a prior history of chest radiation therapy may develop cardiac tamponade as a result of obstruction of lymphatic drainage (Freter & Haddadin, 2014; Lestuzzi, 2010). Primary cancers of the pericardium are rare but account for many of the cases of pericardial effusion leading to cardiac tamponade. Mesothelioma is the most common primary tumor of the heart; other less common tumors include malignant fibrous histiocytoma, rhabdomyosarcoma, and angiosarcoma (Story, 2013).

The cytotoxic treatment of malignancies can lead to the development of pericardial effusion. Thoracic radiation that includes the heart and has a dose greater than 40 Gy can cause chronic pericardial effusions to develop 6–12 months following treatment completion. These effusions may be asymptomatic or cause tamponade and hemodynamic compromise (Curigliano et al., 2012). Chemotherapy and biotherapy can increase the risk of pericardial effusion. Chemotherapy agents associated with pericardial effusion include anthracyclines, especially doxorubicin and daunorubicin (drugs that are most often used in regimens treating breast cancer, sarcomas, lymphomas, and leukemia), and alkylating agents, such as cyclophosphamide (Curigliano et al., 2012). Biotherapy agents can increase capillary permeability and promote the risk of pericardial effusion and include interferon, interleukin-2, interleukin-11, and granulocyte macrophage–colony-stimulating factor (Story, 2013). Targeted agents associated with pericardial effusions and cardiac compromise include monoclonal antibodies, such as trastuzumab, especially when used in an anthracycline-containing regimen for treating breast cancer, and tyrosine kinase inhibitors, especially of the vascular endothelial growth factor (VEGF) receptor, such as sunitinib and sorafenib (Curigliano et al., 2012). Patients treated with antineoplastic therapies may be immunosuppressed and thus at risk for pericardial effusion arising from viral, bacterial, or autoimmune causes (Maisch et al., 2010).

Nonmalignant risk factors for the development of pericardial effusion and cardiac tamponade include pericarditis, which can result from a wide variety of conditions including infections (viral [HIV], bacterial [tuberculosis], and fungal), cardiac surgical procedures (valve repairs), myocardial infarction, chest trauma, connective tissue diseases (systemic lupus erythematosus, rheumatoid arthritis), anticoagulation, hypothyroidism, and uremia (NCI, 2014; Yarlagadda, 2015). Tamponade can result from cardiac perforation caused by penetrating injuries or medical procedures, such as central line placement, pacemaker insertion, cardiac catheterization, sternal bone marrow biopsies, and pericardiocentesis. The right atrium is the most common site of perforation from catheter placement. Cardiac tamponade related to trauma or HIV is more common in young adults, whereas tamponade due to malignancy or renal failure occurs more frequently in older adults (Yarlagadda, 2015).

Pathophysiology

The pericardium is a double-layered fibrous sac surrounding the heart. The outer fibrous layer is the parietal layer, which provides strength and protection for the heart. The inner layer is a serous membrane called the visceral layer and is connected to the surface of the heart. The pericardium functions to support the heart chambers; to protect the heart from friction, infection, and inflammation; and to stabilize the cardiac position against gravity. A small amount of fluid, approximately 10–30 ml, between the two layers in the pericardial space serves as a lubricant to prevent friction between the layers of the heart (Cunningham, Brashers, & McCance, 2013). This fluid normally is reabsorbed and drained by the lymph channels into the mediastinum and right heart chambers.

The intrapericardial pressure normally is lower than the ventricular diastolic pressure and equal to the pleural pressure, thereby allowing the heart chambers to fill. Cardiac tamponade occurs when the accumulating pericardial effusion causes the intrapericardial pressure to rise to the point that filling of the cardiac chambers is impaired (Hoit, 2014). Alterations in the production or clearance of pericardial fluid can cause an effusion to develop. Obstruction of the venous and lymphatic drainage of the heart is the most common cause of fluid buildup (Kaplow, 2013). The type of effusion varies with the causative factor. Most often, the fluid is an exudate that collects as a result of inflammation of the pericardium that may be caused by heart surgery, infections, chemotherapy, or autoimmune conditions (e.g., systemic lupus erythematosus). Serosanguineous fluid may accumulate because of the presence of malignancy, tuberculosis, uremia, or radiation pericarditis (Brashers, 2013). In addition, invasive tumors may bleed into the pericardial space. Blood accumulates quickly, so pericardial effusions caused by bleeding tend to progress more rapidly to cardiac tamponade.

The amount of fluid that causes cardiac tamponade varies depending on how rapidly the fluid collects. With slow, chronic accumulation of fluid, the pericardium has time to stretch and can accommodate fluid volume of 2 L or more before hemodynamic instability occurs (Kwong & Nguyen, 2011). If the accumulation is acute and rapid, tamponade occurs with as little as 100–150 ml of fluid; the intrapericardial pressure rises steeply, resulting in hemodynamic compromise (Kwong & Nguyen, 2011). The initial effect of increased intrapericardial pressure is compression of the right atrium and right ventricle. The compression impairs systemic venous return to the right side of the heart so that filling of the right atrium is decreased during diastole. Blood backs up in the venous circulation, venous pressure increases, and signs and symptoms of right heart failure appear: edema, hepatomegaly, jugular vein distention, and increased diastolic pressure. As compression continues, ventricular filling decreases, leading to decreased stroke volume and cardiac output (Brashers, 2013; Lewis et al., 2011). To compensate, tachycardia occurs in an effort to maintain the cardiac output (Freter & Haddadin, 2014). Without intervention, circulatory collapse can lead to shock, cardiac arrest, and death.

Diagnosis and Assessment

Patient History

A thorough and detailed history is important to help identify the presence of pericardial effusion and the underlying cause. The clinical manifestations of cardiac tamponade will vary based on the volume of fluid, the rapidity of fluid accumulation, and the baseline cardiac function of the patient. Early symptoms are nonspecific and may be overlooked as being caused by progressive disease or pulmonary complications, as dyspnea is the most common symptom. Patients should be assessed for risk factors (such as smoking) for unsuspected cancer or a known history of cancer, focusing on cancers that have a higher risk of causing cardiac tamponade, such as lung or breast cancer (Kaplow, 2013). Information should be gathered about previous therapies that are cardiotoxic, such as thoracic radiation therapy or chemotherapy and biotherapy agents associated with cardiac compromise. Patients also should be questioned about a history of other conditions or risk factors that may cause pericardial effusions or mimic its effects. These include myocardial infarction, uremia caused by renal failure, IV drug abuse or opportunistic infections that could indicate HIV-related effusion, manifestations of tuberculosis (fever, night sweats, weight loss), recent cardiovascular surgery or chest wall trauma, and autoimmune disorders, such as systemic lupus erythematosus (Yarlagadda, 2015).

Physical Examination

The physical examination may reveal tachycardia, tachypnea, jugular venous distension, muffled or distant heart sounds, and a pericardial friction rub. Peripheral edema and abdominal distention indicate venous and visceral congestion. Manifestations of decreased cardiac output resulting in hypoperfusion include peripheral vasoconstriction; cold, clammy extremities; weak pulse; and poor capillary refill (Freter & Haddadin, 2014; Yarlagadda, 2015).

As cardiac tamponade progresses and cardiac output decreases, pulsus paradoxus can occur. The presence of pulsus paradoxus is determined by inflating a blood pressure cuff 20 mm Hg above the systolic pressure and slowly deflating the cuff. The first systolic pressure reading heard during exhalation is noted. The systolic pressure reading heard during both inspiration and exhalation then is noted. If the difference between the two sounds is greater than 10 mm Hg, then the patient has pulsus paradoxus (Story, 2013). However, pulsus paradoxus is not specific to cardiac tamponade. It can occur in other conditions, such as severe chronic obstructive pulmonary disease, asthma, pulmonary embolism, right ventricular infarction, constrictive pericarditis, extreme obesity, or tense ascites, and may be absent or undetectable in patients with severe hypotension, atrial septal defect, left ventricular hypertrophy, aortic regurgitation, or right heart tamponade (Kaplow, 2011; Yarlagadda, 2015).

Hepatojugular reflux, defined as an increase in the jugular venous pressure of 1 cm or more, may appear as a result of increased venous congestion in the liver (Story, 2013). Hepatojugular reflux is assessed by placing the patient supine with the head of the bed elevated at 45° so that the jugular venous pulsations are visible. Pressure is exerted over the right upper quadrant of the abdomen for 30–60 seconds, and the jugular vein is observed for increased jugular venous pressure (Kaplow, 2011). The signs of Beck's triad—hypotension, distant heart sounds, and elevated jugular venous distension—are assessed, but all are not usually present together in cardiac tamponade (Freter & Haddadin, 2014).

Diagnostic Procedures

A routine chest x-ray is not diagnostic of cardiac tamponade but may demonstrate an enlarged cardiac silhouette, known as "water bottle heart," which indicates increased fluid in the pericardial sac and would raise suspicion leading to further testing. The volume of pericardial fluid must be at least 200 ml to be detected on chest x-ray (Lewis et al., 2011). Electrocardiogram (ECG) changes are nonspecific for cardiac tamponade and include tachycardia, low-voltage QRS complex, nonspecific ST-T changes, and premature atrial or ventricular contractions (Grannis et al., 2014). Electrical alternans is a rare ECG finding that indicates pericardial effusion and is due to the swinging motion of the heart within the fluid-filled pericardial sac (Lewis et al., 2011). Alternans of QRS complex alone is not specific for pericardial effusion (Hoit, 2014).

The most precise diagnostic test in cardiac tamponade is a two-dimensional echocardiogram, which can detect as little as 15 ml of effusion (Freter & Haddadin, 2014). It is a painless and noninvasive test that can be performed at the bedside and assesses for the presence, location, and approximate quantity of pericardial fluid, as well as the overall cardiac function. The classic echocardiographic sign of cardiac tamponade is diastolic collapse of the right atrium and ventricle because of the pressure of the pericardial effusion. The sensitivity and specificity of this finding are very high: 38%–60% and 50%–100%, respectively (Chong & Plotnick, 1995). Two-dimensional echocardiogram is the preferred method to guide site selection for percutaneous drainage of the effusion, if indicated (Kwong & Nguyen, 2011). Other findings on echocardiogram include swinging heart, left atrial and ventricular collapse, inspiratory changes in ventricle size, and inferior vena cava distention (Story, 2013).

Other tests that may be used as adjuncts in the diagnosis of cardiac tamponade include CT scan and MRI (Kaplow, 2013). CT scans can detect as little as 50 ml of pericardial fluid, but the motion of the heart and mediastinum can cause artifacts that make it difficult to measure and characterize the effusion. MRI scans may have superior resolution compared to echocardiogram and are useful in characterizing the type of pericardial effusion (e.g., hemorrhagic, transudative, exudative) (Story, 2013). Both CT and MRI may help to distinguish between radiation fibrosis and constrictive pericarditis with effusion. Neither test is better than an echocardiogram; they are both costly and time consuming and do not provide data on cardiac functioning if cardiac tamponade exists (Kaplow, 2011).

A pericardial tap may be performed to obtain pericardial fluid to determine whether the effusion is due to malignancy or other causes if there is sufficient fluid for a safe procedure. The fluid should be examined for gram stain (to distinguish between gram-positive or gram-negative bacilli), acid-fast bacilli stain (tuberculosis), polymerase chain reaction, cytology, carcinoembryonic antigen, and total protein levels (Grannis et al., 2014; Hoit, 2014). The fluid is characterized as transudate or exudate. A transudate has a low protein level and has leaked from the blood vessels as a result of nonmalignant mechanical factors, such as congestive heart failure or cirrhosis. An exudate is rich in protein and has leaked as a result of increased permeability. Malignant effusions often are exudates and contain blood and cellular debris caused by the presence of cancer cells or tumor implants. Biopsies of tissue taken from the pericardium or epicardium can be analyzed for malignancy and infectious agents. Cytology or biology results used alone may be inadequate to diagnose malignancy; the combination of both sets of results has been shown to provide the correct etiology (Maisch et al., 2010).

Differential Diagnosis

The differential diagnosis for cardiac tamponade includes cardiogenic shock, constrictive pericarditis, constrictive-effusive pericarditis, pulmonary embolus, and tension pneumothorax (Yarlagadda, 2015). Tension pneumothorax causes hemodynamic changes that can mimic acute cardiac tamponade. A tension pneumothorax presents with a deviated trachea and unequal breath sounds to distinguish it from cardiac tamponade. A large pleural effusion can transmit elevated intrapleural pressure to the pericardial space, leading to reduced ventricular filling. The resulting hemodynamic changes are the same as with cardiac tamponade (Yarlagadda, 2015). Echocardiogram is increasingly used in the emergency setting as a diagnostic tool to help distinguish between tamponade and other conditions such as myocardial infarction and congestive heart failure (Daley, Bhimji, Bascom, Benninghoff, & Alam, 2014; Spangler & Gentlesk, 2014). In the absence of echocardiography, a central venous pressure (CVP) line may be placed to evaluate pressures in the right side of the heart. CVP measurements greater than 12–14 mm Hg are usually found in cardiac tamponade (Spangler & Gentlesk, 2014).

Evidence-Based Treatment Strategies

Cardiac tamponade is a life-threatening emergency that requires removal of the pericardial fluid to restore hemodynamic stability. The patient's overall condition, presenting symptoms, cancer diagnosis, prognosis, and the risks and benefits of treatment are taken into account when planning interventions. Treatment goals are tailored to the patient's life expectancy and performance status. The immediate goal is removal of pericardial fluid to restore hemodynamic stability and relieve symptoms. The appearance of malignant pericardial effusion often indicates terminal disease, and in critically ill patients, treatment may focus on palliating symptoms and providing supportive care rather than removing fluid. For patients with life expectancies of at least a few months or who have mild symptoms, interventions include supportive care, fluid removal to restore hemodynamic stability, procedures to prevent reaccumulation of fluid, symptom relief, and treatment to control the underlying malignancy (Hoit, 2014; Kwong & Nguyen, 2011; Lewis et al., 2011). A surgical approach usually is necessary to restore hemodynamic stability and is followed by medical management. See Table 16-2 for an overview of surgical approaches for cardiac tamponade.

Pericardiocentesis is the most common initial approach for the management of cardiac tamponade. It provides immediate symptom relief by rapidly removing pericardial fluid and serves as a diagnostic aid to analyze the effusion (Grannis et al., 2014). The most serious complication of pericardiocentesis is bleeding; thus, surgical backup should be available in the event of right ventricle puncture (Story, 2013). A subxiphoid approach is used to insert a needle under echocardiographic or fluoroscopic guidance into the pericardial sac for fluid aspiration. In a truly emergent situation, pericardiocentesis can be performed without localization guidance, such as at the bedside (Maisch et al., 2010). The effusion must be drained slowly over several minutes to prevent right ventricular distention and failure. Once the fluid is drained, a catheter can remain in place over several days to allow for continued drainage and to serve as a route for pericardial sclerosis. Pericardiocentesis is generally a temporary measure, as the effusion reaccumulates rapidly, and more definitive treatments are needed to prevent recurrence

Table 16-2. Surgical Approaches to Cardiac Tamponade

Surgical Procedure	Comments
Pericardiocentesis	• Emergent removal of pericardial fluid at bedside (with surgical backup) • Usually performed in cardiac catheterization laboratory with echocardiogram guidance • Needle inserted via subxiphoid approach toward left shoulder • Catheter can be placed for continued drainage or used for sclerosis • Short-term management
Pericardial sclerosis	• Instillation of sclerosing agent into the pericardial sac to induce scarring and prevent recurrence of fluid accumulation
Percutaneous balloon pericardiostomy	• Insertion of catheter into pericardial space, followed by inflation of balloon to cause tear or hole in pericardium, allowing fluid to drain into the mediastinum • Short-term management
Pericardial window	• Local or general anesthesia with subxiphoid approach; resection of segment of pericardium, allowing fluid to drain into the mediastinum • Allows pericardial biopsies to be obtained • Long-term management in selected patients
Pericardiectomy	• General anesthesia with resection of part or all of the pericardial sac via video-assisted thoracoscopic surgery or thoracotomy to allow drainage and prevent recurrence of fluid accumulation • Long-term management in selected patients

Note. Based on information from Hoit, 2014; Kaplow, 2013; Kwong & Nguyen, 2011; Maisch et al., 2010; Story, 2013.

(Freter & Haddadin, 2014; Grannis et al., 2014). Recommendations for preventing reaccumulation of malignant pericardial effusion include surgical and medical options that proceed in a stepwise fashion depending on the individual patient's performance status and prognosis.

Pericardial sclerosis is attempted once the pericardial fluid is drained. Pericardial sclerosis is the instillation of an agent into the pericardial sac to create inflammation and fibrosis, which seals the pericardial space and prevents fluid reaccumulation. The sclerosing agents selected also provide intrapericardial chemotherapy and include bleomycin, mitomycin C, cisplatin, 5-fluorouracil, mitoxantrone, thiotepa, and radioisotopes (Grannis et al., 2014; Lestuzzi, 2010; Maisch et al., 2010). Radioisotopes such as chromic phosphate have demonstrated high efficacy with no adverse effects, but use is not widespread because of the complexities associated with treatment implementation (Maisch et al., 2010). Pain, fever, nausea, and arrhythmias are common side effects associated with instillation of sclerosing agents.

Percutaneous balloon pericardiotomy is a procedure that may be performed as an alternative to surgical intervention to prevent effusion recurrence (Jones & Jain, 2011). A balloon-tipped catheter is placed across the pericardium under fluoroscopic and echocardiographic guidance and is inflated to tear the pericardium, creating a window for drainage (Grannis et al., 2014). This technique is simple and minimally invasive and may be appropriate for patients who cannot tolerate surgery. Patients who have longer life expectancy and good clinical status, or those who have not responded to pericardiocentesis with sclerosis, may be treated with surgical options that offer more lasting control of pericardial effusion (Lestuzzi, 2010).

Pericardial window is a procedure that is used for patients with recurrent effusions. It can be performed using general anesthesia in the operating room or local anesthesia with thoracoscopy. The procedure also can be performed as a laparoscopic video-assisted thoracoscopic surgery (Kaplow, 2013). The pericardium is exposed, a small incision is made, and a 3 cm diameter piece of pericardium is removed to create a "window" that allows fluid to drain into surrounding tissues. Tube drainage or sclerosis may be combined with this procedure. Chest tubes will remain in place for several days (Story, 2013).

Pericardiectomy is the partial or complete removal of the visceral pericardium. It is considered the definitive treatment for pericardial effusion because it provides immediate relief of pericardial tamponade and allows continuous fluid drainage into the pleural space. General anesthesia is required, leading to a longer recovery time and higher morbidity rate compared to other surgical procedures. Thus, pericardiectomy is reserved for patients with recurrent effusions and a life expectancy longer than one year or to treat patients with radiation-induced constrictive pericarditis (Grannis et al., 2014).

Chemotherapy administered systemically can help prevent recurrence of pericardial effusion in patients with chemotherapy-sensitive cancers, such as lymphoma, leukemia, and germ cell tumors (Freter & Haddadin, 2014; Grannis et al., 2014). Breast cancer may respond to hormone therapy. Systemic chemotherapy to control the precipitating malignancy has been shown to increase survival following pericardial effusion (Lestuzzi, 2010; Lewis et al., 2011). Local instillation of chemotherapy agents with both antineoplastic and sclerosing effects, such as bleomycin or thiotepa, into the pericardial sac is used in conjunction with pericardiocentesis to prevent recurrence of malignant pericardial effusions (Lestuzzi, 2010; Lewis et al., 2011). Chemotherapy also may be used in the setting of a slowly accumulating pericardial effusion when the patient is asymptomatic (Grannis et al., 2014).

Radiation therapy can be used to manage pericardial effusions in patients with radiosensitive tumors who have not had prior radiation or who are refractory to other treatment approaches (Grannis et al., 2014; Lestuzzi, 2010). Response rates of 66%–93% have been reported with radiation therapy, particularly in patients with lymphoma, leukemia, and breast cancer (Grannis et al., 2014). Treatment fields for external beam radiation encompass the heart, pericardial structures, and mediastinum. Total radiation doses range between 2,000 and 4,000 cGy (Grannis et al., 2014).

Supportive care to stabilize the patient's blood pressure and cardiac function and reduce anxiety may be required depending on the extent of the tamponade. Mild cardiac tamponade with minimal or no evidence of hemodynamic compromise may be treated conservatively with careful monitoring, serial echocardiographic studies, avoidance of volume depletion, and therapy aimed at the underlying cause of the pericardial effusion (Hoit, 2014). Oxygen therapy may be needed to reduce the work of the heart, respiratory distress, and anxiety. Blood products, plasma, dextran, or saline may be used to expand circulatory volume but must be used with caution and closely monitored. Volume expansion can significantly increase intracardiac pressures in the intrapericardial space and right atrium and can increase left ventricular end-diastolic pressure, which can precipitate tamponade (Hoit, 2014). Fluid repletion appears to be most effective in patients who are hypovolemic. Inotropic agents, such as dobutamine, may be used in patients with hypotension to increase the strength of cardiac contraction, maintain blood pressure, and improve cardiac output (Story, 2013). The value of inotropic support, whether or not it is given in conjunction with vasodilators, is not clear (Hoit, 2014). An arterial vasodilator, nitroprusside, may be used to decrease the work of the heart and increase blood pressure and cardiac output (Story, 2013). Interventions to avoid include use of alpha-1 agonist drugs, which cause vasoconstriction, increase the work of the heart, and decrease cardiac output; diuretics, which lead to reduced blood volume and ventricular filling and worsen tamponade; and positive-pressure mechanical ventilation, which further reduces cardiac filling (Hoit, 2014; Kaplow, 2011). Placing patients in the semi-Fowler position and reducing their anxiety through use of medications and relaxation techniques help to decrease the work of the heart.

Implications for Oncology Advanced Practice Nurses

Cardiac tamponade is a potentially life-threatening emergency that without rapid intervention can lead to cardiac collapse and death. The symptoms can be vague and occur slowly or acutely. With intervention, rapid improvement is seen. APNs can help to facilitate the appropriate intervention, which is based on the patient's disease, prognosis, expected length of survival, and clinical status.

Nursing management of patients with cardiac tamponade is complex, and APNs must ensure that these patients are assessed and monitored closely. Ongoing assessment of blood pressure, ECG monitoring, and oxygen therapy are critical in patients with cardiac tamponade. Patient and family education along with emotional support is needed to decrease anxiety and maintain optimal cardiac status. Preparation for procedures and monitoring after procedures for complications such as pneumothorax, bleeding, infection, or reaccumulation of pericardial fluid also are needed.

APNs always should consider pericardial effusion in patients with a history of malignancy who present with dyspnea. An echocardiogram should be obtained if pericardial effusion is suspected, as physical examination, chest x-ray, and ECG may be nonspecific (Spangler & Gentlesk, 2014).

Spinal Cord Compression

Spinal cord compression (SCC) is a true oncologic emergency. The most common causes of SCC are invasion or extension of metastatic or local tumor masses into the epidural space that occupy space and compress the spinal cord. Collapsed vertebral bone fragments also may compress the cord (Kaplan, 2013). If unrecognized, SCC has devastating consequences on the patient's neurologic function and ability to maintain functional independence. Without treatment, neurologic impairment progresses from pain to motor weakness, sensory loss, sphincter dysfunction, and ultimately irreversible paralysis (Kaplan, 2013). The longer the SCC goes untreated, the lower the chances for neurologic recovery (Becker & Baehring, 2011b). Early recognition and intervention are critical to preserve function and quality of life.

Incidence

SCC is the second most common neurologic complication of cancer, following brain metastases (Hammack, 2012). SCC affects 5%–14% of the adult cancer population, or about 20,000 people per year (Becker & Baehring, 2011b; Schiff, 2014). Most patients with SCC have a known history of cancer, but in up to 25% of cases, it is the first indication of malignant disease (Lewis et al., 2011; Schiff, 2014). The highest incidence of SCC occurs in patients with solid tumors that commonly metastasize to vertebral bone (Lewis et al., 2011) (see Figure 16-4). Survival following the appearance of SCC is typically limited to a few months (Becker & Baehring, 2011b; Weinstein, 2013).

• Primary cancers of the spinal cord
  – Glioma
  – Astrocytoma
  – Ependymoma
• Cancers with a natural history of bone metastasis
  – Lung
  – Renal
  – Breast
  – Prostate
  – Myeloma
  – Melanoma
• Cancers that metastasize to the spinal cord
  – Seminoma
  – Lymphoma
  – Neuroblastoma

Figure 16-4. Cancer Types at Risk for Spinal Cord Compression

Note. Based on information from Kaplan, 2013.

Signs and Symptoms

The signs and symptoms of SCC depend on the anatomic level and location of the tumor (see Figure 16-5). The thoracic spine is the most common site of spinal metastasis with SCC (60%), followed by the lumbar-sacral spine (25%) and the cervical spine (10%–15%) (Hammack, 2012; Lewis et al., 2011). Signs and symptoms of SCC follow a similar sequence in all patients regardless of the precipitating malignancy. Back pain is the presenting symptom in 90% of the cases, preceding neurologic changes by weeks to months (Huff, 2014; Schiff, 2014). The pain may be localized, radicular (pain in the area of the affected dermatome), referred, or a combination. Acute back pain occurring in the lower back or neck is common among adults and is typically related to benign causes. Pain occurring in the middle or upper back is more likely to herald SCC, especially in patients with a known cancer history (Kaplan, 2013). An urgent neurologic examination is indicated (Schiff, 2014; Weinstein, 2013).

Localized back pain usually is the initial symptom and is described as dull, aching, constant, and progressive. It is the result of expansion, destruction, or fracture of the involved vertebral elements. Unlike the pain from a herniated disc that is relieved by lying down, the pain from SCC worsens when patients are in a supine position and improves with sitting or standing (Iwamoto, Haas, & Gosselin, 2012). Patients report the most pain on arising in the morning, which is due to increased venous stasis and cord edema. Sleeping in a sitting position may provide relief (Becker & Baehring, 2011b; Flaherty, 2011). The intensity of local

Cervical Spine	Thoracic Spine	Lumbar-Sacral Spine
• Breathing difficulties • Loss of sensation in arms • Headache, neck, shoulder, or arm pain • Paralysis involving neck, trunk, arms, and hands • Muscle weakness in neck, trunk, arms, and hands	• Paralysis • Muscle weakness • Chest or back pain • Positive Babinski reflex • Bladder, bowel, and sexual dysfunction • Loss of sensation below the tumor level • Increased sensation above the tumor level	• Paralysis • Foot drop • Weakness in the legs and feet • Loss of sensation in the legs and feet • Bladder, bowel, and sexual dysfunction • Decreased or absent reflexes in the legs • Lower back pain that may radiate down the legs or into the perineal area

Figure 16-5. Signs and Symptoms of Spinal Cord Compression

Note. Based on information from Becker & Baehring, 2011b; Flaherty, 2011; Kaplan, 2013.

pain increases over time, and a radicular component may develop (Schiff, 2014). Compression of the nerve roots or cauda equina causes radicular pain, which follows the pattern of the affected dermatome. Radicular pain can be a constant, dull ache or a burning, shooting pain. Bilateral band-like pain across the chest and abdomen is more common with thoracic cord lesions, whereas unilateral radicular pain is characteristic of lumbar or cervical lesions (Kaplan, 2013). Both localized and radicular pain are exacerbated by coughing, sneezing, moving, and performing the Valsalva maneuver (Huff, 2014; Iwamoto et al., 2012). Nonradicular pain that is referred to other areas in the body may obscure the site of SCC and make diagnosis difficult (Kaplan, 2009). Weakness is the second most common symptom of SCC at presentation and is present in up to 85% of the cases (Hammack, 2012; Kaplan, 2013). Weakness follows pain by weeks to months and may be missed as a symptom of SCC because it is common in patients with advanced cancer. Motor weakness typically begins in the legs regardless of the level of compression. Initially it is more proximal, and patients may have difficulty rising from a chair or toilet and climbing steps. Patients often describe the weakness as a heaviness or stiffness in the legs (Becker & Baehring, 2011b; Kaplan, 2013). Involvement of upper motor neurons leads to weakness associated with increased muscle tone and hyporeflexia. Lower motor neuron involvement leads to weakness caused by decreased muscle tone and hyporeflexia. As SCC progresses, the weakness leads to loss of coordination, difficulty walking, and eventually paralysis (Sun & Nemecek, 2009). Thirty percent of patients will develop irreversible paraplegia within one week of experiencing motor weakness (Weinstein, 2013). The patient's ability to walk at the time of diagnosis is an indicator of neurologic status and the most important predictor of functional outcome (Kaplan, 2013). Patients who can walk prior to treatment generally have good treatment outcomes and at least a one-year survival prognosis. Patients who present with paraplegia are unlikely to walk again, even after treatment, and have a poor survival prognosis (Weinstein, 2013). Figure 16-6 lists prognostic factors predictive for functional outcome following the diagnosis of SCC.

Sensory changes may develop shortly after motor weakness. At the time of SCC diagnosis, 50%–70% of patients demonstrate some sensory deficit (Sun & Nemecek, 2009). Sensory loss depends on the level of cord compression and may include numbness, paresthesias, loss of proprioception, and loss of sensation for touch, pain, temperature, and vibration (Huff, 2014). Sensory loss typically starts in the toes and ascends until it reaches the level of the lesion. Compression of the conus medullaris or cauda equina results in bilateral sensory loss and fol-

Favorable Prognostic Factors	Poor Prognostic Factors
• Early recognition and diagnosis of metastatic spinal cord compression (MSCC) • Prompt initiation of therapy • Able to ambulate at presentation • Slow onset of motor weakness • Single site of cord compression • Radiosensitive tumors—multiple myeloma, lymphoma, breast, prostate, testicular seminoma, neuroblastoma, Ewing sarcoma • Good performance status • Responsive to steroid treatment • Female gender • Long interval between diagnosis of primary tumor and appearance of MSCC	• Paraplegia prior to treatment • Urinary retention • Sphincter incontinence • Rapidly deteriorating neurologic function (in less than 72 hours) • Radioresistant tumors—lung, renal, gastrointestinal, sarcoma, bladder, melanoma • Extensive bone or visceral metastases • Poor performance status

Figure 16-6. Prognostic Factors for Functional Recovery and Survival Following Metastatic Spinal Cord Compression

Note. Based on information from Becker & Baehring, 2011b; Cole & Patchell, 2008; Giglio & Gilbert, 2010; Klimo et al., 2003; Prewett & Venkitaraman, 2010; Weinstein, 2013; Yadav et al., 2009.

From "Spinal Cord Compression" (p. 355) by M. Kaplan in M. Kaplan (Ed.), *Understanding and Managing Oncologic Emergencies: A Resource for Nurses* (2nd ed.), 2013, Pittsburgh, PA: Oncology Nursing Society. Copyright 2013 by Oncology Nursing Society. Reprinted with permission.

lows the dermatome path involving the buttocks, perineal area, posterior thigh, and lateral leg (Dawodu et al., 2014).

Autonomic dysfunction is a common late finding of SCC and is associated with a poor prognosis (Weinstein, 2013). It includes changes in bladder and bowel function and impotence due to decreased sphincter tone and reflex losses. Bladder symptoms include urinary hesitancy and retention followed by incontinence (Flaherty, 2011). In older adults, urinary retention is a more reliable sign of autonomic dysfunction than urinary incontinence, which may occur with increasing age. Bowel dysfunction includes lack of urge to defecate and inability to bear down, leading to constipation, obstipation, and incontinence (Flaherty, 2011). Horner syndrome (drooping eyelid, constricted pupil, and decreased sweating on the affected side of the face) can be seen with tumor involvement around the junction of the cervical and thoracic spines, causing autonomic dysfunction of the sympathetic nerves of the face (Becker & Baehring, 2011b). Autonomic dysreflexia may occur with injury to the spinal cord at or above the level of the sixth or seventh thoracic vertebra. A distended bladder or bowel may be the triggering event. Classic symptoms of autonomic dysreflexia include pounding headache, bradycardia, nasal congestion, hypertension, profuse sweating, and pilomotor erection (goose bumps) above the level of the lesion (Yadav, Shin, Guo, & Konzen, 2009).

Risk Factors and Etiology

The most common risk factor for SCC is the presence of metastatic disease in vertebral bone (Becker & Baehring, 2011b). Solid tumors that metastasize to bone have a high incidence of SCC and include breast, lung, and prostate cancer. Renal cell carcinoma, lymphoma, and multiple myeloma also contribute to the incidence of SCC (Kaplan, 2013) (see Figure 16-4). The location of the cord compression frequently correlates with the volume of vertebral bone, the width of the epidural space, and the patterns of venous blood flow in the region (Kaplan, 2013; Schiff, 2014). Thus, the thoracic spine is the most common site of SCC (60% of cases) because it comprises 12 vertebrae and has the largest volume of bone. The lumbosacral spine (25% of cases) and cervical spine (10%–15% of cases) follow in frequency of SCC location (Hammack, 2012; Lewis et al., 2011). Breast and lung cancers typically involve the thoracic vertebrae but may be more widely distributed among the vertebrae. Malignancies of the prostate, colon, and kidney commonly are the cause of lesions of the lower thoracic and lumbosacral spine (Kaplan, 2013). About 30% of patients with SCC have lesions at multiple levels of the spinal cord (Giglio & Gilbert, 2010). In rare instances, SCC can be caused by primary tumors of the spinal cord, such as ependymoma, astrocytoma, or glioma, which are intramedullary tumors that arise within the spinal cord (Chamberlain & Tredway, 2011).

A study by Lu, Gonzalez, Jolesz, Wen, and Talcott (2005) identified four independent predictors of risk for SCC based on MRI results demonstrating compression of the thecal (dural) sac: abnormal neurologic examination, pain in the middle or upper back, known vertebral metastases, and metastatic disease at initial presentation. APNs can use these factors to be alert for patients who are at increased risk for the development of SCC.

Pathophysiology

The spinal column is composed of 33 vertebrae—7 cervical, 12 thoracic, 5 lumbar, 5 fused sacral (forming the sacrum), and 4 fused coccygeal (forming the coccyx). Between each disc (except the fused ones), an intervertebral disk exists, which functions to absorb shocks and prevent damage to the vertebrae. This forms the spinal canal, which encloses and protects the spinal cord. The spinal cord is a long nerve cable that arises from the medulla oblongata and ends at the level of the first or second lumbar vertebra. The end of the spinal cord, the conus medullaris, is cone shaped, and the lumbar and sacral spinal nerve roots continue outward from it and are called the *cauda equina* because they resemble a horse's tail (Sugerman, 2013).

Three membranes, or *meninges*, cover the brain and spinal cord as a protective mechanism (see Figure 16-7). The innermost layer is the pia mater, which directly adheres to the brain and spinal cord. The subarachnoid space separates the pia mater from the middle membrane and the arachnoid membrane and contains the cerebrospinal fluid (CSF). The subdural space is between the arachnoid membrane and the outermost layer, the dura mater. The dura mater (Latin for "hard mother") is a tough membrane to which the spinal nerves are attached. The space between the dura mater and the vertebral column is the epidural space, which contains the blood vessels and adipose tissue (Sugerman, 2013).

In the majority of cases, SCC results from metastatic disease developing outside the spinal cord (extradural) and invading the epidural space, causing direct com-

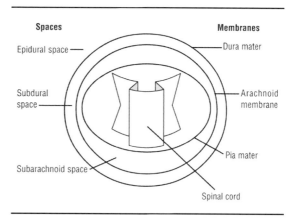

Figure 16-7. Meninges or Membranes Surrounding the Spinal Cord, With Associated Spaces

Note. From "Oncology Emergency Modules: Spinal Cord Compression," by J.A. Flounders and B.B. Ott, 2003, *Oncology Nursing Forum, 30,* p. E18. doi:10.1188/03.ONF.E17-E23. Copyright 2003 by Oncology Nursing Society. Reprinted with permission.

pression of the cord. The main mechanism of tumor invasion of the epidural space is through hematogenous spread of malignant cells that have an affinity for spinal marrow (Prasad & Schiff, 2005). This results in a mass that enlarges and impinges on the thecal sac, anteriorly compressing the spinal cord and leading to collapse of the vertebral body and retropulsion of bony fragments into the epidural space. Primary tumors of the spinal cord are intramedullary and directly invade and destroy the cord. Another cause is lymph node growth from the paraspinal region that extends through the vertebral neural foramen into the epidural space, as seen with lymphoma (Prasad & Schiff, 2005).

Neurologic defects caused by SCC are a result of direct compression of the spinal cord or cauda equina, interruption of the vascular supply to the spinal cord by tumor or bone, or compression from vertebral collapse causing bone fragments to impinge on the spinal cord (Kaplan, 2013). Compression obstructs the normal venous blood flow in the vertebral venous plexus, resulting in vasogenic edema, swelling of the nerve axons, loss of myelin, and ischemia in the areas of compression (Sun & Nemecek, 2009). Additional nerve injury results from the release of neurotoxic substances, including cytokines (interleukin-1 and interleukin-6), inflammatory mediators (prostaglandin E), and excitatory neurotransmitters (serotonin). Hypoxia of the spinal cord stimulates the production of VEGF, which increases vascular permeability and vasogenic edema. Without intervention, the vasogenic edema progresses to ischemia and cytotoxic edema, resulting in irreversible neurologic damage (Prasad & Schiff, 2005).

Diagnosis and Assessment

A thorough history and physical examination are important to detect early indications of SCC. Any complaint of pain in patients with cancer needs a detailed history. Back pain requires careful assessment to determine if any radicular component exists, indicating nerve root compression.

The clinical manifestations of SCC correspond to the location and extent of compression. As pain is the most common presenting symptom, patients can point to the site of pain, and assessment with gentle palpation and percussion can indicate the level of cord compression (Huff, 2014). Straight leg raises will increase radicular pain, indicative of lumbar or thoracic nerve root compression. Pain on neck flexion indicates cervical spine compression, and extreme care is indicated when moving the neck (Weinstein, 2013). A musculoskeletal examination assesses motor function, including evaluation of gait, muscle strength, involuntary movements, and coordination. Difficulty rising from a seated position or climbing stairs is seen with proximal muscle weakness of the legs and often is the first sign of motor weakness associated with SCC (Becker & Baehring, 2011b). Leg strength is assessed by observing heel walking, toe walking, and deep knee bends, if the patient is able, or performing active movements against resistance (Kaplan, 2013). The American Spinal Injury Association (2011) has a standardized form and grading scale to classify motor and sensory function and impairment. The grading categories range from 0 (total paralysis) to 5 (active movement against full resistance) and can be used at baseline and for follow-up assessment.

Reflex assessment is essential to provide information about the patient's neurologic status. Normal reflexes show a brisk response, whereas deep tendon reflexes decrease at the level of cord compression and become hyperactive below (Kaplan, 2013). A positive Babinski sign in adults is always abnormal and indicates dysfunction of the spinal tract (Dawodu et al., 2014). A Babinski sign is elicited by stroking the sole of the foot from the heel to the small toe and then arcing to the great toe. A positive response is dorsiflexion of the great toe with fanning of the other toes, reflecting upper motor neuron disease (Kaplan, 2013).

Sensory assessment should include evaluation of patients' sense of pain, temperature, touch, vibration, and position (proprioception) (Miaskowski, 2009). Careful dermatome mapping of sensory loss can indicate the level of cord damage (Weinstein, 2013). Assessment of autonomic function also is necessary. Taking a careful history of urination is important, and a post-void residual measurement may be needed to assess for neurogenic bladder. Change in bowel habits should be elicited, and digital rectal examination should be performed to assess sphincter tone. Questions about sexual function and recent onset of impotence also are important (Kaplan, 2013).

Imaging of the spine should be performed urgently to document the site of cord compression. Plain films (x-rays) of the spine often are initially obtained in patients with pain but no neurologic changes, as they are easy to obtain. Plain films can show vertebral collapse, erosion, and bone fragment dislocation, but unfortunately, they do not detect early SCC because 50% of the bone must be destroyed before it is evident on plain films (Cole & Patchell, 2008). Plain films also do not detect paraspinal masses that may be extending into the epidural space (Schiff, 2014). Bone scans may be used occasionally. They are more sensitive than plain films but have limitations, as they do not provide structural detail to identify whether an epidural tumor is present (Schiff, 2014).

MRI currently is the gold standard to evaluate SCC because it is the most sensitive, specific, and accurate test for evaluating SCC. MRI allows visualization of the extent of the lesion and anatomy, detects paraspinal masses, and can image multiple levels to assess for areas of disease that are not clinically apparent (Becker & Baehring, 2011b). Myelography with or without CT scanning has largely been replaced by MRI but is still used in certain situations: for patients with metallic implants for whom MRI is contraindicated, for retrieval of CSF to diagnose leptomeningeal metastases, and in conjunction with CT for treatment planning for stereotactic radiosurgery (SRS) (Schiff, 2014). Positron-emission tomography (PET) used in conjunction with CT (PET-CT) can localize the area of cord compression and the extent of tumor involvement. However, it is not recommended as the sole imaging technique for SCC diagnosis because it may miss certain lesions or produce false-positive results (Kaplan, 2013).

Differential Diagnosis

Mechanical back pain associated with trauma, arthritis, muscle strain, old vertebral injury, or lumbar disk disorders, epidural hematoma, epidural or subdural infections, cauda equina syndrome, inflammatory spinal cord injuries, spinal cord damage from exposure to radiation, and neoplastic meningitis are other conditions to consider (Huff, 2014). Most benign causes of SCC generally occur in the cervical or lumbar spine. Pain that worsens with lying down should be considered malignant until proved otherwise (Schiff, 2014). Radiation myelopathy occurs 9–15 months after radiation, and MRI can distinguish it from SCC (Schiff, 2014). MRI is useful to evaluate for most other conditions that may mimic SCC.

Evidence-Based Treatment Strategies

Intervention for SCC needs to begin immediately to prevent permanent damage. Ambulatory status at the time of diagnosis is predictive of ambulation following treatment; 80%–100% of patients who are able to ambulate at diagnosis retain their ability to ambulate (Lewis et al., 2011; Schiff, 2014). Treatment of SCC is individualized and depends on the tumor type, location in the spine, whether it is radiosensitive or chemosensitive, and the patient's prognosis and life expectancy (Huff, 2014). Pain relief is always a priority regardless of the prognosis. The goals of treatment are to optimize quality of life with pain relief and symptom palliation, preserve and restore neurologic function, stabilize the spine, reduce the tumor, and prevent SCC recurrence.

Corticosteroids are administered to all patients as an initial supportive therapy until definitive treatment with radiation or surgery, either alone or in combination, can be instituted (Giglio & Gilbert, 2010). Corticosteroids decrease vasogenic edema in the spinal cord and downregulate VEGF expression, resulting in improvement in neurologic symptoms as well as pain relief. Corticosteroids also have a direct effect on some tumors, particularly lymphoma (Schiff, 2014; Weinstein, 2013). Dexamethasone is the most widely used corticosteroid for SCC. Opinions vary about the optimal loading and maintenance doses. Doses may be tailored to the patient's neurologic status, with symptomatic patients receiving high-dose dexamethasone, and ambulatory patients receiving lower doses (Cole & Patchell, 2008; Lewis et al., 2011). Prospective randomized clinical trials investigating optimal steroid dosing for SCC are lacking, and dose recommendations have been based on evidence gathered from systematic reviews of the literature. In 2003, Klimo, Kestle, and Schmidt conducted an extensive literature review of steroid management of SCC. Based on the review data, they recommended an initial bolus dose of 10 mg of dexamethasone IV, followed by 16 mg/day slowly tapered over several weeks during definitive treatment with radiation therapy or surgery. More recently, Loblaw, Mitera, Ford, and Laperriere (2012) conducted an updated literature review of optimal steroid dosing between January 2004 and May 2011 and proposed guidelines for clinical practice. Their recommendations remain consistent with prior ones: (a) patients with radiographic evidence of SCC but without neurologic deficits do not require steroids; (b) steroids should be administered to any patient with pain or neurologic deficits who has either suspected or confirmed SCC, unless medically contraindicated; (c) patients with minimal neurologic dysfunction are treated with the dexamethasone regimen recommended in 2003 (bolus of 10 mg followed by 16 mg daily in divided doses until taper); and (d) patients with severe neurologic deficits can be started on a high-dose steroid regimen (100 mg bolus followed by maintenance doses of up to 96 mg/day), in spite of increased risk of serious side effects. Once definitive treatment is well established, dexamethasone doses are tapered gradually (Loblaw et al., 2012). Prolonged administration of high-dose dexamethasone has been shown to lead to serious adverse events, particularly in the gastrointestinal tract, including gastric ulcers and bowel perforations that require surgery (Hammack, 2012).

The optimal sequence of definitive treatments for SCC (radiation versus surgery) has not been established (Kaplan, 2013). Based on their literature review, Loblaw et al. (2012) recommended that surgery be reserved for appropriate patients with a good survival prognosis and that other patients with SCC receive radiation therapy alone. Indications for radiation therapy as first-line treatment include radiosensitive tumors (e.g., lymphoma, multiple myeloma, SCLC), expected survival of less than three to four months, multiple levels of compression, and inability to tolerate surgery (Prewett & Venkitaraman, 2010). The optimal radiation dose has not been established. The most frequently used dosing schedule is 30 Gy in 10 daily fractions (Giglio & Gilbert, 2010; Schiff, Brown, & Shaffrey, 2014). Patients with a poor prognosis can be treated with a single fraction of 8 Gy (Loblaw et al., 2012). Radiation therapy provides pain relief (which may take up to two weeks) and controls tumor growth but does not correct spinal instability (Chow, Finkelstein, Saghal, & Coleman, 2011; Georgy, 2008). SBRT, also referred to as radiosurgery, allows delivery of high-dose radiation directly to the vertebrae involved with tumor and spares the spinal cord and surrounding tissue. This technique may be useful as an alternative to conventional external beam radiation to the spine for initial SCC treatment in select patients, for reirradiation following SCC recurrence, or after spinal surgery (Schiff et al., 2014). Early studies have shown that a single fraction of SBRT (median dose 16 Gy) can be safe and effective in relieving mild SCC and controlling tumor growth (Ryu et al., 2010). However, the high doses used in spinal SBRT have the potential to produce severe toxicities in surrounding tissues and structures, and randomized controlled trials are needed (Chow et al., 2011). Delayed side effects following conventional radiation therapy include transient demyelination of spinal posterior columns and white matter necrosis that can develop 12–20 weeks after therapy, causing paresthesias or Lhermitte sign, a sudden, mild, electric shock–like sensation triggered by neck flexion that radiates down the spine into the extremities. Symptoms typically resolve within one year (Giglio & Gilbert, 2010).

Indications for surgical intervention as first-line therapy include rapidly progressing paraplegia, progression of neurologic dysfunction while receiving radiation, spinal instability, pathologic fracture with dislocation of bone fragments, biopsy for unknown tumor type, radioresistant tumors, recurrence after previous radiation therapy, and life expectancy of at least three months (Georgy, 2008). A pivotal randomized controlled trial indicated an advantage for surgical intervention followed by radiation therapy over radiation alone for increasing the chances of regaining and maintaining ambulation (Patchell et al., 2005). The surgical approach depends on the tumor location and extent, type of spinal reconstruction or stabilization planned, and the general condition of the patient. Anterior decompression with mechanical stabilization is the most common surgical approach because 85% of SCC cases are due to epidural metastases located anterior to the spinal cord (Schiff et al., 2014). The anterior surgical approach allows for complete resection of the tumor, thereby relieving pressure on the spinal cord (Schiff et al., 2014; Witham, Khavkin, Gallia, Wolinsky, & Gokaslan, 2006). The resulting defect is filled with polymethyl methacrylate (PMMA, bone cement) that is used in conjunction with internal fixation devices to provide spinal stability for the rest of the patient's life (Witham et al., 2006). Surgery with the use of PMMA is followed by radiation therapy, with a delay of about one week. If a bone graft is used, then radiation must be delayed for six weeks to allow for fusion of the graft (Prasad & Schiff, 2005). Laminectomy has fallen out of favor, as it does not allow for complete tumor resection and increases spinal instability (Becker & Baehring, 2011b). Vertebroplasty and kyphoplasty are minimally invasive procedures that can be used in patients who are poor surgical candidates but have pain without neurologic manifestations related to their SCC (Sun & Nemecek, 2009; Witham et al., 2006). Both procedures involve the percutaneous injection of PMMA into a collapsed vertebral body. In kyphoplasty, a balloon is first inflated to restore vertebral height and reduce kyphosis and is then withdrawn. The cavity created by the balloon is then injected with PMMA for stability. With vertebroplasty, the vertebral body is not re-expanded; only PMMA is injected (Witham et al., 2006). Both procedures can be performed on an outpatient basis, have rare complications, and are highly effective in reducing pain (Witham et al., 2006).

Chemotherapy is a treatment option for SCC in chemosensitive tumors, such as breast cancer, NHL, myeloma, small cell carcinoma, or germ cell tumors. It also is useful in patients with recurrent tumors who have previously been irradiated and cannot tolerate further radiation or in nonsurgical candidates who have not responded to radiation therapy (Abrahm, Banffy, & Harris, 2008; Becker & Baehring, 2011b). Patients generally receive chemotherapy in combination with more rapidly effective interventions such as radiation or surgery (Becker & Baehring, 2011b).

Implications for Oncology Advanced Practice Nurses

Timely recognition of the early signs and symptoms of SCC is critical to preserving patients' quality of life and preventing loss of functional independence. New onset of back or neck pain in a patient with known cancer must be evaluated as potential cord compression. APNs must be aware of the potential for SCC in patients with solid tumors with a propensity to metastasize to bone (e.g., breast, lung, and prostate malignancies) and multiple myeloma (Kaplan, 2013). MRI performed with and without contrast enhancement has become the safest and most accurate method for diagnosing SCC.

Nursing care of patients with SCC is multifactorial. Issues APNs need to address include pain management, prevention of constipation, safety measures, patient and caregiver teaching, emotional support, and referrals to specialists. APNs should be aware that patients with SCC occurring at high levels in the spine (T6 or above) are at risk for autonomic dysreflexia that can be triggered by a distended bladder or bowel and need to be alert for the classic signs: elevated blood pressure, pounding headache, bradycardia, flushing, and profuse sweating above the level of the spinal block (Yadav et al., 2009). APNs have an important role coordinating care with the rehabilitation team and patients and caregivers to prepare patients for discharge to home or hospice. When rehabilitation is possible, goals should be individualized, clear, and attainable (Foulkes, 2010). General rehabilitation goals focus on regaining or retaining functional independence and include improving ambulation, achieving weight bearing and the ability to transfer, and regulating bladder and bowel elimination. Patients with SCC at the end of life require palliative care focusing on pain relief, comfort and safety measures, management of bladder and bowel elimination, and help with coping with the profound functional losses and impending end of life (Abrahm et al., 2008).

Increased Intracranial Pressure

Increased intracranial pressure (ICP) is an elevation in normal brain pressure that occurs as a result of an increase in the volume of the intracranial contents. The skull is a rigid, non-expandable structure, and the presence of edema, hemorrhage, tumor mass, or excess CSF takes up space and can lead to increased ICP (Hickey & Armstrong, 2009). Increased ICP is a life-threatening complication of malignant disease that will result in neurologic complications, brain stem herniation, and death if not treated urgently. A space-occupying lesion, usually a primary brain tumor or metastatic disease, is the most common cause of increased ICP (Shelton, Ferrigno, & Skinner, 2013). The expanding brain tumor and surrounding cerebral edema or blockage of CSF outflow lead to the signs and symptoms of elevated ICP (Armstrong, 2011). Early recognition and intervention are crucial to prevent long-term neurologic complications and death related to increased ICP (Hickey & Armstrong, 2009; Smith & Amin-Hanjani, 2013).

Incidence

According to the American Cancer Society, an estimated 22,850 new cases of primary malignant brain tumors will be diagnosed in 2015 (Siegel, Miller, & Jemal, 2015). However, the majority of intracranial malignancies are metastatic lesions. Brain metastases occur in 24%–45% of all patients with cancer annually and are responsible for 20% of cancer deaths (Tse, 2014). Lung cancer is associated with the greatest incidence of brain metastasis (20%), followed by renal cancer (10%), melanoma (7%), breast cancer (5%), and colorectal cancer (1%) (Lewis et al., 2011). Eighty percent of patients with lung cancer who survive more than two years can be expected to develop brain metastases (Tse, 2014). Primary brain tumors include malignant gliomas and nonmalignant meningiomas, pituitary adenomas, and acoustic neuromas (Huff, 2013). Other causes of increased ICP in patients with cancer are hemorrhage; ischemic stroke; abscesses from viral, bacterial, or fungal infection in immunocompromised patients; or an autoimmune inflammatory process (Becker & Baehring, 2011a; Shelton et al., 2013). Increased ICP is associated with a 20% mortality rate (Gupta & Nosko, 2013).

Signs and Symptoms

The signs and symptoms of increased ICP depend on the location of the lesion within the brain, the extent of pressure increase, and the rate of development of pressure (Armstrong, 2011) (see Figure 16-8). The faster the pathologic processes evolve, the more quickly symptoms appear (Becker & Baehring, 2011a). The constellation of clinical manifestations seen in patients with increased ICP can include headaches, alterations in level of consciousness and cognition, seizures, motor and sensory changes, vomiting, pupillary changes and papilledema, and vital sign alterations (Armstrong, 2011; Gupta & Nosko, 2013).

Headache may be an early symptom of increased ICP (Hickey & Olson, 2009) but also may occur late in the process (Huff, 2013). It typically is a nonspecific tension-type headache and may be accompanied by nausea and vomiting. Patients often describe it as an early-morning headache that improves during the day. Bending over, coughing, or performing the Valsalva maneuver may cause or worsen the headache (Huff, 2013; Lewis et al., 2011). It often is bilateral, located in the frontal or occipital regions, and increases in severity, frequency, and duration with increasing ICP (Hickey & Armstrong, 2009). Patients also may fall readily, particularly backward (Becker & Baehring, 2011a).

Seizures can be the earliest indication of a brain tumor, especially if it is the first occurrence in an adult (Huff, 2013; Tse, 2014). The incidence of seizures in patients with metastatic brain tumors is 30%–40% (Tse, 2014). Hemorrhagic strokes can occur if the tumor bleeds or compresses an artery or if tumor cells obstruct cranial blood flow (Lewis et al., 2011).

Patients' neurologic status is reflected by their level of consciousness. Initially, changes may be so subtle that only family members are aware of the difference (Armstrong, 2011). Other early symptoms include confusion (manifested by progressive disorientation to time, place, and person), restlessness, and lethargy. As ICP rises, lethargy progresses to stupor and coma. Changes in mental status relate to the involved area of the brain and can assist APNs in localizing the affected area. Involvement of the frontal lobe will affect higher-level function, man-

---

Early Signs
- Diplopia
- Blurred vision
- Extremity drifts
- Decreased visual fields
- Decreased visual acuity
- Change in level of consciousness (LOC)
- Headache (most severe in early morning)
- Lethargy, apathy, confusion, restlessness
- Gastrointestinal: Loss of appetite, nausea, occasional/unusual vomiting

Late Signs
- Abnormal posturing
- Temperature elevations
- Cardiovascular: Bradycardia, hypotension, widening pulse pressure
- Respiratory: Slow, shallow respirations, tachypnea, Cheyne-Stokes respirations
- Neurologic: Decreased ability to concentrate, decreased LOC, personality changes, hemiplegia, hemiparesis, seizures, pupil changes, papilledema (cardinal sign)
- Cushing triad (hypertension with a widening pulse pressure, bradycardia, and abnormal respirations)

Figure 16-8. Signs and Symptoms of Increased Intracranial Pressure

Note. Based on information from Armstrong, 2011; Hickey & Olson, 2009; Huff, 2013; Lewis et al., 2011; Shelton, 2013.

ifested as personality changes with emotional lability or flat affect and difficulty in concentration, problem solving, and vigilance. Speech deficits, such as word retrieval, and motor weakness with focal seizure activity can occur with involvement of the posterior frontal lobe. Parietal lobe tumors cause deficits in sensation, inability to recognize common objects, and neglect syndrome (a lack of awareness of the opposite side of the body), as well as seizure activity. Temporal lobe involvement results in short-term memory loss, weakness, and visual field deficits. Cerebellar signs are ataxia, incoordination, nystagmus, vertigo, and nausea (Hickey & Olson, 2009). Visual disturbances associated with increased ICP include diplopia, blurred vision, decreased visual fields, decreased visual acuity, and changes in pupil size and reaction to light. Papilledema (edema and swelling of the optic disk) is a late sign of increased ICP and occurs in approximately 70% of patients with brain tumors (Hickey & Armstrong, 2009). An increase in CSF pressure around the optic nerve that impairs the outflow of venous blood causes papilledema (Armstrong, 2011). Papilledema usually occurs bilaterally and develops within one to five days of ICP increase. If subarachnoid hemorrhage is the cause of increased ICP, then papilledema develops much more rapidly, within two to eight hours (Gupta & Nosko, 2013). Vomiting unrelated to food intake that is sudden and projectile can occur with increased ICP.

Altered vital signs typically are a late finding of increased ICP and indicate brain stem involvement. To compensate for increasing ICP, the blood pressure becomes elevated, leading to increased cardiac output and a stronger heartbeat that causes a widened pulse pressure (Shelton et al., 2013). As the ICP continues to increase, decompensation occurs and the blood pressure falls. The pulse becomes irregular and thready, and profound bradycardia and altered respiratory patterns develop, changing from Cheyne-Stokes respirations to ataxic or agonal breathing (Shelton et al., 2013). Cushing triad, a combination of hypertension with a widening pulse pressure (rising systolic, declining diastolic), bradycardia, and abnormal respirations, is a very late sign of brain stem dysfunction, and patients usually are comatose (Gupta & Nosko, 2013; Hickey & Olson, 2009). These signs appear only when the medulla has been compressed (Gupta & Nosko, 2013), indicating that cerebral herniation may have already occurred (Shelton et al., 2013). With advancing brain stem herniation, patients lose papillary, corneal, and gag reflexes, and motor dysfunction progresses to hemiplegia, decortications, and decerebration (Armstrong, 2011).

Risk Factors and Etiology

Increased ICP is the result of volume changes within the brain tissue, which are caused by increasing edema, hemorrhage, abscess formation, ischemia, excess CSF, or tumor mass. Expanding primary or metastatic brain lesions take up space and often are associated with cerebral edema, intratumoral hemorrhage, and displacement of brain structures that obstruct CSF and venous outflow from the brain (Armstrong, 2011; Becker & Baehring, 2011a). Patients with primary tumors that metastasize to the brain are at greatest risk for increased ICP, especially those with lung cancer and melanoma (Becker & Baehring, 2011a). Metastatic disease spreads to the brain via the bloodstream and generally is distributed within the brain according to blood flow patterns. The cerebrum is the most common site of metastasis in the brain, followed by the cerebellum, and lastly, the brain stem (Lewis et al., 2011). Primary tumors of the brain or spinal cord also can cause increased ICP. Patients with leukemia with high blast counts are at risk for increased ICP because of leukostasis, which can cause diffuse cerebral edema. Hemorrhage resulting from coagulopathy or thrombocytopenia in patients with leukemia may cause increased ICP (Becker & Baehring, 2011a). Tumors compressing the cerebral ventricles can block the flow of CSF, leading to obstructive hydrocephalus and increased ICP

(Huff, 2013). Obstruction to the outflow of CSF also can be caused by the presence of lepto-meningeal metastasis or an occluded Ommaya reservoir (Armstrong, 2011). Tumors can create new blood vessels through angiogenesis, causing disruption of the normal blood-brain barrier and leading to edema (Huff, 2013). Edema following brain irradiation can increase ICP (Shelton et al., 2013). Disseminated intravascular coagulation can lead to increased ICP due to diffuse cerebral hemorrhages (Becker & Baehring, 2011a). The syndrome of inappropriate antidiuretic hormone secretion (SIADH) can cause increased ICP, as dilutional hyponatremia develops with SIADH and causes free water to enter the brain cells leading to cerebral edema (Cope, 2013).

Nonmalignant causes of increased ICP include intracranial hemorrhage that can occur with traumatic brain injury, ruptured aneurysm, arteriovenous malformation, or other vascular anomalies (Smith & Amin-Hanjani, 2013). CNS infections, such as viral encephalitis, toxo-plasmosis, aspergillosis, or candidiasis, or infections from an Ommaya reservoir may cause edema that can result in elevated ICP (Becker & Baehring, 2011a; Hickey & Olson, 2009). Other nonmalignant causes of increased ICP are vasculitis, ischemic infarcts, hydrocephalus, and pseudotumor cerebri (Smith & Amin-Hanjani, 2013).

Pathophysiology

The intracranial cavity is a nonexpandable, closed compartment with a fixed internal volume that contains three components: the brain parenchyma (80%), CSF (10%), and blood (10%) (Smith & Amin-Hanjani, 2013). ICP is the pressure normally exerted by the CSF as it circulates around the brain and spinal cord and within the ventricles. ICP is normally 0–15 mm Hg; pathologic intracranial hypertension (commonly called increased ICP) is present when pressures reach 20 mm Hg or greater (Shelton et al., 2013; Smith & Amin-Hanjani, 2013). Normal ICP briefly rises with coughing or Valsalva maneuvers but is stabilized by homeo-static mechanisms (Becker & Baehring, 2011a). The brain requires about 20% of the cardiac output to meet its metabolic needs for oxygen and glucose. Blood volume within the brain is maintained through autoregulatory mechanisms that control cerebral blood flow (Armstrong, 2011). Autoregulation is achieved through adjustments in the volume of blood within brain arterioles: they can compensate for pressure changes by dilating or constricting to maintain constant cerebral blood volume. Uncontrolled increased ICP compromises cerebral perfusion, leading to ischemia (Gupta & Nosko, 2013).

ICP is directly related to the volume of tissue contained within the skull. The total volume is fixed, and brain tissue, CSF, and blood exist in a state of dynamic equilibrium. An increase in the volume of one compartment must be compensated by a reduction in the volume of another compartment to maintain normal ICP. The brain has a limited capacity to compensate for brief increases in ICP. The first compensatory mechanism related to increased ICP is displacement of CSF out of the cranial vault. If ICP remains high, then cerebral blood volume is reduced through vasoconstriction and compression of intracranial veins (Armstrong, 2011; Boss & Huether, 2013). As compensatory mechanisms are exhausted, autoregulation (the ability of the brain to maintain a constant rate of cerebral blood flow regardless of variations in systemic arterial pressure and venous drainage) fails, and ICP increases. Carbon dioxide accumulates, causing vasodilation and edema and leading to increased blood volume. ICP approaches systemic blood pressure at this stage, thus resulting in a decrease of cerebral pressure and perfusion, causing the brain tissue to experience severe hypoxia and acidosis (Boss & Huether, 2013). If increased ICP is not reversed at this point, the brain tissue shifts or herniates to an area with lower ICP (Huff, 2013). The blood flow in both the herniating tissue and the newly involved area is impaired, causing further ischemia and hypoxia. Herniation leads to a large and rapid increase in ICP. When ICP equals mean systolic arterial pressure, cerebral blood flow ceases, and the damage is irreversible (Becker & Baehring, 2011a; Boss & Huether, 2013).

Diagnosis and Assessment

The clinical manifestations of increased ICP depend on the location of the abnormality and the degree of increased ICP. MRI with gadolinium contrast is the preferred method of neuroimaging (Becker & Baehring, 2011a; Huff, 2013). MRI provides more detail than CT and is more sensitive in differentiating between pathologies that can cause increased ICP—malignancy, infection, inflammation, or ischemia (Armstrong, 2011; Becker & Baehring, 2011a). The blood-brain barrier is frequently disrupted by conditions that cause increased ICP in patients with cancer, and the use of IV gadolinium contrast dye with MRI provides better definition of lesions and edema (Becker & Baehring, 2011a). However, noncontrast head CT is the preferred technique to evaluate for suspected hemorrhage or hydrocephalus because it can quickly image acute changes (Lewis et al., 2011; Shelton et al., 2013). Magnetic resonance angiography is a useful modality to assess vascular abnormalities and has replaced invasive intra-arterial angiography as an imaging tool for increased ICP. PET and specialized MRI techniques, such as proton MRI spectroscopy and functional MRI, may be used to distinguish between tumor and radiation necrosis (Tse, 2014). The fusion of PET and CT scans distinguishes between active disease and scar tissue. Single-photon emission CT can differentiate between infiltrating tumor and solid tumor and between malignant and nonmalignant lesions, such as infection (Armstrong, 2011). A CT-guided stereotactic biopsy may be performed for tissue diagnosis (Tse, 2014). A lumbar puncture can be useful to determine a causative infectious agent or to assess for leptomeningeal metastasis but must be done with caution and after definitive imaging because of the chance of brain herniation with pressure changes (Hickey & Olson, 2009).

Patient History

History taking is important and should include patients' cancer history to assess the potential for metastatic disease or for cerebral edema following prior cranial radiation therapy. Risk factors for unsuspected primaries should be assessed, such as lung cancer, which has a high incidence of brain metastasis. The history of thrombocytopenia, coagulopathies, or traumatic brain injuries that can cause intracranial hemorrhage should be explored (Shelton, 2013). Patients should be questioned regarding changes in mental status and the presence and quality of headaches. Headache is not as common an early complaint in patients with increased ICP as once believed (Hickey & Olson, 2009; Huff, 2013). New-onset headaches or seizures in adults of middle age or older are worrisome and need further evaluation to rule out brain cancer (Huff, 2013).

Physical Examination

Baseline and serial neurologic examinations should be performed to identify changes in patients' neurologic status that indicate rising ICP. The neurologic examination includes assessment of patients' level of consciousness, pupillary size and reaction to light, motor function, and respiratory pattern (Hickey & Armstrong, 2009). Headache, nausea, and vomiting are also evaluated (Gupta & Nosko, 2013).

Assessment of level of consciousness and degree of alertness includes evaluation of patients' cognitive and mental status by asking questions regarding orientation to time and place, short-term memory, and thought processes and observing the patient for language comprehension, flow of speech and articulation, and attention span, as indicated by restlessness, confusion, irritability, or lethargy (Gupta & Nosko, 2013). The Glasgow coma scale (see Table 16-3) can be used to assess neurologic status by evaluating and assigning a score to eye opening response, motor response, and verbal response. A total score of 15 is best and indicates a fully alert person; a score of 3 is the worst and indicates deep coma. Patients with a score lower than 8 are considered to be unconscious (Hickey, 2009).

Assessment of visual acuity and extraocular movements will determine cranial nerve impairment and brain stem functioning (Shelton, 2013). Cranial nerve II (the optic nerve) is evaluated by assessing visual acuity and fields. Pupillary changes often herald increasing ICP and indicate dysfunction of cranial nerve III (the oculomotor nerve). The pupils are assessed for size, shape, and symmetry, and the findings in one pupil are compared with the other (Shelton, 2013). Evaluating extraocular movements assesses cranial nerves IV (trochlear nerve) and VI (abducens nerve), as well as cranial nerve III. Testing extraocular movement involves having the patient follow the clinician's finger

Table 16-3. Glasgow Coma Scale

Response	Score
Eye opening response	
• Spontaneous	4
• To sound	3
• To pain	2
• Never	1
Motor response	
• Obeys commands	6
• Localized pain	5
• Normal flexion (withdrawal)	4
• Abnormal flexion	3
• Extension	2
• None	1
Verbal response	
• Oriented	5
• Confused conversation	4
• Inappropriate words	3
• Incomprehensible sounds	2
• None	1

Note. Based on information from Teasdale & Jennett, 1974.

through the six cardinal gazes as the clinician draws an "H" shape and evaluates for nystagmus in the upward and lateral gazes. Funduscopic examination is the criterion standard in the evaluation of increased ICP (Gupta & Nosko, 2013). Funduscopic examination assesses for papilledema, which is edema and swelling of the optic disk caused by increased pressure on the optic nerve. Papilledema usually is seen bilaterally (Becker & Baehring, 2011a; Gupta & Nosko, 2013).

Assessment of motor defects is necessary, including coordination and balance problems as well as weakness with heel-to-toe walking, Romberg test, finger to nose, and gait (Armstrong, 2011). Motor changes can range from slight weakness to hemiplegia, depending on the location of the lesion and extent of increased ICP. Changes in vital signs occur as increased ICP continues; thus, vital signs should be assessed regularly when ICP is suspected. Cushing triad is a late and ominous finding that indicates brain stem dysfunction and consists of hypertension with a widening pulse pressure, bradycardia, and abnormal respirations (Hickey & Olson, 2009).

Differential Diagnosis

The differential diagnosis for increased ICP includes ruptured aneurysm, arteriovenous malformation, ischemic and hemorrhagic strokes, cerebral abscess, meningitis, trauma, hydrocephalus, encephalitis, epidural and subdural hematomas, pseudotumor cerebri, and vasculitis (Huff, 2013; Smith & Amin-Hanjani, 2013). Any middle-aged or older adult patient presenting with a first seizure should have CNS tumor high on the list of differential diagnoses (Huff, 2013). A thorough history is helpful to begin to distinguish among these entities. Patients with meningitis or abscess are likely to have a fever. Patients with vasculitis usually have an elevated sedimentation rate. Imaging studies are needed to distinguish between the other diagnoses.

Evidence-Based Treatment Strategies

Early recognition and prompt intervention are needed to decrease adverse outcomes related to increased ICP. Reducing cerebral edema and controlling symptoms while determining and treating the cause of increased ICP is the goal of intervention. Initial intervention includes managing factors that can further increase ICP. These factors include hypercapnia, hypoxemia, respiratory procedures (e.g., suctioning and intubation, positive end-expiratory pressure, and Ambu bag not coordinated with respiratory rate), vasodilating drugs, body positioning, Valsalva maneuver, coughing, emotional upset, noxious stimuli (such as invasive procedures), and clustering of nursing activities (Hickey & Olson, 2009).

Corticosteroids are the initial treatment of choice for relieving the acute symptoms of tumor-associated cerebral edema. Corticosteroids rapidly reduce vasogenic edema caused by tumors by decreasing capillary permeability and promoting extracellular fluid resorption (Huff, 2013; Lewis et al., 2011). Although the exact mechanism of action is not clear, corticosteroids have been shown to downregulate VEGF (associated with edema formation) and promote the removal of fluid from edematous tissue surrounding tumors (Lewis et al., 2011). Steroids are initiated prior to radiation therapy or other definitive therapy and tapered to the lowest dose needed to control neurologic symptoms once definitive therapy becomes effective (Shelton et al., 2013). Dexamethasone is the recommended steroid for treating ICP. Dosing is variable but generally is an IV bolus of 10–24 mg of dexamethasone followed by 4 mg every six hours (Huff, 2013; Tse, 2014).

Mannitol and hyperventilation may be used as an alternative or addition to corticosteroids to rapidly reduce cerebral edema in patients with very high ICP (Becker & Baehring, 2011a; Lewis et al., 2011). Mannitol is a hyperosmolar osmotic diuretic that draws free water out of the extracellular space in the edematous brain tissues and into the circulation, where it is excreted by the kidney. Brain volume is reduced because of dehydration of the brain parenchyma (Smith & Amin-Hanjani, 2013). Mannitol is commonly infused as a 20%–25% solution given as an initial IV bolus of 0.75–1 g/kg body weight, followed by 0.25–0.5 g/kg body weight every three to six hours (Becker & Baehring, 2011a). Mannitol therapy is directed at keeping the serum osmolality at 310–315 mOsm; the maximal effect should occur within 15–30 minutes and can last for one to three hours (Hickey & Olson, 2009). Monitoring of serum osmolality is required, and treatment should be stopped if the target serum osmolality is exceeded (Becker & Baehring, 2011a). Mannitol can induce a rebound effect, indicated by elevated ICP, and furosemide, a loop diuretic, may be used to reduce the ICP (Hickey & Olson, 2009). Mechanical hyperventilation is a rapid method to decrease ICP in conjunction with osmotic therapy (Becker & Baehring, 2011a). Mechanical hyperventilation lowers the partial pressure of arterial carbon dioxide ($PaCO_2$) to 25–30 mm Hg, resulting in vasoconstriction and decreased cerebral blood volume. The effect of hyperventilation is transient, lasting 1–24 hours (Smith & Amin-Hanjani, 2013). Elevation of the head of the bed to 30° facilitates jugular venous drainage, thus lowering ICP (Becker & Baehring, 2011a; Hickey & Olson, 2009). The effects of both mannitol and hyperventilation are temporary, and more definitive therapies, such as radiation therapy or surgery, are needed to control the malignancy precipitating the increased ICP (Huff, 2013; Lewis et al., 2011).

Radiation therapy is the standard treatment for brain metastases (Armstrong, 2011; Tse, 2014). Radiation techniques include whole brain radiation therapy (WBRT) and SRS. The technique selected depends on the tumor histology and the size of the lesions (Giglio & Gilbert, 2010). WBRT is used for patients with radiosensitive tumors, such as SCLC and germ cell tumors, and those with multiple brain metastases or tumors that are too large to be treated with surgery or SRS. The recommended radiation dose is 30 Gy delivered in 10 fractions over two weeks (Tse, 2014). WBRT is associated with early cognitive decline, radiation necrosis, and leukoencephalopathy (Giglio & Gilbert, 2010; Tse, 2014) and has been replaced by partial brain irradiation or local-field radiation, such as SRS (Armstrong, 2011). SRS is preferred over WBRT for treating small lesions, especially if they arise from radioresistant tumors, such as NSCLC, renal cell carcinoma, and melanoma (Tse, 2014). Computerized treatment planning and multiple angles are used in SRS to deliver high doses of radiation targeted to the lesion while sparing normal surrounding brain tissue (Huff, 2013). Reactions occur in a small percentage of patients, depending on the volume of normal brain tissue exposed to radiation, and may be acute or delayed. Edema may develop acutely within two weeks of SRS and cause headache and worsen neurologic deficits. Radiation necrosis may develop six months after treatment and be associated with edema and mass effect that may be indistinguishable from tumor. SRS is increasingly being used as an adjunct therapy following surgical resection of brain metastases (Tse, 2014).

Surgical resection or debulking of tumor or hematoma is the most rapid way to alleviate life-threatening increased ICP (Lewis et al., 2011). Ventriculoperitoneal shunt placement also can be performed to provide a pathway for CSF drainage in select patients, such as those with gait apraxia, precipitate micturition, and cognitive decline, who are most likely to respond. Shunting should be avoided in patients with leptomeningeal tumor to prevent seeding of the peritoneum (Becker & Baehring, 2011a).

Chemotherapy can be used when brain metastases arise from highly chemosensitive tumors, such as germ cell tumors, lymphoma, or small cell carcinomas, or in cases in which radiation therapy cannot be used (Lewis et al., 2011). Chemotherapy is an important adjunct in the treatment of primary brain malignancies, the most common of which is malignant glioma (Armstrong, 2011). Alkylating agents, such as temozolomide, and nitrosoureas, including carmustine and lomustine, are used as single agents or in combination regimens because they are able to cross the blood-brain barrier and enter the brain tissue (Armstrong, 2011). Leptomeningeal carcinomatosis is treated with radiation and intrathecal chemotherapy (Becker & Baehring, 2011a). Intrathecal agents are delivered through a lumbar puncture or an Ommaya reservoir, which provides direct access to the CSF through the fourth cerebral ventricle. Agents used for intrathecal treatment include methotrexate and cytarabine (Shelton et al., 2013). Obstruction of CSF outflow precludes use of the intraventricular route for delivery of cytotoxic agents, as it can lead to a severe, irreversible toxic encephalopathy (Becker & Baehring, 2011a). Patients whose neurologic status is depressed because of elevated ICP require monitoring in an intensive care setting (Becker & Baehring, 2011a). Blood pressure fluctuations are avoided, and mean arterial blood pressure should always be above 90 mm Hg. Hypotension leads to reduced cerebral perfusion and oxygenation, ischemia, and secondary brain injury and is managed with immediate fluid bolus. Hypertension does not result in increased cerebral blood flow (Hickey & Olson, 2009). Careful fluid and electrolyte management is important to avoid hypotension and dehydration. Isotonic saline is used for fluid replacement to prevent hyponatremia, which causes cerebral edema and exacerbates increased ICP (Shelton et al., 2013). Hypertonic saline (HTS) may be administered to patients with very high ICP. A preliminary study of 23.4% HTS administered as a rapid IV infusion demonstrated that it was safe and effective in reducing increased ICP secondary to traumatic brain injury in patients who were refractory to mannitol (Ware et al., 2005). A meta-analysis of randomized controlled trials comparing mannitol and HTS in the treatment of elevated ICP concluded that HTS is superior to mannitol for this purpose (Kamel, Navi, Nakagawa, Hemphill, & Ko, 2011). After examining the evidence supporting the use of HTS or mannitol, Marko (2012) concluded that HTS has surpassed mannitol as the gold standard for the medical management of intracranial hypertension. Fever increases cerebral blood flow and brain metabolism and leads to increased ICP and is treated aggressively with antipyretics or cooling devices (Shelton et al., 2013). Analgesics are used to treat pain, and sedation may be necessary to decrease restlessness and anxiety, as all can increase ICP (Shelton et al., 2013). Morphine sulfate and fentanyl are the preferred analgesics for patients who are critically ill. Fentanyl has the benefit of being shorter-acting and allows patients to be quickly wakened for periodic neurologic checks. Lorazepam is the preferred drug for prolonged treatment of anxiety or seizures, and haloperidol is the preferred drug for delirium. Patients receiving these drugs require close monitoring for neurologic changes and sedation side effects (Hickey & Olson, 2009).

Seizures can increase the cerebral metabolic rate and contribute to increased ICP (Hickey & Olson, 2009; Shelton et al., 2013). Patients with status epilepticus receive aggressive anticonvulsant therapy (Tse, 2014). However, prophylactic administration of anticonvulsants to patients with brain metastases and no history of seizures is not supported by data from clinical trials evaluating the effects of phenobarbital, phenytoin, or valproic acid (Sirven, Wingerchuk, Drazkowski, Lyons, & Zimmerman, 2004; Tremont-Lukats, Ratilal, Armstrong, & Gilbert, 2008). In addition, these drugs have significant adverse effects and may interfere with the actions of chemotherapy drugs and targeted agents that are metabolized through the same cytochrome P450 system (Lewis et al., 2011). Prophylaxis is instituted for patients with a known history of seizures. Phenytoin (100 mg three to four times per day) is the most common agent used with increased ICP, although levetiracetam, a newer anticonvulsant agent, also is used (Armstrong, 2011; Olson & Hickey, 2009; Shelton et al., 2013).

ICP can be monitored continuously in the neurologic intensive care unit. The goal of ICP monitoring is to provide data about cerebral perfusion and to initiate therapeutic measures and assess their efficacy (Gupta & Nosko, 2013). Invasive ICP monitoring also allows for therapeutic CSF drainage to improve cerebral perfusion. A variety of ICP monitoring devices are available and are surgically placed into either the brain parenchyma, brain ventricles, or subarachnoid, subdural, and epidural spaces, depending on the device selected (Becker & Baehring, 2011a; Gupta & Nosko, 2013). Infection is the primary complication associated with ICP monitoring and occurs more often in patients with intraventricular catheters. Prophylactic antibiotic use for ventricular catheter placement and routine change of ventricular catheters are not recommended to reduce infection. Randomized trials to provide guidance are lacking. Ventriculostomy catheters are removed promptly when infection occurs. In the event of a new onset of fever in a patient with an intracranial device, a sample of CSF is obtained for a gram stain and culture (Gupta & Nosko, 2013).

Implications for Oncology Advanced Practice Nurses

Increased ICP is an oncologic emergency that can lead to death without prompt intervention. Assessment, recognition, and treatment of early signs and symptoms are critical. Management of increased ICP requires a combined effort with oncology, neurosurgery, and radiation therapy. APNs play an important role in the recognition of early signs and symptoms and coordination of care for patients with increased ICP.

Nursing management of patients with increased ICP is complex. Factors known to increase ICP include many nursing activities. Clustering of nursing activities, such as assessment, turning, bathing, or suctioning, needs to be planned. Safe positioning is important, with the head of the bed elevated to 30° to promote cerebral venous drainage in patients who are not hypovolemic (Becker & Baehring, 2011a; Shelton et al., 2013). Proper alignment is used when turning and positioning patients to avoid precipitating the Valsalva maneuver and to maintain the neck in neutral position at all times. Bowel management is necessary to prevent constipation, which can lead to straining and increased ICP. A quiet room with low lighting is important, along with avoidance of sudden jarring of the bed or other painful stimuli to avoid increases in ICP. Pain, restlessness, and agitation can exacerbate ICP elevation and should be managed with analgesics and/or sedation as appropriate. For the same reason, caregivers should be counseled to avoid stimulating conversations with patients or provoking emotional upset (Hickey & Olson, 2009).

It is important that patients avoid hypotension and dehydration because they can lead to cerebral ischemia, which further increases ICP. Blood pressure must be maintained above 90 mm Hg at all times (Shelton, 2013). Adequate fluid volume is maintained with isotonic saline infusion. Hypotonic solutions are avoided because they can cause fluid to shift into the cells and exacerbate increased ICP (Becker & Baehring, 2011a). Normothermia is important to maintain to avoid increasing the cerebral metabolism. Elevated patient temperatures are treated with antipyretics and cooling devices, and shivering is controlled. Serum levels of anticonvulsant drugs are monitored to ensure therapeutic levels are maintained. Patient and caregiver education and support is an essential need in this setting.

Conclusion

APNs need to have a heightened awareness of who is at risk for developing a structural oncologic emergency. These emergencies can have a devastating impact on patients' functional independence, quality of life, and survival. Early recognition, assessment, and intervention are critical to allow patients to maintain independence. An understanding of the presentation, etiology, pathophysiology, differential diagnosis, and treatment allows APNs to anticipate and intervene early.

Case Study

S.K. is a 23-year-old woman who presents with complaints of shortness of breath and facial swelling, particularly in the morning. She has no past medical or surgical history and works out regularly at the gym. S.K. reports that for the past several weeks she has been fatigued and has not been to the gym. Despite not working out for several weeks, she has lost 10 pounds. She has noticed feeling warm/feverish in the evenings but has not taken her temperature. Upon questioning, she admits that she has had a dry nonproductive cough for the past few days. Initially, the shortness of breath occurred only with exertion, but now at times she is winded even at rest. She has begun to use several pillows at night in order to sleep. She also has noted swelling of her right breast.

The APN examines S.K. and notes that she has a prominent venous pattern on her chest and her right breast is larger than the left breast. Her heart rate is tachycardic. She is unable to lie flat on the examination table without becoming significantly short of breath and developing flushing. S.K. has palpable lymphadenopathy in the supraclavicular areas, more so on the right side than the left, with the largest node measuring 2 cm. She also has bilateral axillary lymphadenopathy.

The APN obtains an immediate chest x-ray, which shows a large anterior mediastinal mass. S.K.'s signs and symptoms most likely indicate lymphoma, either Hodgkin or non-Hodgkin. The APN knows that a tissue sample is necessary to make a definitive diagnosis and to design an appropriate treatment plan and contacts a surgeon to arrange a biopsy. A CT of the chest, abdomen, and pelvis are obtained, as well as an echocardiogram and bone marrow biopsy.

The echocardiogram showed an ejection fraction of greater than 55% and normal wall motion. CT scan revealed edema in the right neck area; enlarged lymph nodes in both neck areas, right greater than left; bilateral axillary lymph nodes; a large mediastinal mass obstructing the SVC; and no obvious abdominal disease. S.K.'s lactate dehydrogenase (LDH) was elevated at 1,235 U/L (normal is less than 600 U/L). The bone marrow biopsy showed no evidence of disease. A right supraclavicular node biopsy showed an anaplastic large cell lymphoma.

S.K. begins a chemotherapy regimen with rituximab, cyclophosphamide, doxorubicin, vincristine, and prednisone (R-CHOP) given intravenously via the left arm. Allopurinol is initiated to prevent tumor lysis. Within a few days S.K. notes a decrease in the size of her right breast, less shortness of breath, and a decrease in the size of the lymph nodes. At the time of her second cycle of chemotherapy, she had clear improvement, and her LDH had returned to normal. She completed six cycles of R-CHOP chemotherapy. Six weeks after treatment completion, a PET-CT scan was negative for disease. Low-dose involved-field radiation was then initiated for consolidation.

At routine follow-up three months after completing therapy, S.K. is doing well. Her chest x-ray is negative and LDH normal. She is scheduled to return in three months to see the APN.

S.K. calls the office three weeks after her visit, stating she is worried that her disease has returned. She is again experiencing shortness of breath and cough. She feels very anxious and is having chest pain when she lies down. The APN is concerned and tells her to come in immediately for evaluation.

On examination, S.K. is tachycardic, hypotensive, and has jugular venous distension. A pulsus paradoxus of 22 mm Hg is noted. An ECG shows low voltage with T-wave inversions. A CT scan shows a moderate to large pericardial effusion and recurrent mediastinal mass with LDH elevated at 960 U/L. An echocardiogram reveals a large pericardial effusion with respiratory flow variation and right atrial and ventricle diastolic collapse.

S.K. is taken emergently to the operating room for a subxiphoid pericardial window, where 700 ml of fluid is removed and sent for cytology. Cytopathology reveals that the fluid is an exudate with elevated protein level and LDH and the presence of recurrent lymphoma.

S.K. begins salvage chemotherapy for recurrence of her disease with etoposide, methylprednisolone, cisplatin, and cytarabine (ESHAP). Her LDH improves after one cycle, and evaluation for autologous stem cell transplantation is initiated. After completion of her second cycle, while her blood counts were still recovering, S.K. notes an enlarged lymph node in the left neck. Her LDH level measures 1,054 U/L. S.K. also complains of pain in her midback. She tells the APN that the pain started 7–10 days earlier while she was in the hospital for the chemotherapy, and she thought it was caused by the hospital bed. The pain has not improved and wraps around to her chest. She describes it as a burning discomfort that is worse with coughing or laughing. She also notes that it is worse if she lies down, so she has been sleeping in a recliner for the past few days.

On examination, S.K. points to the area of T10 and has pain with gentle palpation. The APN arranges for an MRI of S.K.'s entire spine. The APN elects to image the entire spine with an MRI because it is the gold standard and can detect paraspinal masses and multiple involved areas of the spine. The MRI shows a paraspinal mass at T10. The APN starts S.K. on corticosteroids to decrease the edema. Radiation oncology is consulted, as lymphoma is a radiosensitive tumor. S.K. clearly is in a difficult situation because her disease has progressed on therapy. She needs to show a response to some type of therapy (further salvage therapy or experimental therapy) so that she can proceed to stem cell transplantation.

1. What signs and symptoms does S.K. exhibit that may indicate the presence of SVCS?
    *   The signs and symptoms noted include facial swelling in the morning, shortness of breath, prominent venous pattern on her chest, swollen right breast, tachycardia, inability to lie flat on the examination table, and flushing.
    *   All of these manifestations are seen in SVCS, which should make it the top diagnosis the APN needs to evaluate further. The finding of lymphadenopathy adds to the concern because it may indicate lymphoma, which would be a cause of SVCS in a young woman.
2. Why is the APN concerned when S.K. calls complaining of shortness of breath and cough shortly after an office visit?
    *   The APN knows that oncologic emergencies can occur at any time, and the onset of shortness of breath and cough could indicate cardiac tamponade because dyspnea is the most common symptom. S.K. also had reported that she had chest pain when lying down and felt anxious, which increased the APN's concern.
3. Which of the following test results should the APN review to confirm that S.K. has cardiac tamponade?
    D. ECG
    E. MRI
    F. CT scan
    G. Echocardiogram
    *   The answer is D. Echocardiogram is the diagnostic test of choice in cardiac tamponade. The classic finding on echocardiogram that is suggestive of cardiac tamponade is diastolic collapse of the right atrium and right ventricle because of the pressure of the increased pericardial fluid. Other findings on echocardiogram include swinging heart, left atrial and ventricular collapse, inspiratory changes in ventricle size, and inferior vena cava plethora (an excess buildup of fluid in the vena cava). A routine chest x-ray is not diagnostic for cardiac tamponade but may demonstrate an enlarged cardiac silhouette as a result of increased fluid in the pericardial sac and raise suspicion leading to further testing. ECG changes are nonspecific and include low-voltage QRS complex, tachycardia, nonspecific ST-T changes, and premature atrial or ventricular contractions.
4. Why does the APN order an MRI of S.K.'s entire spine when she complains of back pain?
    *   By taking a detailed history, the APN determined that S.K.'s pain is radicular (wrapping around the chest) and worsens with coughing and laughing. It also is worse with lying down, making it more likely to be caused by malignancy. The APN orders a total spine MRI because MRI allows visualization of the extent of the lesion and anatomy, detects paraspinal masses, and can image multiple levels to assess for areas of cord involvement that are not clinically apparent.
5. How does a paraspinal mass cause cord compression?
    *   With lymphoma, lymph nodes in the paraspinal region can grow through the vertebral neural foramen into the epidural space and compress the spinal cord.

Key Points

Superior Vena Cava Syndrome

*   The most common signs and symptoms of SVCS are cough, dyspnea, face or neck swelling, upper extremity swelling, and dilated chest veins.
*   The diagnostic evaluation for SVCS has two components: imaging (chest x-ray initially) and tissue diagnosis to determine the precipitating cause.
*   Treatment of SVCS is based on the etiology, the severity of symptoms, the underlying malignancy, the presence of thrombosis, and the patient's prognosis.

Cardiac Tamponade

- The clinical manifestations of cardiac tamponade depend on the rapidity of fluid accumulation, the amount of fluid, and the patient's baseline cardiac function.
- Echocardiogram is the most precise diagnostic test for cardiac tamponade: It is painless and noninvasive and allows for assessment of the location and quantity of fluid and overall cardiac function.
- The intensity of interventions depends on the patient's life expectancy. Interventions include symptom relief, procedures to remove fluid and prevent reaccumulation, and antineoplastic treatment to control the underlying malignancy, as appropriate.

Spinal Cord Compression

- Pain is the presenting symptom in 90% of the cases of SCC; without intervention, it progresses to motor weakness, sensory loss, autonomic dysfunction, and paralysis.
- The first sign of motor weakness often is difficulty rising from a seated position or climbing stairs because of proximal muscle weakness of the legs.
- The treatment of choice for SCC depends on the tumor type, the location, the rapidity of onset, the radiosensitivity of the tumor, and the mechanism of cord compression.
- The goals of treatment are preservation and restoration of neurologic function, relief of pain, optimization of quality of life, and reduction of tumor.

Increased Intracranial Pressure

- Tumor growth, edema of surrounding tissue, and obstruction of CSF outflow are factors associated with primary and metastatic brain lesions that can cause increased ICP.
- Early-morning headache that worsens with bending over, coughing, or performing the Valsalva maneuver and increases in severity, frequency, and duration is a common sign of increased ICP.
- Treatment focuses on reducing fluid in the brain, providing symptom relief and measures to prevent increased ICP and control seizures, and interventions to reduce tumor mass, as appropriate.

Recommended Resources for Oncology Advanced Practice Nurses

- Cancer.Net (www.cancer.net): This resource for patients is sponsored by the American Society of Clinical Oncology and covers more than 120 types of cancer or cancer-related syndromes, including information on side effects and treatment, and lists links to other reputable sites. This is helpful to guide patients to websites that provide accurate information.
- Kaplan, M. (Ed.). (2013). *Understanding and managing oncologic emergencies: A resource for nurses* (2nd ed.). Pittsburgh, PA: Oncology Nursing Society.
- UpToDate® (www.uptodate.com): A good source for the latest treatment and research on any medical subject. It requires a subscription, but some institutions have an institutional subscription for all employees to use. It covers oncology subjects but also addresses primary care issues that APNs encounter in practice.

The author would like to acknowledge Heather L. Brumbaugh, RN, MSN, ANP, AOCN®, for her contribution to this chapter that remains unchanged from the first edition of this book.

References

Abrahm, J.L., Banffy, M.B., & Harris, M.B. (2008). Spinal cord compression in patients with advanced metastatic cancer. *JAMA, 299,* 937–946. doi:10.1001/jama.299.8.937

Ahmann, F.R. (1984). A reassessment of the clinical implications of the superior vena caval syndrome. *Journal of Clinical Oncology, 2,* 961–969.

American Spinal Injury Association. (2011). ASIA impairment scale. Retrieved from http://www.asia-spinalinjury.org/elearning/ASIA_ISCOS_high.pdf

Armstrong, T. (2011). Central nervous system cancers. In C.H. Yarbro, D. Wujcik, & B.H. Gobel (Eds.), *Cancer nursing: Principles and practice* (7th ed., pp. 1147–1187). Burlington, MA: Jones & Bartlett Learning.

Becker, K.P., & Baehring, J.M. (2011a). Increased intracranial pressure. In V.T. DeVita Jr., S. Hellman, & S.A. Rosenberg (Eds.), *Cancer: Principles and practice of oncology* (9th ed., pp. 2130–2135). Philadelphia, PA: Wolters Kluwer Health/Lippincott Williams & Wilkins.

Becker, K.P., & Baehring, J.M. (2011b). Spinal cord compression. In V.T. DeVita Jr., S. Hellman, & S.A. Rosenberg (Eds.), *Cancer: Principles and practice of oncology* (9th ed., pp. 2136–2141). Philadelphia, PA: Wolters Kluwer Health/Lippincott Williams & Wilkins.

Beeson, M.S. (2014, December 10). Superior vena cava syndrome in emergency medicine. Retrieved from http://emedicine.medscape.com/article/760301-overview

Boss, B.J., & Huether, S.E. (2013). Alterations in cognitive systems, cerebral hemodynamics, and motor function. In K.L. McCance, S.E. Huether, V.L. Brashers, & N.S. Rote (Eds.), *Pathophysiology: The biologic basis for disease in adults and children* (7th ed., pp. 527–580). St. Louis, MO: Elsevier Mosby.

Brashers, V.L. (2013). Alterations in cardiovascular function. In K.L. McCance, S.E. Huether, V.L. Brashers, & N.S. Rote (Eds.), *Pathophysiology: The biologic basis for disease in adults and children* (7th ed., pp. 1129–1193). St. Louis, MO: Elsevier Mosby.

Brumbaugh, H.L. (2011). Superior vena cava syndrome. In C.H. Yarbro, D. Wujcik, & B.H. Gobel (Eds.), *Cancer nursing: Principles and practice* (7th ed., pp. 995–1004). Burlington, MA: Jones & Bartlett Learning.

Chamberlain, M.C., & Tredway, T.L. (2011). Adult primary intradural spinal cord tumors: A review. *Current Neurology and Neuroscience Reports, 11,* 320–328. doi:10.1007/s11910-011-0190-2

Chong, H.H., & Plotnick, G.D. (1995). Pericardial effusion and tamponade: Evaluation, imaging modalities, and management. *Comprehensive Therapy, 21,* 378–385.

Chow, E., Finkelstein, J.A., Saghal, A., & Coleman, R.E. (2011). Metastatic cancer to the bone. In V.T. DeVita Jr., S. Hellman, & S.A. Rosenberg (Eds.), *Cancer: Principles and practice of oncology* (9th ed., pp. 2192–2204). Philadelphia, PA: Wolters Kluwer Health/Lippincott Williams & Wilkins.

Cole, J.S., & Patchell, R.A. (2008). Metastatic epidural spinal cord compression. *Lancet Neurology, 7,* 459–466. doi:10.1016/S1474-4422(08)70089-9

Cope, D.G. (2013). Syndrome of inappropriate antidiuretic hormone secretion. In M. Kaplan (Ed.), *Understanding and managing oncologic emergencies: A resource for nurses* (2nd ed., pp. 411–431). Pittsburgh, PA: Oncology Nursing Society.

Cunningham, S.G., Brashers, V.L., & McCance, K.L. (2013). Structure and function of the cardiovascular and lymphatic systems. In K.L. McCance, S.E. Huether, V.L. Brashers, & N.S. Rote (Eds.), *Pathophysiology: The biologic basis for disease in adults and children* (7th ed., pp. 1083–1128). St. Louis, MO: Elsevier Mosby.

Curigliano, G., Cardinale, D., Suter, T., Plataniotis, G., de Azambuja, E., Sandri, M.T., … Roila, F. (2012). Cardiovascular toxicity induced by chemotherapy, targeted agents and radiotherapy: ESMO clinical practice guidelines. *Annals of Oncology, 23*(Suppl. 7), vii155–vii166. doi:10.1093/annonc/mds293

Daley, B.J., Bhimji, S., Bascom, R., Benninghoff, M.G., & Alam, S. (2014, April 28). Pneumothorax differential diagnoses. Retrieved from http://emedicine.medscape.com/article/424547-differential

Dawodu, S.T., Bechtel, K.A., Beeson, M.S., Hodges, S.D., Humphreys, S.C., & Kellam, J.F. (2014, December 18). Cauda equina and conus medullaris syndromes. Retrieved from http://emedicine.medscape.com/article/1148690-overview

Drews, R.E., & Rabkin, D.J. (2014, June 25). Malignancy-related superior vena cava syndrome [UpToDate version 23.1]. Retrieved from http://www.uptodate.com/contents/malignancy-related-superior-vena-cava-syndrome

Fagedet, D., Thony, F., Timsit, J.-F., Rodiere, M., Monnin-Bares, V., Ferretti, G.R., … Moro-Sibilot, D. (2013). Endovascular treatment of malignant superior vena cava syndrome: Results and predictive factors of clinical efficacy. *Cardiovascular and Interventional Radiology, 36,* 140–149. doi:10.1007/s00270-011-0310-z

Feng, Y., & Pennell, N.A. (2012). Superior vena cava syndrome in lung cancer. *Lung Cancer Management, 1,* 309–315. doi:10.2217/lmt.12.38

Flaherty, A.M. (2011). Spinal cord compression. In C.H. Yarbro, D. Wujcik, & B.H. Gobel (Eds.), *Cancer nursing: Principles and practice* (7th ed., pp. 979–994). Burlington, MA: Jones & Bartlett Learning.

Foulkes, M. (2010). Nursing management of common oncological emergencies. *Nursing Standard, 24*(41), 49–56. doi:10.7748/ns2010.06.24.41.49.c7835

Freter, C.E., & Haddadin, S. (2014, August 1). Oncologic emergencies: Cardiac tamponade. In R. Govindan (Ed.), *InPractice oncology.* Retrieved from http://www.inpractice.com/Textbooks/Oncology/General_Oncology_Topics/ch56_GeneralOnc_Emergencies/Chapter-Pages/Page-3.aspx

Ganeshan, A., Hon, L.Q., Warakaulle, D.R., Morgan, R., & Uberoi, R. (2009). Superior vena caval stenting for SVC obstruction: Current status. *European Journal of Radiology, 71,* 343–349. doi:10.1016/j.ejrad.2008.04.014

Georgy, B.A. (2008). Metastatic spinal lesions: State-of-the-art treatment options and future trends. *American Journal of Neuroradiology, 29,* 1605–1611. doi:10.3174/ajnr.A1137

Giglio, P., & Gilbert, M.R. (2010). Neurologic complications of cancer and its treatment. *Current Oncology Reports, 12,* 50–59. doi:10.1007/s11912-009-0071-x

Grannis, F.W., Jr., Kim, J.Y., & Lai, L. (2014, May 1). Fluid complications: Pericardial effusion. In D.G. Haller, L.D. Wagman, K.A. Camphausen, & W.J. Hoskins (Eds.), *Cancer management: A multidisciplinary approach* (online edition). Retrieved from http://www.cancernetwork.com/cancer-management/fluid-complications/article/10165/1802878?pageNumber=2

Gupta, G., & Nosko, M.G. (2013, May 8). Intracranial pressure monitoring. Retrieved from http://emedicine.medscape.com/article/1829950-overview

Hammack, J.E. (2012). Spinal cord disease in patients with cancer. *Continuum, 18,* 312–327. doi:10.1212/01.CON.0000413660.58045.ae

Hickey, J.V. (2009). Neurological assessment. In J.V. Hickey (Ed.), *The clinical practice of neurological and neurosurgical nursing* (6th ed., pp. 154–180). Philadelphia, PA: Wolters Kluwer Health/Lippincott Williams & Wilkins.

Hickey, J.V., & Armstrong, T.S. (2009). Brain tumors. In J.V. Hickey (Ed.), *The clinical practice of neurological and neurosurgical nursing* (6th ed., pp. 496–520). Philadelphia, PA: Wolters Kluwer Health/Lippincott Williams & Wilkins.

Hickey, J.V., & Olson, D.W.M. (2009). Intracranial hypertension: Theory and management of increased intracranial pressure. In J.V. Hickey (Ed.), *The clinical practice of neurological and neurosurgical nursing* (6th ed., pp. 270–307). Philadelphia: Wolters Kluwer Health/Lippincott Williams & Wilkins.

Hoit, B.D. (2014, October 8). Cardiac tamponade [UpToDate release 23.1]. Retrieved from http://www.uptodate.com/contents/cardiac-tamponade

Huff, J.S. (2013, April 8). Brain neoplasms. Retrieved from http://emedicine.medscape.com/article/779664-overview

Huff, J.S. (2014, April 24). Spinal cord neoplasms. Retrieved from http://emedicine.medscape.com/article/779872-overview

Hunter, W. (1757). History of an aneurysm of the aorta, with some remarks on aneurysms in general. *Medical Observations and Inquiries, 1,* 323–357.

Iwamoto, R.R., Haas, M.L., & Gosselin, T.K. (Eds.). (2012). *Manual for radiation oncology nursing practice and education* (4th ed.). Pittsburgh, PA: Oncology Nursing Society.

Jones, D.A., & Jain, A.K. (2011). Percutaneous balloon pericardiotomy for recurrent malignant pericardial effusion. *Journal of Thoracic Oncology, 6,* 2138–2139. doi:10.1097/JTO.0b013e318230860e

Kamel, H., Navi, B.B., Nakagawa, K., Hemphill, J.C., III, & Ko, N.U. (2011). Hypertonic saline versus mannitol for the treatment of elevated intracranial pressure: A meta-analysis of randomized clinical trials. *Critical Care Medicine, 39,* 554–559. doi:10.1097/CCM.0b013e318206b9be

Kaplan, M. (2009). Back pain: Is it spinal cord compression? *Clinical Journal of Oncology Nursing, 13,* 592–595. doi:10.1188/09.CJON.592-595

Kaplan, M. (2013). Spinal cord compression. In M. Kaplan (Ed.), *Understanding and managing oncologic emergencies: A resource for nurses* (2nd ed., pp. 337–383). Pittsburgh, PA: Oncology Nursing Society.

Kaplow, R. (2011). Cardiac tamponade. In C.H. Yarbro, D. Wujcik, & B.H. Gobel (Eds.), *Cancer nursing: Principles and practice* (7th ed., pp. 915–927). Burlington, MA: Jones & Bartlett Learning.

Kaplow, R. (2013, December 27). Oncologic emergencies: Cardiac tamponade. In D. Camp-Sorrell & R. Hawkins (Eds.), *InPractice oncology nursing.* Retrieved from http://www.inpractice.com/Textbooks/Oncology-Nursing/Oncologic-Emergencies/Cardiac-Tamponade/Chapter-Pages/Page-1.aspx

Klimo, P., Jr., Kestle, J.R.W., & Schmidt, M.H. (2003). Treatment of metastatic spinal epidural disease: A review of the literature. *Neurosurgical Focus, 15*(5), Article 1. Retrieved from http://thejns.org/doi/pdfplus/10.3171/foc.2003.15.5.1 doi:10.3171/foc.2003.15.5.1

Kwong, K.F., & Nguyen, D.M. (2011). Malignant effusions of the pleura and the pericardium. In V.T. DeVita Jr., S. Hellman, & S.A. Rosenberg (Eds.), *Cancer: Principles and practice of oncology* (9th ed., pp. 2205–2213). Philadelphia, PA: Wolters Kluwer Health/Lippincott Williams & Wilkins.

Lanciego, C., Pangua, C., Chacon, J.L., Velasco, J., Boy, R.C., Viana, A., … Garcia, L.G. (2009). Endovascular stenting as the first step in the overall management of malignant superior vena cava syndrome. *American Journal of Roentgenology, 193,* 549–558. doi:10.2214/AJR.08.1904

Laskin, J., Cmelak, A.J., Meranze, S., Yee, J., & Johnson, D.H. (2014). Superior vena cava syndrome. In J.E. Niederhuber, J.O. Armitage, J.H. Doroshow, M.B. Kastan, & J.E. Tepper (Eds.), *Abeloff's clinical oncology* (5th ed., pp. 705–714). Philadelphia, PA: Elsevier Saunders.

Lestuzzi, C. (2010). Neoplastic pericardial disease: Old and current strategies for diagnosis and management. *World Journal of Cardiology, 2,* 270–279. doi:10.4330/wjc.v2.i9.270

Lewis, M.A., Hendrickson, A.W., & Moynihan, T.J. (2011). Oncologic emergencies: Pathophysiology, presentation, diagnosis, and treatment. *CA: A Cancer Journal for Clinicians, 61,* 287–314. doi:10.3322/caac.20124

Loblaw, D.A., Mitera, G., Ford, M., & Laperriere, N.J. (2012). A 2011 updated systematic review and clinical practice guideline for the management of malignant extradural spinal cord compression. *International Journal of Radiation Oncology, Biology, Physics, 84,* 312–317. doi:10.1016/j.ijrobp.2012.01.014

Lu, C., Gonzalez, R.G., Jolesz, F.A., Wen, P.Y., & Talcott, J.A. (2005). Suspected spinal cord compression in cancer patients: A multidisciplinary risk assessment. *Journal of Supportive Oncology, 3,* 305–312.

Maisch, B., Ristic, A., & Pankuweit, S. (2010). Evaluation and management of pericardial effusion in patients with neoplastic disease. *Progress in Cardiovascular Diseases, 53,* 157–163. doi:10.1016/j.pcad.2010.06.003

Marko, N.F. (2012). Commentary: Hypertonic saline, not mannitol, should be considered gold-standard medical therapy for intracranial hypertension. *Critical Care, 16,* 113. Retrieved from http://ccforum.com/content/16/1/113

McKenzie, J.T., McTyre, E., Kunaprayoon, D., & Redmond, K.P. (2013). Stereotactic body radiotherapy for superior vena cava syndrome. *Reports of Practical Oncology and Radiotherapy, 18,* 179–181. doi:10.1016/j.rpor.2012.12.003

Miaskowski, C. (2009). Spinal cord compression. In C.C. Chernecky & K. Murphy-Ende (Eds.), *Acute care oncology nursing* (2nd ed., pp. 492–498). St. Louis, MO: Elsevier Saunders.

National Cancer Institute. (2014, October 21). Cardiopulmonary syndromes (PDQ®). Retrieved from http://www.cancer.gov/cancertopics/pdq/supportivecare/cardiopulmonary/HealthProfessional

National Comprehensive Cancer Network. (2014). *NCCN Clinical Practice Guidelines in Oncology (NCCN Guidelines®): Cancer-associated venous thromboembolic disease* [v.2.2014]. Retrieved from http://www.nccn.org/professionals/physician_gls/pdf/vte.pdf

Nickloes, T.A., Long, C., Mack, L.O., Kallab, A.M., Dunlap, A.B., & Gandhi, S.S. (2014, October 10). Superior vena cava syndrome. Retrieved from http://emedicine.medscape.com/article/460865-overview

Nunnelee, J.D. (2007). Superior vena cava syndrome. *Journal of Vascular Nursing, 25,* 2–5. doi:10.1016/j.jvn.2006.09.004

Patchell, R.A., Tibbs, P.A., Regine, W.F., Payne, R., Saris, S., Kryscio, R.J., … Young, B. (2005). Direct decompressive surgical resection in the treatment of spinal cord compression caused by metastatic cancer: A randomised trial. *Lancet, 366,* 643–648. doi:10.1016/S0140-6736(05)66954-1

Prasad, D., & Schiff, D. (2005). Malignant spinal-cord compression. *Lancet Oncology, 6,* 15–24. doi:10.1016/S1470-2045(04)01709-7

Prewett, S., & Venkitaraman, R. (2010). Overview: Metastatic spinal cord compression: Review of the evidence for a radiotherapy dose fractionation schedule. *Clinical Oncology, 22,* 222–230. doi:10.1016/j.clon.2010.01.006

Roy, C.L., Minor, M.A., Brookhart, M.A., & Choudhry, N.K. (2007). Does this patient with a pericardial effusion have cardiac tamponade? *JAMA, 297,* 1810–1818. doi:10.1001/jama.297.16.1810

Ryu, S., Rock, J., Jain, R., Lu, M., Anderson, J., Jin, J.Y., … Kim, J.H. (2010). Radiosurgical decompression of metastatic epidural compression. *Cancer, 116,* 2250–2257. doi:10.1002/cncr.24993

Schiff, D. (2014, December 24). Clinical features and diagnosis of neoplastic epidural spinal cord compression, including cauda equina syndrome [UpToDate release 23.1]. Retrieved from http://www.uptodate.com/contents/clinical-features-and-diagnosis-of-neoplastic-epidural-spinal-cord-compression-including-cauda-equina-syndrome

Schiff, D., Brown, P., & Shaffrey, M.E. (2014, December 11). Treatment and prognosis of neoplastic epidural spinal cord compression, including cauda equina syndrome [UpToDate release 23.1]. Retrieved from http://www.uptodate.com/contents/treatment-and-prognosis-of-neoplastic-epidural-spinal-cord-compression-including-cauda-equina-syndrome

Schifferdecker, B., Shaw, J.A., Piemonte, T.C., & Eisenhauer, A.C. (2005). Nonmalignant superior vena cava syndrome: Pathophysiology and management. *Catheterization and Cardiovascular Interventions, 65,* 416–423. doi:10.1002/ccd.20381

Shelton, B.K. (2013). Superior vena cava syndrome. In M. Kaplan (Ed.), *Understanding and managing oncologic emergencies: A resource for nurses* (2nd ed., pp. 385–410). Pittsburgh, PA: Oncology Nursing Society.

Shelton, B.K., Ferrigno, C., & Skinner, J. (2013). Increased intracranial pressure. In M. Kaplan (Ed.), *Understanding and managing oncologic emergencies: A resource for nurses* (2nd ed., pp. 157–197). Pittsburgh, PA: Oncology Nursing Society.

Siegel, R.L., Miller, K.D., & Jemal, A. (2015). Cancer statistics, 2015. *CA: A Cancer Journal for Clinicians, 65,* 5–29. doi:10.3322/caac.21254

Sirven, J.I., Wingerchuk, D.M., Drazkowski, J.F., Lyons, M.K., & Zimmerman, R.S. (2004). Seizure prophylaxis in patients with brain tumors: A meta-analysis. *Mayo Clinic Proceedings, 79,* 1489–1494. doi:10.4065/79.12.1489

Smith, E.R., & Amin-Hanjani, S. (2013, July 10). Evaluation and management of elevated intracranial pressure in adults [UpToDate release 21.6]. Retrieved from http://www.uptodate.com/contents/evaluation-and-management-of-elevated-intracranial-pressure-in-adults

Spangler, S., & Gentlesk, P.J. (2014, October 6). Acute pericarditis. Retrieved from http://emedicine.medscape.com/article/156951-overview

Story, K.T. (2013). Cardiac tamponade. In M. Kaplan (Ed.), *Understanding and managing oncologic emergencies: A resource for nurses* (2nd ed., pp. 43–68). Pittsburgh, PA: Oncology Nursing Society.

Sugerman, R.A. (2013). Structure and function of the neurologic system. In K.L. McCance, S.E. Huether, V.L. Brashers, & N.S. Rote (Eds.), *Pathophysiology: The biologic basis for disease in adults and children* (7th ed., pp. 447–483). St. Louis, MO: Elsevier Mosby.

Sun, H., & Nemecek, A.N. (2009). Optimal management of malignant epidural spinal cord compression. *Emergency Medicine Clinics of North America, 27,* 195–208. doi:10.1016/j.emc.2009.02.001

Teasdale, G., & Jennett, B. (1974). Assessment of coma and impaired consciousness: A practical scale. *Lancet, 304,* 81–84. doi:10.1016/S0140-6736(74)91639-0

Theodore, P.R., & Jablons, D. (2010). Thoracic wall, pleura, mediastinum, and lung. In G.M. Doherty (Ed.), *CURRENT diagnosis and treatment: Surgery* (13th ed.). Retrieved from http://www.accesssurgery.com/content.aspx?aID=5214160

Tremont-Lukats, I.W., Ratilal, B.O., Armstrong, T., & Gilbert, M.R. (2008). Antiepileptic drugs for preventing seizures in people with brain tumors. *Cochrane Database of Systematic Reviews, 2008*(2). doi:10.1002/14651858.CD004424.pub2

Tse, V. (2014, April 16). Brain metastases. Retrieved from http://emedicine.medscape.com/article/1157902-overview

Vedantham, S. (2012). Interventional approaches to deep vein thrombosis. *American Journal of Hematology, 87*(Suppl. 1), S113–S118. doi:10.1002/ajh.23145

Ware, M.L., Nemani, V., Meeker, M., Lee, C., Morabito, D., & Manley, G.T. (2005). Effects of 23.4% sodium chloride solution in reducing intracranial pressure in patients with traumatic brain injury: A preliminary study. *Neurosurgery, 57,* 727–736. doi:10.1227/01.NEU.0000175726.08903.0A

Weinstein, S.M. (2013). Management of spinal cord and cauda equina compression. In A.M. Berger, J.L. Shuster Jr., & J.H. Von Roenn (Eds.), *Principles and practice of palliative care and supportive oncology* (4th ed., pp. 514–528). Philadelphia, PA: Wolters Kluwer Health/Lippincott Williams & Wilkins.

Witham, T.F., Khavkin, Y.A., Gallia, G.L., Wolinsky, J.-P., & Gokaslan, Z.L. (2006). Surgery insight: Current management of epidural spinal cord compression from metastatic spine disease. *Nature Clinical Practice Neurology, 2,* 87–94.

Yadav, R., Shin, K.Y., Guo, Y., & Konzen, B. (2009). Cancer rehabilitation. In S.-C.J. Yeung, C.P. Escalante, & R.F. Gagel (Eds.), *Medical care of cancer patients* (pp. 563–570). Shelton, CT: BC Decker.

Yahalom, J. (2011). Oncologic emergencies: Superior vena cava syndrome. In V.T. DeVita Jr., S. Hellman, & S.A. Rosenberg (Eds.), *Cancer: Principles and practice of oncology* (9th ed., pp. 2123–2129). Philadelphia, PA: Wolters Kluwer Health/Lippincott Williams & Wilkins.

Yarlagadda, C. (2015, January 27). Cardiac tamponade. Retrieved from http://emedicine.medscape.com/article/152083-overview

Yu, J.B., Wilson, L.D., & Detterbeck, F.C. (2008). Superior vena cava syndrome—A proposed classification and algorithm for management. *Journal of Thoracic Oncology, 3,* 811–814. doi:10.1097/JTO.0b013e3181804791

CHAPTER 17

Psychosocial Management

Roberta H. Baron, MSN, RN, AOCN®

Introduction

The psychosocial sequelae that challenge patients with cancer and their families are interwoven within all aspects of oncologic care, from diagnosis through terminal care. The psychosocial issues include anxiety and depression; post-traumatic stress disorder (PTSD); fear of recurrence; cognitive changes; sexual health and body image changes; family/caregiver distress; socioeconomic, occupational, and role changes; and, most profoundly, a changed life perspective.

The National Comprehensive Cancer Network® (NCCN®) elected to use the word *distress* to characterize the psychosocial nature of the cancer experience (NCCN, 2015). The term *psychosocial* has a negative connotation, whereas the term *distress* carries less stigma and is more acceptable. NCCN defines distress as a multifactorial, unpleasant experience that is social, emotional, psychological, or spiritual in nature. Distress can range from normal feelings of fear, sadness, and vulnerability to disabling conditions, such as depression, anxiety and panic, isolation, and existential or spiritual crises (NCCN, 2015). How patients cope with and adapt to cancer depends on many intervening variables, such as age, gender, lifestyle, family dynamics, culture and ethnicity, social support, socioeconomic status, religious beliefs, and spirituality.

Family systems theory provides a framework for understanding the impact of cancer on not only the patient but also on the family unit. Coping for patients and families is interdependent—the emotional and behavioral responses of one will always affect the other, positively or negatively. The family, in all its present-day permutations, is the unit of care (Mehta, Cohen, & Chan, 2009; Northouse, 2012; Northouse, Williams, Given, & McCorkle, 2012).

Definitions and Symptoms

Self-Esteem

Sexuality and Cancer, a mainstay of education literature for patients with cancer, shares an analogy used by Wendy Schain, EdD, a psychologist who specializes in counseling patients with cancer (American Cancer Society [ACS], 2011). She likened self-esteem to the total sum of several bank accounts that support an individual's identity. One account is the net worth of the **physical** self—this includes body health and functioning, sexuality, and body image. A second account is the **social** self—this includes personality and character, temperament and outlook on life, and relationships with others. The third account is the **achieving** self—this includes an individual's identity formulated through roles in work, community, and personal and family relationships. The last bank account is the **spiritual** self—this includes an individual's religious and moral beliefs and the strength found in these beliefs.

Throughout life's journey, according to Schain, individuals make deposits into each of these bank accounts. The experience and challenges of cancer draw from each account along the continuum of disease and treatment. Keeping the accounts balanced may require withdrawing from one and depositing into another. It can be analogous to effective coping—having the flexibility to adjust by not defining self-esteem or self-worth on one part of the total self. Yet a person's identity is more than the sum of its interrelated parts. Difficulty in one area of self-esteem (e.g., sexuality) will affect another part of the self (e.g., the social self). A self-image that integrates the physical and psychological changes brought about by the cancer experience is necessary for psychosocial adaptation.

High self-esteem has been associated with better quality of life (QOL). Cancer survivors and caretakers with high self-esteem have been shown to experience lower levels of anxiety and depression and higher QOL scores compared to those with low self-esteem (Costa-Requena, Cristófol, & Cañete, 2012; Kobayashi et al., 2009). In a study of terminally ill patients, those with high self-esteem exhibited fewer psychological symptoms, even in the face of a life-threatening illness (Christianson, Weis, & Fouad, 2013). In a study of Korean women with breast cancer, low self-esteem was directly linked to increased depression. Personal factors (i.e., perceived health status, religious beliefs), environmental factors (i.e., family support, economic status), and disease-related factors (i.e., fatigue) affected depression indirectly and were mediated through self-esteem and hope (Tae, Heitkemper, & Kim, 2012). This highlights the importance of developing strategies to enhance self-esteem and hope, with the goal of decreasing feelings of depression and strengthening coping ability.

Anxiety

Anxiety among patients with cancer is a common response to threats of uncertainty, suffering, and mortality (Traeger, Greer, Fernandez-Robles, Temel, & Pirl, 2012). Prevalence of anxiety in the cancer population can range from 10% during the early course of illness (Mitchell et al., 2011) to as high as 18% in long-term survivors (Mitchell, Ferguson, Gill, Paul, & Symonds, 2013).

Anxiety and depression consist of a cluster of psychological and physiologic symptoms that, if recognized, often are responsive to treatment, but if unrecognized, interfere with coping and QOL. Symptoms of anxiety can range from mild to severe and can fluctuate during periods of increased vulnerability. These vulnerable periods can span the course of the disease from the discovery of a worrisome symptom, to receiving a cancer diagnosis, to recurrence, to the end of life (Holland et al., 2013). Even during long-term remission and survivorship, fears of recurrence and disabilities caused by cancer treatment can continue to promote feelings of uncertainty and anguish. Unrelenting sadness, grief, and loss often occur as a result of the physical and psychosocial losses experienced along the cancer trajectory. The *intensity, duration,* and *extent* to which these symptoms interfere with functioning differentiate abnormal anxiety or a depressive disorder from the normal emotional response to a threatening illness (American Psychiatric Association, 2013).

Fear is a common emotional reaction to a cancer diagnosis. At the beginning of the cancer journey, feelings of fear are related to the unknown and patients' shock that this is really happening to them (Stafford et al., 2013). This response can be especially poignant for asymptomatic patients whose malignancy is discovered unexpectedly (Carrion, Nedjat-Haiem, & Marquez, 2013). Fear is a normal emotional response to an imminent and identifiable threat or danger. Anxiety is a sustained state of apprehension and anticipation of a future threat (American Psychiatric Association, 2013; Schmitz & Grillon, 2012).

Fear and anxiety are interrelated. Fear is associated with surges of autonomic arousal, leading to the stress response of "fight or flight." Anxiety, however, can reduce a person's ability to act. Severe anxiety can cause patients with cancer to feel emotionally paralyzed. The physical symptoms of anxiety are associated with the autonomic response and include muscle tension ranging from generalized aches and pains to autonomic hyperactivity such as palpitations and shortness of breath. Patients may describe feeling restless, trembling, and dizzy, having a lump in their throat, or feeling suffocated. The physical toll of anxiety demands energy, causing patients to feel fatigue and exhaustion when facing the demands of their illness (Lim, Devi, & Ang, 2011). This may be exacerbated by difficulty falling asleep or staying asleep or waking with ruminating thoughts and apprehension about what is happening to them. Patients commonly feel that they are always "on alert" and vigilant for any physical ache or pain that may be interpreted as cancer spread or recurrence.

The psychological symptoms of anxiety are associated with feelings of impending doom. The perceived threat of treatments may increase fear of body image changes and permanent disabilities. Fear and anxiety can range from an acute, transient distress at different stages along the continuum of disease to a major psychiatric illness, such as PTSD, or stress syndromes such as panic attacks or phobias (American Psychiatric Association, 2013; Lim et al., 2011). Therefore, fear and anxiety are normal responses to stressful events, such as cancer, but become pathologic if they persist and interfere with functioning. Certain illness and treatment sequelae (e.g., hyperthyroidism, chronic obstructive pulmonary disease, asthma, hypoxia, infection, pulmonary embolus), alcohol or drug withdrawal (e.g., benzodiazepines, sedatives, opioids), and medications (e.g., steroids, antiemetics) can exacerbate anxiety. This highlights the importance of taking a thorough health and medical history for differential diagnosis (Traeger et al., 2012).

The presence of trauma-related symptoms, such as avoidance behaviors, intrusive thoughts, and heightened arousal, is not uncommon in cancer survivors (Elklit & Blum, 2011; Posluszny, Edwards, Dew, & Baum, 2011). These symptoms are referred to as PTSD and resemble those observed in individuals who have experienced extreme psychological assault, such as with rape, combat, a natural disaster, or a mass catastrophe (Andreasen, 2010). Recurrence of cancer may bring forth traumatic memories for patients who underwent intensive treatments for their cancer. Feelings of dread or doom are not unusual when recurrent disease arouses these memories. People with a history of anxiety disorders that developed in childhood or early adulthood, such as generalized anxiety disorder, panic disorder, and specific phobias, may experience a reemergence or intensification of symptoms with the diagnosis of cancer (Traeger et al., 2012). Phobias such as needle phobia and claustrophobia may interfere with cancer treatment. "Conditioned" or learned responses to repetitive, aversive treatments have been found to contribute to symptoms such as anxiety and anticipatory nausea and vomiting (Rodríguez, 2013).

Gender and ethnicity may influence patterns of anxiety disorders. Research has found that in the United States, women are more likely to have specific phobias than men (American Psychiatric Association, 2013). African Americans, Native Americans, and non-Latino Whites have significantly higher rates of specific phobias compared to Asians and Latinos (American Psychiatric Association, 2013). Comorbid depression also has been found to exacerbate phobic anxiety and increase the risk of suicidal behavior (American Psychiatric Association, 2013). More research is needed in this area to help identify patients who are at greatest risk for comorbidities.

Depression

Although depression has been recognized as one of the most common emotional reactions to the cancer experience, it is also the most overlooked, misunderstood, and misdiagnosed of symptoms (Mitchell et al., 2011; Walker et al., 2013). Prevalence rates vary widely, depending on the definition of depression, diagnostic criteria used, quality of the study, method of assessment, type and stage of cancer, and population demographics (Irwin, Olmstead, Ganz, & Haque, 2013; Li, Fitzgerald, & Rodin, 2012; Mitchell et al., 2011). Estimates of prevalence have ranged from 4% to 49% (Walker et al., 2013).

Depressive symptoms occur on a continuum from normal sadness and grief at the milder end, minor or subthreshold depression in the middle, and major depression at the severe end (American Psychiatric Association, 2013). The diagnoses of anxiety and depression often coexist. Diagnostic criteria for a major depressive disorder must include at least five of the following symptoms that have been present during the same two-week period: At least one of the symptoms must include either a depressed mood most of the day, nearly every day, or a decreased interest or pleasure in all or most activities. The other symptoms include significant weight loss, insomnia, fatigue, agitation, difficulty concentrating, feelings of worthlessness or inappropriate guilt, and recurrent thoughts of death or suicidal ideation (American Psychiatric Association, 2013). Distinguishing between the symptoms related to a depressive disorder and the symptoms related to the cancer can be difficult, as they often overlap or mimic one another. Diagnosing major depression in the palliative care setting is particularly challenging. Symptoms in this population often include weight loss, fatigue, and difficulty sleeping. One study compared the depressive symptoms experienced by patients with incurable disease to the *Diagnostic and Statistical Manual of Mental Disorders*, fourth edition (DSM-IV) criteria for symptoms that constitute depressive disorders. Many of the reported symptoms, such as fatigue, feelings of worthlessness, thoughts of death, and decrease in weight, were reflected in the DSM-IV symptom criteria. The reported symptoms of anxiety, despair, and social withdrawal, which were not part of the criteria, could serve as an indicator of a depressive disorder in this population (Brenne et al., 2013). Sometimes the boundaries between normal sadness, minor or subthreshold depression, and major depression are ambiguous, making it challenging to differentiate among them. The majority of patients with cancer present with subthreshold depression, which is not always easily identified and therefore carries the risk of not being treated (Li, M., et al., 2012). See Table 17-1 for a comparison of symptoms in anxiety and depression.

Growing evidence shows that tumor cell burden and treatment-induced tissue destruction cause a release of proinflammatory cytokines. This cytokine release alters neurotransmitter and neuroendocrine function, which may contribute to depressive symptoms in patients with cancer (Li, M., et al., 2012). A decrease in levels of neurotransmitters (dopamine, norepinephrine, and serotonin) negatively affects homeostasis throughout the body, causing cognitive, behavioral, and systemic symptoms. Thus, a thorough assessment of the cognitive changes associated with depression should be used for definitive diagnosis. Untreated depression places patients at risk for suicide, therefore making diagnosis and treatment imperative (Anguiano, Mayer, Piven, & Rosenstein, 2012).

Individuals often find it difficult to admit to feelings or behaviors related to depression because of fear of being negatively judged as weak in character or because of personal feelings

Table 17-1. Symptoms of Anxiety and Depression[a]

State	Symptoms
Anxiety	Physical symptoms: Sympathetic stimulation, including restlessness, trembling, tremors, muscle tension, heart palpitations, dyspnea, chest tightness, lump in throat, feelings of suffocation, increased perspiration Psychological symptoms: Fear, worry, distress, ruminating thoughts, irritability, apprehension, feelings of inadequacy, feelings of impending doom, hypervigilance
Depression	Physical symptoms[b]: Extreme sadness, crying or despondence, appetite or sleep disturbance, psychomotor agitation or retardation, decreased energy or fatigue, decreased libido Psychological symptoms: Feelings of worthlessness, sense of guilt and failure, hopelessness and emptiness, poor concentration, anhedonia (inability to experience pleasure from activities usually found enjoyable), suicidal ideation

[a] States of anxiety and depression often coexist.

[b] Physical symptoms of depression are similar to side effects of cancer treatment; therefore, psychological symptoms are more indicative of depression in patients with cancer.

Note. Based on information from American Psychiatric Association, 2013; Lim et al., 2011; Traeger et al., 2012.

of failure. Numerous diagnostic tools are available to evaluate mood disorders in the clinical and research settings. For initial diagnosis in the clinical setting, a thorough intake history, physical examination, and psychosocial assessment are appropriate and effective. A single-item screening question (e.g., "Do you feel low in mood or depressed?") has the benefit of being simple and efficient and begins a dialogue that is nonthreatening to both patients and nurses (Anguiano et al., 2012).

Cognitive Dysfunction

Cognitive disorders are those that were not present at birth and therefore show a decline from an individual's previous level of cognitive functioning (American Psychiatric Association, 2013). Mild cognitive disorders are associated with a modest impairment in cognitive performance but still allow an individual to perform daily activities independently, whereas major cognitive disorders represent a significant cognitive decline and interfere with independence (American Psychiatric Association, 2013). Subtle changes may not be apparent and may be confounded with other problems associated with cancer, including depression, anxiety, and fatigue, making detection and management even more challenging (Janelsins et al., 2011). Cognitive dysfunction also can be misdiagnosed as anxiety and depression, or these psychological comorbidities can contribute to changes in cognition (Downing, Caprio, & Lyness, 2013).

Direct/disease-related factors that cause cognitive dysfunction in patients with cancer include primary tumors of the central nervous system (CNS) or brain metastases. Primary and metastatic brain tumors often cause diffuse cognitive dysfunction or focal deficits related to the site of the tumor, such as headaches, seizures, inappropriate behaviors, emotional lability, and focal weakness (Lu-Emerson & Eichler, 2012).

Indirect/treatment-related factors that contribute to cognitive dysfunction include adverse effects of treatment modalities (e.g., medications, radiation therapy, chemotherapy, hormonal therapy, biologic response modifiers) or indirect factors, such as metabolic, endocrine, and nutritional abnormalities that commonly occur with cancer (Holland et al., 2013; Stan,

Loprinzi, & Ruddy, 2013). Radiation therapy is an effective treatment for primary CNS tumors and CNS metastases; however, treatments place patients at risk for cognitive impairment. A recent study examined the molecular pathways that likely contribute to radiation-induced cognitive impairment, including changes in the vascular and glial cell populations, decreased hippocampal neurogenesis, altered neuronal function, and neuroinflammation (Greene-Schloesser, Moore, & Robbins, 2013). Another study showed that it is not the dose of radiation to the whole brain that predicts cognitive impairment, but rather the dose to specific regions in the brain, such as the temporal lobes and hippocampus (Peiffer et al., 2013).

Cognitive impairment caused by chemotherapy agents often is referred to as "chemobrain." Investigators proposed changing the name to "cancer- or cancer therapy–associated cognitive change" because many other factors besides chemotherapy might be contributing to the change in cognitive function (Hurria, Somlo, & Ahles, 2007). Conflicting evidence exists with regard to the type of cognitive changes caused by chemotherapy agents. Cognitive deficits range from having difficulty in the domains of executive function (e.g., planning, decision making), memory, information and processing speed, and attention (Wefel, Saleeba, Buzdar, & Meyers, 2010) to having no deficits other than motor slowing (Tager et al., 2010). A recent meta-analysis in breast cancer survivors who were previously treated with chemotherapy for six months or longer showed a decline in only verbal ability (e.g., difficulty finding words) and visuospatial ability (e.g., getting lost more easily) (Jim et al., 2012). Table 17-2 describes the domains of cognitive function. Drawing definitive conclusions regarding the impact of chemotherapy-induced cognitive dysfunction has been difficult because of the variety of study variables, such as different treatment regimens, patient populations, cognitive tests, and statistical methods (Wefel et al., 2010). Several studies have shown cognitive deficits in patients with cancer prior to chemotherapy, suggesting other causes such as the adverse effects of the cancer itself (e.g., cytokine dysregulation and inflammation) or other treatment-related sequelae (e.g., fatigue and anemia) (Ahles et al., 2010; Nelson & Suls, 2013; Wefel & Schagen, 2012; Wefel, Vardy, Ahles, & Schagen, 2011). Therefore, it is important to inform patients who will be undergoing any can-

Table 17-2. Domains of Cognitive Function

Cognitive Domain	Description
Executive function	Planning, decision making
Attention and concentration	Ability to sustain attention over time Ability to focus on relevant thoughts or actions, while ignoring distractions
Learning and memory	Ability to acquire new information Ability to acquire, store, and recall learned information, differentiated as short term or long term
Information processing speed	Ability to rapidly and efficiently process simple and complex information
Language	Ability to incorporate verbal and written information used to express thoughts
Visuospatial skill	Ability to process and interpret visual information regarding where things are in space
Motor function	Motor performance including speed, strength, and coordination

Note. Based on information from American Psychiatric Association, 2013; Jansen, 2013.

cer treatment modalities that they may experience certain changes in cognition, based on their specific treatment and individual risk factors. Patients and their families should be encouraged to report these changes to their healthcare team (Jansen, 2013).

Age, intelligence, and education level also contribute to the impact of disease- or treatment-related cognitive dysfunction (Bender & Thelen, 2013; Strout & Howard, 2012). Greater intelligence and a higher level of education have been associated with higher cognitive functioning (Bender & Thelen, 2013). Cognitive decline is expected to occur as adults age and may be exacerbated by the decline in hearing and sight. Normal, expected cognitive changes among older adults must be differentiated from psychiatric diagnoses, such as depression, anxiety, dementia, and delirium (Downing et al., 2013). Concurrent use of medications, such as antiemetics and antidepressants, as well as substance abuse, will adversely affect cognitive ability. See Figure 17-1 for potential risk factors that contribute to cognitive dysfunction.

Delirium

Delirium is defined as a disturbance in attention and awareness that represents a change from baseline. It also must be accompanied by an additional disturbance in cognition (e.g., memory, orientation, language, visuospatial ability, perception). These disturbances cannot be better explained by a preexisting or evolving neurocognitive disorder. Evidence also must exist that the disturbance is a physiologic consequence of an underlying medical condition (e.g., brain metastases, pulmonary embolus, urinary tract infection, organ failure, anemia), substance intoxication or withdrawal (e.g., illicit drugs, alcohol), use of a medication (e.g., antiemetics, antidepressants, corticosteroids), exposure to a toxin, or a combination of these factors. Other contributing factors may include an unfamiliar environment or fecal impaction (American Psychiatric Association, 2013) (see Figure 17-2). Delirium is characterized by an acute onset of symptoms (usually within hours to a few days) that can fluctuate in intensity during the course of a day. Patients often exhibit a disturbance in the sleep-wake cycle, such as sleeping all day and staying up all night or becoming agitated at night. Emotional disturbances may include anger, irritability, anxiety, depression, disorganized thinking, and an altered level of consciousness (alertness or arousal). Inappropriate behaviors may be expressed, such as screaming, cursing, or muttering, occurring more often at night. Delirium can be classified as

---

Cancer Treatment
- Concurrent medications
- Local treatment (radiation, surgery)
- Systemic treatment (chemotherapy, hormonal therapy, biologic therapy)
- Treatment location (e.g., treatment administered directly to central nervous system [CNS])
- Treatment regimen, dose, cumulative effects

Direct Disease-Related Factors
- Primary tumors of CNS or CNS metastases

Indirect Disease- or Treatment-Related Factors
- Anemia
- Fatigue
- Hypercalcemia
- Infection
- Metabolic abnormalities
- Multisystem failure
- Nutritional deficiencies
- Pain

Psychological Factors
- Anxiety
- Depression
- Stress

Individual Characteristics
- Age
- Intelligence
- Level of education

Figure 17-1. Potential Factors Contributing to Cognitive Dysfunction

---

Note. Based on information from American Psychiatric Association, 2013; Bender & Thelen, 2013.

Central Nervous System
- Brain metastases
- Head trauma
- Primary brain tumor
- Seizures
- Stroke

Cardiopulmonary
- Congestive heart failure
- Myocardial infarction
- Pulmonary embolus
- Respiratory failure

Infections
- Pneumonia
- Sepsis
- Urinary tract

Metabolic
- Fluid or electrolyte imbalance: Dehydration, hypo-glycemia/hyperglycemia, hypercalcemia, hypona-tremia/hypernatremia
- Organ failure: Renal, hepatic
- Thiamine deficiency

Endocrine
- Adrenal or pituitary insufficiency
- Cushing syndrome
- Hyperparathyroidism
- Hypothyroidism/hyperthyroidism

Hematologic
- Anemia
- Disseminated intravascular coagulation
- Hyperviscosity syndrome
- Leukemic blast cell crisis
- Thrombocytosis

Substance Intoxication or Withdrawal Syndromes
- Illicit drugs and alcohol

Medications
- Analgesics, anesthetics, antidepressants, anti-emetics, antihistamines, antihypertensive agents, antimicrobials, antipsychotics, barbiturates, ben-zodiazepines, corticosteroids, digitalis, diuretics, immunosuppressive agents

Other
- Fecal impaction
- Sensory and/or sleep deprivation
- Temperature dysregulation
- Unfamiliar environment

Figure 17-2. Underlying Causes of Delirium

Note. Based on information from American Psychiatric Association, 2013.

hyperactive, hypoactive, or mixed (Downing et al., 2013). The hyperactive subtype is associated with agitation, restlessness, combative outbursts, mood lability, and hallucinations. With hypoactive delirium, patients may withdraw socially and present as lethargic, sedated, or cognitively detached. The mixed form has characteristics of both and is the most common presentation. Factors that increase the risk of delirium in patients with cancer include advancing age, comorbid conditions, preexisting cognitive impairment, such as prior stroke or dementia, vision or hearing impairment, immobility, dehydration, unfamiliar environment, emotional stress, and depression. Cancer- or treatment-related factors that increase the risk of delirium include infection, major organ failure, use of benzodiazepines, metabolic imbalances, nutritional deficiencies, the use of steroids and opioids, and primary brain tumors or CNS metastases (Downing et al., 2013; LeGrand, 2012).

Delirium often is not recognized or is misdiagnosed by healthcare professionals. In patients with cancer, the symptoms of delirium can be mistaken for depression or other emotional reactions to having cancer (Downing et al., 2013). As many as 83% of patients exhibit delirium at the end of life (American Psychiatric Association, 2013). Most patients will fully recover from delirium regardless of whether they receive treatment. Identifying the cause early, followed by appropriate management, can shorten the course. Early identification also is important because delirium is independently associated with increased morbidity and mortality

(LeGrand, 2012). Some patients will not recover and may experience seizures, coma, or death, especially if the underlying cause remains untreated. It is important for nurses across all settings to recognize delirium in patients with cancer so that treatment can be initiated promptly.

Dementia

Dementia, a disorder that mainly affects older adults, results in a global loss of cognitive and intellectual functioning. Although it is an important risk factor for delirium, it is a distinctly different form of cognitive impairment (Downing et al., 2013). Dementia, in contrast to delirium, is a chronic, irreversible, and progressive decline in cognitive functioning. Diagnostic criteria for dementia include impairment in memory, behavior, and personality, with memory loss being the most common sign. The behavioral components of dementia include apathy, withdrawal, paranoia, wandering, and sleep changes, in contrast to the agitation, restlessness, and fluctuating changes in cognition that are present with delirium. Mood states, such as depression and anxiety, also may occur in patients experiencing dementia and should be diagnosed and treated appropriately (Downing et al., 2013). Because dementia often has an insidious onset, early symptoms may go unrecognized. With disease progression, patients may have more severe cognitive or behavioral deficits along with significant deficits in daily activities. They may become more dependent on others to assist them with activities of daily living (e.g., eating, dressing) and, over time, may require total care. In patients with cancer, dementia may be the result of disease or of treatment-related involvement of the brain and spinal cord, such as with radiation therapy for brain metastases (Khasraw & Posner, 2010). Recognizing the initial signs of dementia can be the key to making the diagnosis. Medical attention should be sought for any signs of memory loss that interferes with a person's daily functioning. This also is true of other cognitive or behavioral problems that prevent people from independently performing their usual activities.

Differential Diagnosis Among Delirium, Dementia, and Depression

Distinguishing among cognitive impairment, delirium, and dementia begins with a clear understanding of the differences in the nature of these separate but sometimes related conditions. Differentiating among delirium, dementia, and depression also can be challenging because the three conditions often overlap and may occur simultaneously (see Table 17-3). Attributes commonly used to distinguish one condition from another include onset, duration, progression, memory, level of orientation, and psychomotor behavior, among others (American Psychiatric Association, 2013).

A wide variety of standardized tools are available to assess cognitive function. The Montreal Cognitive Assessment tool allows for a brief, focused assessment that screens for changes or deficits in cognition (Freitas, Simões, Alves, Duro, & Santana, 2012). Older adult patients suspected of having dementia should be referred for a full evaluation.

Sexuality and Altered Body Image

Sexuality is a broad term that encompasses self-esteem, body image, pleasure, reproduction, and expressions of intimacy, including hugging, kissing, touching, and tenderness (Southard & Keller, 2009). The definition of sexuality must be interpreted individually. What is normal for one person may not be for another, depending on influencing factors such as cultural and

Table 17-3. Comparison of Clinical Features of Delirium, Dementia, and Depression

Clinical Feature	Delirium	Dementia	Depression
Onset	Acute • Hours to days	Chronic, insidious • Months to years	May be acute or chronic • Weeks to months • Situational influences
Course	Fluctuating • Reversible with early treatment of underlying cause	Chronic deterioration • Progression may be slower with treatment, but generally irreversible	Situational fluctuation • Usually reversible with treatment • Often worse in the morning
Mood	Labile	Labile	Extreme sadness May have anxiety/irritability
Memory	Impaired • Immediate and recent	Impaired • Short and long term	May be minimally impaired
Attention	Impaired	Intact	Minimally impaired, but poorly motivated
Alertness	Fluctuates • Hyperactive • Hypoactive • Mixed	Typically not affected until advanced stage	Normal or decreased
Perception	Hallucinations and delusions	May have delusions Usually no hallucinations	May have delusions Often paranoid
Thinking	Disorganized Incoherent speech	Difficulty with abstract thoughts Poor judgment Impaired word finding ability	Intact, but poor concentration Feelings of hopelessness

Note. Based on information from American Psychiatric Association, 2013.

religious norms, value systems, and past and present experiences (Bober & Varela, 2012). The emotional responses to body image changes, such as with mastectomy or hysterectomy, also must be interpreted individually because of these same factors. Internal as well as external body image changes can cause psychological distress related to sexual self-image.

The sexual health of patients with cancer is an important component of psychosocial management, and disturbance in sexual being can negatively affect psychological health and QOL. Sexual dysfunction related to cancer can occur as a result of the disease or treatment-induced side effects. When performing a sexual assessment, clinicians should use an integrated approach that incorporates physical, psychological, relational, social, and cultural components (Bober & Varela, 2012). Pretreatment sexual assessments can be helpful to establish a baseline with which to compare the degree of post-treatment changes (Chen, Clark, & Talcott, 2009). Sexual side effects will vary depending on the type of cancer and the specific treatment modalities used. Female breast cancer survivors often experience vaginal dryness or pain, hot flashes, decreased sexual desire, weight gain, loss of sensation (e.g., nipple), fatigue, and body image concerns. Negative emotions, including anxiety and depression, also are common (Ussher, Perz, & Gilbert, 2012). A major concern in young breast cancer survivors may be related to issues of infertility and delayed childbearing. Contraception is strongly encouraged during systemic or radiation treatment because of possible teratogenic effects to the fetus (Stan et al., 2013). Male prostate cancer survivors often experience prostatectomy-induced erectile dysfunction, loss of penile length, and loss of desire. Hormonal therapy in men can cause loss of libido, hot flashes, fatigue, gynecomastia, and emotional lability (Bober & Varela, 2012; Sadovsky et al., 2010).

Having an open discussion with patients about common sexual health issues is extremely important before, during, and after cancer treatment. Before treatment begins, patients should be educated about the common sexual side effects associated with their treatment. They also should be routinely assessed during and after treatment for any problems that may arise. Healthcare professionals often are reluctant to discuss issues related to sexuality for reasons including embarrassment or discomfort, limited knowledge, lack of time, fear of causing offense or invading privacy, not feeling it is a priority, personal attitudes, and the belief that patients are too sick to be interested (Dyer & das Nair, 2013; Zeng, Liu, & Loke, 2012). Suggestions to help overcome some of these barriers include recognizing that this is an important part of patients' QOL; acknowledging that the discussion may be awkward at first but should become easier with practice; establishing a structure for the conversation; becoming knowledgeable about the topic; and developing an awareness of personal beliefs, opinions, and biases. Figure 17-3 lists tips that APNs may find helpful in communicating with patients about sexual health. Role playing with colleagues is an excellent way to practice communication skills and develop confidence in a safe environment.

Several models have been developed to help nurses communicate more effectively about sexual health and to provide a structure to help guide the conversation. The PLISSIT model (Annon, 1976)—Permission, Limited Information, Specific Suggestions, and Intensive Therapy—provides an intervention framework to guide nurses through sexual counseling. *Permission* encourages nurses to allow patients to express their feelings and concerns by providing an open and trusting environment. *Limited information* refers to patient education regarding the sexual side effects of medication and treatment. At this step, the nurse clarifies any fears and misconceptions that the patient verbalizes and validates specific symptoms that may interfere with sexuality (e.g., fatigue, pain). *Specific suggestions* can be provided after a thorough sexual health history that includes the patient's attitudes, beliefs, and baseline sexual functioning. The nurse can provide the patient with strategies for improving sexual functioning and expression within the physical demands of the illness and treatment. In addition to assessment of treatment-related physical changes, a thorough sexual assessment must take into consideration all the psychological vari-

---

Start with a normalizing statement to open the conversation: "Many patients have questions about sexual activity during cancer treatment," or "Sometimes the medications we use to treat cancer can have an effect on sexual function."

Ask permission to discuss: "There is some information about this topic that I would like to share with you. Is this a good time?"

Respect the patient's privacy: "Would you like your family, partner, friend, etc., to step out of the room?"

Use neutral language: Speak about your patient's "partner" rather than his or her "spouse, husband/wife," etc.

Provide information based on the patient's needs: "I understand you have been experiencing vaginal dryness. I have some information for you on vaginal moisturizers and lubricants."

Convey importance of sexual health and encourage questions at any time: "Do you have any questions or sexual concerns that you would like to discuss? This is an important topic and no question is silly or off limits."

Figure 17-3. Tips to Ease Communication When Discussing Sexual Health

ables that may negatively affect sexuality, such as fear, anxiety, and depression. *Intensive therapy* may be indicated for more severe psychosocial or sexual issues that are beyond the knowledge and comfort level of the nurse and may include referral to a social worker, psychologist, psychiatrist, gynecologist, sexual health specialist, fertility specialist, or physical therapist.

Personal Control

A sense of personal control is the perception that one's behaviors and choices, rather than fate, can bring about positive outcomes and avoid life-threatening situations, such as the diagnosis of cancer (Henselmans, Sanderman, Baas, Smink, & Ranchor, 2009). The perception of personal control may be emotionally shattered for individuals who have made healthy lifestyle choices but find themselves confronting a diagnosis of cancer. Perception of control enables individuals to feel that they can change their life circumstances or their psychological responses to these circumstances. Feelings of control are shaped by individual and situational differences. Understanding the function of control is critical to supporting the coping process (Mystakidou et al., 2012; Wicks & Mitchell, 2010).

Social learning theory and the theory of learned helplessness provide the framework for research on perceived control and the concept of powerlessness (Vollmayr & Gass, 2013). Feelings of powerlessness are situationally determined (e.g., traumatic event such as a cancer diagnosis) but often are influenced by the individual's locus of control. Individuals who have an internal locus of control believe that their choices and behaviors affect outcomes, whereas individuals with an external locus of control believe that outcomes are dependent on the behavior of others or by fate (Wicks & Mitchell, 2010). Behavior is explained by a continuous interaction between internal and external controls (Mystakidou et al., 2012). Patients with cancer with a high internal locus of control regarding the course of their illness are associated with having a positive attitude, higher self-esteem, greater social support, and less anxiety, depression, and physical complaints. Religious control or having a sense of spiritual well-being can serve as a coping mechanism during terminal illness. On the contrary, those who had a low internal locus of control regarding the cause of their disease were associated with feelings of hopelessness and a belief that they caused their illness (Mystakidou et al., 2012).

Other variables, such as age and culture, can affect locus of control. Adolescents and older adults (age 65 and older) with cancer and other chronic illness have been associated with having a more external locus of control (Henninger, Whitson, Cohen, & Ariely, 2012; Wicks & Mitchell, 2010). Japanese people have a more external locus of control compared those in the United States (Mystakidou et al., 2012). By interacting with patients and allowing them to express their feelings, fears, and needs, APNs can help identify their strengths. In addition, by helping them focus attention away from uncontrollable aspects of their illness and direct their energy to aspects they can control, APNs enable patients to become active participants in their care, thus enhancing their sense of personal control. Figure 17-4 provides interventions aimed at enhancing personal control.

Spiritual Distress

In a 2013 International Consensus Conference, spirituality was defined as "a dynamic and intrinsic aspect of humanity through which persons seek ultimate meaning, purpose, and transcendence, and experience relationship to self, family, others, community, society, nature, and the significant or sacred. Spirituality is expressed through beliefs, values, traditions, and

- Involve patients in treatment-related discussions and decision making.
- Openly address patient fears and concerns.
- Provide viable options with comprehensive explanations to allow patients to make optimal choices.
- Respect patients' choices.
- Encourage patients to maintain personal relationships and religious/spiritual beliefs.
- Help patients to identify and focus on their strengths.
- Provide means to enable patients to maintain their independence.

Figure 17-4. Interventions to Enhance Personal Control

practices" (Puchalski, Vitillo, Hull, & Reller, 2014, p. 646). These can include religious practices, meditation, nature, or art (Peteet & Balboni, 2013).

A life-threatening disease such as cancer often challenges the basic components of spirituality. When individuals are forced to confront their own mortality, it may motivate them to question their own spiritual beliefs. Fears brought on by the disease and treatment also may cause spiritual distress in people. Painful or distressing spiritual responses to cancer include feeling abandoned by God, feeling abandoned by spiritual communities, questioning God's love or power, feeling punished, or never working through the anguish and finding meaning in their experience (Alcorn et al., 2010).

Addressing the spiritual needs of patients and families, particularly those approaching the end of life, is an important component of providing holistic care. Studies have shown that many patients facing a life-threatening illness wanted their healthcare team to recognize and support their spiritual and religious needs, but these needs were often not addressed. Failing to address the spiritual needs of patients can lead to depression and a decreased sense of purpose, meaning, and peace (Pearce, Coan, Herndon, Koenig, & Abernethy, 2012; Williams, Meltzer, Arora, Chung, & Curlin, 2011; Winkelman et al., 2011). Alternatively, providing spiritual care has been shown to improve QOL, improve coping with symptoms, and help with decision making near the end of life (El Nawawi, Balboni, & Balboni, 2012). The FICA (Faith, Belief, and Values; Importance and Influence; Community; Address) spiritual assessment tool is based on four domains of spirituality and uses open-ended questions (Borneman, Ferrell, & Puchalski, 2010).

Many patients are able to process their spiritual pain and find positive meaning to the cancer experience. A variety of themes have emerged in patients who have achieved spiritual well-being, including feeling empowered by having a positive attitude; feeling fortunate in life; having faith in their healers; leading an active, full life; gaining strength through religious faith; having a greater appreciation in life (being given a second chance); and gaining personal satisfaction by helping others (Bulkley et al., 2013). Patients with cancer have expressed that the experience has helped them to transcend their own lives, enabling them to understand others better and give back or help others (e.g., empathy and compassion). Taking on this broader life perspective or purpose has been described as *self-transcendence* (Williams, 2012). The experience of self-transcendence often underlies patients' desire to volunteer to help other patients with cancer, for example, becoming an ACS Reach to Recovery® volunteer or participating in clinical trials to support future research.

Risk Factors for Psychosocial Disturbance

All patients diagnosed with cancer are at risk for experiencing psychosocial distress ranging from normal fear resulting from the uncertainty of disease to severe distress such as panic and spiritual crisis. Surveys of people with newly diagnosed and recurrent cancer have demonstrated that 20%–47% of patients show a significant level of distress at some point along the cancer trajectory (NCCN, 2015). Patients are especially vulnerable at major transition points in the disease continuum: workup and diagnosis, treatment cycles, the end of treatment, follow-up office visits, recurrence and progression of disease, treatment failure, and awareness of end of life (Wagner, Spiegel, & Pearman, 2013). Numerous personality characteristics, such as ineffective coping styles, may place patients at an increased risk for distress, as well as disease- or treatment-related stressors, such as body image changes or uncontrolled symptoms. Comorbid conditions also increase patients' risk for psychosocial distress. These include physical illnesses, such as renal, cardiac, pulmonary, and endocrine diseases, or mental illness, such as anxiety, depression, or substance abuse. Additional risk factors include being female, being a younger age, having young children, living alone, and having a history of prior physical or sexual abuse (NCCN, 2015).

Psychosocial distress that goes unrecognized and untreated may negatively affect patients' adherence to treatment, QOL, and survival (Buchmann, Conlee, Hunt, Agarwal, & White, 2013; Kissane, 2009). In August 2012, the American College of Surgeons Commission on Cancer issued new accreditation standards for hospital cancer programs. The standards of care have been developed by the Distress Management Panel of NCCN and include guidelines for recognizing, monitoring, documenting, and promptly treating distress at all stages of disease and in all settings (NCCN, 2015).

All patients should be screened for distress at their initial visit and at appropriate intervals as clinically determined (NCCN, 2015). This initial psychosocial assessment can help to identify those patients who are experiencing moderate to severe distress early on in their care. This is especially important because studies have shown that patients with cancer have a higher rate of suicide than the general population (Crocetti et al., 2012), and this risk peaks within the first year of diagnosis (Anguiano et al., 2012; Johnson, Garlow, Brawley, & Master, 2012).

Symptoms related to disease and treatment must be differentiated from psychological symptoms of distress. Physical side effects of treatment may mimic physical symptoms associated with distress (e.g., anorexia, weight loss, insomnia, fatigue). Signs among older adults will be more complex as a result of comorbid diseases or dementia, anxiety, alcohol or benzodiazepine use, or symptoms of psychosis (Downing et al., 2013). Therefore, in patients with cancer, assessment should focus on symptoms that affect appearance, behavior, or cognition and symptoms that are a change from the patients' previous level of functioning (e.g., guilt, crying, pessimism, hopelessness, flat affect, slowed speech, labile emotions; problems with concentrating and decision making).

Coping and Adaptation

Coping with cancer is a process, and as patients' illness demands change over time, so will their coping methods. Each of the stages of cancer requires different coping skills from patients. Patterns of distress are heightened at major transition points (Artherholt & Fann, 2012). In an investigation of the coping process in adults with leukemia undergoing stem cell transplantation, "fear of death" reached its highest level at diagnosis and immediately before transplantation. After chemotherapy and transplantation, it decreased significantly (Farsi, Nayeri, & Negarandeh, 2012).

Coping has been defined as the thoughts and behaviors people use in an effort to prevent or diminish threat, harm, and loss, or to reduce associated distress (Carver & Connor-Smith, 2010; Folkman, 2010). Coping is a complex, ever-changing dynamic that is influenced by the type and severity of the stressor (context), individual differences (personality traits), and previous coping strategies (Carver & Connor-Smith, 2010). There is no "right" or "wrong" way to cope. Coping and adaptation to illness also depend on patients' psychological makeup, cultural identity, and their available social support resources (Farsi et al., 2012). Each person will respond to the cancer experience based on his or her own reality. Personality characteristics, such as how prone a person is to anxiety and depression, optimism versus pessimism, hardiness and ego strength, and locus of control, will influence coping responses.

Optimism refers to people's generalized positive expectancies about future events (Applebaum et al., 2013). Patients who are optimists suffer fewer emotional consequences from adversity and cope more actively because they reframe stressful events related to a self-image of control and efficacy. Optimism has been linked to better physical well-being, emotional well-being, and more effective coping strategies (Carver, Scheier, & Segerstrom, 2010; Christianson et al., 2013). Optimistic individuals are more likely to engage in proactive coping strategies (e.g., planning, seeking support) rather than avoidance coping strategies (e.g., denial, isolation) when confronted with a threat or challenge (Goodin & Bulls, 2013). *Ego strength* is a resiliency trait that engages the person to master the stress being confronted (Sheppard, Llanos, Hurtado-de-Mendoza, Taylor, & Adams-Campbell, 2013). Individuals with an internal locus of control are more likely to cope by becoming a participant in their care plan and by taking responsibility for their own health (Mystakidou et al., 2012). Positive assets, including self-acceptance, having a purpose in life with hopes and goals, having inner spirituality, maintaining positive relationships, and having a desire for personal growth, can help people with cancer to thrive and maintain resiliency even in the face of a terminal illness.

Lazarus and Folkman's framework commonly is used as a basis for stress and coping research (Lazarus & Folkman, 1984). The theoretical principle underlying this model is that how people evaluate or appraise the challenge at hand determines their emotional and behavioral responses to stress. *Primary appraisal* incorporates the personal meaning of the stressful event as threatening or challenging and is influenced by a person's beliefs, values, and goals. *Secondary appraisal* incorporates a person's evaluation of the options for coping and is determined by the situation and the available resources for coping (physical, psychological, material, and spiritual) (Folkman, 2010). *Self-efficacy*, defined as people's confidence in their ability to carry out the necessary behaviors and skills to overcome a threat, has been shown to positively influence the appraisal process (Schumacher, Sauerland, Silling, Berdel, & Stelljes, 2014). Coping styles, such as taking on a fighting spirit versus a fatalistic or stoic acceptance, also influence the appraisal process.

Once a situation has been appraised, a person may use different styles of coping, including problem-focused, emotion-focused, or meaning-focused coping. While each is an independent category, they often complement one another and are highly interactive (Folkman, 2010). *Problem-focused coping* is directed at taking steps to remove a stressor or to diminish its impact, using strategies such as seeking information about the challenge and decision making. Inherent in taking direct action against the stressor is the individual's need to feel empowered and in control of the situation.

Maintaining emotional equilibrium and safety is another function of coping. Cognitive processes, such as fears, feelings, and worries, influence the emotional responses to stress. *Emotion-focused coping* is aimed at minimizing negative emotions and may include strategies such as crying, seeking emotional support, distancing oneself, accepting responsibility, and performing positive reappraisal (Folkman, 2010). Even denial in the early stages of diagnosis can help individuals from becoming overwhelmed with fear and anxiety. If the intensity and duration of emotion-focused coping causes individuals to disengage mentally or physically from the threatening situation, then this becomes *avoidance-focused coping*. In a study examining the relationship between coping styles and emotional adjustment in patients with cancer, those who used avoidance-style coping strategies, such as behavioral disengagement, were associated with poor emotional adjustment. In contrast, those who used acceptance and humor were associated with high levels of positive emotion (Shapiro, McCue, Heyman, Dey, & Haller, 2010).

Another form of coping, *meaning-focused coping*, was later introduced into the model by findings that positive and negative emotions can occur simultaneously in extremely stressful times, such as when terminal patients are near death. As opposed to emotion-focused coping that regulates negative emotions, meaning-focused coping is one in which people draw on their deeply held values and beliefs to help them focus on the positive aspects of the experience. They may focus on their strengths, reorganize their goals, or reprioritize what is important (Carver & Connor-Smith, 2010; Folkman, 2008, 2010).

The process of adapting to the experience of cancer and treatment requires an adjustment to a changing reality. Each major transition point in the cancer continuum (e.g., diagnosis, recurrence, terminal disease) can be a crisis or an opportunity for growth. At the initial completion of cancer treatment, patients often reflect, "What shall I do with my life now?" A changed reality becomes a catalyst for adaptive adjustment. Integration of a new reality consists of dealing with the stress of uncertainty and ambiguity about the future, reintegration of a new body image and self-image, disruption of sexuality and intimacy, and self-consciousness in relationships and social situations. Returning to normalcy does not mean returning to the same place or identity (Murph, 2010; Street et al., 2010).

The personal meaning of the cancer experience demands that assessment and interventions to support coping must be directed at those variables that strongly affect patients' emotional and behavioral responses. This includes stage of disease and treatment, any comorbid illnesses, management of disease- and treatment-related symptoms, family and social support, gender and developmental life stage, culture and ethnicity, spirituality and hopefulness, and survivorship. Assessment also must include the phase of the disease being experienced along the illness continuum and how coping challenges change over time. Psychosocial interventions should then be both individualized and targeted to points in time when they are most needed (Folkman, 2010). Focusing on individual outcomes rather than on specific coping strategies and aiming interventions at modifiable stressors ensures the most effective way to support adaptation.

Symptoms experienced with cancer and treatment may negatively affect patients' ability to cope. Newly diagnosed younger patients with breast cancer have expressed emotional distress related to menopausal symptoms, such as hot flashes and insomnia, and chemotherapy-related fatigue and neuropathies that interfere with their daily functioning and activity levels (Stan et al., 2013). Women experiencing recurrent ovarian cancer have reported difficulty coping with feelings of hopelessness and helplessness as a result of the side effects of progressive disease and treatments (Price et al., 2013).

As discussed previously, coping is influenced by patients' appraisal of the disease and treatment challenges. This appraisal also may directly affect side effect and symptom experiences. In adults who underwent hematopoietic stem cell transplantation, the use of avoidant style coping significantly predicted that symptoms of the skin, eye, mouth, and gastrointestinal tract, as well as cognitive symptoms (e.g., fear, worry), highly interfered with their lives six months after treatment (Schoulte, Lohnberg, Tallman, & Altmaier, 2011). This highlights the importance for healthcare professionals to not only assess which symptoms are present, but also how much these symptoms interfere with daily activities. Another study showed that "learned resourcefulness," a personality characteristic related to coping, was associated with a decrease in chemotherapy-related fatigue. Learned resourcefulness is the behavioral and cognitive skills acquired to regulate internal events such as emotions (Menshadi, Bar-Tal, & Barnoy, 2013). Resourceful people have more adaptive functioning and enhanced self-help actions.

Gender and Developmental Life Stage

Other contributing factors for psychological distress during the cancer experience include gender and developmental life stage. Rates of depression vary across the life span, and depression occurs differently among men and women. A significantly higher rate of clinical depression has been reported in women as compared to men, with varying reported prevalence rates (Moser, Künzler, Nussbeck, Bargetzi, & Znoj, 2013; Rich, Byrne, Curryer, Byles, & Loxton, 2013). The theoretical basis for this difference is that both biologic and social factors contribute to increased rates of depression in women.

Women have differences in brain structure and function, different genetic factors, and hormonal fluctuations across the reproductive life span that increase their vulnerability to depression. Cancer treatments, such as certain chemotherapy agents, also may contribute to depression by placing women in premature, unnatural menopause. Psychosocial factors that increase women's risk for depression include gender differences in roles, socialization, coping styles, and economic and social status (Leach, Christensen, Mackinnon, Windsor, & Butterworth, 2008).

Men may rely on suppressing their emotions to avoid the risk of appearing "unmanly" and to preserve their masculine image (Hoyt, Stanton, Irwin, & Thomas, 2013). Valued norms of masculinity may include self-reliance, dominance, control, competitiveness, ability to be a provider, and restraint from showing dependence or vulnerability (Zaider, Manne, Nelson, Mulhall, & Kissane, 2012). Of grave concern is that suicide can be a symptom or consequence of depression, and in the United States, men are four times more likely than women to die of suicide. Men found to be at particularly high risk were those 65 years and older who had prostate, lung, head and neck, or pancreatic cancer (Anguiano et al., 2012).

Stereotypes of men and women play a role in gender-based coping. Stereotypes support the beliefs that men are rational, independent, and competitive, whereas women are emotional, dependent, sensitive, and nurturing (Allen & Smith, 2011). Therefore, emotion-focused coping is expected to be used more often by women than men. A cancer diagnosis may bring a display of emotion from a woman, whereas a man may act stoic to remain in control. More often, men use problem-focused coping styles or even denial and avoidance to prevent relinquishing control and independence. Growing evidence shows that in terminally ill patients, the prevalence of depression in men is closer to that in women and may even exceed it. In one palliative care setting, levels of depression were significantly higher in men who were dependent on others to assist them with basic tasks (eating, bathing, using the toilet) compared to women (Hayes et al., 2012). APNs must be aware of and avoid using gender-based stereotypes when assessing coping styles. Assessment and interventions are most effective when based on individuals' personality and methods to cope with crises in the past.

Age and developmental life stage also influence coping and adaptation. The risk of psychological distress increases when life tasks are interrupted at any given age (Maurice-Stam, Verhoof, Caron, & Grootenhuis, 2013). Young adult cancer survivors are often less autonomous, more dependent on their parents, and more socially isolated during transition to adulthood (D'Agostino & Edelstein, 2013). Inherent developmental challenges exist that individuals must resolve at each stage of psychological growth, and cancer can disrupt emotional development and the resolution of life goals (Maurice-Stam et al., 2013; Verhoof, Maurice-Stam, Heymans, & Grootenhuis, 2013).

Disruption of these tasks may negatively affect patients' abilities to cope and to feel hopeful about their future. One study showed that adolescents and young adults experienced psychological distress at the time of cancer diagnosis that exceeded population norms. The symptoms decreased at the 6-month follow-up, but again exceeded population norms at the 12-month follow-up (Kwak et al., 2013), highlighting that at vulnerable transition points (i.e., diagnosis and transition to survivorship), distress can be intensified. In a study of adolescents and young adults (ages 15–30), receiving the news of a cancer diagnosis put them at substantially increased risk of suicidal behavior (completed or attempted suicide), especially within the first year of diagnosis (Lu et al., 2013). Older adults may be less apt to recognize and report psychological symptoms caused by cumulative physical and social losses throughout their life span (e.g., bereavement in older adults increases their risk for chronic depression). Whether patients are young or old, the reordering of priorities and revision of life goals constitute part of the reappraisal of the event as an opportunity for growth, rather than only as a loss.

Culture and Ethnicity

Culture prescribes the beliefs, values, norms, and practices of a group of people, providing identity, meaning, and purpose to their lives. The experience of cancer cannot be understood as an event separate from the cultural context and ethnic identity of the patient. The multidimensional aspects of culture, including language, environment, social structure, religion/worldview, and economy, also can influence the way people choose to be cared for and how they cope with the cancer experience (Lopez-Class et al., 2011). Cultural competency has become a necessity to ensure that quality health care is provided to the nation's increasingly diverse populations and communities. The components of cultural competence include assessment and interventions based on a framework that includes the patient's cultural identity, age, gender, sexual orientation, disabilities, cultural explanations of the patient's illness, cultural factors related to psychosocial functioning and the social environment, and the cultural exchange between the patient and the healthcare provider (Epner & Baile, 2012; Kersey-Matusiak, 2012). Socioeconomic status is an important component. Poverty, unemployment, homelessness, immigration status, lack of social support, and level of education can potentially affect access to care and an individual's understanding and use of available resources and interventions (Kersey-Matusiak, 2012; Marshall et al., 2011).

Symptom assessment and management is an important component of decreasing distress and providing quality care, yet sociocultural factors may influence the way patients perceive and report symptoms, such as pain. Factors may include difficulty communicating, cultural barriers to reporting symptoms, and different cultural norms about expressing pain (Boehmer, Glickman, Winter, & Clark, 2013). Asian patients often view cancer pain as a universal, natural, and inevitable reaction of the body to cancer and also fear that pain medication will cause drug tolerance and addiction. These barriers contribute to a reluctance to report pain and use prescribed analgesics, therefore resulting in inadequate pain control (Chen, Tang, & Chen, 2012; Im, Liu, Kim, & Chee, 2008). This highlights the importance of assessing these patients for perceived pain barriers and providing education to eradicate misconceptions.

Psychosocial assessment within a sociocultural framework may be most effective by considering an individual's or family's perception of a stress or problem, how they are experiencing the problem, and how they express their emotions, rather than searching for distinct entities or definitions of a disorder (Marshall et al., 2011). How the healthcare provider relates to the patient and the provider's own perception and understanding of the problem are important variables (Kersey-Matusiak, 2012). See Figure 17-5 for guidelines for cultural competence.

- Accept that all people have value and are worthy of respect.
- Explore and acknowledge your own beliefs and values, biases, and prejudices.
- Respect religious and cultural norms regarding touch, eye contact, or treatment by the opposite sex.
- Acknowledge and be respectful of patient beliefs regarding alternative treatments or traditional healers.
- Learn the appropriate cultural greeting for patients according to their belief system as a means of establishing rapport and trust.
- Determine patients' preferred language prior to assessment, and arrange for a medical interpreter when appropriate.
- Regardless of education, socioeconomic status, culture, and ethnicity, all people have strengths that can be identified and built upon.
- Negotiate a treatment plan that negotiates patients' value system and lifestyle within acceptable standards of American health care.
- Apply cross-cultural interview techniques to avoid stereotyping. Question patients about beliefs relating to disease causation, treatment, and cure.
- Educate yourself regarding the culture, traditions, rules of interaction, family and social roles, health and illness beliefs, and practices of the populations you serve.
- If legally possible, honor patients' and families' values regarding decision-making practices and preferences regarding the disclosure of bad news and truth-telling.
- Understand that the combined concepts of culture, perceptual worldview, and health and illness beliefs are fundamental to the provision of culturally competent nursing care.

Figure 17-5. Guidelines for Cultural Competence

Note. Based on information from Salimbene, 2006.

Family Systems

Cancer is experienced by patients and families interdependently, and thus, the family is the "unit of care" (Northouse, 2012). Family systems theory provides a framework to assess the impact of cancer on the family (Mehta et al., 2009). A family is defined as a social system with shared goals, beliefs, and history, and within the family, each member acts independently but also as part of the family unit. Therefore, a life-threatening illness such as cancer will affect not only the patient but also family members, particularly those who have direct caregiving responsibilities. Family members of a loved one who has cancer are often so affected by the cancer experience that they also can be considered cancer survivors (Marshall et al., 2011).

An assumption underlying family systems theory is that a homeostatic state or balancing of forces exists within every family—family rules, member roles, subsystems, and boundaries—and expectations exist within the family to ensure internal equilibrium (Mehta et al., 2009). Family homeostasis can be disrupted at any time along the major transition points of the cancer experience, placing the family in a crisis state. Family subsystems and boundaries can be predictive of how patients and family members will cope. If the family is an open system, they will be more adaptable and open to change without losing their unity and will seek out resources and accept contact with other systems more readily. Closed family units are rigid, lack flexibility for adaptation, and are less accepting of contact with other systems (Mehta et al., 2009).

Family roles, rules, and myths are socially, culturally, and gender based. Caregiving has been shown to be more stressful for women (wives or daughters), particularly younger women, than for men (husbands and sons) (Romito, Goldzweig, Cormio, Hagedoorn, & Andersen, 2013). One study showed that men (spouse or partner) in a caregiver role dealt with caregiving issues in a fashion that remained consistent with their masculine role, including being the stronger person in the relationship, focusing on tasks, minimizing disruptions, and keeping their stress to themselves (Lopez, Copp, & Molassiotis, 2012). Older adults, male or female, also are at greater risk for caregiver stress. In addition to the distress associated with caregiving, older adults may be dealing with their own new or worsening comorbidities (Romito et al., 2013). When families are confronting cancer, family roles and rules also will influence communication and decision making. Certain cultures have practices regarding the disclosure of bad news. For example, in China, the decision of whether to disclose a cancer diagnosis to a patient is based on the preference of the family, not the patient (Li, J., et al., 2012). Additionally, a cancer diagnosis will challenge the developmental stage of the family. If cancer occurs during childbearing years, a young couple may face infertility challenges or stressors while balancing work and parenting, in addition to other challenges (Carter, Stabile, Gunn, & Sonoda, 2013).

The impact of cancer on the family will continue as changes in healthcare delivery result in more patients being cared for in the home setting and with family members becoming the primary caregivers. Families must cope not only with the emotional responses to the cancer experience but also with the social, physical, and financial aspects of providing care to their loved ones. Research focused on family caregivers has shown that family members feel ill prepared, have insufficient knowledge, and feel that they receive little support from the healthcare system (Northouse, 2012). The families of long-term cancer survivors have reported that high levels of distress are experienced not only at the initial diagnosis and treatment stage but may last up to five years after diagnosis because of the ongoing challenges of the disease (Kim, Kashy, Spillers, & Evans, 2010). Research is ongoing to identify the impact of distress on families and to identify healthcare interventions that support family coping and adaptation. Guidelines for providing patient and family caregiver support are outlined in Figure 17-6. APNs are in a pivotal role to improve clinical outcomes for patients by identifying the physical, spiritual, and emotional needs of the family unit. Some simple questions to ask the family include "How is this affecting you?", "What information or help do you need?", and "What are you doing to take care of yourself?" (Northouse, 2012).

Social Support

Social support has been shown to buffer the negative effects of cancer by providing direct intervention through physical and emotional support (Applebaum et al., 2013). According to Lazarus and Folkman's cognitive model of stress and coping, when a person is dealing with a stressful event such as cancer, social support can directly influence the person's adjustment

---

- Recognize the importance of the interdependent relationship between patients and their family caregivers.
- Treat patients and caregivers as a single unit of care. This will result in a synergistic effect that will result in improved care for patients and caregivers.
- Identify and acknowledge assets and strengths of patients and caregivers to build confidence and encourage self-efficacy.
- Encourage open communication and mutual support among patients, caregivers, and healthcare professionals. Use three-way communication to simultaneously interact with patients and caregivers to allow each a better understanding of one another's thoughts and concerns.
- Encourage patients and caregivers to set short-term goals.
- Assess physical and emotional symptoms of both patients and caregivers and offer strategies for self-management.
- Encourage active coping strategies, healthy lifestyles, and stress reduction activities to improve overall quality of life for both patients and caregivers.
- Provide information and support to patients and their caregivers. Educate as to specific websites or organizations they can access for information and support.

Figure 17-6. Guidelines for Providing Patient and Family Caregiver Support

---

Note. Based on information from Northouse, 2012.

(Lazarus & Folkman, 1984). Social support consists of two components: structural and functional. The structural component consists of the network of relationships that exist between people (e.g., family, friends, coworkers), which binds them to their community. The functional component includes the type of support provided. This can include emotional, instrumental (tangible), or informational (educational) support (Chou, Stewart, Wild, & Bloom, 2012). Interpersonal relationships, such as family, friends, and spiritual leaders who provide emotional support through love, nurturance, acceptance, and intimacy, can validate to patients that they are valued and that their feelings are accepted and understood. Community and religious resources can provide the person with a social identity and sense of belonging. Instrumental support includes resources such as financial assistance, transportation to medical appointments, physical goods, or services that individuals may receive from their network of relationships (e.g., family, friends, coworkers, church members, ACS). Informational support refers to providing knowledge to individuals that is relevant to the situation. Healthcare providers play a major role in informational support by providing patients with the knowledge and skills needed for effective decision making and coping. Participation in cancer support groups can provide both informational and emotional support. In addition, support groups can help prevent feelings of isolation by providing individuals with the opportunity to share experiences with others (Emilsson, Svensk, Tavelin, & Lindh, 2012). The Internet has become another important vehicle for meeting the psychosocial needs of patients. Internet communications can minimize feelings of isolation, provide a forum to share cancer treatment experiences, and provide hope by making the most current information available. It also is easily accessible and can allow an individual to maintain privacy and anonymity (Yli-Uotila, Rantanen, & Suominen, 2013).

Social support promotes the use of positive coping strategies (Chou et al., 2012), but the effectiveness of social support must be evaluated as to whether it has been tailored to the patient's individual needs and situation, in addition to what, and how strongly, the patient *perceives* his or her social support to be (Drageset, Lindstrøm, Giske, & Underlid, 2012). Perceived social support is the perception of the availability and adequacy of support from close relationships and the satisfaction with the amount and quality of support (Yang et al., 2013). Lower levels of perceived social support have been associated with low QOL (Eom et al., 2013). For example, in a study that identified the predictors of continued smoking in cancer survivors, those with low perceived social support were more likely to continue smoking (Yang et al., 2013).

APNs need to understand and respect the diversity among ethnic populations and be aware that social support will be defined within their cultural perspective. For example, Jordanian women used spiritual meaning to cope with their illness. They did this by talking to God, praying to God, and having their supportive network pray for them (Alqaissi & Dickerson, 2010). In the Latino culture, people have a strong identification and attachment to both their immediate and extended family. While both Latino men and women with cancer benefited from family support, the loss of their traditional gender roles was very distressing. In women, this pertained to the role of caregiver (Lopez-Class et al., 2011), and in men, it was the role of provider (Carrion et al., 2013). Healthcare providers must identify psychosocial support needs in multiethnic populations in order to provide culturally sensitive interventions for these patients.

Spirituality

From the time of initial diagnosis until the end of life, patients are faced with spiritual issues that may lead to spiritual distress or a strengthening of the spirit. Illness heightens spiritual awareness and the use of spiritual coping strategies (Puchalski, 2012). In the realm of suffering, loss, dying, and death, many individuals turn to their faith, religion, or God for comfort (Puchalski, 2012). Therefore, spiritual care is a vital component of quality oncology nursing care throughout the disease trajectory. Spiritual care focuses on meeting the spiritual needs of patients: finding meaning and purpose, hopefulness, relatedness, forgiveness or acceptance, and transcendence (Puchalski, 2012). APNs can provide spiritual care through empathic listening and by helping patients to process the meaning of their illness as it relates to their beliefs, life experiences, and religious practices. Nurses need to validate patients' spiritual needs by encouraging activities of self-expression, such as meditation and prayer; storytelling (e.g., life review); journal writing; music, art, or dance therapy; and being with nature.

Some of the reasons why oncology nurses fail to address their patients' spiritual needs include time restraints, ambiguity about their own spiritual beliefs, lack of confidence, and lack of knowledge regarding the nurse's role in spiritual care (Puchalski, 2012). Oncology APNs are in a prime position to educate other oncology nurses regarding spiritual assessment and the effect that spirituality has on patients' coping with their illness. APNs also are educated to include spiritual assessment as part of overall psychosocial management and refer patients to spiritual counselors, chaplains, and clergy when needed. A quick spiritual screening can entail a few simple questions, such as "Is spirituality or religion important in your life?" and "How well are those resources working for you at this time?" (Puchalski et al., 2009).

The importance of addressing the spiritual concerns of oncology professionals, in addition to those of patients and families, is becoming recognized. Oncology nurses, particularly those who work in palliative care settings and experience many patient deaths, are at personal risk for existential suffering and distress (Ferrell, Otis-Green, & Economou, 2013). Therefore, a support mechanism for the staff should be implemented in oncology settings.

Evidence-Based Treatment Strategies

Management of disease-related and treatment-related symptoms can have a direct impact on patient coping and adaptation. Debilitating symptoms such as pain, fatigue, anxiety, and depression must be effectively managed to provide comprehensive psychosocial care to patients. Uncontrolled physical symptoms, such as pain, account for high rates of suicide and requests for assisted suicide in patients with cancer (Cooke, Gotto, Mayorga, Grant, & Lynn, 2013).

Supportive cancer care has been defined as the necessary services for those people with or affected by cancer to meet a continuum of needs—social, practical, physical, spiritual, emotional, informational, and psychological—throughout the full continuum of living as a cancer survivor (Fitch, 2012). The goals of supportive care are to assist patients in meeting their psychosocial needs, maintaining or improving their QOL, and optimizing their sense of well-being. Supportive care should be directed at the expressed needs of both patients and families and continually monitored and adapted as the course of the disease and treatment unfolds. Each transition point along the cancer continuum will demand new knowledge, new skills, and different networks of support to meet the changing demands of illness, whether it is acute, chronic, or palliative. Supportive care consists of pharmacologic, nonpharmacologic, and programmatic approaches to psychosocial support.

Pharmacologic Interventions

A thorough health history and physical examination must be performed prior to initiation of pharmacologic interventions for psychosocial distress. If possible, assessment should include a family member, as many patients are not aware of changes in their affect or behavior or may minimize their feelings for fear of being stigmatized or viewed as being emotionally weak. If depression, anxiety, or any associated symptom, such as insomnia, is being caused by an underlying problem (e.g., a medical condition, medication side effect, withdrawal from alcohol or narcotics, distressing physical symptoms such as pain), the underlying problem must be identified and treated. The patient can then be assessed for mood disorder before treatments are initiated. Treatment for mood or anxiety disorders should include a multimodality approach: pharmacologic management, individual or family counseling or psychotherapy, cognitive and behavioral interventions, and complementary therapies.

In the cancer population, the medications used most often for depression and anxiety include a class of drugs called the selective serotonin reuptake inhibitors (SSRIs). General side effects of SSRIs include agitation, gastrointestinal disturbance, and sexual dysfunction. However, because SSRIs block the reuptake of only one neurotransmitter in the CNS (serotonin), they frequently are the medication of choice for depression because of their low side effect profile and their low potential for overdose. SSRIs also are the drug of choice for patients experiencing symptoms of both depression and anxiety (Li, M., et al., 2012; Traeger et al., 2012). Citalopram and escitalopram are generally first-line choices because they are well tolerated and have few interactions with other drugs. Paroxetine, fluoxetine, and sertraline should be avoided in patients taking tamoxifen because they inhibit CYP2D6, the enzyme that converts tamoxifen to its active metabolite, endoxifen (Fisher et al., 2013).

Pharmacotherapy also may be chosen to manage some treatment-induced side effects. Venlafaxine, a serotonin-norepinephrine reuptake inhibitor (SNRI), is used to reduce chemotherapy-induced menopausal symptoms, such as mood swings, hot flashes, and insomnia. SNRIs block the reuptake of both serotonin and norepinephrine in the CNS. Duloxetine, a newer antidepressant, is effective against depression, generalized anxiety disorder, and neuropathic pain, which is a fairly common symptom profile in the cancer population. Bupropion, a norepinephrine and dopamine reuptake inhibitor, has proved to be effective for symptoms such as prominent fatigue, cognitive slowing, or pseudodementia, or in patients who are concerned about sexual dysfunction from the SSRIs (Li, M., et al., 2012). These examples point out that for therapeutic results, matching the pharmacologic profile of the drug or drug combination with the patient's clinical profile is an important criterion for successful treatment (Li, M., et al., 2012).

Psychostimulants such as methylphenidate also may have a role in treating depression because of their rapid onset and ability to improve mood, energy levels, concentration, and attention span (Li, M., et al., 2012). Psychostimulants can be effective adjuncts in pain management because they counteract opioid-induced sedation and improve mood (Li, M., et al., 2012). Side effects of psychostimulants include insomnia, tachycardia, and agitation and therefore may exacerbate anxiety associated with depression. Psychostimulants generally are ordered to be given early in the day to avoid insomnia.

Antidepressant therapy is effective for both depressive and anxious states, but benzodiazepines are used most often to treat transient states of anxiety. This classification of drugs also is used for treating insomnia, chemotherapy-related nausea and vomiting, and treatment-related fears and phobias, such as claustrophobia associated with magnetic resonance imaging, and as premedication for unpleasant procedures, such as bone marrow aspiration. Lorazepam usually is the drug of choice because its short half-life is unaffected by age, liver disease, or the concurrent use of an SSRI. The amnesic effect of benzodiazepines may be beneficial for patients who experience anticipatory nausea and vomiting but may be contraindicated in patients who suffer from chemotherapy-related cognitive dysfunction. These medications must be used with extreme caution in older adults because they can increase the risk of confusion, night wandering, and loss of balance, leading to an increase in falls (Traeger et al., 2012). Because episodes of anxiety usually are acute, benzodiazepines can be used to provide immediate relief but should then be discontinued. Figure 17-7 outlines various pharmacologic interventions to treat mood disorders and treatment-related side effects.

Nonpharmacologic Interventions

An integrated and patient-centered approach to psychosocial care is required to provide comprehensive, quality cancer care (Li, M., et al., 2012). This includes both pharmacologic and nonpharmacologic interventions tailored to meet the physical and psychological needs of patients. Initiation of medication is recommended if patients are immobilized by depression or anxiety, as it is difficult for patients to engage in nonpharmacologic activities or programs until their symptoms are controlled and they have adequate energy and focus to learn and participate. Individual counseling or psychotherapy can be very effective to support patients in the initial six to eight weeks until antidepressant therapy becomes fully effective. Individual counseling or psychotherapy should be continued as long as it meets patients' emotional needs.

Integrative oncology is the use of complementary therapies to enhance physical strength and emotional well-being and to manage symptoms, such as pain (Deng & Cassileth, 2013). The term *integrative* implies that standard, conventional care is combined with complementary therapies using a multidimensional and holistic approach to health and healing (Deng & Cassileth, 2013). The acronym *CAM*, for *complementary and alternative medicine*, has been used extensively in the literature to describe this integrative approach; however, the term is misleading. Complementary therapies are used *to supplement* conventional therapies, whereas alternative therapies are used *instead of* conventional therapies (Deng & Cassileth, 2013; Rosenthal & Doherty-Gilman, 2011). Alternative therapies are often unproven and can potentially cause

---

Antidepressants
- Selective serotonin reuptake inhibitors: Block the reuptake of serotonin in the central nervous system. Also useful as an adjunct for the treatment of anxiety.
  - Citalopram (Celexa®), escitalopram (Lexapro®): First-line choices.
  - Paroxetine (Paxil®), fluoxetine (Prozac®), sertraline (Zoloft®): Avoid in patients taking tamoxifen.
- Selective norepinephrine reuptake inhibitors: Block the reuptake of both serotonin and norepinephrine in the central nervous system.
  - Venlafaxine (Effexor®), duloxetine (Cymbalta®): Effective for treatment-induced side effects.
- Bupropion (Wellbutrin®): Activating antidepressant. Weak inhibitor of neuronal reuptake of norepinephrine and dopamine. Does not inhibit reuptake of serotonin. Is effective for fatigue and cognitive slowing. Rarely causes weight gain or sexual dysfunction. Avoid if anxiety accompanies depression.

Psychostimulants
- Have a rapid onset, elevate energy levels, and improve concentration and attention.
- Generally are not first-line treatment but may be beneficial in depression and fatigue.
- Beneficial effects may be limited by side effects of insomnia, agitation, and anxiety.
  - Methylphenidate (Ritalin®)

Anxiolytics (Antianxiety)
- Benzodiazepines: Useful for treatment of transient anxiety, insomnia, and chemotherapy-related nausea and vomiting.
  - Lorazepam (Ativan®), alprazolam (Xanax®): Shortest half-lives.
  - Clonazepam (Klonopin®): Longest half-life.

Figure 17-7. Pharmacologic Interventions for Mood Disorders

Note. Based on information from Li, M., et al., 2012; Traeger et al., 2012.

harm to patients. The deleterious effect of stress and negative mood states on immune function and health outcomes provides the basis for many of these nonpharmacologic interventions (Chandwani et al., 2012). Complementary approaches that can help modulate the immune response include mind-body therapies, which influence interactions among the mind, body, and behavior; manipulative and body-based therapies; and physical activity. Acupuncture, a mind-body therapy, is an effective adjuvant treatment in reducing chemotherapy-induced nausea and vomiting. Studies are ongoing to determine its efficacy in reducing symptoms such as pain, insomnia, anxiety, hot flashes, lymphedema, and radiation-induced xerostomia (Garcia et al., 2013; Lu & Rosenthal, 2013). Alternative approaches include unapproved or harmful cancer prevention diets, herbal and natural products, and miraculous cancer cures (Chandwani et al., 2012; Deng & Cassileth, 2013).

The effective implementation of integrative therapies has been found to relieve physical symptoms and psychological distress in addition to giving patients a feeling of personal control over their illness (Chandwani et al., 2012). However, patients who are using alternative therapies often do not disclose this information to healthcare professionals. Reasons may include that they were never asked about them, an unawareness that the information is important and may affect their cancer treatment, and fear of disapproval from their healthcare team.

It is important that APNs inquire as to whether patients are using complementary or alternative therapies. When asking about their medications, APNs should specifically ask patients if they are using any nonprescription medications, vitamins, or herbal supplements or if they are on a special diet. Patients often think that it is only important to disclose their prescribed medications. APNs also should provide education about any contraindications in the use of these preparations or techniques based on the patient's conventional treatments. Many resources are available for healthcare providers and the public to learn more about therapies such as the National Center for Complementary and Integrative Health, a scientific branch of the National Institutes of Health (Deng & Cassileth, 2013). Figure 17-8 outlines various complementary and alternative therapies.

Programmatic Interventions

Cancer programs provide basic information and practical support to patients with cancer and their families. Programmatic interventions range from one-to-one peer support, such as ACS's Reach to Recovery program, to individual and family support groups, such as those provided by the Cancer Support Community, and support groups accessed via the Internet. Programmatic support for patients with cancer can be found on the local, state, and national levels. These programs form a network of services for social support ranging from instrumental support (e.g., equipment) to informational support (education). ACS has been a leader in providing a broad range of social services to patients with cancer. ACS's I Can Cope® program is an excellent example of an effective programmatic approach that involves both an informational and psychosocial dimension. These types of psychoeducational approaches have been shown to provide patients with the knowledge and skills necessary for problem-focused coping and stress management, in turn increasing their sense of control and competency. A wide variety of types of support programs are available, and all of them can be effective and help patients and families to cope. The choice of the right type of support can be tailored to individual patients based on their needs and preferences.

Hopefulness

Hope is a multidimensional, dynamic life force. Defining hope is a complex endeavor, as the term has many different interpretations, meanings, and usages. Hope has been described in

Definitions
- **Standard Care:** Recommended treatment based on scientific evidence (chemotherapy, radiation, biologic therapy, surgery)
- **Complementary:** Therapies used to *supplement* standard care
- **Alternative:** Therapies used *instead of* standard care

Key Points
- No scientific evidence supports complementary or alternative therapies as curative of cancer.
- Use of alternative therapies that delay standard cancer treatment may decrease chances for remission or cure.
- "Natural" does not mean "safe." Dietary supplements (herbs, supplements, special diets) may cause harm or may interfere with effectiveness of standard therapies.
- Some adjunctive complementary therapies may help patients better tolerate disease symptoms and side effects and improve quality of life.

Examples of Therapies
- Complementary
  - Massage/touch therapies
    * Focus on musculoskeletal system and connective tissue to reduce stress
    * Massage, reflexology, Reiki therapy, manual lymph drainage
  - Mind-body therapies
    * Enable the mind to interact with body and behavior
    * Acupuncture, meditation, relaxation techniques, hypnosis, yoga, tai chi, mindfulness-based therapy, music therapy, art therapy, guided imagery, biofeedback
  - Physical fitness and movement: Aerobics, dance therapy, body conditioning
  - Special diets, vitamins, herbal supplements: As recommended by healthcare team in conjunction with standard therapies
- Alternative
  - "Miraculous cures," "secret ingredients," "ancient remedies"
  - Unapproved or dangerous anticancer diets
  - Dietary supplements, herbs, "natural" products with unproven efficacy or dangerous side effects

Figure 17-8. Standard Versus Complementary and Alternative Therapies

Note. Based on information from Chandwani et al., 2012; Deng & Cassileth, 2013.

the nursing literature as having a dimension of "being" (positive feeling deep inside oneself); a dimension of "doing" (goal setting); a dimension of "becoming" (anticipating future possibilities); and a "relational" dimension (having meaningful relationships, feeling needed and loved) (Hammer, Mogensen, & Hall, 2009).

Hope can be both specific and generalized. Specific hope is connected to time and object. A person may hope that a new treatment will prevent progression of disease. If the treatment is not effective, a more generalized hope, based on faith, personality disposition, or developmental history, can act as a reserve to prevent a person from giving up (e.g., "God will help me through this") (Folkman, 2010; Hammer et al., 2009).

The context of hope may change throughout the cancer trajectory, but its vital force can still exist regardless of disease stage or a patient's care goals. Positive relationships have been found between hope and coping style and effectiveness, regardless of diagnosis, gender, age, marital status, or education. Hope positively influences adaptation to cancer. Hopelessness contributes to anxiety, depression, and feelings that self and life are worthless. At the extreme, hopelessness can contribute to suicide or consideration of physician-assisted suicide toward the end of life (Anguiano et al., 2012).

APNs can foster hope in patients, even at the end of life, by affirming their worth, creating a partnership, allowing them to express their emotions, and encouraging them to share their fears and goals. In interviews to understand the perspectives of palliative care nurses on hope, the nurses reported that having hope themselves helped foster positive relationships, provided comfort, and offered hope to patients and their families (Mok et al., 2010).

Standards of Practice

The NCCN Clinical Practice Guidelines in Oncology are recognized standards for clinical policy and practice in the oncology community. These comprehensive guidelines are based on scientific data and are supported by an expert panel of multidisciplinary physicians and other healthcare professionals from NCCN member institutions. The guidelines address supportive care areas, including distress management (NCCN, 2015). To guide evidence-based practice, NCCN has formulated standards of care for psychosocial management of patients with cancer and has provided algorithms for assessment, treatment, and management. NCCN advises that nurses and all multidisciplinary team members must be responsible for assessing patients with cancer for symptoms of distress.

Other standards of care for assessment and intervention have been provided by the American Psychiatric Association (2013) and the Oncology Nursing Society (Brant & Wickham, 2013). Standards of practice are supported by scientific research, and these guidelines support evidence-based practice for APNs.

Patient and Family Education

Because cancer affects the entire family, education that includes the family unit is an essential role of APNs. Learning who the patient's family is can be accomplished by asking the patient a simple question: "Who do you consider your family?" An initial screening tool such as the NCCN (2015) Distress Thermometer can be useful to help identify a patient's level of distress and whether referral for additional support is needed. If the distress level is high, the APN can determine which referral would be most appropriate based on the problem area specified on the screening tool (e.g., spiritual/religious concerns indicate referral to chaplain).

APNs should educate patients and families about what to expect throughout the cancer experience, including the impact of the disease, treatment, and side effects on patients' physical, psychological, and spiritual health. Evidence-based practice guidelines, such as those from NCCN, can provide APNs with the tools and skills to guide assessment and interventions.

The emotional responses to the diagnosis of cancer often make patients feel as though they are "going crazy" or are out of control. Educating patients and family members regarding the expected emotional reactions to a cancer diagnosis, such as fear, shock, anxiety, and disbelief, will normalize their feelings and give them permission to share. When appropriate, APNs should educate patients and family members regarding the signs and symptoms of anxiety and depression, the risk factors, and the professional resources available to help them. Healthcare providers should involve patients and family members in decision making and problem solving regarding their disease status and treatment to support their sense of control, autonomy, and self-esteem. They also should inform patients that emotional support and peer information are available through programs such as Reach to Recovery and CanSurmount. Patients requiring ongoing counseling or psychotherapy for emotional, spiritual, or psychosocial distress should be referred immediately. One-to-one intervention can provide patients with cognitive behavioral therapy techniques to reframe their experiences and decrease feelings of powerlessness. APNs can encourage patients and family members to participate in psychoeducational programs such as the Cancer Support Community and I Can Cope to gain both educational and emotional support.

The goals of psychosocial education are to enable patients and families to integrate the experience of cancer and maintain a good QOL. Education includes providing a safe and supportive environment for patients to talk about the personal issues important to them. A nonjudgmental approach communicates interest and concern. APNs should take cues from patients and family members and start at a point of factual information and move from less sensitive to more sensitive areas when talking to patients about psychosocial issues. Patients' privacy and respect must be honored to prevent them from feeling embarrassment or self-blame. Patients should receive education regarding ways to increase resilience to psychosocial problems, including nutrition, exercise, good sleeping habits, stress management, and the importance of open communication with healthcare providers and family members regarding their feelings and emotions.

Implications for Oncology Advanced Practice Nurses

Early psychosocial assessment can provide the healthcare team with objective information regarding the general concerns and coping skills of patients and families. Signs and symptoms of emotional or social problems may be less obvious or more difficult to identify than those of a physical nature. A concerted effort to evaluate patients and family members holistically will help to ensure that all their needs can be identified and met. If not identified and supported, emotions can occupy patients' thoughts and expend their mental energy and will not only interfere with coping effectiveness but also may increase somatic complaints and experiences. Early psychosocial interventions can prevent the exacerbation of preexisting levels of distress or psychological illness. Educational programs for APNs provide the theoretical knowledge base and clinical experience to ensure that they have the expertise to perform high-level psychosocial assessments and to plan and provide high-level interventions based on scientific data and standards of practice. APNs also can be effective role models for other nurses, healthcare professionals, and family members in addressing and dealing with patients' strong emotional reactions to a cancer diagnosis. APNs play an integral role in the QOL of patients with cancer and their families by intervening to ensure balance in their emotional, psychological, spiritual, and social lives, as well as in their physical care. Nurses hone these skills over time with consistent application of psychosocial principles of care and by continuing professional education in all aspects of quality patient care. Psychosocial assessment must be a fundamental part of new patient assessments, as well as ongoing interactions. Modeling this assessment behavior and intervention techniques for colleagues and family members will support patients and help to foster a therapeutic healthcare environment.

Conclusion

With technologic advancements in prevention, diagnosis, and treatment, many patients diagnosed with cancer will be long-term survivors of this chronic illness. In addition to extending how long people live with cancer, the goal of providing psychosocial care is to improve how well they live. The importance of addressing the psychosocial needs of patients and their families is now recognized, as evidenced by the hospital accreditation standards released by the American College of Surgeons Commission on Cancer in 2012 that include screening of all patients with cancer for psychosocial distress (Wagner et al., 2013). Developing systems within each hospital setting to successfully implement these standards will be vital to ensure that the psychosocial needs of patients are adequately met.

Case Study

P.B. is a 45-year-old carpenter. He has been married for 15 years and has no children. During the past few months, P.B. has been struggling at his job because of increasing episodes of coughing, fatigue, and shortness of breath with mild exertion. His wife also has noticed that his appetite has been decreasing and all he wants to do at home is lie on the couch and watch TV. His wife finally insists that he make an appointment with his medical doctor. A chest x-ray reveals a lung nodule that also is seen on a subsequent chest computed tomography scan and read as suspicious. A biopsy of the lung nodule reveals a non-small cell lung cancer, and P.B. is referred to an oncologist to discuss treatment options.

When taking the patient's history, the APN learns that P.B. had one son who was killed in an automobile accident at age nine. Since then, P.B. has been suffering from depression but often forgets to take his antidepressant medication. He is an active smoker and has smoked a pack of cigarettes per day since age 25. He also drinks a few beers in the evening to help him unwind. When asked about his current symptoms, P.B. states, "What difference does it make? This is all my fault, and there is nothing I can do about it. God is punishing me because if I was with my son that day, he never would have been in that accident. I deserve to die, so maybe I should just speed up the process. Even God has abandoned me." P.B.'s wife, who is with him, begins to cry and states, "I am here for you." He just shrugs his shoulders and remains silent.

1. What nursing diagnosis would the APN identify from P.B.'s assessment?
   - P.B. has long-standing depression with expressions of guilt and self-blame over his son's death. Other diagnoses include hopelessness and powerlessness, spiritual distress, and risk for suicide. Hopelessness and powerlessness are expressed by the statement "This is all my fault, and there is nothing I can do about it." Spiritual distress is expressed by his feeling of being punished and abandoned by God. Finally, the risk of suicide must be taken seriously when an individual states, "I deserve to die, so maybe I should just speed up the process." This is even more concerning considering his history of depression.

2. What interventions are appropriate to address the identified diagnoses?
   - The APN should set up an immediate referral for psychiatric evaluation. P.B.'s recent diagnosis of lung cancer, guilt over his son's death, spiritual distress over feeling punished and abandoned by God, feelings of hopelessness and powerlessness, and suicidal ideation are all cause for significant concern. In addition, he does not take his antidepressant medication consistently.
   - The APN should assess the physical and emotional symptoms of both P.B. and his wife and offer management strategies for both of them. For example, caregivers often focus on the patient's needs while neglecting their own. Caregivers must be encouraged to take care of their own health needs and take time for themselves.
   - To decrease P.B. and his wife's feelings of hopelessness and powerlessness, the APN can help them identify things they still hope for and enjoy and can help them develop short-term goals. The APN can help foster hope by affirming P.B.'s worth as an individual and encouraging him to express his emotions, fears, and goals. Through empathic listening, the APN can help him process the meaning of the illness and identify spiritual comfort measures, such as praying or talking with a spiritual counselor.
   - Interventions to enhance personal control should be provided, such as encouraging P.B. and his wife to ask questions, maintaining open communication, involving them in treatment-related discussions and decision making, and helping them identify and focus on their

strengths. Providing information about the disease and treatment is important at diagnosis and should be reinforced at each phase of treatment to prevent knowledge deficit. Enabling P.B. to maintain his independence whenever feasible and respecting his choices also can enhance feelings of control.

3. What intervention is necessary when P.B. states that he forgets to take his antidepressant medication?
   • The APN must assess P.B.'s knowledge about the purpose and side effects of the antidepressant and try to understand why he forgets to take it. The patient can then be instructed how it should be taken to ensure effectiveness (i.e., on a daily basis, not once in a while). The APN can provide suggestions to help him remember, for example, putting the medication in a daily pillbox and placing it on top of something he uses every day, such as his keys. The APN can reinforce for P.B. the positive outcomes of pharmacologic treatment for his depression when it is taken correctly.

4. What nonpharmacologic interventions can the APN suggest?
   • In addition to the antidepressant medication prescribed, the APN can help P.B. identify and reach out to his supportive network, which may include his wife, other family members, friends, coworkers, and members of his religious community. The APN could suggest therapeutic resources, such as the Cancer Support Community and Cancer*Care*, for both individual and family support. The APN should encourage P.B. to replace his smoking and beer drinking with healthier habits, and he should be referred to a smoking cessation program. Information should be provided about complementary therapies, such as guided imagery, acupuncture, relaxation techniques, massage, and hypnosis.

Key Points

• Anxiety is a normal emotional response to the cancer experience.
• Anxiety and depression often coexist.
• An individual does not choose to be anxious or depressed; these responses are situational and biologic in nature.
• Delirium is a common acute cognitive dysfunction in the cancer population and must be differentiated from depression and dementia.
• Variables that affect the emotional response to cancer include personal control, self-esteem, sexuality and altered body image, spirituality, and a history of prior anxiety or depressive disorders.
• Variables that influence coping and adaptation to the cancer experience include prior psychosocial risk factors, family systems, social support, culture and ethnicity, and spirituality.
• Both pharmacologic and nonpharmacologic interventions play an important role in the psychosocial support of patients with cancer.
• Psychosocial nursing is holistic care for the body, mind, and spirit.

Recommended Resources for Oncology Advanced Practice Nurses

• ACS (www.cancer.org): ACS provides patient and family services through counseling services and educational programs.
• Cancer*Care* (www.cancercare.org): This organization provides free support, information, and financial assistance to patients and families.

- Cancer Support Community (www.cancersupportcommunity.org): Site provides free psychological help and emotional support to cancer survivors and their family members and caregivers through support groups, psychoeducational workshops, and nutritional and educational guidance.
- CURE: Cancer Updates, Research and Education (www.curetoday.com): CURE combines the science and humanity of cancer by providing education and resources to a half million survivors through its free magazine and publications.
- Livestrong Fertility (www.livestrong.org/we-can-help/fertility-services): This subunit of the Livestrong Foundation website is dedicated to educating patients about fertility issues related to cancer and treatment.
- Livestrong Foundation (www.livestrong.org): This organization assists patients and families through advocacy, education, research, and public education.
- National Cancer Institute (www.cancer.gov): This comprehensive resource site provides information about cancer prevention, treatment, and clinical trials, along with providing links to cancer centers.
- NCCN (www.nccn.org): NCCN is a nonprofit alliance of 26 of the world's leading cancer centers dedicated to the quality of care provided to patients with cancer. NCCN resources include guidelines for psychosocial care.
- National Coalition for Cancer Survivorship (www.canceradvocacy.org): This organization provides advocacy and resources for cancer survivors with a focus on QOL issues.

The author would like to acknowledge Nancy Jo Bush, RN, MN, MA, AOCN®, for her contribution to this chapter that remains unchanged from the first edition of this book.

References

Ahles, T.A., Saykin, A.J., McDonald, B.C., Li, Y., Furstenberg, C.T., Hanscom, B.S., … Kaufman, P.A. (2010). Longitudinal assessment of cognitive changes associated with adjuvant treatment for breast cancer: Impact of age and cognitive reserve. *Journal of Clinical Oncology, 28,* 4434–4440. doi:10.1200/JCO.2009.27.0827

Alcorn, S.R., Balboni, M.J., Prigerson, H.G., Reynolds, A., Phelps, A.C., Wright, A.A., … Balboni, T.A. (2010). "If God wanted me yesterday, I wouldn't be here today": Religious and spiritual themes in patients' experiences of advanced cancer. *Journal of Palliative Medicine, 13,* 581–588. doi:10.1089/jpm.2009.0343

Allen, J., & Smith, J.L. (2011). The influence of sexuality stereotypes on men's experience of gender-role incongruence. *Psychology of Men and Masculinity, 12,* 77–96. doi:10.1037/a0019678

Alqaissi, N.M., & Dickerson, S.S. (2010). Exploring common meanings of social support as experienced by Jordanian women with breast cancer. *Cancer Nursing, 33,* 353–361. doi:10.1097/NCC.0b013e3181d55d33

American Cancer Society. (2011). Sexuality for the woman with cancer. Atlanta, GA: Author.

American Psychiatric Association. (2013). *Diagnostic and statistical manual of mental disorders* (5th ed.). Washington, DC: Author.

Andreasen, N.C. (2010). Posttraumatic stress disorder: A history and a critique. *Annals of the New York Academy of Sciences, 1208,* 67–71. doi:10.1111/j.1749-6632.2010.05699.x

Anguiano, L., Mayer, D.K., Piven, M.L., & Rosenstein, D. (2012). A literature review of suicide in cancer patients. *Cancer Nursing, 35*(4), E14–E26. doi:10.1097/NCC.0b013e31822fc76c

Annon, J.S. (1976). The PLISSIT model: A proposed conceptual scheme for the behavioral treatment of sexual problems. *Journal of Sex Education and Therapy, 2*(1), 1–15. doi:10.1080/01614576.1976.11074483

Applebaum, A.J., Stein, E.M., Lord-Bessen, J., Pessin, H., Rosenfeld, B., & Breitbart, W. (2013). Optimism, social support, and mental health outcomes in patients with advanced cancer. *Psycho-Oncology, 23,* 299–306. doi:10.1002/pon.3418

Artherholt, S.B., & Fann, J.R. (2012). Psychosocial care in cancer. *Current Psychiatry Reports, 14,* 23–29. doi:10.1007/s11920-011-0246-7

Bender, C.M., & Thelen, B.D. (2013). Cancer and cognitive changes: The complexity of the problem. *Seminars in Oncology Nursing, 29,* 232–237. doi:10.1016/j.soncn.2013.08.003

Bober, S.L., & Varela, V.S. (2012). Sexuality in adult cancer survivors: Challenges and intervention. *Journal of Clinical Oncology, 30,* 3712–3719. doi:10.1200/JCO.2012.41.7915

Boehmer, U., Glickman, M., Winter, M., & Clark, M.A. (2013). Long-term breast cancer survivors' symptoms and morbidity: Differences by sexual orientation? *Journal of Cancer Survivorship, 7,* 203–210. doi:10.1007/s11764-012-0260-8

Borneman, T., Ferrell, B., & Puchalski, C.M. (2010). Evaluation of the FICA tool for spiritual assessment. *Journal of Pain and Symptom Management, 40,* 163–173. doi:10.1016/j.jpainsymman.2009.12.019

Brant, J.M., & Wickham, R. (Eds.). (2013). *Statement on the scope and standards of oncology nursing practice: Generalist and advanced practice.* Pittsburgh, PA: Oncology Nursing Society.

Brenne, E., Loge, J.H., Kaasa, S., Heitzer, E., Knudsen, A.K., & Wasteson, E. (2013). Depressed patients with incurable cancer: Which depressive symptoms do they experience? *Palliative and Supportive Care,* 491–501. doi:10.1017/S1478951512000909

Buchmann, L., Conlee, J., Hunt, J., Agarwal, J., & White, S. (2013). Psychosocial distress is prevalent in head and neck cancer patients. *Laryngoscope, 123,* 1424–1429. doi:10.1002/lary.23886

Bulkley, J., McMullen, C.K., Hornbrook, M.C., Grant, M., Altschuler, A., Wendel, C.S., & Krouse, R.S. (2013). Spiritual well-being in long-term colorectal cancer survivors with ostomies. *Psycho-Oncology, 22,* 2513–2521. doi:10.1002/pon.3318

Carrion, I.V., Nedjat-Haiem, F.R., & Marquez, D.X. (2013). Examining cultural factors that influence treatment decisions: A pilot study of Latino men with cancer. *Journal of Cancer Education, 28,* 729–737. doi:10.1007/s13187-013-0522-9

Carter, J., Stabile, C., Gunn, A., & Sonoda, Y. (2013). The physical consequences of gynecologic cancer surgery and their impact on sexual, emotional, and quality of life issues. *Journal of Sexual Medicine, 10*(Suppl. 1), 21–34. doi:10.1111/jsm.12002

Carver, C.S., & Connor-Smith, J. (2010). Personality and coping. *Annual Review of Psychology, 61,* 679–704. doi:10.1146/annurev.psych.093008.100352

Carver, C.S., Scheier, M.F., & Segerstrom, S.C. (2010). Optimism. *Clinical Psychology Review, 30,* 879–889. doi:10.1016/j.cpr.2010.01.006

Chandwani, K.D., Ryan, J.L., Peppone, L.J., Janelsins, M.M., Sprod, L.K., Devine, K., … Mustian, K.M. (2012). Cancer-related stress and complementary and alternative medicine: A review. *Evidence-Based Complementary Alternative Medicine, 2012,* Article 979213. doi:10.1155/2012/979213

Chen, C.H., Tang, S.T., & Chen, C.H. (2012). Meta-analysis of cultural differences in Western and Asian patient-perceived barriers to managing cancer pain. *Palliative Medicine, 26,* 206–221. doi:10.1177/0269216311402711

Chen, R.C., Clark, J.A., & Talcott, J.A. (2009). Individualizing quality-of-life outcomes reporting: How localized prostate cancer treatments affect patients with different levels of baseline urinary, bowel, and sexual function. *Journal of Clinical Oncology, 27,* 3916–3922. doi:10.1200/JCO.2008.18.6486

Chou, A.F., Stewart, S.L., Wild, R.C., & Bloom, J.R. (2012). Social support and survival in young women with breast carcinoma. *Psycho-Oncology, 21,* 125–133. doi:10.1002/pon.1863

Christianson, H.F., Weis, J.M., & Fouad, N.A. (2013). Cognitive adaptation theory and quality of life in late-stage cancer patients. *Journal of Psychosocial Oncology, 31,* 266–281. doi:10.1080/07347332.2013.778936

Cooke, L., Gotto, J., Mayorga, L., Grant, M., & Lynn, R. (2013). What do I say? Suicide assessment and management [Online exclusive]. *Clinical Journal of Oncology Nursing, 17,* E1–E7. doi:10.1188/13.CJON.E1-E7

Costa-Requena, G., Cristófol, R., & Cañete, J. (2012). Caregivers' morbidity in palliative care unit: Predicting by gender, age, burden and self-esteem. *Supportive Care in Cancer, 20,* 1465–1470. doi:10.1007/s00520-011-1233-6

Crocetti, E., Buzzoni, C., Caldarella, A., Intrieri, T., Manneschi, G., Sacchettini, C., … Miccinesi, G. (2012). [Suicide mortality among cancer patients]. *Epidemiologia e Prevenzione, 36,* 83–87.

D'Agostino, N.M., & Edelstein, K. (2013). Psychosocial challenges and resource needs of young adult cancer survivors: Implications for program development. *Journal of Psychosocial Oncology, 31,* 585–600. doi:10.1080/07347332.2013.835018

Deng, G., & Cassileth, B. (2013). Complementary or alternative medicine in cancer care—Myths and realities. *Nature Reviews Clinical Oncology, 10,* 656–664.

Downing, L.J., Caprio, T.V., & Lyness, J.M. (2013). Geriatric psychiatry review: Differential diagnosis and treatment of the 3 D's—delirium, dementia, and depression. *Current Psychiatry Reports, 15,* 365. doi:10.1007/s11920-013-0365-4

Drageset, S., Lindstrøm, T.C., Giske, T., & Underlid, K. (2012). "The support I need": Women's experiences of social support after having received breast cancer diagnosis and awaiting surgery. *Cancer Nursing, 35*(6), E39–E47. doi:10.1097/NCC.0b013e31823634aa

Dyer, K., & das Nair, R. (2013). Why don't healthcare professionals talk about sex? A systematic review of recent qualitative studies conducted in the United Kingdom. *Journal of Sexual Medicine, 10,* 2658–2670. doi:10.1111/j.1743-6109.2012.02856.x

Elklit, A., & Blum, A. (2011). Psychological adjustment one year after the diagnosis of breast cancer: A prototype study of delayed post-traumatic stress disorder. *British Journal of Clinical Psychology, 50,* 350–363. doi:10.1348/014466510X527676

El Nawawi, N.M., Balboni, M.J., & Balboni, T.A. (2012). Palliative care and spiritual care: The crucial role of spiritual care in the care of patients with advanced illness. *Current Opinion in Supportive and Palliative Care, 6,* 269–274. doi:10.1097/SPC.0b013e3283530d13

Emilsson, S., Svensk, A.-C., Tavelin, B., & Lindh, J. (2012). Support group participation during the post-operative radiotherapy period increases levels of coping resources among women with breast cancer. *European Journal of Cancer Care, 21,* 591–598. doi:10.1111/j.1365-2354.2012.01343.x

Eom, C.S., Shin, D.W., Kim, S.Y., Yang, H.K., Jo, H.S., Kweon, S.S., … Park, J.H. (2013). Impact of perceived social support on the mental health and health-related quality of life in cancer patients: Results from a nationwide, multicenter survey in South Korea. *Psycho-Oncology, 22,* 1283–1290. doi:10.1002/pon.3133

Epner, D.E., & Baile, W.F. (2012). Patient-centered care: The key to cultural competence. *Annals of Oncology, 23*(Suppl. 3), 33–42. doi:10.1093/annonc/mds086

Farsi, Z., Nayeri, N.D., & Negarandeh, R. (2012). The coping process in adults with acute leukemia undergoing hematopoietic stem cell transplantation. *Journal of Nursing Research, 20,* 99–109. doi:10.1097/jnr.0b013e318257b5e0

Ferrell, B., Otis-Green, S., & Economou, D. (2013). Spirituality in cancer care at the end of life. *Cancer Journal, 19,* 431–437. doi:10.1097/PPO.0b013e3182a5baa5

Fisher, W.I., Johnson, A.K., Elkins, G.R., Otte, J.L., Burns, D.S., Yu, M., & Carpenter, J.S. (2013). Risk factors, pathophysiology, and treatment of hot flashes in cancer. *CA: A Cancer Journal for Clinicians, 63,* 167–192. doi:10.3322/caac.21171

Fitch, M.I. (2012). Supportive care needs of patients with advanced disease undergoing radiotherapy for symptom control. *Canadian Oncology Nursing Journal, 22,* 84–91. doi:10.5737/1181912x2228491

Folkman, S. (2008). The case for positive emotions in the stress process. *Anxiety, Stress and Coping, 21,* 3–14. doi:10.1080/10615800701740457

Folkman, S. (2010). Stress, coping, and hope. *Psycho-Oncology, 19,* 901–908. doi:10.1002/pon.1836

Freitas, S., Simões, M.R., Alves, L., Duro, D., & Santana, I. (2012). Montreal Cognitive Assessment (MoCA): Validation study for frontotemporal dementia. *Journal of Geriatric Psychiatry and Neurology, 25,* 146–154. doi:10.1177/0891988712455235

Garcia, M.K., McQuade, J., Haddad, R., Patel, S., Lee, R., Yang, P., … Cohen, L. (2013). Systematic review of acupuncture in cancer care: A synthesis of the evidence. *Journal of Clinical Oncology, 31,* 952–960. doi:10.1200/JCO.2012.43.5818

Goodin, B.R., & Bulls, H.W. (2013). Optimism and the experience of pain: Benefits of seeing the glass as half full. *Current Pain and Headache Reports, 17,* 329. doi:10.1007/s11916-013-0329-8

Greene-Schloesser, D.M., Moore, E., & Robbins, M.E. (2013). Molecular pathways: Radiation-induced cognitive impairment. *Clinical Cancer Research, 19,* 2294–2300. doi:10.1158/1078-0432.CCR-11-2903

Hammer, K., Mogensen, O., & Hall, E.O.C. (2009). The meaning of hope in nursing research: A meta-synthesis. *Scandinavian Journal of Caring Sciences, 23,* 549–557. doi:10.1111/j.1471-6712.2008.00635.x

Hayes, R.D., Lee, W., Rayner, L., Price, A., Monroe, B., Hansford, P., … Hotopf, M. (2012). Gender differences in prevalence of depression among patients receiving palliative care: The role of dependency. *Palliative Medicine, 26,* 696–702. doi:10.1177/0269216311416035

Henninger, D.E., Whitson, H.E., Cohen, H.J., & Ariely, D. (2012). Higher medical morbidity burden is associated with external locus of control. *Journal of the American Geriatrics Society, 60,* 751–755. doi:10.1111/j.1532-5415.2012.03904.x

Henselmans, I., Sanderman, R., Baas, P.C., Smink, A., & Ranchor, A.V. (2009). Personal control after a breast cancer diagnosis: Stability and adaptive value. *Psycho-Oncology, 18,* 104–108. doi:10.1002/pon.1333

Holland, J.C., Andersen, B., Breitbart, W.S., Buchmann, L.O., Compas, B., Deshields, T.L., … Freedman-Cass, D.A. (2013). Distress management. *Journal of the National Comprehensive Cancer Network, 11,* 190–209. Retrieved from http://www.jnccn.org/content/11/2/190.long

Hoyt, M.A., Stanton, A.L., Irwin, M.R., & Thomas, K.S. (2013). Cancer-related masculine threat, emotional approach coping, and physical functioning following treatment for prostate cancer. *Health Psychology, 32,* 66–74. doi:10.1037/a0030020

Hurria, A., Somlo, G., & Ahles, T. (2007). Renaming "chemobrain." *Cancer Investigation, 25,* 373–377. doi:10.1080/07357900701506672

Im, E.-O., Liu, Y., Kim, Y.H., & Chee, W. (2008). Asian American cancer patients' pain experience. *Cancer Nursing, 31*(3), E17–E23. doi:10.1097/01.NCC.0000305730.95839.83

Irwin, M.R., Olmstead, R.E., Ganz, P.A., & Haque, R. (2013). Sleep disturbance, inflammation and depression risk in cancer survivors. *Brain, Behavior, and Immunity, 30*(Suppl.), S58–S67. doi:10.1016/j.bbi.2012.05.002

Janelsins, M.C., Kohli, S., Mohile, S.G., Usuki, K., Ahles, T.A., & Morrow, G.R. (2011). An update on cancer- and chemotherapy-related cognitive dysfunction: Current status. *Seminars in Oncology, 38,* 431–438. doi:10.1053/j.seminoncol.2011.03.014

Jansen, C.E. (2013). Cognitive changes associated with cancer and cancer therapy: Patient assessment and education. *Seminars in Oncology Nursing, 29,* 270–279. doi:10.1016/j.soncn.2013.08.007

Jim, H.S.L., Phillips, K.M., Chait, S., Faul, L.A., Popa, M.A., Lee, Y.-H., … Small, B.J. (2012). Meta-analysis of cognitive functioning in breast cancer survivors previously treated with standard-dose chemotherapy. *Journal of Clinical Oncology, 30,* 3578–3587. doi:10.1200/JCO.2011.39.5640

Johnson, T.V., Garlow, S.J., Brawley, O.W., & Master, V.A. (2012). Peak window of suicides occurs within the first month of diagnosis: Implications for clinical oncology. *Psycho-Oncology, 21,* 351–356. doi:10.1002/pon.1905

Kersey-Matusiak, G. (2012). Culturally competent care: Are we there yet? *Nursing Management, 43*(4), 34–39. doi:10.1097/01.NUMA.0000413093.39091.c6

Khasraw, M., & Posner, J.B. (2010). Neurological complications of systemic cancer. *Lancet Neurology, 9,* 1214–1227. doi:10.1016/s1474-4422(10)70220-9

Kim, Y.M., Kashy, D.A., Spillers, R.L., & Evans, T.V. (2010). Needs assessment of family caregivers of cancer survivors: Three cohorts comparison. *Psycho-Oncology, 19,* 573–582. doi:10.1002/pon.1597

Kissane, D. (2009). Beyond the psychotherapy and survival debate: The challenge of social disparity, depression and treatment adherence in psychosocial cancer care. *Psycho-Oncology, 18,* 1–5. doi:10.1002/pon.1493

Kobayashi, M., Ohno, T., Noguchi, W., Matsuda, A., Matsushima, E., Kato, S., & Tsujii, H. (2009). Psychological distress and quality of life in cervical cancer survivors after radiotherapy: Do treatment modalities, disease stage, and self-esteem influence outcomes? *International Journal of Gynecological Cancer, 19,* 1264–1268. doi:10.1111/IGC.0b013e3181a3e124

Kwak, M.Y., Zebrack, B.J., Meeske, K.A., Embry, L., Aguilar, C., Block, R., … Cole, S. (2013). Trajectories of psychological distress in adolescent and young adult patients with cancer: A 1-year longitudinal study. *Journal of Clinical Oncology, 31,* 2160–2166. doi:10.1200/JCO.2012.45.9222

Lazarus, L.S., & Folkman, S. (1984). *Stress, appraisal, and coping.* New York, NY: Springer.

Leach, L.S., Christensen, H., Mackinnon, A.J., Windsor, T.D., & Butterworth, P. (2008). Gender differences in depression and anxiety across the adult lifespan: The role of psychosocial mediators. *Social Psychiatry and Psychiatric Epidemiology, 43,* 983–998. doi:10.1007/s00127-008-0388-z

LeGrand, S.B. (2012). Delirium in palliative medicine: A review. *Journal of Pain and Symptom Management, 44,* 583–594. doi:10.1016/j.jpainsymman.2011.10.013

Li, J., Yuan, X.L., Gao, X.H., Yang, X.M., Jing, P., & Yu, S.Y. (2012). Whether, when, and who to disclose bad news to patients with cancer: A survey in 150 pairs of hospitalized patients with cancer and family members in China. *Psycho-Oncology, 21,* 778–784. doi:10.1002/pon.1979

Li, M., Fitzgerald, P., & Rodin, G. (2012). Evidence-based treatment of depression in patients with cancer. *Journal of Clinical Oncology, 30,* 1187–1196. doi:10.1200/JCO.2011.39.7372

Lim, C.C., Devi, M.K., & Ang, E. (2011). Anxiety in women with breast cancer undergoing treatment: A systematic review. *International Journal of Evidence-Based Healthcare, 9,* 215–235. doi:10.1111/j.1744-1609.2011.00221.x

Lopez, V., Copp, G., & Molassiotis, A. (2012). Male caregivers of patients with breast and gynecologic cancer: Experiences from caring for their spouses and partners. *Cancer Nursing, 35,* 402–410. doi:10.1097/NCC.0b013e318231daf0

Lopez-Class, M., Perret-Gentil, M., Kreling, B., Caicedo, L., Mandelblatt, J., & Graves, K.D. (2011). Quality of life among immigrant Latina breast cancer survivors: Realities of culture and enhancing cancer care. *Journal of Cancer Education, 26,* 724–733. doi:10.1007/s13187-011-0249-4

Lu, D., Fall, K., Sparén, P., Ye, W., Adami, H.-O., Valdimarsdóttir, U., & Fang, F. (2013). Suicide and suicide attempt after a cancer diagnosis among young individuals. *Annals of Oncology, 24,* 3112–3117. doi:10.1093/annonc/mdt415

Lu, W., & Rosenthal, D.S. (2013). Acupuncture for cancer pain and related symptoms. *Current Pain and Headache Reports, 17,* 321. doi:10.1007/s11916-013-0321-3

Lu-Emerson, C., & Eichler, A.F. (2012). Brain metastases. *Continuum, 18,* 295–311. doi:10.1212/01.CON.0000413659.12304.a6

Marshall, C.A., Larkey, L.K., Curran, M.A., Weihs, K.L., Badger, T.A., Armin, J., & García, F. (2011). Considerations of culture and social class for families facing cancer: The need for a new model for health promotion and psychosocial intervention. *Families, Systems, and Health, 29,* 81–94. doi:10.1037/a0023975

Maurice-Stam, H., Verhoof, E.J., Caron, H.N., & Grootenhuis, M.A. (2013). Are survivors of childhood cancer with an unfavourable psychosocial developmental trajectory more likely to apply for disability benefits? *Psycho-Oncology, 22,* 708–714. doi:10.1002/pon.2112

Mehta, A., Cohen, S.R., & Chan, L.S. (2009). Palliative care: A need for a family systems approach. *Palliative and Supportive Care, 7,* 235–243. doi:10.1017/S1478951509000303

Menshadi, N., Bar-Tal, Y., & Barnoy, S. (2013). The relationship between learned resourcefulness and cancer-related fatigue in patients with non-Hodgkin lymphoma. *Oncology Nursing Forum, 40,* 133–138. doi:10.1188/13.ONF .133-138

Mitchell, A.J., Chan, M., Bhatti, H., Halton, M., Grassi, L., Johansen, C., & Meader, N. (2011). Prevalence of depression, anxiety, and adjustment disorder in oncological, haematological, and palliative-care settings: A meta-analysis of 94 interview-based studies. *Lancet Oncology, 12,* 160–174. doi:10.1016/S1470-2045(11)70002-X

Mitchell, A.J., Ferguson, D.W., Gill, J., Paul, J., & Symonds, P. (2013). Depression and anxiety in long-term cancer survivors compared with spouses and healthy controls: A systematic review and meta-analysis. *Lancet Oncology, 14,* 721–732. doi:10.1016/S1470-2045(13)70244-4

Mok, E., Lau, K.P., Lam, W.M., Chan, L.N., Ng, J., & Chan, K.S. (2010). Health-care professionals' perspective on hope in the palliative care setting. *Journal of Palliative Medicine, 13,* 877–883. doi:10.1089/jpm.2009.0393

Moser, M.T., Künzler, A., Nussbeck, F., Bargetzi, M., & Znoj, H.J. (2013). Higher emotional distress in female partners of cancer patients: Prevalence and patient-partner interdependencies in a 3-year cohort. *Psycho-Oncology, 22,* 2693–2701. doi:10.1002/pon.3331

Murph, P. (2010). Psychosocial aspects of cancer care: What does it mean for our patients and families? *Home Healthcare Nurse, 28,* 533–540. doi:10.1097/NHH.0b013e3181f2f3b6

Mystakidou, K., Tsilika, E., Parpa, E., Panagiotou, I., Galanos, A., Gouliamos, A., & Watson, M. (2012). A test of the psychometric properties of the cancer locus of control scale in Greek patients with advanced cancer. *Psycho-Oncology, 21,* 1215–1221. doi:10.1002/pon.2014

National Comprehensive Cancer Network. (2015). *NCCN Clinical Practice Guidelines in Oncology (NCCN Guidelines®): Distress management* [v.1.2015]. Retrieved from http://www.nccn.org/professionals/physician_gls/pdf/ distress.pdf

Nelson, W.L., & Suls, J. (2013). New approaches to understand cognitive changes associated with chemotherapy for non-central nervous system tumors. *Journal of Pain and Symptom Management, 46,* 707–721. doi:10.1016/ j.jpainsymman.2012.11.005

Northouse, L.L. (2012). Helping patients and their family caregivers cope with cancer. *Oncology Nursing Forum, 39,* 500–506. doi:10.1188/12.ONF.500-506

Northouse, L.L., Williams, A.L., Given, B., & McCorkle, R. (2012). Psychosocial care for family caregivers of patients with cancer. *Journal of Clinical Oncology, 30,* 1227–1234. doi:10.1200/JCO.2011.39.5798

Pearce, M.J., Coan, A.D., Herndon, J.E., 2nd, Koenig, H.G., & Abernethy, A.P. (2012). Unmet spiritual care needs impact emotional and spiritual well-being in advanced cancer patients. *Supportive Care in Cancer, 20,* 2269–2276. doi:10.1007/s00520-011-1335-1

Peiffer, A.M., Leyrer, C.M., Greene-Schloesser, D.M., Shing, E., Kearns, W.T., Hinson, W.H., … Chan, M.D. (2013). Neuroanatomical target theory as a predictive model for radiation-induced cognitive decline. *Neurology, 80,* 747–753. doi:10.1212/WNL.0b013e318283bb0a

Peteet, J.R., & Balboni, M.J. (2013). Spirituality and religion in oncology. *CA: A Cancer Journal for Clinicians, 63,* 280–289. doi:10.3322/caac.21187

Posluszny, D.M., Edwards, R.P., Dew, M.A., & Baum, A. (2011). Perceived threat and PTSD symptoms in women undergoing surgery for gynecologic cancer or benign conditions. *Psycho-Oncology, 20,* 783–787. doi:10.1002/ pon.1771

Price, M.A., Bell, M.L., Sommeijer, D.W., Friedlander, M., Stockler, M.R., deFazio, A., … Butow, P.N. (2013). Physical symptoms, coping styles and quality of life in recurrent ovarian cancer: A prospective population-based study over the last year of life. *Gynecologic Oncology, 130,* 162–168. doi:10.1016/j.ygyno.2013.03.031

Puchalski, C.M. (2012). Spirituality in the cancer trajectory. *Annals of Oncology, 23*(Suppl. 3), 49–55. doi:10.1093/ annonc/mds088

Puchalski, C.M., Ferrell, B., Virani, R., Otis-Green, S., Baird, P., Bull, J., … Sulmasy, D. (2009). Improving the quality of spiritual care as a dimension of palliative care: The report of the Consensus Conference. *Journal of Palliative Medicine, 12,* 885–904. doi:10.1089/jpm.2009.0142

Puchalski, C.M., Vitillo, R., Hull, S.K., & Reller, N. (2014). Improving the spiritual dimension of whole person care: Reaching national and international consensus. *Journal of Palliative Medicine, 17,* 642–656. doi:10.1089/ jpm.2014.9427

Rich, J.L., Byrne, J.M., Curryer, C., Byles, J.E., & Loxton, D. (2013). Prevalence and correlates of depression among Australian women: A systematic literature review, January 1999–January 2010. *BMC Research Notes, 6,* 424. doi:10.1186/1756-0500-6-424

Rodríguez, M. (2013). Individual differences in chemotherapy-induced anticipatory nausea. *Frontiers in Psychology, 4,* 502. doi:10.3389/fpsyg.2013.00502

Romito, F., Goldzweig, G., Cormio, C., Hagedoorn, M., & Andersen, B.L. (2013). Informal caregiving for cancer patients. *Cancer, 119,* 2160–2169. doi:10.1002/cncr.28057

Rosenthal, D.S., & Doherty-Gilman, A.M. (2011). Integrative medicine and cancer care. *Virtual Mentor, 13,* 379–383. doi:10.1001/virtualmentor.2011.13.6.msoc1-1106

Sadovsky, R., Basson, R., Krychman, M., Morales, A.M., Schover, L., Wang, R., & Incrocci, L. (2010). Cancer and sexual problems. *Journal of Sexual Medicine, 7,* 349–373. doi:10.1111/j.1743-6109.2009.01620.x

Salimbene, S. (2006). Ten guidelines for culturally and linguistically appropriate care. Retrieved from http://www.medscape.com/viewarticle/544767

Schmitz, A., & Grillon, C. (2012). Assessing fear and anxiety in humans using the threat of predictable and unpredictable aversive events (the NPU-threat test). *Nature Protocols, 7,* 527–532. doi:10.1038/nprot.2012.001

Schoulte, J.C., Lohnberg, J.A., Tallman, B., & Altmaier, E.M. (2011). Influence of coping style on symptom interference among adult recipients of hematopoietic stem cell transplantation. *Oncology Nursing Forum, 38,* 582–586. doi:10.1188/11.ONF.582-586

Schumacher, A., Sauerland, C., Silling, G., Berdel, W.E., & Stelljes, M. (2014). Resilience in patients after allogeneic stem cell transplantation. *Supportive Care in Cancer, 22,* 487–493. doi:10.1007/s00520-013-2001-6

Shapiro, J.P., McCue, K., Heyman, E.N., Dey, T., & Haller, H.S. (2010). Coping-related variables associated with individual differences in adjustment to cancer. *Journal of Psychosocial Oncology, 28,* 1–22. doi:10.1080/07347330903438883

Sheppard, V.B., Llanos, A.A., Hurtado-de-Mendoza, A., Taylor, T.R., & Adams-Campbell, L.L. (2013). Correlates of depressive symptomatology in African-American breast cancer patients. *Journal of Cancer Survivorship, 7,* 292–299. doi:10.1007/s11764-013-0273-y

Southard, N.Z., & Keller, J. (2009). The importance of assessing sexuality: A patient perspective. *Clinical Journal of Oncology Nursing, 13,* 213–217. doi:10.1188/09.CJON.213-217

Stafford, L., Judd, F., Gibson, P., Komiti, A., Mann, G.B., & Quinn, M. (2013). Screening for depression and anxiety in women with breast and gynaecologic cancer: Course and prevalence of morbidity over 12 months. *Psycho-Oncology, 22,* 2071–2078. doi:10.1002/pon.3253

Stan, D., Loprinzi, C.L., & Ruddy, K.J. (2013). Breast cancer survivorship issues. *Hematology/Oncology Clinics of North America, 27,* 805–827. doi:10.1016/j.hoc.2013.05.005

Street, A.F., Couper, J.W., Love, A.W., Bloch, S., Kissane, D.W., & Street, B.C. (2010). Psychosocial adaptation in female partners of men with prostate cancer. *European Journal of Cancer Care, 19,* 234–242. doi:10.1111/j.1365-2354.2008.01012.x

Strout, K.A., & Howard, E.P. (2012). The six dimensions of wellness and cognition in aging adults. *Journal of Holistic Nursing, 30,* 195–204. doi:10.1177/0898010112440883

Tae, Y.S., Heitkemper, M., & Kim, M.Y. (2012). A path analysis: A model of depression in Korean women with breast cancer—mediating effects of self-esteem and hope [Online exclusive]. *Oncology Nursing Forum, 39,* E49–E57. doi:10.1188/12.ONF.E49-E57

Tager, F.A., McKinley, P.S., Schnabel, F.R., El-Tamer, M., Cheung, Y.K., Fang, Y., … Hershman, D.L. (2010). The cognitive effects of chemotherapy in post-menopausal breast cancer patients: A controlled longitudinal study. *Breast Cancer Research and Treatment, 123,* 25–34. doi:10.1007/s10549-009-0606-8

Traeger, L., Greer, J.A., Fernandez-Robles, C., Temel, J.S., & Pirl, W.F. (2012). Evidence-based treatment of anxiety in patients with cancer. *Journal of Clinical Oncology, 30,* 1197–1205. doi:10.1200/JCO.2011.39.5632

Ussher, J.M., Perz, J., & Gilbert, E. (2012). Changes to sexual well-being and intimacy after breast cancer. *Cancer Nursing, 35,* 456–465. doi:10.1097/NCC.0b013e3182395401

Verhoof, E., Maurice-Stam, H., Heymans, H., & Grootenhuis, M. (2013). Health-related quality of life, anxiety and depression in young adults with disability benefits due to childhood-onset somatic conditions. *Child and Adolescent Psychiatry and Mental Health, 7,* 12. doi:10.1186/1753-2000-7-12

Vollmayr, B., & Gass, P. (2013). Learned helplessness: Unique features and translational value of a cognitive depression model. *Cell and Tissue Research, 354,* 171–178. doi:10.1007/s00441-013-1654-2

Wagner, L.I., Spiegel, D., & Pearman, T. (2013). Using the science of psychosocial care to implement the new American College of Surgeons Commission on Cancer distress screening standard. *Journal of the National Comprehensive Cancer Network, 11,* 214–221. Retrieved from http://www.jnccn.org/content/11/2/214.long

Walker, J., Hansen, C.H., Martin, P., Sawhney, A., Thekkumpurath, P., Beale, C., … Sharpe, M. (2013). Prevalence of depression in adults with cancer: A systematic review. *Annals of Oncology, 24,* 895–900. doi:10.1093/annonc/mds575

Wefel, J.S., Saleeba, A.K., Buzdar, A.U., & Meyers, C.A. (2010). Acute and late onset cognitive dysfunction associated with chemotherapy in women with breast cancer. *Cancer, 116,* 3348–3356. doi:10.1002/cncr.25098

Wefel, J.S., & Schagen, S.B. (2012). Chemotherapy-related cognitive dysfunction. *Current Neurology and Neuroscience Reports, 12,* 267–275. doi:10.1007/s11910-012-0264-9

Wefel, J.S., Vardy, J., Ahles, T., & Schagen, S.B. (2011). International Cognition and Cancer Task Force recommendations to harmonise studies of cognitive function in patients with cancer. *Lancet Oncology, 12,* 703–708. doi:10.1016/S1470-2045(10)70294-1

Wicks, L., & Mitchell, A. (2010). The adolescent cancer experience: Loss of control and benefit finding. *European Journal of Cancer Care, 19,* 778–785. doi:10.1111/j.1365-2354.2009.01139.x

Williams, B.J. (2012). Self-transcendence in stem cell transplantation recipients: A phenomenologic inquiry [Online exclusive]. *Oncology Nursing Forum, 39,* E41–E48. doi:10.1188/12.ONF.E41-E48

Williams, J.A., Meltzer, D., Arora, V., Chung, G., & Curlin, F.A. (2011). Attention to inpatients' religious and spiritual concerns: Predictors and association with patient satisfaction. *Journal of General Internal Medicine, 26,* 1265–1271. doi:10.1007/s11606-011-1781-y

Winkelman, W.D., Lauderdale, K., Balboni, M.J., Phelps, A.C., Peteet, J.R., Block, S.D., … Balboni, T.A. (2011). The relationship of spiritual concerns to the quality of life of advanced cancer patients: Preliminary findings. *Journal of Palliative Medicine, 14,* 1022–1028. doi:10.1089/jpm.2010.0536

Yang, H.-K., Shin, D.-W., Park, J.-H., Kim, S.-Y., Eom, C.-S., Kam, S., … Seo, H.-G. (2013). The association between perceived social support and continued smoking in cancer survivors. *Japanese Journal of Clinical Oncology, 43,* 45–54. doi:10.1093/jjco/hys182

Yli-Uotila, T., Rantanen, A., & Suominen, T. (2013). Motives of cancer patients for using the Internet to seek social support. *European Journal of Cancer Care, 22,* 261–271. doi:10.1111/ecc.12025

Zaider, T., Manne, S., Nelson, C., Mulhall, J., & Kissane, D. (2012). Loss of masculine identity, marital affection, and sexual bother in men with localized prostate cancer. *Journal of Sexual Medicine, 9,* 2724–2732. doi:10.1111/j.1743-6109.2012.02897.x

Zeng, Y.C., Liu, X., & Loke, A.Y. (2012). Addressing sexuality issues of women with gynaecological cancer: Chinese nurses' attitudes and practice. *Journal of Advanced Nursing, 68,* 280–292. doi:10.1111/j.1365-2648.2011.05732.x

CHAPTER 18

Cancer Survivorship

Joyce Jackowski, MS, FNP-BC, AOCNP®

Introduction

As cancer survivors live longer after treatment and require ongoing care that focuses on quality of life, efforts are growing to address their needs and provide them with adequate resources. Many survivorship care models have evolved to meet the physical, psychological, social, and spiritual needs of survivors. Employment and insurance issues have presented some unique challenges for oncology advanced practice nurses (APNs). This chapter will address these issues from the historical and present-day perspectives.

Oncology APNs are uniquely prepared to influence survivorship care by applying their knowledge of cancer and health promotion to the period of care beyond active therapy. Oncology APNs can take an active role in rehabilitation and with physicians and mental health colleagues to further education, research, and quality care initiatives, ensuring the best transition for patients after treatment. This chapter also will look at aspects of survivorship, including definition, historical perspective, care models, provision of care, and useful resources for providers and survivors.

Cancer Survivors in the United States

Approximately 1,658,370 Americans will be diagnosed with cancer in 2015 (Siegel, Miller, & Jemal, 2015). This number is predicted to increase with the growing and aging population (Edwards et al., 2002). Advances in early detection and more effective treatments also have resulted in a dramatic increase in the number of cancer survivors (Hewitt, Greenfield, & Stovall, 2006). Statistics show that the majority of people will survive their cancer, with the latest overall relative five-year survival rate from 2005 to 2011 at 66.5% (Howlader et al., 2015). Survival rates for many specific cancers are even higher than that percentage (Siegel et al., 2015). As of January 1, 2014, nearly 14.5 million people with a history of cancer were alive in the United States (American Cancer Society [ACS], 2015b).

The majority of cancer survivors today are older than 65, with the average age slightly higher in women. More than half are survivors of the most common cancers: breast, prostate, and colorectal cancers. Although the numbers on pediatric cancer survivors are even more promising, with 83.4% of children surviving five years from the time of diagnosis (Howlader et al., 2015), this chapter will cover only survivorship of adult-onset cancers.

Historical Development of a Cancer Survivorship Focus

Cancer survivorship was described for the first time in Fitzhugh Mullan's (1985) essay "Seasons of Survival: Reflections of a Physician With Cancer," in the *New England Journal of Medicine*. Mullan identified three "seasons": *acute survival*, which begins with diagnosis, is dominated by testing and therapies, and is accompanied by fear and anxiety; *extended survival*, which is the period when remission occurs, treatment ends, and fear of recurrence is greatest; and *permanent survival*, which is the period when people are facing the adjustment to normal life and dealing with the lasting impact of cancer on their ability to return to previous roles. Mullan's essay promoted recognition of the ongoing needs of individuals with cancer beyond the acute treatment period. Within a short time after publication, Mullan and a group of survivors formed the National Coalition for Cancer Survivorship (NCCS) to raise awareness about quality care for survivors through advocacy. Miller, Merry, and Miller (2008) further categorized long-term survivors into subgroups consisting of: (a) alive, has signs of cancer that require ongoing treatment; (b) alive, in remission, and requires ongoing treatment to maintain remission; or (c) in complete remission without any ongoing treatment. The additional subgroups of long-term survivors address the void for those with metastatic cancer concerned about the inability to achieve a survival period.

As a result of efforts conducted by NCCS and public figures such as Lance Armstrong, increasing attention is being paid to the needs of cancer survivors. In 1996, the National Cancer Institute (NCI) established the Office of Cancer Survivorship for the purpose of funding research that would lead to improved quality of survival for all patients with cancer and educating health professionals, survivors, and caregivers about critical issues for optimal well-being (Rowland, Aziz, Tesauro, & Feuer, 2001). Two reports, *A National Action Plan for Cancer Survivorship: Advancing Public Health Strategies* and *Living Beyond Cancer: Finding a New Balance*, outlined the issues of cancer survivorship and set specific national goals (Centers for Disease Control and Prevention, 2004; Reuben, 2004). The Institute of Medicine (IOM) established a committee in 2005 to examine the range of medical and psychosocial issues that adult cancer survivors face and to make recommendations to improve their health care and quality of life. This resulted in the publication *From Cancer Patient to Cancer Survivor: Lost in Transition* (Hewitt et al., 2006). IOM had produced a similar report in 2003 on pediatric cancer survivorship. Various professional organizations, such as the American Society of Clinical Oncology (ASCO), NCI, NCCS, the Livestrong Foundation, and other advocacy groups, are involved in efforts to promote implementation of the IOM recommendations. The National Comprehensive Cancer Network® (NCCN®) developed guidelines in 2013 and subsequent versions in an attempt to bridge the gap seen in providing survivorship care identified by IOM (Ligibel & Denlinger, 2013).

NCCS and the NCI Office of Cancer Survivorship define someone as a *cancer survivor* "from the time of diagnosis and for the balance of life" (NCCS, n.d.). Family members, friends, and caregivers also are affected by the survivorship experience and therefore are included in this definition (NCCS, n.d.). This definition has increasingly become adopted, but differing opinions exist about the definition of cancer survivors among health professionals, those with a cancer history, and the public. Some believe that survivorship begins at the completion of initial treatment or at the five-year mark from diagnosis. Some survivors reject the term completely, not wanting to be labeled as someone who is different from others (Hewitt et al., 2006).

During the past few years, the post-treatment experience has received greater emphasis. In an editorial in the *Journal of Clinical Oncology*, Ganz (2005) called for the oncology community to "turn its attention" to the period of time at which patients treated with curative intent have completed their initial therapy and require follow-up care that is currently not well studied nor well described. While recognizing the NCCS definition, IOM focused its report on the distinct period in the cancer care trajectory that begins at the end of a primary treatment provided with intention to cure (Hewitt et al., 2006). IOM defined this period as lasting until a cancer recurrence, a second cancer, or death occurs, and it may include some ongoing treatment, such as adjuvant hormonal therapy. The NCI Office of Cancer Survivorship defines a clear focus in its research initiatives on the post-treatment phase of care to include late effects of treatment, development of second cancers, and quality of life in an effort to optimize care following treatment for cancer. This chapter focuses on the patient experience with the intent to cure, with awareness of the paucity of information for those with chronic disease who are being monitored or undergoing active therapy.

Quality of Life and Survivorship

Quality-of-life issues have become a vital concern to cancer survivors, their families, and care providers (Ferrell, Dow, Leigh, Ly, & Gulasekaram, 1995). The affect of a cancer diagnosis and treatment on health-related quality of life can be measured by assessing symptoms and functioning across physical, psychological, social, and spiritual domains. Ferrell (1996) summarized the definitions of these four domains: "Physical well-being is the control or relief of symptoms and the maintenance of function and independence" (p. 911). Psychological well-being is the attempt to maintain "a sense of control in the face of life-threatening illness characterized by emotional distress, altered life priorities, and fears of the unknown, as well as positive life changes" (p. 912). Social well-being is the effort to deal with the affect of cancer on individuals and their roles and relationships; it "provides a way to view not only the cancer or its symptoms but also the person surrounding the tumor" (p. 913). Spiritual well-being, the final domain discussed by Ferrell, is "the ability to maintain hope and derive meaning from the cancer experience that is characterized by uncertainty" (p. 913).

These patient domains represent an established focus of oncology nursing in planning care through the acute phase of treatment. As evidence grows concerning the affect of cancer treatment on survivors' quality of life, these domains must be considered through the post-treatment period (Hewitt et al., 2006). As people live longer, they will need ongoing medical care, psychosocial support, and monitoring for treatment complications and cancer recurrence. Cancer care providers need to develop new follow-up guidelines and systems that address the needs of this growing population so that survivors can be assured the greatest quality of life (Oeffinger & McCabe, 2006).

Physical Effects

The physical effects of cancer and its treatment are described as long-term and late effects according to their onset. Long-term effects, also called persistent or chronic, are adverse effects that begin during treatment and continue beyond the end of treatment. Examples of long-term effects of chemotherapy and radiation therapy are cognitive problems, fatigue, amenorrhea, and peripheral neuropathies. Examples of long-term effects of cancer surgery include lymphedema and chronic pain. Long-term surgical effects also may include structural or functional changes, such as ostomies; limb amputations; sexual dysfunction; urinary incontinence; infertility; difficulty breathing; and impaired vision, hearing, swallowing, eating, or speaking (Ganz,

2006; Khan, Mant, Carpenter, Forman, & Rose, 2011). At least 50% of survivors report some effect from treatment (Valdivieso, Kujawa, Jones, & Baker, 2012), with depression, pain, and fatigue being the most common (Harrington, Hansen, Moskowitz, Todd, & Feuerstein, 2010).

Much of the research on cancer treatment effects does not extend past the acute experience, which contributes to the challenge of designing appropriate interventions. For example, a significant body of research with corresponding management strategies for treatment-related fatigue exists, yet much less is known about fatigue that persists once treatment effects have subsided. Important considerations in planning care for survivors should include being aware of specific long-term effects that may be a problem; preventing or reducing risks during treatment when possible; and providing patients and caregivers with education about symptom management, safety, and compensatory activities (Nail, 2001). NCCN guidelines address ongoing issues with anxiety, depression, cognitive function, fatigue, sexual function, sleep disorders, pain, infections, and exercise in the post-treatment phase (NCCN, 2015c).

Late effects of treatment refer to the unrecognized toxicities that are absent or subclinical at the end of treatment. Manifestation often depends on type of cancer, treatment type, treatment intensity, and an individual's overall health status. The effects may appear months or years following treatment and are related to organ injury that occurs during treatment, manifesting later because of the failure of repair mechanisms over time or organ senescence (Aziz & Rowland, 2003; Ganz, 2006; Khan et al., 2011). Survivors treated with therapy that is less intense or tissue damaging are unlikely to experience a physical late effect, whereas other patients, such as stem cell transplant recipients, have significant risk of future health problems and need careful monitoring (Oeffinger & McCabe, 2006). Late effects from chemotherapy often are drug specific, such as infertility issues and secondary cancers from alkylating agents (Green et al., 2014). See Table 18-1 for a list of possible late or long-term effects of cancer therapy.

As cancer treatment has become more complex, late effects have become more prevalent. A recent report on survivors of hereditary retinoblastoma by Shinohara, DeWees, and Perkins (2014) demonstrated that secondary cancer rate was increased in those with bilateral retinoblastoma compared to unilateral disease.

Risk of death from causes other than cancer recurrence is greatest among those treated with a combination of chemotherapy and radiation (Friedman, 2013). Susceptibility differs for children and younger and older adults. The increased risk of developing a second cancer, either of the same type or of a different type than the original, may be the result of the cancer treatment received, genetic or other susceptibilities such as health behaviors, or some interaction between the two (Hewitt et al., 2006; Travis et al., 2012). In particular, patients surviving Hodgkin lymphoma are at greatest risk for developing a second primary cancer, with risk associated with the age at which treatment was delivered. Solid tumors are more prevalent after treatment at a younger age, and leukemia is more frequent in those treated at an older age (Kattlove & Winn, 2003). The risk of breast cancer is higher in those treated with chest radiation before age 30 and increases with age at the end of follow-up, time since diagnosis, and radiation dosage. These projections are based on older regimens associated with greater risk; more modern treatment approaches include limited-field radiation and chemotherapy with less effect on ovarian function (Travis et al., 2005). Still, NCCN guidelines recommend monitoring for breast cancer as a late effect of chest radiation beginning five to eight years after treatment (NCCN, 2015b).

Psychosocial Effects

Much of the research on the psychosocial effects of cancer is devoted to early diagnosis and treatment and specific cancer sites, particularly breast cancer. Few studies are devoted to the

Table 18-1. Acute, Chronic, and Late Effects of Cancer Treatments

Body System	Chemotherapy Effects	Endocrine Therapy Effects	Biotherapy Effects	Radiation Effects	Surgical Effects
Hematopoietic	Neutropenia, anemia, thrombocytopenia, bone marrow suppression	Anemia	Neutropenia, anemia, thrombocytopenia	Same	Blood loss
Endocrine	Hot flashes, premature menopause, osteoporosis, infertility	Hot flashes, irregular menses, testicular atrophy, adrenal insufficiency		Hypopituitarism, hypothyroidism hot flashes, premature menopause, osteoporosis, infertility	Sexual dysfunction or loss of function, surgical menopause
Gastrointestinal	Nausea, vomiting, taste changes, mucositis, constipation, diarrhea	Nausea, vomiting, diarrhea, liver injury or liver failure	Nausea, vomiting, diarrhea, gastrointestinal bleeding, elevated transaminases, anorexia	Nausea, vomiting, dry mouth, taste changes, swallowing problems, enteritis, proctitis	Short bowel syndrome, ostomy, dumping syndrome, adhesions
Skin/integument	Dry skin, nail changes, pigment changes, hand-foot syndrome, alopecia, radiation recall	Injection-site pain	Rash, hives, pruritus, dry skin	Burns, pigment changes, thickening of tissues, alopecia in radiation field, lymphedema	Scars, infections, lymphedema
Cardiovascular	MI, CHF, cardiomyopathy, coronary artery disease	MI, CVA, DVT, PE, edema, elevated cholesterol	CHF, cardiomyopathy, thromboembolism, hypotension, hypertension	Atherosclerosis, conduction abnormalities	–
Respiratory	Pulmonary fibrosis, interstitial lung disease, hypersensitivity, pneumonitis, pulmonary edema	Shortness of breath	Dyspnea, bronchospasm, hoarseness	Radiation pneumonitis, pulmonary fibrosis	Loss of lung volume after lung resection

(Continued on next page)

Table 18-1. Acute, Chronic, and Late Effects of Cancer Treatments *(Continued)*

Body System	Chemotherapy Effects	Endocrine Therapy Effects	Biotherapy Effects	Radiation Effects	Surgical Effects
Genitourinary	Cystitis, renal failure, impotence, infertility, irregular menses, decreased libido	Irregular menses, vaginal bleeding, loss of libido, impotence, hot flashes, breast pain or tenderness	Proteinuria, renal failure, renal insufficiency	Cystitis, enteritis, proctitis, vaginal stenosis, fistulas, fibrosis of ureters	Altered sexual functioning
Musculoskeletal	Weakness, fatigue	osteopenia, osteoporosis, osteonecrosis of the jaw, bone or joint pain, arthritis, increased fracture risk	Fatigue, asthenia, bone or muscle pain	Decreased function due to induration/scarring	Amputations, scarring, altered body image, phantom limb pain
Nervous system	Peripheral neuropathy, cognitive impairment	Depression, mood swings, insomnia	Peripheral neuropathy	Cognitive problems with brain irradiation	Acute postoperative pain, postmastectomy pain, neuropathic pain
Special senses	Hearing loss, conjunctivitis, tear duct stenosis	Cataracts	–	Vision loss if eye in radiation field	–
Other late effects	Second or higher order cancers	–	Leukemia, myelodysplastic syndromes	Second cancers	–

CHF—congestive heart failure; CVA—cerebrovascular accident; DVT—deep vein thrombosis; MI—myocardial infarction; PE—pulmonary embolism

Note. Based on information from American Society of Clinical Oncology, 2013.

From *Red Flags in Caring for Cancer Survivors*, by T. Baney, H. Belansky, D. Gutaj, C. Hellman-Wylie, H. Mackey, M. Shriner, and S. Vendlinski, 2014. Retrieved from https://www.ons.org/sites/default/files/media/Red%20Flags%20for%20 Cancer%20Survivors.pdf. Copyright 2014 by Oncology Nursing Society. Reprinted with permission.

post-treatment experience, and some question whether these are true late effects of treatment because depression and anxiety occur in the general population (Stanton, 2012; Stein, Syrjala, & Andrykowski, 2008; Vachon, 2006). Psychological effects may include cancer-specific concerns and uncertainties, such as fear of recurrence, or more generalized symptoms of worry, fear of the future, insomnia, fatigue, and difficulty concentrating (Hewitt et al., 2006; Stanton, 2012). Incidence rates of depression, anxiety disorders, and post-traumatic stress disorder (PTSD) are 0%–58%, 6%–23%, and 0%–32%, respectively (Stein et al., 2008). NCCN chose the term *psychosocial distress* in developing guidelines for cancer distress management, defining it as "a multifactorial unpleasant emotional experience of a psychological (cognitive, behavioral, emotional), social, and/or spiritual nature that may interfere with the ability to cope effectively with cancer, its physical symptoms, and its treatment" (NCCN, 2015a, p. DIS-2). Distress reflects a broader set of concerns that range from common feelings of vulnerability, sadness, and fear, to disabling problems of depression, anxiety, panic, social isolation, and existential and spiritual crisis (NCCN, 2015a). Distress may occur as a reaction to the disease and treatment, as well as its consequential effect on social factors, such as employment, insurance, and relationships. Not all psychological effects are negative. Many cancer survivors report feelings of gratitude, good fortune, and an increased sense of self-esteem and mastery (Hewitt et al., 2006; Stanton, 2012). Recent interest has emerged in how cancer survivors derive meaning from their experiences. Qualitative studies report that exploring spirituality is an effective way of coping, restoring sense of self, and finding purpose and meaning (Coward & Kahn, 2004; Ferrell, Smith, Juarez, & Melancon, 2003).

Overall, the majority of long-term cancer survivors do not experience serious psychological problems, having similar adjustment experiences over time following completion of treatment (Hewitt, Rowland, & Yancik, 2003; Stanton, 2012). However, research reports have noted persistent psychological sequelae within subsets of survivors. The criteria for PTSD can be met by 19% of survivors (NCCN, 2015a). Bloom (2002) described variations according to Mullan's phases of survival, with specific issues manifesting during the acute, extended, and permanent survival. In her review article, Stanton (2012) identified risk and protective factors related to psychological adjustment outcomes. Risk factors for poor adjustment and functional limitations include insufficient social support, social seclusion, and lack of intimate partner. Protective factors include having an optimistic outlook, using problem-solving coping strategies, and conveying emotions.

Multiple studies have focused on the psychological distress experienced by older, long-term survivors. One study investigating symptoms of general distress and PTSD did not demonstrate clinical levels of PTSD in survivors; however, it reported a 25% incidence of clinical depression (Deimling, Kahana, Bowman, & Schaefer, 2002). Persistent cancer-related symptoms were the strongest predictors of depression and the PTSD subdimension of hyperarousal. A survey of the cancer-related health worries and related distress of older, long-term survivors in another study revealed that 33% continued to worry about recurrence, a second cancer, and symptoms experienced as a sign of cancer (Deimling, Bowman, Sterns, Wagner, & Kahana, 2006). These worries were significant predictors of anxiety and depression and occurred least commonly among African Americans. Researchers noted that despite the prevalence of continued worries, most survivors reported little impact on overall measures of quality of life. A study of the coping styles of the same population indicated that long-term survivors used planning and acceptance most commonly and that the personal characteristic of optimism was a strong predictor of positive coping. All coping deteriorated with increasing age (Deimling, Wagner, et al., 2006).

Attention also must be given to the informal caregivers for older survivors. Caregivers were more likely to have distress, decreased coping skills, and limited social support when compared to healthy, similarly aged counterparts. The symptoms of distress worsened as the age of the caregiver and survivor increased (Goldzweig et al., 2013). These studies indicate the need for particular attention to assessment for depression and poor coping strategies in older, long-term survivors, particularly those with comorbid or persistent cancer-related effects. Attention to this population is necessary given the current and growing numbers of older survivors.

Survivors' needs and concerns shift over time, and evidence has shown that external sources of support erode, particularly for those most distressed and of older age (Deimling, Wagner, et al., 2006; Goldzweig et al., 2013; Stanton, 2012). Survivors report receiving insufficient information and support once treatment ends. The Livestrong Foundation (2004) surveyed more than 1,000 cancer survivors in 2004 about the affect of the cancer diagnosis and treatment on the quality of their lives. Half of the survey responders reported that their nonmedical needs were unmet. Large cancer centers, hospital systems, and academic facilities tend to offer many patient and family services, but surveys show that these services are inconsistent and frequently dependent on specific individuals (Stanton, 2012; Tesauro, Rowland, & Lustig, 2002). Simple routine assessment of psychological well-being using tools such as the Distress Thermometer (NCCN, 2015a) is an important basic intervention that is becoming required by accrediting agencies and can effectively identify individuals who need referral. Survivors should initially be screened when therapy is completed and reassessed at follow-up visits (Stanton, 2012). Information about psychological support resources based on risk stratification, including individual, group, and web-based formats, should be made available with appropriate referrals for evidence-based care.

The influence of cancer treatment on social functioning includes family issues, such as sexual and marital relationships and adjustment of children, and work-related issues, such as concern over cancer disclosure, stigma, reentry to the workplace, changes in work priorities, discrimination, and health insurance (Ness et al., 2013). These stressors can affect both physical and psychosocial areas of domain with minimal affect on the spiritual domain (Ness et al., 2013). The best way to influence both physical and psychosocial stressors has yet to be determined. However, some studies have evaluated a combination of cognitive behavioral problem-solving interventions with physical training in the time after acute cancer care, with improvement in both physical and psychosocial symptoms (Silver, Baima, & Mayer, 2013). By addressing physical and psychosocial needs, providers are facilitating optimal return to career and economic stability for patients.

Cancer Survivors and Employment

For more than 30 years, the vast majority of working-age adults with cancer want to and are able to perform their jobs and return to work (Hoffman, 2005). Most survivors work to support themselves and their families, and also for the accompanying health insurance, self-esteem, and social support (Hoffman, 2005). A population-based study of cancer survivors compared to matched controls found a substantially increased burden of illness manifested in days lost from work, inability to work, poorer self-rated general health status, and need for help with daily activities (Yabroff, Lawrence, Clauser, Davis, & Brown, 2004). Work limitations are dependent on many factors, including the survivor's age, stage at diagnosis, financial status, education, health insurance, transportation, physical demands of the job, and presence of comorbid health problems (Guy et al., 2013).

Because employers and coworkers often misunderstand work limitations for cancer survivors, laws are required to address these limitations (Valdivieso et al., 2012). Cancer survivors are protected under federal and state laws in the United States as long as they are qualified for and can perform the major responsibilities of their jobs. Federal laws include the Americans With Disabilities Act (ADA), the Federal Rehabilitation Act, the Family and Medical Leave Act, and the Employee Retirement and Income Security Act (Hewitt et al., 2006; Valdivieso et al., 2012) (see Table 18-2).

Most state laws cover cancer survivors because they prohibit discrimination against people with disabilities, but the definition of "disabled" varies in state and federal law. A new focus of attention is protection of information related to genetic susceptibilities of patients. Several federal laws, including the ADA, Health Insurance Portability and Accountability Act (HIPAA), Genetic

Table 18-2. Federal Laws Protecting Cancer Survivors

Federal Law	Description of Coverage	Benefit	Restrictions
Americans With Disabilities Act (ADA)	Prohibits job discrimination by employers, employment agencies, and labor unions against people who have or had cancer and their families. Protects most cancer survivors from the time of diagnosis	Prohibits discrimination in not hiring applicants for a job or training program; firing a worker; providing unequal pay, working conditions, or benefits; punishing an employee for filing discrimination complaint; or screening out disabled employees	Disability definition may not include those without limitations of "major life activity." Does not include employers with fewer than 15 employees Does not cover the military, other than civilian members of the military or people retired from the military
Federal Rehabilitation Act (FRA)	Prohibits public employers and private employers that receive public funding from discriminating based on disability Covers groups not covered by ADA: • Employees of the executive branch of the federal government • Employees of employers receiving federal contracts or federal financial assistance with fewer than 15 employees	Protects survivors regardless of the extent of the disability	Does not cover the military, other than civilian members of the military or people retired from the military
Family and Medical Leave Act (FMLA)	Requires employers with 50 or more employees to provide up to 12 weeks of unpaid, job-protected leave during any 12 month period for employees with a serious health condition that makes them unable to perform the functions of the position	Includes leave for employees with a seriously ill child, parent, or spouse; a healthy newborn; or a newly adopted child Specifies that benefits, including health insurance, are provided Allows intermittent or reduced work schedules or transfer to a different position with equivalent pay	Employees must have worked at least 25 hours per week for one year. Employers may exempt highest-paid workers.

(Continued on next page)

Table 18-2. Federal Laws Protecting Cancer Survivors *(Continued)*

Federal Law	Description of Coverage	Benefit	Restrictions
Employee Retirement and Income Security Act (ERISA)	Prohibits discrimination that prevents employees from collecting benefits under an employee benefit plan	Prohibits setting up conditions related to health status for coverage under health benefits Prohibits termination of employees for the purpose of cutting off benefits Prohibits encouraging employees to retire as a "disabled" person, which can limit benefits	Does not apply to other forms of discrimination Does not protect individuals denied a new job because of medical status, employees experiencing different treatment that does not affect benefits, or employees whose compensation does not include benefits

Note. Based on information from Hoffman, 2005.

Privacy Act, Genetic Information Nondiscrimination Act, and many state laws, protect against genetic discrimination; however, protection can vary widely (Valdivieso et al., 2012).

Health Insurance Challenges

Most Americans with health insurance have coverage that provides for cancer-related care (Hewitt et al., 2006). However, for those survivors who risk losing their insurance because of employment issues or those who are underinsured, the expense of care after treatment can be prohibitive. Even those with good coverage can find it inadequate for the care required for surveillance or management of treatment effects. For survivors aged 18–64, average annual medical expenses for recently diagnosed patients was $17,170, compared to $6,485 for those previously diagnosed with cancer and $3,611 for those with a history of cancer diagnosis (Guy et al., 2013). Most survivors are older than 65 and are covered by Medicare, but gaps related to drug coverage can create high out-of-pocket expenses. In a recent study of people older than age 65, the average annual medical expenses were $23,441 for those recently diagnosed with cancer, $12,357 for those with a previous cancer history, and $8,724 for those without a cancer history (Guy et al., 2013).

Federal laws provide some protection regarding continued insurance coverage for cancer survivors. The Consolidated Omnibus Budget Reconciliation Act (COBRA) allows survivors who lose their jobs to maintain insurance provided through their employer for an additional 18 months (U.S. Department of Labor Employee Benefits Security Administration, 2012). Although COBRA provides protection, the cost of premiums may be cost prohibitive. HIPAA added protection for people changing jobs by eliminating denials for preexisting conditions and denials of eligibility for benefits on the condition of health status. HIPAA provides some reassurance for survivors (and their family members who hold the insurance) who are experiencing *job lock*—the avoidance of changing jobs because of the fear of losing insurance and other health-related benefits (Guy et al., 2013; U.S. Department of Labor Employee Benefits Security Administration, 2004; Valdivieso et al., 2012). Each state regulates health insurance policies, and laws vary significantly. Health insurers have yet to apply consistent policy on survivorship care, and costs can be high and coverage limited (Hewitt et al., 2006).

The Patient Protection and Affordable Care Act, passed into law in 2010, has made changes in healthcare coverage that may help those with cancer (ACS, 2010). Until 2014, those with preexisting conditions could obtain coverage through a state Preexisting Condition Insurance Plan. Starting in 2014, patients were able to purchase insurance through exchanges. The insurance coverage provides cancer screening, treatment, and follow-up care as essential benefits.

Resources on health care and insurance affecting cancer survivors include the following.
- Information on federal laws from the U.S. Department of Labor: www.dol.gov/dol/topic/health-plans/index.htm
- General information about employment and disability available through the U.S. Equal Employment Opportunities Commission: www.eeoc.gov/facts/ada18.html
- Information related to health insurance found through NCCS (www.canceradvocacy.org) and Cancer*Care* (www.cancercare.org/pdf/fact_sheets/fs_entitlements.pdf)
- American Cancer Society, "Medical Insurance and Financial Assistance for the Cancer Patient": www.cancer.org/docroot/MLT/content/MLT_1x_Medical_Insurance_and_Financial_Assistance_for_the_Cancer_Patient.asp?sitearea=&level=1
- American Cancer Society, "The Affordable Care Act: How It Helps People With Cancer and Their Families": http://action.acscan.org/site/DocServer/Affordable_Care_Act_Through_the_Cancer_Lens_Final.pdf?docID=18421

Components of Cancer Follow-Up Care

Care of survivors should incorporate the physical, psychosocial, and spiritual risks and sequelae of a cancer diagnosis and treatment. Care should be coordinated between specialists and primary care providers to ensure that long-term needs are met. The Livestrong Foundation (formerly Lance Armstrong Foundation) held a consensus-building conference in 2011 to develop the essential components for survivorship care (Rechis, Beckjord, Arvey, Reynolds, & McGoldrick, 2011). The group recommended essentials of care delivery, research to establish evidence for care delivery, and the integration of survivorship care into practice. An initial baseline assessment should be completed to establish symptoms that survivors are experiencing (NCCN, 2015c). Follow-up care should include the following components.

Surveillance for cancer recurrence is the periodic assessment beginning at the end of treatment and extending for a period of time that is dependent on the type of cancer, stage at diagnosis, tumor characteristics, and related risk of recurrence. See Table 18-3 for current surveillance recommendations (Baney et al., 2014). Surveillance includes careful review of interval history, physical examination, and appropriate diagnostic testing. The absence of evidence-based practice guidelines for adult survivors makes decision making difficult for clinicians who struggle with underprescribing or overprescribing diagnostic tests and scheduling related follow-up and appropriate intervals for follow-up.

The Children's Oncology Group (COG) has extensive guidelines for follow-up care that can be relevant in the adult population (COG, 2014). Discussion of clinical practice guidelines will be included later in this chapter.

Follow-up visits and testing schedules tend to be frequent during the immediate post-treatment period and generally decrease in frequency over time as the more acute risks diminish (Baney et al., 2014). For example, most recurrences of breast cancer are detected within five years of diagnosis, with the rate of recurrence peaking in the second year (Burstein & Winer,

2000; Emens & Davidson, 2003). However, breast cancer recurrences can occur as late as 20 years after initial diagnosis; no defined time exists for when survivors can be considered definitively cured (Hewitt et al., 2006). Thus, healthcare providers should consider a history of cancer throughout the life of the survivor. As with all survivorship care, the oncology specialist, primary care provider, or a combination of both may provide surveillance for recurrence.

Table 18-3. Recommended Laboratory and Imaging Tests for Surveillance for Selected Cancers

Type of Cancer	Tests	Frequency
Breast	H&P	Every 4–6 months for 5 years then annually
	Mammogram	Yearly
Lymphoma (varies among specific lymphoma types)	H&P with CBCD, LDH	Every 3–6 months for 5 years then annually
	CT, PET/CT	No more than every 6 months for 2 years then annually for a total of 5 years, then as clinically indicated
Colorectal	H&P with CEA	Every 3–6 months for 2 years, then every 6 months for total of 5 years
	Colonoscopy	1 year after completion of treatment (in 3–6 months if no preoperative colonoscopy done due to obstruction lesion), with additional procedures based on findings
	CT chest/abdomen/pelvis	Every 6–12 months for 2 years then annually
	PET/CT	Not routinely recommended
Lung, non-small cell	H&P with CT chest +/- contrast	Every 6–12 months for 2 years then annually
	PET/MRI	Not routinely recommended
Prostate, after initial definitive treatment	H&P with PSA	Every 6–12 months for 5 years then annually
	DRE	Every year but may be omitted if PSA is undetectable
Prostate, node-positive or metastatic	H&P with PSA	Not routinely recommended
Ovarian	H&P	Every 2–4 months for 2 years, then 3–6 months for 3 years, then annually for a total of 5 years
	CA-125	Optional (Salani et al., 2011); every visit if initially elevated

CA—cancer antigen; CBCD—complete blood count with differential; CEA—carcinoembryonic antigen; CT—computed tomography; DRE—digital rectal exam; H&P—history and physical examination; LDH—lactate dehydrogenase; MRI—magnetic resonance imaging; PET—positron-emission tomography; PSA—prostate-specific antigen

Note. From *Red Flags in Caring for Cancer Survivors*, by T. Baney, H. Belansky, D. Gutaj, C. Hellman-Wylie, H. Mackey, M. Shriner, and S. Vendlinski, 2014. Retrieved from https://www.ons.org/sites/default/files/media/Red%20Flags%20 for%20Cancer%20Survivors.pdf. Copyright 2014 by Oncology Nursing Society. Reprinted with permission.

Monitoring for and management of disease and treatment effects, including second cancers, is essential for survivors' long-term health and quality of life. Monitoring requires knowledge of particular treatment effects and related assessments and testing. As with surveillance for recurrence, few published guidelines exist regarding the monitoring of late effects. Examples of monitoring include periodic cardiovascular evaluation for patients treated with anthracyclines, alkylating agents, or taxanes (for which no guidelines exist); breast cancer screening with annual mammography for survivors of Hodgkin lymphoma treated with mantle field radiation eight years following therapy (NCCN, 2015b); screening for hypothyroidism for patients treated with neck radiation; assessment of restoration of ovulation after treatment with alkylating or hormonal agents; and screening for anxiety and depression. Interventions for managing long-term and late treatment effects are important for the recovery and adaptation of survivors. Examples include exploring causes for persistent fatigue after lymphoma, referring patients to specialists if they have urinary incontinence or sexual dysfunction after radical prostatectomy, initiating lymphedema therapy after lymph node dissection, and referring patients to reproduction specialists for infertility. In recent years, design of initial treatment plans that can minimize the risk of late effects has had an affect on quality of life in many cancer types (Hewitt et al., 2006). New methods of tailoring treatment to individual and tumor characteristics have the potential to reduce the risk of late effects and improve outcomes for survivors.

Detection of new cancers includes ongoing screening for cancer as recommended by national guidelines. Frequently, cancer survivors and providers neglect regular cancer screening procedures because of a lack of understanding of increased risk, a feeling that surviving one cancer eliminated the need for concern about others, or fear of finding a new health problem (Hewitt et al., 2006). According to guidelines, such as those published by ACS (2015a), routine screening for breast, colorectal, prostate, cervical, and endometrial cancers should be part of ongoing healthcare recommendations.

Promotion of positive health behaviors includes counseling survivors about lifestyle changes that can reduce comorbid conditions that may be related to age, treatment, genetic susceptibility, or behaviors. For those with a history of cancer, counseling for diet, exercise, and smoking behaviors by primary care providers occurs less often than in healthy counterparts of similar age (Valdivieso et al., 2012). Recommendations should include known risk reduction behaviors, such as initiating smoking cessation, controlling weight, moderating alcohol intake, controlling sun exposure, engaging in regular physical activity, and getting an annual influenza and other appropriate vaccinations.

Summary of Cancer Treatment and Plan for Follow-Up Care

According to Earle (2006), quality survivor care is rooted in a plan for survivorship. Knowing what has been done, what needs to be done, and who will do it is essential for patients completing cancer treatment. The second recommendation of the IOM report states, "Patients completing primary treatment should be provided with a comprehensive care summary and a follow-up care plan that is clearly and effectively explained" (Hewitt et al., 2006, p. 151). A survivorship care plan provides patients and their current and future care providers with a source of information about the treatment they received and related risks and recommendations. It can serve as a tool for counseling survivors about the lifetime significance of this information for their health care. The care plan should be shared with care providers throughout a cancer survivor's life as a blueprint for ongoing medical needs. Patients are advised to maintain a copy of the care plan and treatment summary to make available to future healthcare providers.

An IOM meeting conducted to study the implementation of formalized survivorship care created a report that called for plans that inform patients and their providers of the long-term effects of cancer and its treatment; identify psychosocial support resources in their communities; and provide guidance on follow-up care, prevention, and health maintenance (Hewitt & Ganz, 2007). Barriers to providing these plans include the length of time required and lack of reimbursement for completion, poor access to information over time because of multiple care providers and settings, and absence of evidence-based and consensus-based guidelines for follow-up care (COG, 2014; Earle, 2006; Earle & Ganz, 2012; Haylock, Mitchell, Cox, Temple, & Curtiss, 2007; Hewitt & Ganz, 2007; Hewitt et al., 2006). For a one-hour survivorship visit with a patient, several additional hours of time are needed to prepare for the visit and to complete required documentation after the visit (Earle & Ganz, 2012). ASCO established a committee to address the lack of guidelines for follow-up care and has developed standardized, disease-specific electronic templates for providers to use for breast, colon, small cell lung, and non-small cell lung cancers and lymphoma. Sample templates of the ASCO treatment plans and summaries for cancer are available at ASCO's website (www .asco.org).

Models of Care

The fragmented state of the U.S. healthcare system challenges the delivery of optimal survivorship care. Many barriers exist, including lack of professional education and training, lack of standards or guidelines for care, and difficulties in communication. Overcoming these barriers requires building an integrated systems approach that incorporates a team of primary care providers, oncologists, and other care providers who agree to communicate and develop streamlined transitions in care (Hewitt et al., 2006). Promising models of survivorship care have emerged, including a shared-care model and various forms of specialized follow-up clinics.

A shared-care model is described as a sharing of responsibility for health care between two or more clinicians of different specialties that involves transfer of personal communication about a patient and knowledge about the particular care requirements (Hewitt et al., 2006; Oeffinger & McCabe, 2006). Shared care has become the standard approach to managing chronic illnesses, such as in patients with diabetes, where care is coordinated between an endocrinologist and a primary care physician. Analysis of data collected in the 2001 and 2002 National Ambulatory Medical Care Surveys and the National Hospital Ambulatory Medical Care Survey showed that primary care physicians have a significant role in cancer care, with nearly half of cancer-related ambulatory visits characterized as shared care, although the role of each clinician during these visits is unclear (Hewitt et al., 2006). Formalizing systems, especially communication processes, for facilitating care between oncology specialists and primary care physicians could create a more comprehensive approach to meeting the long-term needs of cancer survivors.

Specialty survivorship programs are evolving in academic institutions around the United States. Initial models were developed for the care of pediatric cancer survivors, where there was early recognition of the need to monitor for late treatment effects. Most of these programs are directed by a pediatric oncologist and coordinated by an oncology nurse practitioner (NP), and about half include other providers of mental health and other specialties (Oeffinger & McCabe, 2006). Disease-specific models were the first examples of adult survivorship care programs. Oeffinger and McCabe (2006) described three distinct care models. The first care model is the most basic and is described as a one-time consultative visit to a survivorship care provider, often an oncology NP. As in pediatric programs, NPs play a central role in care delivery. A summary of cancer treatment and a plan for monitoring late effects are developed, and needs-based counseling and risk reduction recommendations are provided.

The second model is an oncology NP-led clinic that functions as an extension of the care continuum. The NP delivers ongoing care that includes a standard set of services and a follow-up plan. Contact with the primary care provider is reestablished by the oncology NP with sharing of patient information and care guidelines. This begins the transition to shared care and a potential return to community follow-up care based on the patient's risk for recurrence and late effects.

The most complex model is a specialized multidisciplinary survivor program similar to the pediatric programs. This model includes physicians with training and experience in the care of cancer survivors, NPs, and mental health and consulting specialists. The team provides risk-based care. One example of this model is a clinic that provides care for adult survivors of pediatric cancers. This resource-intense model would be challenging to adapt to groups with larger numbers of survivors.

Standards of Care

An organized set of clinical practice guidelines based on the best available evidence would assist clinical decision making and help ensure appropriate care for survivors. COG has developed a model for these guidelines that outlines the long-term follow-up care for pediatric, adolescent, and young adult cancer survivors (COG, 2014). These guidelines are widely available on the Internet with a complementary set of educational materials. Unfortunately, published evidence-based clinical practice guidelines are available for very few adult cancers. The guidelines available are not uniform, primarily because of the absence of adequately powered, well-controlled trials of follow-up after potentially curative initial therapy (Earle & Ganz, 2012; Hewitt et al., 2006). Despite the paucity of research to support clinical guidelines, NCCN first published guidelines for survivorship care in 2013 (NCCN, 2015c). High-quality evidence on the benefits, harms, and relative cost-effectiveness of follow-up strategies is needed to avoid the health and financial hazards of overuse, underuse, and misuse of resources. IOM has called on professional organizations and public and private agencies to support the development of scientific review processes and the necessary research to address this gap in cancer care.

ASCO has published follow-up guidelines for breast (Khatcheressian et al., 2013) and colorectal (Desch et al., 2005) cancers and for fertility preservation (Lee et al., 2006). NCCN also has developed consensus-based treatment guidelines that incorporate follow-up care for some cancers.

Professional Education

Cancer survivorship care is a new specialty, and curricula for health professionals have little, if any, content in this area (Ferrell & Winn, 2006). Few undergraduate nursing programs offer didactic training in cancer care, and the number of programs providing graduate nursing education with an oncology specialty has decreased by half in the past decade (Ferrell, Virani, Smith, & Juarez, 2003). Survivorship training is even less available, as evidenced through a recent survey of oncology nurses that identified knowledge deficits about survivorship care. Less than half of the oncology nurses had an understanding of bone health, genetic risks, financial and employment issues, and partner relationship concerns (Lester, Wessels, & Jung, 2014). Some growth has occurred in continuing education programs offering survivorship content through specialty organizations such as the Oncology Nursing Society (ONS) and a joint five-year educational effort funded by the National Institutes of Health through the City of Hope and Memorial Sloan Kettering Cancer Center; however, far more is needed for nursing and other disciplines. Oncology APNs, particularly clinical nurse specialists, routinely educate and mentor other nurses and students about all aspects of cancer care in formal lectures and in the clinical arena. Incorporating survivorship content when teaching graduate or continuing education courses and mentoring other nurses and APN students can begin to build a workforce that is knowledgeable and prepared to address survivorship as part of the cancer care trajectory. APNs should seek opportunities to participate jointly with their oncology colleagues to develop survivorship practice guidelines and methods to apply them efficiently (e.g., software development). Improving the quality of care for cancer survivors is contingent on having physicians, nurses, and other professionals adequately trained in survivorship care.

Research

Oncology nurses, individually and collectively, have led many initiatives that address the needs of cancer survivors in the areas of pain, fatigue, sexuality, fertility, family coping, long-term sequelae of treatment, and psychosocial concerns (Ferrell, Virani, et al., 2003). Much of the nursing research on cancer survivorship, supported by ONS and the ONS Foundation, the National Institute of Nursing Research, and NCI, addresses the affect of cancer treatment on quality of life (Ferrell, Virani, et al., 2003). With their intimate knowledge and understanding of the cancer treatment experience, oncology APNs can contribute to much-needed evidence building for the development of quality care guidelines and interventions for survivors. Research is needed to determine the affect that providing the treatment summary and survivorship care plan has had on patient morbidity, mortality, and quality of life. Additionally, questions remain as to the best timing of when to provide the survivorship care plan. Through individual research studies and participation in larger initiatives addressing survivorship, such as through the ONS Putting Evidence Into Practice project (www.ons.org/practice-resources/pep), oncology APNs have an opportunity to ensure quality care for survivors and their futures.

Patient and Caregiver Education

Education of patients and their caregivers about treatment modalities, self-care, prevention and reduction of side effects, and management of symptoms to improve quality of life is a cornerstone of oncology nursing care. Yet, nurses are remiss in their preparation of patients and caregivers for the experience following treatment. Historically, celebration with patients ensued at the end of treatment, only to have patients later report feelings of abandonment, as they were unprepared to manage their ongoing needs. Quality of life commonly suffers because patients do not know what to expect (Earle, 2006). As the body of knowledge about the needs and care of cancer survivors grows, education of survivors should take on the same level of importance that is attached to active treatment.

Nurses can begin to incorporate information about survivorship during their first contact with patients. Teaching sessions on the plan of care at the start of therapy can incorporate the importance of long-term follow-up and expand the framework of the cancer care trajectory through the post-treatment period. As patients near the end of treatment, more specific education about what to expect should be introduced and include the following categories of information.

Management Strategies for Long-Term and Late Effects

In addition to the information contained in the treatment summary and care plan, preparing patients for what to expect after treatment and teaching them symptom management strategies is important for their safety and physical and emotional well-being. Preparation can ease the transition during the period when patients see their care providers less frequently and have reduced support. Learning to adapt to these effects is important for recovery. Conversely, it is equally important that patients be made aware of symptoms that could be concerning and should be reported. Symptoms such as a new lump or onset of pain, bleeding, loss of appetite, changes in bowel habits, persistent nausea and vomiting, weight loss of 10 pounds or more, difficulty breathing, or a cough that does not resolve could be signs of a recurrent or new malignancy, another new health problem, or late treatment effect.

Behaviors to Promote Good Health

Cancer survivors are at increased risk for a secondary malignancy and multiple comorbid diseases brought on by cancer treatment, genetic predisposition, or common lifestyle factors. Death rates from noncancer causes are higher for cancer survivors than the general population (Demark-Wahnefried, Aziz, Rowland, & Pinto, 2005; Ganz, 2005; Hewitt et al., 2003). As noted previously, the majority of cancer survivors today are older than 65, adding the burden of age-related comorbid conditions, which carry a poorer prognosis (Edwards et al., 2002). Comorbidities include but are not limited to obesity, cardiovascular disease, osteoporosis, diabetes, and functional decline. Growing evidence shows that positive changes in health behaviors by survivors, including regular exercise regimens, improved nutritional intake, smoking cessation, and sun protection, can aid in disease prevention (Demark-Wahnefried et al., 2005). More research is needed regarding the direct influence of post-treatment behavior changes on cancer-related progression, recurrence, or survival, other health outcomes, and morbidity. In addition, associated interventions targeting primary and secondary prevention of morbidities and new malignancies are needed for the most vulnerable survivors (Demark-Wahnefried et al., 2005; Hewitt et al., 2003).

The end of primary treatment of cancer has been called a *teachable moment,* a term used to describe life transitions or health events that have the potential to motivate individuals to adopt risk-reducing or health-protective behaviors (Ganz, 2005; McBride, Emmons, & Lipkus, 2003). Transition to cancer survivorship is a teachable moment for oncology APNs to introduce healthy lifestyle behaviors. Particular attention is required for specific populations who tend to be less motivated to make healthy behavior changes, such as men, those with limited education, older adults, and urban residents (Demark-Wahnefried et al., 2005). Oncology APNs and other providers should educate patients on existing health guidelines and encourage them to take active roles in general preventive health strategies. These strategies should include smoking cessation, alcohol abstinence, dietary modifications, exercise promotion, use of sunscreen, and cancer screening (Demark-Wahnefried et al., 2005; Hewitt et al., 2003).

Complementary and Alternative Therapies for Cancer Survivors

Complementary and alternative medicine (CAM), as defined by the National Center for Complementary and Integrative Health (NCCIH, 2015), "is a group of diverse medical and healthcare systems, practices, and products that are not generally considered to be part of conventional medicine." See Chapter 8 for further information about CAM use in the oncology setting. CAM use among adult cancer survivors ranges between 43.3% and 66.5% (Mao, Palmer, Healy, Desai, & Amsterdam, 2011). Growing evidence supports that CAM is used among cancer survivors for general health, to boost the immune system, and to control pain (Mao et al., 2012). Cancer survivors were more likely to use CAM than those without a diagnosis of cancer (Mao et al., 2011). CAM use has been primarily investigated in breast cancer, revealing high use during and after treatment (Boon et al., 2000; Humpel & Jones, 2006; Lengacher et al., 2002; Matthews, Sellergren, Huo, List, & Fleming, 2007).

Studies specifically focused on survivors, although limited, also reflect common use of CAM. In a study of colorectal cancer survivors, 75% indicated use of CAM, with younger women and those with poorer perceived quality of life being more likely to participate (Lawsin et al., 2007). Study of breast cancer survivors revealed high usage (69%); patients were younger and diagnosed at younger ages, and those who associated CAM use with cancer had higher trait anxiety (Matthews et al., 2007). However, studies have shown that patients often do not disclose CAM use unless specifically asked; therefore, care providers have a greater need to assess and counsel patients about appropriate use (Ernst, 2015).

Implications for Oncology Advanced Practice Nurses

Oncology APNs are involved in the wide spectrum of cancer care, including direct clinical practice, education of patients and other professionals, and generation of evidence-based practice standards and clinical research. APNs have much to contribute to the design, direction, and delivery of care to cancer survivors by expanding the scope of their influence beyond the end of treatment.

Oncology NPs and clinical nurse specialists need to incorporate routine approaches to designing care for survivors at key intervals, including completion of therapy, preparation for follow-up, and return for surveillance and monitoring. In all cases, the following suggestions for practice and questions to consider can serve as a guide for assessment and intervention.

- Know patient's cancer history. Apply knowledge of treatment effects to identify the long-term risks for patients.
  - What is the cancer type, histology, and stage? What was the age of the patient during treatment? How long ago did it occur? Was there any other cancer history?
  - Did the patient have surgery? What kind and to what site? What are the functional losses and persistent effects?
  - Did the patient receive chemotherapy, biotherapy, hormonal therapy, or targeted agents? Which agents were used? What are the cumulative doses of the anthracyclines? Did the patient receive high doses and multiple cycles of any agents? Did the patient receive bisphosphonates, steroids, or multiple courses of antibiotics/antifungals? Does the patient have persistent symptoms? What are the potential late effects of agents received? Does the patient have any signs or symptoms of late effects?

- – Did the patient receive radiation? What kind, to what site, and at what dosage? Does the patient have persistent symptoms? What are the potential late effects of the radiation? Does the patient have any signs or symptoms of late effects?
  - – Did the patient have a transplant? What kind? What are the potential late effects of the transplant? Does the patient have any signs or symptoms of late effects?
- • Know the surveillance plan for the patient's cancer type. Follow guidelines if they are available.
  - – How often should the person be seen and tested? What are the recommended diagnostic tests, if any?
  - – What other testing should be considered based on the systems review and examination?
- • Know what the patient's risk factors were, if any, both genetic and environmental.
  - – Did the patient undergo genetic susceptibility testing? Does a related screening recommendation exist?
  - – Has the patient eliminated causal behavior, such as smoking, alcohol consumption, or occupational exposure?
- • Screen for other cancers, as indicated.
  - – Has the patient been screened for other cancers?
  - – What are the particular recommendations for cancer screening for this patient?
- • Assess the patient and family for psychosocial and spiritual concerns.
  - – Does the patient report symptoms of anxiety or depression?
  - – Has the patient experienced loss of social functioning, such as with roles, relationships, or employment?
  - – Has the patient experienced discrimination, such as with employment or insurance?
  - – Has the patient experienced serious economic problems?
  - – How are the patient's family members or loved ones coping in this post-treatment period?
- • Know the health behaviors that increase the risk for morbidities and other cancers.
  - – Does the patient smoke or use alcohol or drugs?
  - – Does the patient practice healthy behaviors, such as dietary restriction, weight control, physical exercise, and sun protection?
- • Perform a survivorship-focused history and physical examination, including a review of systems (Friedman, 2013; Ganz, 2006).
  - – Constitutional—weight gain/loss, fatigue, fever and night sweats, pain, changes or limitation in physical exercise ability
  - – Skin and integument—skin changes, lesions; hair loss
  - – Eye, ear, nose, throat, and mouth—hearing loss; dental problems, dry mouth; jaw pain; speech, sight, swallowing disturbance
  - – Pulmonary—dyspnea, cough, pain
  - – Cardiac and vascular—signs and symptoms of congestive heart failure; symptoms of palpitations, coronary, ischemic, or pleuropericardial chest pain; claudication or vascular ischemic attacks; Raynaud disease
  - – Renal—hypertension
  - – Gastrointestinal—chronic diarrhea or constipation; abdominal pain; ostomy function and management, as well as associated sexual functioning; ascites, jaundice
  - – Genitourinary—urinary incontinence, dysuria; erectile dysfunction, infertility; ostomy function and management, related urinary tract infections and sexual functioning
  - – Gynecologic—premature menopause, vaginal dryness or dyspareunia; infertility

- Endocrine—thyroid nodules or symptoms of hypothyroidism, such as unexplained weight gain, increased cholesterol; reproductive history and sexual functioning; symptoms of metabolic syndrome, such as increasing abdominal girth, increasing triglycerides, glucose intolerance
- Hematologic—cytopenia
- Lymphatic—palpable nodules; lymphedema
- Infections—report of chronic infections
- Musculoskeletal—muscular or bone pain, osteoporosis, fracture, decreased bone density, aseptic necrosis
- Neurologic—neuropathic pain, peripheral neuropathy; hearing loss, decreased cognitive function
- Psychiatric/psychosocial—return to previous roles, symptoms of anxiety or depression, difficulty sleeping, disturbed body image; taking psychotropic medication
- Manage symptoms. Apply knowledge of symptom management of acute problems to the chronic presentation. Refer to specialists as needed.
- Provide patients with a treatment summary and care plan.
  - Apply knowledge of the patient's cancer diagnosis and treatment history in developing a comprehensive summary and plan. Review the care plan with patients and emphasize the need to share it with their other healthcare providers.
  - Work with colleagues to develop efficient methods to implement care plan development for all patients. Routinely communicate this plan directly to designated providers.

Conclusion

Cancer survivorship has emerged as an important area of focus in cancer care, largely in response to the demands of cancer survivors in their pursuit of a better quality of life after treatment. Nurses, physicians, and mental health specialists have made significant contributions to the field of research, and NCI has organized a focus for federal sponsorship (Hewitt et al., 2006). Major publications devoted to survivorship have appeared, including the IOM report and entire issues of the *Journal of Clinical Oncology* (November 2006) and the *American Journal of Nursing* (March 2006 supplement). The *Journal of Cancer Survivorship*, established in March 2007, is devoted to publishing information specific to cancer survivorship. ASCO and ONS have incorporated content about survivorship into annual meetings, and NCI sponsors a biannual survivorship research meeting.

Advancing survivorship care will depend on growth in research, education, and clinical practice models. IOM has called on federal agencies, private voluntary organizations, cooperative groups, and registries to urgently support initiatives related to mechanisms, prevalence, and risk of late effects; interventions to alleviate symptoms and improve function and quality of life; care models that are cost effective and address surveillance strategies and interventions; care of the underserved and supportive care and rehabilitation; insurance and employment issues; and methods to overcome barriers and challenges. The challenge lies in the availability of funding for these initiatives in a period of competing national healthcare issues and limited resources (Hewitt et al., 2006).

Oncology APNs coordinate care for patients throughout the cancer care trajectory. Their leadership in clinical practice, education, and research efforts for managing symptoms related to cancer treatment can be expanded beyond the acute survival period. APNs are in a position to influence quality of life in survivors by ensuring that the survivors are prepared with the information that they and their care providers need for the rest of their lives.

Case Study

Three years ago, C.R. was diagnosed at age 52 with invasive ductal carcinoma of the left breast (T1N1M0, stage IIA). The tumor was 1.5 cm, estrogen receptor positive, progesterone receptor negative, and HER2 negative; and 2 out of 10 lymph nodes were positive. Surgical treatment consisted of a left breast lumpectomy, sentinel lymph node biopsy, and axillary node dissection. C.R. received chemotherapy including doxorubicin and cyclophosphamide for four cycles, followed by four cycles of paclitaxel. Her chemotherapy was followed by external beam radiation therapy with 4,500 cGy to the left breast. C.R. was postmenopausal and had stopped hormone replacement therapy at the diagnosis of her breast cancer. At completion of her chemotherapy, she started tamoxifen.

C.R. had no prior surgical history. Her only medication for the past year was atorvastatin for elevated cholesterol. She has two daughters in their early 20s. Her mother was diagnosed with breast cancer at age 68 and died of metastatic disease four years later. C.R.'s only sister has no history of breast cancer. C.R. and her children's father are of Italian American descent.

In the year following her treatment, C.R. experienced "terrible" hot flashes that occurred more than 12 times per day, as well as vaginal dryness and pain during sexual intercourse. She also developed a frozen right shoulder, which caused her pain and made her unable to exercise, especially when playing golf. She received physical therapy for three to four months and regained some of her mobility, although she is still unable to play golf.

C.R. gained mild relief of her hot flashes from acupuncture but continued to experience a marked decrease in her quality of life. Her gynecologist prescribed megestrol acetate 20 mg per day to help with her symptoms of hot flashes. She also received treatment for a chronic yeast infection with several courses of fluconazole. Because of her persistent vaginal complaints, C.R. was referred to a sexual medicine specialist. She was diagnosed with atrophic vaginitis associated with tamoxifen and megestrol acetate. She started vaginal estrogen once daily and low-dose topical estrogen and testosterone ointment. She was counseled about the potential benefits of controlling her symptoms and the breast cancer risks of hormonal therapy.

C.R.'s mammogram and clinical breast examination one year ago were normal, and her bone densitometry dual-energy x-ray absorptiometry scan showed a T-score of −1.5, down from a score of −1.0 the previous year. At that time, she was instructed to take calcium and vitamin D supplements.

C.R. was married just after completing her treatment. She is unable to have vaginal intercourse because of her pain and is unable to play golf with her husband, a favorite shared activity. She also has gained 20 pounds since her treatment and complains she is unable to lose weight despite dieting. She continues to work full time as an accountant, but she recently avoided a promotion because of a reluctance to make career changes for fear of jeopardizing her tenure in the corporation and losing her health insurance.

The APN in an office of a large oncology practice sees C.R. for her biannual follow-up visit. The nurse reviews C.R.'s past history and plan of care for today's visit.

1. According to ASCO guidelines, what testing does C.R. need for surveillance?
   • C.R. requires mammography and clinical breast examination for surveillance.
2. What late effects of treatment is C.R. experiencing?
   • C.R. is experiencing frozen shoulder as a result of radiation, loss of bone density and atrophic vaginitis from tamoxifen, and weight gain from megestrol acetate. C.R. is at risk for continued bone loss and osteoporosis, despite calcium and vitamin D replacement. She has known hypercholesterolemia, and her weight gain and diminished exercise can lead to greater risk. Although her risks for hematologic or cardiac disease from anthracycline and radiation therapy to her left breast are small, they should be considered in overall long-term assessment; cardiac disease can occur as late as 10 years after treatment.

3. C.R. is concerned about her daughters' risks. Should she be referred for genetic counseling and *BRCA* testing?
   - According to ASCO criteria, no indication for genetic testing is present. Indications include Ashkenazi Jewish heritage, history of ovarian cancer at any age in the patient or any first- or second-degree relatives, any first-degree relative with a history of breast cancer diagnosed before age 50, two or more first- or second-degree relatives diagnosed with breast cancer at any age, personal history of or relative with diagnosis of bilateral breast cancer, and history of breast cancer in a male relative.
4. C.R. is experiencing several psychosocial and spiritual sequelae of her disease and treatment. What are they, and what referrals might she benefit from?
   - As a result of her illness, C.R. has experienced relationship changes in her marriage related to painful intercourse and physical limitations that prevent usual joint activities, body image disturbance related to her weight gain, and vocational changes related to anxiety over career and health insurance loss. C.R. could benefit from a session with a social worker or therapist. The APN might also consider whether to change or discontinue megestrol acetate and try other methods to assist with the problem of weight gain, such as a nutritionist for diet advice and physical therapist for activity interventions.
5. What laws would protect C.R. regarding her fears about her employment?
   - C.R. is protected against job discrimination by the ADA and by HIPAA, which guarantees her privacy and portability of health insurance.

Key Points

- Cancer survivors are increasing in numbers, and the complexity of needs is growing as the population ages and the effects of screening, early detection, and improvements in treatment are realized.
- According to NCCS (n.d.), an individual is considered to be a cancer survivor from the time of diagnosis through the balance of his or her life. Family members, friends, and caregivers also are affected by the survivorship experience and therefore are included in this definition.
- Although this definition is widely embraced, increased attention is being focused on the particular needs of those in the period following curative cancer treatment.
- Cancer and its treatment can have a profound lasting effect on quality of life as measured in the assessment of all domains: physical, psychological, social, and spiritual.
- Follow-up care for cancer survivors should incorporate surveillance for signs of a cancer recurrence; monitoring and managing long-term and late treatment effects, including second malignancies; recommendations for cancer screening; counseling about health promotion behaviors; and coordination of care across providers.
- Various models of survivorship care are developing. The shared-care model between the oncology specialist and the primary care provider ensures continuity during the transition to long-term follow-up care. APNs are participating in the implementation of unique clinical programs with the potential to influence care of survivors across varied settings.
- All survivors should be given a written summary of their cancer treatment and a plan for follow-up care.
- APNs are in a unique position to direct and provide care to patients with cancer beyond active treatment throughout the cancer care continuum. Applying their knowledge of cancer and its treatment, APNs can contribute by incorporating the components of survivorship care into their clinical practice and research and education efforts.
- Completion of cancer treatment is a teachable moment and an opportunity to guide patients to adopt behaviors that can reduce their risks of developing comorbid conditions and other cancers.

- Expansion of research and education is key to advancing the quality of life for survivors.
- Survivors treated with less intense or tissue-damaging therapy are unlikely to experience late effects, whereas others who have received more intense or multimodality therapy have significant risk of encountering future health problems and require careful monitoring and risk assessment.

Recommended Resources for Oncology Advanced Practice Nurses

Publications

- For patients: NCI *Facing Forward* series
  - *Facing Forward: Life After Cancer Treatment*
  - *Facing Forward: Making a Difference in Cancer*
  - *Facing Forward: When Someone You Love Has Completed Cancer Treatment*
  - To order or download, visit https://pubs.cancer.gov/ncipl/home.aspx
- Hewitt, M., Greenfield, S., & Stovall, E. (Eds.). (2006). *From cancer patient to cancer survivor: Lost in transition.* Washington, DC: National Academies Press. To order a print copy or download an electronic version, visit www.nap.edu/catalog.php?record_id=11468.
- Reuben, S.H. (2004, May). *Living beyond cancer: Finding a new balance. President's Cancer Panel 2003–2004 annual report.* Bethesda, MD: National Cancer Institute. To view the report, visit http://deainfo.nci.nih.gov/advisory/pcp/annualReports/pcp03-04rpt/Survivorship.pdf.

Organizations/Internet Resources

- American Association for Cancer Research: www.aacr.org
- American Cancer Society Cancer Survivors Network: http://csn.cancer.org
- Association of Cancer Online Resources: www.acor.org
- Cancer*Care*: www.cancercare.org
- Cancer.Net survivorship information: www.cancer.net/survivorship
- Cancer Support Community: www.wellnesscommunitystl.org
- COG: www.survivorshipguidelines.org provides in-depth information on late effects from chemotherapy agents that may be useful in the adult setting
- I'm Too Young For This! Cancer Foundation (formerly Steps for Living): http://stupidcancer.org
- Intercultural Cancer Council: www.iccnetwork.org
- Journey Forward: www.journeyforward.org (survivorship care plan builder)
- Livestrong Fertility: www.livestrong.org/we-can-help/fertility-services
- Livestrong Foundation: www.livestrong.org
- MD Anderson Cancer Center complementary/integrative medicine education resources: www.mdanderson.org/departments/CIMER
- Memorial Sloan Kettering Cancer Center survivorship information: www.mskcc.org/mskcc/html/58022.cfm
- National Lymphedema Network: www.lymphnet.org
- NCCS: www.canceradvocacy.org
- NCI: www.cancer.gov/cancertopics/life-after-treatment
- OncoLink: www.oncolink.com (survivorship care plans)
- Telling Kids About Cancer: www.tellingkidsaboutcancer.com
- Ulman Cancer Fund for Young Adults: www.ulmanfund.org

The author would like to acknowledge Nancy G. Houlihan, RN, MA, AOCN®, for her contribution to this chapter that remains unchanged from the first edition of this book.

References

American Cancer Society. (2010). The Affordable Care Act: How it helps people with cancer and their families. Retrieved from http://action.acscan.org/site/DocServer/Affordable_Care_Act_Through_the_Cancer_Lens_Final.pdf?docID=18421

American Cancer Society. (2015a). American Cancer Society guidelines for the early detection of cancer. Retrieved from http://www.cancer.org/healthy/findcancerearly/cancerscreeningguidelines/american-cancer-society-guidelines-for-the-early-detection-of-cancer

American Cancer Society. (2015b). *Cancer facts and figures 2015*. Retrieved from http://www.cancer.org/research/cancerfactsstatistics/cancerfactsfigures2015/index

American Society of Clinical Oncology. (2013). Long-term side effects of cancer treatment. Retrieved from http://www.cancer.net/survivorship/long-term-side-effects-cancer-treatment

Aziz, N.M., & Rowland, J.H. (2003). Trends and advances in cancer survivorship research: Challenges and opportunity. *Seminars in Radiation Oncology, 13,* 248–266. doi:10.1016/S1053-4296(03)00024-9

Baney, T., Belansky, H., Gutaj, D., Hellman-Wylie, C., Mackey, H., Shriner, M., & Vendlinski, S. (2014). *Red flags in caring for cancer survivors*. Retrieved from https://www.ons.org/sites/default/files/media/Red%20Flags%20for%20Cancer%20Survivors.pdf

Bloom, J.R. (2002). Surviving and thriving? *Psycho-Oncology, 11,* 89–92. doi:10.1002/pon.606

Boon, H., Stewart, M., Kennard, M.A., Gray, R., Sawka, C., Brown, J.B., … Haines-Kamka, T. (2000). Use of complementary/alternative medicine by breast cancer survivors in Ontario: Prevalence and perceptions. *Journal of Clinical Oncology, 18,* 2515–2521.

Burstein, H.J., & Winer, E.P. (2000). Primary care for survivors of breast cancer. *New England Journal of Medicine, 343,* 1086–1094. doi:10.1056/NEJM200010123431506

Centers for Disease Control and Prevention. (2004). A national action plan for cancer survivorship: Advancing public health strategies. Retrieved from http://www.cdc.gov/cancer/survivorship/what_cdc_is_doing/action_plan.htm

Children's Oncology Group. (2014). *Long-term follow-up guidelines for survivors of childhood, adolescent, and young adult cancers* [v.4.0]. Retrieved from http://www.survivorshipguidelines.org

Coward, D.D., & Kahn, D.L. (2004). Resolution of spiritual disequilibrium by women newly diagnosed with breast cancer [Online exclusive]. *Oncology Nursing Forum, 31,* E24–E31. doi:10.1188/04.ONF.E24-E31

Deimling, G.T., Bowman, K.F., Sterns, S., Wagner, L.J., & Kahana, B. (2006). Cancer-related health worries and psychological distress among older adult, long-term cancer survivors. *Psycho-Oncology, 15,* 306–320. doi:10.1002/pon.955

Deimling, G.T., Kahana, B., Bowman, K.F., & Schaefer, M.L. (2002). Cancer survivorship and psychological distress in later life. *Psycho-Oncology, 11,* 479–494. doi:10.1002/pon.614

Deimling, G.T., Wagner, L.J., Bowman, K.F., Sterns, S., Kercher, K., & Kahana, B. (2006). Coping among older-adult, long-term cancer survivors. *Psycho-Oncology, 15,* 143–159. doi:10.1002/pon.931

Demark-Wahnefried, W., Aziz, N.M., Rowland, J.H., & Pinto, B.M. (2005). Riding the crest of the teachable moment: Promoting long-term health after the diagnosis of cancer. *Journal of Clinical Oncology, 23,* 5814–5830. doi:10.1200/JCO.2005.01.230

Desch, C.E., Benson, A.B., III, Somerfield, M.R., Flynn, P.J., Krause, C., Loprinzi, C.L., … Petrelli, N.J. (2005). Colorectal cancer surveillance: 2005 update of an American Society of Clinical Oncology practice guideline. *Journal of Clinical Oncology, 23,* 8512–8521. doi:10.1200/JCO.2005.04.0063

Earle, C.C. (2006). Failing to plan is planning to fail: Improving the quality of care with survivorship care plans. *Journal of Clinical Oncology, 24,* 5112–5116. doi:10.1200/JCO.2006.06.5284

Earle, C.C., & Ganz, P.A. (2012). Cancer survivorship care: Don't let the perfect be the enemy of the good. *Journal of Clinical Oncology, 30,* 3764–3768. doi:10.1200/JCO.2012.41.7667

Edwards, B.K., Howe, H.L., Ries, L.A., Thun, M.J., Rosenberg, H.M., Yancik, R., … Feigal, E.G. (2002). Annual report to the nation on the status of cancer, 1973–1999, featuring implications of age and aging on U.S. cancer burden. *Cancer, 96,* 2766–2792.

Emens, L.A., & Davidson, N.E. (2003). The follow-up of breast cancer. *Seminars in Oncology, 30,* 338–348. doi:10.1016/S0093-7754(03)00094-0

Ernst, E. (2015). Complementary and alternative therapies for cancer [Literature review current through May 2015; topic last updated June 10, 2015]. Retrieved from http://www.uptodate.com/contents/complementary-and-alternative-therapies-for-cancer

Ferrell, B.R. (1996). The quality of lives: 1,525 voices of cancer. *Oncology Nursing Forum, 23,* 909–916.

Ferrell, B.R., Dow, K.H., Leigh, S., Ly, J., & Gulasekaram, P. (1995). Quality of life in long-term cancer survivors. *Oncology Nursing Forum, 22,* 915–922.

Ferrell, B.R., Smith, S.L., Juarez, G., & Melancon, C. (2003). Meaning of illness and spirituality in ovarian cancer survivors. *Oncology Nursing Forum, 30,* 249–257. doi:10.1188/03.ONF.249-257

Ferrell, B.R., Virani, R., Smith, S.L., & Juarez, G. (2003). The role of oncology nursing to ensure quality care for cancer survivors: A report commissioned by the National Cancer Policy Board and Institute of Medicine [Online exclusive]. *Oncology Nursing Forum, 30,* E1–E11. doi:10.1188/03.ONF.E1-E11

Ferrell, B.R., & Winn, R. (2006). Medical and nursing education and training opportunities to improve survivorship care. *Journal of Clinical Oncology, 24,* 5142–5148. doi:10.1200/JCO.2006.06.0970

Friedman, D.L. (2013). Long-term survivorship: Late effects. In A.M. Berger, J.L Shuster Jr., & J.H. Von Roenn (Eds.), *Principles and practice of palliative care and supportive oncology* (4th ed., pp. 854–867). Philadelphia, PA: Wolters Kluwer Health/Lippincott Williams & Wilkins.

Ganz, P.A. (2005). A teachable moment for oncologists: Cancer survivors, 10 million strong and growing! *Journal of Clinical Oncology, 23,* 5458–5460. doi:10.1200/JCO.2005.04.916

Ganz, P.A. (2006). Monitoring the physical health of cancer survivors: A survivorship-focused medical history. *Journal of Clinical Oncology, 24,* 5105–5111. doi:10.1200/JCO.2006.06.0541

Goldzweig, G., Merims, S., Ganon, R., Peretz, T., Altman, A., & Baider, L. (2013). Informal caregiving to older cancer patients: Preliminary research outcomes and implications. *Annals of Oncology, 24,* 2635–2640. doi:10.1093/annonc/mdt250

Green, D.M., Nolan, V.G., Goodman, P.J., Whitton, J.A., Srivastava, D., Leisenring, W.M., … Robison, L.L. (2014). The cyclophosphamide equivalent dose as an approach for quantifying alkylating agent exposure: A report from the childhood cancer survivor study. *Pediatric Blood and Cancer, 61,* 53–67. doi:10.1002/pbc.24679

Guy, G.P., Jr., Ekwueme, D.U., Yabroff, K., Dowling, E.C., Li, C., Rodriguez, J.L., … Virgo, K.S. (2013). Economic burden of cancer survivorship among adults in the United States. *Journal of Clinical Oncology, 31,* 3749–3757. doi:10.1200/JCO.2013.49.1241

Harrington, C.B., Hansen, J.A., Moskowitz, M., Todd, B.L., & Feuerstein, M. (2010). It's not over when it's over: Long-term symptoms in cancer survivors—A systematic review. *International Journal of Psychiatry in Medicine, 40,* 163–181. doi:10.2190/PM.40.2.c

Haylock, P.J., Mitchell, S.A., Cox, T., Temple, S.V., & Curtiss, C.P. (2007). The cancer survivor's prescription for living. *American Journal of Nursing, 107*(4), 58–70. doi:10.1097/01.NAJ.0000271186.82445.b6

Hewitt, M., & Ganz, P.A. (2007). *Implementing cancer survivorship care planning* [Institute of Medicine Report]. Washington, DC: National Academies Press.

Hewitt, M., Greenfield, S., & Stovall, E. (Eds.). (2006). *From cancer patient to cancer survivor: Lost in transition.* Washington, DC: National Academies Press.

Hewitt, M., Rowland, J.H., & Yancik, R. (2003). Cancer survivors in the United States: Age, health, and disability. *Journals of Gerontology, Series A: Biological Sciences and Medical Sciences, 58,* M82–M91. doi:10.1093/gerona/58.1.M82

Hoffman, B. (2005). Cancer survivors at work: A generation of progress. *CA: A Cancer Journal for Clinicians, 55,* 271–280. doi:10.3322/canjclin.55.5.271

Howlader, N., Noone, A.M., Krapcho, M., Garshell, J., Miller, D., Altekruse, S.F., … Cronin, K.A. (Eds.). (2015). SEER cancer statistics review, 1975–2012. Retrieved from http://seer.cancer.gov/csr/1975_2012

Humpel, N., & Jones, S.C. (2006). Gaining insight into the what, why, and where of complementary and alternative medicine use by cancer patients and survivors. *European Journal of Cancer Care, 15,* 362–368. doi:10.1111/j.1365 -2354.2006.00667.x

Kattlove, H., & Winn, R.J. (2003). Ongoing care of patients after primary treatment for their cancer. *CA: A Cancer Journal for Clinicians, 53,* 172–196. doi:10.3322/canjclin.53.3.172

Khan, N.F., Mant, D., Carpenter, L., Forman, D., & Rose, P.W. (2011). Long-term health outcomes in a British cohort of breast, colorectal and prostate cancer survivors: A database study. *British Journal of Cancer, 105*(Suppl. 1), S29–S37. doi:10.1038/bjc.2011.420

Khatcheressian, J.L., Hurley, P., Bantug, E., Esserman, L., Grunfeld, E., Halburg, F., … Davidson, N.E. (2013). Breast cancer follow-up and management after primary treatment: American Society of Clinical Oncology clinical practice guideline update. *Journal of Clinical Oncology, 31,* 961–965. doi:10.1200/JCO.2012.45.9859

Lawsin, C., DuHamel, K., Itzkowitz, S.H., Brown, K., Lim, H., Thelemaque, L., & Jandorf, L. (2007). Demographic, medical, and psychosocial correlates to CAM use among survivors of colorectal cancer. *Supportive Care in Cancer, 15,* 557–564. doi:10.1007/s00520-006-0198-3

Lee, S.J., Schover, L.R., Partridge, A.H., Patrizio, P., Wallace, W.H., Hagerty, K., … Oktay, K. (2006). American Society of Clinical Oncology recommendations on fertility preservation in cancer patients. *Journal of Clinical Oncology, 24,* 2917–2931. doi:10.1200/JCO.2006.06.5888

Lengacher, C.A., Bennett, M.P., Kip, K.E., Keller, R., LaVance, M.S., Smith, L.S., & Cox, C.E. (2002). Frequency of use of complementary and alternative medicine in women with breast cancer. *Oncology Nursing Forum, 29,* 1445–1452. doi:10.1188/02.ONF.1445-1452

Lester, J.L., Wessels, A.L., & Jung, Y. (2014). Oncology nurses' knowledge of survivorship care planning: The need for education [Online exclusive]. *Oncology Nursing Forum, 41,* E35–E43. doi:10.1188/14.ONF.E35-E43

Ligibel, J.A., & Denlinger, C.S. (2013). New NCCN Guidelines® for survivorship care. *Journal of the National Comprehensive Cancer Network, 11,* 640–644.

Livestrong Foundation. (2004). Livestrong poll finds nearly half of people living with cancer feel their non-medical needs are unmet by the healthcare system. Retrieved from http://www.prnewswire.com/news-releases/livestrongtm-poll-finds-nearly-half-of-people-living-with-cancer-feel-their-non-medical-needs-are-unmet-by-the-healthcare-system-75593032.html

Mao, J., Palmer, C., Healy, K., Desai, K., & Amsterdam, J. (2011). Complementary and alternative medicine use among cancer survivors: A population-based study. *Journal of Cancer Survivorship, 5,* 8–17. doi:10.1007/s11764-010-0153-7

Matthews, A.K., Sellergren, S.A., Huo, D., List, M., & Fleming, G. (2007). Complementary and alternative medicine use among breast cancer survivors. *Journal of Alternative and Complementary Medicine, 13,* 555–562. doi:10.1089/acm.2007.03-9040

McBride, C.M., Emmons, K.M., & Lipkus, I.M. (2003). Understanding the potential of teachable moments: The case of smoking cessation. *Health Education Research, 18,* 156–170. doi:10.1093/her/18.2.156

Miller, K., Merry, B., & Miller, J. (2008). Seasons of survivorship revisited. *Cancer Journal, 14,* 369–374. doi:10.1097/PPO.0b013e31818edf60

Mullan, F. (1985). Seasons of survival: Reflections of a physician with cancer. *New England Journal of Medicine, 313,* 270–273. doi:10.1056/NEJM198507253130421

Nail, L.M. (2001). Long-term persistence of symptoms. *Seminars in Oncology Nursing, 17,* 249–254. doi:10.1053/sonu.2001.27916

National Center for Complementary and Integrative Health. (2015, February). Terms related to complementary and integrative health. Retrieved from https://nccih.nih.gov/health/providers/camterms.htm?nav=gsa

National Coalition for Cancer Survivorship. (n.d.). About us: History of NCCS. Retrieved from http://www.canceradvocacy.org/about/org

National Comprehensive Cancer Network. (2015a). *NCCN Clinical Practice Guidelines in Oncology (NCCN Guidelines®): Distress management* [v.1.2015]. Retrieved from http://www.nccn.org/professionals/physician_gls/PDF/distress.pdf

National Comprehensive Cancer Network. (2015b). *NCCN Clinical Practice Guidelines in Oncology (NCCN Guidelines®): Hodgkin lymphoma* [v.2.2015]. Retrieved from http://www.nccn.org/professionals/physician_gls/PDF/hodgkins.pdf

National Comprehensive Cancer Network. (2015c). *NCCN Clinical Practice Guidelines in Oncology (NCCN Guidelines®): Survivorship* [v.1.2015]. Retrieved from http://www.nccn.org/professionals/physician_gls/pdf/survivorship.pdf

Ness, S., Kokal, J., Fee-Schroeder, K., Novotny, P., Satele, D., & Barton, D. (2013). Concerns across the survivorship trajectory: Results from a survey of cancer survivors. *Oncology Nursing Forum, 40,* 35–42. doi:10.1188/13.ONF.35-42

Oeffinger, K.C., & McCabe, M.S. (2006). Models for delivering survivorship care. *Journal of Clinical Oncology, 24,* 5117–5124. doi:10.1200/JCO.2006.07.0474

Rechis, R., Beckjord, E.B., Arvey, S.R., Reynolds, K.A., & McGoldrick, D. (2011). *The essential elements of survivorship care: A Livestrong brief.* Retrieved from http://images.livestrong.org/downloads/flatfiles/what-we-do/our-approach/reports/ee/EssentialElementsBrief.pdf?_ga=1.40847786.966852371.1430504857

Reuben, S.H. (2004, May). *Living beyond cancer: Finding a new balance: President's Cancer Panel 2003–2004 annual report.* Bethesda, MD: National Cancer Institute.

Rowland, J.H., Aziz, N.M., Tesauro, G., & Feuer, E.J. (2001). The changing face of cancer survivorship. *Seminars in Oncology Nursing, 17,* 236–240. doi:10.1053/sonu.2001.27912

Salani, R., Backes, F., Fung, M., Holschneider, C., Parker, L., Bristow, R., & Goff, B. (2011). Posttreatment surveillance and diagnosis of recurrence in women with gynecologic malignancies: Society of Gynecologic Oncologists recommendations. *Journal of Obstetrics and Gynecology, 204,* 466–478. doi:10.1016/j.ajog.2011.03.008

Shinohara, E.T., DeWees, T., & Perkins, S. (2014). Subsequent malignancies and their effect on survival in patients with retinoblastoma. *Pediatric Blood and Cancer, 61,* 116–119. doi:10.1002/pbc.24714

Siegel, R.L., Miller, K.D., & Jemal, A. (2015). Cancer statistics, 2015. *CA: A Cancer Journal for Clinicians, 65,* 5–29. doi:10.3322/caac.21254

Silver, J., Baima, J., & Mayer, R. (2013). Impairment-driven cancer rehabilitation: An essential component of quality care and survivorship. *CA: A Cancer Journal for Clinicians, 63,* 295–317. doi:10.3322/caac.21186

Stanton, A. (2012). What happens now? Psychosocial care for cancer survivors after medical treatment completion. *Journal of Clinical Oncology, 30,* 1215–1220. doi:10.1200/JCO.2011.39.7406

Stein, K.D., Syrjala, K., & Andrykowski, M. (2008). Physical and psychological long-term and late effects of cancer. *Cancer, 112*(Suppl. 11), 2577–2592. doi:10.1002/cncr.23448

Tesauro, G.M., Rowland, J.H., & Lustig, C. (2002). Survivorship resources for post-treatment cancer survivors. *Cancer Practice, 10,* 277–283. doi:10.1046/j.1523-5394.2002.106007.x

Travis, L.B., Hill, D., Dores, G.M., Gospodarowicz, M., van Leeuwen, F.E., Holowaty, E., … Gail, M.H. (2005). Cumulative absolute breast cancer risk for young women treated for Hodgkin lymphoma. *Journal of the National Cancer Institute, 97,* 1428–1437. doi:10.1093/jnci/dji290

Travis, L.B., Ng, A.K., Allan, J.M., Pui, C., Kennedy, A.R., Xu, G., … Boice, J.D., Jr. (2012). Second malignant neoplasms and cardiovascular disease following radiotherapy. *Journal of the National Cancer Institute, 104,* 357–370. doi:10.1093/jnci/djr533

U.S. Department of Labor Employee Benefits Security Administration. (2004, December). The Health Insurance Portability and Accountability Act (HIPAA). Retrieved from http://www.dol.gov/ebsa/newsroom/fshipaa.html

U.S. Department of Labor Employee Benefits Security Administration. (2012, November). *An employee's guide to health benefits under COBRA: The Consolidated Omnibus Budget Reconciliation Act of 1986.* Retrieved from http://www.dol.gov/ebsa/pdf/cobraemployee.pdf

Vachon, M. (2006). Psychosocial distress and coping after cancer treatment. *American Journal of Nursing, 106*(Suppl. 2), 26–31. doi:10.1097/00000446-200603003-00011

Valdivieso, M., Kujawa, A.M., Jones, T., & Baker, L.H. (2012). Cancer survivors in the United States: A review of the literature and a call to action. *International Journal of Medical Sciences, 9,* 163–173. doi:10.7150/ijms.3827

Yabroff, K.R., Lawrence, W.F., Clauser, S., Davis, W.W., & Brown, M.L. (2004). Burden of illness in cancer survivors: Findings from a population-based national sample. *Journal of the National Cancer Institute, 96,* 1322–1330. Retrieved from http://jnci.oxfordjournals.org/content/96/17/1322.full.pdf

CHAPTER 19

Palliative and End-of-Life Care

Debra E. Heidrich, MSN, RN, ACHPN

Introduction

Although great strides have been made in the diagnosis and treatment of cancer, it still accounts for 1 of every 4 deaths in the United States and is the second leading cause of death (Siegel, Miller, & Jemal, 2015). Progressive cancer and cancer treatments are associated with significant physical, psychosocial, and spiritual symptoms. These symptoms frequently are not managed optimally (Rainbird, Perkins, Sanson-Fisher, Rolfe, & Anseline, 2009; Teunissen et al., 2007). With this in mind, palliative care has become an essential component of quality care for both patients and their family members throughout the trajectory of an advanced or progressive illness, especially for those with advanced cancer (National Comprehensive Cancer Network® [NCCN®], 2015). Oncology advanced practice nurses (APNs) serve key roles in providing quality, cost-effective palliative care by applying advanced skills in assessment, diagnosis, and management of symptoms, as well as by communicating and coordinating care with all members of the interdisciplinary team.

Definition and Key Components of Palliative Care

Palliative care is defined by the Centers for Medicare and Medicaid Services (CMS) and the National Quality Forum as "patient and family-centered care that optimizes quality of life by anticipating, preventing, and treating suffering. Palliative care throughout the continuum of illness involves addressing physical, intellectual, emotional, social, and spiritual needs and to facilitate patient autonomy, access to information, and choice" (National Consensus Project for Quality Palliative Care [NCP], 2013, p. 7). The key features of palliative care are listed in Figure 19-1.

Palliative care is viewed as a continuum of care from diagnosis through death and includes hospice care and bereavement counseling, as illustrated in Figure 19-2. At diagnosis of a life-

- The patient and family are the focus of care.
- Symptoms are anticipated, prevented, and treated skillfully.
- Psychosocial, emotional, and spiritual symptoms are as important as physical symptoms.
- Patient autonomy is respected, requiring access to information to assist with decision making.
- Care is provided by an interdisciplinary team of providers.
- Life is affirmed and death is accepted as a normal process.
- Bereavement counseling for both the patient and the family are included as part of the plan of care.

Figure 19-1. Key Features of Palliative Care

Note. Based on information from National Comprehensive Cancer Network, 2015; National Consensus Project for Quality Palliative Care, 2013; World Health Organization, n.d.

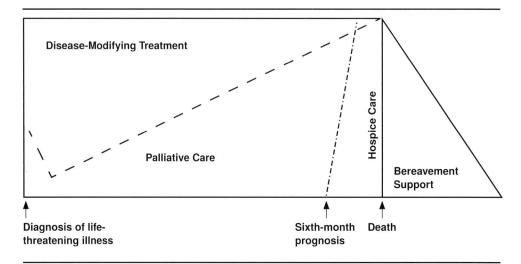

Figure 19-2. The Palliative Care Continuum

Note. Based on information from Ferris et al., 2009; National Consensus Project for Quality Palliative Care, 2009.

threatening illness, palliative care is provided along with disease-directed, life-prolonging therapies. The foci of palliative care at this time are management and anticipation of symptoms and communication about treatment goals. This also is an ideal time to initiate a discussion of advance care planning. See Chapter 20 for more information on code status, advance directives, and competency for decision making.

These palliative interventions may be initiated by the primary oncology team and augmented by palliative care experts based on patient and family needs. Because of the positive affect of specialized palliative care programs, expert palliative care services are increasingly being integrated into oncology care settings, providing continuity of care throughout the disease trajectory (Gilbert et al., 2012; Muir et al., 2010).

In settings where palliative care services are not integrated into the routine care of patients at diagnosis, the oncology clinician should consider consultation with palliative care experts when the patient has (a) advanced disease with a prognosis of less than one year, (b) significant symptom burden from disease or from treatment, (c) significant social or psychosocial distress, or (d) impaired performance status (Ramchandran & von Roenn, 2013). Impaired performance status is defined as Eastern Cooperative Oncology Group Performance Status grade

3 or higher or a Karnofsky Performance Status score of less than 50%. These scales are shown in Tables 19-1 and 19-2.

Palliative symptom management becomes the main focus of care when disease-directed, life-prolonging therapies are no longer effective, appropriate, or desired. At this time, referral may be made to hospice care programs.

Palliative care is a growing specialty. The number of palliative care programs in hospitals has more than doubled in the past 10 years. As of 2011, 85% of hospitals with more than 300 beds

Table 19-1. Eastern Cooperative Oncology Group (ECOG) Performance Status

Grade	ECOG
0	Fully active, able to carry on all predisease performance without restriction
1	Restricted in physically strenuous activity but ambulatory and able to carry out work of a light or sedentary nature (e.g., light housework, office work)
2	Ambulatory and capable of all self-care, but unable to carry out any work activities; up and about more than 50% of waking hours
3	Capable of only limited self-care, confined to bed or chair more than 50% of waking hours
4	Completely disabled; cannot carry on any self-care; totally confined to bed or chair
5	Dead

Note. From "Toxicity and Response Criteria of the Eastern Cooperative Oncology Group," by M.M. Oken, R.H. Creech, D.C. Tormey, J. Horton, T.E. Davis, E.T. McFadden, and P.P. Carbone, 1982, *American Journal of Clinical Oncology, 5,* p. 654. Reprinted with permission of Eastern Cooperative Oncology Group, Robert Comis, MD, Group Chair.

Table 19-2. Karnofsky Performance Status

Percentage of Normal Performance Status	Karnofsky Definitions
100	Normal; no complaints; no evidence of disease
90	Able to carry on normal activity; minor signs or symptoms of disease
80	Normal activity with effort; some signs or symptoms of disease
70	Cares for self; unable to carry on normal activity or do active work
60	Requires occasional assistance, but is able to care for most of needs
50	Requires considerable assistance and frequent medical care
40	Disabled; requires special care and assistance
30	Severely disabled; hospitalization is indicated although death not imminent
20	Very sick; hospital admission necessary; active supportive treatment necessary.
10	Moribund; fatal processes progressing rapidly
0	Dead

Note. Based on information from Karnofsky et al., 1948.

have palliative care services available (Center to Advance Palliative Care [CAPC], 2011). Certification in hospice and palliative care is available for physicians, nurses of all levels (i.e., nursing assistants, licensed practical nurses, RNs, APNs), social workers, and chaplains (CAPC, n.d.). Palliative care programs are found in multiple settings, including (a) consultative teams in acute care settings, such as intensive care and emergency department, (b) ambulatory care clinics, as a separate entity or integrated within other specialty practices or clinics (e.g., oncology, heart failure, chronic lung disease), (c) home-based care programs, usually associated with a homecare or hospice agency, and (d) long-term care or nursing home programs.

Studies support that palliative care programs have a positive influence on outcomes in patients with cancer. People being treated by palliative care teams report lower symptom intensity, improved quality of life, longer survival, less aggressive end-of-life care, and improved patient and family satisfaction when compared to standard care without palliative care consultation (Bakitas et al., 2009; Bischoff, Weinberg, & Rabow, 2013; Bükki et al., 2013; Follwell et al., 2009; Temel et al., 2010).

Standards for Palliative Care

NCP covers eight domains of quality palliative care in their clinical practice guidelines, as outlined in Figure 19-3. These guidelines are based on the tenets of "patient and family centered palliative care; comprehensive palliative care with continuity across health settings; early introduction of palliative care at diagnosis of a serious disease or life-threatening condition;

Domain 1: Structure and Processes of Care—includes guidelines on interdisciplinary assessment; patient and family–focused care planning; interdisciplinary services; education, training and support of team members; quality assessment and improvement; continuity of care across settings; and patient and family–focused environment of care.
Domain 2: Physical Aspects of Care—includes assessment and management of pain and other symptoms within the context of the disease status.
Domain 3: Psychological and Psychiatric Aspects of Care—includes assessment and interventions to address psychological and psychiatric needs to maximize patient and family coping and quality of life, as well as addressing grief and bereavement needs.
Domain 4: Social Aspects of Care—includes comprehensive person-centered assessment and interventions to address patient and family needs, promote patient and family goals, and maximize patient and family strengths and well-being.
Domain 5: Spiritual, Religious, and Existential Aspects of Care—includes comprehensive spiritual screening and assessment to identify preferences, beliefs, rituals, and practices; identification of spiritual distress and related issues; and facilitation of desired religious or spiritual practices.
Domain 6: Cultural Aspects of Care—includes serving the patient, family, and community in a culturally and linguistically appropriate manner and enhancing the program's cultural and linguistic competence.
Domain 7: Care of Patients at the End of Life—includes identifying, communicating, and managing the signs and symptoms of patients at the end of life; developing a plan of care to prevent and immediately treat symptoms in accordance with the patient and family preferences for site of care; providing respectful post-death care that honors cultural and religious practices; and initiating an immediate bereavement plan.
Domain 8: Ethical and Legal Aspects of Care—includes respecting patient and family goals, preferences, and choices within the limits of the law, current standards of care, and professional practice standards; and identifying, acknowledging, and addressing complex ethical issues that may arise.

Figure 19-3. Domains for Quality Palliative Care

Note. Based on information from National Consensus Project for Quality Palliative Care, 2013.

interdisciplinary collaborative palliative care; clinical and communication expertise within palliative care team members; relief of physical, psychological, emotional, and spiritual suffering and distress of patients and families; a focus on quality; and equitable access to palliative care services" (NCP, 2013, pp. 9–10).

NCCN (2015) updated its clinical practice guidelines for palliative care in oncology programs in 2015, listing the following standards:

- Institutions should develop processes for integrating palliative care into cancer care, both as part of usual oncology care and for patients with specialty palliative care needs.
- All cancer patients should be screened for palliative care needs at their initial visit, at appropriate intervals, and as clinically indicated.
- Patients and families should be informed that palliative care is an integral part of their comprehensive cancer care.
- Educational programs should be provided to all healthcare professionals and trainees so that they can develop effective palliative care knowledge, skills, and attitudes.
- Palliative care specialists and interdisciplinary palliative care teams, including board-certified palliative care physicians, advanced practice nurses, physician assistants, social workers, chaplains, and pharmacists, should be readily available to provide consultative or direct care to patients/families who request or require their expertise.
- Quality of palliative care should be monitored by institutional quality improvement programs. (p. PAL-1)

Hospice Palliative Care

Hospice is the part of the palliative care continuum that focuses on care within the final six months of life. Hospice is both a philosophy of care and a regulated insurance benefit. As a philosophy, it is a model of high-quality, compassionate care that helps patients and families live as fully as possible when cure is not possible (National Hospice and Palliative Care Organization [NHPCO], n.d.-a). It is based on the understanding that dying is part of the life cycle and that meticulous management of physical, psychosocial, and spiritual symptoms will promote quality of living for the patient and family system.

The term *hospice* has been around for centuries, but the modern concept began in the 1960s and 1970s as a grassroots movement. A dissatisfaction with the care of dying patients, along with the growing knowledge of symptom management, death and dying, and grief, fueled this movement. Dame Cicely Saunders is considered the founder of the modern hospice approach to care. She established St. Christopher Hospice in London, England, in 1967 after two decades of caring for dying patients and their loved ones. She lectured extensively on the improved symptom management and patient and family satisfaction achieved at St. Christopher Hospice and the importance of an interdisciplinary approach to care of physical, emotional, psychological, and spiritual well-being. After hearing Saunders speak, Dr. Florence Wald, RN, MSN, FAAN, took a sabbatical from her job as dean of Yale School of Nursing to work at St. Christopher Hospice. Wald then pioneered the movement in the United States, establishing the Connecticut Hospice in 1974 (NHPCO, n.d.-b).

Throughout the 1970s, many hospice organizations sprouted up in the United States. At the same time, psychiatrist Elisabeth Kübler-Ross's publications and talk show appearances discussing death, dying, and grief helped provide added momentum to the hospice movement. However, growth was ultimately stymied by the lack of a recognized mechanism for payment for hospice services. After demonstration projects showed that interdisciplinary care focused on quality of living and improved outcomes over usual care were possible at lower cost if multiple symptoms of terminal illness were addressed, Congress approved the Medicare hospice benefit in 1982. This benefit became permanent in 1986. With a stable source of payment for hospice care, there was a steady growth of hospice programs throughout the United States (NHPCO, n.d.-b). In 2013, there were more than 5,800 hospices in the country (NHPCO, 2014).

Because hospice care is part of the palliative care continuum (see Figure 19-2), the same key features of palliative care (see Figure 19-1) apply to hospice care. The difference is that the patient has reached a point on the continuum where life-prolonging treatments are no longer contributing to quality of life. The Medicare hospice benefit stipulates that the patient must have a prognosis of six months or less to be eligible for this benefit. In the United States, this six-month prognosis is often used to define hospice care.

It is important to note that the eligibility criteria for hospice should not be confused with length of service; patients can receive hospice care for as long as they meet eligibility criteria, even if they are enrolled in a hospice program for more than six months (NHPCO, n.d.-a). Late referrals to hospice are much more common than prolonged lengths of stay. The median length of stay in 2013 was only 18.5 days, with 34.5% of patients dying or discharged within seven days of admission (NHPCO, 2014). When patients are referred so late, they do not have time to get the full benefit of the interdisciplinary services available to them. For example, they may not have sufficient energy or the cognitive function to address important psychosocial and spiritual issues.

Barriers to Hospice Care

Multiple factors likely contribute to late referrals, including both healthcare provider barriers and patient and family barriers. Healthcare provider barriers include difficulty in predicting six-month prognosis, discomfort discussing end-of-life issues with patients, lack of time to discuss emotional issues with patients, concern that referral to hospice will lead to a loss of hope, difficulty identifying when life-prolonging therapies are no longer helping, real or perceived requirement that all life-prolonging therapies must be discontinued in hospice, concern that discontinuing therapies will hasten death, and lack of knowledge about hospice care and palliative symptom management (Brickner, Scannell, Marquet, & Ackerson, 2004; Friedman, Harwood, & Shields, 2002; Hui & Bruera, 2013; Kreuter & Herth, 2011).

Physicians often are overly optimistic when estimating prognoses, which may contribute to late referrals to hospice programs. On average, studies show physicians overestimate survival time by a factor of four to five (Christakis & Lamont, 2000; Krishnan et al., 2013; Stiel et al., 2010). In their classic study, Christakis and Lamont (2000) found that the closer the relationship between the physician and the patient, the less accurate the prediction. Until better objective measures to assist in making accurate prognoses are available, a recommended subjective measure is to ask the "surprise" question: Would you be surprised if this patient died in the next year? If it would not be a surprise, the patient is likely appropriate for a hospice referral (Moss et al., 2010).

Interventions in hospice care are aimed at relieving distressing symptoms and enhancing quality of life for the patient and the family. Life-prolonging therapies often are not part of the hospice plan of care, but no therapies are specifically excluded in hospice. Disease-modifying or life-prolonging therapies may be part of the plan of care if these therapies are the best approach for relieving distressing symptoms or enhancing quality of life (City & Labyak, 2010). Decisions about what disease-modifying medications should be discontinued are difficult for patients, healthcare providers, and hospice agencies. These therapies often are very expensive, making it difficult for hospice programs to afford the therapy. The true risks and benefits for people with advanced disease often are unknown. Some clinicians feel that carefully selected individuals may benefit from chemotherapy or targeted therapies even at advanced stages of an illness (Hui & Bruera, 2013). However, investigational studies showing some survival advantage with certain treatments rarely include the typical hospice patients (i.e., older adults or those with multiple medical problems). Therefore, the survival advantages shown in these studies may not be generalizable. Well-designed, controlled trials are needed to evaluate the trade-offs between benefits and risks in people who would otherwise meet hospice admission criteria (Alvarez, Westeel, Cortés-Jofré, & Cosp, 2013). Hospice programs must evaluate the goals of disease-modifying therapies on a case-by-case basis to determine if they are consistent with the hospice plan of care.

Patient and family barriers to hospice referral include being uncomfortable with confronting end-of-life issues, equating the word hospice with "giving up," and having misinformation about hospice services (Friedman et al., 2002).

Reimbursement for Hospice and Palliative Care Services

The Medicare hospice benefit is the primary source of reimbursement for hospice palliative care. Most private insurance companies model their hospice benefit after the Medicare model. To be eligible for the Medicare hospice benefit, (a) the patient must be eligible for Medicare Part A, (b) the referring physician and hospice medical director must certify, to the best of their knowledge, that the patient has a six-month or less prognosis if the disease runs its natural course, and (c) the patient must elect hospice care for the treatment of the terminal illness (i.e., waives right to traditional Medicare for the treatment of the terminal illness and its symptoms) (CMS, 2015). The patient may continue to get treatment under traditional Medicare for conditions not related to the terminal illness. For example, a person with limited life expectancy from a cancer diagnosis who had previously been treated for multiple sclerosis could continue to receive treatment for the multiple sclerosis under traditional Medicare.

Hospice services are interdisciplinary and are provided based on patient and family needs. A list of services that all hospices must have available is provided in Figure 19-4. The Medicare hospice benefit includes four different levels of care, reflecting the variations in care intensity required to meet patient and family needs (City & Labyak, 2010):
- Routine home care: Care provided in the patient's place of residence, including private home, nursing home, or residential care setting.
- Continuous home care: Care provided in the patient's place of residence during a time of crisis requiring predominantly continuous nursing care.
- General inpatient care: Care provided in an inpatient facility for pain or symptom control when the symptom cannot be managed at home.
- Inpatient respite care: Care provided in an approved facility on a short-term basis to give respite to the family caregiver.

• Nursing care	• Home health and homemaker services
• Physician services	• Physical, occupational, and speech therapies
• Social services	• Dietary/nutrition counseling
• Counseling services, including but not limited to bereavement counseling, dietary counseling, and spiritual counseling	• Grief and loss counseling
	• Volunteers
	• Short-term inpatient care for pain and symptom control
• Medical equipment and supplies	
• Medications for symptom control	• Short-term respite care

Figure 19-4. Services Included in the Medicare Hospice Benefit

---

Note. Based on information from Centers for Medicare and Medicaid Services, 2015.

Hospices are paid at a fixed daily rate based on the level of care to cover interdisciplinary team care, medications related to the terminal illness, and medical supplies and equipment. It is recognized that some care will cost more than what the hospice will receive in reimbursement. The financial viability of a hospice program is based on maintaining a large enough census that includes patients who require less expensive care to balance the costs of the few who require more expensive care.

It is important to note that the Medicare hospice benefit does not pay for room and board, treatment or medications aimed at curing the terminal illness, or any care for the terminal illness that is not arranged by the hospice and part of the hospice plan of care (CMS, 2015). For example, an emergency room visit may not be covered if it is not arranged by the hospice. Patients and families are taught to call the hospice 24-hour on-call service in urgent situations. Should they decide they want to pursue therapies that are not part of the hospice plan of care, patients always have the right revoke the Medicare hospice benefit and go back to traditional Medicare at any time.

Reimbursement for nonhospice palliative care varies with the setting. Physicians and APNs may be able to bill for consultations under insurance plans, such as Medicare Part A for inpatient care or Part B for ambulatory or home-based care. Often, palliative care physicians and APNs use symptom management codes to bill for services, allowing the provider who is managing the disease process to bill under the diagnosis code. The care provided by other members of the interdisciplinary team often is not eligible for reimbursement. Many palliative care programs do not receive enough in reimbursements to cover the salaries of the providers. However, the cost savings to hospitals by transitioning patients to less expensive levels of care, discontinuing unnecessary and expensive interventions (e.g., laboratory studies and scans), and facilitating earlier discharges is significant, often considerably more than the salaries of the palliative care team (Morrison et al., 2008). Hospitals support palliative care programs because palliative care teams (CAPC, 2014)

- Lower costs for hospitals and payers
- Provide a systematic approach to patients with high-intensity needs
- Support primary care providers
- Increase patient and family satisfaction
- Assist the hospital to meet Joint Commission standards
- Ease the burdens on staff, promoting retention
- Meet the needs of an aging population.

Grief and Bereavement

Many losses are experienced by people with advanced, progressive cancer. These include anything from the loss of hair and how that body image change affects the individual, the loss of control over time and schedules, the loss of social roles, or the loss of life. Grief is a normal and expected reaction to loss; the intensity of the grief response is related to the significance of the loss to the individual. Key definitions related to loss and grieving are listed in Figure 19-5. Because people with cancer and their family members experience multiple kinds of grief throughout the cancer experience, oncology APNs must support individuals through the normal grieving process and be able to identify complicated grief reactions that may require additional levels of support.

Two major types of complicated grief are prolonged grief and disenfranchised grief. Prolonged grief is defined as persistent and severe yearning for the deceased beyond 6–12 months after the loss (Bryant, 2013). Prolonged grief disorder is recognized as a mental disorder causing significant distress and disability and is included in the *Diagnostic and Statistical Manual of Mental Disorders* (5th ed.) (American Psychiatric Association, 2013; Bryant, 2013; Waldrop

- Loss: The absence of an object, position, ability, or attribute
- Grief: The psychological, social, and somatic responses to loss
- Anticipatory grief: The psychological, social, and somatic responses to an anticipated loss
- Mourning: The outward and active expression of grief through participation in various death and bereavement rituals that vary by culture (i.e., the cultural response to grief)
- Bereavement: The state of having suffered a loss; the period of time during which grief and mourning occur. The first year after a loss is generally the most difficult.
- Complicated grief: A disturbance in the normal process of grief

Figure 19-5. Loss and Grief Definitions

Note. Based on information from Buglass, 2010; Corless, 2015.

& Kutner, 2013). Disenfranchised grief occurs when a loss cannot be openly acknowledged. Examples include death of a person in a "nonsanctioned" relationship, such as an extramarital affair or homosexual relationship; loss resulting from miscarriage or abortion; or the loss of the essence of the individual before actual death, such as with severe dementia.

Manifestations of grief include social, physical, and cognitive-emotional reactions and vary widely from one individual to another, as illustrated in Table 19-3. There is no right way to grieve. Mourning and bereavement are influenced by religious practices, the nature of the relationship with the deceased, the age of the deceased, and the manner of death (Corless, 2015).

Grief Theories

Theories of the grief process help explain the reactions and responses to grief and have evolved over time. Kübler-Ross (1969) described five phases or stages of grief: denial, anger, bargaining, depression, and acceptance. This theory assists in understanding the kinds of reactions observed in people experiencing loss. These stages are not linear; there is often overlap. They also do not necessarily occur sequentially. Building on the concepts introduced by Kübler-Ross and others, Worden (2008) described grief work in terms of four tasks to accomplish to resolve grief: accepting the reality of the loss (i.e., letting go of denial), experiencing the pain of the grief, adjusting to the environment without the deceased person, and withdrawing emotionally from the deceased by forming an ongoing relationship with the memories of the deceased in a way that allows the bereaved person to continue with life. Worden referred to this process as *relocation*.

The Dual Process Model of Coping with Bereavement, introduced in 1999, was built upon previously introduced theories of grieving. It was developed to show the dynamic nature of grief and explain variations in the ways individuals come to terms with bereavement (Stroebe & Schut, 2010). According to this model, the bereaved person oscillates between loss-oriented coping and restoration-oriented coping; both loss-oriented and restoration-oriented processes are necessary for adjustment to the loss. Loss-oriented coping includes concentrating on and working through some aspect of the loss experience itself (e.g., crying, yearning, relocation). Restoration-oriented coping involves mastering new tasks, reorganizing life, and developing a new identity.

Addressing Grief

Too often, discussions with patients about their losses are avoided. Losses require time and emotional energy for everyone—patients, family members, and healthcare providers. The fear exists that discussing death may lead to loss of hope and somehow hasten death. Patients may

Table 19-3. Normal Manifestations of Grief

Domain	Behaviors
Social	• Restlessness and inability to sit still • Uncomfortable around other people/social withdrawal • Feeling of not wanting to be alone • Lack of ability to initiate and maintain organized patterns of activity
Physical	• Anorexia and weight loss; or the opposite, overeating and weight gain • Heart palpitations; nervousness, tension, panic • Shortness of breath • Tightness in throat • Inability to sleep • Lack of energy and feelings of physical exhaustion • Headaches, muscular aches, gastrointestinal distress
Cognitive-emotional	• Sadness and crying • Forgetfulness or difficulty concentrating • Feelings of anger or guilt • Mood swings • Sense of helplessness • Yearning for the deceased • Dreams of the deceased

Note. Based on information from Corless, 2015; Rando, 1984.

avoid discussing fears and concerns with family members, believing that these topics will upset them. This pattern of avoidance can contribute to anxiety, depression, and guilt.

It is important to counsel patients and families to express feelings and heal relationships while patients have the physical and mental capacity to participate in these conversations. Byock (1997) introduced the "five things" of relationship completion that have been used by many hospice professionals: forgiving others, seeking forgiveness, thanking others, expressing love, and saying good-bye. Encouraging patients and families to address these "five things" may assist with finding meaning and assuaging guilt.

Another helpful intervention is to encourage individuals to participate in mourning practices (i.e., the cultural practices and rituals associated with death, dying, and burial) that are meaningful to them. Death and funeral practices vary among cultures and religions; it is important to ask what practices are important to individuals. Some patients may want to plan their own funerals, including meeting with a funeral home professional and discussing the service with a religious leader. The healthcare team can help arrange these meetings.

Bereavement involves processing many thoughts and emotions. Grief support groups help some people by providing a safe place to tell their story and enabling them to hear how others are dealing with their own grief. Some people find expressing themselves in groups to be difficult. They may benefit from one-on-one support from family members, friends, faith community members and leaders, or mental health professionals. When it is appropriate for the setting and relationship, the APN can plan a bereavement visit or telephone call. This follow-up not only provides an opportunity for bereaved patients to tell their stories again, but it also can be used to assess the need for additional bereavement services.

Corless (2015) identified several counseling interventions that may be helpful for the bereaved. When individuals are harboring thoughts or feelings that were never expressed to the deceased, they may find it helpful to express them in a letter or journal or talk to an empty chair or picture. Anger may be vented by banging a pillow on a mattress, screaming at home or in a parked car, or crying loudly in a private location. Interventions to assist individuals in finding meaning in past or current events include guided imagery, journal writing, analyzing role changes, and drawing pictures.

Community Resources for Palliative and Hospice Care

Patients who meet the eligibility criteria for hospice and accept the hospice philosophy of care should be referred to a Medicare-certified hospice care program. Although programs not certified for Medicare payments may be available in some communities, certification ensures that the program meets the standards defined by CMS. Hospice organizations range from small, independent organizations, to organizations affiliated with larger healthcare systems, to very large corporations with multiple offices throughout a region or across the United States.

Most hospital discharge planners and social workers maintain lists of hospices available in their communities. Hospice organizations that are members of NHPCO may be found by searching by zip code on the NHPCO website (www.nhpco.org).

In 2012, hospital-based palliative care programs were available in 66% of hospitals with more than 50 beds and 85% of hospitals with more than 300 beds (CAPC, 2012). These programs range from single-professional consultations (usually nurse or physician), to interdisciplinary consultation teams, to programs that include specialty palliative care units. The Joint Commission launched a certification process for hospice inpatient palliative care programs in 2011. This certification set standards for information management, access to services, communication, patient-directed interdisciplinary care, coordination of services, and performance improvement (CAPC, 2011). While certification ensures that programs meet these standards, many palliative care programs are not yet certified.

Outpatient provision of palliative care in practices and clinics is in early development, and the prevalence of ambulatory palliative care programs is unknown. Most of the highly evaluated practices are part of a cancer center (Rabow, 2013). The structure and function of the outpatient programs vary depending on such factors as affiliation with an established inpatient palliative care program, number of disciplines involved in the care, referral sources, and model of care (consultative versus co-management of patients). Currently, no certification process exists for ambulatory palliative care.

Home-based, hospice-based, and nursing home–based palliative care programs are available in some communities (Sefcik, Rao, & Ersek, 2013; Zhang et al., 2013). These models have the potential to increase quality of care for people with chronic, progressive illnesses, especially for those who do not meet hospice eligibility criteria but have significant symptom burden.

No certification process exists for nonhospice community-based palliative care. Programs that are homecare certified may be able to bill for services if the patient meets homecare criteria, but no separate insurance benefit exists for home palliative care at this time.

APNs caring for patients with advanced, progressive illnesses who are not discharged to interdisciplinary hospice or palliative care programs must be aware of community resources that may help address patient and family needs and work with social workers and discharge planners to assist in coordinating care. Community resources may include
• Homecare services for those with a skilled home need for nursing care or therapies
• Home health aide or homemaker services, which may or may not be covered by insurance depending on identified needs and insurance plan
• Social services agencies
• Area Agency on Aging services, which may include meal delivery, home health/homemaker services, caregiver support, legal advice, transportation, and equipment such as wheelchairs

- Agencies that provide support specifically to people with a cancer diagnosis, such as the American Cancer Society or the Cancer Support Community
- Lay-led and professional-led grief support programs. (Hospices often accept families into their grief support programs even if the patient was not enrolled in a hospice.)

Interdisciplinary Team

Interdisciplinary care is an essential component of comprehensive palliative care programs and required for certification of hospice and palliative care services (CAPC, 2011; CMS, 2015; NCCN, 2015; NCP, 2013). The expertise of several disciplines is required to meet the varied physical, psychological, emotional, and spiritual needs of the patient and family system (City & Labyak, 2010). Interdisciplinary care differs from multidisciplinary care. Multidisciplinary care is when professionals from each discipline assess the patient and formulates a plan in their specific area of expertise (i.e., the traditional consultation model of care in acute care settings). The interdisciplinary approach requires collaboration of all disciplines involved to create a patient- and family-directed plan of care. In palliative care settings, the patient and family are a part of the palliative care interdisciplinary team (City & Labyak, 2010). Interdisciplinary care requires that each discipline expand and blend its traditional role in care with those of other disciplines. Specifically, the physical, functional, and interpersonal well-being and transcendent dimensions of care are addressed by the physician, nurse, pharmacist, therapist, nutritionist, volunteers, nursing assistants, homemakers, counselors, social workers, psychologists, and chaplains.

Patient and Family Education

The patient and family have multiple educational needs throughout the continuum of palliative cancer care. Initial education of patients and families includes telling them about palliative care and how it is integrated with cancer care throughout the course of the illness. This also includes clarifying any misperceptions about palliative care, noting that many people often equate palliative care with hospice care.

The palliative care APN assists the patient and family in identifying goals of care throughout the course of the illness. In order to have these discussions, the APN must provide and clarify information about the patient's current condition, options for care and likely outcomes, and anticipated symptoms. When the patient's desires for the care they want and do not want if prognosis is limited are discussed, the APN is able to assist the patient to develop clear advance directives or update existing advance directives.

Throughout the course of the illness, patient and family teaching is essential for optimal symptom management. APNs provide information about anticipated physical, psychological, emotional, and spiritual symptoms; symptom prevention; early indicators of symptoms; the importance of prompt management; and the appropriate use of pharmacologic and nonpharmacologic interventions to manage symptoms. Skills required for the care of the patient (e.g., administering medications, changing dressings, caring for catheters, using medical equipment) also must be taught. Patients and families need information on resources available in the community for assistance and support.

Education of the patient and family also includes information about how response to treatment and quality of life are monitored. When signs and symptoms indicate disease progression or poor quality of life on treatment, the options of discontinuing interventions that are not helpful and enrolling in a hospice program are discussed. Whether or not the patient chooses hospice care, education includes expected disease progression; signs and symptoms of approaching death; appropriate symptom management in the final weeks, days, and hours before death; and dealing with grief and bereavement.

Implications for Oncology Advanced Practice Nurses

As discussed previously, integration of palliative care into the care of the cancer patient has a positive impact on quality of life, mood, symptom intensity, and end-of-life care (Ramchandran & von Roenn, 2013). The oncology APN needs to have an understanding of palliative care and how it is integrated into oncology care throughout the illness continuum. Palliation of symptoms is every nurse's role, and oncology APNs provide this general palliative care as part of routine care. Oncology APNs play a key role in ordering a specialized palliative care consult when appropriate (i.e., for those with advanced disease with a prognosis less than one year, those with significant symptom burden or psychosocial distress, those with poor performance status) (Ramchandran & von Roenn, 2013).

If a specialty palliative care service is not available in the setting where the APN practices, the oncology APN's plan of care for the patient should specifically include advance care planning; symptom identification and management; patient and family support for psychoemotional needs, including grief counseling; and referral to hospice care, when appropriate. This plan of care includes referrals to other members of the interdisciplinary team and to community resources to assist in addressing these multiple needs. When specialty palliative care services are not available in the community or agency, oncology APNs may serve as advocates for starting a palliative care program.

Future Directions

The specialty of palliative care has grown exponentially since the early 1990s (Goldstein & Morrison, 2013). The aging population and research showing the positive influence of palliative care programs on quality, satisfaction, and cost-effectiveness have contributed to the growth of palliative care programs. Palliative care will continue to be integrated into healthcare specialties and subspecialties, including oncology. APNs will be integral in identifying models for delivering optimal palliative care throughout the continuum of cancer care. It is not enough to have a palliative care program in the hospital; palliative care must be provided in all cancer care settings, with communication among all settings to ensure continuity of care.

Many interventions used in end-of-life care settings are based more on clinical experiences than research. As more and more physicians and APNs specialize in palliative care and more research is conducted, the evidence base for symptom management in the advanced stages of illness will continue to grow (Goldstein & Morrison, 2013).

Conclusion

Palliative care is a continuum of care initiated at the time of diagnosis of a serious disease or life-threatening condition that continues throughout disease progression, death, and bereavement. Palliative care is an essential component of comprehensive, quality oncology care and has been demonstrated to improve symptom management, quality of life, survival, and patient and family satisfaction. This quality, cost-effective care is provided through an interdisciplinary team that focuses on exquisite symptom management and patient- and family-centered, goal-directed care.

Key Points

- Palliative care focuses on quality of life by anticipating, preventing, treatment symptoms that affect quality of life.
- The patient and family are the major focus of care.
- Hospice is a part of the palliative care continuum but focuses on individuals no longer eligible for curative treatments.
- Hospice is a Medicare benefit for most people and can be administered in a patient's home, a nursing home, an assisted living facility, or a private home or hospice residence.

Case Study

J.B. is a 57-year-old woman with late-stage colon cancer. She has been divorced for 10 years with little contact with her former husband. She has three children aged 17, 19, and 21.

J.B. was diagnosed with colon cancer with extensive liver metastasis one year ago. She underwent a colectomy to remove the bulk of the tumor and started treatment with FOLFOX. The oncology APN discussed palliative care with J.B. and made a referral to the inpatient palliative care team.

J.B. met with the palliative care APN before being discharged from the hospital. An advance care planning discussion was initiated and J.B.'s goals for care and concerns were discussed. J.B. was aware that cure was not possible but hoped to live to see her youngest child graduate from high school. She and her children were overwhelmed with the diagnosis. J.B. was very concerned about the future of her children's education and emotional and financial support. She identified her three sisters and her church community as her support system. The palliative care APN made a referral to the palliative care social worker, who initiated a visit with J.B. and then planned follow-up telephone calls with her every other week during J.B.'s chemotherapy treatment. The palliative care APN consulted with both the surgical team and the oncology APN to address the patient's postoperative pain and bowel protocol. A follow-up appointment with the palliative care APN was planned as an outpatient in the palliative care clinic to continue advance care planning and ensure optimal symptom management.

After six months of treatment and several outpatient palliative care visits in addition to her oncology care, J.B. had completed her advance directives. She had been taught how to complete a symptom distress screening tool and instructed to contact the oncology APN with symptom issues during treatment. The social worker had supported J.B. in discussing her illness and prognosis with her children, sisters, and minister. An attorney also was consulted to assist with guardianship issues should J.B. die before her youngest son turned 18 (neither the son nor his father wanted a closer relationship with each other) and to assist with estate planning. The oncology APN coordinated symptom management during cancer treatment. The palliative care interdisciplinary team reviewed J.B.'s case at monthly team meetings.

Follow-up scans indicated disease progression despite treatments. The oncologist met with J.B. to review the scans and the options for second-line therapy versus comfort care. A meeting between J.B., the oncology APN, and the palliative care team was planned to review the patient's understanding of her prognosis and options and to discuss her care goals.

J.B. reported that she had felt increasingly weak and was not able to do as much. She had anticipated the news that her disease was progressing. J.B. had discussed this with the social worker over the past several weeks and had been thinking about what she would do with either good or bad reports. Given the disease progression, J.B. was very clear that she did not want any additional cancer treatment. Her son had graduated from high school the previous month and all three children were staying at home for the summer. J.B. wanted to be cared for at home, but she did not want her boys to be burdened by her care needs. J.B.'s sisters had agreed to take turns caring for her when she needed more assistance. J.B. agreed to meet with a hospice agency. Her self-report symptom inventory indicated that symptoms were well controlled with current interventions.

The palliative care social worker helped J.B. and her family transition counseling and social support to the hospice social worker, bereavement counselor, volunteers, and their minister. The palliative APN reviewed the current symptom management plan of care with the hospice interdisciplinary team to ensure continuity of care.

1. When should J.B. have been referred for palliative care?
   A. When her prognosis was believed to be six months or less
   B. When scans indicated progression of disease despite treatment
   C. When the advanced-stage disease was diagnosed
   D. When she asked for a palliative care consult

   The correct answer is C. Palliative care should be initiated at the time of diagnosis of any life-threatening illness. The palliative care team assists with symptom management and discussion of care goals. As the disease progresses, less focus is on disease-directed therapies and more is put on palliative care (i.e., physical, psychological, emotional, and spiritual symptom management and quality-of-life issues).

2. True/False: J.B.'s palliative care needs could have been optimally addressed by an APN working within the full scope of the APN's practice.

   The statement is false. Optimal palliative care requires the expertise of an interdisciplinary team. While excellent symptom management, psychosocial and spiritual support, and advance care planning needs are addressed by the APN, J.B.'s case illustrates the importance of a social worker on the team. In addition, this case illustrates the importance of collaboration between the oncology team, the palliative care team, and the hospice interdisciplinary team.

3. List at least four key features of palliative care.
   • The patient and family are the focus of care.
   • Symptoms are anticipated, prevented, and treated skillfully.
   • Psychosocial, emotional, and spiritual symptoms are as important as physical symptoms.
   • Patient autonomy is respected, requiring access to information to assist with decision making.
   • Care is provided by an interdisciplinary team of providers.
   • Life is affirmed and death is accepted as a normal process.
   • Bereavement counseling for both the patient and the family is included as part of the plan of care.

4. If J.B.'s insurance benefit for hospice care is modeled after the Medicare hospice benefit, which of the following is true?
   A. The hospice will bill the insurance company based on the services provided each day.
   B. The hospice reimbursement covers all members of the interdisciplinary team, as specified in the plan of care, except for physician care, which is billed separately.
   C. If the hospice interdisciplinary team determines that J.B. needs hospitalization to manage an acute symptom, the insurance reverts back to traditional care and the hospital will bill the insurance company for that stay.
   D. If J.B.'s family needs a break from care, the hospice can arrange a five-day stay in a contracted facility for respite care. The hospice will receive a different level of payment for those respite days.

   The best answer to this is D. *Respite* is an accepted level of care under the Medicare hospice benefit. The length of a respite stay is five days and the hospice is reimbursed at a rate slightly higher than the routine homecare rate. In this example, answer A is not correct. A hospice receives a daily rate for routine home care no matter how many services are provided on a particular day. Answer B is also not correct. Hospice payments include all interdisciplinary team services; however, if J.B. were to see a physician or APN for services unrelated to the terminal illness, it would be billed separately. Answer C is not correct. If a hospital stay is required for acute symptom management and it is arranged by the hospice, the hospice will receive a higher daily rate for this level of care. Hospices that do not have their own inpatient units to use for acute symptom management will have a contract with a local hospital for this level of care that includes the daily rate the hospice will pay the hospital.

The author would like to acknowledge Deborah A. Boyle, RN, MSN, AOCN®, FAAN, and Regina M. Fink, RN, PhD, AOCN®, FAAN, for their contributions to this chapter that remain unchanged from the first edition of this book.

References

Alvarez, M.P., Westeel, V., Cortés-Jofré, M., & Cosp, X.B. (2013). Chemotherapy versus best supportive care for extensive small cell lung cancer. *Cochrane Database of Systematic Reviews, 2013*(11). doi:10.1002/14651858.CD001990.pub3

American Psychiatric Association. (2013). *Diagnostic and statistical manual of mental disorders* (5th ed.). Washington, DC: Author.

Bakitas, M., Lyons, K.D., Hegel, M.T., Balan, S., Barnett, K.N., Brokaw, F.C., … Ahles, T.A. (2009). The project ENABLE II randomized controlled trial to improve palliative care for rural patients with advanced cancer: Baseline finding, methodological challenges, and solutions. *Palliative and Supportive Care, 7*, 75–86. doi:10.1017/S1478951509000108

Bischoff, K., Weinberg, V., & Rabow, M.W. (2013). Palliative and oncologic co-management: Symptom management for outpatients with cancer. *Supportive Care in Cancer, 21*, 3031–3037. doi:10.1007/s00520-013-1838-z

Brickner, L., Scannell, K., Marquet, S., & Ackerson, L. (2004). Barriers to hospice care and referrals: Survey of physicians' knowledge, attitudes, and perceptions in a health maintenance organization. *Journal of Palliative Medicine, 7*, 411–418. doi:10.1089/1096621041349518

Bryant, R.A. (2013). Is pathological grief lasting more than 12 months grief or depression? *Current Opinions in Psychiatry, 26*, 41–46. doi:10.1097/YCO.0b013e32835b2ca2

Buglass, E., (2010). Grief and bereavement theories. *Nursing Standard, 24*(41), 44–47. doi:10.7748/ns2010.06.24.41.44.c7834

Bükki, J., Scherbel, J., Stiel, S., Klein, C., Meidenbauer, N., & Ostgathe, C. (2013). Palliative care needs, symptoms, and treatment intensity along the disease trajectory in medical oncology outpatients: A retrospective chart review. *Supportive Care in Cancer, 21*, 1743–1750. doi:10.1007/s00520-013-1721-y

Byock, I. (1997). *Dying well.* New York, NY: Riverhead Books.

Center to Advance Palliative Care. (n.d.). Certification and licensing. Retrieved from https://www.capc.org/providers/palliative-care-resources/palliative-care-resources-certification-licensing

Center to Advance Palliative Care. (2011). *America's care of serious illness: A state-by-state report card on access to palliative care in our nation's hospitals.* Retrieved from http://reportcard.capc.org/pdf/state-by-state-report-card.pdf

Center to Advance Palliative Care. (2012). *Growth of palliative care in U.S. hospitals 2012 snapshot.* Retrieved from http://reportcard.capc.org/pdf/capc-growth-analysis-snapshot-2011.pdf

Center to Advance Palliative Care. (2014). *The case for hospital palliative care.* Retrieved from https://www.capc.org/media/filer_public/06/90/069053fe-12bf-4485-b973-d290f7c2ecbf/thecaseforhospitalpalliativecare_capc.pdf

Centers for Medicare and Medicaid Services. (2015, January). *Medicare hospice benefits* (CMS Product No. 02154). Retrieved from http://www.medicare.gov/Pubs/pdf/02154.pdf

Christakis, N.A., & Lamont, E.B. (2000). Extent and determinants of error in doctors' prognoses in terminally ill patients: Prospective cohort study. *BMJ, 320*, 469–473. doi:10.1136/bmj.320.7233.469

City, K.A.E., & Labyak, M.J. (2010). Hospice palliative care for the 21st century: A model for quality end-of-life care. In B.R. Ferrell & N. Coyle (Eds.), *Oxford textbook of palliative nursing* (3rd ed., pp. 13–52). New York, NY: Oxford University Press.

Corless, I.B. (2015). Bereavement. In B.R. Ferrell, N. Coyle, & J.A. Paice (Eds.), *Oxford textbook of palliative nursing* (4th ed., pp. 487–499). New York, NY: Oxford University Press.

Ferris, F.D., Bruera, E., Cherny, N., Cummings, C., Currow, D., Dudgeon, D., … Von Roenn, J.H. (2009). Palliative cancer care a decade later: Accomplishments, the need, next steps—From the American Society of Clinical Oncology. *Journal of Clinical Oncology, 27,* 3052–3058. doi:10.1200/JCO.2008.20.1558

Follwell, M., Burman, D., Le, L.W., Wakimoto, K., Seccareccia, D., Bryson, J., … Zimmermann, C. (2009). Phase II study of an outpatient palliative care intervention in patients with metastatic cancer. *Journal of Clinical Oncology, 27,* 206–213. doi:10.1200/JCO.2008.17.7568

Friedman, B.T., Harwood, M.K., & Shields, M. (2002). Barriers and enablers to hospice referrals: An expert overview. *Journal of Palliative Medicine, 5,* 73–84. doi:10.1089/10966210252785033

Gilbert, J.E., Howell, D., King, S., Sawka, C., Hughes, E., Angus, H., & Dudgeon, D. (2012). Quality improvement in cancer symptom assessment and control: The Provincial Palliative Care Integration Project (PPCIP). *Journal of Pain and Symptom Management, 43,* 663–678. doi:10.1016/j.jpainsymman.2011.04.028

Goldstein, N.E., & Morrison, R.S. (2013). Preface. In N.E. Goldstein & R.S. Morrison (Eds.), *Evidence-based practice of palliative medicine* (p. i). Philadelphia, PA: Elsevier. doi:10.1016/B978-1-4377-3796-7.09983-3

Hui, D., & Bruera, E. (2013). Personalizing treatment decisions for cancer patients at the end of life: Reply to Soh and Wong. *Journal of Pain and Symptom Management, 45,* e4–e5. doi:10.1016/j.jpainsymman.2013.02.001

Karnofsky, D.A., Abelmann, W.H., Craver, L.F., & Burchenal, J.H. (1948). The use of the nitrogen mustards in the palliative treatment of carcinoma. *Cancer, 1*(4), 634–656. doi:10.1002/1097-0142(194811)1:4<634::AID-CNCR2820010410>3.0.CO;2-L

Kreuter, M., & Herth, F.J. (2011). Supportive and palliative care of advanced nonmalignant lung disease. *Respiration, 82,* 307–316. doi:10.1159/000330730

Krishnan, M., Temel, J.S., Wright, A.A., Bernacki, R., Selvaggi, K., & Balboni, T. (2013). Predicting life expectancy in patients with advanced incurable cancer: A review. *Journal of Supportive Oncology, 11,* 68–74. doi:10.12788/j.suponc.0004

Kübler-Ross, E. (1969). *On death and dying.* New York, NY: Macmillan.

Morrison, R.S., Penrod, J.D., Cassel, B., Caust-Ellenbogen, M., Litke, A., Spragens, L., & Meier, D.E. (2008). Cost savings associated with US hospital palliative care consultation programs. *Archives of Internal Medicine, 168,* 1783–1790. doi:10.1001/archinte.168.16.1783

Moss, A.H., Lunney, J.R., Culp, S., Auber, M., Kurian, S., Rogers, J., … Abraham, J. (2010). Prognostic significance of the 'surprise' question in cancer patients. *Journal of Palliative Medicine, 13,* 837–840. doi:10.1089/jpm.2010.0018

Muir, J.C., Daly, F., Davis, M.S., Weinberg, R., Heintz, J.S., Paivanas, T.A., & Beveridge, R. (2010). Integrating palliative care into the outpatient, private practice oncology setting. *Journal of Pain and Symptom Management, 40,* 126–135. doi:10.1016/j.jpainsymman.2009.12.017

National Comprehensive Cancer Network. (2015). *NCCN Clinical Practice Guidelines in Oncology (NCCN Guidelines®): Palliative care* [v.2.2015]. Retrieved from http://www.nccn.org/professionals/physician_gls/pdf/palliative.pdf

National Consensus Project for Quality Palliative Care. (2009). *Clinical practice guidelines for quality palliative care* (2nd ed.). Pittsburgh, PA: Author.

National Consensus Project for Quality Palliative Care. (2013). *Clinical practice guidelines for quality palliative care* (3rd ed.). Pittsburgh, PA: Author.

National Hospice and Palliative Care Organization. (n.d.-a). History of hospice care. Retrieved from http://www.nhpco.org/history-hospice-care

National Hospice and Palliative Care Organization. (n.d.-b). Key hospice messages. Retrieved from http://www.nhpco.org/press-room/key-hospice-messages

National Hospice and Palliative Care Organization. (2014). *NHPCO's facts and figures: Hospice care in America* (2014 edition). Retrieved from http://www.nhpco.org/sites/default/files/public/Statistics_Research/2014_Facts_Figures.pdf

Oken, M.M., Creech, R.H., Tormey, D.C., Horton, J., Davis, T.E., McFadden, E.T., & Carbone, P.P. (1982). Toxicity and response criteria of the Eastern Cooperative Oncology Group. *American Journal of Clinical Oncology, 5,* 649–655. doi:10.1097/00000421-198212000-00014

Rabow, M.W. (2013). What new models exist for ambulatory palliative care? In N.E. Goldstein & R.S. Morrison (Eds.), *Evidence-based practice of palliative medicine* (pp. 468–473). doi:10.1016/B978-1-4377-3796-7.00079-3

Rainbird, K., Perkins, J., Sanson-Fisher, R., Rolfe, I., & Anseline, P. (2009). The needs of patients with advanced, incurable cancer. *British Journal of Cancer, 101,* 759–764. doi:10.1038/sj.bjc.6605235

Ramchandran, K.J., & von Roenn, J.H. (2013). What is the role for palliative care in patients with advanced cancer? In N.E. Goldstein & R.S. Morrison (Eds.), *Evidence-based practice of palliative medicine* (pp. 276–280). doi:10.1016/B978-1-4377-3796-7.00048-3

Rando, T.A. (1984). *Grief, dying, and death: Clinical interventions for caregivers.* Champaign, IL: Research Press Publishers.

Sefcik, J.S., Rao, A., & Ersek, M. (2013). What models exist for delivering palliative care and hospice in nursing homes? In N.E. Goldstein & R.S. Morrison (Eds.), *Evidence-based practice of palliative medicine* (pp. 450–457). doi:10.1016/B978-1-4377-3796-7.00077-X

Siegel, R.L., Miller, K.D., & Jemal, A. (2015). Cancer statistics, 2015. *CA: A Cancer Journal for Clinicians, 65,* 5–29. doi:10.3322/caac.21254

Stiel, S., Bertram, L., Neuhaus, S., Nauck, F., Ostgathe, C., Elsner, F., & Radbruch, L. (2010). Evaluation and comparison of two prognostic scores and the physicians' estimate of survival in terminally ill patients. *Supportive Care in Cancer, 18,* 43–49. doi:10.1007/s00520-009-0628-0

Stroebe, M., & Schut, H. (2010). The dual process model of coping with bereavement: A decade on. *Omega, 61,* 273–289.

Temel, J.S., Greer, J.A., Muzikansky, A., Gallagher, E.R., Admane, S., Jackson, V.A., ... Lynch, T.J. (2010). Early palliative care for patients with metastatic non-small-cell lung cancer. *New England Journal of Medicine, 363,* 733–742. doi:10.1056/NEJMoa1000678

Teunissen, S.C., Wesker, W., Kruitwagen, C., de Haes, H.C., Voest, E.E., & de Graeff, A. (2007). Symptom prevalence in patients with incurable cancer: A systematic review. *Journal of Pain and Symptom Management, 34,* 94–104. doi:10.1016/j.jpainsymman.2006.10.015

Waldrop, D., & Kutner, J.S. (2013). What is prolonged grief disorder and how can its likelihood be reduced? In N.E. Goldstein & R.S. Morrison (Eds.), *Evidence-based practice of palliative medicine* (pp. 436–442). doi:10.1016/B978-1-4377-3796-7.00074-4

Worden, J.W. (2008). *Grief counseling and grief therapy: A handbook for the mental health practitioner* (4th ed.). New York, NY: Springer Publishing Company.

World Health Organization. (n.d.). WHO definition of palliative care. Retrieved from http://www.who.int/cancer/palliative/definition/en

Zhang, M., Smith, K.L., Cook-Mack, J., Wajnberg, A., DeCherrie, L.V., & Soriano, T.A. (2013). How can palliative care be integrated into home-based primary care programs? In N.E. Goldstein & R.S. Morrison (Eds.), *Evidence-based practice of palliative medicine* (pp. 458–467). doi:10.1016/B978-1-4377-3796-7.00078-1

CHAPTER 20

Roles of the Oncology Advanced Practice Nurse

Wendy H. Vogel, MSN, FNP, AOCNP®

Introduction

Today's healthcare environment is characterized by increasingly complex and expensive treatments for cancer in a setting of significant cost constraints and intense pressure to contain these costs. Complicating this are drug shortages and rising personnel shortages. Many private oncology practices are affiliating with hospital systems, and community practices are closing. The population continues to age, and the demand for services is increasing.

Against this backdrop, the skill set of the oncology advanced practice nurse (APN) seems ideally suited to enhance care quality and clinical outcomes. This improvement occurs through the delivery of advanced nursing services together with program development, consultation and education, and evidence-based practice development. This chapter outlines the components of the oncology APN role, examines cross-cutting skills that oncology APNs need to optimize role outcomes, and highlights challenges in role development.

Background

Advanced practice nursing in oncology can be characterized as the delivery of services to patients, families, care providers, and organizations based on expanded and specialized knowledge and skills concerning the care of individuals with a risk of or a diagnosis of cancer. APNs require theoretical knowledge and advanced clinical skills to provide expert care to patients with cancer, their families, and the community (Brant & Wickham, 2013).

Oncology APN roles encompass several elements, including that of expert clinician, mentor/coach, consultant, educator, author, researcher, administrator, and case manager/coordinator. The functional emphasis depends on the specific advanced practice role (nurse practitioner [NP] or clinical nurse specialist [CNS]), the organizational structure, the setting (inpatient, ambulatory care, office-based practice, home care, or educational institution), the needs of patients and staff, and the expectations and goals of the APN. A distinction exists between specialized nursing practice and advanced nursing practice. *Specialized* nursing practice involves concentration in a selected clinical nursing area and may be developed from clinical experience and continuing education. *Advanced* nursing practice employs advanced education and specialized practice preparation that integrates theoretical, empirical, and practice knowledge at the graduate level. Particular advanced practice roles may have additional specific competency requirements. State boards of nursing may regulate and govern advanced practice role titles, scopes of practice, and role responsibilities (see Chapter 21 for additional information).

The Robert Wood Johnson Foundation and the Institute of Medicine (IOM) recently published recommendations based on a two-year initiative for the assessment and transformation of the nursing profession (IOM, 2011). This report, *The Future of Nursing: Leading Change, Advancing Health*, set forth four key messages. The first recommendation from this report is that nurses should practice to the full extent of their education and training. Because of the inconsistency of scope-of-practice laws from state to state, many APNs cannot practice to the full scope of their licensure and training. Unfortunately, at a time when the numbers of physicians and oncologists are declining and healthcare resources are dwindling, some physician colleagues continue to challenge any expansion of the APN scope of practice.

The Consensus Model for Advanced Practice Registered Nurse (APRN) Regulation: Licensure, Accreditation, Certification, and Education (LACE) should address this problem. LACE will further the role of nursing leadership in the healthcare environment, allowing APNs to practice to the fullest scope of their education (APRN Consensus Work Group & National Council of State Boards of Nursing APRN Advisory Committee, 2008; Stanley, 2012). The goal of LACE is to eliminate inconsistencies in scope of practice between states, thus allowing greater mobility of advanced practice clinicians to meet the rising healthcare needs of the nation (Rounds, Zych, & Mallary, 2013). The Oncology Nursing Society (ONS) and the Oncology Nursing Certification Corporation have endorsed the consensus statement.

The IOM report noted that nurses should achieve higher levels of education and training and that the education system must promote seamless academic progression (IOM, 2011). Debate continues about the need for APNs to be educated at the doctoral level (Brar, Boschma, & McCuaig, 2010; Chism, 2009) and the regulation and certification of APN practice (Gormley & Glazer, 2012; Lugo, O'Grady, Hodnicki, & Hanson, 2010). Many of the APN roles as well as those of other advanced practitioners (such as physician assistants) overlap, making it difficult to logically differentiate roles as distinct and unique entities. A lack of clarity exists regarding terminology such as *scope of practice*, *advanced practice nursing*, and *nursing practice*, among others (Dowling, Beauchesne, Farrelly, & Murphy, 2013; Stasa, Cashin, Buckley, & Donoghue, 2014). The IOM report recommended doubling the number of doctorate-prepared nurses by 2020 (IOM, 2011). The nursing profession must come to a universal agreement on terminology, educational requirements, and regulatory authority to promote advanced practice roles nationally and internationally (Dowling et al., 2013).

The IOM report also noted that nurses should be educated with other health professionals, such as physicians or pharmacists, as students and through their careers (IOM, 2011). Nurse residency programs also were recommended. With the influx of non-oncology APNs into the oncology field, the development of oncology APN residency programs is needed. A need exists for lifelong learning opportunities as well. Support by employers in providing these opportunities and funding is crucial.

The National Association of Clinical Nurse Specialists (NACNS) issued a practice statement outlining the core competencies and outcomes for CNS practice. NACNS conceptualizes the CNS role as the use of clinical expertise with a specialty focus to improve clinical and economic outcomes within three spheres of influence or practice domains: patients/clients, nursing, and the organization/system (NACNS, 2010). The National Organization of Nurse Practitioner Faculties (NONPF) identified core competencies of the NP role, endorsing the evolution of the doctorate of nursing practice as the entry level for NP practice (NONPF, 2012). These new competencies build on existing master's degrees and doctorate of nursing practice core competencies. Core NP competencies that encompass all populations include (a) scientific foundation, (b) leadership, (c) quality, (d) practice inquiry, (e) technology and information, (f) policy, (g) health delivery systems, (h) ethics, and (i) independent practice (NONPF, 2012). ONS has published a position statement on the role of the APN in oncology care (ONS, 2015b), as well as a statement on the scope and standards of advanced oncology nursing practice (Brant & Wickham, 2013). ONS also offers guidance for the educational preparation and role development of the oncology APN (Jacobs & Mayer, 2015).

Although APN role functions and priorities may be setting specific, the practice of APNs is characterized by several common features, including the use of advanced specialty knowledge in practice; critical thinking; autonomous clinical judgment and ethical decision making; application of evidence to improve practice; and professional leadership (NACNS, 2010; NONPF, 2012). Regardless of the specific APN roles, essential APN skills include leadership, collaboration, management of change, scholarly practice, mentorship, negotiation, and conflict resolution. Factors that influence the implementation of advanced nursing roles are summarized in Figure 20-1. These factors include professional relationships, employer and colleague support, mentorship, professional and educational support, and adequate resources, as well as personal characteristics and experiences of the APN.

Current and future challenges for oncology APN role development include refining role definitions, advanced specialty education, certification and regulation, prescriptive authority, reimbursement, relationships with other staff groups, and evaluation of advanced nursing practice effectiveness (Brar et al., 2010; Brooten, Youngblut, Deosires, Singhala, & Guido-Sanz, 2012; Lugo et al., 2010; Sullivan-Bentz et al., 2010). Critical skills for the APN will assist in overcoming these challenges, such as collaborative and negotiation skills and the ability to act as a change agent.

Expert Direct Practitioner

APNs integrate and apply specialty knowledge to improve outcomes for patients. They take a holistic approach to clinical practice with an emphasis on communication, counseling, conflict resolution, and coordination. The ONS position statement on access to quality care notes that oncology nurses should have a substantial role in planning and implementing cancer care services (ONS, 2015a).

Studies suggest that the expert practice of APNs results in better patient education and adherence, decreased length of stay, and fewer hospital readmissions, as well as improved quality of life, patient satisfaction, and access to care (Bauer, 2010; Donald et al., 2013; Kapu, Kleinpell, & Pilon, 2014; Kim, 2011; Moore & McQuestion, 2012). Evidence also shows that APNs improve perceptions of the overall healthcare team in addition to decreasing cost (Kapu et al., 2014; Kilpatrick, 2013; Moore & McQuestion, 2012). The results of these studies and other literature such as the *Future of Nursing* report (IOM, 2011) support the use of APNs in workforce solutions for physician shortages (Morgan, Abbott, McNeil, & Fisher, 2012; Newhouse et al., 2012). The IOM report also commented that APNs are not physician "extenders" or "sub-

Characteristics of the APN
- Adaptability, stamina, creativity
- Confident, assertive, patient, optimistic, proactive
- Strong decision-making, problem-solving, and time management skills
- Strong skills in negotiation, conflict resolution, and relationship building
- Accepts personal accountability for quality of relationships and achievement of outcomes

Previous Experience of the APN
- Specialty experience
- Previous experience as a staff nurse
- Previous experience as an APN

Quality of APN Relationships
- Effective working relationships with managers and supervisors, nursing staff colleagues, APN colleagues, physicians, and other key stakeholders

Professional and Educational Issues
- Job autonomy
- Sustained mentoring
- Performance measurement
- Adequate orientation to the role
- Maintenance of clinical competence
- Clear regulatory framework for APN practice
- Effective role modeling during educational preparation
- Compensation package commensurate with responsibilities
- Availability of professional and educational resources and collegial consultations
- Familiarity of colleagues, staff, and employers with APN role and scope of practice
- Educational preparation encompasses both generic APN skills (e.g., evidence-based practice skills, research skills, time management) and specialty skills

Organizational Issues
- Organizational positioning and status of the APN role within the organization
- Proactive and inclusive planning; transparent decision-making processes
- Clear, flexible, evolving, and responsive APN role definitions and boundaries
- Highly valued interdisciplinary teamwork, expertise, outcomes management, and evidence-based practice
- Clearly articulated goals and priorities that include employee satisfaction and individual and team productivity
- APN role expectations that encourage autonomy and are realistic, compatible with those of the APN, and well matched to the resources provided to the APN

Available Resources
- Office space
- Nursing assistant support
- Continuing education support
- Computer, appropriate software, and technologic support
- Secretarial support, transcription services, billing management
- Seed funding and expert consultative support for research projects
- Knowledgeable, timely, and supportive guidance and advocacy from other nurse leaders

Figure 20-1. Factors Influencing Advanced Practice Nurse (APN) Role Development

Note. Based on information from Doerksen, 2010; Hill & Sawatzky, 2011; Paplanus et al., 2014; Pron, 2013; Stewart et al., 2010; Sullivan-Bentz et al., 2010; Szanton et al., 2010.

stitutes" but are healthcare providers who address the full health continuum from the promotion of health and disease prevention to diagnosis and treatment, as well as incorporating a range of services from other disciplines (IOM, 2011). The report observed that no studies have shown that APNs give lesser care than physicians or that care is superior in states with more restricted APN practice.

Unique APN roles have been described in the oncology setting, such as in bone marrow transplantation (Knopf, 2011); oncology critical care (D'Agostino & Halpern, 2010); breast specialty (National Breast Cancer Centre's Specialist Breast Nurse Project Team, 2003); genetic counseling (Britell, 2010; Swiderski, 2011); high-risk cancer clinics (Vogel, 2003); neuro-oncology (Bartolo et al., 2012; Zwinkels et al., 2009); palliative care (Fox, 2014); patient navigation (Crockett-Maillet, 2008); prostate cancer clinics (Madsen, Craig, & Kuban, 2009); radiation oncology (Hollis & McMenamin, 2014; Moore-Higgs et al., 2003); survivorship (Economou, Edgington, & Deutsch, 2010; O'Brien et al., 2014); symptom management clinics (Mason, DeRubeis, Foster, Taylor, & Worden, 2013); and urgent care centers (Ruegg, 2013), among many more.

For APNs in the NP role, expert practice includes comprehensive assessment, diagnosis, and care management in collaboration with physicians and other healthcare team members. NPs also promote wellness and health maintenance, prevent complications, and provide acute and chronic care. Responsibilities of the NP role include conducting physical examinations and other health assessment and screening activities; diagnosing and treating acute and chronic conditions; performing, ordering, and interpreting laboratory and diagnostic studies; and prescribing pharmacologic and nonpharmacologic therapies. Delivery of these services requires that NPs enter into an explicit collaborative practice with physician colleagues while simultaneously achieving and maintaining a high degree of autonomy in their practice. The requirements, limitations, scope, and regulation of prescriptive authority vary widely from state to state (see Chapter 21). Acquisition of advanced technical skills often is a requirement for NP practice but may be restricted by specific state or facility regulations. These procedures can include chest tube insertion, bone marrow aspiration, skin biopsy, lumbar puncture, or access of an Ommaya reservoir for administration of intrathecal chemotherapy. It is important that these skills be gained under the appropriate supervision and direction and that methods for demonstrating continuing competence to perform these procedures are in place. ONS has developed standards for the oncology APN role (Brant & Wickham, 2013). These standards complement and extend the core competencies for all NP practice (NONPF, 2012). ONS has also developed competencies for both NPs (ONS, 2007) and CNSs (ONS, 2008). These competencies describe the roles of the oncology NP and the oncology CNS in regard to improvement of health and nursing-sensitive patient outcomes; promotion of the nursing profession; leadership/mentorship; ensuring quality of care and decreasing cost; and system improvements.

CNS expert practice includes the delivery of interventions to patients and their families to prevent or ameliorate symptom distress and functional limitations, provide emotional support, and enhance comfort. CNSs also intervene to reduce behaviors such as nonadherence; promote effective coping, problem solving, and self-care management; and enhance physical, psychological, and spiritual well-being (NACNS, 2010; Viele, 2010). The delivery of these interventions is based on a systematic assessment, including health history, physical examination, and relevant laboratory and diagnostic studies. Many CNSs provide direct care to high-risk, multiproblem patients and their families, as well as patients who are at highest risk for adverse outcomes, whereas others improve outcomes for patients by influencing the direction and quality of staff nurses' problem solving. Even when providing direct care, CNSs may simultaneously address other role components and spheres of influence, for example, by educating staff or gathering information needed to address a system problem that is adversely affecting care delivery. CNS practice often focuses on populations of patients rather than individual patients.

Documentation of services is a key component of the direct practice role. Clear and precise documentation of APN services is important for several reasons. First, documentation of the assessment, diagnosis, and interventions assists in ensuring coordination of care and achieving desired clinical outcomes. Second, it reflects the achievement of outcomes in important areas of APN practice, including comprehensive evaluation and holistic intervention. Quality documentation supports an image of the APN as a knowledgeable and effective member of the care team and reinforces visibility of the role. Documentation of services also is necessary to meet qualifications for reimbursement of APN services. Lastly, documentation allows appropriate utilization review and quality-of-care evaluation, as well as collection of data useful for research and education. Figure 20-2 lists elements that should be included in an APN consultation note.

Barriers to reimbursement for delivery of expert clinical services may exist for APNs practicing in either the NP or CNS role. Although the federal government provides for reimbursement for all healthcare providers in its programs, individual states and private payers control which providers are eligible for reimbursement and may limit reimbursement for services not provided directly by physicians.

- Reason for consultation
- History of present illness, past medical history, current concerns, review of systems
- Limited physical examination
- Current medications
- Relevant laboratory studies
- Assessment and recommendations
- Plans for reevaluation and follow-up
- Signature

Figure 20-2. Elements of an Advanced Practice Nurse Consultation Note

Case Manager

Case management is recognized as an important aspect of the care continuum. Although operationalized differently in various settings, case management is a practice framework designed to integrate quality, productivity, safety, and cost to achieve desired patient-centric and organizational outcomes, improve access to healthcare services, and achieve enhanced care coordination among providers and continuity across settings (Leonard & Miller, 2012). Case management requires knowledge of the disease process and treatment options together with expertise and skills that optimize quality and cost-effectiveness across the continuum of care. At the advanced level, case management is a process frequently encompassing a broad range of activities, such as disease management or population-based case management, but still includes the core functions of assessment, planning, implementation, coordination/interaction, monitoring/evaluation, and promotion of positive outcomes (Leonard & Miller, 2012). Organizational goals supporting the use of an APN may include reducing the length of stay, preventing readmission, optimizing resource use and costs, increasing access to services, and creating desire to become a recognized center of excellence for a particular service. The case manager's accountability typically extends across repeated episodes of care and beyond traditional geographic boundaries (Stachowiak & Bugel, 2013).

APN case management functions align closely with the traditional APN roles (clinical practice, consultation, education, and research) and incorporate APN skills in clinical leadership, collaboration, communication, and change management. The American Nurses Credentialing Center defines case management as a dynamic and systematic collaborative approach to providing and coordinating healthcare services to a defined population and contends that the framework for nursing case management includes five components: assessment, planning, implementation, evaluation, and interaction (Leonard & Miller, 2012). This mirrors the advanced practice role that requires competency in directing expert care, providing guidance and coaching, consulting with staff, interpreting research, coordinating multidisciplinary collaboration, and acting as a change agent.

Treadwell and Giardino (2014) described the role of the case manager in a medical home team. This could have application in oncology medical homes with the APN in the case manager role. A medical home is a patient-focused system for the delivery of quality health care and is emerging as a potential solution to the currently fragmented healthcare delivery system.

Coordinator

Because cancer is often a long-term or chronic illness, patients experience an extended period of contact with an increasingly specialized and complex healthcare system. Achieving integration across settings and among members of the interdisciplinary cancer care team is paramount to quality cancer care. The role of APN as coordinator may be a role in itself or encompassed within another role such as case manager, patient navigator, or direct caregiver.

Although continuity of care has been variously defined in the literature (Uijen, Schers, Schellevis, & van den Bosch, 2012), most definitions suggest that continuity of care is a philosophy and a quality standard of care. Continuity of care includes the themes of personal relationship, communication among providers, and cooperation among providers (Uijen et al., 2012). It also involves patients, lay caregivers, and healthcare providers working together to provide a coordinated, comprehensive continuum that meets the needs of patients, provides for transitions between settings, results in improved clinical outcomes, and promotes a cost-effective use of healthcare resources. *Coordination* is a term used in many definitions of continuity of care. Coordination suggests a smooth and efficient operation. Discharge planning models, multidisciplinary planning teams, formalized communication and referral mechanisms among providers, survivorship plans, and integrated documentation tools and case management plans across settings are examples of models that emphasize continuity of plan.

However, barriers to continuity of care exist. Barriers may include a sense of threat regarding the involvement of healthcare providers outside of one's own institution, together with interagency and interprofessional competition and territoriality. Lack of knowledge regarding the services of other disciplines and resources is compounded when accompanied by hesitancy or resistance to collaborate. Suboptimal communication between providers and healthcare settings is magnified by the fact that health records are not easily shared among agencies and providers (Han & Rayson, 2010). Reimbursement issues also affect the range, intensity, duration, and location of services that are available to patients, at the expense of both quality and continuity of care (Houlihan, 2009; Natale-Pereira, Enard, Nevarez, & Jones, 2011). High caseloads, lack of preparation time, inadequate staffing, and absence of clear system guidelines are additional barriers. Patient factors also exist, such as illiteracy, unrecognized cognitive impairment, distrust of the system, language barriers, access disparity, and cultural differences (Belling et al., 2011; Chugh, Williams, Grigsby, & Coleman, 2009; Han & Rayson, 2010).

Continuity of care aims to achieve and maintain a maximum level of functional health while simultaneously optimizing physical and psychospiritual comfort, facilitating transitions between settings and caregivers, and optimizing the use of healthcare resources (Uijen et al., 2012). Factors exist that facilitate the continuity of care. An interdisciplinary approach to care that acknowledges the whole person, including the family, and addresses the highly technical and often complex problems of cancer care is essential. Although team composition and leadership may shift over time, mutual respect and recognition of each provider's unique contribution are fundamental characteristics of an interdisciplinary approach. Case conferences, shared documentation tools, and interdisciplinary care standards can be effective strategies to facilitate communication and collaboration. A comprehensive, systematic assessment of patient and family needs contributes to continuity of care. Once the needs for care are identified, three key questions should be posed to promote goal setting, teaching, and resource coordination: (a) What activities are to be performed to maintain or enhance individual and family functioning? (b) Who will perform these activities, and who is the designated alternate? and (c) What health teaching, referrals, and equipment and supplies are required?

Successful continuity of care requires active participation of patients and families; therefore, another required element of continuity of care is patient and family education and involvement in decision making. The identification of measurable goals, development of the plan together with patients and family members, and coordination of supplemental resources (such as home nursing care, laboratory services, medications, rehabilitation, and respite care) also are essential.

Lastly, care must be integrated through each transition in care setting or care providers. An area that can cause particular difficulties for patients with cancer is the transfer of specific care measures into the community (Belling et al., 2011; Han & Rayson, 2010). It is essential to determine whether the community setting has the necessary educational, procedural, financial, and material support to effectively transfer care into the community. Careful exploration of these issues, along with referral to agencies well in advance of the transition of care, provision of copies of clinic procedures and protocols, and an opportunity to observe the care procedure, are essential to ensure a smooth transition in care.

APN interventions to promote continuity of care also include efforts to help patients and families verbalize feelings of fear, vulnerability, and helplessness; build trust and confidence in new caregiver personnel; and develop realistic problem solving and contingency planning. Outcome indicators of continuity of care include optimal patient functioning (including physical, psychological, and social function), adherence to prescribed medical regimens, patient safety, patient comfort, and patient and family satisfaction (Haggerty, Roberge, Freeman, Beaulieu, & Bréton, 2011; Uijen et al., 2012). Continuity of care outcomes are now incorporated into existing quality measurement and accreditation programs.

Consultant

Although consultation is a core competency of advanced practice, the term itself may be used in different ways in various situations. Consultation refers to a two-way interaction designed to solicit, provide, and receive help. The consultant is recognized as having specialized expertise. The consultee requests the assistance of that expert in management of a problem that he or she believes to be within the expertise of the consultant. Consultants try to aid an individual, group, or organization in identifying and using resources to deal with problems and manage change. Internal consultants are part of the system with which they are consulting, whereas external consultants function from outside the system.

Consultation has several fundamental principles. First, the problem focus is always identified by the consultee. Furthermore, the professional responsibility for patients always remains with the consultee, and the consultant is not responsible for the consultee's work. The consultee remains free to accept or reject the ideas and recommendations of the consultant. Salerno, Hurst, Halvorson, and Mercado (2007) updated the long-used "Ten Commandments for Effective Consultations" (Goldman, Lee, & Rudd, 1983). The consultant determines the specific needs of the consultee and establishes the timeline for the consultation. The consultant conducts his or her own assessment of the patient or situation by reviewing the medical record or relevant data. Additional information or medical testing may be required based on the consultant's expertise.

Based on the information gathered during assessment, the consultant makes recommendations and offers options. The recommendations are specific and thorough and should anticipate potential problems. The focus of the consultation must then be identified and may or may not be the problem for which help was initially sought. Reframing of the problem focus for the consultation requires discernment, skill, and tact, particularly if the problem is the consultee's lack of expertise. Respecting professional boundaries is critical (Geppert & Shelton, 2012). When reframing a consultation request, both the consultant and the consultee must agree that the reframed issue is the one on which they will work and must mutually agree to their roles and responsibilities.

Once the specific issue is identified, the consultant and consultee jointly consider interventions, negotiate how the interventions will be carried out and by whom, and come to consensus on each participant's ongoing responsibilities. Contingency plans also are developed (Salerno et al., 2007). It is advantageous for the consultant to tactfully offer choices rather than forcing a specific kind of help onto a consultee. Using the phrase "Would that be helpful?" can invite clarification and feedback about a suggested action, plan, or advice. Resistance often means the consultant is pressing solutions onto others or that the consultee desires more control in the situation. Dialogue such as "I'm sensing that these suggestions are not fitting well for you; what would you rather be doing?" will facilitate feedback about resistance. Following the intervention, the consultant and consultee engage in follow-up and evaluation, examining both the process of consultation and the achieved outcomes. Thoughtful negotiation of roles and responsibilities, together with strong communication and relationship development skills, will improve the consultant's effectiveness. Figure 20-3 further develops these core principles of effective APN consultation.

The medical consultation is often more streamlined than the previously described process. The medical consultation, based on Goldman's Ten Commandments (Goldman et al., 1983), is a request for help in the care of a patient by another with specialized expertise. The consultation is for the patient's benefit, not the consultee's benefit (although the consultee may acquire specific and specialized knowledge during the process) (Geppert & Shelton, 2012). Figure 20-4 demonstrates this process. The process requires clarification of the consultation request, assessment, recommendations, and follow-up communication. The continued involvement of the consultant may vary from situation to situation. Oncology APNs may provide expert consultations to various populations.

The aforementioned consultation process is formal, but consultation also may be informal. Informal consultations include brief interactions around a circumscribed problem, quick questions to the consultant, or a brief and simple request for specific information. The consultant considers whether meeting these informal requests for information fully addresses the problem or whether the request signals a broader problem requiring a more comprehensive approach. In the latter situation, the APN still may meet the informal consultation request, while at the same time suggesting a more comprehensive and thorough investigation of the problem and potential solutions.

It is necessary to distinguish consultation from clinical and administrative supervision and from comanagement, collaboration, and referral. Clarity regarding the differences among these processes is important in APN consultation, in part because the APN role includes expert practice. Although consultation and clinical and administrative supervision share the goal of developing the knowledge, skills, self-esteem, and autonomy of another (referred to as the *subordinate*), a hierarchical relationship exists. The supervisor is responsible for safeguarding the care of the subordinate's patients, and the supervisor is accountable for the subordinate's work. Comanagement, collaboration, and referral may result from a consultation, but they are not considered to be consultative activities. Comanagement of

The consultant remains self-aware.
- The consultant remains conscious of whether, instead of consulting, he or she is operating in another role (such as avenger, rescuer, bully, nag, friend, disciplinarian, confidante, confederate, or playmate).
- The consultant regularly evaluates his or her own performances and uses that evaluation as an opportunity for learning.

Consultation requires developed communication and relationship-building skills.
- Consultation always is about relationships, particularly listening and valuing.
- Consultation begins when the objectives of the consultee and the type of consultation desired are clarified, and agreement about roles and responsibilities exists.
- Consultation respects professional boundaries.
- Consultation should be deferred if the consultant or consultee is upset or frustrated.

The consultant helps consultees to develop their own solutions.
- Consultation is based on the belief that people want to do a good job; consultants should communicate high expectations and trust in the consultee's abilities.
- The consultant provides options and contingency plans, recommends resources, and gives opinions, but ultimately, the consultee must decide upon the final solution.
- The consultant solicits ideas from the consultee using active listening and without critiquing, prior to offering his or her own ideas.
- Inviting feedback about an action plan or advice the consultant has offered allows the consultee to be in control of the process.
- Sometimes consultation provides solutions, and sometimes it provides assistance that helps consultees to find the solution themselves. The consultant should consider the difficulty of the task and the experience and preferences of the consultee.
- The consultant should consider whether the consultee is essentially seeking reassurance and confirmation. The consultant can use this as an opportunity to offer validation and strengthen competence.

Consultation should focus on strengths and opportunities, not weaknesses and problems.
- The consultee may see the question of "why" as a blaming or fault-finding question.
- The consultant should avoid giving advice, but rather should provide information the consultee can use to solve the problem.
- The consultant and consultee should acknowledge and show appreciation for each person's contribution.

The consultant always is an educator.
- The consultant should educate people as a supportive partner and coach, promoting self-sufficiency.
- The consultant should provide consultees with the tools needed to build skills for success in their goals.

Figure 20-3. Principles of Effective Consultation

Note. Based on information from Block, 2011; Geppert & Shelton, 2012; Lippitt & Lippitt, 1986; Yoder-Wise & Kowalski, 2006.

patients or referral of patients to the APN for specific services may occur during the delivery of care. For example, the APN may manage some aspects of care for a patient (such as providing complex teaching, running a family meeting, or performing a complex dressing change) while the staff nurse manages other aspects of that same patient's care. The staff nurse may refer a patient to the APN for sexual counseling, and the APN may refer a patient to the staff nurse for management of a potentially occluded central venous catheter. Given the multidimensional nature of their roles, APNs are engaged in all of these activities, but what differentiates the activities is the issue of responsibility for the outcome of care. In comanagement, collaboration, and referral, the APN and the RN each share specific responsibilities for delivering the intervention and evaluating its effects. With consultation, the staff nurse retains responsibility for delivering the intervention to the patient under his or her

- Clarify the need/request from the consultee.
- Establish a timeline for completion of the consultation.
- Assemble relevant information.
- Perform assessment.
- Synthesize the data from the assessment.
- Make clear, concise, brief recommendations, including contingency plans.
- Respect professional boundaries.
- Determine who will be responsible for particular aspects of care.
- Provide direct follow-up communication, preferably through personal contact.
- Provide resources, education, and references for the patient and the consultee.
- Determine with the consultee and the patient when the consultation services should cease.

Figure 20-4. The Medical Consultation Process

Note. Based on information from Geppert & Shelton, 2012; Goldman et al., 1983; Salerno et al., 2007.

care, and the APN is responsible for the quality of the recommendations to the RN and for clearly managing and documenting the process of consultation.

RNs' resistance to change, complacency or apathy, feelings of implied threat or criticism, and unfamiliarity of seeking consultation with an APN can impede development of the consultant role. As APNs enter a new organization or team as a consultant, it is important that they meet with administrators, physicians, nurses, and leaders and members of the interdisciplinary team to learn more about the needs of the team, identify key players, and describe their role and areas of expertise. Visibility is essential to develop the consultant role. For example, in an inpatient setting, making regular unit rounds and attending interdisciplinary team meetings, shift reports, and family conferences will help APNs to identify patients with complex clinical needs who could benefit from consultation. With each consultation request, APNs have an opportunity to demonstrate their areas of expertise and to provide informal education about the types of cases that are appropriate for future consultations.

Educator

Delivering education to patients and families, serving as an educator and preceptor for nurses in graduate nursing education, and providing specialty education to staff nurses and other members of the healthcare team are key components of the APN role. In educating patients, families, students, and staff, APNs must apply a systematic process to the development, implementation, and evaluation of education. The educational process begins with a learning needs assessment, followed by development of learning objectives, selection of the method or methods of instruction, and design of the program, and concludes with program evaluation. Each of these steps is guided by one or more learning theories and by adult learning principles.

Theoretical Perspectives Relevant to Learning

Educational interventions are guided by a number of different theoretical orientations. Some interventions are drawn from the disciplines of educational, social, cognitive, behavioral, or developmental psychology, whereas others are based on stress and coping, change, or systems theories. In an educator role, APNs may apply several of these theoretical frameworks simultaneously.

Integrating new information at a time of vulnerability, crisis, anxiety, and fear presents challenges. Shortened length of inpatient hospital stays, the shifting of care to outpatient settings, the aging of the population, and the costs and complexities of technologically advanced treatment modalities compound these challenges. Increasing diversity within the U.S. population creates an imperative that educators incorporate theoretical knowledge of cultural, ethnic, and religious diversity in healthcare beliefs, lifestyle practices, and communication styles into adult learning theory (Chachkes & Christ, 1996). Table 20-1 summarizes theoretical perspectives that can be applied to explain and understand the process of teaching and motivating health behavior change in adults.

Patient and Family Education

To be active participants in their health care, patients and families must possess necessary knowledge and skill. Knowledge enables patients to take necessary self-care actions to prevent the development of complications, to intervene quickly when problems develop, and to comply with needed procedures and therapies. It also assists them in interacting effectively with healthcare personnel, making decisions that are congruent with their preferences, and taking the necessary steps to maintain or regain health. From a cognitive behavioral perspective, knowledge promotes a constructive understanding of the illness process, eliminates erroneous beliefs, enhances coping and problem solving, and mitigates anxiety, fear, uncertainty, and worry. The entire family unit, including any people who are significant to the patient's daily life, must be included in education.

The process begins with an evaluation of patient and family learning needs. A significant body of literature examines the information needs of patients and families across the process of diagnosis and treatment of various cancers and through recovery or end of life (Collins, McClimens, Mekonnen, & Wyld, 2014; Danesh, Belkora, Volz, & Rugo, 2014; Feldman-Stewart et al., 2013; Goldfarb & Casillas, 2014; James-Martin, Koczwara, Smith, & Miller, 2014; McNair, Brookes, Kinnersley, & Blazeby, 2013; Milbury, Rosenthal, El-Naggar, & Badr, 2013; Rüesch et al., 2014; Volk et al., 2014; Warren, Footman, Tinelli, McKee, & Knai, 2014). Techniques for gleaning the information needs of patients include advisory groups, critical incident technique, focus groups, interviews, professional standards, questionnaires, and surveys. To establish priorities for delivery of patient and family education, the clinician begins by focusing on the patient's learning needs. The ONS *Standards of Oncology Education: Patient/Significant Other and Public* (Blecher, Ireland, & Watson, 2016) provides APNs with comprehensive guidelines for the development of formal and informal oncology educational programs for patients and families.

A variety of factors influence patients' information-seeking behaviors and readiness for learning, including coping style, education level, motivation, learning style, health literacy, expectations, values, culture, decision-making preferences, physical and psychological comfort, energy level, developmental stage, and physical, physiologic, and cognitive capabilities. Each of these factors is considered in the development of objectives for individual or group education, as well as in the design and evaluation of educational materials. Many commercially prepared educational materials are available for teaching patients. Prepared materials can be used to teach new information and to augment or reinforce previously taught information. Use of prepared materials can be effective and efficient, but the materials must be evaluated for their relevance to learning need, content accuracy, and readability. Language differences between patients and nurses present an obvious obstacle to communication and patient education. Professional interpreters, bilingual staff members, and volunteers may facilitate communication. Many prepared materials are available in languages other than English, although these should be similarly evaluated. When preparing or evaluating educational materials, APNs need to consider many factors (Carson et al., 2012; Charvet-Berard, Chopard, & Perneger, 2008; Doak, Doak, & Root, 1996; Hagopian, 1996; Moult, Franck, & Brady, 2004; Rees,

Table 20-1. Theoretical Perspectives for Teaching and Motivating Healthy Behavior

Theory	Major Concept(s)	Key Principles	Application to Teaching, Motivating, and Health Behavior Change
Operant/conditioned learning behavioral models	Stimulus-response linkages are conditioned by reinforcements (rewards).	Reinforced behaviors will occur frequently. Desired behaviors can be elicited through shaping and reinforcement.	Assessment of learner includes consideration of • Factors reinforcing undesirable health behaviors • Factors for motivating and reinforcing desired health behaviors.
Cognitive/information processing	Behavior and affect result from insights, principles, concepts, relationships, generalizations, rules, or theories held by the individual, and effecting change in one or more of these dimensions mediates all behavior change.	Teaching-learning occurs by reorganizing perceptual or cognitive fields (including principles, relationships, concepts, theories, or rules) through purposive involvement, cooperative and interactive inquiry, problem solving, and problem raising.	Suggests importance of insights, memory, outlook, and thought patterns for cognitive, affective, and psychomotor learning and problem solving.
Mastery learning	Any behavior or task can be broken down into its component behaviors.	Breaks down complex units of instruction into the smallest component parts and then builds complex behaviors/tasks by putting the smaller units together.	Offers helpful principles when learning requires mastery of several skills.
Social learning	Beliefs that one is capable of performing a certain behavior and that performance of that behavior will produce the desired outcome.	Four sources of information influence the process of learning: personal mastery, vicarious experiences, verbal persuasion, and physiologic feedback.	Suggests that health education should include strategies to build self-confidence and enhance self-efficacy as a means to achieve sustained behavior change.
Compliance model	The extent to which a patient's health behaviors (e.g., taking medication, following a diet) coincides with the recommendations and/or prescriptions of healthcare providers.	Control of health and illness is associated directly with compliance with provider-directed regimens. An individual's noncompliance with the provider's recommendations/prescriptions may be the result of a lack of knowledge, defiance/opposition/denial, or emotional distress.	Emphasizes importance of interventions to motivate patients to accept treatment plans as valuable and provides them with knowledge, skills, and encouragement to change behavior patterns to fit the requirements of the regimen.

(Continued on next page)

Table 20-1. Theoretical Perspectives for Teaching and Motivating Healthy Behavior (*Continued*)

Theory	Major Concept(s)	Key Principles	Application to Teaching, Motivating, and Health Behavior Change
Health belief model	Contrast of compliers and noncompliers relative to • Their perceptions of the severity of illness • Their susceptibility to illness and its consequences • The value of the benefits of treatment • The barriers to and costs of treatment • The cues that stimulate health-related actions.	Identifies factors that influence compliance or noncompliance with a health professional's recommendations for care. Emphasizes an avoidance orientation related to seeking preventive care to decrease the probability of negative health and illness outcomes.	Helps in identifying barriers to and costs of prevention, early detection, and treatment as prominent factors associated with preventive health practices or maintenance of illness regimens.
Health promotion model	Individuals strive for health, well-being, enjoyment, and fulfillment, and they self-initiate behaviors directed toward attaining higher levels of health.	Cognitive-perceptual factors that determine health promotion activities include the importance of health, perceived self-efficacy, and perceived benefits and barriers. These cognitive-perceptual factors are modified by demographic variables, expectations, past experiences with health professionals and with other behavioral change, biologic variables, and situational variables, such as access. The likelihood of engaging in health promotion behaviors depends on cues to action, including a desire for increased well-being, interaction with others interested in health promotion, advice, and information.	Identifies the essential role of the health-care professional in assisting individuals to overcome barriers to health-promoting activities, increasing the importance of positive consequences of preferred behaviors, and reducing the frequency of negative consequences.
Transtheoretical model of the stages of change	Change is a series of stages, each with its own characteristics and each amenable to different interventions.	Stages of change are precontemplation, contemplation, preparation, action, and maintenance.	Can be used to guide assessment of stage of change and to tailor interventions.

(Continued on next page)

Table 20-1. Theoretical Perspectives for Teaching and Motivating Healthy Behavior *(Continued)*

Theory	Major Concept(s)	Key Principles	Application to Teaching, Motivating, and Health Behavior Change
Stress and coping theory	Evaluation of a stimulus as stressful depends on the individual's cognitive appraisal of the situation as exceeding available personal resources within one's environment. Cognitive appraisal includes two dimensions: (1) Does this situation threaten me? and (2) What can I do about it?	Coping consists of cognitive and behavioral efforts to manage specific demands that are appraised as stressful or exceeding personal resources. Coping resources include positive beliefs, problem-solving skills, and social skills. Coping styles in responding to stressful or threatening situations lie along a continuum from monitoring (a tendency to seek information, worry, and remain vigilant) to blunting (a tendency to avoid or distract oneself).	Healthcare providers can assist patients in managing stress by providing educational interventions to enhance problem-solving and social skills and strengthen positive beliefs.
Self-regulation or common sense theory	An individual's understanding of an illness is the critical factor in his or her decisions about compliance with recommendations, self-care management, and coping response.	Illness representations are constructed from accumulated experiences over time and are an integration of knowledge gathered from the media, personal contacts, health professionals' input, symptoms and body sensations, and past experiences with illness. An illness representation has four features: identity of concrete symptoms, the cause of the problem, the timeline of the problem (how long it will last), and the consequences of the problem.	Assessment of learners should include an evaluation of their illness representation and consideration of how this representation shapes behavior, self-care management, and coping responses.
Explanatory models of health and illness	In an attempt to attribute meaning to seemingly disordered events, patients and families interpret the events, symptoms, and illnesses they experience into explanatory models.	Explanatory models of health and illness are shaped by cultural factors. Explanatory models of health and illness shape individuals' understanding of what caused their health problem, why it started, what the illness is doing to their body, how long the illness will occur, and what kind of treatment they should be given.	Assists healthcare professionals to tailor educational interventions to harmonize with patients' explanatory model and/or to evolve with the patients a mutual representation of the healthcare problem that promotes healthy behaviors and progress toward improved health and well-being.

(Continued on next page)

Table 20-1. Theoretical Perspectives for Teaching and Motivating Healthy Behavior (Continued)

Theory	Major Concept(s)	Key Principles	Application to Teaching, Motivating, and Health Behavior Change
Ecological systems theory	Individuals can only be understood in reciprocity with their environmental context. Environmental contexts are nested within each other and include the chronosystem (the developmental processes and life transitions experienced by the individual), the microsystem (activities, family relationships, and material environment of the home), the mesosystems (e.g., school, work, social network), exosystems (social systems, institutions, government), and macrosystems (cultures, larger society).	Individuals and their behavior can only be understood with the context of their chronosystem, microsystem, mesosystem, exosystem, and macrosystem.	Individual behavior is shaped, restricted, and reinforced by a variety of systems, and thus, much less "individual choice" may exist than other theories of learning suggest.
Life span developmental frameworks	The interrelationships among chronologic age, normative developmental trajectories, cohort experiences, and non-normative life events	Biologic, environmental, and behavioral determinants, in conjunction with specified developmental influences, shape the life span of individuals and families.	In developing patient education, factors that should be considered include normative chronologic or age-graded factors (e.g., reading ability), historical events that influence particular birth cohorts (e.g., war, natural disasters), and life events that occur asynchronously with the life course (e.g., illness in young adults).

(Continued on next page)

Table 20-1. Theoretical Perspectives for Teaching and Motivating Healthy Behavior (Continued)

Theory	Major Concept(s)	Key Principles	Application to Teaching, Motivating, and Health Behavior Change
Motivational interviewing	Fears of, need for, and commitment to behavior change	Emphasizes resolution of ambivalence regarding change. Includes respectful and individualized discussion that addresses six key elements: (a) feedback about personal risk factors, (b) personal responsibility for change, (c) advice to change, (d) suggestions or a menu of approaches by which change might be achieved, (e) empathy and listening style of counseling, and (f) messages that support self-efficacy for change.	Details principles for the delivery of interventions to help patients to resolve ambivalence about changing health-related behaviors and adhering to health professional recommendations.

Note. Based on information from Leventhal & Cameron, 1987; Rankin & Stallings, 1996; Rankin et al., 2005; Saarmann et al., 2000.

Ford, & Sheard, 2002). The accuracy, breadth, and depth of the content are assessed. The content is assessed for balance or bias and whether the source of the material is reputable. The material must be readable, organized, and visually appealing. The reading level must be appropriate for the audience. Any technical terms must be clearly defined. The healthcare provider's contact information should be included.

Staff Education

Providing specialty staff education can enhance provision of competent patient care, improve job satisfaction, and promote recruitment and retention. The format of education delivered to staff nurses and other healthcare team members can range from brief unit-based in-services focusing on a specific aspect of diagnosis or treatment to a formal presentation at a national conference. Creative teaching and learning strategies include case study discussions, journal clubs, computer-assisted instruction, programmed instructional modules, games, and simulations. Demonstrations enhance variety, encourage learning at one's own pace, reinforce content, and build critical-thinking skills. In developing curriculum and evaluating continuing education programs for oncology nurses, the ONS *Standards of Oncology Nursing Education: Generalist and Advanced Practice Levels* (Jacobs & Mayer, 2015) is a useful guide for oncology APNs. Adult learning principles, as summarized in Figure 20-5, can be incorporated into the design, delivery, and evaluation of learning activities. Barriers to staff participation in educational programs are addressed as part of the planning process. APNs can overcome some of these barriers by keeping content relevant to the audience, by considering financial, geographic, and timing issues in program logistics, and by ensuring that educational program faculty members are credible, knowledgeable, experienced, flexible, and skilled.

The development of educational programs is guided by specific and measurable objectives that describe what cognitive, affective, or psychomotor learning will result from the educational program. Objectives describe what the learners are expected to do and how well they must perform if they have mastered the objective. Table 20-2 provides a taxonomy of educational objectives along with verbs that can be used in developing objectives that reflect each dimension of learning.

- Adult learners must perceive a need for information based on knowledge or skills needed to perform more effectively.
- Learning objectives must be relevant and timely.
- Commitment to the learning experience increases with learner engagement.
- Adults are problem or task oriented. Educational activities need to focus on the resolution of problems or completion of tasks.
- The educator is more of a facilitator and resource person and less of an instructor/transmitter of knowledge; emphasis is on partnership to clearly define learning goals and the means to achieve them.
- Learning activities should recognize and build upon the significant body of experiences that adult learners possess.
- Adult learners have multiple demands on their time. Therefore, education should be self-paced, efficient, and self-directed and should allow for flexibility in scheduling.
- The learning environment should be physically and psychologically comfortable, reflect mutual respect, and allow for freedom of expression.
- Feedback is necessary for adult learners, and positive reinforcement can facilitate learning.
- Adults are motivated to learn by both extrinsic (pay, promotion) and intrinsic (self-esteem, personal achievement) rewards.

Figure 20-5. Adult Learning Principles

Note. Based on information from McCorkle et al., 1996.

Table 20-2. Developing Specific and Measurable Educational Objectives

Domain	Level	Definition	Descriptors/Verbs
Cognitive	Knowledge	Recalls previous material	Identifies
	Comprehension	Grasps meaning of material	Describes
	Application	Comprehends material	Recognizes
	Analysis	Applies material	Recalls Exemplifies
	Synthesis	Breaks down material into components, understanding structure	Classifies Summarizes
	Evaluation	Puts components into a new whole	Compares Contrasts
		Judges value of material based on defined criteria	Explains Generates Plans Produces
Affective	Receiving	Aware of and listens to new information	Discusses
	Responding	Reacts to phenomenon	Responds Manifests
	Valuing	Attaches value to phenomenon	Expresses Reflects Behaves in accord with value
Psychomotor	Imitation	Begins skill after observation	Executes Implements
	Manipulation	Practices to improve performance	Demonstrates
	Precision	Performs accurate skill	Performs Coordinates
	Articulation	Coordinates skill with other activities	
	Naturalization	Is proficient with skill on cue	

Note. Based on information from Anderson & Krathwohl, 2001; Reilly & Oermann, 1992.

Evaluation strategies, a component of program planning, are chosen to match the learning objectives. Examples include tests of knowledge, performance checklists, return demonstrations, peer evaluation, case presentations, and expert review or audit of performance. Evaluation strategies can be formative or summative. *Formative evaluation* is a method of judging the worth of a program while the program activities are forming or happening. It gives information about the process of learning and what additional information might be needed. In contrast, *summative evaluation* occurs at the end of a learning activity and is focused on the extent to which the stated objectives or outcomes were achieved. When testing of knowledge or a competency is used for summative evaluation, those tests may be criterion-referenced (i.e., achievement of criterion of 85% of questions correct) or norm-referenced (i.e., achievement is compared with a larger group of learners, for example, with national standardized examinations).

Evaluation of educational programs includes a determination of progress toward meeting the learning objectives (i.e., outcomes evaluation) and how effectively the educational program was delivered (i.e., process evaluation). *Process evaluation* refers to a systematic method of assessing implementation. The goal is to use data to provide a description of how a program is operating compared with the manner in which the program was intended to operate. Some questions that process evaluations might address include the following: How many nurses attended the educational session? What are their characteristics? How long did it take for participants to complete the program? Were the educational facilities acceptable? Were the objectives met? An *outcome evaluation*, on the other hand, provides a picture of the results or effectiveness of a program in achieving its intended goals. Depending on the goals, questions addressed by an outcome evaluation might include the following: Did program participants learn how to effectively perform a particular procedure? Did the educational program result in satisfactory scores on a test of chemotherapy administration knowledge?

Oncology nurses need to develop and sustain a commitment to lifelong learning. APNs can role-model this for staff in a variety of ways, including demonstrating clinical curiosity, showing responsibility for one's own learning and for the need to remain current with an ever-expanding scientific knowledge base in oncology, actively participating in a professional organization's activities, and regularly reading professional journals.

Researcher

The APN's role in research includes participation in all phases of the research process, research evaluation and critique, research utilization, and the conduct and dissemination of research (Bruner & O'Mara, 2014; Hansen, Moinpour, & Ermete, 2014). Oncology APN competencies include research involvement (ONS, 2007, 2008). Oncology APNs should possess certain research skills. These include the identification of research questions, actual participation in research, and the translation of research findings to current practice. Publication and presentation of research findings is included in these competencies. Oncology APNs may have various levels of involvement in research at different times in practice. Oncology nursing research is not limited to the academic setting; community oncology nursing research activity is vital, as the majority of oncology care is delivered in the community setting (Klinger, Figueras, Beney, Armer, & Levy, 2014). Oncology APNs also use research by providing evidence-based management of patients.

An understanding of good clinical practices for the conduct of research (American Society of Clinical Oncology [ASCO], 2003) and thorough knowledge of critical appraisal are core skills needed to achieve research competencies. Also needed are skills in posing a clinical question that is answerable with evidence and the ability to locate and retrieve evidence. At a higher level of research engagement, APNs evaluate practice by examining the extent to which desired clinical, system, and fiscal outcomes are achieved. This requires familiarity with the various outcomes that may be measured, as well as an ability to critically assess outcome measurement tools for their reliability, validity, and sensitivity to change. Additional research competencies include the ability to distinguish research from quality improvement; knowledge of the principles of the design, conduct, statistical analysis, and interpretation of outcome evaluation research; and effective written and oral presentation skills. APNs prepared at the doctoral level are more likely to have the skills necessary to perform research and interpret findings (Currey, Considine, & Khaw, 2011). Other APNs may need some degree of expert consultation in statistical analysis or collaboration with a nurse researcher in selecting an outcome measure, designing the study, and interpreting and disseminating the results (Donovan, Nolte, Edwards, & Wenzel, 2014).

Goldberg and Moch (1998) described an APN–nurse researcher collaborative model. In this model, the APN offers a strong clinical base in nursing with advanced practice skills and detailed knowledge of the clinical institution. Both of these are necessary to the design and conduct of a clinical research study. The nurse researcher brings a strong theoretical base in nursing, together with skills in research design and statistical analysis and expertise in disseminating findings through publications and presentations. This model is designed to assist APNs in being involved in the generation and dissemination of new knowledge and in receiving the additional expert support and coaching necessary to achieve higher research competencies without doctoral preparation. Academic-service partnerships between nurses in practice and academic settings may be an effective mechanism to establish such APN–nurse researcher collaborations (Donovan et al., 2014; Edwards, Webber, Mill, Kahwa, & Roelofs, 2009).

Factors exist that may hinder APN research. Some of these factors include turf disagreements among disciplines, inadequate funding, inadequate graduate education, organizational barriers, competing commitments, and lack of mentors (Edwards et al., 2009; MacDonald, Newburn-Cook, Allen, & Reutter, 2013; McMaster, Jammali-Blasi, Andersson-Noorgard, Cooper, & McInnes, 2013). Research is discussed further in Chapter 9.

Challenges in Advanced Practice Nurse Role Implementation

The process of implementing an APN role is complex, dynamic, and varied. Hardy and Hardy (1988) differentiated role stress, role strain, role conflict, role ambiguity, and role incongruity. *Role stress* is a condition in which role obligations are conflicting, ambiguous, incongruous, excessive, or unpredictable. *Role strain* is the feeling of frustration, tension, or anxiety that results from the experience of role stress. *Role conflict* occurs when the role expectations held by the APN, supervisors, or other members of the interdisciplinary team are incompatible. APNs may experience interprofessional (e.g., between APNs and physicians) and intraprofessional (e.g., between APNs and other nurses) role conflicts. *Role ambiguity* occurs when a lack of clarity exists regarding the expectations of the APN role or when uncertainty exists about how the APN will meet those expectations. On the other hand, *role incongruity* occurs when a discrepancy exists between the role expectations held by the APN and those held by stakeholders, such as the supervisor or colleagues on the clinical team.

Hardy and Hardy (1988) maintained that role strain accompanies major role transitions and may actually facilitate role transition by increasing awareness of gaps in knowledge and skill. The development of strategies to cope with role stress can minimize role strain. Factors contributing to role stress include role ambiguity, role conflict, and role incongruity (Cranford, 2013; Smith, 2011; Specht, 2013; Tarrant & Sabo, 2010). Role ambiguity results when a lack of clarity about role definition and expectations, a blurring of responsibilities, or uncertainty about role implementation exists, or when there is lack of prior insight into the current role (Smith, 2011). For many APNs, role ambiguity exists in terms of how to operationalize various roles, who is or should be the primary customer of APN services (patients or staff), where APNs should target their interventions, the amount of autonomy, and the lack of optimal reporting structure. Role conflict develops when role expectations are perceived as contradictory or mutually exclusive. Role conflict may occur between APNs and other members of the nursing profession. For example, the staff nurse may perceive that discharge planning is the role of the APN, whereas the APN believes it is the staff nurses' responsibility to coordinate discharge planning and that the APN contribution is as an expert on the team for difficult cases. Role conflict also can develop between the APN and other disciplines, including social workers or physicians. Role incongruity may emerge when a mismatch occurs between one's skills and the obligations of the role. An example of role incongruity is a new APN who has not yet developed strong skills in invasive procedures but is mandated to fulfill this role expectation without sufficient additional training, support, and mentoring. Role incongruity also develops when role expectations are not well matched with strengths, talents, and expected role behaviors. For example, role incongruity can develop if the APN has strong skills in communication and education but must spend most of his or her time developing practice protocols or attending committee meetings.

Characteristics of the work setting (e.g., office location; resources available; time pressures; competing objectives; size, complexity, and distribution of the patient population) and the administrative structure (e.g., structural placement of APNs within the organization; reporting structure; autonomy; consonance between goals and expectations of individual APNs, supervisors, and the organization) have a major influence on APN role definition and expectation (DiCenso et al., 2010). A thoroughly developed strategic plan for APN role implementation is essential. This plan should include role clarity, acceptance by other team members, and involvement of other providers in the implementation process (DiCenso et al., 2010; Sangster-Gormley, Martin-Misener, & Burge, 2013; McNamara, Giguère, St-Louis, & Boileau, 2009; Yeager, 2010). Bryant-Lukosius and DiCenso (2004) offered a framework to guide the development, implementation, utilization, and evaluation of APN roles. They suggested that APN role implementation and utilization should include an examination by all stakeholders of how well the model of care and relationships among team members and services are meeting patients' health needs. Based on an understanding of gaps in met needs, priority problems and goals are identified, and then a revised model of care that notes the APN's role in that model is defined.

Various strategies exist to promote APN role implementation. During role acquisition, APN students benefit from identification with a role model and the opportunity to have realistic clinical experiences, develop competency profiles, and gain direct experience with all core skills. Faculty practice, panel discussions, and self and peer evaluation can facilitate role implementation as APNs transition into practice (Spoelstra & Robbins, 2010). As APNs transition to their initial role, a structured, goal-oriented plan for the first two years of role function and identification of a role model are essential. These goals and the structured plan ideally are negotiated and supported with nursing/medical leadership, and progress is reviewed at each supervisory meeting (Carter et al., 2010; Yeager, 2010). The emphasis in the first phase of role development is on developing role clarity and resolving role incongruity; networking; building effective relationships within the interdisciplinary team and the organization; clinical mastery; and participation in key committees and strategic initiatives (Hollis & McMenamin, 2014; McNamara et al., 2009; Sangster-Gormley et al., 2013; Sangster-Gormley, Martin-Misener, Downe-Wamboldt, & DiCenso, 2011). To minimize role ambiguity and conflict, it is important to clarify the purpose and multidimensionality of the APN role in terms of expert practice, practice development, education, research, and leadership. Definition of the relationship between the APN role and the role of other care providers and clarification of issues of accountability, autonomy, collaboration, communication, reporting mechanisms, and reimbursement also are important aspects of developing a new APN role (Bryant-Lukosius & DiCenso, 2004; Hollis & McMenamin, 2014).

Once the APN role is established, efforts focus on managing priorities, developing and implementing small-scale projects to demonstrate effectiveness, and gradual broadening of organizational impact (Catania et al., 2012). A formal process of goal setting with the supervisor and regular review of progress remain essential to APN success. Development of a support system that allows periodic self-evaluation; a place to manage anger, frustration, or dissatisfaction; and a mechanism to prevent complacency are fundamental to maximize outcomes once the APN role is implemented and integrated within the organization (Bryant-Lukosius & DiCenso, 2004; Sangster-Gormley et al., 2013). Mechanisms to ensure continued professional development and sustain clinical competency may be accomplished through continuing education, publication, quality measurements, and a network of peer and informational support for management of ongoing role challenges (Hollis & McMenamin, 2014; Sangster-Gormley et al., 2013).

Advanced Practice Nurse Skills That Contribute to Improved Outcomes

Evidence-Based Clinical Decision Making, Critical Thinking, and Scholarly Practice

Evidence-based practice is an essential component of quality nursing care and an essential competency for all healthcare professionals. APNs have a fundamental role in building capacity for evidence-based practice in staff and in promoting the translation of new research into clinical practice. Assisting staff in this process is accomplished by communicating and actively disseminating research findings and promoting system readiness to adopt innovations (Catania et al., 2012; D'Agostino & Halpern, 2010; Sommers, 2010). The process of evidence-based clinical decision making begins by posing an answerable clinical question, searching the literature for relevant information, and then performing a critical appraisal. If change is warranted by the research evidence and fits with clinician skills, resource availability, and patient preferences, the process follows with implementation of the change in practice and outcomes evaluation (Irwin, Bergman, & Richards, 2013; Sommers, 2010; Underhill, Boucher, Roper, & Berry, 2012).

Translating research evidence into clinical decisions, tools, and programs improves outcomes for patients and staff (Fineout-Overholt, Melnyk, Stillwell, & Williamson, 2010). This process begins with a critical appraisal of the available literature. The steps in critical appraisal are summarized in Figure 20-6. The goal of critical appraisal is to evaluate the scientific merit and potential clinical applicability of each study's findings. This can be applied to a group of studies covering similar problem areas to determine what findings have a strong enough basis to be used in clinical practice. Users of research need to know how much confidence they can place in the underlying evidence and recommendations. Critical appraisal is balanced and respectful, and if contradictory evidence exists, the full scope of the controversy is considered. Critical appraisal is like any other skill: it is learned through practice and dialogue with others. Journal clubs, colleague discussions, problem-based learning, clinical mentoring, and structured debates are ideal ways to develop skills and discernment in critical appraisal (Facchiano & Snyder, 2012; Fowler, Gottschlich, & Kagan, 2013; Jenicek, Croskerry, & Hitchcock, 2011; Pinnock & Welch, 2014).

The first step in critical appraisal is to determine the level of evidence a particular study represents. Different levels of evidence should be critiqued using somewhat different criteria, and the strength of one's conclusions across studies is influenced by the level of evidence. Figure 20-7 presents an example of an evidence hierarchy, with expert opinion representing the weakest evidence and meta-analysis and systematic reviews of randomized trials repre-

- Acquire overall perspective and identify the level of evidence (systematic review, randomized controlled trial, uncontrolled trial, case series, qualitative study, expert opinion).
- Apply critique criteria based on level of evidence:
  - Quantitative
  - Qualitative
  - Guidelines or systematic review.
- Summarize major study elements and findings using a standardized comparative template.
- Identify the strengths and weaknesses.
- Determine the potential applicability of the study to practice.
  - Are setting and sample comparable to your population?
  - Are study findings positive? Equivocal? Negative?
- Is the effect size balanced with potential side effects, cost, feasibility, and patient preferences?
- Determine collective weight of the evidence of this study in comparison to other studies, balancing study quality, findings, and applicability to practice.
- Synthesize the evidence for dissemination to influence practice and improve patient outcomes (protocol, practice standard, policy and procedure, guidelines, patient and family education, integrated review, publication/presentation).

Figure 20-6. Steps in Critical Appraisal of Research

Note. Based on information from Cope, 2014a, 2014b; DiCenso et al., 2005.

senting the strongest evidence (Gopalakrishnan & Ganeshkumar, 2013; Rutledge, DePalma, & Cunningham, 2004). Next, a table is prepared that organizes, summarizes, and synthesizes the individual pieces of evidence. This evidence profile highlights what is known, identifies gaps, and gives direction to the application of evidence in clinical practice. The next step is to examine the strengths and weaknesses of the study. Guidelines are available for identifying methodological weaknesses and limitations of quantitative and qualitative studies (Cope, 2014a; Craig & Smyth, 2011; Creswell, 2013; Denzin & Lincoln, 2011; DiCenso, Guyatt, & Ciliska, 2005; Melnyk & Fineout-Overholt, 2014). In evaluating clinical practice guidelines, APNs should consider why the guideline was developed, the composition (expertise and disciplinary perspective) of the panel that developed the guideline, and the entity of financial sponsorship (Graham, Mancher, Wolman, Greenfield, & Steinberg, 2011; Reames, Krell, Ponto, & Wong, 2013; Sargent, 2010). The decision-making process (expert opinion, consensus opinion, systematic review of evidence, or some combination) used in developing the guideline is determined. The clinical question for which the guideline was developed to address is verified. Other questions to pose in critically evaluating guidelines include: Were gaps in the evidence explicitly identified? How explicitly is the evidence linked to the recommendations in the guideline? If lower levels of evidence are incorporated (e.g., expert opinion), how explicitly is this labeled? Are the reasons for the inclusion of expert opinion, the line of reasoning, and the strength of extrapolation from other data clearly identified? How are patient preferences incorporated into the guideline? Is cost-effectiveness considered? What is the mechanism and interval for updating the guideline?

Next, the study's potential applicability to practice is determined, taking into consideration several factors: Are the setting and sample comparable to the practice's population? Are study findings positive, equivocal, or negative? Does the effect size (the strength of the relationship between intervention and outcome) balance the potential side effects and costs of the intervention? Is the intervention feasible and consistent with patient preferences? If multiple studies of a given intervention exist, the weight of evidence across studies must be determined, balancing study quality, findings, and the applicability to practice. The last step in the critical appraisal of research is synthesis of the evidence for dissemination to influence practice and improve patient outcomes. This can occur through development of protocols, practice standards, policies, guidelines, patient and family educational materials, or integrated reviews of the literature developed for journal publication.

In summary, oncology APNs make essential contributions to improved outcomes by role-modeling a systematic, evidence-based approach to clinical decision making and through the leadership of initiatives that translate research into practice. With responsibilities for expert practice, education, research, and consultation, oncology APNs are ideally positioned to support clinical staff in identifying, critically appraising, and synthesizing the literature and to direct organizational initiatives to disseminate evidence and to promote widespread adoption of best practices based on evidence.

Collaboration

Providing quality care involves interprofessional collaboration. The World Health Organization (WHO) defined interprofessional collaboration as multiple and varied healthcare professionals working together with patients, families, caregivers, and communities "to deliver the highest quality of care" (WHO, 2010, p. 7).

Collaboration is the process of working together within the negotiated framework to achieve the goal of the partnership. In collaboration, collective values are acknowledged, individuals are respected, and power is shared equally. The building blocks of an effective partnership include frequent face-to-face meetings, role clarity, a shared agenda and mutually beneficial goals, mutual

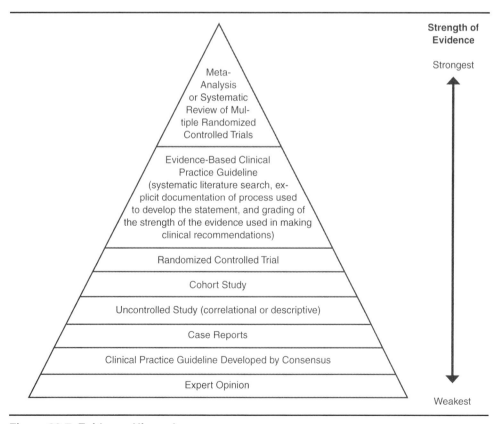

Figure 20-7. Evidence Hierarchy

accountability, trust, and understanding co-collaborators' roles (Adams, Orchard, Houghton, & Ogrin, 2014; Stringer, Curran, & Asghari, 2013). Clark and Greenawald (2013) noted that for effective collaboration between medicine and nursing to occur, there must be organizational support, shared expectations, relationships between individuals, and effective communication. Interprofessional collaboration also requires confidence, and this may be lacking in those new to the profession (Pfaff, Baxter, Jack, & Ploeg, 2014). APN collaboration with others to improve patient outcomes encompasses working with other members of the nursing team and those in other disciplines (Price, Doucet, & Hall, 2014). IOM recommends interprofessional teams to address patients' complex needs (Roett & Coleman, 2013). Improving interprofessional collaboration will improve patient outcomes (Buscemi, Steglitz, & Spring, 2012).

Baggs (1994) defined six critical elements for effective collaborative practice: trust, cooperation, assertiveness, shared decision making, communication, and coordination. At the center of the interprofessional and interdisciplinary collaborative practice models are two tenets: (a) patient needs are the foremost priority in the provision of care, and (b) patients require expertise and skills of different types of providers simultaneously during each encounter or hospital admission (Graham et al., 2011; Roett & Coleman, 2013). Collaboration requires developing relationships, building trust, and establishing an atmosphere of candor in communication. Barriers to collaboration include misunderstanding of roles; incongruent expectations; competition; territoriality; imbalance of power; devaluing of the contributions, intentions, or integrity of others; inexperience; poor communication; inadequate administrative support; and a lack of mutuality in resolving challenges and disappointments (Adams et al., 2014; Clark & Greenawald, 2013; Pfaff et al., 2014; Price et al., 2014; Susilo, van den Eertwegh, van Dalen, & Scherpbier, 2013).

A certain amount of duplication and role overlap exists among members of the healthcare team, which can result in territorial behaviors. With territoriality, the focus is on the professionals' role, knowledge base, or authority rather than the patient. Simply defining pieces of care provision that individual team members are uniquely trained to provide is not consistent with a focus on the needs of the patient and does not contribute to coordination of care, cooperation, or shared decision making. Collaboration provides opportunities for team members to develop a shared purpose, recognize divergent and complementary skills and contributions, and promote effective communication (Graham et al., 2011; Stringer et al., 2013). Paradoxically, territoriality may be increased by efforts to artificially define which role components or intervention approaches are the exclusive responsibility or expertise of any one role or one discipline. Establishing credibility often is a matter of time, patience, and mutual respect that evolves as team members share common patient-related experiences. Although successful professional collaboration requires effort, it ultimately enhances continuity and reduces care fragmentation (Buscemi et al., 2012; Graham et al., 2011).

Through collaboration with others, APNs not only influence care that patients and families receive, but they also shape the environment of care for patients and families and foster a healthy work environment for staff. These objectives are achieved through forming partnerships with nursing staff; collaborating with nursing administration; establishing strong interdisciplinary care teams with other advanced practitioners, physicians, and other caregivers; and networking with colleagues across the institution, health system, or community. Collaborating as colleagues and partners, APNs assist staff to develop greater expertise in patient care, strengthen their ability to function effectively as part of the team, frame their work and contributions within the context of the organization, and foster pride in their accomplishments.

Leadership

To successfully navigate the healthcare system for patients, guide multidisciplinary teams, advocate for practice improvements, strategically manage change, accept risks, garner credibility, inspire others to achieve excellence, and communicate and negotiate effectively, oncology APNs require strong leadership skills. NONPF has identified leadership as a core competency, and descriptions of the oncology APN role place an emphasis on leadership.

Leadership is variously defined, however. Rigolosi (2012) suggested that leadership is the use of communication processes to influence the activities of an individual or group toward attainment of a goal. Management theory designates two basic components of leader behavior: a concern for the task and outcomes to be achieved, and a concern for the people responsible for the task. A leader's behavioral style is not one component or another but rather a composite of behaviors that provides a balance of the two components. For example, as task behavior decreases, relationship behavior increases. Leadership theory develops these two components further by differentiating *transactional leadership* (how leaders motivate followers to accomplish goals and solve problems) and *transformational leadership* (how leaders inspire followers by creating a vision and promoting energetic movement toward making that vision a reality) (Burns, 2004).

Leadership must be seen as a dimension of practice for all APNs (Scott & Miles, 2013). Leadership also must be differentiated from management and better defined in the nursing profession. The IOM *Future of Nursing* report calls upon the Centers for Medicare and Medicaid Services, healthcare organizations, nursing education programs, and nursing associations to support the development of models of care that include nurses in leadership capacities and to provide opportunities for nursing leadership initiatives (IOM, 2011). Scott and Miles (2013) noted that leadership is both a process and a role, thus applicable to all nurses, not just those in administrative positions. For oncology APNs, clinical leadership denotes quality management of patients with cancer. Scott and Miles also noted five dimensions of clinical leadership that are foundational skills: clinical expertise, effective communication, collaboration, coordination, and interpersonal understanding. Leadership uses the collective wisdom of colleagues to optimize patient outcomes.

ONS (2012) has developed leadership competencies. The competencies are represented through five domains: personal mastery, vision, knowledge, interpersonal effectiveness, and systems thinking. This competency model notes leadership transitions between three levels as required, depending on current role needs. The three levels are individual, group, and governance levels. The individual level addresses skills for personal growth, while the group level addresses competencies needed in the leadership of groups, such as a clinical unit or professional group. The competencies demonstrate how oncology APNs might adapt these competencies at the governance level. The governance-level competencies are expanded skills that might reach outside of the oncology setting.

Leadership skill development is a lifelong learning process (Scott & Miles, 2013). Leadership skill development may occur through life events or deliberate activities and education. Self-confidence, or belief in one's ability to lead, is essential for successful leadership (Scott & Miles, 2013). The ONS leadership competencies reflect that leadership development evolves continually throughout one's nursing practice (ONS, 2012). Oncology APNs can foster leadership skills in colleagues and nursing staff by role-modeling and encouraging leadership activities (Nevidjon, 2014).

Change Agent

A key skill set and potentially one of the most complex to acquire and refine is that of a change agent. A theoretical framework can be helpful in strategically guiding the process. One of the most frequently applied conceptual frameworks, particularly for change processes that are designed to translate new knowledge into practice, is the Diffusion of Innovation Model proposed by Everett Rogers. Rogers (2003) described five stages in the change process: knowledge (learning about the existence and function of the innovation), persuasion (becoming convinced of its value), decision (committing to the adoption of the innovation), implementation (putting it into practice), and confirmation (accepting the innovation).

Change efforts focus on strategies and communication channels specific to each stage in the process of innovation adoption. For example, in the knowledge stage, it is important to publicize the innovation. In the persuasion phase, one-on-one discussion with opinion leaders might be helpful. At the beginning of a change process, two kinds of information are needed: information about current practices, and evidence showing why and how current practice could change. At the persuasion stage, when people are starting to think about the pros and cons of a change, gaining the involvement and visible participation of champions and opinion leaders—people who control resources, influence decisions, and have expert and referent power—can be key. In the persuasion stage, it also is important to link the innovation to improvements in outcomes and to address fears, concerns, and barriers. These strategies build a sense of competency and enthusiasm to handle the change.

In the decision phase, success is based on the involvement and input of a wide range of stakeholders in making decisions. Decisions may include how to implement the change, how to overcome logistical challenges, and how to define the essential ingredients for success. It is helpful if the stakeholder group includes individuals who are early adopters and strong proponents of organizational change.

The implementation plan includes the pace and scope of change, who will drive the change (whether from the bottom up or top down), and what support structures are needed. Throughout implementation, continued communication, involvement, and honesty are necessary, both in reinforcing the message regarding the need for change and in responding to concerns and resistance.

In the last stage, the confirmation stage, it is important to reinforce new behaviors and to capture and disseminate the benefits of the change. An evaluation process can provide data showing that the change is producing the anticipated effects. Acceptance of the innovation and integration into daily practice is enhanced by dissemination efforts. Reports to upper management, presentations, newsletter articles, a poster presentation, or a fact sheet can aid in describing the process and outcomes achieved.

Negotiation

Negotiation, an essential skill for APNs, is the mutual discussion and arrangement of the terms of a transaction or agreement. In any negotiation, each party desires basic human needs of security, economic well-being, and a sense of belonging, recognition, and control over one's life (Cornelius, 2000). Negotiation involves analyzing the problem, generating ideas and potential actions that offer a mutually acceptable solution to the problem, understanding the role that each side will play, and identifying criteria that indicate a successful outcome.

Donaldson (2007) divided the negotiating process into six basic skills: preparing, setting limits and goals, listening, communicating clearly, knowing when to pause, and closing the deal. Preparation is essential in conducting a successful negotiation (Hake & Shah, 2011). Before the negotiation, consideration is given to what each party wants from the negotiation. Parties examine what each has that the other might want, as well as what each is comfortable giving away. Hake and Shah (2011) described this as "creating value"—in other words, developing solutions that meet the needs of both parties. It is important to reflect on potential alternatives if agreement is not reached. The past relationship of the parties involved may influence the negotiation. It is helpful to understand what the expected outcomes are, what the results of previous negotiations were, and what, if any, precedents were set. Both parties consider the consequences of winning or losing the negotiation. Other questions to be considered include: Who has what power in the relationship? Who controls resources? Who stands to lose the most if agreement is not reached? What power does one party have to deliver what the other hopes for? Based on this fact-finding, possible solutions and compromises are identified. In a negotiation that is "win-win," both parties feel positive about the negotiation at its conclusion. This promotes good working relationships afterward. The negotiation itself is a careful exploration of each party's position, with the goal of finding a mutually acceptable compromise. In an ideal situation, one party finds that the other party wants what the first is prepared to trade, and vice versa (Hake & Shah, 2011; Susilo et al., 2013). Regardless of whether this ideal situation exists, ultimately, both sides feel comfortable with the final solution if the agreement is considered win-win. Win-lose outcomes are considered only if an ongoing relationship with the other party is not required, because having lost, the losing party may be uncooperative or resistant in future mutual endeavors.

When preparing for a negotiation, APNs need to have thorough knowledge of themselves, an understanding of their preferred outcome, and an awareness of their minimally acceptable outcome (Hake & Shah, 2011). This allows the APN to determine in advance what can and cannot be accepted. It may be helpful to discuss the preferred outcome and the minimally acceptable outcome with a mentor or experienced colleague and to benchmark these expectations.

Three skills are essential for successful negotiation: a clear understanding of the other's perception of the problem and style of negotiation, a level of comfort in dealing with highly charged emotions, and communication skills to resolve misunderstandings and maintain a supportive and respectful relationship (Hake & Shah, 2011). Strong emotions, such as fear, anxiety, anger, frustration, and hurt, often arise during high-stakes negotiations. These emotions could interfere with optimal functioning and therefore must be effectively managed. Strong preparation helps to build confidence, which can help with managing emotions.

Active listening is a communication skill that is essential to obtain the most complete information about the goals and position of the other party. Therapeutic communication techniques, such as restating, paraphrasing, reflecting, and asking for more information, are all necessary to effective negotiation. It is important for APNs to know their own negotiation style and limitations. Hake and Shah (2011) described several types of negotiation styles, defined in Table 20-3. Looking for a win-win solution is a type of negotiation called cooperative, whereas competitive negotiators will attempt to obtain as much of their own agenda as possible with as little compromise as possible. In any negotiation, the APN must create and sustain mutual respect while at the same time maintaining an attitude of confidence and competence.

Outcomes Evaluation

A number of authors have proposed frameworks for the evaluation of outcomes of APN practice (Begley et al., 2013; Bourbonniere et al., 2009; Brooten et al., 2012; Comiskey, Coyne, Lalor, & Begley, 2014; Elliott, Begley, Kleinpell, & Higgins, 2014; Imhof, Naef, Wallhagen, Schwarz, & Mahrer-Imhof, 2012; Kapu & Kleinpell, 2013; Neville & Swift, 2012). Although each of these frameworks varies somewhat in its definition and grouping of variables, most are based on a consideration of structure, process, and patient and family outcome variables. *Structure outcomes* are contributions of the APN to patient, staff, and organizational system improvements that influence the processes and outcomes of care. Examples of structure outcomes include the number of workshops given for staff and the number of staff who attend each workshop, time spent in each APN role component, patient education resources and

Table 20-3. Negotiating Styles

Negotiating Style	Description
Cooperative	Desire is for a win-win situation, in which both parties are able to get the best possible result.
Competitive	Aim is to win regardless of what the other party needs or desires.
Inductive	Negotiating begins with small details and works upward until agreement is obtained.
Deductive	Negotiating begins with an agreed-upon strategy.
Mixed	Negotiating is a blend of both inductive and deductive methods.
Soft	Negotiator seeks agreement despite the cost, offering concessions to preserve a positive relationship with other side.
Hard	Negotiator is determined to seek own interests; is competitive, hides the bottom line, and offers few concessions.
Principled	Negotiations rely on interests of both parties rather than positions.

Note. Based on information from Hake & Shah, 2011.

critical pathways developed, or the number of patients seen in a nurse-led symptom management clinic. *Process outcomes* evaluate the human and technical aspects of the APN role, including clinician, educator, researcher, and administrator, and may include staff nurse satisfaction with the APN, peer review, and the degree to which the APN's goals and productivity levels established by the organization have been met. Evaluation of the APN's direct influence on patient and family outcomes may include an evaluation of role impact on symptom distress, functional status, knowledge for self-management, patient satisfaction, adherence, length of stay, hospital admission, prevention of adverse events, resource use, and cost.

The selection of outcome measures for APN practice is problematic, in part because traditional medical outcomes may not fully capture the contribution of APNs (Neville & Swift, 2012). Because patient care is multidisciplinary, isolating the effect of APNs on patient and family outcomes may be challenging. Simultaneously evaluating multiple dimensions of APN functioning, including structure, process, and outcome variables, contributes to describing the full affect of the APN role (Brooten et al., 2012). APN practice improves the quality, safety, and cost-effectiveness of patient care (Bergman, Perhed, Eriksson, Lindblad, & Fagerström, 2013; Blackmore et al., 2013; Dyar, Lesperance, Shannon, Sloan, & Colon-Otero, 2012; Kapu et al., 2014; Morgan et al., 2012; Newhouse et al., 2012; Reuben et al., 2013; Sangster-Gormley et al., 2013; Sawatzky, Christie, & Singal, 2013).

Initial evaluations of the APN role may focus on outcomes related to acceptance and satisfaction, whereas continued evaluation may emphasize safety, efficacy, and cost savings (Bryant-Lukosius & DiCenso, 2004). Prospective data collection in each domain related to the established goals of the APN is essential in documenting the diversity of the APN's contributions. Data elements may include time spent in each of the role components; number of referrals and types of patients seen; staff programs delivered; standards of practice developed; quality of care; scholarly presentations and publications; contributions to committees and organizational initiatives; and participation in research (Fulton, 2013; Kapu et al., 2014; MacNeil & MacKinnon, 2011; Morgan et al., 2012; Sawatzky et al., 2013). Activities are linked to specific outcomes, such as the prevention of complications or improvements in staffing patterns; practice quality and consistency; length of stay and readmission; costs; resource utilization; generated revenue; and satisfaction (Blackmore et al., 2013; Bryant-Lukosius & DiCenso, 2004). Continued study of APN outcomes to develop a more refined understanding of the roles and cost-effectiveness of APNs as providers of quality health care is urgently needed.

Oncology APNs are uniquely positioned to provide expertise and leadership in the identification and implementation of nursing-sensitive and multidisciplinary outcome indicator sets. Nursing-sensitive indicators have inconsistent evidence because of varying definitions and data collection and analysis methods (Burston, Chaboyer, & Gillespie, 2014). However, across the continuum of healthcare settings, some nursing-sensitive indicators include symptom control and management; functional status (including physical and psychosocial functioning and self-care abilities); fiscal concerns; safety (which includes adverse incidents and complications); and perceptual status (which includes patient satisfaction with nursing care and with the results of nursing care) (Burston et al., 2014; Griffiths, Richardson, & Blackwell, 2012; Milani, Mauri, Gandini, & Magon, 2013).

The ONS Putting Evidence Into Practice initiative (www.ons.org/practice-resources/pep) provides helpful tools to identify and measure oncology nursing-sensitive patient outcomes and provides summaries of evidence-based interventions to improve patient and family outcomes (Gobel, Beck, & O'Leary, 2006). Organizations, such as the American Nurses Association, which developed the National Database of Nursing Quality Indicators, recommend quality indicators for hospitals and long-term care facilities that are sensitive to outcomes affected by nursing care. ONS (Given & Sherwood, 2005) published a white paper on nursing-sensitive patient outcomes. This paper describes patient outcomes that are responsive to nursing interventions.

ASCO has developed a system for measuring and improving the delivery of quality cancer services (Campion, Larson, Kadlubek, Earle, & Neuss, 2011; Jacobson, Neuss, & Hauser, 2012). The quality metrics may be applied to community practices (Hendricks, 2013; Peterson, 2012), outpatient oncology settings (Gilmore, Schulmeister, & Jacobson, 2013), or university cancer centers (Blayney et al., 2009). Compensation for physicians or practices may be based on quality metrics (Makari-Judson, Wrenn, Mertens, Josephson, & Stewart, 2014).

Also, the Centers for Medicare and Medicaid Services is engaged in new initiatives to identify and measure key indicators of quality of care and to link the achievement of specific quality benchmarks to provider reimbursement incentives (Berg, 2008; Wilensky, 2011). Disease-specific standards of care developed by the National Comprehensive Cancer Network® and quality measures for breast and colorectal cancer developed by the American College of Surgeons Commission on Cancer (www.facs.org/quality-programs/cancer/ncdb/qualitymeasures) can be used to inform the development of APN outcome measures. No one set of outcome measures is appropriate for all situations.

In selecting and introducing standardized outcome measures, APNs need to consider immediate and long-term outcomes that are measurable, valued by decision makers, and sensitive to changes in nursing care (Brooten et al., 2012). Valid, reliable, and clinically useful tools for documenting the key aspects of patient care (e.g., pain assessment, prevention and management of oral complications, maintenance of functional status) can be used to promote efficient and systematic documentation of care delivery and retrieval of data useful for clinical and programmatic improvements.

Conclusion

The challenges and complexity of delivering effective cancer care will continue to grow. Earlier diagnosis and the burgeoning array of effective treatment modalities are transforming cancer into a chronic illness. Patients and their families will have an even greater need for expert guidance and coaching, as well as effective case management, to support them in making well-informed decisions about treatment options and to optimize their self-management and continuity of care across this extended chronic illness continuum. Moreover, because of the aging of the population, the number of individuals living with cancer is expected to continue to grow. These challenges underscore the importance of the advanced clinical practice role to ensure access to quality cancer care and to optimize clinical and fiscal outcomes. The advent of individualized and customized treatment plans (tailored to individual preferences and increasingly to unique genetic characteristics and biologic disease features) also will require oncology nurses at the bedside to have access to consultative expertise and specialty education programs that oncology APNs are uniquely prepared to offer. Exponential growth in the science of cancer care and in supportive care research emphasizes the essential contribution of oncology APNs' skills in critical appraisal, synthesis, and research translation.

As with all healthcare professionals, oncology APNs will continue to be challenged to measure and describe the outcomes for patients, staff, and system capacity achieved through their activities. Public demand exists for such accountability, and increasingly, reimbursement mechanisms and hospital recognition may be based on a documented achievement of quality outcomes. The knowledge, expertise, broad skill set, flexibility, and public credibility of oncology APNs strongly position this advanced nursing role to lead the continued evolution of cancer care, to address dilemmas surrounding access to care, and to enhance outcomes for patients and families experiencing the diagnosis of cancer.

Case Study

A.S. is a 71-year-old woman admitted two days ago for vertebroplasty and to receive her first cycle of chemotherapy for newly diagnosed stage IIIA IgG kappa multiple myeloma complicated by compression fractures of thoracic vertebrae T4–T8. She has severe bone pain, which is currently well managed with controlled-release long-acting narcotic agents. A staff nurse on the unit mentions in patient care rounds that the patient is quite nauseated, and as the APN is leaving rounds with the nurse, the staff nurse asks whether the patient's nausea is normal, given that the patient has not yet received her chemotherapy treatment.

1. What type of consultation does this represent?
   - Consultation may be formal or informal, may be client or consultee centered, and may focus on patients or administrative issues. In this situation, the question represents an informal, client-centered, case consultation request.
2. Describe how the APN would proceed in handling this consultation request.
   - In responding to this question, the APN must decide whether the question can be answered immediately or whether more information is required. In addition, it is not clear whether the nurse is asking for consultative assistance in managing the nausea and exactly what she is seeking from the APN. The APN needs more information about the patient's situation before answering the question, but it is unclear if the nurse wishes to involve the APN in direct evaluation of the patient. More information is needed about the kind of assistance the staff nurse is requesting.
   - The APN responds by saying, "That is interesting, and there are a few different possibilities for her nausea that I can think of—can you tell me more about her status and the other medications she is taking?" The nurse explains that A.S. moves about with the assistance of a walker, has no standing order for antiemetics, and has not had a bowel movement since admission. The nurse admits that she has been too busy to further evaluate the patient.

3. If the nurse chooses to ask the APN to evaluate the patient with her, who is ultimately responsible for the patient's care and outcome?

    • The APN could offer to evaluate the patient with the nurse or could suggest that the nurse evaluate the patient and that they discuss the case further in the afternoon. The first option promotes direct APN consultative involvement in the case, whereas the second option provides the staff nurse with more independence and responsibility. Regardless of which option the nurse chooses, control of the consultation and responsibility for the patient's care must remain with the staff nurse, and the staff nurse must be provided with the opportunity to clarify the kind of assistance she is seeking from the APN.

    • The patient is returning to the community, and her primary nurse consults with the APN because he recognizes that A.S. is at high risk for readmission and has a complex medical regimen to manage at home. The patient is somewhat frail. The consultation request is to help to evaluate the adequacy of the discharge plan.

4. What elements should the APN include in the evaluation and management plan to ensure continuity of care?

    • The plan to ensure continuity of care begins with a comprehensive assessment of the patient and family's needs and strengths. That assessment addresses three key questions: (a) What self-care activities are to be performed to maintain or enhance function, comfort, and well-being? (b) Who will perform those activities now, who will perform those over time, and who is the designated alternate? (c) What health teaching, referrals, equipment, devices, or supplies are required? Elements of continuity include an interdisciplinary approach to care, comprehensive assessment of patient and family needs and strengths, patient and family education and involvement in decision making, identification and coordination of supplemental resources, integration of care through each transition, and a documented plan of care.

    • The APN receives an email from the supervisor that because of shortages in the staff development division, the APN will be required to assist with teaching cardiopulmonary resuscitation (CPR) to staff nurse orientees and with recertifying current staff in CPR. The APN sees this responsibility as inconsistent with the specialty role, perceives that the nurse educators should have primary responsibility for helping staff to meet this basic competency, and worries that to incorporate this responsibility, less time will be devoted to working with the staff in the development of evidence-based care standards for symptom management. The supervisor closed the email by saying that she will discuss this further with the APN at their next regular meeting.

5. Describe how the APN would prepare for this negotiation.

    • Although it is not completely apparent from the email alone that there is room for negotiation on this issue, the fact that the supervisor is willing to discuss it at the next meeting suggests that she may be willing to negotiate the scope or the terms of the APN's involvement in CPR training. Negotiation is the mutual discussion and arrangement of the terms of a transaction or agreement and involves analyzing the problem, generating ideas and potential actions that offer a mutually acceptable solution to the problem, understanding the role that each side will play, and identifying criteria that indicate a successful outcome. The APN prepares for the discussion by considering the desired outcome of the negotiation and what the supervisor anticipates. The APN also should consider what the APN and the supervisor each has that the other might want, and what each might be comfortable giving away. Alternatives must be considered if agreement cannot be obtained, as well as the future implications of disagreement. The history of the APN-supervisor relationship is contemplated, along with how that history might affect the negotiation. The APN then considers possible solutions and compromises. Were other individuals in the system also recruited to assist with CPR training? Is this a temporary solution until additional educators are recruited to meet the demand? What responsibilities might be shifted from the APN to another team member so that the APN can accommodate this request? If the APN accommodates this request, what resources (e.g., secretarial support, research assistant, equipment, conference attendance, compensatory time off, additional salary support) might be provided to the APN to assist in managing the total workload, to reward teamwork, or to offset the additional time commitment? If the APN agrees to this request, what is the time frame of the commitment to assist with teaching, and when can that commitment be renegotiated? It also may be helpful to discuss the preferred and the minimally acceptable outcomes, as well as the potential solutions and compromises with a colleague or mentor to gain another perspective.

Key Points

- The APN role includes the functions of clinician, consultant, educator, researcher, and coordinator. Essential APN skills include leadership, collaboration, change management, scholarly practice, mentorship, negotiation, and conflict resolution.
- The educational process begins with a learning needs assessment, followed by development of learning objectives, selection of the methods of instruction, and design of the program, and concludes with program evaluation. Learning objectives are specific and measurable with two components: performance and criterion.
- The following adult learning principles may be incorporated into educational programming.
  - Adults are self-directed and require involvement in all stages of the learning process, from planning through evaluation.
  - Adults have significant life experiences and a diverse skill set upon which to base education.
  - Adults like feedback about progress toward goals, learn best in a comfortable environment, and value information that helps them to solve immediate problems.
- The APN's role in research includes participation in research evaluation and critique, research utilization, and the conduct and dissemination of research. APNs have a fundamental responsibility for the translation of research into clinical decisions, tools, and programs to improve patient outcomes.
- Leadership is the use of communication processes to influence the activities of an individual or group toward the attainment of a goal. It includes both concern for the task and outcomes to be achieved and the concerns for the people who are responsible for the task.

Recommended Resources for Oncology Advanced Practice Nurses

- Advanced Practitioner Society for Hematology and Oncology: www.apsho.org
- Blanchard, K., Edington, D.W., & Blanchard, M. (1999). *The one minute manager balances work and life* (1st Quill ed.). New York, NY: HarperCollins.
- Block, P. (2011). *Flawless consulting: A guide to getting your expertise used* (3rd ed.). San Francisco, CA: Pfeiffer.
- Edelman, J., & Crain, M.B. (1993). *The Tao of negotiation: How you can prevent, resolve, and transcend conflict in work and everyday life.* New York, NY: HarperBusiness.
- Fulton, J.S., Lyon, B.L., & Goudreau, K.A. (2014). *Foundations of clinical nurse specialist practice* (2nd ed.). New York, NY: Springer.
- *Journal of the Advanced Practitioner in Oncology* (*JADPRO*): www.advancedpractitioner.com

- Kritek, P.B. (1994). *Negotiating at an uneven table: A practical approach to working with difference and diversity.* San Francisco, CA: Jossey-Bass.
- Maxwell, J.C. (2013). *The 5 levels of leadership: Proven steps to maximize your potential.* New York, NY: Center Street.
- Shell, G.R., & Moussa, M. (2008). *The art of woo: Using strategic persuasion to sell your ideas.* New York, NY: Penguin Group (USA) Incorporated.
- Stewart, J.G., & DeNisco, S.M. (2013). *Role development for the nurse practitioner.* Burlington, MA: Jones & Bartlett Learning.
- Stone, D., Patton, B., & Heen, S. (2010). *Difficult conversations: How to discuss what matters most.* New York, NY: Penguin.
- Sullivan-Marx, E.M., McGivern, D.O., Fairman, J.A., & Greenberg, S.A. (Eds.). (2010). *Nurse practitioners: The evolution and future of advanced practice* (5th ed.). New York, NY: Springer.

The author would like to acknowledge Sandra A. Mitchell, CRNP, PhD, AOCN®, for her contribution to this chapter that remains unchanged from the first edition of this book.

References

Adams, T.L., Orchard, C., Houghton, P., & Ogrin, R. (2014). The metamorphosis of a collaborative team: From creation to operation. *Journal of Interprofessional Care, 28,* 339–344. doi:10.3109/13561820.2014.891571

American Society of Clinical Oncology. (2003). American Society of Clinical Oncology policy statement: Oversight of clinical research. *Journal of Clinical Oncology, 21,* 2377–2386. doi:10.1200/JCO.2003.04.026

Anderson, L.W., & Krathwohl, D.R. (Eds.). (2001). *A taxonomy for learning, teaching, and assessing: A revision of Bloom's taxonomy of educational objectives.* New York, NY: Longman.

APRN Consensus Work Group & National Council of State Boards of Nursing APRN Advisory Committee. (2008). *Consensus model for APRN regulation: Licensure, accreditation, certification and education.* Retrieved from http://www.aacn.nche.edu/education-resources/APRNReport.pdf

Baggs, J.G. (1994). Development of an instrument to measure collaboration and satisfaction about care decisions. *Journal of Advanced Nursing, 20,* 176–182. doi:10.1046/j.1365-2648.1994.20010176.x

Bartolo, M., Zucchella, C., Pace, A., De Nunzio, A.M., Serrao, M., Sandrini, G., & Pierelli, F. (2012). Improving neuro-oncological patients care: Basic and practical concepts for nurse specialist in neuro-rehabilitation. *Journal of Experimental and Clinical Cancer Research, 31,* 82. doi:10.1186/1756-9966-31-82

Bauer, J.C. (2010). Nurse practitioners as an underutilized resource for health reform: Evidence-based demonstrations of cost-effectiveness. *Journal of the American Academy of Nurse Practitioners, 22,* 228–231. doi:10.1111/j.1745-7599.2010.00498.x

Begley, C., Elliott, N., Lalor, J., Coyne, I., Higgins, A., & Comiskey, C. (2013). Differences between clinical specialist and advanced practitioner clinical practice, leadership, and research roles, responsibilities, and perceived outcomes (the SCAPE study). *Journal of Advanced Nursing, 69,* 1323–1337. doi:10.1111/j.1365-2648.2012.06124.x

Belling, R., Whittock, M., McLaren, S., Burns, T., Catty, J., Jones, R., ... Wykes, T. (2011). Achieving continuity of care: Facilitators and barriers in community mental health teams. *Implementation Science, 6,* 23. doi:10.1186/1748-5908-6-23

Berg, T.L. (2008). The Centers for Medicare and Medicaid Services (CMS) EHR demonstration project. *South Dakota Medicine, 61,* 282.

Bergman, K., Perhed, U., Eriksson, I., Lindblad, U., & Fagerström, L. (2013). Patients' satisfaction with the care offered by advanced practice nurses: A new role in Swedish primary care. *International Journal of Nursing Practice, 19,* 326–333. doi:10.1111/ijn.12072.

Blackmore, C.C., Edwards, J.W., Searles, C., Wechter, D., Mecklenburg, R., & Kaplan, G.S. (2013). Nurse practitioner-staffed clinic at Virginia Mason improves care and lowers costs for women with benign breast conditions. *Health Affairs, 32,* 20–26. doi:10.1377/hlthaff.2012.0006

Blayney, D.W., McNiff, K., Hanauer, D., Miela, G., Markstrom, D., & Neuss, M. (2009). Implementation of the Quality Oncology Practice Initiative at a university comprehensive cancer center. *Journal of Clinical Oncology, 27,* 3802–3807. doi:10.1200/JCO.2008.21.6770

Blecher, C.S., Ireland, A.M., & Watson, J.L. (2016). *Standards of oncology education: Patient/significant other and public* (4th ed.). Pittsburgh, PA: Oncology Nursing Society.

Block, P. (2011). *Flawless consulting: A guide to getting your expertise used* (3rd ed.). San Francisco, CA: Pfeiffer.

Bourbonniere, M., Mezey, M., Mitty, E.L., Burger, S., Bonner, A., Bowers, B., … Nicholson, N.R., Jr. (2009). Expanding the knowledge base of resident and facility outcomes of care delivered by advanced practice nurses in long-term care: Expert panel recommendations. *Policy, Politics, and Nursing Practice, 10,* 64–70. doi:10.1177/1527154409332289

Brant, J.M., & Wickham, R. (Eds.). (2013). *Statement on the scope and standards of oncology nursing practice: Generalist and advanced practice.* Pittsburgh, PA: Oncology Nursing Society.

Brar, K., Boschma, G., & McCuaig, F. (2010). The development of nurse practitioner preparation beyond the master's level: What is the debate about? *International Journal of Nursing Education Scholarship, 7,* Article 9. doi:10.2202/1548-923X.1928

Britell, J.C. (2010). Role of advanced nurse practitioners and physician assistants in Washington State. *Journal of Oncology Practice, 6,* 37–38. doi:10.1200/JOP.091068

Brooten, D., Youngblut, J.M., Deosires, W., Singhala, K., & Guido-Sanz, F. (2012). Global considerations in measuring effectiveness of advanced practice nurses. *International Journal of Nursing Studies, 49,* 906–912. doi:10.1016/j.ijnurstu.2011.10.022

Bruner, D.W., & O'Mara, A. (2014). Nurse scientists in cancer cooperative groups. *Seminars in Oncology Nursing, 30,* 4–10. doi:10.1016/j.soncn.2013.12.002

Bryant-Lukosius, D., & DiCenso, A. (2004). A framework for the introduction and evaluation of advanced practice nursing roles. *Journal of Advanced Nursing, 48,* 530–540. doi:10.1111/j.1365-2648.2004.03235.x

Burns, J.M. (2004). *Transforming leadership: The new pursuit of happiness.* New York, NY: Atlantic Monthly Press.

Burston, S., Chaboyer, W., & Gillespie, B. (2014). Nurse-sensitive indicators suitable to reflect nursing care quality: A review and discussion of issues. *Journal of Clinical Nursing, 23,* 1785–1795. doi:10.1111/jocn.12337

Buscemi, J., Steglitz, J., & Spring, B. (2012). The impact of team science collaborations in health care: A synopsis and comment on "Interprofessional collaboration: Effects of practice-based interventions on professional practice and healthcare outcomes." *Translational Behavioral Medicine, 2,* 378–379. doi:10.1007/s13142-012-0169-9

Campion, F.X., Larson, L.R., Kadlubek, P.J., Earle, C.C., & Neuss, M.N. (2011). Advancing performance measurement in oncology: Quality Oncology Practice Initiative participation and quality outcomes. *Journal of Oncology Practice, 7*(Suppl. 3), 31s–35s. doi:10.1200/JOP.2011.000313

Carson, S.S., Vu, M., Danis, M., Camhi, S.L., Scheunemann, L.P., Cox, C.E., … Nelson, J.E. (2012). Development and validation of a printed information brochure for families of chronically critically ill patients. *Critical Care Medicine, 40,* 73–78. doi:10.1097/CCM.0b013e31822d7901

Carter, N., Martin-Misener, R., Kilpatrick, K., Kaasalainen, S., Donald, F., Bryant-Lukosius, D., … DiCenso, A. (2010). The role of nursing leadership in integrating clinical nurse specialists and nurse practitioners in healthcare delivery in Canada. *Nursing Leadership, 23*(Spec. No. 2010), 167–185. doi:10.12927/cjnl.2010.22274

Catania, K., Askew, T., Birkhimer, D., Courtney, L., Hanes, D., Lamprecht, M., … Vendlinski, S. (2012). From unit based to population focused: Transforming the role of the oncology clinical nurse specialists. *Clinical Nurse Specialist, 26,* 103–106. doi:10.1097/NUR.0b013e31824590d0

Chachkes, E., & Christ, G. (1996). Cross cultural issues in patient education. *Patient Education and Counseling, 27,* 13–21. doi:10.1016/0738-3991(95)00785-7

Charvet-Berard, A., Chopard, P., & Perneger, T.V. (2008). Measuring quality of patient information documents with an expanded EQIP scale. *Patient Education and Counseling, 70,* 407–411. doi:10.1016/j.pec.2007.11.018

Chism, L.A. (2009). Toward clarification of the doctor of nursing practice degree. *Advanced Emergency Nursing Journal, 31,* 287–297. doi:10.1097/TME.0b013e3181be0fd6

Clark, R.C., & Greenawald, M. (2013). Nurse-physician leadership: Insights into interprofessional collaboration. *Journal of Nursing Administration, 43,* 653–659. doi:10.1097/NNA.0000000000000007

Chugh, A., Williams, M.V., Grigsby, J., & Coleman, E.A. (2009). Better transitions: Improving comprehension of discharge instructions. *Frontiers of Health Services Management, 25*(3), 11–32.

Collins, K., McClimens, A., Mekonnen, S., & Wyld, L. (2014). Breast cancer information and support needs for women with intellectual disabilities: A scoping study. *Psycho-Oncology, 23,* 892–897. doi:10.1002/pon.3500

Comiskey, C., Coyne, I., Lalor, J., & Begley, C. (2014). A national cross-sectional study measuring predictors for improved service user outcomes across clinical nurse or midwife specialist, advanced nurse practitioner and control sites. *Journal of Advanced Nursing, 70,* 1128–1137. doi:10.1111/jan.12273

Cope, D.G. (2014a). Analysis and use of different research review approaches in nursing. *Oncology Nursing Forum, 41,* 207–208. doi:10.1188/14.ONF.207-208

Cope, D.G. (2014b). Method and meanings: Credibility and trustworthiness of qualitative research. *Oncology Nursing Forum, 41,* 89–91. doi:10.1188/14.ONF.89-91

Cornelius, H. (2000). *The gentle revolution: Men and women at work, what goes wrong and how to fix it.* New South Wales, Australia: Simon & Schuster.

Craig, J.V., & Smyth, R.L. (Eds.). (2011). *The evidence-based practice manual for nurses* (3rd ed.). Philadelphia, PA: Elsevier Churchill Livingstone.

Cranford, J.S. (2013). Bridging the gap: Clinical practice nursing and the effect of role strain on successful role transition and intent to stay in academia. *International Journal of Nursing Education Scholarship, 10,* 99–105. doi:10.1515/ijnes-2012-0018

Creswell, J.W. (2013). *Qualitative inquiry and research design: Choosing among five approaches* (3rd ed.). Thousand Oaks, CA: Sage Publications.

Crockett-Maillet, G. (2008). The breast cancer navigator: A new role for nurse practitioners. *Advance for Nurse Practitioners, 16*(1), 53–54, 56.

Currey, J., Considine, J., & Khaw, D. (2011). Clinical nurse research consultant: A clinical and academic role to advance practice and the discipline of nursing. *Journal of Advanced Nursing, 67,* 2275–2283. doi:10.1111/j.1365-2648.2011.05687.x

D'Agostino, R., & Halpern, N.A. (2010). Acute care nurse practitioners in oncologic critical care: The Memorial Sloan-Kettering Cancer Center experience. *Critical Care Clinics, 26,* 207–217. doi:10.1016/j.ccc.2009.09.003

Danesh, M., Belkora, J., Volz, S., & Rugo, H.S. (2014). Informational needs of patients with metastatic breast cancer: What questions do they ask, and are physicians answering them? *Journal of Cancer Education, 29,* 175–180. doi:10.1007/s13187-013-0566-x

Denzin, N.K., & Lincoln, Y.S. (Eds.). (2011). The Sage *handbook of qualitative research* (4th ed.). Thousand Oaks, CA: Sage.

DiCenso, A., Bryant-Lukosius, D., Martin-Misener, R., Donald, F., Abelson, J., Bourgeault, I., … Harbman, P. (2010). Factors enabling advanced practice nursing role integration in Canada. *Nursing Leadership, 23*(Spec. No. 2010), 211–238. doi:10.12927/cjnl.2010.22279

DiCenso, A., Guyatt, G., & Ciliska, D. (2005). *Evidence-based nursing: A guide to clinical practice.* St. Louis, MO: Elsevier Mosby.

Doak, C.C., Doak, L.G., & Root, J.H. (1996). *Teaching patients with low literacy skills* (2nd ed.). Philadelphia, PA: J.B. Lippincott.

Doerksen, K. (2010). What are the professional development and mentorship needs of advanced practice nurses? *Journal of Professional Nursing, 26,* 141–151. doi:10.1016/j.profnurs.2009.04.005

Donald, F., Martin-Misener, R., Carter, N., Donald, E.E., Kaasalainen, S., Wickson-Griffiths, A., … DiCenso, A. (2013). A systemic review of the effectiveness of advanced practice nurses in long-term care. *Journal of Advanced Nursing, 69,* 2148–2161. doi:10.1111/jan.12140

Donaldson, M.C. (2007). *Negotiating for dummies* (2nd ed.). Hoboken, NJ: Wiley Publishing.

Donovan, H.S., Nolte, S., Edwards, R.P., & Wenzel, L. (2014). Nursing research in the Gynecologic Oncology Group. *Seminars in Oncology Nursing, 30,* 44–52. doi:10.1016/j.soncn.2013.12.008

Dowling, M., Beauchesne, M., Farrelly, F., & Murphy, K. (2013). Advanced practice nursing: A concept analysis. *International Journal of Nursing Practice, 19,* 131–140. doi:10.1111/ijn.12050

Dyar, S., Lesperance, M., Shannon, R., Sloan, J., & Colon-Otero, G. (2012). A nurse practitioner directed intervention improves the quality of life of patients with metastatic cancer: Results of a randomized pilot study. *Journal of Palliative Medicine, 15,* 890–895. doi:10.1089/jpm.2012.0014

Economou, D., Edgington, A., & Deutsch, A. (2010). Roles of the clinical nurse specialist and nurse practitioner in survivorship care. *Journal of the Advanced Practitioner in Oncology, 1,* 87–94. doi:10.6004/jadpro.2010.1.2.11

Edwards, N., Webber, J., Mill, J., Kahwa, E., & Roelofs, S. (2009). Building capacity for nurse-led research. *International Nursing Review, 56,* 88–94. doi:10.1111/j.1466-7657.2008.00683.x

Elliott, N., Begley, C., Kleinpell, R., & Higgins, A. (2014). The development of leadership outcome-indicators evaluating the contribution of clinical specialists and advanced practitioners to health care: A secondary analysis. *Journal of Advanced Nursing, 70,* 1078–1093. doi:10.1111/jan.12262

Facchiano, L., & Snyder, C.H. (2012). Evidence-based practice for the busy nurse practitioner: Part three: Critical appraisal process. *Journal of the American Academy of Nurse Practitioners, 24,* 704–715. doi:10.1111/j.1745-7599.2012.00752.x

Feldman-Stewart, D., Madarnas, Y., Mates, M., Tong, C., Grunfeld, E., Verma, S., … Brundage, M. (2013). Information needs of post-menopausal women with hormone receptor positive early-stage breast cancer considering adjuvant endocrine therapy. *Patient Education and Counseling, 93,* 114–121. doi:10.1016/j.pec.2013.03.019

Fineout-Overholt, E., Melnyk, B.M., Stillwell, S.B., & Williamson, K.M. (2010). Evidence-based practice, step by step: Critical appraisal of the evidence: Part III. *American Journal of Nursing, 110*(11), 43–51. doi:10.1097/01.NAJ.0000390523.99066.b5

Fowler, L., Gottschlich, M.M., & Kagan, R.J. (2013). Burn center journal club promotes clinical research, continuing education, and evidence-based practice. *Journal of Burn Care and Research, 34,* e92–e98. doi:10.1097/BCR.0b013e3182839b03

Fox, K. (2014). The role of the acute care nurse practitioner in the implementation of the Commission on Cancer's standards on palliative care. *Clinical Journal of Oncology Nursing, 18*(Suppl. 1), 39–44. doi:10.1188/14.CJON.S1.39-44

Fulton, J.S. (2013). Making outcomes of clinical nurse specialist practice visible [Editorial]. *Clinical Nurse Specialist, 27*, 5–6. doi:10.1097/NUR.0b013e31827caca1

Geppert, C.M.A., & Shelton, W.N. (2012). A comparison of general medical and clinical ethics consultations: What can we learn from each other? *Mayo Clinic Proceedings, 87*, 381–389. doi:10.1016/j.mayocp.2011.10.010

Gilmore, T.R., Schulmeister, L., & Jacobson, J.O. (2013). Quality Oncology Practice Initiative certification program: Measuring implementation of chemotherapy administration safety standards in the outpatient oncology setting. *Journal of Oncology Practice, 9*(Suppl. 2), 14s–18s. doi:10.1200/JOP.2013.000886

Given, B.A., & Sherwood, P.R. (2005). Nursing-sensitive patient outcomes—A white paper. *Oncology Nursing Forum, 32*, 773–784. doi:10.1188/05.ONF.773-784

Gobel, B.H., Beck, S.L., & O'Leary, C. (2006). Nursing-sensitive patient outcomes: The development of the Putting Evidence Into Practice resources for nursing practice. *Clinical Journal of Oncology Nursing, 10*, 621–624. doi:10.1188/06.CJON.621-624

Goldberg, N.J., & Moch, S.D. (1998). An advanced practice nurse–nurse researcher collaborative model. *Clinical Nurse Specialist, 12*, 251–255. doi:10.1097/00002800-199811000-00015

Goldfarb, M., & Casillas, J. (2014). Unmet information and support needs in newly diagnosed thyroid cancer: Comparison of adolescents/young adults (AYA) and older patients. *Journal of Cancer Survivorship, 8*, 394–401. doi:10.1007/s11764-014-0345-7

Goldman, L., Lee, T., & Rudd, P. (1983). Ten commandments for effective consultations. *Archives of Internal Medicine, 143*, 1753–1755. doi:10.1001/archinte.1983.00350090131022

Gopalakrishnan, S., & Ganeshkumar, P. (2013). Systematic reviews and meta-analysis: Understanding the best evidence in primary healthcare. *Journal of Family Medicine and Primary Care, 2*, 9–14. doi:10.4103/2249-4863.109934

Gormley, D.K., & Glazer, G. (2012). Legislative: Nursing distance learning programs and state board of nursing authorizations. *Online Journal of Issues in Nursing, 17*(3), 10. doi:10.3912/OJIN.Vol17No03LegCol01

Graham, R., Mancher, M., Wolman, D.M., Greenfield, S., & Steinberg, E. (Eds.). (2011). *Clinical practice guidelines we can trust.* Retrieved from http://www.nap.edu/catalog/13058/clinical-practice-guidelines-we-can-trust

Griffiths, P., Richardson, A., & Blackwell, R. (2012). Outcomes sensitive to nursing service quality in ambulatory cancer chemotherapy: Systematic scoping review. *European Journal of Oncology Nursing, 16*, 238–246. doi:10.1016/j.ejon.2011.06.004

Haggerty, J.L., Roberge, D., Freeman, G.K., Beaulieu, C., & Bréton, M. (2011). Validation of a generic measure of continuity of care: When patients encounter several clinicians. *Annals of Family Medicine, 10*, 443–451. doi:10.1370/afm.1378

Hagopian, G.A. (1996). Patient and family education. In R. McCorkle, M. Grant, M. Frank-Stromborg, & S.B. Baird (Eds.), *Cancer nursing: A comprehensive textbook* (2nd ed., pp. 1223–1234). Philadelphia, PA: Elsevier Saunders.

Hake, S., & Shah, T. (2011). Negotiation skills for clinical research professionals. *Perspectives in Clinical Research, 2*, 105–108. doi:10.4103/2229-3485.83224

Han, P.K.J., & Rayson, D. (2010). The coordination of primary and oncology specialty care at the end of life. *Journal of the National Cancer Institute Monographs, 2010*(40), 31–37. doi:10.1093/jncimonographs/lgq003

Hansen, L.K., Moinpour, C.M., & Ermete, R.B. (2014). Enhancing nurse contributions to SWOG clinical trials. *Seminars in Oncology Nursing, 30*, 26–31. doi:10.1016/j.soncn.2013.12.005

Hardy, M.E., & Hardy, W.L. (1988). Role stress and role strain. In M.E. Hardy & M.E. Conway (Eds.), *Role theory: Perspectives for health professionals* (2nd ed., pp. 159–239). Norwalk, CT: Appleton & Lange.

Hendricks, C.B. (2013). Re-engineering a small oncology practice for quality using the ASCO Quality Oncology Practice Initiative. *Journal of Oncology Practice, 9*, 169–170. doi:10.1200/JOP.2013.000972

Hill, L.A., & Sawatzky, J.V. (2011). Transitioning into the nurse practitioner role through mentorship. *Journal of Professional Nursing, 27*, 161–167. doi:10.1016/j.profnurs.2011.02.004

Hollis, G., & McMenamin, E. (2014). Integrating nurse practitioners into radiation oncology: One institution's experience. *Journal of the Advanced Practitioner in Oncology, 5*, 42–46. doi:10.6004/jadpro.2014.5.1.9

Houlihan, N.G. (2009). Transitioning to cancer survivorship: Plans of care. *Oncology, 23*(Suppl. 8), 42–48.

Imhof, L., Naef, R., Wallhagen, M.I., Schwarz, J., & Mahrer-Imhof, R. (2012). Effects of an advanced practice nurse in-home health consultation program for community-dwelling persons aged 80 and older. *Journal of the American Geriatrics Society, 60*, 2223–2231. doi:10.1111/jgs.12026

Institute of Medicine. (2011). *The future of nursing: Leading change, advancing health.* Retrieved from http://www.nap.edu/catalog/12956/the-future-of-nursing-leading-change-advancing-health

Irwin, M.M., Bergman, R.M., & Richards, R. (2013). The experience of implementing evidence-based practice change: A qualitative analysis. *Clinical Journal of Oncology Nursing, 17*, 544–549. doi:10.1188/13.CJON.544-549

Jacobs, L.A., & Mayer, D.K. (Ed.). (2015). *Standards of oncology nursing education: Generalist and advanced practice levels* (4th ed.). Pittsburgh, PA: Oncology Nursing Society.

Jacobson, J.O., Neuss, M.N., & Hauser, R. (2012). Measuring and improving value of care in oncology practices: ASCO programs from Quality Oncology Practice Initiative to the Rapid Learning System. *American Society of Clinical Oncology Education Book, 32*, e70–e76. doi:10.14694/EdBook_AM.2012.32.e70

James-Martin, G., Koczwara, B., Smith, E.L., & Miller, M.D. (2014). Information needs of cancer patients and survivors regarding diet, exercise and weight management: A qualitative study. *European Journal of Cancer Care, 23*, 340–348. doi:10.1111/ecc.12159

Jenicek, M., Croskerry, P., & Hitchcock, D.L. (2011). Evidence and its uses in health care and research: The role of critical thinking. *Medical Science Monitor, 17*(1), RA12–RA17. doi:10.12659/MSM.881321

Kapu, A.N., & Kleinpell, R. (2013). Developing nurse practitioner associated metrics for outcomes assessment. *Journal of the American Association of Nurse Practitioners, 25*, 289–296. doi:10.1111/1745-7599.12001

Kapu, A.N., Kleinpell, R., & Pilon B. (2014). Quality and financial impact of adding nurse practitioners to inpatient care teams. *Journal of Nursing Administration, 44*, 87–96. doi:10.1097/NNA.0000000000000031

Kilpatrick, K. (2013). How do nurse practitioners in acute care affect perceptions of team effectiveness? *Journal of Clinical Nursing, 22*, 2636–2647. doi:10.1111/jocn.12198

Kim, M.Y. (2011). Effects of oncology clinical nurse specialists' interventions on nursing-sensitive outcomes in South Korea [Online exclusive]. *Clinical Journal of Oncology Nursing, 15*(5), E66–E74. doi:10.1188/11.ONF.E66-E74

Klinger, K., Figueras, C., Beney, K.M., Armer, J.M., & Levy, S. (2014). Nursing contributions in community clinical oncology research programs. *Seminars in Oncology Nursing, 30*, 38–43. doi:10.1016/j.soncn.2013.12.007

Knopf, K.E. (2011). Core competencies for bone marrow transplantation nurse practitioners. *Clinical Journal of Oncology Nursing, 15*, 102–105. doi:10.1188/11.CJON.102-105

Leonard, M., & Miller, E. (2012). *Nursing case management review and resource manual* (4th ed.). Silver Spring, MD: American Nurses Credentialing Center.

Leventhal, H., & Cameron, L. (1987). Behavioral theories and the problem of compliance. *Patient Education and Counseling, 10*, 117–138. doi:10.1016/0738-3991(87)90093-0

Lippitt, G., & Lippitt, R. (1986). *The consulting process in action* (2nd ed.). San Diego, CA: University Associates.

Lugo, N.R., O'Grady, E.T., Hodnicki, D., & Hanson, C. (2010). Are regulations more consumer-friendly when boards of nursing are the sole regulators of nurse practitioners? *Journal of Professional Nursing, 26*, 29–34. doi:10.1016/j.profnurs.2009.09.001

MacDonald, S.E., Newburn-Cook, C.V., Allen, M., & Reutter, L. (2013). Embracing the population health framework in nursing research. *Nursing Inquiry, 20*, 30–41. doi:10.1111/nin.12017

MacNeil, J., & MacKinnon, K. (2011). Making visible the contributions of the clinical nurse specialist. *Nursing Leadership, 24*(4), 88–98. doi:10.12927/cjnl.2012.22737

Madsen, L.T., Craig, C., & Kuban, D. (2009). A multidisciplinary prostate cancer clinic for newly diagnosed patients: Developing the role of the advanced practice nurse. *Clinical Journal of Oncology Nursing, 13*, 305–309. doi:10.1188/09.CJON.305-309

Makari-Judson, G., Wrenn, T., Mertens, W.C., Josephson, G., & Stewart, J.A. (2014). Using Quality Oncology Practice Initiative metrics for physician incentive compensation. *Journal of Oncology Practice, 10*, 58–62. doi:10.1200/JOP.2013.000953

Mason, H., DeRubeis, M.B., Foster, J.C., Taylor, J.M.G., & Worden, F.P. (2013). Outcomes evaluation of a weekly nurse practitioner-managed symptom management clinic for patients with head and neck cancer treated with chemoradiotherapy. *Oncology Nursing Forum, 40*, 581–586. doi:10.1188/13.ONF.40-06AP

McCorkle, R., Preston, F., & Volker, D.L. (1996). Cancer nursing education today. In R. McCorkle, M. Grant, M. Frank-Stromborg, & S.B. Baird (Eds.), *Cancer nursing: A comprehensive textbook* (2nd ed., pp. 1247–1260). Philadelphia, PA: Elsevier Saunders.

McMaster, R., Jammali-Blasi, A., Andersson-Noorgard, K., Cooper, K., & McInnes, E. (2013). Research involvement, support needs, and factors affecting research participation: A survey of mental health consultation liaison nurses. *International Journal of Mental Health Nursing, 22*, 154–161. doi:10.1111/j.1447-0349.2012.00857.x

McNair, A.G.K., Brookes, S.T., Kinnersley, P., & Blazeby, J.M. (2013). What surgeons should tell patients with oesophago-gastric cancer: A cross sectional study of information needs. *European Journal of Surgical Oncology, 39*, 1278–1286. doi:10.1016/j.ejso.2013.08.005

McNamara, S., Giguère, V., St-Louis, L., & Boileau, J. (2009). Development and implementation of the specialized nurse practitioner role: Use of the PEPPA framework to achieve success. *Nursing and Health Sciences, 11*, 318–325. doi:10.1111/j.1442-2018.2009.00467.x

Melnyk, B.M., & Fineout-Overholt, E. (2014). *Evidence-based practice in nursing and healthcare: A guide to best practice* (3rd ed.). Philadelphia, PA: Wolters Kluwer Health/Lippincott Williams & Wilkins.

Milani, A., Mauri, S., Gandini, S., & Magon, G. (2013). Oncology nursing minimum data set (ONMDS): Can we hypothesize a set of prevalent nursing sensitive outcomes (NSO) in cancer patients? *Ecancermedicalscience, 7*, 345. doi:10.3332/ecancer.2013.345

Milbury, K., Rosenthal, D.I., El-Naggar, A., & Badr, H. (2013). An exploratory study of the informational and psycho-social needs of patients with human papillomavirus-associated oropharyngeal cancer. *Oral Oncology, 49,* 1067–1071. doi:10.1016/j.oraloncology.2013.07.010

Moore, J., & McQuestion, M. (2012). The clinical nurse specialist in chronic diseases. *Clinical Nurse Specialist, 26,* 149–163. doi:10.1097/NUR.0b013e3182503fa7

Moore-Higgs, G.J., Watkins-Bruner, D., Balmer, L., Johnson-Doneski, J., Komarny, P., Mautner, B., & Velji, K. (2003). The role of licensed nursing personnel in radiation oncology part A: Results of a descriptive study. *Oncology Nursing Forum, 30,* 51–58. doi:10.1188/03.ONF.51-58

Morgan, P.A., Abbott, D.H., McNeil, R.B., & Fisher, D.A. (2012). Characteristics of primary care office visits to nurse practitioners, physician assistants and physicians in United States Veterans Health Administration facilities, 2005 to 2010: A retrospective cross-sectional analysis. *Human Resources for Health, 10,* 42. doi:10.1186/1478-4491-10-42

Moult, B., Franck, L.S., & Brady, H. (2004). Ensuring quality information for patients: Development and preliminary validation of a new instrument to improve the quality of written health care information. *Health Expectations, 7,* 165–175. doi:10.1111/j.1369-7625.2004.00273.x

Natale-Pereira, A., Enard, K.R., Nevarez, L., & Jones, L.A. (2011). The role of patient navigators in eliminating health disparities. *Cancer, 117,* 3543–3552. doi:10.1002/cncr.26264

National Association of Clinical Nurse Specialists. (2010). *Clinical nurse specialist core competencies.* Retrieved from http://www.nacns.org/docs/CNSCoreCompetenciesBroch.pdf

National Breast Cancer Centre's Specialist Breast Nurse Project Team (2003). An evidence-based specialist nurse role in practice: A multicentre implementation study. *European Journal of Cancer Care, 12,* 91–97. doi:10.1046/j.1365-2354.2003.00331.x

National Organization of Nurse Practitioner Faculties. (2012). *Nurse practitioners' core competencies.* Retrieved from http://c.ymcdn.com/sites/www.nonpf.org/resource/resmgr/competencies/npcorecompetenciesfinal2012.pdf

Nevidjon, B. (2014). A seat at the table: Redesigning cancer care [Guest editorial]. *Clinical Journal of Oncology Nursing, 18,* 13–14. doi:10.1188/14.CJON.13-14

Neville, L., & Swift, J. (2012). Measuring the impact of the advanced practitioner role: A practical approach. *Journal of Nursing Management, 20,* 382–389. doi:10.1111/j.1365-2834.2012.01356.x

Newhouse, R.P., Weiner, J.P., Stanik-Hutt, J., White, K.M., Johantgen, M., Steinwachs, D., … Bass, E.B. (2012). Policy implications for optimizing advanced practice registered nurse use nationally. *Policy, Politics, and Nursing Practice, 13,* 81–89. doi:10.1177/1527154412456299

O'Brien, M., Stricker, C.T., Foster, J.D., Ness, K., Arlen, A.G., & Schwartz, R.N. (2014). Navigating the seasons of survivorship in community oncology. *Clinical Journal of Oncology Nursing, 18*(Suppl. 1), 9–14. doi:10.1188/14.CJON.S1.9-14

Oncology Nursing Society. (2007). *Oncology nurse practitioner competencies.* Retrieved from https://www.ons.org/sites/default/files/npcompentencies.pdf

Oncology Nursing Society. (2008). *Oncology clinical nurse specialist competencies.* Retrieved from https://www.ons.org/sites/default/files/cnscomps.pdf

Oncology Nursing Society. (2012). *Oncology Nursing Society leadership competencies.* Retrieved from https://www.ons.org/sites/default/files/leadershipcomps.pdf

Oncology Nursing Society. (2015a). *Access to quality cancer care.* Retrieved from https://www.ons.org/advocacy-policy/positions/policy/access

Oncology Nursing Society. (2015b). *The role of the advanced practice nurse in oncology care.* Retrieved from https://www.ons.org/advocacy-policy/positions/education/apn

Paplanus, L.M., Bartley-Daniele, P., & Mitra, K.S. (2014). Knowledge translation: A nurse practitioner clinical ladder advancement program in a university-affiliated, integrated medical center. *Journal of the American Association of Nurse Practitioners, 26,* 424–437. doi:10.1002/2327-6924.12082

Peterson, J. (2012). Implementing Quality Oncology Practice Initiative (QOPI) participation in a community oncology practice. *Journal of Registry Management, 39,* 154–157.

Pfaff, K.A., Baxter, P.E., Jack, S.M., & Ploeg, J. (2014). Exploring new graduate nurse confidence in interprofessional collaboration: A mixed methods study. *International Journal of Nursing Studies, 51,* 1142–1152. doi:10.1016/j.ijnurstu.2014.01.001

Pinnock, R., & Welch, P. (2014). Learning clinical reasoning. *Journal of Paediatrics and Child Health, 50,* 253–257. doi:10.1111/jpc.12455

Price, S., Doucet, S., & Hall, L.M. (2014). The historical social positioning of nursing and medicine: Implications for career choice, early socialization, and interprofessional collaboration. *Journal of Interprofessional Care, 28,* 103–109.

Pron, A.L. (2013). Job satisfaction and perceived autonomy for nurse practitioners working in nurse-manage health centers. *Journal of the American Academy of Nurse Practitioners, 25,* 213–221. doi:10.1111/j.1745-7599.2012.00776.x

Rankin, S.H., & Stallings, K.D. (1996). *Patient education: Issues, principles, practices* (3rd ed.). Philadelphia, PA: Wolters Kluwer Health/Lippincott Williams & Wilkins.

Rankin, S.H., Stallings, K.D., & London, F. (2005). *Patient education in health and illness* (5th ed.). Philadelphia, PA: Wolters Kluwer Health/Lippincott Williams & Wilkins.

Reames, B.N., Krell, R.W., Ponto, S.N., & Wong, S.L. (2013). Critical evaluation of oncology clinical practice guidelines. *Journal of Clinical Oncology, 31,* 2563–2568. doi:10.1200/JCO.2012.46.8371

Rees, C.E., Ford, J.E., & Sheard, C.E. (2002). Evaluating the reliability of DISCERN: A tool for assessing the quality of written patient information on treatment choices. *Patient Education and Counseling, 47,* 273–275. doi:10.1016/S0738-3991(01)00225-7

Reilly, D.E., & Oermann, M.H. (1992). *Clinical teaching in nursing education* (2nd ed.). New York, NY: National League for Nursing.

Reuben, D.B., Ganz, D.A., Roth, C.P., McCreath, H.E., Ramirez, K.D., & Wenger, N.S. (2013). Effect of nurse practitioner comanagement on the care of geriatric conditions. *Journal of the American Geriatrics Society, 61,* 857–867. doi:10.1111/jgs.12268

Rigolosi, E.L.M. (2012). *Management and leadership in nursing and health care: An experiential approach* (3rd ed.). New York, NY: Springer.

Roett, M.A., & Coleman, M.T. (2013). Practice improvement, part II: Collaborative practice and team-based care. *FP Essentials, 414,* 11–18.

Rogers, E.M. (2003). *Diffusion of innovations* (5th ed.). New York, NY: Free Press.

Rounds, L.R., Zych, J.J., & Mallary, L.L. (2013). The consensus model for regulation of APRNs: Implications for nurse practitioners. *Journal of the American Academy of Nurse Practitioners, 25,* 180–185. doi:10.1111/j.1745-7599.2013.00812.x

Ruegg, T.A. (2013). A nurse practitioner-led urgent care center: Meeting the needs of the patient with cancer [Online exclusive]. *Clinical Journal of Oncology Nursing, 17,* E52–E57. doi:10.1188/13.CJON.E52-E57

Rüesch, P., Schaffert, R., Fischer, S., Feldman-Stewart, D., Ruszat, R., Spörri, P., … Schmid, H.-P. (2014). Information needs of early-stage prostate cancer patients: Within- and between-group agreement of patients and health professionals. *Supportive Care in Cancer, 22,* 999–1007. doi:10.1007/s00520-013-2052-8

Rutledge, D.N., DePalma, J.A., & Cunningham, M. (2004). A process model for evidence-based literature syntheses. *Oncology Nursing Forum, 31,* 543–550. doi:10.1188/04.ONF.543-550

Saarmann, L., Daugherty, J., & Riegel, B. (2000). Patient teaching to promote behavioral change. *Nursing Outlook, 48,* 281–287. doi:10.1067/mno.2000.107277

Salerno, S.M., Hurst, F.P., Halvorson, S., & Mercado, D.L. (2007). Principles of effective consultation: An Update for the 21st-century consultant. *Archives of Internal Medicine, 167,* 271–275. doi:10.1001/archinte.167.3.271

Sangster-Gormley, E., Martin-Misener, R., & Burge, F. (2013). A case study of nurse practitioner role implementation in primary care: What happens when new roles are introduced? *BMC Nursing, 12,* 1. doi:10.1186/1472-6955-12-1

Sangster-Gormley, E., Martin-Misener, R., Downe-Wamboldt, B., & DiCenso, A. (2011). Factors affecting nurse practitioner role implementation in Canadian practice settings: An integrative review. *Journal of Advanced Nursing, 67,* 1178–1190. doi:10.1111/j.1365-2648.2010.05571.x

Sargent, D. (2010). What constitutes reasonable evidence of efficacy and effectiveness to guide oncology treatment decisions? *Oncologist, 15*(Suppl. 1), 19–23. doi:10.1634/theoncologist.2010-S1-19

Sawatzky, J.V., Christie, S., & Singal, R.K. (2013). Exploring outcomes of a nurse practitioner-managed cardiac surgery follow-up intervention: A randomized trial. *Journal of Advanced Nursing, 69,* 2076–2087. doi:10.1111/jan.12075

Scott, E.S., & Miles, J. (2013). Advancing leadership capacity in nursing. *Nursing Administration Quarterly, 37,* 77–82. doi:10.1097/NAQ.0b013e3182751998

Smith, A.C. (2011). Role ambiguity and role conflict in nurse case managers: An integrative review. *Professional Case Management, 16,* 182–196. doi:10.1097/NCM.0b013e318218845b

Sommers, R.M. (2010). Translating evidence-based research into practice. *Journal of the Advanced Practitioner in Oncology, 1,* 235–244. doi:10.6004/jadpro.2010.1.4.2

Specht, J.A. (2013). Mentoring relationships and the levels of role conflict and role ambiguity experienced by novice nursing faculty. *Journal of Professional Nursing, 29,* e25–e31. doi:10.1016/j.profnurs.2013.06.006

Spoelstra, S.L., & Robbins, L.B. (2010). A qualitative study of role transition from RN to APN. *International Journal of Nursing Education Scholarship, 7*(1). doi:10.2202/1548-923X.2020

Stachowiak, M.E., & Bugel, M.J. (2013). The clinical nurse leader and the case manager: Are both roles needed? *American Journal of Nursing, 113*(1), 59–63. doi:10.1097/01.NAJ.0000425754.43827.14

Stanley, J.M. (2012). Impact of new regulatory standards on advanced practice registered nursing: The APRN Consensus Model and LACE. *Nursing Clinics of North America, 47,* 241–250. doi:10.1016/j.cnur.2012.02.001

Stasa, H., Cashin, A., Buckley, T., & Donoghue, J. (2014). Advancing advanced practice: Clarifying the conceptual confusion. *Nurse Education Today, 34,* 356–361. doi:10.1016/j.nedt.2013.07.012

Stewart, J.G., McNulty, R., Griffin, M.T.Q., & Fitzpatrick, J.J. (2010). Psychological empowerment and structural empowerment among nurse practitioners. *Journal of the American Academy of Nurse Practitioners, 22,* 27–34. doi:10.1111/j.1745-7599.2009.00467.x

Stringer, K., Curran, V., & Asghari, S. (2013). Pharmacists and family physicians: Improving Interprofessional collaboration through joint understanding of our competencies. *Frontiers in Pharmacology, 4,* 151. doi:10.3389/fphar.2013.00151

Sullivan-Bentz, M., Humbert, J., Cragg, B., Legault, F., Laflamme, C., Bailey, P.H., & Doucette, S. (2010). Supporting primary health care nurse practitioners' transition to practice. *Canadian Family Physician, 56,* 1176–1182. Retrieved from http://www.cfp.ca/content/56/11/1176.long

Susilo, A.P., van den Eertwegh, V., van Dalen, J., & Scherpbier, A. (2013). Leary's Rose to improve negotiation skills among health professionals: Experiences from a Southeast Asian culture. *Education for Health, 26,* 54–59. Retrieved from http://www.educationforhealth.net/text.asp?2013/26/1/54/112803

Swiderski, M. (2011). Predictive genetic testing: Can specialized advanced practitioners quell consumer confusion? *Journal of the Advanced Practitioner in Oncology, 2,* 71–85. doi:10.6004/jadpro.2011.2.2.2

Szanton, S.L., Mihaly, L.K., Alhusen, J., & Becker, K.L. (2010). Taking charge of the challenge: Factors to consider in taking your first nurse practitioner job. *Journal of the American Academy of Nurse Practitioners, 22,* 356–360. doi:10.1111/j.1745-7599.2010.00522.x

Tarrant, T., & Sabo, C.E. (2010). Role conflict, role ambiguity, and job satisfaction in nurse executives. *Nursing Administration Quarterly, 34,* 72–82. doi:10.1097/NAQ.0b013e3181c95eb5

Treadwell, J., & Giardino, A. (2014). Collaborating for care: Initial experience of embedded case managers across five medical homes. *Professional Case Management, 19,* 86–92. doi:10.1097/NCM.0000000000000017

Uijen, A.A., Schers, H.J., Schellevis, F.G., & van den Bosch, W.J.H.M. (2012). How unique is continuity of care? A review of continuity and related concepts. *Family Practice, 29,* 264–271. doi:10.1093/fampra/cmr104

Underhill, M.L., Boucher, J., Roper, K., & Berry, D.L. (2012). Symptom management excellence initiative: Promoting evidence-based oncology nursing practice. *Clinical Journal of Oncology Nursing, 16,* 247–250. doi:10.1188/12.CJON.247-250

Viele, C.S. (2010). Role of the oncology clinical nurse specialist. *Journal of the Advanced Practitioner in Oncology, 1,* 48–50. doi:10.6004/jadpro.2010.1.1.6

Vogel, W.H. (2003). The advanced practice nursing role in a high-risk breast cancer clinic. *Oncology Nursing Forum, 30,* 115–122. doi:10.1188/03.ONF.115-122

Volk, R.J., Linder, S.K., Leal, V.B., Rabius, V., Cinciripini, P.M., Kamath, G.R., … Bevers, T.B. (2014). Feasibility of a patient decision aid about lung cancer screening with low-dose computed tomography. *Preventive Medicine, 62,* 60–63. doi:10.1016/j.ypmed.2014.02.006

Warren, E., Footman, K., Tinelli, M., McKee, M., & Knai, C. (2014). Do cancer-specific websites meet patient's information needs? *Patient Education and Counseling, 95,* 126–136. doi:10.1016/j.pec.2013.12.013

Wilensky, G.R. (2011). Lessons from the Physician Group Practice Demonstration—A sobering reflection. *New England Journal of Medicine, 365,* 1659–1661. doi:10.1056/NEJMp1110185

World Health Organization. (2010). *Framework for action on interprofessional education and collaborative practice.* Retrieved from http://www.who.int/hrh/resources/framework_action/en

Yeager, S. (2010). Detraumatizing nurse practitioner orientation. *Journal of Trauma Nursing, 17,* 85–101. doi:10.1097/JTN.0b013e3181e73607

Yoder-Wise, P.S., & Kowalski, K.E. (2006). *Beyond leading and managing: Nursing administration for the future.* St. Louis, MO: Elsevier Mosby.

Zwinkels, H., Roon, K., Jeurissen, F.J.F., Taphoorn, M.J.B., Hop, W.C.J., & Vecht, C.J. (2009). Management of temozolomide toxicity by nurse practitioners in neuro-oncology. *Oncology Nursing Forum, 36,* 225–231. doi:10.1188/09.ONF.225-231

CHAPTER 21

Professional Practice of Advanced Practice Nurses

Kathy Sharp, MSN, FNP-BC, AOCNP®, CCD

Introduction

This chapter presents a review of the fundamental principles that are part of advanced practice nursing. Demonstration of this knowledge, via successful completion of the advanced oncology certified nurse practitioner (AOCNP®) or the advanced oncology certified clinical nurse specialist (AOCNS®) certification examination, is an integral part of the journey to excellence in professional oncology practice (Oncology Nursing Certification Corporation [ONCC], n.d.). These principles include information on licensure, certification, scope of practice, standards, credentialing, practice regulation and reimbursement, and ethics. The information is not comprehensive and is intended to be a guide for the AOCNS and AOCNP in oncology practice.

Advanced Practice Nursing

In the *Consensus Model for APRN Regulation: Licensure, Accreditation, Certification and Education*, the National Council of State Boards of Nursing (NCSBN) APRN Advisory Committee recognized four distinct advanced practice roles: certified registered nurse anesthetist (CRNA), certified nurse midwife (CNM), clinical nurse specialist (CNS), and certified nurse practitioner (CNP). These all are under the title umbrella of advanced practice registered nurses (APRNs) (APRN Consensus Work Group & NCSBN APRN Advisory Committee, 2008). Likewise, the Oncology Nursing Society (ONS) recognized that the CNS and CNP have unique roles and areas of specialization within the oncology healthcare arena: "APRN practice in oncology nursing includes CNSs, NPs, and dually prepared (CNS and NP) nurses who are prepared at the graduate level (i.e., master's or doctorate) with a specialty focus in oncology practice" (ONS, 2015a). ONS defined each role and, through ONCC, created separate certifications for each, including AOCNP and AOCNS (ONCC, n.d.).

Regulation of Practice

APN practice is regulated at two levels: a second licensure, which is at the state level, and certification, which is through national organizations. Other factors that may influence or guide practice are credentialing and privileging, scopes of practice, and standards of practice. Agencies, such as NCSBN, also contribute to regulation of practice. In 1978, NCSBN was founded to provide a vehicle through which boards of nursing could ensure that nurses in the workforce have the skills and knowledge needed to practice, thus safeguarding the public. In the years since its inception, NCSBN also has made recommendations regarding APN practice, and in 2007 adopted a list of guiding principles regarding regulation. As of January 1, 1997, all states regulate APN practice in some manner. Eighteen states currently license APNs. Thirty-two jurisdictions grant authority to practice through certificates, recognition, registration, or similar means. In granting authority to practice beyond the RN scope of practice, boards rely on conventional authority mechanisms, including graduation from approved educational programs or certification examinations. Thirty-eight jurisdictions currently rely on national certification programs to measure competency (NCSBN, 2015a, 2015b, 2015e).

Registration

Registration is a historical term and was originally used in the early days of nursing when nurses registered with their state boards. In the present time, registration generally is synonymous with licensure. Regardless of and apart from certification requirements, all oncology APNs must be licensed in their state(s) as a registered nurse and are subject to that state's legal regulations for recognition and licensure of advanced practice nursing. Although the American Nurses Association (ANA) and ONS have defined the scope of advanced nursing practice, the state boards of nursing and federal laws are ultimately responsible for regulation (NCSBN, 2015e).

Licensure

NCSBN (2015c) defined licensure as "the process by which boards of nursing grant permission to an individual to engage in nursing practice after determining that the applicant has attained the competency necessary to perform a unique scope of practice." The licensing requirements of each state differ according to the state nurse practice act. All states require a license as an RN, and some states require second licensure as an APN. Some states use different terms for the APN (such as APRN, APNP, ARNP, etc.), so it is prudent for new APNs to investigate the board of nursing website for the state in which they will be practicing prior to graduation. Experienced APNs who may be moving to another state to practice should likewise make use of these sites to see if new requirements must be met (NCSBN, 2015c). The Advanced Practice Registered Nurse Compact, approved May 4, 2015, allows an advanced practice registered nurse to hold one multistate license with a privilege to practice in other compact states. NCSBN's compact model included proposed legislation and rules to guide state regulation of APN practice (NSCBN, 2015d). The complete document is available at www.ncsbn.org/APRN_Compact_Final_050415.pdf.

Certification

Unlike the legal scope of practice, which is defined by the laws of each state, certification is not a governmental process. Certification is regulated by a professional agency, such as ONCC. Certification is established to determine individual competence based on achievement of specific predetermined criteria. ONCC provides two advanced oncology certifications. Nurses who have the educational preparation to function in the role of CNS and meet the eligibility requirements for testing may receive certification by passing the AOCNS examination. Successful scores result in receiving the AOCNS credential. Likewise, those who are educated in an NP graduate program and meet eligibility requirements for testing may sit for the NP examination to earn the AOCNP credential. A previous credential, advanced oncology certified nurse (AOCN®), also is recognized but is available for renewal only to those who already hold this certification, as this was the original oncology advanced credential before the development of separate certifications for the CNS and NP (ONCC, n.d.).

The separate examinations came about after a role delineation study commissioned by ONCC in 2003. More than 625 APNs participated and rated tasks and knowledge in order of importance to their job. The results provided evidence that although CNSs and NPs needed much core knowledge, definite differences existed in work responsibilities. ONCC also received input about areas of professional development and education that participants desired. As a result, ONCC introduced the separate certification examinations in 2005 (ONCC, 2015).

Also worth noting is that some states grant APN licensure on the basis of national certification but do not specify the type. Generally, states are moving toward certification as a mechanism to grant an APN license. Many states do not specify which type of certification is acceptable, but not all states recognize the AOCNP or AOCNS credential. APNs must be thoroughly familiar with the rules and regulations of the state in which they plan to practice (see Table 21-1).

Credentialing and Privileging

Credentialing is one method of ensuring credibility and protecting the public (Brant & Wickham, 2013). The term is often used interchangeably with *certification* as well as *privi-*

Table 21-1. Understanding Certification Credentialing Privileging and Licensure

Term	Who Typically Confers	Scope of Practice	Requirements
Certification	National organizations	According to certifying agency	Meet education criteria (i.e., coursework, clinical hours, pass exam from national organization)
Credentialing	Healthcare institutions	Practice Prescription privileges Application for Medicare NPI (National Provider Identifier) number for reimbursement Other as defined by workplace	Meet educational criteria and obtain successful certification from recognized certifying body
Privileging	Workplace	As approved by workplace	Complete application process in workplace and be approved by medical staff
Licensure	State board	Defined by state law	Defined by state law

leging. Credentialing generally is a term that applies to institutional governing bodies, such as those that oversee hospital medical staff, managed care organizations, or insurance providers, and used by those who have the authority to decide if an APN may be included (i.e., credentialed) on their list of healthcare providers. Credentialing is a way of ensuring that the APN has met all the licensure, certification, and any other federal- or state-mandated regulations for advanced nursing practice. *Privileging* is a term that typically applies to services the APN can provide within an institution, such as a hospital, and defines the limits of APN practice. The privileges requested may change over time as the APN acquires new skills. In general terms, the APN is credentialed and then completes a list of privileges, oftentimes procedure based, which are approved by the institution (Brassard & Smolenski, 2013; Hittle, 2010).

Scope of Practice

The scope of practice of oncology APNs integrates both medical and nursing paradigms, which benefits the care of patients with cancer and their families. The oncology APN's scope of practice is defined by federal regulations, state nurse practice acts, ONS guidelines, and practice agreements with the employer. ONS has developed a statement on the scope of practice, which may serve as a guide to both new graduates and APNs with years of experience. It may be used to develop a job description and clinical collaborative practice agreement, both of which will affect the practice privileges of APNs in their particular setting. The scope of practice may be independent of or in collaboration with a physician, depending on state regulations. Variances of state law may specify physician supervision, delegation, or collaboration with APNs (Brant & Wickham, 2013; Edmunds, 2010).

Standards

Standards are authoritative statements that define responsibilities of APNs, provide direction and evaluation for APN practice, and reflect the values of advanced practice nursing in oncology. The *Statement on the Scope and Standards of Oncology Nursing Practice: Generalist and Advanced Practice*, the *Oncology Nurse Practitioner Competencies*, and the *Oncology Clinical Nurse Specialist Competencies* may serve as guides for APNs' self-evaluation and for peer or employer evaluation. Standards also may help the lay public understand the role of the APN and can provide a resource for health policy makers (Brant & Wickham, 2013; ONS, 2007, 2008).

In 1990, ONS first published the *Standards of Advanced Practice in Oncology Nursing*. This document was revised and retitled in 1997 and again in 2003. The latest publication—*Statement on the Scope and Standards of Oncology Nursing Practice*—addresses generalist and advanced practice (Brant & Wickham, 2013). The standards of care follow the nursing process: assessment, diagnosis, planning, implementation, and evaluation. The standards of professional performance relate to quality of care, self-evaluation, education, leadership ethics, multidisciplinary collaboration, and research. The oncology standards also mirror those of the American Association of Nurse Practitioners (AANP), which developed a list of standards of practice (AANP, 2013b; Brant & Wickham, 2013).

Reimbursement

Effective January 1998, the provisions of the Balanced Budget Act of 1997 expanded to include reimbursement to NPs and CNSs by authorizing them to bill Medicare directly for their services if they have a National Provider Identifier (NPI) number and are credentialed as an APNP or APRN. Reimbursement is set at 85% of the level of physician reimbursement or 80% of the actual charge, whichever is smaller. Starting in 2007, all providers were required to obtain an NPI number. This number will remain the same no matter where the provider practices. Each practice site also must obtain an NPI number, which is unique to the site. Each APN must go through the credentialing process with each individual commercial insurance company to bill for reimbursement (AANP, 2013a).

Medicare Standards for Advanced Practice Nurses

Obtaining an NPI number is the first step in being credentialed by Medicare or commercial insurance companies as a provider. The NPI is a unique 10-digit number assigned to each healthcare provider. The use of the NPI officially began in October 2006 and replaced the Medicare Provider Identification Number, the Unique Physician Identification Number, and the Medicaid Provider Number. As of May 2007, only the NPI is accepted for billing. The NPI also replaced identifying numbers that were assigned to providers by individual commercial insurers. Information and applications may be found online at https://nppes.cms.hhs.gov (Centers for Medicare and Medicaid Services [CMS], n.d.).

APNs may qualify for reimbursement under Medicare Part B if they
- Are legally authorized to provide services in the state where the service is provided
- Are licensed as an RN in the state where they practice
- Hold a master's degree or a doctor of nursing practice
- Are certified as an NP or a CNS by a national certifying body that has established standards for NPs or CNSs. (This also applies to CNMs and CRNAs; however, those roles are not pertinent to oncology.)

Services will be covered if they are medically necessary and reasonable, comparable to those provided by a medical doctor (MD) or a doctor of osteopathy (DO), furnished in collaboration with the MD or DO as required by state law, and not excluded by Medicare. As of December 2003, Medicare pays for an NP in hospice if the NP is selected as the attending provider. However, the NP is prohibited from certifying or recertifying that the patient has a terminal illness. CNSs are not eligible to serve as attending providers (CMS, 2013). Hospice NPs may conduct face-to-face encounters as described in § 20.1(5) as part of the recertification process, but documentation must attest that the findings were provided to the certifying physician (CMS, 2013, 2015a).

To enroll as a Medicare provider, individuals must complete a form provided by CMS, which can be obtained at www.cms.gov/Medicare/Provider-Enrollment-and-Certification/Medicare-ProviderSupEnroll/EnrollmentApplications.html. The information requested includes the clinician's name, date of birth, contact information, the location of the practice and address where payments are sent, the year of graduation, and the name of the collaborating or supervising physician. CMS also will request information about the location of patient medical records, practice management organization information, billing agency information, and information about any electronic claims transmissions companies that the APN may use. Any legal actions or judgments previously imposed on the APN must be reported. By signing and submitting the form, the applicant is agreeing to abide by Medicare regulation (CMS, 2014a).

APNs must employ accurate coding and documentation of services to receive reimbursement from Medicare and other insurers. *Coding* is the assignment of a numeric or alphanumeric classification to indicate the diagnosis or procedure. Level I of the Healthcare Common Procedure Coding System (HCPCS) refers to current procedural terminology (CPT) coding and is used to identify procedures, such as paracentesis, biopsy, and injections. Level II

HCPCS coding primarily is used to identify products, supplies, and services not included in CPT codes, such as durable medical equipment. The International Statistical Classification of Diseases and Related Health Problems, 10th Revision (ICD-10) is used to identify the disease or symptom that is treated and went into effect October 2014, with a compliance date of October 1, 2015 (CMS, 2015b).

According to general principles of medical record documentation set forth by Medicare (CMS, 2014b), the following information should be included with each patient encounter.
• Reason(s) for the patient's visit and relevant history, including appropriate health risks
• Physical examination findings and prior diagnostic test results
• The patient's response to previous interventions
• Assessment and diagnosis
• Plan of care, including written or inferred rationale for diagnostic or other services
• Date and identity of provider
• Documentation to substantiate the CPT and ICD-10 codes that were reported and billed.
   Visit www.cms.gov/Medicare/Coding/icd10 for more information about ICD-10

Nurse Practitioner Versus Clinical Nurse Specialist Role in Advanced Practice

Delineation and Recognition

In an environment where NP and CNS roles increasingly are being blended under the title of APN, ONS took a firm stance that each of the roles remain separate and distinct entities with unique domains of practice, based on the 2003 role delineation study, which revealed discernable differences in the work responsibilities of NPs and CNSs in oncology. In 2006, ONS further solidified the distinction of each role by dividing the previous certification test with the credential AOCN® into two separate examinations, one for NPs and one for CNSs. Although the AOCN examination has been eliminated as of 2008, people who have received AOCN certification in the past may continue to maintain that title through continuing education (ONCC, n.d., 2015).

Scope of Practice Comparison

ONS identified five functional roles for the APN: direct care provider or caregiver, administrator/coordinator, consultant, researcher, and educator. Although NPs and CNSs are both recognized as clinical experts, ONS states that the domain of care, the scope of practice, and the spheres of influence distinguish the NP and CNS roles (ONS, 2007, 2008, 2015a).

CNSs' scope of practice includes providing clinical expertise in cancer care, assisting patients and families with symptom and palliative care needs, and serving as a patient advocate. CNSs participate in staff and healthcare team development via education, role modeling, and dissemination of research findings. NPs' scope of practice comprises comprehensive health assessments; diagnosis (including ordering, supervising, and interpreting diagnostic tests); prescribing pharmacologic and nonpharmacologic treatments; and screening to prevent illness and promote wellness (ONS, 2007, 2008, 2015a).

Competencies

CNS competencies are based on three spheres of influence (see Table 21-2). These are the patient/client sphere, the nurse/nursing sphere, and the organization/system sphere. The

Table 21-2. Clinical Nurse Specialist Competencies

Sphere of Influence	Competency	Description
Patient/client	Health assessment Diagnosis of health status and plan of care Intervention Evaluation	Knowledge and skills are used to assess, diagnose, and manage illness and risk behaviors in patients with a past, current, or potential diagnosis of cancer and improve nursing-sensitive outcomes.
Nurse/nursing practice	Assessment/definition of problems Diagnosis, outcome identification, and plan of care Intervention Evaluation Professional role	Nursing practice is advanced and nursing-sensitive patient outcomes are improved by updating and improving norms and standards of oncology nursing practice.
Organization/ system	Assessment Diagnosis, outcome identification, and plan of care Intervention Evaluation	Competencies in this sphere advocate for professional nursing; provide skills, leadership, knowledge, and behaviors to influence changes at the system level; and improve quality, cost-effective outcomes.

Note. Based on information from Oncology Nursing Society, 2008.

patient/client sphere includes demonstration of quality patient outcomes through assessment and intervention by CNSs. The nurse/nursing sphere acknowledges the contributions of CNSs to nurses and nursing through their leadership and staff development activities, including the creation of evidence-based policies, procedures, and protocols. The organizational/system sphere recognizes CNSs' contributions to health care via informational, educational, and other activities that involve healthcare team members, communities, and healthcare systems. The ONS CNS core competencies are available at www.ons.org/sites/default/files/cnscomps .pdf (ONS, 2008).

NP competencies are divided into seven parts that represent the core knowledge required for entry into practice as an oncology NP (see Table 21-3). These are health promotion, protection, and disease prevention; the nurse-patient relationship; teaching/coaching; professional role; healthcare delivery systems; monitoring and ensuring quality healthcare practice; and caring for diverse populations. Oncology NPs are recognized as clinical experts and provide direct, episodic health care to patients with cancer, including management of acute and chronic problems, symptom management, and palliative care. NPs influence the patients' family members, other healthcare providers, nursing staff, hospital and other healthcare systems, and the community through direct and indirect interaction; individual, group, and community education; and legislative and political activism. The ONS NP competencies are available at www.ons.org/sites/default/files/npcompentencies.pdf (ONS, 2007).

Professional Responsibilities

Healthcare Legislation

ONS standards and competencies state that oncology APNs participate in activities that enhance practice, and the arena of healthcare legislation provides multiple opportunities for

Table 21-3. Nurse Practitioner Competencies

Standard	Competency
Health promotion, health protection, disease prevention and treatment	Assesses all aspects of patient health, including those for health promotion, health protection, and disease prevention; uses evidence-based clinical practice guidelines to guide screening, health promotion, and counseling.
Nurse practitioner–patient relationship	Demonstrates personal, collaborative, and therapeutic approaches to patient care.
Teaching-coaching function	Includes functions such as imparting knowledge to the patient for self-care; coaching involves advocacy, support, and reinforcement.
Professional role	Demonstrates a commitment to the implementation, preservation, and evolution of the oncology nurse practitioner role.
Negotiating healthcare delivery systems	Oversees and directs the delivery of clinical services within the healthcare system.
Monitoring and ensuring quality of healthcare practice	Ensures quality of care via consultation, collaboration, continuing education, certification, and evaluation; engages in interdisciplinary peer and systems review.
Caring for diverse populations	Involves provision of culturally competent care with respect to cultural and spiritual beliefs and making healthcare resources available for people from diverse cultures.

Note. Based on information from Oncology Nursing Society, 2007.

such participation. APNs should be aware of and promote passage of legislation supporting cancer care and should serve as a liaison to legislative bodies and individuals regarding issues related to oncology nursing and advanced oncology nursing practice. Oncology APNs may be involved in healthcare legislation by serving as a resource or researcher for specific healthcare issues, especially those involving cancer care. Simply corresponding with policy makers regarding current legislation and providing factual information from the viewpoint of the APN oftentimes can make a positive impact on critical issues (ONS, 2007, 2008, 2015a).

Continuous Quality Improvement

Continuous quality improvement (CQI) may be known by other names, such as quality improvement (QI), quality assurance (QA), or quality improvement process, although some fundamental differences exist in each. The word *continuous* implies an ongoing or constant course of action, unlike QA, which may involve a retrospective review of an event or procedure. The CQI process in a facility such as a hospital usually entails people from different but interactive areas coming together to review a systems process. The end result usually is focused on improving patient care or cost-saving measures and generally is more process oriented than individual oriented. The ONS CNS competencies outline opportunities for CQI participation within the organization/system sphere (ONS, 2008).

CQI for the APN is a multifaceted process involving self-evaluation, patient evaluation, peer evaluation, systems evaluation, and the use and promotion of evidence-based practice (EBP). The ONS standards of professional performance outline the APN's obligation to be engaged in each level of CQI (ONS, 2007).

Self-evaluation can be achieved by seeking feedback from patients, professional colleagues, members of the healthcare team, and employers and by modifying practice in response to their evaluation. Attainment of professional learning or performance goals can be other measurable self-improvement tools. Finally, a comparison of patient treatment plans to nationally established guidelines may provide valuable feedback for APNs' self-evaluation of performance (i.e., benchmarking) (ONS, 2007, 2008).

Patient evaluation is a continuous process that includes complete patient assessment, diagnosis, planning, and review of response to the treatment plan. Measuring patient outcomes and modifying plans according to research and benchmarks also are part of patient evaluation and the CQI process (ONS, 2007, 2008).

Several agencies monitor, recommend, and publish standards for healthcare quality. Some of these, along with their mission, are listed in Table 21-4.

Evidence-Based Practice

EBP uses the most current evidence to make decisions regarding the care of patients. This requires performing ongoing evaluation of findings from well-designed research or designing

Table 21-4. Missions of Agencies Dedicated to Healthcare Quality

Agency	Mission
Agency for Healthcare Research and Quality	Agency that supports research designed to improve healthcare quality, decrease cost, and create more access to essential services. www.ahrq.gov
Institute for Healthcare Improvement	Independent, nonprofit organization dedicated to accelerating healthcare system improvement. www.ihi.org
Institute for Safe Medication Practices	Nonprofit organization with the mission of providing education for healthcare professionals and consumers regarding safe practices for medications. http://ismp.org
Joint Commission	Agency that provides accreditation for hospitals, managed care entities, and healthcare facilities. Its mission is improved safety and quality of care. www.jointcommission.org
National Association for Healthcare Quality	Organization that supports education and knowledge acquisition for healthcare quality professionals; publishes the *Journal for Healthcare Quality*. www.nahq.org
National Committee for Quality Assurance	Independent, nonprofit organization whose twofold mission is to improve the quality of health care delivered to consumers and to educate the public to make more informed decisions. www.ncqa.org
National Quality Forum	Organization that published a report identifying 19 measurable standards for assessing the quality of cancer care in breast and colorectal cancer, symptom management, and end-of-life care. www.qualityforum.org/Publications/2009/05/National_Voluntary_Consensus _Standards_for_Quality_of_Cancer_Care.aspx

and conducting research to supplement evidence that is missing. The ONS NP and CNS competencies mandate use of current evidence for decision making and evaluation by APNs.

ONS has created the Putting Evidence Into Practice (PEP) resources www.ons.org/practice-resources/pep to assist oncology nurses in identifying, appraising, and using evidence. ONS (2015b) has categorized evidence into seven levels:

- Recommended for Practice
- Likely to Be Effective
- Benefits Balanced With Harm
- Effectiveness Not Established
- Effectiveness Unlikely
- Not Recommended for Practice
- Expert Opinion.

Several online resources are available for APNs to access nationally recognized guidelines (see Figure 21-1). Each of the organizations is committed to quality cancer care and all include participation by experts in oncology.

Community Involvement

APNs are in a unique position to support improvement in cancer care through involvement in national organizations focused on cancer, cancer research, or advanced oncology practice. Examples include the American Cancer Society (ACS), ONS, or any of the specialty organizations such as Susan G. Komen (www.komen.org), the Leukemia and Lymphoma Society (www.leukemia-lymphoma.org), or the Livestrong Foundation (www.livestrong.org). Involvement may take the form of acting as a resource for factual information or offering to serve on local, community, or national boards.

Media

The media is a great conduit for the distribution of information. By fostering a relationship with local or national media personalities, APNs can open the door of opportunity for disseminating education to the public. That education may be about a disease process, APN practice, or healthcare legislative concerns. Media-savvy APNs have the opportunity to affect public policy and policy makers, as well as heighten awareness of the importance of the APN role. Resources may be found on the Media Center page of the ONS website (www.ons.org/newsroom/media-center).

Research

Standard IX of the standards of professional performance in the *Statement on the Scope and Standards of Oncology Nursing Practice: Generalist and Advanced Practice* (Brant & Wickham, 2013) outlines oncology APNs' involvement in research. An important research obligation of

---

Agency for Healthcare Research and Quality: www.ahrq.gov
American Society of Clinical Oncology: www.asco.org
National Comprehensive Cancer Network: www.nccn.org
Oncology Nursing Society: www.ons.org/practice-resources/pep

Figure 21-1. Resources for Oncology Evidence-Based Guidelines

APNs is the dissemination of research to others. This involves ongoing review and analysis of current research reported in the literature, which requires understanding of research design, statistical data analysis, and application of research findings. Notable findings then may be translated into practice through staff education or changing of policies and procedures (Brant & Wickham, 2013).

APNs also may be directly involved in performing research through participation in nationally sponsored clinical trials. If so, some of their responsibilities may include enrollment of patients, collection of data, education of participants and their families or significant others, and observation of participants for side effects or response to treatment.

Ethics

The Merriam-Webster online dictionary defines *ethics* as a set of principles or values of good or right behavior or as a standard of conduct made by members of a profession ("Ethics," n.d.). Ethical dilemmas exist when a situation requires a choice about right behavior or conduct between two equal and opposing alternatives. With each patient encounter, APNs incorporate ethical principles and values into their practice. For the purposes of this chapter, principles and values are identified as separate elements, but much overlap exists. Regardless, they should be used as a guide for individual oncology APN practice. The Ethics and Compliance Initiative defines values as "the core beliefs we hold regarding what is right and fair in terms of our actions and our interactions with others" (Ethics and Compliance Initiative, 2009b). A *principle,* as defined by an online dictionary, is a basic truth, law, or code of conduct ("Principle," n.d.).

A majority of the time, these principles are such a fundamental part of APN behavior and patient interaction that they are not readily identified as entities unto themselves. However, to understand their importance as an integral part of professional practice, it is necessary to identify and define each principle and value and to understand their specific meaning.

Ethical Principles

Four basic ethical principles exist, although some authors may include more. These are autonomy, beneficence, nonmaleficence, and justice (ANA, 2011).

Autonomy describes patients' ability to self-rule and make decisions regarding their care. Each patient has a right to self-determination, including the ability to choose among medically indicated treatments as well as to refuse any unwanted treatments. This principle is the moral basis for obtaining informed consent and accepting informed refusal. Autonomy also is a trait ascribed to the APN, and the development of autonomy is essential to successful role implementation (ANA, 2011).

Beneficence simply means doing good. Some people may confuse doing good with the intent to do good. All interactions with patients should be based on the intent toward the patient. For instance, chemotherapy is known to have many harmful, painful, or even life-threatening complications; thus, giving chemotherapy might not be considered beneficial in the eyes of some. Although APNs know chemotherapy has negative side effects, it is intended to help rid the patient of cancer cells. The key here is the intent to act in the best interest of the patient while not forgetting that patients have the autonomy to decide what is good for themselves. APNs should not allow internal conflicts to arise because of a paternalistic ideation toward the patient (i.e., deciding what is best for the patient) (ANA, 2011).

Nonmaleficence means to do no harm. This principle has its origins in the Hippocratic oath and commands that APNs do not cause injury to patients. This term also includes the implication to individually evaluate anticipated treatments to ensure that the potential harm or negative side effects do not outweigh the anticipated benefit (ANA, 2011).

Justice is the duty to be fair in all interactions and also applies to the allocation of sometimes-meager resources. Institutional or insurance allocation policies may define the benefits dispensed to each person, thus affecting oncology APNs' just actions to patients. Justice implies that each person will receive what he or she is due. Often, justice is based on need, but in the arena of scarce personnel and fiscal resources, justice often is based on the distribution of what is available (ANA, 2011).

Ethical Values

In addition to ethical principles, APNs use ethical values, including confidentiality, fidelity, compassion, integrity, and veracity, in their professional practice. These ethical values are not unique to oncology practice but should be an integral part of oncology care.

Confidentiality is the respect for patients' private information. The term applies to information shared with the healthcare provider in one-to-one interactions and to information contained in patients' records. Healthcare Insurance Portability and Accountability Act (HIPAA) regulations spell out how patients' personal information must be handled in order to provide the optimum security. HIPAA laws allow patients to designate which family members, friends, or others may be privy to information contained in their medical record. According to these laws, patients also may specify how agencies, such as a hospital billing department, may use or share information. If patient permission is not obtained, only what is necessary for continuity of care may be shared (U.S. Department of Health and Human Services, 2003).

Fidelity is the obligation to keep one's promise and commitments, both to others and to oneself. Patients expect APNs to be meticulous in their follow-through and depend on APNs' conscientious attention to detail. Fidelity is a value that supports patients' trust and confidence. Time spent advocating for patients with insurance companies and championing healthcare issues are examples of fidelity in action (ANA, 2011; Ethics and Compliance Initiative, 2009a).

Compassion is a deep awareness of the patient's situation and suffering and is accompanied by a desire to act in a kind and helpful manner. Sister Simone Roach stated that the philosophy of caring (which includes compassion) guides interactions with patients, families, and communities and is the very essence of nursing (Hagedorn & Quinn, 2004). According to Schantz (2007), compassion impels and empowers people to not just acknowledge, but also to act. *Caring*, often used interchangeably with *compassion*, drives nurses to develop relationships with patients, evoking trust and compelling behaviors to improve the physical, spiritual, and psychological state of patients (ANA, 2011; Lachman, 2012).

Integrity refers to individuals being true to and adhering to a moral set of values, with honesty being among those values. Integrity and veracity overlap to some degree. *Veracity* refers to the duty or obligation to be truthful and honest with patients. Although it is known that honesty includes telling the truth, honesty also includes avoiding deception, misrepresentation, and nondisclosure unless the patient indicates a desire to not know certain information. Integrity demands that the patient's informed request to not know certain information must be honored, even if this causes conflict with the oncology APN's sense of values (ANA, 2011; Ethics and Compliance Initiative, 2009b).

Informed Consent

Informed consent requires effective communication and represents a joint venture between the patient and the healthcare professional. It is not just an episodic event but rather a continuous process of information exchange. Informed consent includes disclosure, adequate patient understanding, voluntariness, competence, and recognition of barriers to informed consent. APNs need to recognize that patients have the right to refuse or withdraw consent at any time (U.S. Department of Health and Human Services, n.d.).

Disclosure is an explanation of the procedure, treatment, or other intervention intended for the patient. Complete disclosure includes all the positive and negative effects associated with the intervention, and it is clearly presented in language that is educationally appropriate for the patient. It also includes the potential outcome without the intended treatment (Hall, Prochazka, & Fink, 2012).

The patient's understanding may depend on many factors, including the type of disclosure, the surroundings in which the disclosure takes place, the stress of the individual hearing or presenting of information, the presence of pain or anxiety, the proper education level of the information being presented, and the presence or absence of other individuals, such as family members or additional members of the healthcare team. The presenter must evaluate whether the patient's understanding is adequate. One effective method of doing this is to have the patient repeat back a summary of what was explained. A signed consent is not always an informed consent. *Voluntariness* refers to the willingness of the patient to give consent without coercion.

Competence should not be confused with capacity when referring to the patient's ability to make decisions. *Competence* is a legal term that refers to one's mental ability to understand the information presented and make decisions after weighing the pros and cons of a situation. *Capacity* is only the ability to make a decision and is not necessarily based on competent, rational thought. For instance, a patient with Alzheimer dementia has the capacity to make a decision but not the cognitive prowess to make a competent decision. Decision-making capacity is determined by the person's ability to understand the diagnosis and treatment; to deliberate and weigh options, risks, and benefits; and to communicate a choice to another person. Decision making also is influenced by personal belief systems, societal norms, and the belief systems of family and friends. A person may make a poor decision, but that does not indicate that the person is not competent.

Oncology APNs should be mindful that barriers and exceptions to informed consent exist. Language can be a barrier if the patient and the informer do not speak the same language or if the patient has difficulty understanding or comprehending the informer's language because of education level or because of physical or psychological trauma or illness, such as receptive aphasia. Alterations in level of consciousness from sedation or effects of illness or pain also can be a temporary or permanent barrier. Although often not identified as a barrier, presenting information in a way that implies a bias by the informer can hamper informed consent.

Exceptions for informed consent include emergency situations or the inability to give informed consent because of the presence of mind-altering substances, such as alcohol or drugs. Patients also may waive consent and authorize others to receive information.

Do-Not-Resuscitate Orders

Do-not-resuscitate (DNR) orders also may be known as "no code," "no CPR" (cardiopulmonary resuscitation), or the newer term "DNAR" (do not attempt resuscitation). ANA (2012) recommends that the DNR decision should be explicitly discussed by patients, family members, and the healthcare team. A designated surrogate or durable power of attorney also should be included in the absence of family or if patients are unable to act in their own best interests. Having family members present during these discussions may avoid problems in the future.

When spouses/family are not present for these discussions and do not agree with the outcome of the decision on code status, significant distress may result for all.

Healthcare providers must be careful to differentiate that "no code" does not mean "no care," as many patients and families often believe. It can present a barrier for patients in making a good decision. Patients who are DNR can receive full and aggressive care. Furthermore, it is not a requirement for patients admitted to hospice to have a DNR order.

In many states, the MD alone may decide if the patient is a DNR, but this often does not promote satisfaction with care on the part of families or patients and is not a recommended practice. It is advisable for APNs to check the statutes of the state in which they practice if there are questions about this issue. DNR orders should be clearly documented in the patient's record and should not contain implications regarding withdrawal of care. It is a good idea to document who was present for the DNR discussion (ACS, 2015b; ANA, 2012).

Patient Self-Determination Act

The Patient Self-Determination Act became federal law in 1991 and requires healthcare agencies to inform patients about advance directives upon admission. It does not require that patients complete advance directives, only that they are aware of their right to make decisions about these issues (ACS, 2015b; ANA, 2012).

Advance Directives

Advance directives are mechanisms that provide a way for patients to make their wishes regarding health care known in the event that they lose their decision-making capability. Advance directives may include a legal power of attorney, a durable power of attorney for health care, and a living will. APNs are in a unique position to serve as patient advocates by educating patients who do not understand advance directives (ACS 2015b; National Cancer Institute, 2015). Advance directive forms may vary by state. Forms for each state are available by following the "Advance Care Planning" link on the Caring Connections website at www.caringinfo.org (see Table 21-5).

Durable Power of Attorney for Health Care

A legal power of attorney also may be called a *durable power of attorney*, which can cause confusion. No matter what the name, a legal power of attorney or durable power of attorney

Table 21-5. Types of Advance Directives

Advance Directive	Description
Durable power of attorney for health care; may also be called a healthcare proxy or healthcare surrogate	A legal document giving a specific individual the authority to make healthcare decisions if the patient is incapable of making his or her wishes known
Living will	Written document that specifies what types of medical treatment the individual desires
Legal power of attorney; may also be called a durable power of attorney	A legal document designating a specific individual to act for the patient in financial/legal matters such as making bank transactions and signing checks and legal documents for the patient

should not be confused with a *durable power of attorney for health care*. The durable power of attorney for health care also may be known as a *healthcare surrogate* or *healthcare proxy*. By contrast, the legal power of attorney for finance is a signed and notarized legal document giving an individual, who is appointed by the patient, the authority to conduct the patient's business affairs. In some states, in the absence of a durable power of attorney for health care, the legal power of attorney may also make healthcare decisions for the patient if the patient becomes unable to make these decisions and has no next of kin. The individual who is appointed by the patient as the durable power of attorney for health care is authorized to make healthcare decisions for the patient if the patient becomes incapable of doing so. The durable power of attorney for health care does not have any authority for legal transactions; this person's job is limited to healthcare decision making. The durable power of attorney for health care is a legal document, and although it does not have to be notarized, it must be witnessed, and notarization is recommended. Notarization is a legal verification that the patient was of a competent mind when the document was signed and that the document was not coerced in any way. A copy of this document should be given to the patient's healthcare provider and to the healthcare facility where the patient may be treated. The patient should keep the original document (ACS, 2015a). In comparison, the legal power of attorney document must be notarized to be considered authorized.

Each state may use slightly different forms. Visit http://uslwr.com/formslist.shtm to see the forms for each state (see Table 21-6).

Living Will

A living will is a document written while the patient is competent to make decisions. It may include the patient's preferences about life-prolonging procedures and equipment and whether to withhold treatments. A living will usually specifies the extent of resuscita-

Table 21-6. Advance Directive Specifics

Document	Spokesperson	Cost If Done Without Attorney	Notary/ Witness	Legal Assistance Required	Activation Required to Use	Governs
Durable power of attorney (POA) for finance	POA(s)	No	Notary	No	No	Finances
Durable POA for health care	POA(s)	No	Witness	No	Yes	Health care
Living will	MD	No	Witness	No	Yes	Health care
Five Wishes®	MD	No	Witness; notary in some states	No	Yes	Health care
Guardianship	Court-appointed guardian	Yes	Court	Yes	No	Health care and finances

tion efforts and what is included, such as whether to administer defibrillation, CPR, artificial respiration via a ventilator, and so on. A living will may be as specific as the patient desires. Forms are readily available at all healthcare facilities and on the Internet (e.g., the U.S. Living Will Registry at www.uslivingwillregistry.com). Living wills also can be initiated through an attorney. Although a living will can be a list of handwritten directions by the patient, a typed and notarized document indicating that the patient was competent at the time the document was written is preferable. As with the durable power of attorney for health care, a copy of this document should be given to and discussed with the patient's healthcare providers. A copy should also be filed at the patient's healthcare facility of choice. The patient will keep the original document. Patients have the right to rescind or verbally revise their living will at any time. A written living will never overrides the desires of a competent patient (ACS, 2015a).

Ethical Controversies

Terminating or Withholding Treatment

The decision to terminate or withhold treatment should be directed by the patient if he or she is competent to do so. In the absence of the patient's competence, the patient's advance directive will provide direction. If no advance directive exists, the next of kin will be placed in the position of making decisions about treatment based on information provided by the healthcare provider. In cases of conflict about decisions, or if no one is available to make decisions for the patient or if a skilled nursing facility admission is imminent in some states, a court-appointed guardian will make decisions for the patient. APNs can rely on a number of resources to assist in this process. Ethical guidance may be found in the *Code of Ethics for Nurses* from ANA (2015), as well as multiple online resources (see Table 21-7). Most hospitals also have ethics committees and ethical experts who can provide consultation for families and healthcare providers. Ethical standards for APNs can be found on the ANA website (www.nursingworld.org), in the ONS *Statement on the Scope and Standards of Oncology Nursing Practice* (Brant & Wickham, 2013), and on the ONS website (www.ons.org).

Euthanasia

The word *euthanasia* means "gentle and easy death" or "good death." It often has been called "mercy killing." Generally, it means putting to death someone who is suffering from a painful or prolonged illness or injury. The difference between euthanasia and patient-assisted suicide is patient involvement. Euthanasia actively involves someone other than the patient. Euthanasia may take three forms:
- Voluntary—with the consent of the patient
- Involuntary—without the consent of the patient
- Nonvoluntary—in cases where the patient is incapacitated or unable to choose.

Euthanasia differs from the act of withholding life-sustaining treatment. If life-sustaining treatment is withheld, death occurs as the result of the disease. With euthanasia, death is caused by the physician, another healthcare provider, or another person. Voluntary and physician-assisted suicide are alike in that both involve patient choice. Euthanasia is equivalent to homicide in the eyes of the legal system and is illegal in the United States (ANA, 2013).

Table 21-7. Ethics Resources

Organization	Resource
American Nurses Association	*Code of Ethics for Nurses*: www.nursingworld.org/MainMenuCategories/Ethics Standards/CodeofEthicsforNurses End-of-life issues: www.nursingworld.org/MainMenuCategories/EthicsStandards/End-of-Life *Euthanasia, Assisted Suicide, and Aid in Dying* position statement: www.nursing world.org/MainMenuCategories/EthicsStandards/Ethics-Position-Statements/Euthanasia-Assisted-Suicide-and-Aid-in-Dying.pdf *Nursing Care and Do Not Resuscitate (DNR) and Allow Natural Death (AND) Decisions*: www.nursingworld.org/MainMenuCategories/EthicsStandards/Ethics-Position-Statements/Nursing-Care-and-Do-Not-Resuscitate-DNR-and-Allow-Natural-Death-Decisions.pdf
Ethics and Compliance Initiative	www.ethics.org
Kennedy Institute of Ethics	https://kennedyinstitute.georgetown.edu
National Hospice and Palliative Care Organization	www.nhpco.org
Oncology Nursing Society	Ethical standards in the *Statement on the Scope and Standards of Oncology Nursing Practice: Generalist and Advanced Practice* (Brant & Wickham, 2013) *Role of the Nurse When Hastened Death Is Requested (Endorsed Position Statement, Hospice and Palliative Nurses Association)*: www.ons.org/advocacy-policy/positions/ethics/hastened-death

Healthcare Professional–Assisted Suicide

Assisted suicide is any act that entails making a means of suicide available to a patient with knowledge of the patient's intention. Assisted suicide has been intensely debated in recent years, and physician-assisted suicide has been legalized in Oregon, Washington, Vermont, and Montana (ProCon.org, 2014). Oncology APNs and other nurses are prohibited from participation in assisted suicide/euthanasia because it is a violation of the Code of Ethics. Nurses should refrain from using judgmental language in the presence of the patient, family, significant others, and professional colleagues if assisted suicide is requested (ANA, 2013; ONS, 2011). Most workplaces have policies on this issue as well.

Another subject that lies in the gray area between euthanasia/assisted suicide and terminal comfort measures is the term *double effect*. This is defined as the administration of medications to alleviate or suppress pain, which, when given to terminal patients, may indirectly shorten their lives. These medications are not given with the intent to hasten or cause death but may result in death. This subject has been debated in the literature and in the media; therefore, APNs, especially those employed in oncology and hospice, should be well versed in this issue (Allmark, Cobb, Liddle, & Tod, 2010; United States Conference of Catholic Bishops, 2009).

Access to Care

Access to health care has been on the political forefront for many years, and the public regards unequal access to health care as a social injustice. APNs have been given credit for providing health care to rural areas that traditionally have been underserved. Unfortunately, APNs, because of a variety of barriers, may find themselves placed in a position where they cannot provide care because of financial reimbursement issues or restrictions from third-party payers. State scope-of-practice barriers, physician supervision issues, and prescriptive authority limitations also play a part in access-to-care difficulties for patients. All APNs must be cognizant of state regulations and the presence of access-to-care barriers in the state in which they are employed, as well as in bordering states if appropriate (Brant & Wickham, 2013; ONS, 2015a).

Access to hospice care is another end-of-life issue that oncology APNs may encounter. Issues such as insurance coverage, the legal inability of APNs to certify patients for hospice, narrow definitions of eligibility criteria, limitations of hospice care, and discontinuation of hospice have the potential to create barriers and ethical dilemmas for patients and APNs (Bouton, 2005).

Ethical Decision Making

Many models exist to guide or assist in the ethical decision-making process, each with a variety of steps or phases. Most, however, are expanded versions of the nursing process.

The first step is recognition of an ethical dilemma or problem and the need for intervention. Ideally, early recognition and intervention minimizes the severity of the issue (Cohen & Erickson, 2006; Resnick, 2011).

The second step is to gather relevant information and facts. This stage may include identification of key players. Obviously, the physician or physicians, the oncology APN, and the patient are all primary participants. The patient's family and/or significant others, the primary nurse or nurses, and a durable power of attorney for health care may be members of the discussion group as well (Cohen & Erickson, 2006; Resnick, 2011).

Third, a thorough assessment of the problem is required, which includes identification and clarification of the ethical principles and values at stake and a clarification of each key player's viewpoint of the situation. Although input from all affected parties is important, the patient's and/or power of attorney's values and thoughts take top priority. It is important for new oncology APNs to be self-aware regarding ethical dilemmas. Sometimes the dilemma is the oncology APN's response to moral distress. Because the response to conflict is highly individualized, it is always wise to openly discuss the perceived dilemma with peers, other team members, or more experienced colleagues to help to separate individual distress from an actual ethical dilemma involving the patient. APNs also must note that conflicts or dilemmas exist on numerous levels and may involve nurses, other healthcare providers, pastoral care, hospital administration, patients, family members, and significant others (Cohen & Erickson, 2006).

Once the conflict is assessed and connected to an ethical value violation, a range of options for resolution are proposed and discussed. At this point, options are only being discussed. If deliberations by all parties do not result in a reasonable set of options, an ethics consult may be needed. Most hospitals have an ethics committee and an ethics consultant available to assist in problem resolution. Ethics committees may comprise people with special training and interest in bioethics, seasoned clinicians with expert decision-making and leadership skills, and people with expertise in conflict mediation. A well-balanced ethics committee contains a mix of people from a wide variety of healthcare and other backgrounds, as well as community members who have been invited because of excellent communication or management skills (McLennon, Uhrich, Lasiter, Chamness, & Helft, 2013; Resnick, 2011). Ideally, an ethics consultant is available 24 hours a day, seven days a week for crisis situations; however, a formal ethics committee usually will handle decision making for the majority of ethical dilemmas. A study by Jansky, Marx, Nauck, and Alt-Epping (2013) explored expectations and attitudes regarding ethics consultation. The study results suggested that past experiences in dealing with ethical conflicts might reflect preexisting patterns of interprofessional communication. The study revealed differences in how physicians and nurses rated ethical conflicts and indicated that staff tended to discuss issues with peers.

Steps five and six are synchronous, with the selection of an option and presentation of reasons to support the choice usually occurring in concert. Again, this step may involve the assistance of ethical experts to facilitate selection. Finally, as with any problem intervention, the outcome must be evaluated. Questions for review may include the following (Cohen & Erickson, 2006; Resnick, 2011): Are all the involved parties satisfied with the resolution? Could this dilemma have been avoided, and if so, how? Will this intervention require ongoing intervention, as well as evaluation and follow-up? For resources regarding ethics, refer to Table 21-7.

Conclusion

The professional roles, responsibilities, and ethical issues are integral to oncology APNs' practice. Oncology APNs must be thoroughly familiar with these concepts and resources if they are to successfully apply them to their practice. The implications of using these concepts will benefit patients as well as oncology APNs.

Case Study

M.S. is a 70-year-old woman admitted for febrile neutropenia after one cycle of carboplatin and paclitaxel for stage IV ovarian cancer. The patient had febrile-induced delirium on admission, which resolved as the fever abated. Prior to her diagnosis of ovarian cancer, M.S. was in fair health with controlled hypertension. Her daughter had mentioned that M.S. was experiencing some forgetfulness, and the oncology APN noted this in the medical record as questionable early-stage Alzheimer disease. Despite the severity of her response to the first cycle, M.S. expressed her desire to her daytime nurse to continue chemotherapy. M.S. was not asked about advance directives on admission because of her confused mental state; however, her daughter reported that she is her mother's durable power of attorney for health care. Once the fever resolved and her mental status cleared, M.S. verified that her daughter was indeed her durable power of attorney for health care and denied having any other advance directives. The daughter is an only child and has no other close relatives for emotional support. The daughter wants her mother to discontinue treatment and does not feel that her mother is competent to make decisions regarding her health care, so her advance directive for health care has been activated. The staff caring for M.S. are divided in their opinions about her continuing therapy. They have expressed their views only to each other and the oncology APN, not to the patient or her daughter.

1. How can the oncology APN intervene to assist the patient, the family, and the healthcare providers?
   • Using the steps of the ethical decision-making process, the APN
     – Identifies the problem: Conflict between the patient and her daughter
     – Gathers information. (This step may initiate more questions.)
       * The daughter and the physician are questioning the patient's competency. The APN would discern if M.S. might be making competent but poor decisions versus incompetent decisions.

* The patient is in reasonable health, but can she physically tolerate more chemotherapy? What is her performance status? What is potential response rate of chemotherapy? What are M.S.'s goals of care?
* What is the likelihood of a repeat episode of febrile neutropenia?
- The nurses are divided in their opinions and have expressed their opinions.

2. What ethical principles and values are implicated in this situation?
   - M.S.'s autonomy is paramount in this case. She has the right to self-determination despite her daughter's status as durable power of attorney for health care as long as she has been apprised of all the pros and cons of continuing treatment.
   - From the standpoint of the healthcare providers, the principles of nonmaleficence, beneficence, and justice are all important in this situation. The healthcare providers do not want to cause harm to the patient with chemotherapy, but at the same time they realize that ultimately chemotherapy may be good by treating M.S.'s cancer. They realize that their decisions must be fair for all people involved.
   - As part of the information-gathering process, the oncology APN talks privately with M.S. and then her daughter to glean an understanding of why each person is approaching the situation in her particular manner. The oncology APN also meets with the staff to gather their input. The oncology APN realizes from her conversations that M.S. wants treatment because she believes it will improve her chances of survival. Conversely, her daughter believes that her mother may die quicker from the side effects of chemotherapy than she would from the cancer. She is also concerned that further chemotherapy will destroy her mother's quality of life. The oncology APN also realizes that M.S.'s daughter is frightened of being alone because she has no other living relatives and no emotional support. She also realizes that the daughter may be having difficulty with the new role of caregiver to her mother.

3. At this point, how could the APN further utilize the steps in the ethical decision-making process for successful resolution of the situation?
   - Identify options: The APN identifies the following needs and interventions.
     - The patient's goals and performance status
     - Emotional support for the daughter (i.e., community support group, counseling by a trained professional)
     - Education both for M.S. and her daughter and for the hospital staff regarding National Comprehensive Cancer Network clinical practice guidelines for ovarian cancer, survivorship statistics for patients with ovarian cancer, incidence of febrile neutropenia, and chemotherapy-induced side effects. The APN uses her knowledge of learning theory to assess the learning ability of all the parties and how to present the material to each.
     - Through evidence, the oncology APN identifies that an increased risk of febrile neutropenia exists with the current treatment of carboplatin and paclitaxel; however, this may be treated with a colony-stimulating factor such as pegfilgrastim.
     - Discussion with M.S.'s primary care physician and oncologist regarding the question of mental competency
   - Make a choice: After discussions with the primary care physician and the oncologist and evaluation of M.S.'s mental status and decision-making capability, all the providers believe M.S. to be quite capable of making an autonomous decision. Following the oncology APN's educational interventions and demonstrations of active listening and compassion, M.S.'s daughter begins to recognize and understand her fears. She also feels hopeful that the colony-stimulating factor will decrease the likelihood of a repeat episode of febrile neutropenia. M.S. and her daughter also understand that ovarian cancer is more of a chronic disease with remissions and relapses, and both decide that treatment really is the best option. The APN also educated the staff and facilitated open discussion of their feelings regarding the situation.

- Identify reasons to support choices: The oncology APN's excellent oncology education, as well as her knowledge of research findings, has helped to resolve this situation and avert a potentially difficult ethical dilemma.
- Evaluate outcomes and need for further follow-up: The oncology APN is aware that continued evaluation of this situation is needed. If the patient develops febrile neutropenia again, further discussions with the patient and her daughter, as well as with the rest of the healthcare team, will be necessary.

Key Points

- Oncology APNs should be familiar with
  - Licensing, registration, and certification requirements and scope of practice of the state in which they practice
  - Content in the *Statement on the Scope and Standards of Oncology Nursing Practice: Generalist and Advanced Practice* (Brant & Wickham, 2013)
  - The application of EBP guidelines
  - The ethical principles and values that are used every day to guide interactions with patients, families, healthcare providers, healthcare agencies, suppliers, insurers, and others who may be involved in the provision of patient care
  - The ethical issues and purpose of DNR orders, informed consent, patient self-determination, and advance directives
  - Ethical controversies of euthanasia, physician-assisted suicide, termination or withholding of life support, and access-to-care issues
  - APN professional practice mandates regarding monitoring of and involvement in healthcare legislation, particularly that which affects the provision of cancer care
  - The steps to ethical decision making and how to obtain assistance in decision making.

Recommended Resources for Oncology Advanced Practice Nurses

- Camp-Sorrell, D., & Hawkins, R.A. (Eds.). (2014). *Clinical manual for the oncology advanced practice nurse* (3rd ed.). Pittsburgh, PA: Oncology Nursing Society.
- Individual state Nurse Practice Act information via links on the NCSBN website: www.ncsbn.org
- ONCC: www.oncc.org
- ONS: www.ons.org

References

Allmark, P., Cobb, M., Liddle, B.J., & Tod, A.M. (2010). Is the doctrine of double effect irrelevant in end-of-life decision making? *Nursing Philosophy, 11,* 170–177. doi:10.1111/j.1466-769X.2009.00430.x

American Association of Nurse Practitioners. (2013a). Fact sheet: Medicare reimbursement. Retrieved from http://www.aanp.org/component/content/article/68-articles/325-medicare-reimbursement

American Association of Nurse Practitioners. (2013b). *Standards of practice for nurse practitioners.* Retrieved from http://www.aanp.org/images/documents/publications/standardsofpractice.pdf

American Cancer Society. (2015a). Advance directives. Retrieved from http://www.cancer.org/acs/groups/cid/documents/webcontent/002016-pdf.pdf

American Cancer Society. (2015b). The Patient Self-Determination Act (PSDA). Retrieved from http://www.cancer.org/treatment/findingandpayingfortreatment/understandingfinancialandlegalmatters/advancedirectives/advance-directives-patient-self-determination-act

American Nurses Association. (2011). Short definitions of ethical principles and theories: Familiar words, what do they mean? Retrieved from http://nursingworld.org/MainMenuCategories/EthicsStandards/Resources/Ethics-Definitions.pdf

American Nurses Association. (2012). Nursing care and do not resuscitate (DNR) and allow natural death (AND) decisions [Position statement]. Retrieved from http://www.nursingworld.org/MainMenuCategories/EthicsStandards/Ethics-Position-Statements/Nursing-Care-and-Do-Not-Resuscitate-DNR-and-Allow-Natural-Death-Decisions.pdf

American Nurses Association. (2013). Euthanasia, assisted suicide, and aid in dying [Position statement]. Retrieved from http://www.nursingworld.org/euthanasiaanddying

American Nurses Association. (2015). Code of ethics for nurses. Retrieved from http://www.nursingworld.org/codeofethics

APRN Consensus Work Group & National Council of State Boards of Nursing APRN Advisory Committee. (2008). Consensus model for APRN regulation: Licensure, accreditation, certification and education. Retrieved from https://www.ncsbn.org/Consensus_Model_for_APRN_Regulation_July_2008.pdf

Bouton, B.L. (2005). Ethical "hot buttons" in hospice care. Retrieved from http://www.medscape.com/viewarticle/505225

Brant, J.M., & Wickham, R. (2013). Statement on the scope and standards of oncology nursing practice: Generalist and advanced practice. Pittsburgh, PA: Oncology Nursing Society.

Brassard, A., & Smolenski, M. (2013). Removing barriers to advanced practice registered nurse care: Hospital privileges. INSIGHT on the Issues, 55. Retrieved from http://assets.aarp.org/rgcenter/ppi/health-care/insight55.pdf

Centers for Medicare and Medicaid Services. (n.d.). National Provider Identifier. Retrieved from https://nppes.cms.hhs.gov/NPPES/Welcome.do

Centers for Medicare and Medicaid Services. (2013). Hospice certification/recertification requirements. Retrieved from http://www.cgsmedicare.com/hhh/coverage/Coverage_Guidelines/CERT_ReCERT_Requirements.html

Centers for Medicare and Medicaid Services. (2014a). Enrollment applications. Retrieved from http://www.cms.gov/Medicare/Provider-Enrollment-and-Certification/MedicareProviderSupEnroll/EnrollmentApplications.html

Centers for Medicare and Medicaid Services. (2014b). Evaluation and management services guide. Retrieved from https://www.cms.gov/Outreach-and-Education/Medicare-Learning-Network-MLN/MLNProducts/downloads/eval_mgmt_serv_guide-ICN006764.pdf

Centers for Medicare and Medicaid Services. (2015a). Chapter 9—Coverage of hospice services under hospital insurance regulations. In Medicare benefit policy manual. Retrieved from http://www.cms.gov/Regulations-and-Guidance/Guidance/Manuals/downloads/bp102c09.pdf

Centers for Medicare and Medicaid Services. (2015b). ICD-10. Retrieved from http://www.cms.gov/Medicare/Coding/icd10

Cohen, J.S., & Erickson, J.M. (2006). Ethical dilemmas and moral distress in oncology nursing practice. Clinical Journal of Oncology Nursing, 10, 775–780. doi:10.1188/06.CJON.775-780

Edmunds, M.W. (2010). NPs must adhere to state scope-of-practice regulations. Journal for Nurse Practitioners, 6, 664. doi:10.1016/j.nurpra.2010.08.006

Ethics. (n.d.). In Merriam-Webster online dictionary. Retrieved from http://www.merriam-webster.com/dictionary/ethics

Ethics and Compliance Initiative. (2009a). Definitions of values. Retrieved from http://www.ethics.org/?q=resource/definitions-values

Ethics and Compliance Initiative. (2009b). Ethics glossary. Retrieved from http://esc.webair.com/resource/ethics-glossary

Hagedorn, S., & Quinn, A.A. (2004). Theory-based nurse practitioner practice: Caring in action. Topics in Advanced Practice Nursing eJournal, 4(4). Retrieved from http://www.medscape.com/viewarticle/496718_4

Hall, D.E., Prochazka, A.V., & Fink, A.S. (2012). Informed consent for clinical treatment. CMAJ, 184, 533–540. doi:10.1503/cmaj.112120

Hittle, K. (2010). Understanding certification, licensure, and credentialing: A guide for the new nurse practitioner. Journal of Pediatric Health Care, 24, 203–206. doi:10.1016/j.pedhc.2009.09.006

Jansky, M., Marx, G., Nauck, F., & Alt-Epping, B. (2013). Physicians' and nurses' expectations and objections toward a clinical ethics committee. Nursing Ethics, 20, 771–783. doi:10.1177/0969733013478308

Lachman, V.D. (2012). Applying the ethics of care to your nursing practice. MEDSURG Nursing, 21, 112–114, 116. Retrieved from http://nursingworld.org/MainMenuCategories/EthicsStandards/Resources/Applying-the-Ethics-of-Care-to-Your-Nursing-Practice.pdfe-Era-of-Health-Care-Reform.pdf

McLennon, S.M., Uhrich, M., Lasiter, S., Chamness, A.R., & Helft, P.R. (2013). Oncology nurses' narratives about ethical dilemmas and prognosis-related communication in advanced cancer patients. *Cancer Nursing, 36,* 114–121. doi:10.1097/NCC.0b013e31825f4dc8

National Cancer Institute. (2015). Advance directives. Retrieved from http://www.cancer.gov/about-cancer/managing-care/advance-directives

National Council of State Boards of Nursing. (2015a). Guiding principles. Retrieved from https://www.ncsbn.org/1325.htm

National Council of State Boards of Nursing. (2015b). History. Retrieved from http://www.ncsbn.org/181.htm

National Council of State Boards of Nursing. (2015c). Licensure. Retrieved from https://www.ncsbn.org/licensure.htm

National Council of State Boards of Nursing. (2015d). Licensure compacts. Retrieved from https://www.ncsbn.org/compacts.htm

National Council of State Boards of Nursing. (2015e). Nurse practice act, rules and regulations. Retrieved from https://www.ncsbn.org/nurse-practice-act.htm

Oncology Nursing Certification Corporation. (n.d.). Certifications. Retrieved from http://www.oncc.org/certifications

Oncology Nursing Certification Corporation. (2015). About ONCC. Retrieved from http://www.oncc.org/about-oncc

Oncology Nursing Society. (2007). *Oncology nurse practitioner competencies.* Retrieved from https://www.ons.org/sites/default/files/npcompentencies.pdf

Oncology Nursing Society. (2008). *Oncology clinical nurse specialist competencies.* Retrieved from https://www.ons.org/sites/default/files/cnscomps.pdf

Oncology Nursing Society. (2011). Role of the nurse when hastened death is requested (endorsed position statement, Hospice and Palliative Nurses Association). Retrieved from https://www.ons.org/advocacy-policy/positions/ethics/hastened-death

Oncology Nursing Society. (2015a). The role of the advanced practice nurse in oncology care [Position statement]. Retrieved from https://www.ons.org/advocacy-policy/positions/education/apn

Oncology Nursing Society. (2015b). PEP rating system overview. Retrieved from https://www.ons.org/practice-resources/pep

Principle. (n.d.). In *The Free Dictionary.* Retrieved from www.thefreedictionary.com/principle

ProCon.org. (2014, April 17). State-by-state guide to physician-assisted suicide. Retrieved from http://euthanasia.procon.org/view.resource.php?resourceID=000132

Resnick, D.B. (2011). What is ethics in research and why is it important? Retrieved from http://www.niehs.nih.gov/research/resources/bioethics/whatis

Schantz, M.L. (2007). Compassion: A concept analysis. *Nursing Forum, 42,* 48–55. doi:10.1111/j.1744-6198.2007.00067.x

United States Conference of Catholic Bishops. (2009). *Ethical and religious directives for Catholic health care services* (5th ed.). Retrieved from http://www.usccb.org/issues-and-action/human-life-and-dignity/health-care/upload/Ethical-Religious-Directives-Catholic-Health-Care-Services-fifth-edition-2009.pdf

U.S. Department of Health and Human Services. (n.d.). Informed consent FAQs. Retrieved from http://www.hhs.gov/ohrp/policy/faq/informed-consent/index.html

U.S. Department of Health and Human Services. (2003). Summary of the HIPAA privacy rule. Retrieved from http://www.hhs.gov/ocr/privacy/hipaa/understanding/summary/privacysummary.pdf

CHAPTER 22

Test Questions

Wendy H. Vogel, MSN, FNP, AOCNP®,
Shirley Triest-Robertson, PhD, AOCNS®, ACHPN, ACNSBC, RN-BC (Pain),
and Barbara Holmes Gobel, MS, RN, AOCN®

1. Which of the following patients is at the highest risk for significant bone marrow suppression?
   a. 70-year-old woman with non-small cell carcinoma of the lung, metastatic to the liver with a 10% weight loss prior to diagnosis. Other comorbidities include diabetes and rheumatoid arthritis. Planned treatment with carboplatin, paclitaxel, and bevacizumab.
   b. 22-year-old man with Hodgkin lymphoma, stage II, bulky disease. No comorbidities. Planned treatment with ABVD (doxorubicin, bleomycin, vinblastine, and dacarbazine).
   c. 65-year-old woman with breast cancer, stage II. Comorbidities include hypertension. Planned treatment with CMF (cyclophosphamide, methotrexate, and 5-fluorouracil).
   d. 58-year-old man with colorectal cancer, stage IIIA (Dukes C). Comorbidities include cardiovascular disease with a history of myocardial infarction and hypertension. Planned treatment with FOLFOX (5-fluorouracil, leucovorin, and oxaliplatin).

   Answer: A. The risk factors for significant bone marrow suppression in this patient include age, poor nutritional status (indicated by weight loss prior to diagnosis), history of rheumatoid arthritis (an autoimmune disease), and diabetes (National Comprehensive Cancer Network® [NCCN®], 2014). Her chemotherapy also is associated with a greater than 20% risk of febrile neutropenia. In the patient with Hodgkin lymphoma, ABVD has a moderate risk of febrile neutropenia (10%–20%) (NCCN, 2014). Age is a risk factor for bone marrow suppression in the patient with breast cancer. FOLFOX has a moderate risk of febrile neutropenia.

2. Which of the following chemotherapy agents puts patients at risk for severe and prolonged myelosuppression?
   a. Cyclophosphamide
   b. Doxorubicin
   c. Carmustine
   d. Paclitaxel

   Answer: C. Carmustine is a nitrosourea. This class of drugs is cell cycle nonspecific and has the most potent and prolonged effect on myelosuppression. Carmustine may cause severe myelosuppression that may last up to 85 days. The nadir of carmustine occurs in 26–60 days (Polovich, Olsen, & LeFebvre, 2014). Cyclophosphamide and paclitaxel produce moderate myelosuppression. Although doxorubicin, an alkylating agent, may produce severe myelo-suppression, the duration is generally only about 21 days (Polovich et al., 2014).

3. A patient will begin radiation therapy to marrow-producing fields for about six weeks. The most appropriate time for the advanced practice nurse (APN) to begin assessment for myelosuppression is
   a. Week 3.
   b. Week 4.
   c. Week 6.
   d. One week after radiation.
   Answer: A. The APN would assess for myelosuppression beginning at week 3 and con-tinuing regularly until bone marrow recovery. Myelosuppression secondary to radiation therapy peaks at week 3. Suppression may occur in all cell lines simultaneously rather than sequentially as seen with chemotherapy. The recovery period also may be less pre-dictable because radiation treatments will be required for several weeks after suppression peaks (Gosselin, 2011).

4. The oncology APN is educating a patient who is neutropenic on strategies to prevent infection. Which of the following strategies to prevent infection during neutropenia has the lowest level of research evidence?
   a. Avoidance of exposure to crowds and small children
   b. Avoidance of fresh flowers in standing water or soil
   c. Compliance with prophylactic antimicrobial therapy
   d. Avoidance of tap water and drinking bottled water only
   Answer: D. Drinking only bottled water or processed drinks as a method of avoiding infection during neutropenic episodes has low supporting evidence. The other sugges-tions all have high supporting evidence and should be encouraged (Irwin, Erb, Williams, Wilson, & Zitella, 2013).

5. Which of the following patient presentations is the most likely to represent a second malignancy caused by treatment of a first malignancy?
   a. Breast cancer presenting in a patient previously treated for Hodgkin lymphoma with chemotherapy and mantle field radiation
   b. Medullary carcinoma of the breast in a patient previously treated for basal carcinoma of the face and upper back by resection and topical 5-fluorouracil
   c. Prostate cancer in a patient previously treated for lung cancer with radiation to the apex of the left lung
   d. Ovarian cancer in a patient previously treated for adenocarcinoma of the breast with mastectomy and AC (doxorubicin and cyclophosphamide)
   Answer: A. Females between 10–15 years of age treated for Hodgkin lymphoma have a great risk of developing second malignancies (Jazbec, Todorovski, & Jereb, 2007; Ottavi-ani, Robert, Huh, Palla, & Jaffe, 2013). Mantle field radiation increases the risk of a subse-quent breast or lung cancer. Ovarian cancer occurring in a patient previously diagnosed with breast cancer, regardless of treatment, is more suggestive of a hereditary genetic mutation as the causative factor rather than the treatment. Medullary breast cancer and prostate cancer in patients previously treated for another cancer do not appear to be sec-ond malignancies caused by treatment of the first malignancy.

6. Which of the following is NOT a risk factor for myelosuppression?
   a. Poor nutritional status
   b. Autoimmune disease
   c. Age younger than 30
   d. Liver disease

   Answer: C. Age younger than 30 is not a risk factor for myelosuppression. Specific health factors increase the risk for significant bone marrow suppression when concomitant with cancer or its therapy. These risks include advanced age (older than 65 years); poor nutritional status; preexisting autoimmune disease, diabetes mellitus, gastrointestinal disorders, liver disease, and hematopoietic diseases; and substance abuse (NCCN, 2015g; Shelton, 2013).

7. Which of the following is usually the first indicator of bone marrow suppression and usually has the quickest response rate?
   a. Leukocytes
   b. Erythrocytes
   c. Platelets
   d. Immunoglobulins

   Answer: A. Leukopenia usually is the earliest indicator of bone marrow suppression and recovers more rapidly than other cell lines. Leukopenia occurs about 7–15 days after treatment. Depletion of the cell line is directly related to the normal turnover rate of the cell line after the antineoplastic agent destroys normal regrowth mechanisms. Granulocytes typically live only six to eight hours; platelets survive an average of 5–7 days; and erythrocytes live approximately 120 days. Platelets have the longest nadir, persisting for more than 20 days in many patients. Red cells generally only present serious problems in patients receiving highly suppressing erythrocytic agents such as anthracyclines or platinols (Polovich et al., 2014; Shelton, 2013).

8. The APN notes that a patient's complete blood count shows leukopenia, thrombocytopenia, and anemia. No obvious reason is noted in the patient history, annual physical examination, or initial blood tests for this abnormality (such as history of immunosuppressive drugs, bleeding, or drug abuse). The patient's chemistry panel and iron studies are essentially normal. What would be the appropriate diagnostic test to determine the etiology of these deficits?
   a. Chemistry panel and lactate dehydrogenase
   b. Bone survey and beta-2 microglobulin
   c. Positron-emission tomography (PET) scan
   d. Bone marrow aspiration and biopsy with peripheral smear

   Answer: D. In a patient with an abnormal complete blood count with all cell lines diminished and without evidence for a specific disorder and in whom an error in cell production is suspected, a bone marrow aspiration and biopsy should be performed. In many settings, oncology APNs perform this diagnostic test. If the APN suspects that cell destruction is likely, cell survival studies (e.g., red blood cell survival studies may be performed with nuclear-tagged red blood cells infused and followed by body scans), as well as hemolysis studies (e.g., direct bilirubin, schistocytes by smear) may be performed (Erb & Vogel, 2013; Shelton, 2012).

9. A patient presents with lethargy, decreased level of consciousness, a subnormal temperature, and no clinical signs of infection. The hemoglobin is 10 g/dl, platelets are 124,000/

mm³, and the absolute neutrophil count is 300/mm³. The patient's blood counts have been suppressed for about two weeks. What should the APN suspect?

a. Myocardial infarction
b. Sepsis
c. Metastatic disease to the brain
d. Cardiac tamponade

Answer: B. Sepsis should be suspected in this patient. Although fever is the cardinal symptom of infection, the degree of immune suppression may blunt the patient's ability to mount a fever response (NCCN, 2015g). A subnormal body temperature may indicate a leukopenia-related infection, a more severe sepsis, or the presence of gram-negative organisms (NCCN, 2015g; Shelton, 2011). Inflammatory symptoms, such as erythema-enhanced capillary permeability, swelling, or pus formation, may not always be present in patients with leukopenia because of the absence of white blood cells to produce inflammation. Fatigue is common even without infectious complications. Leukopenia beyond 7 days is thought to significantly increase the risk of infection, and virtually all who are leukopenic beyond 21 days become infected (NCCN, 2015g).

10. The new APN graduate approaches her mentor because of a conflict with a collaborating physician. Which of the following would be the mentor's best response?

a. "You would be better off just letting this issue lie, because that physician is difficult to deal with."
b. "How have you handled conflict with coworkers in the past?"
c. "I will be happy to intervene for you; I know that physician well."
d. "Deal with the situation, then come back to me and we will discuss how your method worked."

Answer: B. The new APN graduate is undergoing role acquisition, and a mentor or role model will assist in this process (Spoelstra & Robbins, 2010). Role acquisition is facilitated by a successful mentor. In asking the new APN how she has handled conflict in the past, the seasoned APN is performing the teacher/coach/trainer role and is assisting the new APN in the evaluation of past conflicts and the success of her previous attempts at resolution. From this evaluation, the seasoned APN can assist the new graduate in formulating a successful response. The APN mentor also can explore the sources of the conflict that have developed between the APN and the physician (e.g., differing expectations, assumptions, priorities, role conflict) that might be intensifying the conflict. Additionally, the mentor could review negotiation strategies with the new APN (Hake & Shah, 2011).

11. Which of the following demonstrates a successful collaborative practice between the APN and a physician?

a. The physician orders the plan of care, and the APN carries out the order.
b. The APN has developed protocols based on previous practice and uses these for practice.
c. The physician and APN jointly develop protocols and hold patient conferences weekly.
d. The physician provides the APN with reference books on which to base APN practice.

Answer: C. Collaboration is the process of working together within the negotiated framework to achieve the goal of the partnership. In collaboration, values are shared, respect is mutual, and power is equal (Baggs, 1994). An effective collaborative partnership includes a shared agenda and mutually beneficial goals (Adams, Orchard, Houghton, & Ogrin, 2014; Stringer, Curran, & Asghari, 2013). Effective collaborative practice consists of six critical elements: trust, cooperation, assertiveness, shared decision making, communication, and coordination (Baggs, 1994). The APN and physician developing protocols together demonstrates cooperation, communication, coordination, and shared decision making. By holding weekly patient conferences, information is shared and decisions that are in the patient's best interest may be made.

12. The APN decides to establish a cancer risk consultative practice. What should the APN consider first?
    a. How to write a business plan
    b. Personal strengths and areas of expertise
    c. Whether insurers will reimburse for this service
    d. Ways to gain community buy-in to the new practice
    Answer: B. Many things need to be considered before opening a consultative practice. One of the most important questions is what are the APN's personal strengths and areas of expertise (Block, 2011). It also is important to consider whether cancer risk consultative services are desired by the APN's potential "customers" (i.e., patients, administrators, collaborating/referring healthcare providers). Consultation refers to a two-way interaction designed to solicit, provide, and receive help, and the consultant is recognized as having specialized expertise. The nurse also must identify areas in which personal growth is needed. The other issues, although important, are secondary to the APN's ability to offer this service. Resistance to change, complacency or apathy, feelings of implied threat or criticism, and unfamiliarity of seeking consultation with an APN can impede development of the consultant role. In every consultative situation, the APN has an opportunity to demonstrate areas of expertise and to provide informal education about the types of cases that are appropriate for future consultations (Geppert & Shelton, 2012).

13. Which of the following resources would be the most useful for oncology advanced practice faculty members in planning and evaluating advanced-level education offered in master's programs?
    a. NCCN guidelines for clinical oncology practice
    b. Oncology Nursing Society's (ONS's) *Statement on the Scope and Standards of Oncology Nursing Practice: Generalist and Advanced Practice*
    c. Comprehensive texts covering oncology diagnosis, management, and follow-up care
    d. ONS's *Standards of Oncology Nursing Education: Generalist and Advanced Practice Levels*
    Answer: D. ONS's *Standards of Oncology Nursing Education: Generalist and Advanced Practice Levels* (Jacobs & Mayer, 2016), in conjunction with the *Statement on the Scope and Standards of Oncology Nursing Practice* (Brant & Wickham, 2013), provides educational guidelines for oncology nurse educators to enhance the quality of oncology nursing education, improve the quality of care, and promote the standardization of oncology nursing academic preparation (Blecher, 2004). The standards were developed to reflect the structure, process, and outcomes of educational offerings. Standards are included for faculty, resources, curriculum, the teaching-learning process, and the student.

14. The oncology APN is designing a survey for patients to assess the continuity of care from hospital discharge to the home setting. All of the following could be outcome indicators of continuity of care EXCEPT

    a. The patient indicates that he is able to perform self-care in his own environment.

    b. At the patient's subsequent healthcare visit, a medication review indicates that the patient is correctly taking all prescribed medications.

    c. The patient has access to a medical alert system designed for fall detection.

    d. The patient reports satisfaction with the hospital admission process.

Answer: D. All of the answers except for D could be useful indicators in the assessment of continuity of care from the hospital to the home setting. Continuity-of-care outcomes are now incorporated into existing quality measurement and accreditation programs. Outcome indicators of continuity of care include optimal patient functioning (including physical, psychological, and social function), adherence to the prescribed medical regimen, patient safety, patient comfort, and patient and family satisfaction (Haggerty, Roberge, Freeman, Beaulieu, & Bréton, 2012; Uijen, Schers, Schellevis, & van den Bosch, 2012). The hospital admission process would not indicate continuity of care in this case.

15. The oncology APN is providing a medical consultation for a patient referred to her high-risk cancer clinic for risk reduction, screening, and management recommendations. An appointment is made prior to a pending surgical consultation for consideration of a prophylactic mastectomy. The APN has requested and reviewed the patient's medical records from other healthcare providers. She has taken a thorough history and performed a physical assessment. She recommends screening tests and frequencies, as well as potential risk reduction interventions. What else should the oncology APN do?

    a. Determine who is responsible for ordering recommended screening tests.

    b. Communicate with the referring healthcare provider about recommendations

    c. Provide the patient with educational resources and references as well as community supports.

    d. All of the above.

Answer: D. All of the above should be included in the medical consultation. The APN clarified the reason for the consultation and made a timely appointment. The APN then gathered and reviewed pertinent information, performed a thorough history and physical assessment, synthesized the data, and made recommendations. Patient education is a key part of the consultation. It is then essential that the APN consultant, the patient, and the referring provider agree about who will be responsible for following through on the recommendations, respecting the boundaries of each other's professional practice. The APN should communicate with the referring provider. The referring practitioner also may require references and resources for the medical recommendations (Geppert & Shelton, 2012).

16. The transtheoretical model of the stages of change operates on the premise that

    a. Change is a series of stages, each with its own characteristics and each amenable to different interventions.

    b. Change occurs in response to a stressful stimulus as individuals see that their situation exceeds their available resources.

    c. Change occurs while striving toward health, well-being, enjoyment, and fulfillment.

    d. Change occurs because of a common sense factor—as individuals understand more about an illness, compliance with healthcare recommendations increases.

Answer: A. The transtheoretical model of the stages of change theorizes that change is a series of stages, each with its own characteristics and each amenable to different interventions (Leventhal & Cameron, 1987; Saarmann, Daugherty, & Riegel, 2000). The stages include precontemplation, contemplation, preparation, action, and maintenance.

This model can be used to guide healthcare interventions and education. The stress and coping theory views healthcare change as occurring in response to a stressful stimulus as individuals see that their situation exceeds their available resources. Healthcare changes that occur while striving toward health, well-being, enjoyment, and fulfillment is the premise of the health promotion model. And lastly, the self-regulation theory (common sense theory) presumes that as individuals understand more about an illness, compliance with healthcare recommendations increases.

17. The oncology APN is developing educational objectives for an educational talk for other advanced practitioners about incorporating a tobacco cessation program into their practice. Which of the following objectives indicates achievement of learning in the affective domain?
    a. The participant will identify the four critical steps in tobacco cessation counseling.
    b. The participant will discuss application of the tobacco cessation program with his or her own patient population.
    c. The participant will implement the program in his or her own practice within two months of class completion.
    d. The participant will recognize pharmaceutical approaches based on his or her practice formulary.

    Answer: B. Assessment of the affective domain involves receiving information and responding or interpreting this in accordance with one's own value system, that of the organization, or that of the population being served. The participant assesses the patient population and considers how the newly acquired information would be applied so that it would have value to the population (Anderson & Krathwohl, 2001). Identification of critical steps and the recognition of various pharmaceutical approaches involves the cognitive domain, which is the recall and understanding of material. Implementation of a tobacco cessation program involves the psychomotor domain.

18. Which of the following is an accurate statement regarding cancer risk assessment tools?
    a. The Claus model estimates the risk of breast or ovarian cancer based on age, race, and number of breast biopsies.
    b. The majority of cancers have reliable risk assessment tools, and existing risk assessment tools have weaknesses.
    c. Risk assessment tools enable clinicians to convey a cancer risk estimate to individuals to motivate screening activities and behavior changes.
    d. The Gail model, one of the most commonly used breast cancer risk assessment tools, estimates the risk of a genetic mutation that could cause breast cancer.

    Answer: C. Cancer risk assessment tools help clinicians to convey cancer risk to patients, with the intention to motivate patients to perform screening activities and behavior changes. Most cancers do not have reliable, validated risk assessment tools, and no known existing tool encompasses all known risk factors or is without weaknesses. The Gail model is one of the most commonly used risk assessment tools. It estimates a woman's five-year risk and overall lifetime risk for breast cancer. It does not take into account the age at breast cancer diagnosis in affected family members, history of bilateral breast cancer, second-degree relatives affected with breast cancer, or history of ovarian cancer or lobular carcinoma in situ. It does not evaluate hereditary risk and in fact may be falsely low in people with hereditary breast and ovarian cancer syndrome (Quante, Whittemore, Shriver, Strauch, & Terry, 2012). The Claus model estimates breast cancer risk based on first- and second-degree relatives with breast or ovarian cancer.

19. Which of the following is an example of primary cancer prevention?
    a. Teaching breast self-examination technique to a 25-year-old woman
    b. Ordering a yearly mammogram and performing a yearly clinical breast examination in a 52-year-old woman
    c. Advising a 47-year-old woman with a Gail model risk of 2.1% to stop smoking and that taking tamoxifen for five years could lower her breast cancer risk
    d. Ordering carcinoembryonic antigen testing every three months in an individual following successful treatment for colorectal cancer

    Answer: C. Primary cancer prevention aims to reverse or inhibit cancer by modification of a person's environment or behaviors or through pharmacologic mechanisms (Spratt, 1981). APNs assist in the achievement of primary cancer prevention by promoting health and wellness and assisting patients to reduce risks known to contribute to cancer development, such as smoking.

20. Which of the following studies about cancer risk reduction showed potential for harm by an agent thought to be a candidate for chemoprevention?
    a. The STAR trial (Study of Tamoxifen and Raloxifene)
    b. The SELECT trial (Selenium and Vitamin E Cancer Prevention Trial)
    c. The CARET trial (Beta-Carotene and Retinol Efficacy Trial)
    d. The BCPT trial (Breast Cancer Prevention Trial)

    Answer: C. In the CARET study, beta-carotene showed no benefit in men at high risk for lung cancer. In fact, 28% more lung cancers were diagnosed and 17% more deaths occurred in participants taking beta-carotene and vitamin A than in those taking placebos (Clark et al., 1996). The oncology APN must be familiar with current evidence when advising individuals about cancer risk reduction.

21. Which of the following is NOT an evidence-based method for promoting tobacco cessation?
    a. Increased tobacco costs and taxes
    b. Use of gum or hard candy as an oral substitute for tobacco
    c. Use of a combination of behavioral counseling and pharmacotherapy
    d. Limits on tobacco advertisements and marketing directed at children and teenagers

    Answer: B. All of these methods, with the exception of oral substitutes for tobacco, have evidence that proves effectiveness in decreasing the number of new smokers and increasing smoking cessation rates. Studies show that adolescents are three times more sensitive to tobacco advertising than adults and are more likely to be influenced to smoke by advertisements for cigarettes than by peer pressure (Campaign for Tobacco-Free Kids, 2015), so controlling the marketing of tobacco to children and teenagers will decrease the number of smokers. A comprehensive tobacco control program that includes excise tax increases results in greater reductions in cigarette smoking (Messer & Pierce, 2010). The combined use of behavioral counseling and pharmacotherapy will increase cessation rates (Fiore et al., 2008; Harrill-Smith, Ripley-Moffitt, & Goldstein, 2013).

22. Guidelines for lung cancer screening include patients who are all the following EXCEPT those who
    a. Have a 10–20-pack-year smoking history.
    b. Are current or former smokers.
    c. Are in reasonably good health, other than smoking.
    d. Are 55–74 years old.

Answer: A. People screened for lung cancer should have at least a 30-pack-year smoking history. In 2011, results from the National Lung Screening Trial were published, citing a 20% reduction in lung cancer deaths with annual low-dose helical CT (LDCT) in smokers with at least a 30-pack-year smoking history (one pack per day for 30 years). Since then, the American Cancer Society (ACS) and NCCN have updated their lung cancer screening guidelines, which are summarized in Table 1-6. ACS (2015a) and NCCN (2015e) recommend screening for lung cancer with annual LDCT in patients who are aged 55–74, are current or former smokers (30 pack-years or greater), and are otherwise in good health. NCCN also has made screening recommendations for those who smoke less but have additional risk factors. It is noted that smoking cessation counseling should not be eliminated in lieu of lung cancer screening.

23. Which of the following statements about screening is false?
    a. Smoking cessation counseling should not be eliminated in lieu of lung cancer screening.
    b. Recommendations for colorectal cancer include screening at age 50 with either annual fecal occult blood test (FOBT) or fecal immunochemical testing (FIT), sigmoidoscopy every five years, annual FOBT or FIT in combination with sigmoidoscopy every five years, or a full colonoscopy every 10 years.
    c. Recommendations for cervical screening generally include initiation of Pap test alone by age 21, and by age 30, co-testing with Pap and HPV testing every year until age 70.
    d. ACS and NCCN recommend annual breast screening with MRI as an adjunct to mammography in women with a high risk for breast cancer.
    Answer: C. This statement is false. Recommendations for cervical cancer generally include initiation of Pap test alone by age 21. By age 30, co-testing with Pap and HPV testing every five years is preferred over Pap testing alone every three years. Annual screening with any test in any age group is not recommended (ACS, 2015b; Saslow et al., 2012). The other three statements are true.

24. The Prostate, Lung, Colorectal, and Ovarian (PLCO) Cancer Screening Trial found which of the following?
    a. Early detection of low-risk disease results in decreased morbidity and increased quality of life if men with prostate cancer are treated with aggressive therapy.
    b. Early detection of low-risk disease results in decreased mortality and morbidity if men with prostate cancer are treated with moderate to aggressive therapy.
    c. Early detection of low-risk disease may ultimately result in increased morbidity and diminished quality of life if men with prostate cancer are treated with aggressive therapy.
    d. Early detection of low-risk disease does not benefit men unless aggressive therapy is rapidly initiated.
    Answer: C. In 2009, a large U.S. randomized study called the Prostate, Lung, Colorectal and Ovarian (PLCO) Cancer Screening Trial found that early detection of low-risk disease may ultimately result in increased morbidity and diminished quality of life if men with prostate cancer are treated with aggressive therapy (Croswell, Kramer, & Crawford, 2011). In fact, routine screening may lead to overdiagnosis and overtreatment in a large part of the screened population.

25. The oncology APN is asked to give a lecture about hereditary predisposition testing to a group of medical residents. Which of the following statements would accurately reflect the use of genetic testing in oncology?

    a. Genetic testing is now readily and commercially available for most cancers.

    b. Genetic testing is best used to help individuals at high risk for developing cancer to make good decisions about cancer screening and prevention strategies.

    c. Genetic testing could be used in routine population screening because recent scientific advances have decreased costs of testing and insurance policies will readily cover testing.

    d. Individuals who have genetic testing require knowledge about the testing process and plan of care following testing, but few negative psychosocial issues have been encountered in clinical practice.

Answer: B. Genetic testing is best used to help individuals at high risk for developing cancer to make good decisions about cancer screening and prevention strategies. It is not a tool to be used in routine population screening because most cancers are sporadic and not hereditary in nature. The clinician also must consider the expense of testing and the complex counseling needs of these families (Robson, Storm, Weitzel, Wollins, & Offit, 2010). Individuals with expertise in cancer genetics are necessary to educate those at risk about the strengths, limitations, and risks associated with genetic testing. The process of testing can lead to ethical, legal, and social issues, and nurses need to safeguard patients and families from these potential risks.

26. Which of the following best describes germ-line mutations?

    a. Germ-line mutations cause 85% of all cancers.

    b. Primary treatment of cancers often is based on the detection of germ-line mutations.

    c. Germ-line mutations affect one cell line and all subsequent cells derived from that cell division.

    d. Germ-line mutations occur in the sperm or egg cell initially and may be noted in every cell of an individual.

Answer: D. Germ-line mutations occur in hereditary cancer predisposition syndromes, affecting only around 10% of people with cancer. These mutations occur in the egg or sperm and affect every cell in the body and may be passed on to subsequent generations. A common example is a mutation in the *BRCA1* or *BRCA2* gene, which may lead to hereditary breast and ovarian cancer. Detection of a germ-line mutation most often alters prevention and screening strategies (Gunder & Martin, 2011).

27. The oncology APN is caring for a patient with a known *MSH2* mutation. Which of the following recommendations would be suggested for cancer prevention or early detection specific for people with this mutation?

    a. Annual mammography beginning at age 35

    b. Annual chest x-rays and sputum cultures

    c. Annual colonoscopy with prompt removal of polyps starting between ages 20–25

    d. Annual full-body skin examination with prompt removal of any suspicious skin lesions

Answer: C. Patients with a mutation in *MLH1* and *MSH2* have an 80% lifetime risk of developing colorectal cancer compared with a 6% risk in the general population. Women with mutations in these genes have a 60% lifetime risk for developing endometrial cancer and a 12% lifetime risk for developing ovarian cancer (Weissman et al., 2012). Therefore, a biannual pelvic examination beginning at age 25 with transvaginal ultrasound at ages 30–35 every 6–12 months would be recommended. A prophylactic hysterectomy with bilateral salpingo-oophorectomy could be discussed when childbearing is complete. Breast cancer risk is not known to increase in people with this mutation.

28. The oncology APN is caring for four different families who are all requesting genetic testing. Which of these families should be counseled that current available genetic tests are NOT likely to identify a hereditary predisposition?
    a. A family with three members with melanoma, one of whom also has pancreatic cancer
    b. A family with a 65-year-old grandmother with breast cancer, an uncle with prostate cancer diagnosed at age 80, and a son with lung cancer diagnosed at age 48
    c. A family with a grandmother with endometrial cancer diagnosed at age 49, her son with colorectal cancer diagnosed at age 49, and her daughter with renal cancer diagnosed at age 42
    d. A family with a woman who had breast cancer at age 49 and ovarian cancer at age 61 and who has a paternal cousin with bilateral breast cancer diagnosed at age 50

    Answer: B. Although several cancers are present in this family, the breast cancer and prostate cancer were both diagnosed after age 50. The first family's history (a) is suggestive of hereditary melanoma because of the incidence of melanoma in three family members, as well as the pancreatic cancer, which also can be found in this syndrome (Lindor, McMaster, Lindor, & Greene, 2008). The third family (c) has cancers associated with hereditary nonpolyposis colorectal cancer (HNPCC) syndrome. This family also has cancers diagnosed before age 50 and first-degree relatives affected with an HNPCC cancer (Kohlmann & Gruber, 2012). The fourth family (d) is suggestive of a hereditary cancer syndrome because of the woman with two primary cancers and an individual with a cancer that is bilateral in a paired organ (Petrucelli, Daly, & Feldman, 2013).

29. The definition of a previvor is a person who is
    a. Diagnosed with a cancer that was subsequently found to be hereditary.
    b. Diagnosed with a hereditary mutation but does not have a cancer diagnosis.
    c. Living with a terminal cancer diagnosis.
    d. Diagnosed with a cancer that is suspected to be hereditary but not confirmed.

    Answer: B. A previvor is an individual who has a genetic predisposition for developing cancer but does not have a cancer diagnosis (Hoskins, Roy, & Greene, 2012).

30. The oncology APN is consulted by a family practice APN colleague who wants to know what hereditary predisposition test should be ordered for a certain patient. Understanding that the colleague has little knowledge about genetic testing, what would be the oncology APN's best response?
    a. Give basic information, including the strengths, limitations, risks, and psychosocial limitations associated with genetic testing and encourage the family practice APN to refer to a hereditary genetics professional.
    b. Refuse to discuss this, as the family practice APN should not be ordering these types of tests.
    c. Give the family practice APN the information needed to order the test for the patient.
    d. Tell the family practice APN that ordering a genetic test is outside the APN's scope of practice.

    Answer: A. Genetic testing is best used to help individuals at high risk for developing cancer to make good decisions about cancer screening and prevention strategies. It is not a tool to be used in routine population screening because of the expense of testing and the complex counseling needs associated with it. Because of the increasing availability of testing, individuals with expertise in cancer genetics are needed to educate at-risk individuals about the strengths, limitations, and risks associated with genetic testing. The

Essentials of Genetic and Genomic Nursing: Competencies, Curricula Guidelines, and Outcome Indicators (Jenkins, 2009) define the minimum genetic and genomic competencies for all nurses in the United States. One of the biggest risks and liabilities that occur when genetic testing is ordered outside of the formal genetic testing process by a credentialed genetic healthcare provider is that care may not be appropriately coordinated and offered to the entire family at risk. Credentialed genetic professionals are trained in using the pedigree to identify those at risk and coordinating care for the entire family.

31. Which of the following statements regarding performance status is correct?
    a. Performance status has prognostic but not therapeutic implications.
    b. The Karnofsky Performance Status (KPS) scale and the Eastern Cooperative Oncology Group (ECOG) scale, although frequently used, are not yet validated.
    c. Obtaining baseline performance status and then monitoring periodically is not an accurate assessment of changes resulting from disease; thus, making treatment modifications based on this would be inappropriate.
    d. The ECOG performance scale has six levels (0–5) to evaluate patients and their behaviors, from fully ambulatory and functional to fully bedridden and nonfunctional.
    Answer: D. The ECOG performance scale has six levels (0–5), with level 0 indicating fully ambulatory and functional and level 4 indicating fully bedridden and nonfunctional (Oken et al., 1982). The ECOG and KPS scales are the most frequently used, validated measurement tools for performance status both in clinical practice and in clinical trials (Karnofsky, Abelmann, Craver, & Burchenal, 1948). By obtaining a baseline score and then periodic assessments of performance status, clinicians can predict the initial affect of disease on patients, their tolerance of treatment, and the progression or regression of disease burden. The information gleaned from this assessment will influence initial and ongoing therapeutic interventions.

32. For which patient would a plain radiograph (x-ray) be most appropriate?
    a. An obese man with a suspected sacral tumor
    b. A 55-year-old woman with multiple myeloma
    c. An obese woman with a suspected intestinal obstruction
    d. A 72-year-old man with a scapular lesion
    Answer: B. Plain radiographs still play a significant role in cancer diagnosis by demonstrating suspicious areas in two-dimensional imaging. They also have the advantage of being relatively quick and inexpensive. Purely lytic bone metastases, such as in multiple myeloma, are best evaluated by plain bone films (skeletal surveys), so the 55-year-old woman with multiple myeloma could be evaluated by x-ray. In patients with a peripheral lung lesion, x-ray is ideal for evaluation and also is excellent for pneumonias and intestinal obstructions. Radiographs of the chest can provide information regarding the size of lesions in the lung, the presence or absence of calcifications, and the growth rate of lung nodules (Chen & Whitlow, 2011). Radiography may be limited by obesity because of reduced contrast imaging. Interpretation of x-rays can be hindered because of location, particularly in areas such as the sacrum, sternum, and scapula, which have obscured views (Chen & Whitlow, 2011).

33. In which of the following is the choice of diagnostic scanning most appropriate?
    a. PET scan for staging in renal cancer
    b. Magnetic resonance imaging (MRI) evaluation of an upper abdominal lesion

c. Computed tomography (CT) scan to evaluate a musculoskeletal malignancy

d. PET scan in the workup of a solitary pulmonary nodule

Answer: D. PET scanning involves the injection of a positron-labeled (radioactive) tracer, usually glucose (F-fluorodeoxyglucose). Metabolically active areas, such as tumors, will take up the glucose and will show up as "hot" spots on images produced by gamma camera tomography (Chen & Whitlow, 2011). Certain tissues, such as kidney and brain, take up glucose, limiting evaluation by PET scanning. PET scanning is considered the gold standard for evaluating a solitary pulmonary nodule or mass (Kanne et al., 2012). CT scanning for evaluating musculoskeletal malignancies can be difficult because the CT may produce image artifact where cortical bone is present (Zoga et al., 2012). MRI can be limited in chest and upper abdominal scanning because of respiratory motion artifact.

34. The pathology report on a 42-year-old woman following lumpectomy reveals the following: 2.5 cm tumor, estrogen receptor/progesterone receptor negative, HER2 2+ by immunohistochemistry (IHC), 1 of 15 lymph nodes positive. The oncology APN recognizes that the next appropriate step is to

a. Recommend referral for chemotherapy.

b. Order repeat testing to ensure that the tumor is not hormonally reactive.

c. Order further testing by fluorescence in situ hybridization (FISH) on the tumor to reassess HER2 status.

d. Recommend proceeding with mastectomy because of the aggressiveness of the tumor.

Answer: C. IHC testing of HER2 reported at 2+ is considered equivocal; therefore, further testing by FISH is indicated to detect overexpression. FISH is the more accurate test to assess HER2 status (Wolff et al., 2013).

35. An HIV-infected individual is diagnosed with Kaposi sarcoma and asks the APN why he developed this cancer. Which of the following is NOT true?

a. HIV-infected individuals have a 10-fold increased risk of cancer.

b. The increased risk in HIV-infected individuals may be due to chronic immunosuppression as well as chronic viral infection.

c. Viruses like HIV also increase the risk for solid tumors, such as breast and colon cancer.

d. HIV infection could increase the risk for a lymphoma.

Answer: C. HIV is not known to increase the risk of solid tumors but does increase the risk of several cancers, including Kaposi sarcoma, cervical cancer, non-Hodgkin lymphoma, and ocular cancers. HIV-infected individuals have a 10-fold increased risk of cancer (Serraino et al., 2007). This increased risk in HIV-infected individuals may be a result of chronic immunosuppression as well as chronic viral infection.

36. Which of the following is a contraindication for colonoscopy?

a. International normalized ratio of 4.0

b. Esophageal varices

c. History of colorectal cancer

d. Need to visualize the small intestine

Answer: A. Colonoscopy can visualize the entire colon with a flexible scope and can facilitate biopsy of any suspicious areas, removal of polyps, and collection of stool specimens. Contraindications to colonoscopy include acute diverticulitis, significant adhesions in the pelvis or abdomen, acute exacerbations of inflammatory bowel disease, suspected bowel perforation, recent pulmonary embolus or myocardial infarction, and blood coagulation abnormalities.

37. Following a mediastinoscopy, a patient reports a significant increase in shortness of breath, anxiety, and chest pain. Upon examination, tachycardia and pulsus paradoxus are noted. Pulse oximetry is 85%. What must be ruled out first?
    a. Pneumothorax
    b. Pneumonia
    c. Chronic obstructive pulmonary disease
    d. Asthma exacerbation
    Answer: A. Complications of mediastinoscopy may include hemorrhage, pneumothorax, recurrent or phrenic nerve injury, tracheal or esophageal injury, wound infection, or difficulties with anesthesia (Silvestri et al., 2013). This patient is presenting with signs and symptoms of a pneumothorax, which could potentially be life threatening. When the patient history notes a recent mediastinoscopy, pneumothorax must be included in the differential.

38. Which of the following is a genetic test performed on tumor cells that has prognostic and predictive uses?
    a. Circulating tumor cells (CTCs)
    b. Oncotype DX®
    c. CA 27.29
    d. *BRCA1* test
    Answer: B. Oncotype DX is a 21-gene reverse transcription polymerase chain reaction expression assay performed on breast tumor cells' RNA (Harris et al., 2007). It has both prognostic and predictive uses. CTCs are used to detect microscopic evidence of metastases and may be prognostic of recurrence (Compton et al., 2012). The CA 27.29 is a breast cancer tumor marker, a substance secreted by the tumor, and is used in the workup of many different cancers and plays a significant role in staging and diagnosis (Febbo et al., 2011). The *BRCA1* is a genetic test; however, it is performed on the blood, not tumor cells. If present, this genetic mutation would be found in all cells of the body, not just in tumor cells (see Chapter 2 for more information).

39. Which of the following is a risk factor for postoperative nausea and vomiting?
    a. Older age
    b. Male sex
    c. Surgical procedure involving the ear
    d. Short duration of surgery
    Answer: C. Male sex, shorter surgery, and older age are not considered to be risk factors for postoperative nausea and vomiting. Female sex, surgeries of longer duration, and surgical procedures involving the ear do increase the risk of postoperative nausea and vomiting. Other risk factors might include ingesting food too quickly following surgery; surgeries of the nose, throat, or breast; long duration of surgery; and being of pediatric-patient age (Sharma & Jamal, 2013).

40. Which of the following statements about surgical biopsy is accurate?
    a. An incisional biopsy removes the entire nonvisible mass.
    b. An excisional biopsy removes a visible mass in its entirety.
    c. A negative core needle biopsy reading ensures a benign lesion.
    d. The disadvantage of needle biopsy is difficult access to tumor.

Answer: B. An excisional biopsy removes a visible mass in its entirety. An incisional biopsy removes part of a visible mass. A negative biopsy reading obtained via a fine or core needle does not ensure a benign lesion. If a lesion is highly suspicious for malignancy and a needle biopsy yields negative or inconclusive results, an open biopsy is necessary to obtain enough tissue to verify a diagnosis (Bugalho et al., 2013). In the case of precursor neoplastic findings, as in lobular carcinoma in situ of the breast, a needle biopsy is insufficient for diagnosis or management. A follow-up surgical excision removes additional tissue for pathologic examination to exclude adjacent malignant cells (Atkins, Cohen, Nicholson, & Rao, 2013). Needle biopsies have the advantages of easy access, minimal or no scarring, and minimal discomfort.

41. Each of the following comorbid conditions increases the risk for intraoperative or postoperative complications EXCEPT
    a. Personal history of congestive heart failure.
    b. Personal history of gastroesophageal reflux.
    c. Obesity.
    d. Recent personal history of herpes zoster infection.
    Answer: D. All of the comorbid conditions listed have a potential for causing intraoperative or postoperative complications except for a personal history of herpes zoster infection (Robinson et al., 2013). A personal history of congestive heart failure confers a 12% increase in hospital stay. Obesity increases the risk for intraoperative and postoperative respiratory events by fourfold, and a history of uncontrolled reflux allows for an eightfold increase in intubation events, including aspiration (Amri, Bordeianou, Sylla, & Berger, 2014).

42. All of the following presurgical conditions would increase the risk of postsurgical infection EXCEPT
    a. Malnutrition.
    b. Being a current smoker.
    c. Uncontrolled diabetes.
    d. Past personal history of hepatitis.
    Answer: D. A past personal history of hepatitis is not known to increase the risk of postoperative infection. Abstinence from smoking for as little as one week before surgery can have a positive influence on tissue oxygenation. Suboptimal nutritional states increase the risk of infection. Nutritional supplements or enteral feedings may be necessary to ready the body for surgery and improve nitrogen balance and protein stores (Hennessey et al., 2010). Tight control of serum blood sugars with sliding-scale insulin may improve the infection threshold (Kiran, Turina, Hammel, & Fazio, 2013).

43. The oncology APN is performing a preoperative assessment. The assessment reveals that the patient is on the following medications. Which of these should be discontinued more than 24 hours preoperatively?
    a. St. John's wort
    b. Benazepril
    c. Lorazepam
    d. Sertraline
    Answer: A. St. John's wort is an herbal preparation with reported uses for anxiety, depression, and insomnia. The concentration of active ingredients in herbal products varies widely among preparations. Adverse reactions of St. John's wort include an antiplate-

let effect. Abrupt cessation of this alternative medication may initiate withdrawal symptoms. Therefore, it is recommended that St. John's wort be discontinued two weeks before surgery (Savina & Couturaud, 2011). Sertraline, lorazepam, and benazepril should not be discontinued more than 24 hours preoperatively.

44. Which of the following biopsy techniques will likely require further and a more definitive tissue biopsy?
    a. Fine needle aspiration
    b. Open biopsy
    c. Excisional biopsy
    d. Incisional biopsy
    Answer: A. A fine needle aspiration biopsy can obtain cells from a palpable mass for identification of the presence or absence of malignant cells in the sample. However, a fine needle aspiration often does not indicate histologic differences necessary for treatment; therefore, patients typically require a more definitive tissue biopsy. Additional pathologic markers may be required, such as when neoadjuvant chemotherapy is under consideration, to obtain adequate information for cancer treatment planning. A larger-gauge core needle biopsy may be an appropriate method to obtain additional tissue that provides a diagnosis with histologic detail. Furthermore, a negative biopsy reading obtained by fine needle aspiration or core needle biopsy does not ensure a benign lesion. If a lesion is highly suspicious for malignancy and a needle biopsy yields negative or inconclusive results, another technique (Bugalho et al., 2013) or open biopsy is necessary to obtain enough tissue to verify a diagnosis.

45. Which of the following is NOT a goal of cancer surgical therapy?
    a. Maximizing potential for control or cure of disease
    b. Minimizing comorbidities
    c. Treating micrometastases
    d. Maintaining patient and family active participation
    Answer: C. The goals of cancer surgical therapy should be reviewed with the patient and family. These goals include maximizing potential for control or cure of cancer, minimizing comorbidities, and retaining active participation of patients and families (Rizk, 2013).

46. All of the following are core measures of the Surgical Care Improvement Project EXCEPT
    a. Administration of broad-spectrum prophylactic antibiotics within one hour of surgical incision.
    b. Close glucose monitoring postoperatively.
    c. Removal of urinary catheter on postoperative day 1 or 2.
    d. Thorough preoperative hair removal with a safety razor.
    Answer: C. It is recommended to avoid preoperative hair removal with a razor (Joint Commission, 2014). Clipping of the hair is preferred. If complete removal of body hair surrounding the surgical site is necessary, removal just prior to the skin incision in surgery is preferred instead of hours prior to surgery. This reduces potential areas of inflammation and subsequent superficial infection caused by trauma to the skin. Other core measures of the Surgical Care Improvement Project include
    • Administration of broad-spectrum prophylactic antibiotics within one hour of surgical incision and discontinuation within 24 hours following surgery
    • Close glucose monitoring with 6 am sample on postoperative day 1

- Removal of urinary catheter on postoperative day 1 or 2
- Maintenance of perioperative core temperature with warming blankets
- Administration of beta-blockers the morning of surgery and repeated in the perioperative phase
- Implementation of venous thromboembolic prophylaxis measures with lower limb compression pumps and anticoagulant prophylaxis using heparin or low-molecular-weight blood thinners.

47. Which of the following surgeries is considered "dirty" and requires preoperative and intraoperative administration of antibiotics?
    a. Partial resection of the sigmoid colon
    b. Mastectomy
    c. Resection of a cervical lymph node
    d. Amputation of the great toe
    Answer: A. Surgeries involving the alimentary tract, including oral and digestive organs, are designated as "dirty" cases. These procedures, as well as abscess drainage and overt infections, require preoperative and intraoperative administration of antibiotics. Surgical procedures involving the upper or lower digestive tracts (e.g., colon resection) also may require preoperative sterilization with multiple doses of oral agents (Roos et al., 2013). The other surgeries may benefit from administration of an IV broad-spectrum antibiotic just prior to skin incision, unless other risk factors are present, such as known infection, immunocompromised state, significant cardiac valvular disease, or artificial valves or joints or if surgical time may extend beyond two hours.

48. Which of the following represents a true statement about margins?
    a. Removal of all cancerous tissues is indicative of a cure.
    b. Resection of cancerous tissue is always adjuvant therapy to the primary systemic therapy.
    c. The goal of debulking a metastatic tumor is to remove all micrometastatic evidence of the tumor to provide a late-stage cure.
    d. Adequate surgical margins vary by cancer type.
    Answer: D. Adequate margins vary from cancer to cancer. The important work of clinical trials serves to document what constitutes a "negative" or adequate margin with each individual cancer (Diaz et al., 2014; Thompson et al., 2014). Micrometastatic disease is always a possibility after what seems to be a complete resection of tumor; therefore, the phrase "we got it all" does not indicate a "cure" of the cancer. Systemic treatment of the cancer is indicated for the treatment of micrometastasis. Neoadjuvant chemotherapy or radiation therapy may precede surgery in an effort to decrease the overall size of the tumor and potentially allow a less aggressive surgical approach (Larentzakis & Theodorou, 2014). Debulking involves surgically removing visible or palpable tumor to decrease overall tumor burden in metastatic disease, but the goal is not necessarily to achieve clean margins or remove all microscopic evidence of disease. Instead, debulking aims to improve quality of life and enhance the ability of systemic therapy to treat advanced cancer (Robinson & Cantillo, 2014).

49. Which of the following is a potential drawback of robotic-assisted or minimally invasive surgeries?
    a. Increased rate of infection
    b. Increased duration of surgical procedure

    c. Increased risk of internal bleeding

    d. Longer recovery time

Answer: B. The APN must often remind patients that even with minimally invasive procedures, such as laparoscopy, robotic-assisted surgery, or minimally invasive surgery, there is still a need to heal, and there may be side effects of prolonged anesthesia that result from longer procedure times. Other disadvantages for the surgeon related to minimally invasive surgery compared to traditional open surgery include decreased depth perception, lack of tactile feedback with the surgical field, and decreased intracavitary ease of suturing. Robotic-assisted laparoscopy surgery often can take 1.5 times longer than traditional open surgery (Sooriakumaran et al., 2014). Appropriate patient selection is important to avoid additional surgical and anesthesia time.

50. The most common sources of postoperative fever come from all of the following EXCEPT

    a. Urinary tract.

    b. Gastrointestinal tract.

    c. Respiratory system.

    d. Operative site.

Answer: B. The most common sites of postoperative fever arise in the pulmonary system, urinary tract, or operative site and also can be related to medications or occur as a result of phlebitis. Bacterial infections in postoperative patients can be endogenous or exogenous and can originate from preexisting conditions, the surgical procedure, or nosocomial risk from rotating staff (Godfrey, Villa, Dawson, Swindells, & Schouten, 2013).

51. All of the following statements accurately define breakthrough pain EXCEPT

    a. Breakthrough pain may be somatic, visceral, neuropathic, or a combination of these types of pain.

    b. The definition of breakthrough pain is a transitory pain that "breaks through" a well-controlled pain plan.

    c. Breakthrough pain is quantified easily, is of limited duration, has an identifiable cause, and functions to warn and protect from tissue damage.

    d. Breakthrough pain may occur without stimulus or as a result of certain activities or biologic events and is associated with decreased quality of life and increased cost and hospitalizations.

Answer: C. Breakthrough pain is defined as transitory pain that "breaks through" a well-controlled pain plan (Wengström et al., 2014). It may be somatic, visceral, neuropathic, or a combination of these. It results from certain activities or biologic events or may occur without a precipitating factor. Breakthrough pain is associated with decreased quality of life and increased cost and hospitalizations. However, breakthrough pain is not easily quantified and, unlike acute pain, does not function to warn of or protect from tissue damage.

52. Which of the following is associated with genetic, psychological, and environmental factors and causes a state of dependency on a substance?

    a. Addiction

    b. Tolerance

    c. Pseudoaddiction

    d. Physical dependence

Answer: A. Addiction is a disease that has genetic, psychosocial, and environmental influences, causing a state of dependence on a substance and is a result of habitual use of this substance for nonmedical reasons. Addiction is associated with deviant behavior, such as inadequate self-control over drug use, continued use despite harm, drug craving, and drug-seeking behaviors (Oliver et al., 2012). Opioid addiction is rare among patients with cancer (Anghelescu, Ehrentraut, & Faughnan, 2013).

53. A patient with chronic pain is currently taking acetaminophen 325 mg and oxycodone 5 mg, two tablets every four hours. The patient's pain rating is 7, which is unacceptable to him. During the workup for the increase in pain, the APN should
    a. Consider the use of an interventional strategy such as nerve block or neurostimulation.
    b. Consider the addition of a neuropathic agent such as an antidepressant, anticonvulsant, or topical anesthetic.
    c. Instruct the patient to increase the acetaminophen and oxycodone combination to three tablets every four hours for up to a week.
    d. Calculate the 24-hour analgesic dose and increase it by 50%, and then administer the equianalgesic dose in a controlled-release form, using oxycodone-acetaminophen for breakthrough pain.
    Answer: D. According to the NCCN guidelines, when pain intensity is rated higher than a 4, the total 24-hour dose should be calculated. The new scheduled dose is determined by the previous total 24-hour dose and is increased by 50%. If the patient has reached the maximum daily limit of the nonsteroidal anti-inflammatory drug (NSAID), the clinician should consider a sustained-release medication. A new breakthrough dose is calculated at 10%–20% of this new 24-hour dose and is given every one hour as needed (NCCN, 2015a). Increasing the acetaminophen and oxycodone combination to three tablets every four hours would give the patient an acetaminophen dose of 5,850 mg per 24 hours, which is over the recommended 4 g/day maximum dose. Although an interventional strategy or addition of a neuropathic agent might eventually be helpful, until the cause of the increased pain is determined, neither of these is appropriate.

54. The incidence of fatigue subjectively reported in patients with cancer undergoing active treatment is estimated to be
    a. 25%.
    b. 75%.
    c. 100%.
    d. 25%–50%.
    Answer: C. Subjective reports of fatigue in patients with cancer approach 100% in patients receiving chemotherapy, radiation therapy, stem cell transplant, or biologic therapy (Mitchell, 2011).

55. Which of the following pharmacologic interventions is approved by the U.S. Food and Drug Administration (FDA) for the treatment of chemotherapy-associated cognitive impairment?
    a. Erythropoietin
    b. Modafinil
    c. Methylphenidate
    d. No approved treatments are available.
    Answer: D. No treatment is currently approved to prevent or decrease any of the cognitive symptoms associated with chemotherapy (Mulrooney, 2010; Von Ah, Jansen, &

Allen, 2014). Various treatments are proposed based on potential etiologies and are under study. The passage of time may relieve cognitive impairment.

56. The APN is assessing a patient who complains of neuropathic pain symptoms. The patient's pain is not controlled on the current pain management plan of extended-release oxycodone. Which of the following could be added to the patient's current medications to address the neuropathic pain?
    a. Methadone
    b. Acetaminophen
    c. Ketoprofen
    d. Buprenorphine

    Answer: A. Methadone is an excellent choice for neuropathic pain (Aiello-Laws et al., 2009; NCCN, 2015a). Methadone accumulates with repetitive dosing. After a few days, the interval of administration can be increased while maintaining analgesic effects (Aiello-Laws et al., 2009). Careful titration and follow-up is necessary. Acetaminophen and ketoprofen are both NSAIDs and are not effective in neuropathic pain. Partial agonists, such as buprenorphine, have limited use in cancer pain because of their ceiling effects and their ability to precipitate withdrawal syndrome in patients on pure agonist agents (NCCN, 2015a).

57. Which of the following nonpharmacologic interventions is likely to be an effective intervention for both fatigue and cognitive impairment?
    a. Erythropoietin
    b. Acupuncture
    c. Dexamethasone
    d. Exercise

    Answer: D. Evidence suggests that exercise could be an effective intervention for both fatigue and cognitive dysfunction (Mitchell et al., 2014; Mustian, Sprod, Janelsins, Peppone, & Mohile, 2012; Von Ah et al., 2014). However, more research is needed to document a consistent positive effect of exercise. The other answers are not likely to be effective interventions in both fatigue and cognitive dysfunction.

58. The APN is assessing a patient with breast cancer who is three years out from her diagnosis. The patient is complaining of tightness and burning pain in her mastectomy site, axilla, and back of her arm. This pain worsens with arm movements. Examination shows no signs of local recurrence, rashes, or adenopathy. Her cancer treatment consisted of mastectomy, axillary dissection, chemotherapy, radiation to the cancer site and axilla, and hormonal therapy. She is currently on an aromatase inhibitor. CT scan of the chest is negative. Her CA 27.29 is normal. What is a likely cause of her pain?
    a. Bone metastasis
    b. Postmastectomy pain syndrome
    c. Radiation dermatitis
    d. Aromatase inhibitor–induced arthralgia

    Answer: B. This patient's pain is likely postmastectomy pain syndrome, which occurs in 25%–60% of mastectomy patients. Postoperative radiation and extensive axillary dissection are risk factors. Symptoms include tight, burning pain in mastectomy site, axilla, and back of arm; paresthesia, dysesthesia, allodynia, hyperalgesia, or loss of shoulder function; neuroma pain (scar pain); and phantom breast pain (Ripamonti, Santini, Maranzano, Berti, & Roila, 2012). Her breast cancer tumor marker, CA 27.29, is normal, as is her CT scan of the chest, making bone metastasis less likely. Radiation dermatitis is an acute condition, and this patient is three years out from her diagnosis. Aromatase inhibitors can cause arthralgias; however, the pain this patient describes is more neuropathic in nature.

59. A patient with metastatic breast cancer consults the oncology APN regarding treatment with paclitaxel rather than paclitaxel protein-bound particles. The patient has experienced peripheral neuropathy with past treatment and has read that paclitaxel causes less peripheral neuropathy. How should the APN respond?
    a. "Neurotoxicity with paclitaxel protein-bound particles will reverse itself in three to six months."
    b. "The incidence of peripheral neuropathies is equal in paclitaxel and paclitaxel protein-bound particles."
    c. "The incidence of arthralgias is equal for both drugs, but protein-bound paclitaxel neuropathies are more quickly reversible."
    d. "Paclitaxel protein-bound particles is not approved for metastatic breast cancer and is not a choice at this time."
    Answer: C. Paclitaxel protein-bound particles does not use Cremophor® to deliver the drug to the cancer cell, which increases the neurotoxicity. However, the higher incidence of neurotoxicity with paclitaxel protein-bound particles occurs because higher doses (71% vs. 56%) can be used. This side effect is more quickly reversible, but if the toxicity exceeds grade 3, dose interruption is required. Paclitaxel protein-bound particles is approved for metastatic breast cancer (Abraxis Oncology, 2013).

60. The APN notes that a patient is taking St. John's wort for depression and is currently receiving irinotecan for metastatic colorectal cancer. The APN's best response is to
    a. Recommend that the patient stop taking St. John's wort, as it is not a scientifically supported treatment for depression.
    b. Allow the patient to continue taking St. John's wort, as it is a relatively harmless complementary therapy.
    c. Tell the patient to not alter the dose of St. John's wort so that the effectiveness of the chemotherapy will not change.
    d. Recommend an alternative drug because St. John's wort may decrease the effectiveness of chemotherapy.
    Answer: D. Strong evidence shows that St. John's wort may have some effectiveness in relieving mild to moderate depression. Multiple side effects, however, are possible, including gastrointestinal distress, skin reactions, fatigue, sedation, restlessness, anxiety, sexual dysfunction, dizziness, headache, dry mouth, weight loss, and increased thyroid levels. It also is metabolized by the cytochrome P450 systems and therefore interacts with many drugs, including warfarin, digoxin, antidepressants, antibiotics, loperamide, and irinotecan. St. John's wort decreases the effectiveness of the active metabolite SN-38 of irinotecan by almost 50% (Rahimi & Abdollahi, 2012).

61. The APN gathers the following information from a new patient who is a highly educated Caucasian woman and a former smoker with existing comorbidities and newly diagnosed lung cancer. Family history reveals that the patient's mother died of breast cancer after receiving multiple chemotherapy protocols. The patient is reluctant to receive conventional therapy or prescription medication. The APN recognizes that the patient is at high risk for

a. Depression and anxiety disorders.
b. Addiction to opioids and benzodiazepines.
c. Suicide from lack of coping skills.
d. Taking complementary and alternative medications.

Answer: D. Information from several studies has begun to describe the characteristics of people who would be more likely to use complementary and alternative medicine (CAM). These characteristics include higher educated women who have taken CAM previously; have had recent hospitalization; have family who failed conventional medication; are former smokers (as opposed to current smokers or those who have never smoked); suffer from conditions such as back or neck pain, colds, joint pain and stiffness, anxiety, and depression; and have strong beliefs in CAM and the values of mind-body healing (Prasad, Ziegenfuss, Cha, Sood, & Tilburt, 2013; Saghatchian et al., 2014).

62. Which of the following best describes the Dietary Supplement Health and Education Act (DSHEA) of 1994?
    a. It is voluntary for all supplements, herbals, other botanicals, vitamins, and minerals.
    b. It verifies the accuracy of the individual ingredients listed within each supplement.
    c. It verifies that claims are not made regarding diagnosis, prevention, treatment, or cure.
    d. It prohibits the use of literature that describes the use of and outcome of using supplements.

Answer: C. Claims must not be made about the diagnosis, prevention, treatment, or cure for a specific disease. This is not a voluntary process. If the DSHEA determines that unfounded claims have been made, the manufacturer is liable. Literature that explains the use of the supplement and the outcome is allowed but is monitored. Manufacturers of supplements may say, for example, that a supplement improves the respiratory status, but not that it prevents colds (DSHEA, 1994).

63. The Federation of State Medical Boards approved the Model Guidelines for the Use of Complementary and Alternative Therapies in Medical Practice, of which the major emphasis was to
    a. Encourage the use of only CAM with level 1–based evidence such as meta-analyses.
    b. Discourage the use of interventions that are not scientifically supported and that may harm the patient.
    c. Encourage APNs to recommend scientifically supported CAM therapy to their patients.
    d. Balance evidence-based practice with compassion and respect for the autonomy and dignity of the patient.

Answer: D. The guidelines for the use of CAM in medical practice are used to educate and regulate physicians and those who co-manage patients, such as APNs, who use CAM in their practices and may not be currently licensed by a governing body with licensed or state-regulated CAM providers. The guidelines affirm that all healthcare providers have a duty to avoid harm and a duty to act in a patient's best interest. The initiative encourages the medical community to adopt clinically responsible and ethically appropriate standards that promote public safety, and at the same time educates healthcare providers on safeguards to ensure that services are provided within professional practice boundaries (Chase, Gibson, Sumner, Bea, & Alberts, 2014; Deng & Cassileth, 2014; Institute of Medicine, 2005).

64. Which of the following statements reflects the most significant contribution to the further success of CAM therapy?
    a. Most CAM therapy has an established billing code to obtain reimbursement.
    b. Safe and effective CAM modalities exist for some common conditions.
    c. Acupuncturists, naturopaths, and massage therapists are licensed in every state.
    d. Many certification programs exist for APN practitioners in the area of CAM.

    Answer: B. Evidence exists for safe and effective CAM modalities for several medical conditions. However, very few established billing codes exist, which necessitates out-of-pocket expenses for most patients who participate in CAM. Licensure for specific people who practice CAM is the responsibility of each individual state; not all states choose to license acupuncturists, naturopaths, and other CAM practitioners (American Holistic Nurses' Certification Corporation, 2014; BlueCross BlueShield of North Carolina, 2015; Find-A-Code, n.d.; National Center for Complementary and Integrative Health [NCCIH], 2015).

65. Which of the following should be included in post-treatment surveillance for patients with breast cancer?
    a. Complete blood count and liver function tests
    b. Chest x-ray, bone scan, MRI scan, PET scan
    c. Mammogram within six months after radiation therapy
    d. Close follow-up at three- to six-month intervals for at least three years

    Answer: D. According to the American Society of Clinical Oncology (ASCO) clinical practice guidelines (Khatcheressian et al., 2013), the only recommended breast cancer surveillance of the available answers is a history and physical examination every 3–6 months for the first three years after primary therapy; every 6–12 months for years 4 and 5; and then annually. Other recommendation schedules are given for breast self-examination, mammography at least six months after radiation therapy and preferably one year after the initial diagnostic mammogram, and regular pelvic examinations (Khatcheressian et al., 2013).

66. Which of the following would be a comprehensive resource that examines the medical and psychosocial issues that adult cancer survivors face, with recommendations to improve health care and quality of life?
    a. *National Action Plan for Cancer Survivorship*
    b. *Living Beyond Cancer: Finding a New Balance*
    c. *From Cancer Patient to Cancer Survivor: Lost in Transition*
    d. "Seasons of Survival: Reflections of a Physician With Cancer"

    Answer: C. Two reports, the *National Action Plan for Cancer Survivorship*, published in 2003 by the U.S. DHHS, the Centers for Disease Control and Prevention, and the Livestrong Foundation, and *Living Beyond Cancer: Finding a New Balance*, published in 2004 by the President's Cancer Panel, outlined the issues of cancer survivorship and set specific national goals. The Institute of Medicine (IOM) established a committee in 2005 to examine the range of medical and psychosocial issues faced by adult cancer survivors and to make recommendations to improve their health care and quality of life. This resulted in the comprehensive publication *From Cancer Patient to Cancer Survivor: Lost in Transition* (Hewitt, Greenfield, & Stovall, 2006). A recent update on this classic comprehensive resource was presented in the *Lancet* by Kirsch (2012).

67. A 35-year-old patient is seen in the follow-up clinic. The patient received radiation therapy to the chest for Hodgkin lymphoma 10 years ago. The surveillance test the APN would order during this visit is

    a. Bone scan.
    b. Brain scan.
    c. Mammogram/MRI.
    d. Bone marrow biopsy.
Answer: C. The risk of breast cancer is increased in those treated with chest radiation before age 30 and increases with age at the end of follow-up, time since diagnosis, and radiation dose. These projections are based on older regimens associated with greater risk; more modern treatment approaches include limited-field radiation and chemotherapy with less effect on ovarian function (Schellong et al., 2014). Monitoring for breast cancer as a late effect of chest or axilla radiation is recommended in the NCCN guidelines, using MRI and mammography for women who received radiation between the ages of 10 and 30. This screening should be initiated 8–10 years after radiation or at age 40, whichever occurs first (NCCN, 2015d). In particular, those surviving Hodgkin lymphoma are at greatest risk for second primary cancers, with the degree of risk associated with the age at which treatment was delivered. Solid tumors are more prevalent after treatment at a younger age, and leukemia is more frequent in those treated at an older age (Schellong et al., 2014).

68. Which statistical procedure is used to determine the time until an event occurs?
    a. Blinding
    b. Survival analysis
    c. Analysis of variance
    d. Statistical significance
Answer: B. Survival analysis is the collection of statistics that deal with analyzing the time from treatment until an event occurs, such as death. Examples of events include duration of response or survival. Blinding is a process by which the patient, and sometimes the researcher, is unaware of which treatment is being administered. Analysis of variance is a method to statistically compare means of several groups or observations. Statistical significance refers to the probability that the results of research could have occurred by chance (Goel, Khanna, & Kishore, 2010).

69. Which principle of risk-benefit analysis ensures that benefits are maximized and harm is minimized during clinical trial research?
    a. Justice (Declaration of Helsinki)
    b. Beneficence (Belmont Report)
    c. Voluntary consent (Nuremberg Code)
    d. Protection of human subjects (Code of Federal Regulations)
Answer: B. The Belmont Report actually covers three basic ethical principles: respect, beneficence, and justice (National Commission for the Protection of Human Subjects of Biomedical and Behavioral Research, 1979). *Beneficence* describes the principle of doing no harm and maximizing benefits while minimizing harm. *Justice* means giving each person an equal share and according to need, individual effort, societal contribution, or merit. *Respect* describes the need to treat individuals and their decisions as autonomous and, if that autonomy is compromised, the obligation to protect that individual. The Declaration of Helsinki contains the recommendations for the process of clinical research (World Medical Association, 2013). The Nuremberg Code established voluntary consent and required justification for research (National Institutes of Health Office of Human Subjects Research, n.d.). The *Code of Federal Regulations* contains guidelines for the conduct of institutional review boards (U.S. DHHS, 2009).

70. The participant's signature on the informed consent form for a clinical trial signifies
    a. The individual's agreement to participate in the clinical research based on the treatment group to which he or she is randomized.
    b. If it is a phase III clinical trial, the realization that no other acceptable treatment is available.
    c. That the participant has agreed to release the investigator, sponsor, institution, and its agents from liability for negligence.
    d. Acknowledgment that the consenting process was adequate for the participant to make a decision to participate in the clinical research.

    Answer: D. The informed consent process begins the first time that clinical research is mentioned to potential research participants. The process continues beyond the signing of the informed consent document to the formalization or documentation that the consenting process has been adequate for the person to make a decision to participate in the clinical research. Participants are discouraged from beginning participation in a clinical trial if they are likely to withdraw based on the arm to which they are randomized. Phase III clinical trials usually are randomized controlled trials that compare the outcomes of the usual standard of care to the research treatment. The patient can be randomized to an acceptable standard of care or research treatment. One of the requirements of informed consent is that it must not release or appear to release the investigator, sponsor, institution, or its agents from liability for negligence (U.S. FDA, 2014).

71. The International Committee of Medical Journal Editors (ICMJE) will only consider publishing clinical trial results if the clinical trial is
    a. Conducted through a national oncology study group.
    b. Registered before enrolling the first human subject.
    c. Powered for detecting a significant difference at 80%.
    d. At least a phase II clinical trial with significant results.

    Answer: B. ICMJE is interested in providing clinical trial information for all potential participants that will increase their access to medical information and contribute to their decision making. This includes but is not limited to phase III clinical trials (ICMJE, n.d.). ICMJE's goal is to provide full knowledge of and access to clinical trials for potential participants. Additionally, ICMJE supports the publication of both negative and positive clinical trial results in the spirit of full disclosure to the scientific and public community.

72. Which of the following has the strongest level of evidence when conducted with multiple randomized controlled clinical trials?
    a. Correlational descriptive study
    b. Well-conducted case-control study
    c. Expert opinions from an international group
    d. Meta-analysis of randomized controlled studies

    Answer: D. Although meta-analyses may be conducted with studies having similar hypotheses or variables, they have the strongest level of evidence when conducted with multiple randomized controlled clinical trials. A meta-analysis of studies with small samples or poorly designed studies does not provide the same level of evidence as that of a meta-analysis of randomized controlled studies. Correlational descriptive studies and case-control studies provide mid-level evidence. Expert opinion is the weakest level of evidence (ONS, n.d.).

73. Which two levels regulate APN practice?
    a. Licensure and certification
    b. Credentialing and privileging
    c. Certification and credentialing
    d. Scope of practice and standards of practice

    Answer: A. Licensure, which is at the state level, and certification, which is given by national organizations, provides APN regulation. Other factors that may influence or guide practice in individual settings of care are credentialing and privileging, scopes of practice, and standards of practice. Credentialing is one method of ensuring credibility to and protection of the public. The oncology APN's scope of practice is defined by federal regulations, state nurse practice acts, ONS guidelines, and practice agreements with the employer. ONS has developed a statement on the scope of practice, which may serve as a guide to both new graduates and APNs with years of experience. Standards are authoritative statements that define responsibilities of APNs, provide direction and evaluation for APN practice, and reflect the values of advanced practice in oncology (Brant & Wickham, 2013).

74. One of the qualifications required by APNs to obtain Medicare Part B reimbursement is to
    a. Hold a minimum of a bachelor's degree in nursing.
    b. Provide a service included by Medicare or secondary insurance.
    c. Provide service in collaboration with a medical doctor (MD) or doctor of osteopathy (DO) as required by state law.
    d. Be certified in specialty area of oncology such as advanced oncology certified clinical nurse specialist (AOCNS®) or advanced oncology certified nurse practitioner (AOCNP®).

    Answer: C. APNs may qualify for reimbursement under Medicare Part B if applicants meet the following requirements: legally authorized to provide services in the state where the service is provided; licensed as a registered nurse in the state where they practice; hold a master's degree in a defined clinical area of nursing from an accredited institution; and certified as a nurse practitioner (NP) or a clinical nurse specialist (CNS) by a national certifying body that has established standards for NPs or CNSs. Recognized certifying organizations include the American Academy of Nurse Practitioners; the American Nurses Credentialing Center; the National Certification Corporation for Obstetric, Gynecologic, and Neonatal Nursing; the Pediatric Nursing Certification Board; the Oncology Nursing Certification Corporation; and the American Association of Critical-Care Nurses (AACN) Certification Corporation. Services will be covered if they are comparable to those provided by an MD or DO, furnished in collaboration with the MD or DO as required by state law, and not excluded by Medicare (Centers for Medicare and Medicaid Services [CMS], n.d.-a).

75. The sphere of influence in which the CNS contributes to the development of evidence-based nursing care policies is
    a. Patient/client.
    b. Nurse/nursing.
    c. Patient/family.
    d. Organizational/systems.

    Answer: B. The nurse/nursing sphere acknowledges the contributions of CNSs to nurses and nursing through their leadership and staff development activities, including the development of evidence-based policies, procedures, and protocols. The organizational/

systems sphere recognizes CNS contributions to health care via information, education, and other activities that involve healthcare team members, communities, and healthcare systems (AACN, n.d.).

76. The APN observes that the bed rest instruction to patients after intrathecal methotrexate administration is different among practitioners. The APN intends to gather and document information on the current practice. This is an example of
    a. Benchmarking.
    b. Quality assurance.
    c. Evidence-based practice.
    d. Quality improvement.
    Answer: B. All of these answers are examples of continuous quality improvement and imply an ongoing or constant course of action, but quality assurance usually involves a retrospective review of an event or procedure and compares compliance with accepted standards. Quality improvement in a facility such as a hospital usually entails people from different but interactive areas coming together to review a systems process. The end result usually is focused on improving patient care or cost-saving measures and generally is more process-oriented than individual-oriented (U.S. DHHS, n.d.). Continuous quality improvement for the APN is a multifaceted process involving self-evaluation, patient evaluation, peer evaluation, systems evaluation, and the use and promotion of evidence-based practice (U.S. DHHS, n.d.).

77. What does the Patient Self-Determination Act require hospitals to do?
    a. Require patients to complete a living will
    b. Inform patients about advance directives
    c. Require patients to complete an advance directive
    d. Inform patients about a durable power of attorney for health care
    Answer: B. The Patient Self-Determination Act became federal law in 1991 and requires healthcare agencies to inform patients about advance directives upon admission. It does not require patients to fill out advance directives, only to be aware of their right to make decisions about these issues (Pope, 2013).

78. A patient diagnosed with colorectal cancer is on a continuous infusion of 5-fluorouracil. The patient calls to report symptoms of angina-like chest pain. Past medical history includes arteriosclerotic disease with associated renal and cardiac compromise. The APN recognizes the chest pain is most likely caused by
    a. Congestive heart failure.
    b. Ventricular arrhythmias.
    c. Arterial vasocontractions.
    d. Decreased left ventricular ejection fraction.
    Answer: C. 5-Fluorouracil is known to produce arterial vasocontractions that could cause chest pain. In addition, risk factors for the development of cardiotoxicity identified in a group of 668 patients receiving 5-fluorouracil or capecitabine included preexisting cardiac and renal disease. When cardiotoxicity from 5-fluorouracil does occur, it most frequently is associated with the first course of a continuous infusion of the drug (Francis, 2014).

79. Which of the following best describes heart disease risk for patients who received radiation to the left breast?

a. It is no greater in women who received radiation therapy to the right breast.

b. It continues to rise each year after treatment has ended for the patient's entire lifetime.

c. It continues to decrease annually, reaching equal risk as having radiation therapy to the right breast.

d. It remains greater than for women who had radiation therapy to the right breast at 20 years after treatment.

Answer: D. Even 20 years after treatment, the risk of heart disease appears to be greater in women who received radiation to the left breast as compared to the right breast (Goody et al., 2013).

80. A patient presents to the APN with a headache, confusion, and some visual and neurologic disturbances. The patient has colorectal cancer and is currently being treated with bevacizumab, irinotecan, leucovorin, and 5-fluorouracil. The most appropriate diagnostic test for the APN to order is

a. A CT scan.

b. An MRI.

c. An electroencephalogram.

d. A lumbar puncture.

Answer: B. The incidence of reversible posterior leukoencephalopathy syndrome (RPLS) in patients receiving bevacizumab has been reported to be less than 0.5%. The signs of RPLS include headache, seizure, lethargy, confusion, blindness, and other visual and neurologic disturbances. Mild to severe hypertension may be present but is not necessary. An MRI is used to confirm a diagnosis. Symptoms have been reported to begin from 16 hours to one year after start of bevacizumab. If RPLS occurs, discontinue bevacizumab and treat hypertension, if present. Symptoms usually resolve or improve within days, but patients may experience ongoing neurologic sequelae. No data exist that demonstrate safety of reinitiating bevacizumab therapy in patients previously experiencing RPLS (Genentech, Inc., 2015; Wang, Zhao, Lin, & Feng, 2014).

81. A woman with non-small cell lung cancer is being treated with docetaxel and is nearing a cumulative dose of 400 mg/m^2. The patient describes constant tearing in her right eye for the last several days. After a baseline ophthalmic examination is completed, the APN must

a. Rule out canalicular inflammation associated with canalicular duct stenosis and begin topical antibiotics and steroids.

b. Rule out conjunctivitis from a compromised immune system and order topical antibiotics.

c. Rule out a blocked tear duct and consider whether surgical removal of the canalicular and nasolacrimal ducts may be necessary.

d. Rule out trichomegaly irritating the cornea and recommend trimming of the eyelashes.

Answer: A. For patients who are undergoing weekly docetaxel therapy, epiphora is an expected side effect and is seen at median doses of 400 mg/m^2. Docetaxel is secreted in tears, causing irritation of the eye, and may cause canalicular inflammation and blockage of tear ducts with epiphora. Weekly docetaxel is associated with a 64% incidence rate of development of epiphora and canalicular stenosis. Erosive conjunctivitis may be reversible, but punctal stenosis may not be (Esmaeli et al., 2006). Patients on weekly docetaxel should be seen by an ophthalmologist at baseline and then every four to six weeks or more often as needed. Assess patients for excess tearing at baseline and prior to each dose. Topical antibiotics and dexamethasone may be useful. Surgery with silicone intubation of canalicular and nasolacrimal ducts may be needed to manage stenosis. Docetaxel may need to be discontinued. If the patient is still tearing, it is doubtful that the tear duct is blocked, but treatment is necessary to minimize the occurrence of this side effect (Ho & Mackey, 2014; Yamagishi, Ochi, Yamane, Hasebe, & Takigawa, 2014).

82. Which of the following characterizes quality-of-life interventions that are designed to prevent, anticipate, and treat suffering and are driven by patient- and family-centered care?
    a. Hospice care
    b. Intensive care
    c. Palliative care
    d. Supportive care
    Answer: C. Palliative care is the overriding construct that characterizes care driven by the patient and/or family and focuses on quality of life. Palliative care uses interventions to provide symptom management to patients (CMS, 2013; National Consensus Project for Quality Palliative Care, 2013).

83. An important nursing strategy in the management of cluster symptoms is to
    a. Assess the symptoms with one assessment scale.
    b. Assess the symptoms using multiple assessment approaches.
    c. Treat each symptom one by one to bring about a positive response.
    d. Treat the symptom that the patient identifies as the most burdensome.
    Answer: B. An important nursing strategy related to the management of symptoms in clusters is to assess the symptoms using multiple assessment approaches according to their complexity (Aktas, 2013). Treating each symptom one by one may not have a positive effect on another symptom.

84. The focus of care in palliative care is
    a. The family.
    b. The patient.
    c. The healthcare team.
    d. The patient and family.
    Answer: D. The patient and family are the unit of care in palliative care. The family is expected to provide "hands on" care and may experience more deleterious effects of caregiving during the time of advanced disease and require more assistance from palliative care at that time (NCCN, 2015f).

85. The wife of a patient being cared for by hospice tells the APN, "I just can't take this. I am exhausted and can't take care of my husband anymore." The APN's most appropriate response to the wife is
    a. "You are the only one who is able to take care of your husband."
    b. "We will have to change your husband's benefits so that he can go back in the hospital."
    c. "Tell me more about how you are feeling, and let's try to identify ways that we can get you more support."
    d. "Your comments are very selfish. I am sure that your husband would have taken care of you if you were dying."

Answer: C. Family caregiver vulnerability has become a well-acknowledged aspect of palliative care (Davies & Steele, 2010; Harding et al., 2012). Family members often are responsible for decision making about palliative care services, completing household tasks, working outside of the home, and intervening with multiple healthcare providers (Grant et al., 2013). These demands may impart considerable challenges onto an existing stressful situation. Family members caring for patients who are dying require significant support and guidance in their role as caregiver.

86. The major role of the APN with a doctor of nursing practice (DNP) degree as opposed to a PhD is to
    a. Close the long-standing gap between research and practice.
    b. Perform clinical research at the point of care.
    c. Perform rigorous scientific research.
    d. Remain mostly focused on academics.
    Answer: B. Closing the long-standing gap between research and practice is the responsibility of all oncology APNs with advanced degrees. But the oncology APN with a DNP has more of a clinical research focus and is not expected to remain academically focused (Edwardson, 2010; Rolfe & Davies, 2009; Vincent, Johnson, Velasquez, & Rigney, 2010).

87. A patient is considering enrolling in a phase II clinical trial. Which of the following statements demonstrates that the patient has an accurate understanding of the purpose of this clinical trial?
    a. "I hope I can help someone else someday by taking part in this clinical trial."
    b. "I hope my cancer will be cured by this new treatment."
    c. "I hope I am not in the treatment group that receives the placebo."
    d. "I hope this new treatment will help me live to see my daughter's graduation."
    Answer: A. The purpose of phase I and II clinical trials is to evaluate the safety of the drug by determining the correct dosage and to determine efficacy for specific cancer(s). It is not known whether participants in phase I or II clinical trials will benefit from the drugs because the main outcome assessed is tolerability of the drug at various doses and efficacy in certain cancers. Phase III clinical trials can offer more hope to participants that their cancer may actually be treated more successfully than with the current treatments available. Phase III trials also typically use a comparison group of standard of care or placebo (National Cancer Institute [NCI], 2013).

88. The purpose of an institutional review board (IRB) is to
    a. Design clinical trials based on input from leading researchers in the institution.
    b. Ensure that consent is obtained and documented as appropriate.
    c. Protect the rights and welfare of researchers.
    d. Ensure that participants in clinical trials are paid fairly for their participation.
    Answer: B. IRBs have four major purposes: (a) protect the rights and welfare of research participants, (b) determine that potential benefits are greater than the risks, (c) ensure that research participant recruitment is equitable, and (d) ensure that consent is obtained and documented when appropriate (U.S. FDA, 2015). If clinical trial participants are being paid, IRBs would be concerned as to whether this presents an ethical conflict.

89. A patient is considering using essential oils to treat pain. The APN is concerned that untoward effects associated with CAM may affect the patient's current conventional medical treatment. Which of the following websites would provide both the APN and

patient with current and comprehensive evidence-based information on CAM treatment?

    a. Micromedex Solutions

    b. WebMD

    c. Wikipedia

    d. NCCIH

Answer: D. Although Micromedex Solutions is a good resource to obtain information on medication interactions with CAM, it will not provide comprehensive information on other characteristics of each CAM or detailed information on the research. WebMD and Wikipedia tend to be more patient focused and may not be as current. The NCCIH website is comprehensive, current, and a valuable resource for APNs and patients alike (NCCIH, 2015).

90. Which of the following is a reason why patients might not discuss CAM with their provider?

    a. There are always too many other issues to discuss during the office visit.

    b. Patients are too embarrassed to admit they are taking CAM.

    c. Providers never ask their patients if they were using CAM.

    d. Patients are not interested in using CAM.

Answer: C. Rizzo and Xie (2006) surveyed 1,559 patients about their reasons for not discussing CAM with their providers. The number-one response was that their providers never asked about their CAM use. Many CAM therapies support a health- and wellness-focused lifestyle and are of interest to patients, especially if they are thought to be beneficial in treating symptoms or disease. CAM use is increasing. The 2007 National Center for Health Statistics/NCCIH survey indicated that 38% of adults in the United States had used some form of CAM therapy during the previous 12 months (Barnes, Bloom, & Nahin, 2008).

91. The APN is frustrated with the billboards and newspapers advertising Curamin® and its ability to treat pain. The APN considers this false advertising and is concerned that patients may be misled by it. What resource should the APN use to report this and determine if laws have been broken?

    a. MedWatch

    b. Better Business Bureau

    c. American Cancer Society

    d. National Cancer Institute

Answer: A. MedWatch allows healthcare professionals and consumers to report problems that they experience or suspect related to certain FDA-regulated products. This, in turn, compiles a list of recalls and other information that is available to the public. Although the Better Business Bureau may offer beneficial information on how to stop scams and other fraud and promote honest advertising, the official government agency designed for this specific example is a division of FDA, MedWatch (Better Business Bureau, n.d.; U.S. FDA, n.d.). ACS has a hotline to report fraud and abuse, but the MedWatch program is designed to handle fraud reports in relation to CAM (ACS, n.d.). Although NCI is designed to monitor fraud, it is more so in the context of research that it sponsors.

92. The APN is discussing code status with a patient. The patient is leaning toward instituting a do-not-resuscitate (DNR) order but asks for further clarification, ask-

ing "If I have a DNR order, will I still receive chemotherapy?" How should the APN respond?

a. "No, because if you decide to have a DNR order, the team will call hospice."
b. "No, you are no longer eligible to receive further chemotherapy."
c. "Yes, if you are eligible to receive further chemotherapy."
d. "Yes, but a DNR order would not be recommended then."

Answer: C. The patient can receive full and aggressive care. A DNR order does not mean that a patient has six months or less to live, which is a criterion for entry into hospice care. Eligibility for chemotherapy and contemplation of DNR status should be considered separately. More importantly, if the patient is eligible for chemotherapy, code status has little bearing on continuation of treatment. Patients often do make the decision to forgo further treatment when they are discussing DNR, but those decisions do not have to be dependent on one another (American Nurses Association [ANA], 2012).

93. The intent to benefit the patient by prescribing chemotherapy even though the patient will likely experience side effects is an example of what?

a. Autonomy
b. Beneficence
c. Nonmaleficence
d. Justice

Answer: B. Beneficence is the intent to do good, even when it is known that adverse effects may result from the action. The overriding thought in this situation is that the APN knows chemotherapy is intended to control or cure the cancer. Autonomy describes patients' ability to make their own decisions regarding their care. Nonmaleficence is defined as doing no harm. Justice is the obligation to be fair in all interactions and distribution of resources with patients (ANA, 2011).

94. A patient has requested a palliative referral while in the hospital with challenging pain. What is one of the major factors that would influence the APN's decision?

a. Patients seen by palliative care have shorter survivals.
b. Patients in palliative care are usually treated more aggressively, especially at the end of life.
c. Patients seen by palliative care are more likely to be enrolled in hospice.
d. Patients in palliative care have lower symptom intensity.

Answer: D. Unlike A, B, and C, answer D is supported by the findings in the literature. Because the patient is experiencing pain that is not well controlled, this would be a great opportunity to optimize pain control by including palliative care on the treatment team (Bakitas et al., 2009; Bischoff, Weinberg, & Rabow, 2013; Bükki et al., 2013; Follwell et al., 2009; Temel et al., 2010).

95. A patient is confused about the difference between palliative care and hospice care. Which of the following might clarify this for the patient?

a. Hospice is the same as palliative care.
b. Palliative care is a part of hospice care.
c. Palliative care and hospice care are entirely different with different purposes.
d. Hospice care is a part of palliative care.

Answer: D. According to the National Quality Forum's consensus report, "Palliative care refers to patient- and family-centered care that optimizes quality of life by anticipating, preventing, and treating suffering. Palliative care throughout the continuum of illness involves addressing physical, intellectual, emotional, social, and spiritual needs and facilitating patient autonomy, access to information, and choice" (National Quality Forum, 2006, p. 3). In that same report, hospice care is defined as "a service delivery system that provides palliative care for patients who have a limited life expectancy and require comprehensive biomedical, psychosocial, and spiritual support as they enter the terminal stage of an illness or condition. It also supports family members coping with the complex consequences of illness, disability, and aging as death nears. Hospice care further addresses the bereavement needs of the family following the death of the patient" (p. 3).

96. A patient is hesitant to enroll in hospice because of the belief that life-prolonging therapies will be discontinued. What is an appropriate response?
    a. "This is correct. Patients first need to decide to discontinue the therapies."
    b. "Therapies that are discontinued in hospice are evaluated and discussed with the patient."
    c. "All treatments are allowed in hospice, so there is no need to worry."
    d. "All treatments are allowed if the prognosis is less than two weeks."
    Answer: B. Treatments or prescription drugs intended to cure a terminal illness are not covered by the hospice benefit. It is sometimes difficult to determine whether an intervention is being used to cure a disease or provide symptom management. Many of these interventions intended to provide only symptom management can also be very expensive and are therefore a limiting factor for the hospice's budget. Other interventions that are not covered include room and board, emergency department visits, inpatient care, and ambulance transportation unless it is arranged by hospice (CMS, n.d.-c). If the intervention is related to a diagnosis other than the reason the patient is on hospice, then the patient's Medicare or usual insurance may continue to cover the medications and other therapies as they have in the past (CMS, n.d.-b).

97. What is the primary source of reimbursement for hospices?
    a. Private insurance carriers
    b. Self-pay
    c. Social Security
    d. Medicare Hospice Benefit
    Answer: D. Since it was established in 1982, the primary source of payment for hospice services in the United States is the Medicare Hospice Benefit. In 2011, the program paid for 84% of hospice costs while private insurance paid for 7.7% and self-pay accounted for 1.1% (National Hospice and Palliative Care Organization, 2012).

98. The patient has just died, and the patient's lifelong partner is hesitant to acknowledge the death because the couple had been very careful to keep their homosexual relationship a secret. This fact is making it hard for the partner to heal emotionally. This is an example of what type of grief?
    a. Disenfranchised
    b. Prolonged
    c. Anticipatory
    d. Normal
    Answer: A. Disenfranchised grief occurs when loss cannot be openly acknowledged. Examples of these type of situations include the death of a person in a "nonsanctioned" relationship such as extramarital affairs or homosexual relationships (Jenkins, Edmund-

son, Averett, & Yoon, 2014). Prolonged grief is persistent, severe yearning for the deceased beyond 6–12 months after the loss (Bryant, 2013). Anticipatory grief describes the psychological, social, and somatic responses to an anticipated loss (Buglass, 2010; Corless, 2010).

99. What is the government agency established to fund research on improving the quality and length of survival for all patients with cancer and to educate healthcare professionals, survivors, and caregivers about critical issues for optimal well-being?
    a. Livestrong Foundation
    b. Office of Cancer Survivorship
    c. Institute of Medicine
    d. American Society of Clinical Oncology
    Answer: B. The Office of Cancer Survivorship was created in 1996 to further educate healthcare professionals and caregivers on the needs of cancer survivors and determine how to better meet those needs. This program is part of the Division of Cancer Control and Population Sciences at NCI (n.d.). The Livestrong Foundation, formerly known as the Lance Armstrong Foundation, has programs that serve to bring awareness to the cancer experience and encourage ways to address unmet needs of survivors (Livestrong Foundation, n.d.). IOM is not a government agency. It was designed to create and share "unbiased and authoritative advice" (IOM, n.d.). ASCO is a society of medical professionals who offer research and education, prevention strategies, and quality care to "conquer cancer" (ASCO, 2015).

100. According to NCCN guidelines, what are the most common long-term effects of cancer treatment?
    a. Pain, infertility, impaired hearing
    b. Fatigue, depression, anxiety, pain
    c. Dyspnea, impaired vision and swallowing
    d. Structural/functional changes, urinary incontinence
    Answer: B. The most commonly reported symptoms in cancer survivors are fatigue, depression, anxiety, and pain. These symptoms also interfere most with patients' ability to perform activities of daily living (NCCN, 2015c).

101. A 69-year-old woman presents for her two-year follow-up after treatment for breast cancer. She is still not sleeping well or motivated to perform her usual activities of daily living. She experiences fatigue throughout the day. Based on this information, what additional questions should the APN ask?
    a. What are the patient's social supports? What social activities is the patient involved in? Does the patient have a close friend she can confide in?
    b. Does the patient have trouble falling asleep or staying asleep? Does the patient take sleep aids?
    c. When was the last time the patient had a complete blood count done? How is the patient eating?
    d. Has the patient been exposed to anyone who is ill? Did the patient receive a flu vaccine?
    Answer: A. Stanton (2012) determined that risk factors for poor adjustment and functional limitations include insufficient social support, social seclusion, and lack of intimate partner. Protective factors include optimistic outlook, using problem-solving strategies, and conveying emotions. Also, coping deteriorates with age (Goldzweig et al., 2013).

102. Which of the following is a useful psychological well-being screening tool consisting of a single item?
    a. State-Trait Anxiety Inventory (STAI)
    b. Hospital Anxiety and Depression Scale (HADS)
    c. Mini-Mental State Examination (MMSE)
    d. NCCN Distress Thermometer

    Answer: D. The NCCN Distress Thermometer has demonstrated validity and concordance with HADS. Unlike HADS, however, it only has one item that is required to determine distress level (NCCN, 2015c). STAI is a diagnostic tool that identifies anxiety versus depression. It has been used to identify caregiver distress as well (American Psychological Association, n.d.). The MMSE consists of 11 items that were designed to briefly screen for cognitive impairment and cognitive changes over time (Velayudhan et al., 2014).

103. The Americans With Disabilities Act states that a cancer survivor is protected from being terminated from a job as long as
    a. The survivor is qualified for and can perform all responsibilities of the job.
    b. The survivor does not require any special accommodations.
    c. The employer has no one else qualified to do the survivor's job.
    d. The employer has more than three employees.

    Answer: A. Cancer survivors are protected under federal and state laws as long as they are qualified for and can perform the major responsibilities of the job. The employer is responsible for providing reasonable accommodations for the cancer survivor to perform the job (Valdivieso, Kujawa, Jones, & Baker, 2012).

104. A 56-year-old man is being treated with sunitinib for renal cell cancer. He has been receiving scheduled ondansetron for nausea and vomiting. He is having chronic escalating pain that requires a long-acting, inexpensive opioid. In addition, he has a history of atrial fibrillation. Which opioid would NOT be a good choice for him?
    a. Extended-release morphine
    b. Methadone
    c. Extended-release oxycodone
    d. Transdermal fentanyl

    Answer: B. Sunitinib therapy increases the risk for QT interval prolongation and appears to be dose dependent (Bello et al., 2009). Although methadone is a very inexpensive opioid, its risk can increase when combined with other medications that also increase QT interval, such as ondansetron. Prolongation of QT interval can lead to fatal torsades de pointes (Miranda, McMain, & Smith, 2011).

105. The patient has been on androgen deprivation therapy for several years for prostate cancer. Which of the following diseases is the patient at high risk for?
    a. A second cancer
    b. Hypothyroidism
    c. Idiopathic lung disease
    d. Coronary heart disease

    Answer: D. Although it is not certain if androgen deprivation therapy actually increases mortality, it does increase the risk for cardiovascular events. Careful monitoring of cardiovascular risk and clinical management is recommended (Allan, Collins, Frydenberg, McLachlan, & Matthiesson, 2014).

106. A 49-year-old man presents to the oncology APN with heart failure. He received his first dose of docetaxel the day before. He has no history of heart failure. He asks if his heart failure can be reversed. What would be the best response?
    a. Yes. Heart failure caused by acute toxicity is usually reversible.
    b. Yes. Heart failure is reversible if the patient has low-risk factors for congestive heart failure (CHF).
    c. No. Docetaxel causes irreparable heart damage.
    d. No. It is advised that patients continue their docetaxel. CHF will continue to be a problem.

    Answer: C. Heart failure may occur with anthracycline administration as an acute, early-onset, or late-onset toxicity. Heart failure caused by acute toxicity usually is reversible. Early onset occurs within the first year following treatment. Late onset occurs more than one year after treatment and can occur as late as 10 years following completion of therapy (Bonita & Pradhan, 2013; Bowles et al., 2012; Yeh & Bickford, 2009).

107. A 66-year-old man will be initiating gemcitabine treatment for his pancreatic cancer. Past medical history includes hypercholesterolemia, hypertension, diabetes, chronic obstructive pulmonary disease, and 30-pack-year smoking. Which prevention recommendation would be most valuable for him at this time?
    a. Stop smoking.
    b. Increase antihypertensive medication.
    c. Decrease daily insulin.
    d. Increase use of inhaler.

    Answer: A. Gemcitabine is a risk factor for interstitial pneumonitis. Synergistic personal risk factors include cigarette smoking, age older than 70 or very young age, prior radiation therapy to the lungs, preexisting pulmonary disease, and high fraction of inspired oxygen. The major preventable risk factor for interstitial pneumonitis is to counsel the patient to stop smoking (Dang et al., 2013; Hamid & Carvajal, 2013; Kharofa, Cohen, Tomic, Xiang, & Gore, 2012; Venkatramani et al., 2013).

108. A 64-year-old woman with lung cancer is currently on bevacizumab. She presents with fever, chills, breathlessness, unproductive cough, and severe dyspnea. The chest x-ray and CT scan demonstrate ground-glass linear opacities. The oncology APN has ordered a complete blood count, urinalysis, virology test, and cultures of blood and sputum. These tests are all negative. The APN's next consideration may be to order
    a. A bronchoscopy with bronchoalveolar lavage.
    b. An open lung biopsy.
    c. Pulmonary function tests.
    d. A brain scan.

    Answer: A. The symptoms that this patient is experiencing could lead to a diagnosis of pneumonitis, especially after having received bevacizumab, but this diagnosis is one of exclusion. The differentials of infection or disease progression should be ruled out. An open lung biopsy may be risky with bevacizumab therapy. Pulmonary function tests characterize the pattern of obstructive versus restrictive abnormality and severity of respiratory impairment and probably would not be directly helpful in making a conclusive diagnosis. A brain scan also is not directly helpful in determining the differential at this point. The bronchoscopy would yield the best information to help rule out disease progression, infection, or pneumonitis (Grünwald et al., 2013).

109. Glucocorticoid therapy may be initiated for diagnosis of pneumonitis. When should the oncology APN expect to see clinical and also radiographic improvement?
    a. Weeks for clinical, months for radiographic
    b. Hours for clinical, weeks for radiographic
    c. Months for clinical, weeks to months for radiographic
    d. Days for clinical, weeks to months for radiographic

    Answer: D. Although pneumonitis can be a potentially fatal complication, if it is successfully treated, clinical improvement will be seen within days. Radiographic improvement, however, will take weeks to months. Steroid therapy cannot reverse damage caused by fibrosis but will stop further inflammation and damage it may cause (Hadjinicolaou, Nisar, Parfrey, Chilvers, & Östör, 2012).

110. A 68-year-old woman presents with multiple myeloma and will be starting bortezomib therapy. She is diabetic and has baseline peripheral neuropathies manifested as numbness in her feet. She is able to perform all of her ADLs. What dose of bortezomib should the oncology APN initiate for this patient?
    a. Reduced dose of 1 mg/m^2 and administer subcutaneously (SC)
    b. Normal dose of 1.3 mg/m^2 and administer IV
    c. Normal dose of 1.3 mg/m^2 and administer SC
    d. Reduced dose of 1 mg/m^2 and administer IV

    Answer: C. There is no dose adjustment for grade 1 peripheral neuropathy, but clinical trials with SC administration of bortezomib support reduced risk of peripheral neuropathy. Because the patient is at higher risk for peripheral neuropathy at baseline, SC administration is recommended. If the patient's peripheral neuropathy progresses to grade 2, then a dose reduction to 1 mg/m^2 will be advised. It is much easier to prevent peripheral neuropathy than to treat it (Millennium Pharmaceuticals, Inc., 2012).

111. A 67-year-old patient is receiving capecitabine and presents with pain and tingling of the hands and feet. The oncology APN also notes edema, erythema, tenderness, and desquamation. The patient is most likely experiencing
    a. Peripheral neuropathy.
    b. Chemotherapy extravasation.
    c. Cellulitis.
    d. Hand-foot syndrome.

    Answer: D. Peripheral neuropathy may present with pain and tingling but usually does not accompany any overt skin changes. Tingling, burning, pain, erythema, and swelling may be present with early chemotherapy extravasation and blistering and later signs of necrosis and ulceration. Because capecitabine is not a vesicant, extravasation would not be in the differential (Fidalgo et al., 2012). Cellulitis could certainly be in the differential with its erythema, swelling, pain, and warmth but may also be accompanied by fever and elevated white blood cell count. Because the symptoms occurred shortly after the administration of capecitabine, it is likely that the patient is experiencing hand-foot syndrome (Miller, Gorcey, & McLellan, 2014).

112. Treatment of acneform rashes in an individual taking cetuximab includes
    a. Tetracycline.
    b. Chlorpromazine.
    c. Cimetidine.
    d. NSAIDs.

Answer: A. Tetracycline and minocycline have been cited as effective for early phases of exanthema. They reportedly assist in the management of pruritus, burning, stinging, and overall skin irritation (Wehler et al., 2013).

113. What treatment should the oncology APN recommend for xerosis cutis?
    a. Nondrying soaps
    b. Bath soaks
    c. Moisturizing ointments
    d. Emollients with urea
    Answer: D. Xerosis cutis, or dry skin, is a common side effect of many systemic cancer therapies. It can be accentuated with older age. Recommendations to avoid all soaps is the standard of care with xerosis cutis. Bath soaks may aggravate dry skin. Ointments may cause follicular occlusion and lead to folliculitis. Standard emollients, especially those containing urea, are suggested as a treatment for xerosis cutis (Bensadoun et al., 2013).

114. Drug regimens combine drugs that have synergy but minimal overlapping toxicities, such as CHOP: cyclophosphamide, doxorubicin, vincristine, and prednisone. In the CHOP regimen, what are the two drugs with myelosuppressive side effects?
    a. Cyclophosphamide and doxorubicin
    b. Cyclophosphamide and vincristine
    c. Doxorubicin and vincristine
    d. Vincristine and prednisone
    Answer: A. The myelosuppression with cyclophosphamide occurs in 7–10 days, whereas that of doxorubicin occurs in 10–14 days. Vincristine and prednisone are nonmyelosuppressive, but vincristine is neurotoxic, and prednisone causes hyperglycemia and other side effects. The regimens were developed to be given in the ambulatory setting and commonly are dosed in schedules with a cycle every 21 days so that normal cells can recover before the next cycle (Wilkes, 2011).

115. A common side effect of irinotecan is
    a. Cardiomyopathy.
    b. Peripheral neuropathy.
    c. Persistent, delayed diarrhea.
    d. Severe nausea and vomiting.
    Answer: C. A common side effect of irinotecan is persistent, delayed diarrhea. Patients should be taught to take an aggressive regimen of loperamide—4 mg at the first sign of diarrhea and then 2 mg every two hours until 12 hours have passed without any diarrhea (should not exceed 48 hours of loperamide at these doses)—and should be monitored closely. Patients should receive IV hydration if they are unable to maintain oral hydration, should be given antidiarrheals (e.g., octreotide) for grade 3 or 4 diarrhea and should be started on antibiotics if the diarrhea persists after 24 hours or if ileus, fever, or neutropenia develops (Pharmacia & Upjohn Co., 2014).

116. Cardiotoxicity is known to occur with the use of trastuzumab. Because of this toxicity, how often is monitoring for left ventricular ejection fraction (LVEF) recommended?
    a. Baseline only
    b. Baseline and after each treatment
    c. Baseline and at completion of treatment
    d. Baseline, every three months during treatment, and upon completion of treatment

Answer: D. Monitoring for LVEF when administering trastuzumab is recommended at baseline, every three months during treatment, and upon completion of treatment. The drug should be held for at least four weeks for (a) 16% or greater absolute decrease in LVEF from pretreatment values or (b) an LVEF value below institutional limits of normal and 10% or greater absolute decrease in LVEF from pretreatment values. Resume drug if, within four to eight weeks, the LVEF returns to within normal limits and the absolute decrease from baseline is 15% or less. Permanently discontinue trastuzumab for persistent (longer than eight weeks) decline in LVEF or for suspension of trastuzumab dosing on more than three occasions for cardiomyopathy (Genentech, Inc., 2014).

117. Which of the following is considered to be an absolute contraindication for breast-conserving therapy requiring radiation therapy?
    a. Tumors larger than 5 cm
    b. Tumors with focally positive margins
    c. Prior radiation therapy to the breast or chest wall
    d. Patients with connective tissue disease involving the skin
    Answer: C. A history of prior radiation therapy to the breast or chest wall is an absolute contraindication for breast-conserving therapy requiring radiation therapy. The other three contraindications are relative and are considered on an individual basis (NCCN, 2015b).

118. Which monoclonal antibody would be more likely to cause a hypersensitivity reaction when administered?
    a. Cetuximab
    b. Alemtuzumab
    c. Panitumumab
    d. Ibritumomab tiuxetan
    Answer: D. Monoclonal antibodies are made to be totally human (human, suffix -*umab*), mostly human and only a small part mouse (humanized, suffix -*zumab*), some mouse and some human (chimeric, suffix -*ximab*), or entirely mouse protein (murine, suffix -*momab*). The more mouse protein a monoclonal antibody contains, the greater the risk of hypersensitivity reactions when administered (Scott, Wolchok, & Old, 2012).

119. After completing her first infusion of rituximab, a patient informs the APN of difficulty breathing. The O_2 saturation on room air is 90% (baseline 99%). Physical assessment reveal crackles in the bases of both lungs. The APN's priority intervention would be to
    a. Initiate emergency medical system response.
    b. Obtain an electrocardiogram to rule out myocardial infarction.
    c. Order blood gases to determine the cause of dyspnea.
    d. Obtain a chest x-ray to rule out capillary leak syndrome.
    Answer: A. Rituximab has been implicated in rare sudden death within 24 hours of administration (symptom constellation includes hypoxia, pulmonary infiltrates, acute respiratory distress syndrome, myocardial infarction, ventricular fibrillation, or cardiogenic shock); 80% of fatal reactions occur after the first infusion. If symptoms appear, the drug must be stopped and lifesaving treatment begun. Because this is potentially an emergency situation, the patient should be supported through an emergency response approach until symptoms stabilize (Biogen Idec, Inc., & Genentech, Inc., 2014; Clifford et al., 2011).

120. The APN is doing medication teaching for a patient who has just been started on selective serotonin reuptake inhibitors (SSRIs) for cancer-related depression. What side effects will the APN review with the patient related to SSRIs?
    a. Agitation, gastrointestinal disturbance, and sexual dysfunction
    b. Agitation, gastrointestinal disturbance, and cognitive dysfunction
    c. Agitation, genitourinary disturbance, and cognitive dysfunction
    d. Agitation, genitourinary disturbance, and neuropathic pain

    Answer: A. General side effects of SSRIs include agitation, gastrointestinal disturbance, and sexual dysfunction. However, because SSRIs block the reuptake of only one neurotransmitter in the central nervous system (serotonin), they frequently are the medication of choice for depression because of their low side effect profile and low potential for overdose. SSRIs also are the drug of choice for patients experiencing symptoms of both depression and anxiety (Li, Fitzgerald, & Rodin, 2012; Traeger, Greer, Fernandez-Robles, Temel, & Pirl, 2012).

121. A patient presents to the APN with edema, muscle and joint aches, pruritus, ecchymosis, headache, and low-grade fever. The patient has completed chemotherapy for breast cancer and has been on tamoxifen for more than six months. Which laboratory test result would the APN expect to be abnormal?
    a. Complete blood count
    b. Alanine aminotransferase, aspartate aminotransferase
    c. Albumin
    d. Creatinine

    Answer: B. The most common presenting signs and symptoms of drug-induced liver injury include edema, pruritus, jaundice, malaise, headache, anorexia, ecchymosis, low-grade fever, muscle and joint aches, and urine and stool color changes. Hepatotoxicity is influenced by the chemical property of the drug, such as with tamoxifen; individual genetics, such as obesity and diabetes, which are common in women with breast cancer; and environmental factors. Because most liver test abnormalities occur 5–90 days after drug ingestion, the patient must be considered for drug-induced liver injury. Serum aminotransferases, alanine aminotransferase, and aspartate aminotransferase would be most frequently elevated with liver damage. Serum albumin and coagulation factors detect abnormalities of liver metabolism and synthesis. A decrease in serum albumin is seen in patients with cirrhosis and ascites. Serum albumin levels typically are normal in viral hepatitis, drug-induced liver injury, and obstructive jaundice (Mehta, 2012).

122. Which of the following represents the diagnostic criteria for dementia?
    a. Impairment in memory, orientation, and perception of an acute nature
    b. Impairment in memory, orientation, and perception of a chronic nature
    c. Impairment in memory, behavior, and personality of an acute nature
    d. Impairment in memory, behavior, and personality of a chronic nature

    Answer: D. Dementia, in contrast to delirium, is a chronic, irreversible, and progressive decline in cognitive functioning. Diagnostic criteria for dementia include impairment in memory, behavior, and personality, with memory loss being the most common sign (Downing, Caprio, & Lyness, 2013). Delirium is defined as a disturbance in attention and awareness that represents a change from baseline. It also must be accompanied by an additional disturbance in cognition (e.g., memory, orientation, language, visuospatial ability, perception) (American Psychiatric Association, 2013).

123. Cognitive deficits related to chemotherapy include all of the following EXCEPT
    a. Feelings of euphoria.
    b. Difficulty in planning.
    c. Difficulty with memory.
    d. Difficulty in decision making.

    Answer: A. Cognitive deficits related to chemotherapy administration range from having difficulty in the domains of executive function (e.g., planning, decision making), memory, information and processing speed, and attention (Wefel, Saleeba, Buzdar, & Meyers, 2010) to having no deficits other than motor slowing (Tager et al., 2010).

124. Which of the following nitrosoureas crosses the blood-brain barrier and acts as a radiosensitizer?
    a. Cisplatin
    b. Carmustine
    c. Lomustine
    d. Temozolomide

    Answer: D. Carmustine and lomustine are lipid soluble and cross the blood-brain barrier. Cisplatin is a radiosensitizer but does not cross the blood-brain barrier. Temozolomide crosses the blood-brain barrier and is a radiosensitizer (Merck & Co., Inc., 2015).

125. The most common acute side effects related to radiation therapy for breast cancer include
    a. Fatigue and alopecia.
    b. Fatigue and skin reaction.
    c. Fatigue and telangiectasia.
    d. Atrophy and fibrosis of the skin.

    Answer: B. The two most common acute side effects related to radiation therapy for breast cancer are fatigue and skin reaction (dermatitis). It is estimated that approximately 63% of women with breast cancer have fatigue at the onset of chemotherapy (Liu et al., 2009), reaching up to 80% while receiving treatment (de M Alcântara-Silva, Freitas-Junior, Freitas, & Machado, 2013). Late effects of radiation therapy to the skin include atrophy, scaling, fibrosis, telangiectasia, necrosis, and pigmentation changes (Archambeau, Pezner, & Wasserman, 1995; Davis et al., 2003; Harper, Franklin, Jenrette, & Aguero, 2004). These side effects arise months to years after treatment, typically are not reversible, and occur with dose ranges of 2.5–3 Gy/day.

126. A patient with small cell lung cancer comes into the office with complaints of cough, dyspnea, and a feeling of fullness in the head that is worse in the morning. The APN recognizes the symptoms may indicate
    a. Pleural effusion.
    b. Cardiac tamponade.
    c. Spinal cord compression.
    d. Superior vena cava syndrome (SVCS).

    Answer: D. The most common signs and symptoms related to SVCS include face or neck swelling (82%), upper extremity swelling (68%), dyspnea (66%), cough (50%), and dilated chest vein collaterals (38%) (Brumbaugh, 2011). Symptoms related to SVCS frequently are worse in the morning because the patient has been lying supine during the night.

127. A newly graduated nurse asks the APN when a patient with lymphoma may begin to experience relief of symptoms of SVCS after radiation therapy has been initiated. The APN's most appropriate response is which of the following?
    a. Within 24 hours
    b. Within three weeks
    c. Within two months
    d. Within three to four days

    Answer: D. Overall, patients may notice improvement in venous congestion within three to four days of treatment as a result of improved venous blood flow. Radiation therapy provides maximum symptom relief within three to four weeks in 70% of patients with lung cancer and 95% of patients with lymphoma (Drews & Rabkin, 2014; Nickloes et al., 2014).

128. The most common symptom of cardiac tamponade is
    a. Cough.
    b. Dyspnea.
    c. Chest pain.
    d. Hoarseness.

    Answer: B. Symptoms of cardiac tamponade can include cough, chest pain, and hoarseness, but the most common symptom of cardiac tamponade is dyspnea (Freter & Haddadin, 2014; Grannis, Kim, & Lai, 2014).

129. Of the following, which cancer is most likely to result in spinal cord compression (SCC)?
    a. Prostate cancer
    b. Acute myelocytic leukemia
    c. Acute lymphocytic leukemia
    d. Chronic lymphocytic leukemia

    Answer: A. Prostate cancer is the most likely to result in SCC, as the highest incidence of SCC occurs in patients with solid tumors that commonly metastasize to vertebral bone (Lewis, Hendrickson, & Moynihan, 2011).

130. A patient who is newly diagnosed with cancer complains of pain in the lower back that radiates around to the chest and a heaviness of the legs. The most appropriate test for the APN to order is
    a. Plain film x-rays.
    b. A lumbar puncture.
    c. An electromyography.
    d. An MRI.

    Answer: D. Pain and weakness are two of the most common symptoms related to SCC. MRI currently is the gold standard to evaluate for SCC because it allows visualization of the extent of the lesion and anatomy, detects paraspinal masses, and can image multiple levels to assess for areas of disease that are not clinically apparent (Becker & Baehring, 2011).

131. A patient newly diagnosed with acute promyelocytic leukemia complains of a headache and experiences vomiting unrelated to food intake. The APN recognizes these symptoms as
    a. Hypercalcemia.
    b. SVCS.
    c. Increased intracranial pressure.
    d. Disseminated intravascular coagulation.

Answer: C. Patients with acute promyelocytic leukemia often have a high blast cell count on diagnosis and are at risk for increased intracranial pressure (ICP). Increased ICP associated with leukemia also may be a result of hemorrhage caused by coagulopathy or thrombocytopenia (Rodriguez, 2014).

132. What is the most important strategy in treating a patient for disseminated intravascular coagulation (DIC)?
    a. Treat the clotting.
    b. Treat the bleeding.
    c. Treat the underlying cause.
    d. Treat the electrolyte imbalance.
    Answer: C. The first priority in managing DIC is to treat the underlying disorder. All other treatments will provide only temporary relief of the symptoms associated with DIC (Kaplan, 2013a).

133. The characteristic metabolic disturbances associated with tumor lysis syndrome (TLS) include
    a. Hyperkalemia, hyperuricemia, hypophosphatemia, and hypocalcemia.
    b. Hypokalemia, hyperuricemia, hyperphosphatemia, and hypercalcemia.
    c. Hyperkalemia, hyperuricemia, hyperphosphatemia, and hypocalcemia.
    d. Hyperkalemia, hyperuricemia, hyperphosphatemia, and hypercalcemia.
    Answer: C. When a cell is lysed as a result of chemotherapy or other precipitating factors, intracellular contents are released into the vascular system. These intracellular contents include potassium, nucleic acids (which are converted into uric acid in the kidneys), and phosphorus. The phosphorus binds to calcium in the circulation, which causes hypocalcemia (Lydon, 2011).

134. Which of the following patients has the greatest risk for the development of TLS?
    a. A patient with stage I breast cancer
    b. A patient with stage IIB colon cancer
    c. A patient with acute promyelocytic leukemia
    d. A patient with chronic myeloid leukemia
    Answer: C. Tumor lysis syndrome occurs most frequently in patients with lymphoproliferative malignancies or in patients with elevated white blood cell counts, such as high-grade lymphomas or acute leukemias (Fojo, 2011).

135. A patient is admitted to the hospital for treatment of a newly diagnosed Burkitt lymphoma. The patient has a large mediastinal tumor and positive retroperitoneal nodes. Which of the following medications is most important to order?
    a. Allopurinol
    b. Rasburicase
    c. Fluconazole
    d. Itraconazole
    Answer: B. For patients thought to be at high risk for TLS, prevention strategies include prophylactic hydration to maintain a urine output greater than 150–200 ml/hr and prophylactic rasburicase (Coiffier, Altman, Pui, Younes, & Cairo, 2008; Gobel, 2013).

136. A patient with metastatic breast cancer is admitted to the hospital with weakness, confusion, and serum calcium level of 13.5 mg/dl. What nonpharmacologic interventions are appropriate for this patient?

a. Encourage fluid intake, and put the patient on strict fall precautions.
b. Encourage fluid intake, and do not allow the patient to get out of bed.
c. Encourage fluid intake, and put the patient on standard fall precautions.
d. Encourage fluid intake, and allow the patient to walk without assistance.

Answer: A. The management of hypercalcemia requires improved renal calcium excretion that may be enhanced by good fluid intake (Kaplan, 2013b). Neurologic manifestations of hypercalcemia that include weakness and confusion can progress to coma and obtundation; thus, it is critical to provide for the patient's safety by instituting measures such as strict fall precautions.

137. Fifteen minutes into an infusion of asparaginase for the treatment of acute lymphocytic leukemia, the patient experiences flushing, dyspnea, wheezing, angioedema, and urticaria. The APN recognizes the symptoms as
    a. Sepsis.
    b. Anaphylaxis.
    c. Tumor lysis syndrome.
    d. Disseminated intravascular coagulation.

Answer: B. Presenting signs and symptoms of anaphylaxis vary significantly among patients. The most common are urticaria, angioedema, flushing, and pruritus (Eisenberg, 2013). Hypersensitivity reactions to asparaginase are common.

138. Sources of hematopoietic stem cells (HSCs) for allogeneic transplantation include all of the following EXCEPT
    a. Umbilical cord blood.
    b. HSCs from self.
    c. Matched sibling donor.
    d. Matched unrelated donor.

Answer: B. HSCs for allogeneic transplantation can be harvested from umbilical cord blood, matched sibling donors, and matched unrelated donors. Harvesting HSCs from the intended recipient is an autologous transplantation (Sureda et al., 2015).

139. How long must a transplant recipient be monitored for a delayed immune hemolysis response after receiving marrow from an ABO-mismatched donor?
    a. The rest of the patient's life
    b. One year after transplant
    c. The first 100 days after transplant
    d. Approximately four months after transplant

Answer: D. Because the life span of red blood cells is approximately 120 days, patients who have received marrow from an ABO-mismatched donor should be monitored for delayed immune hemolysis for approximately four months following transplant (AABB, American Red Cross, America's Blood Centers, & Armed Services Blood Program, 2013).

140. Graft-versus-host disease is best defined as
    a. A histocompatibility reaction that occurs between the recipient cells and the donor human leukocyte antigen cells
    b. An immune reaction that occurs between the recipient cells and the immunologically competent donor eosinophils
    c. An immune reaction that occurs between the recipient cells and the immunologically competent donor T lymphocytes

d. An immune reaction that occurs between the recipient cells and the immunologically competent donor B lymphocytes

Answer: C. Graft-versus-host disease is an immune reaction that occurs between the recipient cells and the immunologically competent donor T lymphocytes (Raza & Vierling, 2014).

141. The most common virus associated with oral mucositis in a patient who has received stem cells is
    a. Cytomegalovirus.
    b. Epstein-Barr virus.
    c. Herpes simplex virus.
    d. Human immunodeficiency virus-6.

Answer: C. The most common virus associated with oral mucositis in the stem cell recipient is herpes simplex virus (Kedia et al., 2013; Liu et al., 2013).

142. Sulfonamides are used prophylactically in patients undergoing stem cell transplantation to prevent
    a. *Aspergillus.*
    b. *Varicella zoster.*
    c. *Clostridium difficile.*
    d. *Pneumocystis jiroveci* pneumonia.

Answer: D. The prophylactic administration of sulfonamides (e.g., pentamidine, dapsone) is used in patients undergoing stem cell transplantation to prevent *Pneumocystis jiroveci* pneumonia (Kedia et al., 2013; Tomblyn et al., 2009).

143. A patient who had undergone breast-conserving treatment with a lumpectomy is scheduled for boost radiation. What should the APN include as part of the teaching regarding the boost radiation?
    a. Boost radiation is delivered to the entire breast and is given to eliminate a recurrence of the cancer.
    b. Boost radiation is given to the surgical scar and is given to decrease the risk of recurrence of the cancer.
    c. Boost radiation is given to the surgical scar and is given to eliminate the risk of recurrence of the cancer.
    d. Boost radiation is delivered to the localized area where the tumor was removed and is given to eliminate a recurrence of the cancer.

Answer: B. Patients undergoing breast-conserving treatment commonly receive treatment to what is known as a *boost field*. This field usually is treated alone once the patient has completed treatment to the entire breast. This treatment field is around the surgical scar, and treatment is aimed at local tissues, as this area has a high chance for recurrence. Treatment is commonly given to women who are younger than age 50 and in those who have high-grade disease (NCCN, 2015b).

144. Which of the following are considered common side effects related to radiation therapy for breast cancer?
    a. Fatigue and infection
    b. Fatigue and skin reaction
    c. Alopecia and pancytopenia
    d. Anemia and thrombocytopenia

Answer: B. The two most common acute side effects related to RT for breast cancer are fatigue and skin reaction (dermatitis). It is estimated that approximately 63% of women with breast cancer have fatigue at the onset of chemotherapy (Liu et al., 2009), reaching up to 80% while receiving treatment (de M Alcântara-Silva et al., 2013). Significant amounts of bone marrow are not included in the fields for radiation therapy for breast cancer; thus, low blood counts and infection are not common side effects.

145. A patient with colorectal cancer is receiving concomitant 5-fluorouracil and radiation therapy. Which of the following is an important teaching strategy to explain to this patient?
    a. Diarrhea typically occurs toward the end of treatment and generally is not a problem for most patients.
    b. Constipation typically occurs toward the end of treatment and generally is not a problem for most patients.
    c. Diarrhea typically occurs one to two weeks into treatment, and the amount and duration of diarrhea should be assessed routinely.
    d. Constipation typically occurs one to two weeks into treatment, and the patient should contact the healthcare provider, as it often can be serious.
    Answer: C. Diarrhea typically occurs one to two weeks into treatment and can worsen with the administration of chemotherapy. The amount and duration of diarrhea are patient dependent and should be routinely assessed. Dietary modifications, such as a low-residue diet, and over-the-counter and prescription medications may be necessary, as well as IV fluids, depending on the patient's vital signs at the time of assessment. A dietitian may work with the team, particularly if probiotics are incorporated into the patient's diet (Delia et al., 2007; Visich & Yeo, 2010).

146. Late effects of radiation therapy to the colorectal area include
    a. Fatigue and skin reactions.
    b. Fatigue and sexuality issues.
    c. Enteritis and sexuality issues.
    d. Enteritis and delayed immunosuppression.
    Answer: C. Late effects in this population may include enteritis and sexuality issues. Enteritis is characterized by dysmotility and malabsorption (Shadad, Sullivan, Martin, & Egan, 2013). Sexuality issues include dyspareunia, vaginal dryness, and vaginal stenosis in women, and weakened orgasm and erectile dysfunction in men.

147. An important teaching strategy for a patient receiving radiation therapy to the breast is that the patient will
    a. Have the entire breast exposed during the radiation therapy.
    b. Need to be completely exposed during the radiation therapy.
    c. Be able to be covered by a gown during the radiation therapy.
    d. Have the entire breast exposed during the radiation therapy, but no one will see the patient during this time.
    Answer: A. Because it can cause emotional distress, women must understand that during the radiation treatments to the breast, the entire breast will be exposed (see Chapter 6). They also need to know that a camera and microphone will be present in the treatment area so that the radiation therapy technician can see the patient and know that the patient is safe.

148. Which of the following assessment criteria takes priority when caring for a patient with cancer and depression?
    a. Anger
    b. Delirium
    c. Suicidal ideation
    d. Unrelenting pain

    Answer: C. Too often, healthcare professionals assume that psychological distress is normal for patients with cancer and overlook its significant impact. Patients with cancer have a higher rate of depression than the general population, and depressive states place patients at a higher risk for suicide (Anguiano, Mayer, Piven, & Rosenstein, 2012).

149. A patient appears anxious and inquires about the next doctor's visit for the patient's first chemotherapy treatment. Which response by the APN would be most appropriate to help alleviate the patient's fears?
    a. "Didn't the doctor already review the treatment with you?"
    b. "Chemotherapy is not your enemy; it is to try to cure you."
    c. "Everyone is scared of chemotherapy, but everyone survives."
    d. "It is normal to feel anxious about chemotherapy. Let me tell you what to expect."

    Answer: D. Fear and anxiety result from a perceived threat or apprehension regarding the unknown. Educating patients about what to expect when undergoing tests, procedures, or a new treatment such as chemotherapy helps them to regain a sense of control over their cancer and cancer treatment (Stafford et al., 2013) (see Chapter 17).

150. Which of the following statements regarding sexuality is true?
    a. Changes in body image are the only predictors of sexual self-image.
    b. A person is considered asexual if he or she is not able to engage in intercourse.
    c. The emotional responses to body image changes such as mastectomy are consistent among all patients.
    d. Emotions such as fear, anxiety, and depression can exacerbate feelings of loss related to changes in body image.

    Answer: D. Emotional responses to body image changes are personal; what is normal for one person may be considered abnormal for another. Many factors influence the emotional responses to body image changes, including the patient's values, cultural and religious norms, and past and present life experiences (Bober & Varela, 2012).

151. The APN is meeting with a patient who is starting treatment for breast cancer. Which of the following conveys the importance of sexual health and encourages the patient to ask questions at any time?
    a. "I can have the physician see you if you have any questions about your sexual health."
    b. "Is there anything that I have not reviewed with you that you would like to know?"
    c. "If you have any questions about infertility related to your breast cancer treatment, I can give you a referral to a fertility specialist."
    d. "Do you have any questions or sexual concerns that you would like to discuss? This is an important topic and no question is silly or off limits."

    Answer: D. The sexual health of patients with cancer is an important component of psychosocial management, and disturbance in sexual being can negatively affect psychological health and quality of life. Sexual dysfunction related to cancer can occur as a result of the disease or treatment-induced side effects. When performing a sexual assessment, clinicians should use an integrated approach that incorporates physical, psychological, relational, social, and cultural components (Bober & Varela, 2012). Pretreatment sexual assessments can be helpful to establish a baseline with which to compare the degree of post-treatment changes (Chen, Clark, & Talcott, 2009). Having an open discussion with patients about common sexual health issues is extremely important before, during, and after cancer treatment. Before treatment begins, patients should be educated about the common sexual side effects associated with their treatment. They also should be routinely assessed during and after treatment for any problems that may arise.

152. Which of the following factors has been shown to positively affect coping?
    a. Marital status
    b. Social support
    c. Age and gender
    d. Culture and ethnicity
    Answer: B. Social support such as family, friends, and community and religious resources, as well as the healthcare team, can positively affect the patient's coping responses by changing the person's appraisal of the event or emotional response to it. Variables such as marital status, age, gender, and culture and ethnicity do not directly affect coping styles (Chou, Stewart, Wild, & Bloom, 2012).

153. A patient with metastatic lung cancer is actively dying and expresses fear that he will not go to heaven when he dies. Which of the following would be the most appropriate response from the APN?
    a. "What's done is done."
    b. "Don't worry about those things; it will all work out."
    c. "Do you want to share with me why you feel this way?"
    d. "Should I ask a chaplain to come and discuss this concern with you?"
    Answer: C. Spiritual care is a vital component of oncology nursing care, and the nurse can provide spiritual care through empathic listening and by helping patients to process the meaning of their illness as it relates to their beliefs, life experiences, and religious beliefs. One outcome of a spiritual assessment may be to have a chaplain see the patient (Puchalski, 2012).

154. A patient with lung cancer receiving radiation therapy for two weeks presents with the following vital signs: a temperature of 101.5°F (38.6°C), a blood pressure of 90/50 mm Hg, pulse of 116 bpm, and respirations of 24 breaths per minute. What is most likely the cause of the patient's change in vital signs?
    a. Sepsis
    b. Infection
    c. Radiation fibrosis
    d. Radiation pneumonitis
    Answer: B. Based on the time the patient has been receiving radiation therapy, infection is the most likely cause of the change in vital signs. Sepsis would be ruled out by observing the patient's response to fluids and antimicrobial therapy. Patients with pneumonitis usually present with shortness of breath with or without cough (Yirmibesoglu et al., 2012). Depending on the severity, patients may have a low-grade fever and the cough may be productive. Fibrosis is a late effect of radiation therapy in which patients present with cough, dyspnea, and tachypnea. Management is similar to that of patients with pneumonitis.

References

AABB, American Red Cross, America's Blood Centers, & Armed Services Blood Program. (2013). *Circular of information for the use of human blood and blood components.* Retrieved from http://www.aabb.org/tm/coi/Documents/coi1113.pdf

Abraxis Oncology. (2013). *Abraxane® (paclitaxel protein-bound particles)* [Package insert]. Retrieved from http://www.abraxane.com/downloads/Abraxane_PrescribingInformation.pdf

Adams, T.L., Orchard, C., Houghton, P., Ogrin, R. (2014). The metamorphosis of a collaborative team: From creation to operation. *Journal of Interprofessional Care, 28,* 339–344. doi:10.3109/13561820.2014.891571

Aiello-Laws, L., Reynolds, J., Deizer, N., Peterson, M., Ameringer, S., & Bakitas, M. (2009). Putting evidence into practice: What are the pharmacologic interventions for nociceptive and neuropathic cancer pain in adults? *Clinical Journal of Oncology Nursing, 13,* 649–655. doi:10.1188/09.CJON.649-655

Aktas, A. (2013). Cancer symptom clusters: Current concepts and controversies. *Current Opinion in Supportive and Palliative Care, 7,* 38–44. doi:10.1097/SPC.0b013e32835def5b

Allan, C.A., Collins, V.R., Frydenberg, M., McLachlan, R.I, & Matthiesson, K.L. (2014). Androgen deprivation therapy complications. *Endocrine-Related Cancer, 21*(4), T119–T129. doi:10.1530/ERC-13-0467

American Association of Critical-Care Nurses. (n.d.). The Synergy Model in practice. Retrieved from http://www.aacn.org/wd/certifications/content/syninpract.pcms?menu=certification

American Cancer Society. (n.d.). Report fraud or abuse. Retrieved from http://www.cancer.org/aboutus/whoweare/governance/report-fraud-or-abuse

American Cancer Society. (2015a). American Cancer Society guidelines for the early detection of cancer. Retrieved from http://www.cancer.org/healthy/findcancerearly/cancerscreeningguidelines/american-cancer-society-guidelines-for-the-early-detection-of-cancer

American Cancer Society. (2015b). *Cancer facts and figures 2015.* Retrieved from http://www.cancer.org/research/cancerfactsstatistics/cancerfactsfigures2015/index

American Holistic Nurses' Certification Corporation. (2014). List of endorsed schools. Retrieved from http://www.ahncc.org/home/endorsedschools.html

American Nurses Association. (2011). Short definitions of ethical principles and theories: Familiar words, what do they mean? Retrieved from http://nursingworld.org/MainMenuCategories/EthicsStandards/Resources/Ethics-Definitions.pdf

American Nurses Association. (2012, March). Nursing care and do not resuscitate (DNR) and allow natural death (AND) decisions [Position statement]. Retrieved from http://www.nursingworld.org/MainMenuCategories/EthicsStandards/Ethics-Position-Statements/Nursing-Care-and-Do-Not-Resuscitate-DNR-and-Allow-Natural-Death-Decisions.pdf

American Psychiatric Association. (2013). *Diagnostic and statistical manual of mental disorders* (5th ed.). Washington, DC: Author.

American Psychological Association. (n.d.). The State-Trait Anxiety Inventory (STAI). Retrieved from http://www.apa.org/pi/about/publications/caregivers/practice-settings/assessment/tools/trait-state.aspx

American Society of Clinical Oncology. (2015). ASCO profile and mission statement. Retrieved from http://www.asco.org/about-asco/asco-profile-and-mission-statement

Amri, R., Bordeianou, L.G., Sylla, P., & Berger, D.L. (2014). Obesity, outcomes and quality of care: Body mass index increased the risk of wound-related complications in colon cancer surgery. *American Journal of Surgery, 207,* 17–23. doi:10.1016/j.amjsurg.2013.05.016

Anderson, L.W., & Krathwohl, D. (Eds.). (2001). *A taxonomy for learning, teaching, and assessing: A revision of Bloom's taxonomy of educational objectives.* New York, NY: Longman.

Anghelescu, D.L., Ehrentraut, J.H., & Faughnan, L.G. (2013). Opioid misuse and abuse: Risk assessment and management in patients with cancer pain. *Journal of the National Comprehensive Cancer Network, 11,* 1023–1031.

Anguiano, L., Mayer, D.K., Piven, M.L., & Rosenstein, D. (2012). A literature review of suicide in cancer patients. *Cancer Nursing, 35*(4), E14–E26. doi:10.1097/NCC.0b013e31822fc76c

Archambeau, J.O., Pezner, R., & Wasserman, T. (1995). Pathophysiology of irradiated skin. *International Journal of Radiation Oncology, Biology, Physics, 31,* 1171–1185. doi:10.1016/0360-3016(94)00423-I

Atkins, K.A., Cohen, M.A., Nicholson, B., & Rao, S. (2013). Atypical lobular hyperplasia and lobular carcinoma in situ at core breast biopsy: Use of careful radiologic-pathologic correlation to recommend excision or observation. *Radiology, 269,* 340–347. doi:10.1148/radiol.13121730

Baggs, J.G. (1994). Development of an instrument to measure collaboration and satisfaction about care decisions. *Journal of Advanced Nursing, 20,* 176–182. doi:10.1046/j.1365-2648.1994.20010176.x

Bakitas, M., Lyons, K.D., Hegel, M.T., Balan, S., Barnett, K.N., Brokaw, F.C., … Ahles, T.A. (2009). The project ENABLE II randomized controlled trial to improve palliative care for rural patients with advanced cancer: Baseline findings, methodological challenges, and solutions. *Palliative and Supportive Care, 7,* 75–86. doi:10.1017/S1478951509000108

Barnes, P.M., Bloom, B., & Nahin, R.L. (2008). Complementary and alternative medicine use among adults and children: United States, 2007. *National Health Statistics Reports, 12,* 1–23.

Becker, K.P., & Baehring, J.M. (2011). Spinal cord compression. In V.T. DeVita Jr., S. Hellman, & S.A. Rosenberg (Eds.), *Cancer: Principles and practice of oncology* (9th ed., pp. 2136–2141). Philadelphia, PA: Wolters Kluwer Health/Lippincott Williams & Wilkins.

Bello, C.L., Mulay, M., Huang, X., Patyna, S., Dinolfo, M., Levine, S., … Rosen, L. (2009). Electrocardiographic characterization of the QTc interval in patients with advanced solid tumors: Pharmacokinetic-pharmacodynamic evaluation of sunitinib. *Clinical Cancer Research, 15,* 7045–7052. doi:10.1158/1078-0432.CCR-09-1521

Bensadoun, R., Humbert, P., Krutman, J., Luger, T., Triller, R., Rougier, A., … Dreno, B. (2013). Daily baseline skin care in the prevention, treatment, and supportive care of skin toxicity in oncology patients: Recommendations from a multinational expert panel. *Cancer Management and Research, 5,* 401–408. doi:10.2147/CMAR.S52256

Better Business Bureau. (n.d.). About. Retrieved from http://www.bbb.org/wisconsin/get-to-know-us/about-us

Biogen Idec, Inc., & Genentech, Inc. (2014). *Rituxan® (rituximab)* [Package insert]. South San Francisco, CA: Author.

Bischoff, K., Weinberg, V., & Rabow, M.W. (2013). Palliative and oncologic co-management: Symptom management for outpatients with cancer. *Supportive Care in Cancer, 21,* 3031–3037. doi:10.1007/s00520-013-1838-z

Blecher, C.S., Ireland, A.M., & Watson, J.L. (2016). *Standards of oncology education: Patient/significant other and public* (4th ed.). Pittsburgh, PA: Oncology Nursing Society.

Block, P. (2011). *Flawless consulting: A guide to getting your expertise used* (3rd ed.). San Francisco, CA: Pfeiffer.

BlueCross BlueShield of North Carolina. (2015). Corporate medical policy: Complementary and alternative medicine. Retrieved from http://www.bcbsnc.com/assets/services/public/pdfs/medicalpolicy/complementary_and_alternative_medicine.pdf

Bober, S.L., & Varela, V.S. (2012). Sexuality in adult cancer survivors: Challenges and intervention. *Journal of Clinical Oncology, 30,* 3712–3719. doi:10.1200/JCO.2012.41.7915

Bonita, R., & Pradhan, R. (2013). Cardiovascular toxicities of cancer chemotherapy. *Seminars in Oncology, 40,* 156–167. doi:10.1053/j.seminoncol.2013.01.004

Bowles, E.J., Wellman, R., Feigelson, H.S., Onitilo, A.A., Freedman, A.N., Delate, T., … Wagner, E.H. (2012). Risk of heart failure in breast cancer patients after anthracycline and trastuzumab treatment: A retrospective cohort study. *Journal of the National Cancer Institute, 104,* 1293–1305. doi:10.1093/jnci/djs317

Brant, J.M., & Wickham, R. (Eds.). (2013). *Statement on the scope and standards of oncology nursing practice: Generalist and advanced practice.* Pittsburgh, PA: Oncology Nursing Society.

Brumbaugh, H.L. (2011). Superior vena cava syndrome. In C.H. Yarbro, D. Wujcik, & B.H. Gobel (Eds.), *Cancer nursing: Principles and practice* (7th ed., pp. 995–1004). Burlington, MA: Jones & Bartlett Learning.

Bryant, R.A. (2013). Is pathological grief lasting more than 12 months grief or depression? *Current Opinion in Psychiatry, 26,* 41–46. doi:10.1097/YCO.0b013e32835b2ca2

Bugalho, A., Ferreira, D., Eberhardt, R., Dias, S.S., Videira, P.A., Herth, F.J., & Carreiro, L. (2013). Diagnostic value of endobronchial and endoscopic ultrasound-guided fine needle aspiration for accessible lung cancer lesions after nondiagnostic conventional techniques: A prospective study. *BMC Cancer, 13,* 130. doi:10.1186/1471-2407-13-130

Buglass, E. (2010). Grief and bereavement theories. *Nursing Standard, 24*(41), 44–47. doi:10.7748/ns2010.06.24.41.44.c7834

Bükki, J., Scherbel, J., Stiel, S., Klein, C., Meidenbauer, N., & Ostgathe, C. (2013). Palliative care needs, symptoms, and treatment intensity along the disease trajectory in medical oncology outpatients: A retrospective chart review. *Supportive Care in Cancer, 21,* 1743–1750. doi:10.1007/s00520-013-1721-y

Campaign for Tobacco-Free Kids. (2015, May 6). Toll of tobacco in the United States of America. Retrieved from http://www.tobaccofreekids.org/research/factsheets/pdf/0072.pdf

Centers for Medicare and Medicaid Services. (n.d.-a). Documentation guidelines for evaluation and management (E/M) services. Retrieved from http://www.cms.gov/Outreach-and-Education/Medicare-Learning-Network-MLN/MLNEdWebGuide/EMDOC.html

Centers for Medicare and Medicaid Services. (n.d.-b). How hospice works. Retrieved from http://www.medicare.gov/what-medicare-covers/part-a/how-hospice-works.html

Centers for Medicare and Medicaid Services. (n.d.-c). Your Medicare coverage. Is my test, item, or service covered? Retrieved from http://www.medicare.gov/coverage/hospice-and-respite-care.html

Centers for Medicare and Medicaid Services. (2013). *Medicare hospice benefits* (CMS Product No. 02154). Retrieved from http://www.medicare.gov/Pubs/pdf/02154.pdf

Chase, D.M., Gibson, S.J., Sumner, D.A., Bea, J.W., & Alberts, D.S. (2014). Appropriate use of complementary and alternative medicine approaches in gynecologic cancers. *Current Treatment Options in Oncology, 15,* 14–26. doi:10.1007/s11864-013-0269-x

Chen, M.Y.M., & Whitlow, C.T. (2011). Scope of diagnostic imaging. In M.Y.M. Chen, T.L. Pope, & D.J. Ott (Eds.), *Basic radiology* (2nd ed.). New York, NY: McGraw-Hill Medical. Retrieved from http://www.accessmedicine.com

Chen, R.C., Clark, J.A., & Talcott, J.A. (2009). Individualizing quality-of-life outcomes reporting: How localized prostate cancer treatments affect patients with different levels of baseline urinary, bowel, and sexual function. *Journal of Clinical Oncology, 27,* 3916–3922. doi:10.1200/JCO.2008.18.6486

Chou, A.F., Stewart, S.L., Wild, R.C., & Bloom, J.R. (2012). Social support and survival in young women with breast carcinoma. *Psycho-Oncology, 21,* 125–133. doi:10.1002/pon.1863

Clark, L.C., Combs, G.F., Jr., Turnbull, B.W., Slate, E.H., Chalker, D.K., Chow, J., … Taylor, J.R. (1996). Effects of selenium supplementation for cancer prevention in patients with carcinoma of the skin: A randomized controlled trial. *JAMA, 276,* 1957–1963. doi:10.1001/jama.1996.03540240035027

Clifford, D.B., Ances, B., Costello, C., Rosen-Schmidt, S., Andersson, M., Parks, D., … Tyler, K.L. (2011). Rituximab-associated progressive multifocal leukoencephalopathy in rheumatoid arthritis. *Archives of Neurology, 68,* 1156–1164. doi:10.1001/archneurol.2011.103

Coiffier, B., Altman, A., Pui, C.-H., Younes, A., & Cairo, M.S. (2008). Guidelines for the management of pediatric and adult tumor lysis syndrome: An evidence-based review. *Journal of Clinical Oncology, 26,* 2767–2778. doi:10.1200/JCO.2007.15.0177

Compton, C.C., Byrd, D.R., Garcia-Aguilar, J., Kurtzman, S.H., Olawaiye, A., & Washington, M.K. (Eds.). (2012). *AJCC cancer staging atlas: A companion to the seventh editions of the AJCC Cancer Staging Manual and Handbook* (2nd ed.). New York, NY: Springer.

Corless, I.B. (2010). Bereavement. In B.R. Ferrell & N. Coyle (Eds.), *Oxford textbook of palliative nursing* (3rd ed., pp. 597–611). New York, NY: Oxford University Press.

Croswell, J.M., Kramer, B.S., & Crawford, E.D. (2011). Screening prostate cancer with PSA testing: Current status and future directions. *Oncology, 25,* 452–460, 463. Retrieved from http://www.cancernetwork.com/oncology-journal/screening-prostate-cancer-psa-testing-current-status-and-future-directions

Dang, J., Li, G., Ma, L., Diao, R., Zang, S., Han, C., … Yao, L. (2013). Predictors of grade ≥ 2 and ≥ 3 radiation pneumonitis in patients with locally advanced non-small cell lung cancer treated with three-dimensional conformal radiotherapy. *Acta Oncologica, 52,* 1175–1180. doi:10.3109/0284186X.2012.747696

Davies, B., & Steele, R. (2010). Supporting families in palliative care. In B.R. Ferrell & N. Coyle (Eds.), *Oxford textbook of palliative nursing* (3rd ed., pp. 587–618). New York, NY: Oxford University Press.

Davis, A.M., Dische, S., Gerber, L., Saunders, M., Leung, S.F., & O'Sullivan, B. (2003). Measuring postirradiation subcutaneous soft-tissue fibrosis: State-of-the-art and future directions. *Seminars in Radiation Oncology, 13,* 203–213. doi:10.1016/S1053-4296(03)00022-5

de M Alcântara-Silva, T.R., Freitas-Junior, R., Freitas, N.M.A., & Machado, G.D.P. (2013). Fatigue related to radiotherapy for breast and/or gynaecological cancer: A systematic review. *Journal of Clinical Nursing, 22,* 19–20. doi:10.1111/jocn.12236

Delia, P., Sansotta, G., Donato, V., Frosina, P., Messina, G., De Renzis, C., & Famularo, G. (2007). Use of probiotics for prevention of radiation-induced diarrhea. *World Journal of Gastroenterology, 13,* 912–915. doi:10.3748/wjg.v13.i6.912

Deng, G., & Cassileth, B. (2014). Integrative oncology: An overview. *American Society of Clinical Oncology Educational Book, 34,* 233–242. doi:10.14694/EdBook_AM.2014.34.233

Diaz, E.S., Aoyama, C., Baquing, M.A., Beavis, A., Silva, E., Holschneider, C., & Cass, I. (2014). Predictors of residual carcinoma or carcinoma-in-situ at hysterectomy following cervical conization with position margins. *Gynecology Oncology, 132,* 76–80. doi:10.1016/j.ygyno.2013.11.019

Dietary Supplement Health and Education Act of 1994, Pub. L. No. 103-417. Retrieved from http://www.health.gov/dietsupp/ch1.htm

Downing, L.J., Caprio, T.V., & Lyness, J.M. (2013). Geriatric psychiatry review: Differential diagnosis and treatment of the 3 D's—delirium, dementia, and depression. *Current Psychiatry Reports, 15,* 365. doi:10.1007/s11920-013-0365-4

Drews, R.E., & Rabkin, D.J. (2014, June 25). Malignancy-related superior vena cava syndrome [UpToDate version 23.1]. Retrieved from http://www.uptodate.com/contents/malignancy-related-superior-vena-cava-syndrome

Edwardson, S.R. (2010). Doctor of philosophy and doctor of nursing practice as complementary degrees. *Journal of Professional Nursing, 26,* 137–140. doi:10.1016/j.profnurs.2009.08.004

Eisenberg, S. (2013). Infusion reactions. In M. Kaplan (Ed.), *Understanding and managing oncologic emergencies: A resource for nurses* (2nd ed., pp. 199–255). Pittsburgh, PA: Oncology Nursing Society.

Erb, C.H., & Vogel, W.H. (2013). Management of the complications of hematologic malignancy and treatment. In M. Olsen & L.J. Zitella (Eds.), *Hematologic malignancies in adults* (pp. 537–647). Pittsburgh, PA: Oncology Nursing Society.

Esmaeli, B., Amin, S., Valero, V., Adinin, R., Arbuckle, R., Banay, R., … Rivera, E. (2006). Prospective study of incidence and severity of epiphora and canalicular stenosis in patients with metastatic breast cancer receiving docetaxel. *Journal of Clinical Oncology, 24,* 3619–3622. doi:10.1200/JCO.2005.04.4453

Febbo, P.G., Ladanyi, M., Aldape, K.D., De Marzo, A.M., Hammond, M.E., Hayes, D.F., … Birkeland, M.L. (2011). NCCN Task Force report: Evaluating the clinical utility of tumor markers in oncology. *Journal of the National Comprehensive Cancer Network, 9*(Suppl. 5), S-1–S-32. Retrieved from http://www.jnccn.org/content/9/Suppl_5/S-1.long

Fidalgo, J.A.P., Fabregat, L.G., Cervantes, A., Margulies, A., Vidall, C., & Roila, F. (2012). Management of chemotherapy extravasation: ESMO-EONS clinical practice guidelines. *Annals of Oncology, 23*(Suppl.), vii167–vii173. doi:10.1093/annonc/mds294

Find-A-Code. (n.d.). ABC code set. Retrieved from http://www.findacode.com/abc-codes-set.html

Fiore, M.C., Jaén, C.R., Baker, T.B., Bailey, W.C., Benowitz, N.L., Curry, S.J., … Wewers, M.E. (2008). *Treating tobacco use and dependence: 2008 update* (Clinical practice guideline). Rockville, MD: U.S. Department of Health and Human Services.

Fojo, A.T. (2011). Metabolic emergencies. In V.T. DeVita Jr., T.S. Lawrence, & S.A. Rosenberg (Eds.), *Cancer: Principles and practice of oncology* (9th ed., pp. 2142–2152). Philadelphia, PA: Wolters Kluwer Health/Lippincott Williams & Wilkins.

Follwell, M., Burman, D., Le, L.W., Wakimoto, K., Seccareccia, D., Bryson, J., … Zimmermann, C. (2009). Phase II study of an outpatient palliative care intervention in patients with metastatic cancer. *Journal of Clinical Oncology, 27,* 206–213. doi:10.1200/JCO.2008.17.7568

Francis, N. (2014). The need for routine monitoring of cardiac function in patients receiving 5-fluorouracil infusion. *Clinical Journal of Oncology Nursing, 18,* 360–362. doi:10.1188/14.CJON.360-362

Freter, C.E., & Haddadin, S. (2014, August 1). Oncologic emergencies: Cardiac tamponade. In R. Govindan (Ed.), *InPractice oncology.* Retrieved from http://www.inpractice.com/Textbooks/Oncology/General_Oncology_Topics/ch56_GeneralOnc_Emergencies/Chapter-Pages/Page-3.aspx

Genentech, Inc. (2014). *Herceptin® (trastuzumab)* [Package insert]. South San Francisco, CA: Author.

Genentech, Inc. (2015). *Avastin® (bevacizumab)* [Package insert]. South San Francisco, CA: Author.

Geppert, C.M.A., & Shelton, W.N. (2012). A comparison of general medical and clinical ethics consultations: What can we learn from each other? *Mayo Clinic Proceedings, 87,* 381–389. doi:10.1016/j.mayocp.2011.10.010

Gobel, B.H. (2013). Tumor lysis syndrome. In M. Kaplan (Ed.), *Understanding and managing oncologic emergencies: A resource for nurses* (2nd ed., pp. 433–459). Pittsburgh, PA: Oncology Nursing Society.

Godfrey, C., Villa, C., Dawson, L., Swindells, S., & Schouten, J.T. (2013). Controlling healthcare-associated infections in the international research setting [Letter to the editor]. *Journal of Acquired Immune Deficiency Syndromes, 62,* e115–e118. doi:10.1097/QAI.0b013e3182845b95

Goel, M.K., Khanna, P., & Kishore, J. (2010). Understanding survival analysis: Kaplan-Meier estimate. *International Journal of Ayurveda Research, 1,* 274–278.

Goldzweig, G., Merims, S., Ganon, R., Peretz, T., Altman, A., & Baider, L. (2013). Informal caregiving to older cancer patients: Preliminary research outcomes and implications. *Annals of Oncology, 24,* 2635–2640. doi:10.1093/annonc/mdt250

Goody, R.B., O'Hare, J., McKenna, K., Dearey, L., Robinson, J., Bell, P., … Hanna, G.G. (2013). Unintended cardiac irradiation during left-sided breast cancer radiotherapy. *British Journal of Radiology, 86,* 20120434. doi:10.1259/bjr.20120434

Gosselin, T.K. (2011). Principles of radiation therapy. In C.H. Yarbro, D. Wujcik, & B.H. Gobel (Eds.), *Cancer nursing: Principles and practice* (7th ed., pp. 249–268). Burlington, MA: Jones & Bartlett Learning.

Grannis, F.W., Jr., Kim, J.Y., & Lai, L. (2014, May 1). Fluid complications: Pericardial effusion. In D.G. Haller, L.D. Wagman, K.A. Camphausen, & W.J. Hoskins (Eds.), *Cancer management: A multidisciplinary approach* (online edition). Retrieved from http://www.cancernetwork.com/cancer-management/fluid-complications/article/10165/1802878?pageNumber=2

Grant, M., Sun, V., Fujinami, R., Sidhu, R., Otis-Green, S., Juarez, G., … Ferrell, B. (2013). Family caregiver burden, skills preparedness, and quality of life in non-small-cell lung cancer. *Oncology Nursing Forum, 40,* 337–346. doi:10.1188/13.ONF.337-346

Grünwald, V., Weikert, S., Pavel, M.E., Hörsch, D., Lüftner, D., Janni, W., …. Weber, M.M. (2013). Practical management of everolimus-related toxicities in patients with advanced solid tumors. *Onkologie, 36,* 295–302. doi:10.1159/000350625

Gunder, L.M., & Martin, S.A. (2011). *Essentials of medical genetics for health professionals.* Burlington, MA: Jones & Bartlett Learning.

Hadjinicolaou, A.V., Nisar, M.K., Parfrey, H., Chilvers, E.R., & Östör, A.J. (2012). Non-infectious pulmonary toxicity of rituximab: A systematic review. *Rheumatology, 51,* 653–662. doi:10.1093/rheumatology/ker290

Haggerty, J.L., Roberge, D., Freeman, G.K., Beaulieu, C., & Bréton, M. (2012). Validation of a generic measure of continuity of care: When patients encounter several clinicians. *Annals of Family Medicine, 10,* 443–451. doi:10.1370/afm.1378

Hake, S., & Shah, T. (2011). Negotiation skills for clinical research professionals. *Perspectives in Clinical Research, 2,* 105–108. doi:10.4103/2229-3485.83224

Hamid, O., & Carvajal, R.D. (2013). Anti-programmed death-1 and anti-programmed death-ligand 1 antibodies in cancer therapy. *Expert Opinion on Biological Therapy, 13,* 847–861. doi:10.1517/14712598.2013.770836

Harding, R., Epiphaniou, E., Hamilton, D., Bridger, S., Robinson, V., George, R., … Higginson, I.J. (2012). What are the perceived needs and challenges of informal caregivers in home cancer palliative care? Qualitative data to construct a feasible psycho-educational intervention. *Supportive Care in Cancer, 20,* 1975–1982. doi:10.1007/s00520-011-1300-z

Harper, J.L., Franklin, L.E., Jenrette, J.M., & Aguero, E.G. (2004). Skin toxicity during breast irradiation: Pathophysiology and management. *Southern Medical Journal, 97,* 989–993. doi:10.1097/01.SMJ.0000140866.97278.87

Harrill-Smith, C., Ripley-Moffitt, C., & Goldstein, A.O. (2013). Tobacco cessation in 2013: What every clinician should know. *North Carolina Medical Journal, 74,* 401–405.

Harris, L., Fritsche, H., Mennel, R., Norton, L., Ravdin, P., Taube, S., … Bast, R.C., Jr. (2007). American Society of Clinical Oncology 2007 update of recommendations for the use of tumor markers in breast cancer. *Journal of Clinical Oncology, 25,* 5287–5312. doi:10.1200/JCO.2007.14.2364

Hennessey, D.B., Burke, J.P., Ni-Dhonochu, T., Shields, C., Winter, D.C., & Mealy, K. (2010). Preoperative hypoalbuminemia is an independent risk factor or the development of surgical site infection following gastrointestinal surgery: A multi-institutional study. *Annals of Surgery, 252,* 325–329. doi:10.1097/SLA.0b013e3181e9819a

Hewitt, M., Greenfield, S., & Stovall, E. (Eds.). (2006). *From cancer patient to cancer survivor: Lost in transition.* Washington, DC: National Academies Press.

Ho, M.Y., & Mackey, J.R. (2014). Presentation and management of docetaxel-related adverse effects in patients with breast cancer. *Cancer Management and Research, 6,* 253–259. doi:10.2147/CMAR.S40601

Hoskins, L.M., Roy, K.M., & Greene, M.H. (2012). Toward a new understanding of risk perception among young female *BRCA1/2* "previvors". *Families, Systems, and Health, 30,* 32–46. doi:10.1037/a0027276

Institute of Medicine. (n.d.). About the IOM. Retrieved from http://www.iom.edu/About-IOM.aspx

Institute of Medicine. (2005). *Complementary and alternative medicine in the United States.* Washington, DC: National Academies Press.

International Committee of Medical Journal Editors. (n.d.). About the recommendations. Retrieved from http://www.icmje.org/recommendations/browse/about-the-recommendations

Irwin, M.M., Erb, C., Williams, C., Wilson, B.J., & Zitella, L.J. (2013). *Putting evidence into practice: Improving oncology patient outcomes; Prevention of infection.* Pittsburgh, PA: Oncology Nursing Society.

Jacobs, L.A., & Mayer, D.K. (2016). *Standards of oncology nursing education: Generalist and advanced practice levels* (4th ed.). Pittsburgh, PA: Oncology Nursing Society.

Jazbec, J., Todorovski, L., & Jereb, B. (2007). Classification tree analysis of second neoplasms in survivors of childhood cancer. *BMC Cancer, 7,* 27. doi:10.1186/1471-2407-7-27

Jenkins, C.L., Edmundson, A., Averett, P., & Yoon, I. (2014). Older lesbians and bereavement: Experiencing the loss of a partner. *Journal of Gerontological Social Work, 57,* 273–287. doi:10.1080/01634372.2013.850583

Jenkins, J.F. (Ed.). (2009). *Essentials of genetic and genomic nursing: Competencies, curricula guidelines, and outcome indicators* (2nd ed.). Silver Spring, MD: American Nurses Association.

Joint Commission. (2014, October). Surgical Care Improvement Project. Retrieved from http://www.jointcommission.org/surgical_care_improvement_project

Kanne, J.P., Jensen, L.E., Mohammed, T.-L.H., Kirsch, J., Amorosa, J.K., Brown, K., … Shah, R.D. (2012). American College of Radiology ACR Appropriateness Criteria®: Radiographically detected solitary pulmonary nodule. Retrieved from http://www.acr.org/~/media/ACR/Documents/AppCriteria/Diagnostic/SolitaryPulmonaryNodule.pdf

Kaplan, M. (2013a). Disseminated intravascular coagulation. In M. Kaplan (Ed.), *Understanding and managing oncologic emergencies: A resource for nurses* (2nd ed., pp. 69–102). Pittsburgh, PA: Oncology Nursing Society.

Kaplan, M. (2013b). Hypercalcemia of malignancy. In M. Kaplan (Ed.), *Understanding and managing oncologic emergencies: A resource for nurses* (2nd ed., pp. 103–155). Pittsburgh, PA: Oncology Nursing Society.

Karnofsky, D.A., Abelmann, W.H., Craver, L.F., & Burchenal, J.H. (1948). The use of the nitrogen mustards in the palliative treatment of carcinoma. With particular reference to bronchogenic carcinoma. *Cancer, 1,* 634–656. doi:10.1002/1097-0142(194811)1:4<634::AID-CNCR2820010410>3.0.CO;2-L

Kedia, S., Acharya, P.S., Mohammad, F., Nguyen, H., Asti, D., Mehta, S., … Mobarakai, N. (2013). Infectious complications of hematopoietic stem cell transplantation. *Journal of Stem Cell Research and Therapy.* doi:10.4172/2157-7633.S3-002

Kharofa, J., Cohen, E.P., Tomic, R., Xiang, Q., & Gore, E. (2012). Decreased risk of radiation pneumonitis with incidental concurrent use of angiotensin-converting enzyme inhibitors and thoracic radiation therapy. *International Journal of Radiation Oncology, Biology, Physics, 84,* 238–243. doi:10.1016/j.ijrobp.2011.11.013

Khatcheressian, J.L., Hurley, P., Bantug, E., Esserman, L.J., Grunfeld, E., Halberg, F., … Davidson, N.E. (2013). Breast cancer follow-up and management after primary treatment: American Society of Clinical Oncology clinical practice guideline update. *Journal of Clinical Oncology, 31,* 961–965. doi:10.1200/JCO.2012.45.9859

Kiran, R.P., Turina, M., Hammel, J., & Fazio, V. (2013). The clinical significance of an elevated postoperative glucose value in nondiabetic patients after colorectal surgery: Evidence for the need for tight glucose control? *Annals of Surgery, 258,* 599–604. doi:10.1097/SLA.0b013e3182a501e3

Kirsch, B. (2012). Many US cancer survivors still lost in transition. *Lancet, 379,* 1865–1866. doi:10.1016/S0140 -6736(12)60794-6

Kohlmann, W., & Gruber, S.B. (2012). Lynch syndrome. In R.A. Pagon, M.P. Adam, H.H. Ardinger, S.E. Wallace, A. Amemiya, L.J.H. Bean, … K. Stephens (Eds.), *GeneReviews.* Seattle, WA: University of Washington. Retrieved from http://www.ncbi.nlm.nih.gov/books/NBK1211

Larentzakis, A., & Theodorou, D. (2014). A multicenter study of survival after neoadjuvant radiotherapy/chemotherapy and esophagectomy for ypT0N0M0R0 esophageal cancer. *Annals of Surgery, 259,* e67. doi:10.1097/ SLA.0000000000000364

Leventhal, H., & Cameron, L. (1987). Behavioral theories and the problem of compliance. *Patient Education and Counseling, 10,* 117–138. doi:10.1016/0738-3991(87)90093-0

Lewis, M.A., Hendrickson, A.W., & Moynihan, T.J. (2011). Oncologic emergencies: Pathophysiology, presentation, diagnosis, and treatment. *CA: A Cancer Journal for Clinicians, 61,* 287–314. doi:10.3322/caac.20124

Li, M., Fitzgerald, P., & Rodin, G. (2012). Evidence-based treatment of depression in patients with cancer. *Journal of Clinical Oncology, 30,* 1187–1196. doi:10.1200/JCO.2011.39.7372

Lindor, N.M., McMaster, M.L., Lindor, C.J., & Greene, M.H. (2008). Concise handbook of familial cancer susceptibility syndromes—Second edition. *Journal of the National Cancer Institute, Monographs, 2008*(38), 3–93. doi:10.1093/ jncimonographs/lgn001

Liu, L., Fiorentino, L., Natarajan, L., Parker, B.A., Mills, P.J., Sadler, G.R., … Ancoli-Israel, S. (2009). Pre-treatment symptom cluster in breast cancer patients is associated with worse sleep, fatigue and depression during chemotherapy. *Psycho-Oncology, 18,* 187–194. doi:10.1002/pon.1412

Liu, Q., Lin, R., Liu, C., Wu, M., Xuan, L., Jiang, X., … Sun, J. (2013, December). Epstein-Barr virus infection in recipient of allogeneic hematopoietic stem cell transplantation: The role of cytomegalovirus (Abstract No. 4555). Abstract presented at the 55th ASH Annual Meeting and Exposition, New Orleans, LA. Retrieved from https:// ash.confex.com/ash/2013/webprogram/Paper60324.html

Livestrong Foundation. (n.d.). Our approach. Retrieved from http://www.livestrong.org/What-We-Do/Our-Approach

Lydon, J. (2011). Tumor lysis syndrome. In C.H. Yarbro, D. Wujcik, & B.H. Gobel (Eds.), *Cancer nursing: Principles and practice* (7th ed., pp. 1014–1028). Burlington, MA: Jones & Bartlett Learning.

Mehta, N. (2012). Drug-induced hepatotoxicity. Retrieved from http://emedicine.medscape.com/article/169814- overview

Merck & Co., Inc. (2015). *Temodar® (temozolomide)* [Package insert]. Whitehouse Station, NJ: Author.

Messer, K., & Pierce, J.P. (2010). Changes in age trajectories of smoking experimentation during the California Tobacco Control Program. *American Journal of Public Health, 100,* 1298–1306. doi:10.2105/AJPH.2009 .160416

Millennium Pharmaceuticals, Inc. (2012). *Velcade® (bortezomib)* [Package insert]. Cambridge, MA: Author.

Miller, K.K., Gorcey, L., & McLellan, B.N. (2014). Chemotherapy-induced hand-foot syndrome and nail changes: A review of clinical presentation, etiology, pathogenesis, and management. *Journal of the American Academy of Dermatology, 71,* 787–794. doi:10.1016/j.jaad.2014.03.019

Miranda, D.G., McMain, C.L., & Smith, A.J. (2011). Medication-induced QT-interval prolongation and torsades de pointes. *U.S. Pharmacist, 36,* HS-2–HS-8. Retrieved from http://www.uspharmacist.com/content/d/ feature/c/26648

Mitchell, S.A. (2011). Cancer-related fatigue. In C.H. Yarbro, D. Wujcik, & B.H. Gobel (Eds.), *Cancer nursing: Principles and practice* (7th ed., pp. 772–791). Burlington, MA: Jones & Bartlett Learning.

Mitchell, S.A., Hoffman, A.J., Clark, J.C., DeGennaro, R.M., Poirier, P., Robinson, C.B., & Weisbrod, B.L. (2014). Putting evidence into practice: An update of evidence-based interventions for cancer-related fatigue during and following treatment. *Clinical Journal of Oncology Nursing, 18*(Suppl. 6), S38–S58. doi:10.1188/14.CJON.S3.38-58

Mulrooney, T. (2010). Cognitive impairment. In C.G. Brown (Ed.), *A guide to oncology symptom management* (pp. 123–137). Pittsburgh, PA: Oncology Nursing Society.

Mustian, K.M., Sprod, L.K., Janelsins, M., Peppone, L.J., & Mohile, S. (2012). Exercise recommendations for cancer -related fatigue, cognitive impairment, sleep problems, depression, pain, anxiety, and physical dysfunction: A review. *Oncology and Hematology Review, 8,* 81–88.

National Cancer Institute. (2013). Cancer clinical trials at the NIH Clinical Center. Retrieved from http://www.cancer .gov/about-nci/organization/clinical-center-fact-sheet

National Cancer Institute Office of Cancer Survivorship. (n.d.). About cancer survivorship. Retrieved from http://cancercontrol.cancer.gov/ocs/about/index.html

National Center for Complementary and Integrative Health. (2015). Research results. Retrieved from http://nccam.nih.gov/research/results

National Commission for the Protection of Human Subjects of Biomedical and Behavioral Research. (1979). *The Belmont report: Ethical principles and guidelines for the protection of human subjects of research*. Bethesda, MD: Author.

National Comprehensive Cancer Network. (2014). *NCCN Clinical Practice Guidelines in Oncology (NCCN Guidelines®): Myeloid growth factors* [v.2.2014]. Retrieved from http://www.nccn.org/professionals/physician_gls/pdf/myeloid_growth.pdf

National Comprehensive Cancer Network. (2015a). *NCCN Clinical Practice Guidelines in Oncology (NCCN Guidelines®): Adult cancer pain* [v.2.2015]. Retrieved from http://www.nccn.org/professionals/physician_gls/pdf/pain.pdf

National Comprehensive Cancer Network. (2015b). *NCCN Clinical Practice Guidelines in Oncology (NCCN Guidelines®): Breast cancer* [v.2.2015]. Retrieved from http://www.nccn.org/professionals/physician_gls/pdf/breast.pdf

National Comprehensive Cancer Network. (2015c). *NCCN Clinical Practice Guidelines in Oncology (NCCN Guidelines®): Distress management* [v.1.2015]. Retrieved from http://www.nccn.org/professionals/physician_gls/pdf/distress.pdf

National Comprehensive Cancer Network. (2015d). *NCCN Clinical Practice Guidelines in Oncology (NCCN Guidelines®): Hodgkin lymphoma* [v.2.2015]. Retrieved from http://www.nccn.org/professionals/physician_gls/pdf/hodgkins.pdf

National Comprehensive Cancer Network. (2015e). *NCCN Clinical Practice Guidelines in Oncology (NCCN Guidelines®): Lung cancer screening* [v.2.2015]. Retrieved from http://www.nccn.org/professionals/physician_gls/pdf/lung_screening.pdf

National Comprehensive Cancer Network. (2015f). *NCCN Clinical Practice Guidelines in Oncology (NCCN Guidelines®): Palliative care* [v.2.2015]. Retrieved from http://www.nccn.org/professionals/physician_gls/pdf/palliative.pdf

National Comprehensive Cancer Network. (2015g). *NCCN Clinical Practice Guidelines in Oncology (NCCN Guidelines®): Prevention and treatment of cancer-related infections* [v.2.2015]. Retrieved from http://www.nccn.org/professionals/physician_gls/pdf/infections.pdf

National Consensus Project for Quality Palliative Care. (2013). *Clinical practice guidelines for quality palliative care* (3rd ed.). Retrieved from https://www.hpna.org/multimedia/NCP_Clinical_Practice_Guidelines_3rd_Edition.pdf

National Hospice and Palliative Care Organization. (2012). *NHPCO facts and figures: Hospice care in America*. Retrieved from http://www.nhpco.org/sites/default/files/public/Statistics_Research/2012_Facts_Figures.pdf

National Institutes of Health Office of Human Subjects Research. (n.d.). *Nuremberg code*. Retrieved from https://www.research.buffalo.edu/rsp/irb/forms/Nuremberg_Code.pdf

National Quality Forum. (2006). *A national framework and preferred practices for palliative and hospice care quality. A consensus report*. Washington, DC: Author.

Nickloes, T.A., Long, C., Mack, L.O., Kallab, A.M., Dunlap, A.B., & Gandhi, S.S. (2014, October 10). Superior vena cava syndrome. Retrieved from http://emedicine.medscape.com/article/460865-overview

Oken, M.M., Creech, R.H., Tormey, D.C., Horton, J., Davis, T.E., McFadden, E.T., & Carbone, P.P. (1982). Toxicity and response criteria of the Eastern Cooperative Oncology Group. *American Journal of Clinical Oncology, 5,* 649–656. doi:10.1097/00000421-198212000-00014

Oliver, J., Coggins, C., Compton, P., Hagan, S., Matteliano, D., Stanton, M., … Turner, H.N. (2012). American Society for Pain Management Nursing position statement: Pain management in patients with substance use disorders. *Pain Management Nursing, 13,* 169–183. doi:10.1016/j.pmn.2012.07.001

Oncology Nursing Society. (n.d.). PEP rating system overview. Retrieved from https://www.ons.org/practice-resources/pep

Oncology Nursing Society. (2015). The role of the advanced practice nurse in oncology care [Position statement]. Retrieved from https://www.ons.org/advocacy-policy/positions/education/apn

Ottaviani, G., Robert, R.S., Huh, W.W., Palla, S., & Jaffe, N. (2013). Sociooccupational and physical outcomes more than 20 years after the diagnosis of osteosarcoma in children and adolescents: Limb salvage versus amputation. *Cancer, 119,* 3727–3736. doi:10.1002/cncr.28277

Petrucelli, N., Daly, M.B., & Feldman, G.L. (2013, September 26). *BRCA1* and *BRCA2* hereditary breast and ovarian cancer. In R.A. Pagon, M.P. Adam, H.H. Ardinger, S.E. Wallace, A. Amemiya, L.J.H. Bean, … K. Stephens (Eds.), *GeneReviews*. Seattle, WA: University of Washington. Retrieved from http://www.ncbi.nlm.nih.gov/books/NBK1247

Pharmacia & Upjohn Co. (2014). *Camptosar® (irinotecan)* [Package insert]. New York, NY: Author.

Polovich, M., Olsen, M., & LeFebvre, K.B. (Eds.). (2014). *Chemotherapy and biotherapy guidelines and recommendations for practice* (4th ed.). Pittsburgh, PA: Oncology Nursing Society.

Pope, T.M. (2013). Legal briefing: The new Patient Self-Determination Act. *Journal of Clinical Ethics, 24,* 156–167.

Prasad, K., Ziegenfuss, J.Y., Cha, S.S., Sood, A., & Tilburt, J.C. (2013). Characteristics of exclusive users of mind-body medicine versus other alternative medicine approaches in the United States. *Explore, 9,* 219–225. doi:10.1016/j.explore.2013.04.001

Puchalski, C.M. (2012). Spirituality in the cancer trajectory. *Annals of Oncology, 23*(Suppl. 3), 49–55. doi:10.1093/annonc/mds088

Quante, A.S., Whittemore, A.S., Shriver, T., Strauch, K., & Terry, M.B. (2012). Breast cancer risk assessment across the risk continuum: Genetic and nongenetic risk factors contributing to differential model performance. *Breast Cancer Research, 14,* R144. doi:10.1186/bcr3352

Rahimi, R., & Abdollahi, M. (2012). An update on the ability of St. John's wort to affect the metabolism of other drugs. *Expert Opinion on Drug Metabolism and Toxicology, 8,* 691–708. doi:10.1517/17425255.2012.680886

Raza, A., & Vierling, J.M. (2014). Graft-versus-host disease. In M.E. Gershwin, J.M. Vierling, & M.P. Manns (Eds.), *Liver immunology: Principles and practice* (2nd ed., pp. 425–441). doi:10.1007/978-3-319-02096-9_29

Ripamonti, C.I., Santini, D., Maranzano, E., Berti, M., & Roila, F. (2012). Management of cancer pain: ESMO clinical practice guidelines. *Annals of Oncology, 23*(Suppl. 7), vii139–vii154. doi:10.1093/annonc/mds233

Rizk, N. (2013). Surgery for esophageal cancer: Goals of resection and optimizing outcomes. *Thoracic Surgery Clinics, 23,* 491–498. doi:10.1016/j.thorsurg.2013.07.009

Rizzo, J.A., & Xie, Y. (2006). Managed care, consumerism, preventive medicine: Does a causal connection exist? *Managed Care Interface, 19,* 46–50.

Robinson, T.N., Wu, D.S., Pointer, L., Dunn, C.L., Cleveland, J.S., Jr., & Moss, M. (2013). Simple frailty score predicts postoperative complications across surgical specialties. *American Journal of Surgery, 206,* 544–550. doi:10.1016/j.amjsurg.2013.03.012

Robinson, W., & Cantillo, E. (2014). Debulking surgery and intraperitoneal chemotherapy are associated with decreased morbidity in women receiving neoadjuvant chemotherapy for ovarian cancer. *International Journal of Gynecological Cancer, 24,* 43–47. doi:10.1097/IGC.0000000000000009

Robson, M.E., Storm, C.D., Weitzel, J., Wollins, D.S., & Offit, K. (2010). American Society of Clinical Oncology policy statement update: Genetic and genomic testing for cancer susceptibility. *Journal of Clinical Oncology, 28,* 893–901. doi:10.1200/JCO.2009.27.0660

Rodriguez, A.L. (2014). Bleeding and thrombotic complications. In C.H. Yarbro, D. Wujcik, & B.H. Gobel (Eds.), *Cancer symptom management* (4th ed., pp. 287–316). Burlington, MA: Jones & Bartlett Learning.

Rolfe, G., & Davies, R. (2009). Second generation professional doctorates in nursing. *International Journal of Nursing Studies, 46,* 1265–1273. doi:10.1016/j.ijnurstu.2009.04.002

Roos, D., Dijksman, L.M., Tijssen, J.G., Gouma, D.J., Gerhards, M.F., Oudemans-van Straaten, H.M. (2013). Systematic review of perioperative selective decontamination of the digestive tract in elective gastrointestinal surgery. *British Journal of Surgery, 100,* 1579–1588. doi:10.1002/bjs.9254

Saarmann, L., Daugherty, J., & Riegel, B. (2000). Patient teaching to promote behavioral change. *Nursing Outlook, 48,* 281–287. doi:10.1067/mno.2000.107277

Saghatchian, M., Bihan, C., Chenailler, C., Mazouni, C., Dauchy, S., & Delaloge, S. (2014). Exploring frontiers: Use of complementary and alternative medicine among patients with early-stage breast cancer. *Breast, 23,* 279–285. doi:10.1016/j.breast.2014.01.009

Saslow, D., Solomon, D., Herschel, H.W., Killackey, M., Kulasingam, S.L., Cain, J., … Myers, E.R. (2012). American Cancer Society, American Society for Colposcopy and Cervical Pathology, and American Society for Clinical Pathology screening guidelines for the prevention and early detection of cervical cancer. *American Journal of Clinical Pathology, 137,* 516–542. doi:10.1309/AJCPTGD94EVRSJCG

Savina, E.N., & Couturaud, F. (2011). [Optimal duration of anticoagulation of venous thromboembolism]. *Journal des Maladies Vasculaires, 36*(Suppl. 1), S28–S32. doi:10.1016/S0398-0499(11)70005-1

Schellong, G., Riepenhausen, M., Ehlert, K., Brämswig, J., Dörffel, W., Schmutzler, R.K., … Bick, U. (2014). Breast cancer in the young women after treatment for Hodgkin disease during childhood or adolescence. *Deutsches Arzteblatt International, 111,* 3–9. doi:10.3238/arztebl.2014.0003

Scott, A.M., Wolchok, J.D., & Old, L.J. (2012). Antibody therapy of cancer. *Nature Reviews Cancer, 12,* 278–287.

Serraino, D., Piselli, P., Busnach, G., Burra, P., Citterio, F., Arbustini, E., … Franceschi, S. (2007). Risk of cancer following immunosuppression in organ transplant recipients and in HIV-positive individuals in southern Europe. *European Journal of Cancer, 43,* 2117–2123.

Shadad, A.K., Sullivan, F.J., Martin, J.D., & Egan, L.J. (2013). Gastrointestinal radiation injury: Symptoms, risk factors and mechanisms. *World Journal of Gastroenterology, 19,* 185–198. doi:10.3748/wjg.v19.i2.185

Sharma, A., & Jamal, M.M. (2013). Opioid induced bowel disease: A twenty-first century physicians' dilemma. Considering pathophysiology and treatment strategies. *Current Gastroenterology Reports, 15,* 334. doi:10.1007/s11894-013-0334-4

Shelton, B.K. (2011). Infection. In C.H. Yarbro, D. Wujcik, & B.H. Gobel (Eds.), *Cancer nursing: Principles and practice* (7th ed., pp. 713–744). Burlington, MA: Jones & Bartlett Learning.

Shelton, B.K. (2012). Hematology and oncology problems. In J.G.W. Foster. & S.S. Prevost (Eds.), *Advanced practice nursing of adults in acute care* (pp. 591–651). Philadelphia, PA: F.A. Davis.

Shelton, B.K. (2013). The hematologic and immunologic systems. In R.D. Dennison (Ed.), *Pass CCRN* (4th ed., pp. 636–684). Philadelphia, PA: Elsevier.

Silvestri, G.A., Gonzalez, A.V, Jantz, M.A., Margolis, M.L., Gould, M.K., Tanoue, L.T., … Detterbeck, F.C. (2013). Methods for staging non-small cell lung cancer: Diagnosis and management of lung cancer, 3rd ed: American College of Chest Physicians evidence-based clinical practice guidelines. *CHEST Journal, 143*(Suppl. 5), e211S–e250S. doi:10.1378/chest.12-2355

Sooriakumaran, P., Srivastava, A., Shariat, S.F., Stricker, P.D., Ahlering, T., Eden, C.G., … Tewari, A.K. (2014). A multinational, multi-institutional study comparing positive surgical margin rates among 22,393 open, laparoscopic, and robotic-assisted radical prostatectomy patients. *European Urology, 66,* 450–456. doi:10.1016/j.eururo.2013.11.018

Spoelstra, S.L., & Robbins, L.B. (2010). A qualitative study of role transition from RN to APN. *International Journal of Nursing Education Scholarship, 7*(1). doi:10.2202/1548-923X.2020

Spratt, J.S. (1981). The primary and secondary prevention of cancer. *Journal of Surgical Oncology, 18,* 219–230. doi:10.1002/jso.2930180302

Stafford, L., Judd, F., Gibson, P., Komiti, A., Mann, G.B., & Quinn, M. (2013). Screening for depression and anxiety in women with breast and gynaecologic cancer: Course and prevalence of morbidity over 12 months. *Psycho-Oncology, 22,* 2071–2078. doi:10.1002/pon.3253

Stanton, A. (2012). What happens now? Psychosocial care for cancer survivors after medical treatment completion. *Journal of Clinical Oncology, 30,* 1215–1220. doi:10.1200/JCO.2011.39.7406

Stringer, K., Curran, V., & Asghari, S. (2013). Pharmacists and family physicians: Improving interprofessional collaboration through joint understanding of our competencies. *Frontiers in Pharmacology, 4,* 151. doi:10.3389/fphar.2013.00151

Sureda, A., Bader, P., Cesaro, S., Dreger, P., Duarte, R.F., Dufour, C., … Madrigal, A. (2015). Indications for allo- and auto-SCT for haematological diseases, solid tumours and immune disorders: Current practice in Europe, 2015. *Bone Marrow Transplantation.* Advance online publication. doi:10.1038/bmt.2015.6

Tager, F.A., McKinley, P.S., Schnabel, F.R., El-Tamer, M., Cheung, Y.K., Fang, Y., … Hershman, D.L. (2010). The cognitive effects of chemotherapy in post-menopausal breast cancer patients: A controlled longitudinal study. *Breast Cancer Research and Treatment, 123,* 25–34. doi:10.1007/s10549-009-0606-8

Temel, J.S., Greer, J.A., Muzikansky, A., Gallagher, E.R., Admane, M.B.S., Jackson, V.A., … Lynch, T.J. (2010). Early palliative care for patients with metastatic non–small-cell lung cancer. *New England Journal of Medicine, 363,* 733–742. doi:10.1056/NEJMoa1000678

Thompson, J.E., Egger, S., Böhm, M., Haynes, A.-M., Matthews, J., Rasiah, K., & Stricker, P.D. (2014). Superior quality of life and improved surgical margins are achievable with robotic radical prostatectomy after a long learning curve: A prospective single-surgeon study of 1552 consecutive cases. *European Urology, 65,* 521–531. doi:10.1016/j.eururo.2013.10.030

Tomblyn, M., Chiller, T., Einsele, H., Gress, R., Sepkowitz, K., Storek, J., … Boeckh, M.J. (2009). Guidelines for preventing infectious complications among hematopoietic cell transplantation recipients: A global perspective. *Biology of Blood and Marrow Transplantation, 15,* 1143–1238. doi:10.1016/j.bbmt.2009.06.019

Traeger, L., Greer, J.A., Fernandez-Robles, C., Temel, J.S., & Pirl, W.F. (2012). Evidence-based treatment of anxiety in patients with cancer. *Journal of Clinical Oncology, 30,* 1197–1205. doi:10.1200/JCO.2011.39.5632

Uijen, A.A., Schers, H.J., Schellevis, F.G., & van den Bosch, W.J.H.M. (2012). How unique is continuity of care? A review of continuity and related concepts. *Family Practice, 29,* 264–271. doi:10.1093/fampra/cmr104

U.S. Department of Health and Human Services. (n.d.). What is the difference between quality improvement and quality assurance? Retrieved from http://www.hrsa.aquilentprojects.com/healthit/toolbox/HealthITadoptiontoolbox/QualityImprovement/whatarediffbtwqinqa.html

U.S. Department of Health and Human Services. (2009). Code of federal regulations (Title 45, Part 46). Retrieved from http://www.hhs.gov/ohrp/policy/ohrpregulations.pdf

U.S. Food and Drug Administration. (n.d.). MedWatch: The FDA safety information and adverse event reporting program. Retrieved from http://www.fda.gov/safety/medwatch/default.htm

U.S. Food and Drug Administration. (2014). Title 21—Food and Drugs—Chapter I—Food and Drug Administration Department of Health and Human Services. Subchapter A—General. Part 50. Sec. 50.25: Elements of informed consent. Retrieved from http://www.accessdata.fda.gov/scripts/cdrh/cfdocs/cfcfr/CFRSearch.cfm?fr=50.25

U.S. Food and Drug Administration. (2015). Clinical trials and human subject protection. Retrieved from http://www .fda.gov/ScienceResearch/SpecialTopics/RunningClinicalTrials/default.htm

Valdivieso, M., Kujawa, A.M., Jones, T., & Baker, L.H. (2012). Cancer survivors in the United States: A review of the literature and a call to action. *International Journal of Medical Sciences, 9,* 163–173. doi:10.7150/ijms.3827

Velayudhan, L., Ryu, S.-H., Raczek, M., Philpot, M., Lindesay, J., Critchfield, M., & Livingston, G. (2014). Review of brief cognitive tests for patients with suspected dementia. *International Psychogeriatrics, 26,* 1247–1262. doi:10.1017/S1041610214000416

Venkatramani, R., Kamath, S., Wong, K., Olch, A.J., Malvar, J., Sposto, R., … Mascarenhas, L. (2013). Correlation of clinical and dosimetric factors with adverse pulmonary outcomes in children after lung irradiation. *International Journal of Radiation Oncology, Biology, Physics, 86,* 942–948. doi:10.1016/j.ijrobp.2013.04.037

Vincent, D., Johnson, C., Velasquez, D., & Rigney, T. (2010). DNP-prepared nurses as practitioner-researchers: Closing the gap between research and practice. *American Journal of Nurse Practitioners, 14*(11/12), 28–34. Retrieved from http://www.doctorsofnursingpractice.org/wp-content/uploads/2014/08/Vincet_et_al.pdf

Visich, K.L., & Yeo, T.P. (2010). The prophylactic use of probiotics in the prevention of radiation therapy-induced diarrhea. *Clinical Journal of Oncology Nursing, 14,* 467–473. doi:10.1188/10.CJON.467-473

Von Ah, D., Jansen, C.E., & Allen, D.H. (2014). Evidence-based interventions for cancer- and treatment-related cognitive impairment. *Clinical Journal of Oncology Nursing, 18*(Suppl. 6), S17–S25. doi:10.1188/14.CJON.S3.17-25

Wang, W., Zhao, L.R., Lin, X.Q., & Feng, F. (2014). Reversible posterior leukoencephalopathy syndrome induced by bevacizumab plus chemotherapy in colorectal cancer. *World Journal of Gastroenterology, 20,* 6691–6697. doi:10.3748/wjg.v20.i21.6691

Wefel, J.S., Saleeba, A.K., Buzdar, A.U., & Meyers, C.A. (2010). Acute and late onset cognitive dysfunction associated with chemotherapy in women with breast cancer. *Cancer, 116,* 3348–3356. doi:10.1002/cncr.25098

Wehler, T.C., Graf, C., Möhler, M., Herzog, J., Berger, M.R., Gockel, I., … Schimanski, C.C. (2013). Cetuximab-induced skin exanthema: Prophylactic and reactive skin therapy are equally effective. *Journal of Cancer Research and Clinical Oncology, 139,* 1667–1672. doi:10.1007/s00432-013-1483-4

Weissman, S., Burt, R., Church, J., Erdman, S., Hampel, H., Holter, S., … Senter, L. (2012). Identification of individuals at risk for Lynch Syndrome using targeted evaluations and genetic testing: National Society of Genetic Counselors and the Collaborative Group of the Americas on Inherited Colorectal Cancer Joint Practice Guideline. *Journal of Genetic Counseling, 21,* 484–493. doi:10.1007/s10897-011-9465-7

Wengström, Y., Rundström, C., Geerling, J., Pappa, T., Weisse, I., Williams, S., … Rustøen, T. (2014). The management of breakthrough cancer pain—Educational needs a European nursing survey. *European Journal of Cancer Care, 23,* 121–128. doi:10.1111/ecc.12118

Wilkes, G.M. (2011). Chemotherapy administration. In C.H. Yarbro, D. Wujcik, & B.H. Gobel (Eds.), *Cancer nursing: Principles and practice* (7th ed., pp. 390–458). Burlington, MA: Jones & Bartlett Learning.

Wolff, A.C., Hammond, M.E.H., Hicks, D.G., Dowsett, M., McShane, L.M., Allison, K.H., … Hayes, D.F. (2013). Recommendations for human epidermal growth factor receptor 2 testing in breast cancer: American Society of Clinical Oncology/College of American Pathologists clinical practice guideline update. *Journal of Clinical Oncology, 31,* 3997–4013. doi:10.1200/JCO.2013.50.9984

World Medical Association. (2013). *WMA Declaration of Helsinki—Ethical principles for medical research involving human subjects.* Retrieved from http://www.wma.net/en/30publications/10policies/b3

Yamagishi, T., Ochi, N., Yamane, H., Hasebe, S., & Takigawa, N. (2014). Epiphora in lung cancer patients receiving docetaxel: A case series. *BMC Research Notes, 7,* 322. doi:10.1186/1756-0500-7-322

Yeh, E.T., & Bickford, C.L. (2009). Cardiovascular complications of cancer therapy: Incidence, pathogenesis, diagnosis, and management. *Journal of the American College of Cardiology, 53,* 2231–2247. doi:10.1016/j.jacc.2009.02.050

Yirmibesoglu, E., Higginson, D.S., Fayda, M., Rivera, M.P., Halle, J., Rosenman, J., … Marks, L.B. (2012). Challenges scoring radiation pneumonitis in patients irradiated for lung cancer. *Lung Cancer, 76,* 350–353. doi:10.1016/j.lungcan.2011.11.025

Zoga, A.C., Weissman, B.N., Kransdorf, M.J., Adler, R., Appel, M., Bancroft, L.W., … Ward, R.J. (2012). American College of Radiology ACR Appropriateness Criteria®: Soft-tissue masses. Retrieved from http://www.acr.org/~/media/ACR/Documents/AppCriteria/Diagnostic/SoftTissueMasses.pdf

Index

The letter *f* after a page number indicates that relevant content appears in a figure; the letter *t,* in a table.